Essential Family Medicine

Essential Family Medicine

Fundamentals and Case Studies

Third Edition

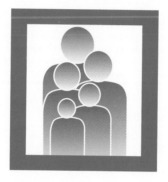

Robert E. Rakel, MD

Professor
Department of Family and Community Medicine
Baylor College of Medicine
Houston, Texas

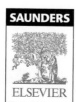

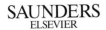

1600 John F. Kennedy Boulevard
Suite 1800
Philadelphia, Pennsylvania 19103-2899

ESSENTIAL FAMILY MEDICINE
Fundamentals and Case Studies, *Third Edition*
Copyright © 2006, 1998, 1993 by Elsevier Inc.

ISBN-13: 978-1-4160-2377-7
ISBN-10: 1-4160-2377-1

NOTICE

Library of Congress Cataloging-in-Publication Data

Essential family medicine : fundamentals and case studies / [edited by] Robert E. Rakel. — 3rd ed.
    p. ; cm.
  Rev. ed. of: Essentials of family practice. 2nd ed. c1998.
  Includes bibliographical references and index.
  ISBN-13: 978-1-4160-2377-7
  ISBN-10: 1-4160-2377-1
  1. Family medicine. 2. Family medicine—Case studies. I. Rakel, Robert E II. Essentials of family practice.
  [DNLM: 1. Family Practice—Case Reports. WB 110 E782 2006]
RC49.E87 2006
610—dc22

             2006048302

Acquisitions Editor: Rolla Couchman
Developmental Editor: Joanie Milnes
Senior Project Manager: Cecelia Bayruns
Design Direction: Karen O'Keefe Owens
Cover Designer: Louis Forgione
Marketing Manager: Laura Meiskey

Printed in the United States of America.

Last digit is the print number: 9 8 7 6 5 4 3 2 1

Contributors

Allan V. Abbott, MD
Associate Dean for Curriculum and CME, Family
Medicine, Keck School of Medicine, University of
Southern California, Los Angeles, California
Elbow Pain (Epicondylitis)

Thomas Agresta, MD
University of Connecticut, St. Francis Hospital, Hartford,
Connecticut
Tender Swelling of Hands and Feet (Sickle Cell Disease)

Virginia D. Aguila, MD
Assistant Professor, Department of Family Medicine,
Creighton University Medical Center, Omaha, Nebraska
Breast Cancer

Janet R. Albers, MD
Program Director and Associate Chair, Department of
Family and Community Medicine, Southern Illinois
University, Springfield, Illinois
Irregular Menses (Dysfunctional Uterine Bleeding)

Michael Altman, MD
Assistant Professor, Family and Community Medicine,
University of Texas, Houston Medical School; Family
Medicine, Memorial-Hermann Hospital, Houston, Texas
Acne

Mark Andrews, MD
Assistant Professor, Family and Community Medicine,
Wake Forest University School of Medicine, Winston-
Salem, North Carolina
*Red Area on Left Temple (Basal Cell Carcinoma); Rash
on Right Shoulder (Actinic Keratosis)*

Ann M. Aring, MD
Assistant Clinical Professor, Department of Family
Medicine, Ohio State University; Assistant Program
Director, Riverside Family Practice Residency Program,
Riverside Methodist Hospital, Columbus, Ohio
Lower Abdominal Pain (Pelvic Inflammatory Disease)

Brian S. Bacak, MD
Assistant Professor of Family Medicine, University of
Colorado Health Science Center; Rose Family Medicine
Residency, Denver, Colorado
Heartburn (Gastroesophageal Reflux Disease)

Bruce Bagley, MD
Medical Director, Quality Improvement, American
Academy of Family Physicians, Leawood, Kansas
The Electronic Medical Record

Robert A. Baldor, MD
Professor and Vice-Chairman, Family Medicine and
Community Health, University of Massachusetts Medical
School; Vice-Chairman, Family Medicine, University of
Massachusetts Memorial Health Center, Worcester,
Massachusetts
Cough (Possible Asthma); Breast Mass

David M. Barclay III, MS, MPH
Associate Professor, Department of Family and
Community Medicine, Temple University School of
Medicine, Philadelphia, Pennsylvania
*Ringing in Ears (Tinnitus); Irregular Menstruation and
Fatigue (Cushing's Syndrome)*

Amber Barnhart, MD
Director of Predoctoral Education; Associate Professor,
Department of Family and Community Medicine,
Southern Illinois University School of Medicine;
Residency Faculty, Department of Family Medicine,
Memorial Medical Center; Residency Faculty,
Department of Family Medicine, St. John's Hospital,
Springfield, Illinois
Clumsiness and Difficulty Walking (Brain Tumor)

Wendy Brooks Barr, MD, MPH
Instructor, Department of Family Practice and
Community Medicine, University of Pennsylvania,
Philadelphia, Pennsylvania
Cervical Cancer Screening

Bruce Barrett, MD, PhD
Assistant Professor, Department of Family Medicine,
University of Wisconsin-Madison, Madison, Wisconsin
Productive Cough (Acute Bronchitis)

Max Bayard, MD
Associate Professor and Program Director, Department of
Family Medicine, East Tennessee State University James
H. Quillen College of Medicine, Johnson City, Tennessee
*Restless Legs Syndrome; Bleeding Peptic Ulcer (Alcohol
Withdrawal Syndrome)*

J. Mark Beard, MD
Assistant Professor, Family Medicine, University of
Washington; Active Staff, Family Medicine, University of
Washington Medical Center; Associate Staff, Family
Medicine, Seattle Cancer Care Alliance, Seattle, Washington
*Selecting Radiographic Tests: Radiographs, Computed
Tomography, Magnetic Resonance Imaging, Ultrasound,
and Nuclear Imaging*

Ian M. Bennett, MD, PhD
Assistant Professor, Family Practice and Community Medicine, University of Pennsylvania, Philadelphia, Pennsylvania
Contraception

Baruch A. Brody, PhD
Leon Jaworski Professor of Biomedical Ethics; Director, Center for Medical Ethics and Health Policy, Baylor College of Medicine, Houston, Texas
Ethics in Family Medicine

Leslie Brott, MD
Staff Physician, Medicine/Pediatrics, Williamette Valley Medical Center, McMinnville, Oregon
Pancreatitis (Acute Pancreatitis); Bizarre Behavior (Schizophrenia); Influenza

Chester R. Burns, MD, PhD
James Wade Rockwell Professor of Medicine, University of Texas Medical Branch at Galveston, Institute for the Medical Humanities, Galveston, Texas
The Relevance of Medical History to Family Medicine

Kara L. Cadwallader, MD
Assistant Clinical Professor, Family Practice Residency of Idaho, Boise, Idaho
Dyspnea on Exertion (Congestive Heart Failure)

Jon C. Calvert, MD
Clinical Professor, Department of Family Practice, University of Oklahoma College of Medicine; Active Staff, Department of Obstetrics and Gynecology, Hillcrest Medical Center; Active Staff, Department of Obstetrics and Gynecology, Saint John Medical Center, Tulsa, Oklahoma
Cervical Dysplasia: Diagnosis and Management

Roberto Cardarelli, DO, MPH
Assistant Professor; Director, Center for Evidence-Based Medicine, Department of Family Medicine, University of North Texas Health Science Center at Fort Worth; Network Research Director, North Texas Primary Care Practice-Based Research Network (NorTex), University of North Texas Health Science Center at Fort Worth, Fort Worth, Texas
Sore Throat (Acute Pharyngitis); High Blood Pressure (Hypertension)

Cheng-Chieh Chuang, MD
Clinical Instructor, Family Medicine, Brown University School of Medicine, Providence, Rhode Island; President, Lakeside Family Medicine, Raynham, Massachusetts
Swollen Foreskin (Diabetes Mellitus Type 2); Changing Nevus (Melanoma)

Heidi Chumley, MD
Director of Predoctoral Education, Unviersity of Kansas School of Medicine, Kansas City, Kansas
Genital Warts (Condyloma Acuminata)

Richard D. Clover, MD
Dean, School of Public Health and Information Sciences, University of Louisville; Associate Vice President for Health Informatics, University of Louisville, Louisville, Kentucky
Nasal Congestion in a 15-Month-Old Girl (Immunization)

Stephen G. Cook, MD
Community Health Clinic, Lakewood, Washington
Hiccups; Cold and Numb Hands and Feet (Frostbite); Gallstones

Jane E. Corboy, MD
Associate Professor and Director of Graduate Medical Education, Family and Community Medicine, Baylor College of Medicine, Houston, Texas
Chest Pain (Angina Pectoris)

Peter F. Cronholm, MD, MSCE
Assistant Professor, Department of Family Medicine and Community Health; Adjunct Scholar, Center for Clinical Epidemiology and Biostatistics; Senior Fellow, Leonard Davis Center for Healthcare Economics; Associate, Firearm and Injury Center at Penn, University of Pennsylvania, Philadelphia, Pennsylvania
Sexually Transmitted Diseases (Gonorrhea); Domestic Violence

Michael Crouch, MD, MSPH
Associate Professor, Family and Community Center Medicine, Baylor College of Medicine; Active Staff, Family Medicine, St. Lukes Episcopal; Active Staff, Family Medicine Division of Medicine Department, The Methodist Hospital, Houston, Texas
Abdominal Pain and Loose Bowel Movements (Hypercholesterolemia)

Loren A. Crown, MD
Clinical Professor, Department of Family Medicine, University of Tennessee, Covington, Tennessee
Snakebite

Timothy P. Daaleman, DO, MPH
Associate Professor, Department of Family Medicine, University of North Carolina; Attending Physician, Department of Family Medicine, University of North Carolina Hospitals; Research Associate, Program on Aging, Disability and Long-Term Care, Cecil G. Sheps Center for Health Services Research, Chapel Hill, North Carolina
Terminal Illness

James M. Daniels, MD, MPH
Professor, Department of Family and Community Medicine, Southern Illinois University School of Medicine; Director, Southern Illinois University School of Medicine, Quincy, Illinois
Upper Extremity Numbness and Pain (Double Crush Syndrome); Low Back Pain

Lloyd A. Darlow, MD
Clinical Assistant Professor of Family Practice, Weill
Medical College of Cornell University, New York,
New York; Chairman, Department of Family Practice,
Cayuga Medical Center at Ithaca, Ithaca, New York
*Difficulty Paying Attention (Attention-
Deficit/Hyperactivity Disorder)*

Darwin Deen, MD, MS
Director, Undergraduate Medical Education, Department
of Family and Social Medicine, Albert Einstein College of
Medicine, Bronx, New York
Abdominal Obesity (Metabolic Syndrome)

Jennifer DeVoe, MD, DPhil
Instructor, Department of Family Medicine, Oregon
Health and Science University (OHSU), Portland, Oregon
*Leg Pain and Swelling (Venous Thrombosis); Bedwetting
(Childhood Nocturnal Enuresis)*

Lisa Dolovich, MD, BScPham, PharmD, MSc
Associate Professor, Departments of Family Medicine,
Medicine, and Clinical Epidemiology and Biostatistics,
McMaster University, Hamilton, Ontario, Canada
Patient Compliance

Frank J. Domino, MD
Associate Professor and Clerkship Professor, Department
of Family Medicine and Community Health, University of
Massachusetts Medical School, Worchester, Massachusetts
Cough (Possible Asthma)

Marguerite R. Duane, MD
Clerkship Director and Associate Professor, Department
of Medicine, Georgetown University Medical Center,
Washington, D.C.
*Fever and Cough (Influenza); Shortness of Breath in a
12-Year-Old Girl (Asthma)*

Charles B. Eaton, MD, MS
Professor, Family Medicine, Brown Medical School,
Providence, Rhode Island; Director, Center for Primary
Care and Prevention, Memorial Hospital of Rhode Island,
Pawtucket, Rhode Island
Hyperlipidemia (Mixed Lipid Disorder)

John W. Ely, MD, MSPH
Associate Professor, Family Medicine, University of Iowa,
Roy J. and Lucille A. Carver College of Medicine, Iowa
City, Iowa
Sinus Congestion (Sinusitis)

Bernard Ewigman, MD, MSPH
University of Chicago Pritzker School of Medicine,
Chicago, Illinois
Evidence-Based Medicine

Ruth Falik, MD
Assistant Professor of Medicine, Baylor College of
Medicine; Attending Physician, General Internal
Medicine, Ben Taub General Hospital, Houston, Texas
*Episodic Chest Pain (Angina Pectoris); Palpitations
(Atrial Fibrillation)*

Robert S. Fawcett, MD, MS
Assistant Clinical Professor, Family Medicine, Penn State
Hershey Medical Center, Hershey, Pennsylvania; Medical
Director, Thomas Hart Family Medicine; Active Staff
Member, Family Medicine, York Hospital, York,
Pennsylvania
Pigmented Thumbnail (Nail Lentigo)

Jeanne M. Ferrante, MD
Associate Professor, Department of Family Medicine,
University of Medicine and Dentistry of New Jersey,
Newark, New Jersey
Dizziness (Vestibular Neuritis)

Matthew J. Fleig, MD
Assistant Professor, Family Medicine, University of
Rochester; Attending Family Medicine, Highland
Hospital, Rochester, New York
Newborn Distress (Neonatal Resuscitation)

Robert S. Freelove, MD
Associate Director, Smoky Hill Family Medicine
Residency Program; Clinical Instructor, University of
Kansas School of Medicine–Wichita, Salina, Kansas
*Delirium (Hypomagnesemia); Hand Swollen and Red
(Spider Bite)*

David L. Gaspar, MD
Associate Professor, Director of Predoctoral Education,
Department of Family Medicine, University of Colorado
at Denver Health Sciences Center, Denver, Colorado
Vesicular Rash (Varicella); Pruritic Rash (Urticaria)

James M. Gill, MD, MPH
Associate Professor, Family and Community Medicine,
Thomas Jefferson University; Senior Scholar, Health
Policy, Philadelphia, Pennsylvania; Director, Health
Services Research, Family and Community Medicine,
Wilmington, Delaware
Shoulder and Back Pain (Fibromyalgia)

Gary R. Gray, DO
Assistant Clinical Professor, Family and Community
Medicine, University of California, San Francisco,
California; Program Director, Family Practice Residency,
Natividad Medical Center, Salinas, California
Toe Pain and Swelling (Gout); Ear Pain (Bell's Palsy)

Larry A. Green, MD
Professor of Family Medicine and Director of the
National Program Office for Prescription for Health,
University of Colorado Health Sciences Center, Denver,
Colorado; Senior Scholar in Residence, Robert Graham
Center: Policy Studies in Family Medicine and Primary
Care, Washington, D.C.
The Future of Family Medicine

Kenneth J. Grimm, MD, MS
Associate Program Director, Family Medicine, Oakwood
Hospital and Medical Center, Dearborn, Michigan;
Clinical Instructor, Family Medicine, University of
Michigan, Ann Arbor, Michigan
*Abdominal Pain (Endometriosis); Back Pain
(Osteoporosis)*

Rahul Gupta, MD
Assistant Professor of Medicine, Internal Medicine, University of Alabama at Birmingham, Huntsville Regional Medical Campus; Attending Physician, Medicine, Huntsville Hospital, Huntsville, Alabama
Widespread Pruritic Rash (Adverse Drug Reaction); Headache

R. Brian Haynes, MD, PhD
Michael Gent Professor and Chair, Department of Clinical Epidemiology and Biostatistics, DeGroote School of Medicine at McMaster University; Active Staff, Section of General Internal Medicine, Hamilton Health Sciences; Professor, Department of Medicine, DeGroote School of Medicine at McMaster University, Hamilton, Ontario, Canada
Patient Compliance

Valerie L. Hearns, MD
Associate Professor and Vice Chair, Department of Family Medicine, University of South Dakota School of Medicine; Medical Staff, Family Medicine, Sioux Valley Hospital, University of South Dakota Medical Center; Medical Staff, Family Medicine, Avera McKennan Hospital, Sioux Falls, South Dakota
Nausea and Vomiting (Pyelonephritis); Vaginal Itching and Discharge (Vaginitis); Left Lower Abdominal Pain (Ectopic Pregnancy)

Joel J. Heidelbaugh, MD
Clinical Assistant Professor, Department of Family Medicine, University of Michigan, Ann Arbor, Michigan; Medical Director, Ypsilanti Health Center, Ypsilanti, Michigan
Right Upper Quadrant Abdominal Pain (Cholelithiasis); Peptic Ulcer Disease; Gastroesophageal Reflux Disease

David Henderson, MD
Assistant Professor, Department of Family Medicine, Family Medicine Residency Program, University of Connecticut School of Medicine, Hartford, Connecticut; Saint Francis Hospital and Medical Center, Farmington, Connecticut
Tender Swelling of Hands and Feet (Sickle Cell Disease)

Charles E. Henley, DO, MPH
Professor and Founders and Associates Research Chair in Family Medicine, Department of Family Medicine, University of Oklahoma College of Medicine, Tulsa; Active Staff, Family Medicine, Hillcrest Medical Center; Active Staff and Chair, Family Medicine, Tulsa Regional Medical Center, Tulsa, Oklahoma
Disease Prevention

Warren L. Holleman, PhD
Assistant Professor, Department of Family and Community Medicine, Baylor College of Medicine, Houston, Texas
Ethics in Family Medicine

Keith B. Holten, MD
Clinical Professor, Family Medicine, University of Cincinnati College of Medicine, Cincinnati, Ohio; Residency Director, Family Medicine, Clinton Memorial Hospital, University of Cincinnati, Wilmington, Ohio
Evaluating the Medical Literature; Diagnosis and Management of an Acute Exacerbation (Chronic Obstructive Pulmonary Disease)

William Y. Huang, MD
Associate Professor, Department of Family and Community Medicine, Baylor College of Medicine, Houston, Texas
Problem Solving in Family Medicine

Matthew L. Hunsaker, MD
Director, Rural Medical Education Program (RMED), National Center for Rural Health Professions, University of Illinois College of Medicine at Rockford, Rockford, Illinois; Physician, Family Medicine, KSB Hospital, Dixon, Illinois; Medical Director, Family Medicine, Tri-County Clinic, Northern Illinois University, Malta, Illinois
Type 2 Diabetes Mellitus

David Q. Hutcheson-Tipton, MD
Lieutenant Commander, Medical Corps, United States Navy; Department Head, Family Practice Department, Makalapa Clinic, Naval Health Clinic Hawaii, Pearl Harbor, Hawaii
Nasal Congestion (Allergic Rhinitis); Difficulty Maintaining an Erection (Erectile Dysfunction)

David M. Jester, MD
Associate Professor and Predoctoral Director, Department of Family Medicine, Medical College of Georgia, Augusta, Georgia
Confusion in a Man 70 Years Old (Sepsis); Ankle Edema and Superficial Ulcer Stasis (Venus Stasis Ulcer)

Norman B. Kahn, Jr., MD
Vice President, Science and Education, American Academy of Family Physicians, Leawood, Kansas
The Future of Family Medicine

Victoria S. Kaprielian, MD
Clinical Professor, Community and Family Medicine, Duke University Medical Center; Attending Staff, Community and Family Medicine, Duke University Hospital; Attending Staff, Family Medicine, Durham Regional Hospital, Durham, North Carolina
Urinary Frequency and Dysuria (Urinary Tract Infection)

Michael G. Kavan, MD
Associate Dean for Student Affairs, Associate Professor of Family Medicine, Associate Professor of Psychiatry, Creighton University School of Medicine, Omaha, Nebraska
Multiple Somatic Complaints (Generalized Anxiety Disorder)

Louis A. Kazal, Jr., MD
Chief Clinical Officer, Department of Community and
Family Medicine, Dartmouth Medical School, Hanover,
New Hampshire
Arm Laceration (Laceration Repair)

David Kibbe, MD, MBA
Director, Center for Health Information Technology,
American Academy of Family Physicians, Leawood, Kansas
The Electronic Medical Record

Sanford R. Kimmel, MD
Professor of Family Medicine, Department of Family
Medicine; Associate Residency Director; Family Practice
Residency, Medical University of Ohio, Toledo, Ohio
Short Child (Constitutional Growth Delay)

T. Alex King, MD
Assistant Professor, Department of Family Practice and
Community Medicine, University of Texas Southwestern
Medical Center at Dallas, Dallas, Texas
Skin Papule (Basal Cell Carcinoma)

Scott Kinkade, MD, MSPH
Assistant Professor of Family Medicine, Director of
Predoctoral Education, Department of Family and
Community Medicine, University of Texas Southwestern
Medical School, Dallas, Texas
Acne (Acne Vulgaris); Disorientation (Heat Stroke)

Kurt Kurowski, MD
Associate Professor, Department of Family and Preventive
Medicine, The Chicago Medical School at RFUMS, North
Chicago, Illinois; Staff Physician, Family Medicine,
Swedish Covenant Hospital, Chicago, Illinois; Staff
Physician, Family Practice, ENH-Highland Park Hospital,
Highland Park, Illinois
*Dysuria and Urinary Frequency (Urinary Tract
Infection); Alzheimer's Disease*

Elizabeth Laffey, MD
Assistant Professor, Department of Community and
Family Medicine, Saint Louis University School of
Medicine, Belleville, Illinois
*Lymphadenopathy (HIV Infection); Abnormal Liver
Function Tests (Chronic Viral Hepatitis)*

Frederick Lambert, MD
Assistant Professor, Department of Family Medicine,
Albert Einstein College of Medicine, MMG-Castle Hill
Family Practice, Bronx, New York
*Worsening Low Back Pain (Metastatic Cancer Pain
Management)*

Greg L. Ledgerwood, MD
Clinical Assistant Professor, Department of Family
Medicine, University of Washington School of Medicine,
Seattle, Washington; Private Practice, Omak,
Washington
Multiple Allergies (Allergic Rhinitis Asthma)

Sarah Ellen Lesko, MD
Family Physician, Carolyn Downs Family Medical Center,
Seattle, Washington
*Fatigue (Hypothyroidism); Irregular Bowel Movements
(Colon Cancer)*

Walter D. Leventhal, MD
Clinical Associate Professor of Family Medicine, Medical
University of South Carolina, Charleston, South Carolina;
Senior Partner, Dorchester Medical Associates,
Summerville, South Carolina
Rash and Fever (Rocky Mountain Spotted Fever)

Kenneth Lin, MD
Assistant Professor, Department of Family Medicine,
Georgetown University, Washington, D.C.
Behavior Problem in a 2-Year-Old Boy (Autism)

Kurt A. Lindberg, MD
Pisacano Leadership Foundation Alumnus, Lakewood
Family Medicine, Holland, Michigan
*Nausea, Vomiting, and Lethargy (Acute Renal Failure);
Pain "Everywhere" (Fibromyalgia); Diarrhea*

Jennifer E. Lochner, MD
Assistant Professor, Department of Family Medicine,
Oregon Health and Science University, Portland, Oregon
*Fever without Source in Children (Fever); Pruritus
(Atopic Dermatitis)*

David P. Losh, MD
Professor, Department of Family Medicine, University of
Washington, Seattle, Washington
*Selecting Radiographic Tests: Radiographs, Computed
Tomography, Magnetic Resonance Imaging, Ultrasound,
and Nuclear Imaging*

Linda Lou, MD, MPH
Practicing Physician, Community Health Center,
Tucson, Arizona
Right Flank Pain (Nephrolithiasis)

Barbara A. Majeroni, MD
Associate Clinical Professor of Family Medicine,
University at Buffalo School of Medicine and Biomedical
Sciences, State University of New York, Buffalo, New York
Unexplained Weight Loss (Hyperthyroidism)

Geoffrey Margo, MD, PhD
Clinical Associate Professor, Psychiatry, University of
Pennsylvania Health System; Director,
Consultation/Liaison Psychiatry Service, Psychiatry,
Pennsylvania Hospital, Philadelphia, Pennsylvania
Anxiety (Social Phobia)

Katherine Margo, MD, PhD
Director of Student Activities; Assistant Professor,
Department of Family Practice and Community
Medicine, University of Pennsylvania School of Medicine,
Philadelphia, Pennsylvania
Chest Pain and Fatigue (Anxiety Disorder)

James C. Martin, MD
Program Director, Family Practice Residency Program, CHRISTUS Santa Rosa Health Care; Clinical Professor, University of Texas Health Science Center, San Antonio, Texas
The Future of Family Medicine

Jeffrey Alan May, MD
Clinical Instructor, Family Medicine, University of Tennessee-Memphis College of Health Sciences, Covington, Tennessee
Spider Bites

Eugene A. Merzon, MD
Department of Family Medicine, Sackler School of Medicine, Tel Aviv University, Tel Aviv, Israel; Tutor, Department of Family Medicine and Family Practice Residency, Leumit Health Fund, Israel; Family Physician, Jonathan Clinic, Leumit Health Fund, Ariel, Israel
Vitamin B$_{12}$ Deficiency

James S. Millar, MD, MPH
Associate Professor and Medical Director, Department of Family Medicine, University of Oklahoma–Tulsa, Tulsa, Oklahoma
Penile Discharge (Gonorrhea)

Karl E. Miller, MD
Professor and Vice Chair, Family Medicine, Chattanooga Unit, University of Tennessee College of Medicine, Chattanooga, Tennessee
Vaginal Discharge (Vulvovaginal Candidiasis)

Eugene Mochan, PhD, DO
Associate Dean, Primary Care and Continuing Education; Professor, Philadelphia College of Osteopathic Medicine, Philadelphia, Pennsylvania
Bilateral Knee Pain (Osteoarthritis)

Venita W. Morell, MD
Affiliate Associate Professor, Family and Community Medicine, Wake Forest University School of Medicine, Winston-Salem, North Carolina; Medical Director, Okaloosa County Health Department, Fort Walton Beach, Florida
Insomnia

R. Michael Morse, MD
Founders and Associates Professor, Chair of Family Medicine, Department of Family Medicine, University of Oklahoma, College of Medicine, Tulsa, Oklahoma
Disease Prevention

Scott E. Moser, MD
Associate Professor, Family and Community Medicine, The University of Kansas School of Medicine–Wichita, Wichita, Kansas
Cramping Abdominal Pain (Irritable Bowel Syndrome); Hyperactive Child (Attention-Deficit/Hyperactivity Disorder)

Donald E. Nease, Jr., MD
Associate Professor, Department of Family Medicine, University of Michigan; Attending Physician, Family Medicine, University of Michigan Hospitals and Health Centers, Ann Arbor, Michigan
Fatigue and Difficulty Concentrating (Depression)

Giang T. Nguyen, MD, MPH
Clinical Instructor, Family Practice and Community Medicine, University of Pennsylvania School of Medicine; Attending Physician, Family Practice and Community Medicine, Hospital of the University of Pennsylvania, and Pennsylvania Presbyterian Medical Center, Philadelphia, Pennsylvania
Vaginal Bleeding (Endometrial Cancer)

Melissa Nothnagle, MD
Assistant Professor, Department of Family Medicine, Brown Medical School, Providence, Rhode Island
Third-Trimester Vaginal Bleeding (Placenta Previa); Severe Menstrual Cramps (Primary Dysmenorrhea)

Alice Anne O'Donell, MD
Professor, Department of Family Medicine, John Sealy Hospital, The University of Texas Medical Branch, Galveston, Texas
The Relevance of Medical History to Family Medicine

John G. O'Handley, MD
Mount Carmel Family Practice, Columbus, Ohio
Fever and Fussiness in a 22-Month-Old Child (Acute Otitis Media)

Trish Palmer, MD
Assistant Professor, Family Medicine, Midwest Orthopaedics at Rush, Chicago, Illinois
Ankle Injury (Ankle Sprain); Persistent Productive Cough (Mountain Sickness)

Jon S. Parham, DO, MPH
Associate Professor, Predoctoral Director, Family Medicine, University of Tennessee Graduate School of Medicine; Active Staff Member, Family Medicine, University of Tennessee Medical Center, Knoxville, Tennessee; Active Staff Member, Consulting, Family Medicine, Peninsula Hospital, Louisville, Tennessee
Skin "Spots" and Bruising (Thrombocytopenia)

Paul Paulman, MD
Professor and Predoctoral Director, Family Medicine, University of Nebraska Medical Center, Omaha, Nebraska
Tiredness (Anemia)

Layne A. Prest, PhD
Director of Behavioral Medicine and Associate Professor of Family Medicine, University of Nebraska Medical Center; Medical Family Therapist, Department of Family Medicine, Nebraska Medical Center, Omaha, Nebraska
Chest Pain and Shortness of Breath (Panic Disorder)

David P. Rakel, MD
Director, University of Wisconsin Integrative Medicine;
Assistant Professor, Department of Family
Medicine, University of Wisconsin Medical School;
University of Wisconsin Hospitals and Clinics,
Department of Family Medicine,
University of Wisconsin; Saint Mary's Hospital and
Medical Center, Madison, Wisconsin
Integrative Medicine

Robert E. Rakel, MD
Professor, Department of Family and Community
Medicine, Baylor College of Medicine, Houston, Texas
*The Family Physician; The Problem-Oriented Medical
Record*

Kalyanakrishnan Ramakrishnan, MD
Associate Professor of Family and Preventive Medicine,
University of Oklahoma Health Sciences Center,
Oklahoma City, Oklahoma
*Bilateral Leg Pain (Peripheral Arterial Disease);
Hyperthyroidism*

Dino William Ramzi, MD
Medical Director, Community Clinic, Inc., Rockville,
Maryland
Dyspnea and Confusion (Pulmonary Embolism)

Anna Mies Richie, MD
Assistant Professor, Department of Family and
Community Medicine, Springfield Family Medicine
Residency Program, Southern Illinois University School
of Medicine; Southern Illinois University Family and
Community Medicine, Springfield, Illinois
*Obesity and Elevated Blood Pressure (Metabolic
Syndrome); Shoulder and Wrist Pain (Rheumatoid
Arthritis)*

Rodney Riedel, MD
Primary Care Sports Medicine Fellow, University of
Connecticut, St. Francis Hospital, Hartford, Connecticut
Right Elbow Pain (Tendinosis)

Patrick Riley, MD
Resident, Saint Louis University School of Medicine,
Belleville, Illinois
Abnormal Liver Function Tests (Chronic Viral Hepatitis)

Adam Rindfleisch, MD
Family Medicine Physician, University of Wisconsin
Northeast Family Medical Center; St. Mary's Hospital,
Madison, Wisconsin
Integrative Medicine

John C. Rogers, MD, MPH
Professor and Vice Chair for Education, Family and
Community Medicine, Baylor College of Medicine,
Houston, Texas
Problem Solving in Family Medicine

Timothy Scanlan, MD, MBA
Associate Clinical Professor, Family and Community
Medicine, University of Kansas School of Medicine;
Medical Director, Addiction Specialists of Kansas,
Wichita, Kansas
*Feeling Depressed (Drug Dependency); Heartburn
(Alcohol Problem)*

Stephen Scott, MD
Assistant Professor, Family and Community Medicine,
Baylor College of Medicine, Houston, Texas
Interpreting Laboratory Tests

John W. Sellors, MSc, MD
Visiting Professor, Department of Family Medicine,
University of Washington; Senior Medical Advisor,
Reproductive Health, Program for Appropriate
Technology in Health, Seattle, Washington; Clinical
Professor, Department of Family Medicine, McMaster
University, Hamilton, Ontario, Canada
Patient Compliance

Douglas R. Smucker, MD, MPH
Associate Professor, Family Medicine, University of
Cincinnati, Cincinnati, Ohio
Evaluating the Medical Literature

Daniel L. Stulberg, MD
Associate Professor, Family Medicine, University of
Colorado; Chair, Department of Family Medicine, Rose
Medical Center; Residency Director, Rose Family Medical
Residency, University of Colorado, Denver, Colorado
Thorn in Bottom of Foot (Plantar Wart)

Jeffrey Susman, MD
Professor and Chair, Family Medicine, University of
Cincinnati; Chair, Family Medicine, University Hospital;
Family Medicine, The Christ Hospital, Cincinnati, Ohio;
Family Medicine, Clinton Memorial Hospital,
Wilmington, Ohio
Evaluating the Medical Literature

Richard R. Terry, DO
Director, Wilson Family Practice Residency; Director,
Osteopathic Medical Education, United Health Services
Hospitals; Associate Clinical Professor, SUNY Upstate
Medical University, Clinical Campus at Binghamton,
Johnson City, New York
Overweight (Obesity)

Barbara Thompson, MD
Sealy Hutchings and Lucille Wright Hutchings Chair and
Professor, Family Medicine; Assistant Dean for Faculty
Practice, University of Texas Medical Branch; Medical
Director, University of Texas Medical Branch Hospitals
and Clinics, Galveston, Texas
The Relevance of Medical History to Family Medicine

Pamela H. Tietze, MD
Associate Professor, Family Medicine, University of Oklahoma College of Medicine, Tulsa, Oklahoma
  Perianal Itching (Pinworms)

John W. Tipton, MD
Associate Professor and Vice Chair, Department of Family Medicine, University of Oklahoma College of Medicine, Tulsa, Oklahoma
  Giardiasis

Richard P. Usatine, MD
Professor and Vice Chair for Medical Student Education, Department of Family and Community Medicine, University of Texas Health Science Center at San Antonio, San Antonio, Texas
  Genital Warts (Condyloma Acuminata)

Miriam Vincent, MD, PhD
Professor and Chair, Department of Family Medicine, SUNY–Downstate Medical Center; University Hospital of Brooklyn, Brooklyn, New York
  Sore Throat (Pharyngitis)

Randy Wertheimer, MD
Associate Professor, Department of Family Medicine and Community Health, University of Massachusetts School of Medicine, Worcester, Massachusetts; Chair of Family Medicine, Cambridge Health Alliance, Cambridge, Massachusetts
  Fatigue, Nausea, Breast Tenderness (Normal Pregnancy)

Veronica Wilbur, RN, MSN
Assistant Professor, Nursing, Wilmington College, New Castle, Delaware
  Type 1 Diabetes Mellitus

W. Michael Woods, MD
Associate Professor, Program Director, University of Oklahoma College of Medicine, Tulsa, Oklahoma; Department of Family Medicine, Rural Program, Ramona, Oklahoma
  Chest Pain and Shortness of Breath (Iron Deficiency Anemia)

Therese Zink, MD, MPH
Assistant Professor, Department of Family and Community Medicine, University of Minnesota, Minneapolis, Minnesota
  Family Dynamics and Health

Kira Zwygart, MD
Assistant Professor, Family Medicine, University of South Florida College of Medicine; Family Medicine, Tampa General Hospital, Tampa, Florida
  Tremor (Parkinson's Disease)

Preface

This third edition is designed as were the first two: to serve as a resource for medical students and others learning the essentials of our discipline. Although the title has been modified to reflect the name change of the American Board of Family Practice to the American Board of Family Medicine, the focus remains the same as in previous editions.

A number of significant changes have been made in this edition:

- Advancing technology has made it possible to make the entire text plus valuable additional material available electronically.
- Online access provides not only the text but also additional cases and links to other Elsevier publications.
- The printed version and the additional material can be downloaded to a personal computer or a PDA (personal digital assistant).
- Evidence-based ratings are used throughout the text to indicate the strength of the evidence presented.
- Color is used to highlight important features.
- Key Points are boxed for easy retrieval of essential information.
- Evidence-based medicine content is enhanced through a relationship with FPIN (Family Physicians Inquiries Network), a national consortium dedicated to using information technology to improve healthcare.

In this edition there are six new chapters in the Fundamentals section:

- **The Future of Family Medicine.** The authors are among leaders from the seven U.S. family medicine organizations that participated in the Future of Family Medicine Project.
- **The Relevance of Medical History to Family Medicine.** Those who ignore history are destined to repeat it.
- **Evidence-Based Medicine.** This chapter is written by the president and executive editor of FPIN, who is also Chairman of Family Medicine at the University of Chicago.
- **Evaluating the Medical Literature.** This chapter outlines how to understand and evaluate studies published in the medical literature.
- **Integrative Medicine.** This chapter presents a thorough approach to the use of complementary and alternative medicine techniques that make family physicians truly comprehensive primary care physicians.
- **The Electronic Medical Record.** This information is essential to the future practice of modern family medicine.

Following the Fundamentals section are 138 case studies covering the entire spectrum of family medicine. These cases illustrate the variety of challenges in family medicine and the rewards of managing patients over time. Of the problems presented, 82 are in the printed version and 56 more in the electronic version. Patients present just as they would to a family physician and a differential diagnosis is developed using problem solving techniques typical of those used in family medicine.

Additional material that is available in the electronic version includes:

- Integrative Medicine–21 tables, including Popular Herbal Remedies: Key Facts for Primary Providers, Points to Consider When Advising Patients about Herbal Remedies, Important Considerations Regarding Supplementation of Specific Nutrients, Points to Consider When Referring Patients for Manipulative Therapies, and Mind Body Techniques and Therapies.
- Evidence-Based Medicine–Three appendixes that include five Critical Appraisal Worksheets, a glossary of EBM terms, and a list of EBM electronic resources.
- Disease Prevention—39 tables, including Actual causes of Death in the United States in 1990 and 2000, Eating Plan for Healthy Americans, and Probability of Developing Invasive Cancers by Age and Sex, 1998–2000.
- 56 additional case studies.
- ABFM Board (American Board of Family Medicine) style questions.

Primary care is unique in that diseases present in their early undifferentiated stage when it is most difficult to make a specific diagnosis. The fact that family physicians feel comfortable with a variety of often vague presenting complaints distinguishes them from physicians in a narrow specialty. It is this variety that keeps the family physician professionally stimulated and perpetually challenged, and that sustains the excitement of practicing medicine.

My special thanks to colleagues who have taken the time to share their knowledge and experience with us by providing cases drawn from their practices. My thanks also to the excellent staff at W.B. Saunders for their attention to detail and insistence on quality, and to my wife Peggy, who for more than 50 years has supported my passion for the written word.

Robert E. Rakel, MD

Contents

Contents

Contents

Student Consult Contents

Part I

Fundamentals

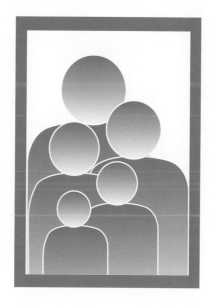

1 The Family Physician

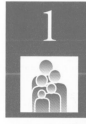

Robert E. Rakel

KEY POINTS

1. The American Board of Family Practice was established in 1969 and changed its name to the American Board of Family Medicine in 2004.
2. The AAFP is the American Academy of Family Physicians, not the American Academy of Family Practice.
3. Primary care is the provision of continuing, comprehensive care to a population undifferentiated by gender, disease, or organ system.
4. The most cost-effective health care systems depend on a strong primary care base. The United States has the most expensive health care system in the world but ranks among the worst in overall quality of care because of its weak primary care base.
5. The most challenging diagnoses are those that present in their early, undifferentiated stage when there are often only subtle differences between serious disease and minor ailments.
6. The family physician is the quarterback, orchestrating the skills of a variety of health professionals who may be involved in the care of a seriously ill patient.

The family physician provides continuing, comprehensive care in a personalized manner to patients of all ages and to their families, regardless of the presence of disease or the nature of the presenting complaint. Family physicians accept responsibility for managing an individual's total health needs while maintaining an intimate, confidential relationship with the patient.

Family medicine emphasizes responsibility for total health care—from the first contact and initial assessment through the ongoing care of chronic problems. Prevention and early recognition of disease are essential features of the discipline. Coordination and integration of all necessary health services with the least amount of fragmentation and the skills to manage most medical problems allow family physicians to provide cost-effective health care.

Family medicine is a specialty that shares many areas of content with other clinical disciplines, incorporating this shared knowledge and using it uniquely to deliver primary medical care. In addition to sharing content with other medical specialties, family medicine emphasizes knowledge from areas such as family dynamics, interpersonal relations, counseling, and psychotherapy. The specialty's foundation, however, remains clinical, with the primary focus on the medical care of people who are ill.

Devotion to continuing, comprehensive, personalized care, early detection and management of illness, prevention of disease and maintenance of health, and the ongoing management of patients in a community setting uniquely qualify the family physician to deliver primary care.

The curriculum for training family physicians is designed to represent realistically the skills and body of knowledge that the physicians will require in practice. This curriculum relies heavily on an accurate analysis of the problems seen and the skills used by family physicians in their practices. Unfortunately, the content of residency training programs for the primary care specialties has not always been appropriately directed toward solving the problems most commonly encountered by physicians practicing in these specialties. The almost randomly educated primary physician of previous years is being replaced by one specifically prepared to address the kinds of problems likely to be encountered in practice. For this reason, the "model office" is an essential component of all family practice residency programs.

THE JOY OF FAMILY PRACTICE

If you cannot work with love but only with distaste, it is better that you should leave your work and sit at the gate of the temple and take alms from those who work with joy.

Kahlil Gibran (1883–1931)

The rewards in family medicine come largely from knowing patients intimately over time and sharing their trust, respect, and friendship. The thrill is the close bond (actually friendship) that develops with patients. This bond is strengthened with each physical or emotional crisis in a person's life, when he or she turns to the family physician for help.

It is especially rewarding when the family physician cares for a newly married couple, delivers their first baby, sees them frequently for well-child care, and provides ongoing care for the parents, the growing child, and any subsequent children. No other medical specialty is so privileged. To participate in a family's life in such a close and intimate manner is uniquely rewarding.

The practice of family medicine involves the joy of greeting old friends in every examining room, and the variety of problems encountered keeps the physician professionally stimulated and perpetually challenged. In contrast, physicians practicing in narrow specialties often lose their enthusiasm for medicine after seeing the same problems every day. The variety in family practice sustains the excitement and precludes boredom.

PHYSICIAN AND PATIENT SATISFACTION

Physician satisfaction is associated with quality of care, particularly as measured by patient satisfaction. The strongest factor associated with a physician's satisfaction is not personal income but the ability to provide high-quality care to his or her patients. Physicians are most satisfied with their practice when they can have an ongoing relationship with their patients, the freedom to make clinical decisions without financial conflicts of interest, adequate time with patients, and sufficient communication with specialists (DeVoe et al., 2002). DeVoe et al. also found that general internists were more dissatisfied with their careers than family physicians (20.6% vs. 17.3%). Not only can such dissatisfaction lead to health problems in the physicians themselves, but it is difficult to imagine a patient being satisfied with care provided by a dissatisfied physician. Women have a greater chance of burnout than men.

Landon et al. (2003) found that rather than declining income, the strongest predictor of decreasing satisfaction in practice is loss of clinical autonomy. This includes the inability of physicians to obtain services for their patients, control their time with patients, and maintain the freedom to provide high-quality care.

In an analysis of 33 specialties, Leigh et al. (2002) found surprisingly that physicians in high-income "procedural" specialties such as obstetrics/gynecology, otolaryngology, ophthalmology, and orthopedics were the most dissatisfied. Physicians in these specialties and those in internal medicine were more likely than family physicians to be dissatisfied with their careers. Among the specialty areas most satisfying according to the Leigh et al. study was geriatrics. Because the population of those older than age 65 in the United States has doubled since 1960 and will double again between 2000 and 2030 to more

Table 1-1	Physician Attributes Contributing to Patient Satisfaction

1. Does not judge but understands and supports
2. Always honest and direct
3. Acts as partner in maintaining health
4. Treats both serious, and nonserious conditions
5. Attends to emotional/physical health
6. Listens to me
7. Encourages me to lead healthier lifestyle
8. Tries to get to know me
9. Can help with any problem
10. Someone I can stay with as I grow older

From Stock Keister MC, Green LA, Kahn NB, Phillips RL, McCann J, Fryer GE. What people want from their family physician. Am Fam Physician 2004b;69:2310.

than 70 million, it is important that we have sufficient primary care physicians to care for them. The need and the rewards of this type of practice must be communicated to students before they decide how to spend the rest of their professional lives.

Overall, 70% of U.S. physicians are satisfied with their career, with 40% being very satisfied and only 20% dissatisfied (Leigh et al., 2002).

Personal attributes of physicians considered most important for patient satisfaction are listed in rank order in Table 1-1. In addition, people want their primary care doctor to meet five basic criteria: "to be in their insurance plan, to be in a location that is convenient, to be able to schedule an appointment within a reasonable period of time, to have good communication skills, and to have a reasonable amount of experience in practice." They especially want "a physician who listens to them, who takes the time to explain things to them, and who is able to effectively integrate their care" (Stock Keister et al., 2004a,b).

DEVELOPMENT OF THE SPECIALTY

As long ago as 1923, Francis Peabody commented that the swing of the pendulum toward specialization had reached its apex and that modern medicine had fragmented the health care delivery system to too great a degree. He called for a rapid return of the generalist physician who would give comprehensive, personalized care.

Dr. Peabody's declaration proved premature; society and the medical establishment were not ready for such a proclamation. The trend toward specialization gained momentum through the 1950s, and fewer physicians entered general practice. In the early 1960s, leaders in the field of general practice began advocating a seemingly paradoxical solution to reverse the trend and correct the scarcity of general practitioners—the creation of still another specialty. These physicians envisioned a specialty that embodied the knowledge, skills, and ideals that they knew as primary care. In 1966, the concept of a new specialty in primary care received official recognition in two separate reports published 1 month apart. The first of these was the report of the Citizens' Commission on Graduate Medical Education of the American Medical Association (1966), also known as the Millis Commission Report. The second report came from the Ad Hoc Committee on Education for Family Practice of the Council of Medical Education of the American Medical Association (1996), also called the Willard Committee. Three years later, in 1969, the American Board of Family Practice came into being as the 20th medical specialty board, thus giving birth to the specialty of family practice. The name of the specialty board was changed in 2004 to the American Board of Family Medicine (ABFM).

Much of the impetus for the Millis and Willard reports came from the American Academy of General Practice, which was renamed the American Academy of Family Physicians in 1971. The name change reflected a desire to increase emphasis on family-oriented health care and to gain academic acceptance for the new specialty of family practice.

The ABFM has distinguished itself by being the first specialty board to require recertification (every 7 years), now called maintenance of certification, to ensure the ongoing competence of its members. Among basic requirements for certification and recertification, the ABFM has included continuing education, the foundation on which the American Academy of General Practice had been built when organized in 1947. A diplomate of the ABFM must complete 300 hours of acceptable continuing education activity every 6 years and one self-assessment module per year over the Internet to be eligible for recertification. Once eligible, a candidate's competence is examined by cognitive testing and performance in practice evaluation. The ABFM's emphasis on quality of education, knowledge, and performance has facilitated the rapid increase in prestige for the family physician in our health care system. The obvious logic of the ABFM's emphasis on continuing education to maintain required knowledge and skills has been adopted by other specialties and state medical societies. Now, all specialty boards are committed to the concept of recertification to ensure that their diplomates remain current with advances in medicine.

DEFINITIONS

Family Medicine

Family medicine is the medical specialty that provides continuing and comprehensive health care for the individual and the family. It is the specialty in breadth that integrates the biologic, clinical, and behavioral sciences. The scope of family medicine encompasses all ages, both sexes, each organ system, and every disease entity (AAFP, 1993).

In many countries, the term general practice is synonymous with family medicine. The Royal New Zealand College of General Practitioners emphasizes that a general practitioner provides care that is "anticipatory as well as responsive, and is not limited by the age, sex, race, religion or social circumstances of patients, nor by their physical or mental states." The general practitioner must be available and must provide care that is personal, comprehensive, continuing, and coordinated in the context of family and community. He or she must be the patient's advocate; be competent, caring, and compassionate; be able to live with uncertainty; and be willing to recognize limitations and refer when necessary (Richards, 1997).

Both the Council on Graduate Medical Education and the Association of American Medical Colleges define generalist physicians as those who have completed 3-year training programs in family medicine, internal medicine, or pediatrics and do not subspecialize. The Council on Graduate Medical Education emphasizes that this definition should be "based on an objective analysis of training requirements in disciplines that provide graduates with broad capabilities for primary care practice" (Graduate Medical Education National Advisory Committee, 1980).

Family Physician

The family physician is a physician who is educated and trained in the discipline of family medicine, a broadly encompassing medical specialty. Family physicians possess unique attitudes, skills, and knowledge that qualify them to provide continuing and comprehensive medical care, health maintenance, and preventive services to each member of a family regardless of sex, age, or type of problem, be it biologic, behavioral, or social. These specialists, because of their background and interactions with the family, are best qualified to serve as each patient's advocate in all health-related matters, including the appropriate use of consultants, health services, and community resources (American Academy of Family Physicians, 1993).

The World Organization of Family Doctors (World Organization of National Colleges, Academies, and Academic Associations of General Practitioners/ Family Physicians [WONCA]) defines the family doctor in part as

the physician who is primarily responsible for providing comprehensive health care to every individual seeking medical care, and arranging for other health personnel to provide services when necessary. The family physician functions as a generalist who accepts everyone seeking care whereas other health providers limit access to their services on the basis of age, sex, and/or diagnosis. (World Organization of National Colleges, Academies, and Academic Associations of General Practitioners/Family Physicians, 1991, p. 2)

Of Americans reporting an individual provider as their usual source of care in 1996, 62% named a family physician compared with 16% naming an internist and 15% naming a pediatrician. Of those without a primary care physician, twice as many (12%) went without needed services when compared with those with a primary care physician (6%) (Robert Graham Center for Policy Studies in Family Practice and Primary Care, 2000).

Primary Care

Primary care is that care provided by physicians specifically trained for and skilled in comprehensive first-contact and continuing care for ill persons or those with an undiagnosed sign, symptom, or health concern (the "undifferentiated" patient) not limited by problem origin (biologic, behavioral, or social), organ system, or gender.

Primary care includes, in addition to diagnosis and treatment of acute and chronic illnesses, health promotion, disease prevention, health maintenance, counseling, and patient education, in a variety of health care settings such as office, inpatient, critical care, long-term care, home care, and day care. Primary care is performed and managed by a personal physician, using other health professionals for consultation or referral as appropriate.

Primary care provides patient advocacy in the health care system to accomplish cost-effective care by coordination of health care services. Primary care promotes effective doctor-patient communication and encourages the role of the patient as a partner in health care (American Academy of Family Physicians, 1994).

The Institute of Medicine defines primary care as the provision of integrated, accessible health care services by clinicians who are accountable for addressing a large majority of personal health care needs, developing a sustained partnership with patients, and practicing in the context of family and community (Stock Keister et al., 2004a,b).

Because many physicians deliver primary care in different ways and with varying degrees of preparation, the staff of the ABFM has further clarified the definition. According to the ABFM, primary care is a form of delivery of medical care that encompasses the following functions:

1. It is first-contact care, serving as a point of entry for the patient into the health care system.
2. It includes continuity by virtue of caring for patients over a period of time, both in sickness and in health.
3. It is comprehensive care, drawing from all the traditional major disciplines for its functional content.
4. It serves a coordinative function for all the health care needs of the patient.
5. It assumes continuing responsibility for individual patient follow-up and community health problems.
6. It is a highly personalized type of care.

Primary Care Physician

A primary care physician is a generalist physician who provides definitive care to the undifferentiated patient at the point of first contact and takes continuing responsibility for providing the patient's care. Such a physician must be trained specifically to provide primary care services.

Primary care physicians devote the majority of their practice to providing primary care services to a defined population of patients. The style of primary care practice is such that the personal primary care physician serves as the entry point for substantially all the patient's medical and health care needs, not limited by problem origin, organ system, gender, or diagnosis. Primary care physicians are advocates for the patient in coordinating the use of the entire health care system to benefit the patient (American Academy of Family Physicians, 1994).

The ABFM and the American Board of Internal Medicine have agreed on a definition of the generalist physician and that "providing optimal generalist care requires broad and comprehensive training that cannot be gained in brief and uncoordinated educational experiences" (Kimball and Young, 1994, p. 316). They define the generalist physician as one "who provides continuing, comprehensive, and coordinated medical care to a population undifferentiated by gender, disease, or organ system" (p. 315).

Physicians who provide primary care should be trained specifically to manage the problems encountered in a primary care practice. Rivo et al. (1994) identified the common conditions and diagnoses that generalist physicians should be competent to manage in a primary care practice and compared these with the training of the various "generalist" specialties. They recommended that the training of generalist physicians include at least 90% of the key diagnoses. By comparing the content of residency programs, they found that this goal was met by family practice (95%), internal medicine (91%), and pediatrics (91%) but that obstetrics and gynecology

(47%) and emergency medicine (42%) fell far short of this goal.

PERSONALIZED CARE

> *It is much more important to know what sort of patient has a disease than what sort of disease a patient has.*
>
> Sir William Osler (1904)

Family physicians do not just treat patients; they care for people. This caring function of family medicine emphasizes the personalized approach to understanding the patient as a person, respecting the person as an individual, and showing compassion for his or her discomfort. The best illustration of a caring and compassionate physician is "The Doctor" by Sir Luke Fieldes (Fig. 1-1), showing a physician at the bedside of an ill child in the preantibiotic era. This painting has become the symbol for medicine as a caring profession.

> *Caring without science is well-intentioned kindness, but not medicine. On the other hand, science without caring empties medicine of healing and negates the great potential of an ancient profession. The two complement and are essential to the art of doctoring. (Lown, 1996, p. 223)*

Compassion means co-suffering and reflects the physician's willingness somehow to share the patient's anguish and understand what the sickness means to that person. Compassion is an attempt to "feel" along with the patient. Pellegrino (1979, p. 161) stated that "we can never feel with another person when we pass judgment as a superior, only when we see our own frailties as well as his." Pellegrino goes on to comment that a compassionate authority figure is effective only when others can receive the "orders" without being humiliated. The physician must not "put down" the patients but must be ever ready, in Galileo's words, "to pronounce that wise, ingenuous, and modest statement—'I don't know.'" Compassion, practiced in these terms in each patient encounter, obtunds the inherent dehumanizing tendencies of today's highly institutionalized and technologically oriented patterns of patient care.

> *The treatment of a disease may be entirely impersonal; the care of a patient must be completely personal. (Peabody, 1930)*

If an intimate relationship with patients remains our primary concern as physicians, high-quality medical care will persist, regardless of the way in which it is organized and financed. For this reason, family medicine emphasizes consideration of the individual patient in the full context of his or her life, rather than the episodic care of a presenting complaint. The Millis Commission Report stressed that the family physician "focuses not upon individual organs and systems but upon the whole man who lives in a complex social setting, and knows that diagnosis or treatment of a part often overlooks major causative factors and therapeutic opportunities" (Citizens' Commission on Graduate Medical Education, American Medical Association [Millis Commission], 1966, p. 35).

Family physicians assess the illnesses and complaints presented to them, dealing personally with the majority and arranging special assistance for a few. The family physician serves as the patients' advocate, explaining the causes and implications of illness to the patients and their families, and serves as an advisor and confidant to the family, both individually and collectively. The family physician receives many intellectual satisfactions from this practice, but the greatest reward arises from the depth of human understanding and personal satisfaction inherent in family practice.

Patients have adjusted somewhat to a more impersonal form of health care delivery and frequently look to institutions rather than to individuals for their health care; yet, their need for personalized concern and compassion remains. Tumulty (1970) found that patients consider a good physician to be one who (1) shows genuine interest in them, (2) thoroughly evaluates their problem, (3) demonstrates compassion, understanding, and warmth, and (4) provides clear insight into what is wrong and what must be done to correct it.

The family physician's relationship with each patient should reflect compassion, understanding, and patience combined with a high degree of intellectual

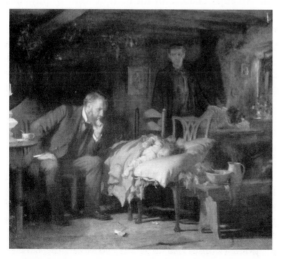

Figure 1-1 *The Doctor* by Sir Luke Fieldes, 1891. (Tate Gallery, London, UK)

honesty. The physician must be thorough in approaching problems but also possess a keen sense of humor. He or she must be capable of encouraging in each patient optimism, courage, insight, and the self-discipline necessary for recovery.

Bulger (1998) addressed the threats to scientific compassionate care in today's managed care environment. "With health care time inordinately rationed today in the interest of economy, Americans could organize themselves right out of compassion. . . . It would be a tragedy, just when we have so many scientific therapies at hand, for scientists to negotiate away the element of compassion, leaving this crucial dimension of healing to nonscientific healers" (p. 106). Time for patient care is becoming increasingly threatened. Bulger described a study involving a "Good Samaritan" principle, showing that the decision of whether to stop and care for a person in distress is predominantly a function of having the time to do so. Even those with the very best intentions require time to be of help to a suffering person.

Ludmerer (1999) focused on the problems facing medical education in this environment.

> *Some managed care organizations have even urged that physicians be taught to act in part as advocates of the insurance payer rather than the patients for whom they care. . . . Medical educators would do well to ponder the potential long-term consequences of educating the nation's physicians in today's commercial atmosphere in which the good visit is a short visit, patients are 'consumers,' and institutional officials speak more often of the financial balance sheet than of service and the relief of patients' suffering.*

Cranshaw et al. (1995) raised similar concerns:

> *Our first obligation must be to serve the good of those persons who seek our help and trust us to provide it. Physicians, as physicians, are not, and must never be, commercial entrepreneurs, gate-closers, or agents of fiscal policy that runs counter to our trust. Any defection from primacy of the patient's well-being places the patient at risk by treatment that may compromise quality of or access to medical care. . . . Only by caring and advocating for Fthe patient can the integrity of our profession be affirmed. (p. 1553)*

CHARACTERISTICS AND FUNCTIONS OF THE FAMILY PHYSICIAN

Attributes of the Family Physician

The following characteristics are certainly desirable for all physicians, but they are of greatest importance for the physician in family practice:

1. A strong sense of responsibility for the total ongoing care of the individual and the family during health, illness, and rehabilitation
2. Compassion and empathy, with a sincere interest in the patient and the family
3. A curious and constantly inquisitive attitude
4. Enthusiasm for the undifferentiated medical problem and its resolution
5. An interest in the broad spectrum of clinical medicine
6. The ability to deal comfortably with multiple problems occurring simultaneously in one patient
7. A desire for frequent and varied intellectual and technical challenges
8. The ability to support children during growth and development and during their adjustment to family and society
9. The ability to assist patients in coping with everyday problems and in maintaining stability in the family and community
10. The capacity to act as coordinator of all health resources needed in the care of a patient
11. A continuing enthusiasm for learning and for the satisfaction that comes from maintaining current medical knowledge through continuing medical education
12. The ability to maintain composure in times of stress and to respond quickly with logic, effectiveness, and compassion
13. A desire to identify problems at the earliest possible stage (or to prevent disease entirely)
14. A strong wish to maintain maximal patient satisfaction, recognizing the need for continuing patient rapport
15. The skills necessary to manage chronic illness and to ensure maximal rehabilitation following acute illness
16. An appreciation for the complex mix of physical, emotional, and social elements in holistic and personalized patient care
17. A feeling of personal satisfaction derived from intimate relationships with patients that naturally develop over long periods of continuous care, as opposed to the short-term satisfaction gained from treating episodic illnesses
18. A skill for and commitment to educating patients and families about disease processes and the principles of good health

The ideal family physician is an explorer, driven by a persistent curiosity and the desire to know more. The family physician is required to be part theologian, as was Paracelsus, part politician, as was Benjamin Rush, and part humorist, as was Oliver Wendell Holmes. At all times, however, the care of the patient—the whole patient—is the primary goal.

Continuing Responsibility

One of the essential functions of the family physician is the willingness to accept ongoing responsibility for managing a patient's medical care. Once a patient or a family has been accepted into the physician's practice, responsibility for care is both total and continuing. The Millis Commission chose the term *primary physician* to emphasize the concept of primary responsibility for the patient's welfare; however, the term *primary care physician* is more popular and refers to any physician who provides first-contact care.

The family physician's commitment to patients does not cease at the end of illness but is a continuing responsibility, regardless of the patient's state of health or the disease process. There is no need to identify the beginning or endpoint of treatment because care of a problem can be reopened at any time, even though a later visit may be primarily for another problem. This prevents the family physician from focusing too narrowly on one problem and helps maintain a perspective on the total patient in his or her environment. Peabody (1930) believed that much patient dissatisfaction results from the physician's neglecting to assume personal responsibility for supervision of the patient's care: "For some reason or other, no one physician has seen the case through from beginning to end, and the patient may be suffering from the very multitude of his counselors" (p. 8).

The greater the degree of continuing involvement with a patient, the more capable the physician is in detecting early signs and symptoms of organic disease and differentiating it from a functional problem. Patients with problems arising from emotional and social conflicts can be managed most effectively by a physician who has intimate knowledge of the individual and of his or her family and community background. This knowledge comes only from insight gained by observing the patient's long-term patterns of behavior and responses to changing stressful situations. This longitudinal view is particularly useful in the care of children and allows the physician to be more effective in assisting children to reach their full potential. The closeness that develops between physicians and young patients increases a physician's ability to aid the patients with problems that occur during later periods in life, such as adjustment to puberty, problems with employment, or marriage and changing social pressures. As the family physician maintains this continuing involvement with successive generations within a family, the ability to manage intercurrent problems increases with knowledge of the total family background.

By virtue of this ongoing involvement and intimate association with the family, the family physician develops a perceptive awareness of a family's nature and style of operation. This ability to observe families over time allows valuable insight that improves the quality of medical care provided to an individual patient. One of the greatest challenges in family medicine is the need to be alert to the changing stresses, transitions, and expectations of family members over time and to the effect that these and other family interactions have on the health of individuals.

Although the family is the family physician's primary concern, his or her skills are equally applicable to the individual living alone or to people in other varieties of family living. Individuals with alternative forms of family living interact with others who have a significant effect on their lives. The principles of group dynamics and interpersonal relationships that affect health are equally applicable to everyone.

The family physician must assess an individual's personality so that presenting symptoms can be appropriately evaluated and given the proper degree of attention and emphasis. A complaint of abdominal pain may be treated lightly in one patient who frequently presents with minor problems, but the same complaint would be investigated immediately and in depth in another individual who has a more stoic personality. The decision regarding which studies to perform and when is influenced by knowledge of the patient's lifestyle, personality, and previous response pattern. The greater the degree of knowledge and insight into the patient's background, which is gained through years of ongoing contact, the more capable the physician is of making an appropriate early and rapid assessment of the presenting complaint. The less background information the physician has to rely on, the greater is the need to depend on costly laboratory studies and the more likely is overreaction to the presenting symptom. Families receiving continuing, comprehensive care have fewer incidences of hospitalization, fewer operations, and fewer physician visits for illnesses compared with those having no regular physician. This is due, at least in part, to the physician's knowledge of the patients, to the physician's seeing them earlier for acute problems and thus preventing complications that would require hospitalization, to the physician's being available by telephone, and to the physician's seeing them more frequently in the office for health supervision. Care is also less expensive because there is less need to rely on radiographic and laboratory procedures and visits to emergency departments.

Collusion of Anonymity

The need for a primary physician who accepts continuing responsibility for patient care was emphasized by Michael Balint (1965) in his concept of "collusion of anonymity." In this situation, the patient is seen by a variety of physicians, not one of whom is willing to accept total management of the problem. Important decisions are made—some good, some bad—but without anyone feeling fully responsible for them.

Peabody (1930) examined the futility of a patient's making the rounds from one specialist to another without finding relief, because the patient

lacked the guidance of a sound general practitioner who understood his physical condition, his nervous temperament and knew the details of his daily life. And many a patient who on his own initiative has sought out specialists, has had minor defects accentuated so that they assume a needless importance, and has even undergone operations that might well have been avoided. Those who are particularly blessed with this world's goods, who want the best regardless of the cost and imagine that they are getting it because they can afford to consult as many renowned specialists as they wish, are often pathetically tragic figures as they veer from one course of treatment to another. Like ships that lack a guiding hand upon the helm, they swing from tack to tack with each new gust of wind but get no nearer to the Port of Health because there is no pilot to set the general direction of their course. (pp. 21–22)

Chronic Illness

The family physician must also be committed to managing the common chronic illnesses that have no known cure but for which continuing management by a personal physician is all the more necessary to maintain an optimal state of health for the patient. It is a difficult and often trying job to manage these continuing, unresolvable, and progressively crippling problems, control of which requires a remodeling of the lifestyle of the entire family.

Almost half (45%) of all Americans have a chronic condition. The costs both to individuals and to the health care system are enormous. In 2000, care of chronic illness consumed 75 cents of every health care dollar spent in the United States (The Robert Wood Johnson Foundation Annual Report, 2002).

Quality of Care

Primary care provided by physicians specifically trained to care for the problems presenting to personal physicians, who know their patients over a span of time, is of higher quality than care provided by other physicians. This has been confirmed by a variety of studies comparing the care given by physicians in different specialties.

Following a review of the literature on quality and cost of care, Boex et al. (1993) noted that

the quality of clinical outcomes of primary care practitioners is comparable to that of specialists or subspecialists in similar, clinically appropriate situations. . . . Practitioners working within their domains of practice have higher quality outcomes than those working outside their regular domains. . . . Physicians and advance practice nurse generalists trained in and practicing generalist competencies provide a higher quality of primary care to their patients than those whose domains of practice are by definition restricted to specialized areas.

When hospitalized patients with pneumonia are cared for by family physicians or full-time specialist hospitalists, the quality of care is comparable, but the hospitalists incur higher hospital charges, longer lengths of stay, and use more resources (Smith et al., 2002).

In the United States, a 20% increase in the number of primary care physicians is associated with a 5% decrease in mortality (40 fewer deaths per 100,000), but the benefit is even greater if the primary care physician is a family physician. Adding one more family physician per 10,000 people is associated with 70 fewer deaths per 100,000, which is a 9% reduction in mortality. Specialists practicing outside their specialty area have increased mortality rates for acquired pneumonia, acute myocardial infarction, congestive heart failure, and upper gastrointestinal hemorrhage. Specialists are trained to look for zebras instead of horses, and specialty care usually means more tests, which can lead to a cascade effect and consequently greater likelihood of adverse effects. A study of the major determinants of health outcomes in all 50 U.S. states found that when the number of specialty physicians increase, outcomes are worse, whereas mortality rates are lower where there are more primary care physicians (Starfield, 2005).

McGann and Bowman (1990) compared the morbidity and mortality of patients hospitalized by family physicians and by internists. They found that, even though the family physicians' patients were older and more severely ill, there was no significant difference in morbidity and mortality. In addition, the total charges for their hospital care were lower.

A comparison of family physicians and obstetricians/gynecologists in the management of low-risk pregnancies showed no difference with respect to neonatal outcomes. However, women cared for by family physicians had fewer cesarean sections and episiotomies and were less likely to receive epidural anesthesia (Hueston et al., 1995).

Patients of subspecialists practicing outside their specialty have longer lengths of hospital stay and higher mortality rates than patients of subspecialists practicing within their specialty or patients of general internists (Weingarten et al., 2002).

The quality of our health care system is being eroded by physicians' being extensively trained, at great expense, to practice in one area and instead practicing in another, such as anesthesiologists practicing in emergency departments and surgeons practicing as generalists. Primary care, to be done well, requires extensive training specifically tailored to problems frequently seen in primary care. These include the early detection, diagnosis, and treatment of depression; the early diagnosis of cancer (especially of the breast and the colon); the management of gynecologic problems; and the care of those with chronic or terminal illness.

As much-needed changes in the American medical system are implemented, it would be wise to keep some perspective on the situation regarding physician distribution. Beeson (1974) has commented:

> I have no doubt at all that a good family doctor can deal with the great majority of medical episodes quickly and competently. A specialist, on the other hand, feels that he must be thorough, not only because of his training but also because he has a reputation to protect. He, therefore, spends more time with each patient and orders more laboratory work. The result is a waste of doctors' time and patients' money. This not only inflates the national health bill, but also creates an illusion of doctor shortage when the only real need is to have the existing doctors doing the right things. (p. 48)

Cost-effective Care

The physician who is well acquainted with the patient not only provides more personal and humane medical care but does so more economically than does the physician involved in only episodic care. The physician who knows his or her patients well can assess the nature of their problems more rapidly and accurately. Because of the intimate, ongoing relationship, the family physician is under less pressure to exclude diagnostic possibilities by use of expensive laboratory and radiographic procedures than is the physician who is unfamiliar with the patient.

The United States has the most expensive health care system in the world. The cost of health care in the United States was just under 6% of the gross domestic product in 1965. It shot up 9.3% in 2002, the largest increase in 11 years, to a total of $1.55 trillion, which is 15% of the gross domestic product, and continues to increase. Projections put health spending at almost 18% of the gross domestic product by 2012.

Although the rhetoric suggests that this cost is worth it to have the best health care system in the world, the truth is that we are far from that goal. In a comparison of the quality of health care in 13 countries using 16 different health indicators, the United States ranked 12th, second from the bottom. A wealth of evidence indicates that quality of health care is associated with primary care performance. Of the seven countries at the top of the average health ranking, five have strong primary care infrastructures. "The higher the primary care physician-to-population ratio in a state, the better most health outcomes are" (Starfield, 2000, p. 485).

Similarly, the greater the number of primary care physicians practicing in a country, the lower is the cost of health care. Figure 1-2 shows that in Great Britain, Canada, and the United States, the cost of health care is inversely proportional to the percentage of generalists practicing in that country.

Countries with strong primary care have lower overall health care costs, improved health outcomes, and healthier populations (Starfield, 2001). In a comparison of 11 features of primary care in 11 Western countries, the United States ranked lowest in terms of primary care ranking and per capita health care expenditures and also performed poorly on public satisfaction, health indicators, and the use of medication (Starfield, 1994).

The Uninsured

In 2004, the total number of uninsured in the United States was approximately 44 million, and contrary to widespread belief, the problem is not confined simply to unemployed or poor persons. More than half of the uninsured have annual incomes greater than $75,000 and eight of 10 are in working families.

The number of Americans without health insurance has been increasing by 1 million per year. In 1995, 14% were without health insurance, and in 2003, the number rose by 1.4 million to 16% of the population. The number of those who are underinsured is growing

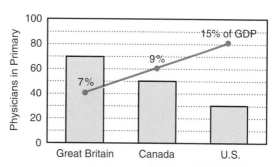

Figure 1-2 Inverse relationship between percentage of primary care physicians and cost of health care in Great Britain, Canada, and the United States.

even more rapidly. "Will we try to save our skins by delivering minimally adequate care on the cheap or will we stand up and be counted in the fight for universal health insurance?" (Eisenberg, 1999, p. 2256). The United States is the only developed country that does not have universal health care coverage for all its citizens. In 1997, the United States had only 33% of the population covered by government-insured health insurance, the lowest percentage of any Organization for Economic Cooperation and Development country (Anderson et al., 1999).

Clearly, the increasing complexity of our health care system multiplies expense and wastefulness when a patient self-diagnoses his or her problems or selects his or her own specialist rather than developing a firm and ongoing relationship with a family physician. The most efficient and cost-effective system involves one personal physician who ensures the most logical and economic management of a problem.

Medical care should be available to patients in the precise degree needed, neither too extensive nor too limited. This ensures that simple problems will not be magnified out of proportion. The more complex and involved a diagnostic process is, the more costly it becomes and the greater is the potential for error. Specialists generally treat their patients more resource intensively than do generalists, resulting in increased cost of care. Cherkin et al. (1987) showed that internists were 1.7 times more likely to hospitalize patients than were family physicians and 1.3 times more likely to refer.

Family physicians order fewer tests than do specialists, perhaps because they know their patients well. MacLean (1993) compared the hospital care given by family physicians with that of all other specialties for patients with gastrointestinal bleeding, nonsurgical back pain, and nutritional, metabolic, or dehydration disorders. He found that the effectiveness of the care was comparable but that the cost of care provided by family physicians was less.

The Institute of Medicine report on the uninsured, Insuring America's Health: Principles and Recommendations, called for "health care coverage by 2010 that is universal, continuous, affordable, sustainable, and enhancing of high-quality care that is effective, efficient, safe, timely, patient centered, and equitable. . . . While stopping short of advocating a specific approach, the IOM's Committee on the Consequences of Uninsurance acknowledges that the single payer model is the most effective in ensuring continuous universal coverage that would remain affordable for individuals and for society" (Geyman, 2004, p. 635).

Comprehensive Care

The term *comprehensive medical care* spans the entire spectrum of medicine. The effectiveness with which a physician delivers primary care depends on the degree of involvement attained during training and practice. The family physician must be trained comprehensively to acquire all the medical skills necessary to care for the majority of patient problems. The greater the number of skills omitted from the family physician's training and practice, the more frequent is the need to refer minor problems to another physician. A truly comprehensive primary care physician adequately manages acute infections, performs biopsies of skin and other lesions, repairs lacerations, treats musculoskeletal sprains and minor fractures, removes foreign bodies, treats vaginitis, provides obstetric care and care for the newborn infant, gives supportive psychotherapy, and supervises diagnostic procedures. The needs of a family physician's patient range from a routine physical examination, when the patient feels well and wishes to identify potential risk factors, to a problem that calls for referral to one or more narrowly specialized physicians with highly developed technical skills. The family physician must be aware of the variety and complexity of skills and facilities available to help manage patients and must match these to the individual's specific needs, giving full consideration to the patient's personality and expectations.

Management of an illness involves much more than a diagnosis and an outline for treatment. It also requires an awareness of all the factors that may aid or hinder an individual's recovery from illness. This requires consideration of religious beliefs; social, economic, or cultural problems; personal expectations; and heredity. The outstanding clinician recognizes the effects that spiritual, intellectual, emotional, social, and economic factors have on a patient's illness.

The family physician's ability to confront relatively large numbers of unselected patients with undifferentiated conditions and carry on a therapeutic relationship over time is a unique primary care skill. The skilled family physician will have a higher level of tolerance for the uncertain than will his or her consultant colleague.

Society will benefit more from a surgeon who has a sufficient volume of surgery to maintain proficiency through frequent use of well-honed skills than from one who has a low volume of surgery and serves also as a primary care physician. The early identification of disease while it is in its undifferentiated stage requires specific training and is not a skill that can be automatically assumed by someone whose training has been mostly in hospital intensive care units. It is unfortunate that, when the number of procedures is inadequate to fully occupy specialists skilled in complex technical procedures, their remaining time is spent providing care (frequently primary care) in areas where their training was limited and often deficient.

Many physicians eventually enter a type of practice different from what their residency prepared them for; the question remains whether many, especially those entering primary care, will undergo the difficult and costly retraining necessary to do the job well.

Interpersonal Skills

One of the foremost skills of the family physician is the ability to use effectively the knowledge of interpersonal relations in the management of patients. This powerful element of clinical medicine is perhaps the specialty's most useful tool. Modern society considers the medical care system inadequate in those situations in which understanding and compassion are important to the patient's comfort and recovery from illness. Physicians too often are seen as lacking this personal concern and as being unskilled in understanding personal anxiety and feelings. There is an obvious need to nourish the seed of compassion and concern for sick people with which students enter medical school.

Family medicine emphasizes the integration of compassion, empathy, and personalized concern to a greater degree than does a more technical or task-oriented specialty. Some of the earnest solicitude of the old country doctor and his or her untiring compassion for people must be incorporated as effective yet impersonal modern medical procedures are applied. The patient should be viewed compassionately as a person in distress who needs to be treated with concern, dignity, and personal consideration. He or she has a right to be given some insight into his or her problems, a reasonable appraisal of the potential outcome, and a realistic picture of the emotional, financial, and occupational expenses involved in his or her care. The greatest deterrents to filing malpractice claims are patient satisfaction, good patient rapport, and active patient participation in the health care process.

To relate well to patients, a physician must develop compassion and courtesy, the ability to establish rapport and to communicate effectively, the ability to gather information rapidly and to organize it logically, the skills required to identify all significant patient problems and to manage these problems appropriately, the ability to listen, the skills necessary to motivate people, and the ability to observe and detect nonverbal clues.

Much of the family physician's effectiveness in interpersonal relationships depends on his or her charisma. Charisma is a personal magic of leadership, a magnetic charm or appeal that arouses special loyalty or enthusiasm. The charismatic physician is most likely to engender maximal patient compliance and satisfaction. The physician must be aware of his or her own feelings, however, and their effect on the patient. Charisma can be a useful therapeutic tool, but one must learn how and when to use it effectively because it can also rebound with unfavorable consequences. The physician should be aware that the patient's needs are paramount. The temptation to "take an ego trip" is frequent and hazardous.

Accessibility

Just as charisma is therapeutic, so too is the mere availability of the physician. The feeling of security that the patient gains just by knowing that he or she can "touch" the physician, either in person or by phone, is in itself therapeutic and has a comforting and calming influence. Accessibility is an essential feature of primary care. Services must be available when needed and should be within geographic proximity. When primary care is not available, many individuals turn to hospital emergency departments. Emergency department care is, of course, fine for emergencies, but it is no substitute for the personalized, long-term, comprehensive care that a family physician can provide.

Many practices are going to open-access scheduling in which patients can be seen the day they call, as has been advocated in the Future of Family Medicine report (see Chapter 2, "Future of Family Medicine"). Open-access scheduling permits patients to be seen the day they wish to. This tells the patient that he or she is the highest priority and his or her problem will be handled immediately. It also is more efficient for the physician who cares for a problem early, before it progresses in severity and becomes complicated, requiring more physician time and patient disability.

Diagnostic Skills: Undifferentiated Problems

The family physician must be, above all, an outstanding diagnostician. Skills in this area must be honed to perfection because problems are usually seen in their early, undifferentiated state and without the degree of resolution that is usually present by the time patients are referred to consulting specialists. This is a unique feature of family medicine because symptoms seen at this stage are often vague and nondescript, with signs being either minimal or absent. Unlike the consulting specialist, the family physician does not evaluate the case after it has been preselected by another physician, and the diagnostic procedures used by the family physician must be selected from the entire spectrum of medicine.

At this stage of disease, there are often only subtle differences between the early symptoms of serious disease and those of self-limiting, minor ailments. To the inexperienced person, the clinical pictures may appear identical, but to the astute and experienced family physician, one symptom will be more suspicious than another because of the greater probability that it signals a potentially serious illness. Diagnoses are frequently made based on probability, and the likelihood that a specific disease is present frequently depends on the incidence of the disease relative to the symptom seen in the physician's community during a given time of year. Approximately one fourth of all patients seen will never be assigned a final, definitive diagnosis because the resolution of a presenting symptom or complaint will come before a specific diagnosis can be made. Pragmatically, this is an efficient method that is less costly and achieves high patient satisfaction, even though it may be disquieting to the purist physician who believes a thorough workup and specific diagnosis always should be obtained. Similarly, family physicians are more likely to use a therapeutic trial to confirm the diagnosis.

The family physician is an expert in the rapid assessment of a problem presented for the first time. He or she evaluates its potential significance, often making a diagnosis by exclusion rather than by inclusion, after making certain that the symptoms are not those of a serious problem. Once assured, some time is allowed to elapse. Time is used as an efficient diagnostic aid. Follow-up visits are scheduled at appropriate intervals to watch for subtle changes in the presenting symptoms. The physician usually identifies the symptom that has the greatest discriminatory value and watches it more closely than the others. The most significant clue to the true nature of the illness may depend on subtle changes in this key symptom. The family physician's effectiveness is often determined by his or her knack for perceiving the hidden or subtle dimensions of illness and following them closely.

The maxim that an accurate history is the most important factor in arriving at an accurate diagnosis is especially appropriate to family medicine because symptoms may be the only obvious feature of an illness at the time that it is presented to the family physician. Further inquiry into the nature of the symptoms, time of onset, extenuating factors, and other unique subjective features may provide the only diagnostic clues available at such an early stage. Above all, the family physician must be a skilled clinician with the ability to evaluate symptoms, verbal and nonverbal communication, and early signs of illness to choose those diagnostic tests that are of greatest value in diagnosing a problem early.

The family physician must be a perceptive humanist, alert to early identification of new problems. Arriving at an early diagnosis may, in fact, be of less importance than determining the real reason the patient came to the physician. The symptoms may be the result of a self-limiting or acute problem, but anxiety or fear may be the true precipitating factor. Although the symptom may be hoarseness that has resulted from postnasal drainage accompanying an upper respiratory tract infection, the patient may fear it is caused by a laryngeal carcinoma similar to that recently found in a friend. Clinical evaluation must rule out the possibility of laryngeal carcinoma, but the patient's fears and apprehension regarding this possibility must also be allayed. Similarly, a 42-year-old man with influenza and pleuritic chest pain may be anxious and apprehensive because his father died at age 45 years of an acute myocardial infarction. (In fact, a frequent reason for a patient's requesting a complete checkup and electrocardiogram is the recent heart attack of an acquaintance at work.) Mild thrombophlebitis in a 35-year-old woman could bring her to the physician in a more anxious state than is warranted because her mother died of a pulmonary embolus, or a woman's anxiety about breast cancer may well stem from a friend's recent breast surgery.

Every physical problem has an emotional component, and although this factor is usually minimal, it can be extremely significant. A patient's personality, fears, and anxieties all play a role in every illness and are important factors in all primary care.

The Family Physician as Coordinator

Francis Peabody, Professor of Medicine at Harvard Medical School from 1921 to 1927, was a man ahead of his time; his comments remain appropriate today:

> *Never was the public in need of wise, broadly trained advisors so much as it needs them today to guide them through the complicated maze of modern medicine. The extraordinary development of medical science, with its consequent diversity of medical specialism and the increasing limitations in the extent of special fields—the very factors, indeed, which are creating specialists, in themselves create a new demand, not for men who are experts along narrow lines, but for men who are in touch with many lines. (Peabody, 1930, p. 20)*

The family physician, by virtue of his or her breadth of training in a wide variety of medical disciplines, has unique insights into the skills possessed by physicians in the more limited specialties. The family physician is best prepared to select specialists whose skills can be applied most appropriately to a given case, as well as to coordinate the activities of each, so that they are not counterproductive.

As medicine becomes more specialized and complex, the family physician's role as the integrator of health services becomes increasingly important. The family physician not only facilitates the patient's access to the whole health care system but also interprets the activities of this system to the patient, explaining the nature of the illness, the implication of the treatment, and the effect of both on the patient's way of life. The following statement from the Millis Commission Report concerning expectations of the patient is especially appropriate:

> The patient wants, and should have, someone of high competence and good judgment to take charge of the total situation, someone who can serve as coordinator of all the medical resources that can help solve his problem. He wants a company president who will make proper use of his skills and knowledge of more specialized members of the firm. He wants a quarterback who will diagnose the constantly changing situation, coordinate the whole team, and call on each member for the particular contributions that he is best able to make to the team effort. (Citizens' Commission on Graduate Medical Education, American Medical Association [Millis Commission], 1966, p. 39)

Such breadth of vision is important for a coordinating physician. He or she must have a realistic overview of the problem and an awareness of the many alternative routes to select the one that is most appropriate. A physician familiar with one form of treatment tends to rely on it excessively, whereas the family physician can select the best approach from all possible alternatives. As stated:

> It should be clear, too, that no simple addition of specialties can equal the generalist function. To build a wall one needs more than the aimless piling up of bricks, one needs an architect. Every operation which analyzes some part of the human mechanism requires to be balanced by another which synthesizes and coordinates. (Pellegrino, 1966, p. 542)

The complexity of modern medicine frequently involves a variety of health professionals, each with highly developed skills in a particular area. In planning the patient's care, the family physician, having established rapport with a patient and family and having knowledge of the patient's background, personality, fears, and expectations, is best able to select and coordinate the activities of appropriate individuals from the large variety of medical disciplines. He or she can maintain effective communication among those involved as well as function as the patient's advocate and interpret to the patient and family the many unfamiliar and complicated procedures being used. This prevents any one consulting physician, unfamiliar with the concepts or actions of all others involved, from ordering a test or medication that would conflict with other treatment. Dunphy (1964) described the value of the surgeon and the family physician working closely as a team:

> It is impossible to provide high quality surgical care without that knowledge of the whole patient which only a family physician can supply. When their mutual decisions . . . bring hope, comfort and, ultimately, health to a gravely ill human being, the total experience is the essence and the joy of medicine. (p. 12)

The ability to orchestrate the knowledge and skills of diverse professionals is a skill to be learned during training and cultivated in practice. It is not an automatic attribute of all physicians or merely the result of exposure to a large number of professionals. These coordinator skills extend beyond the traditional medical disciplines into the many community agencies and allied health professions as well. Because of his or her close involvement with the community, the family physician is ideally suited to be the integrator of the patient's care, coordinating the skills of consultants when appropriate and involving community nurses, social agencies, the clergy, or other family members when needed. Knowledge of community health resources and personal involvement with the community can be used to maximal benefit, not only for diagnostic and therapeutic purposes but also to achieve the best possible level of rehabilitation.

THE FAMILY PHYSICIAN IN PRACTICE

The advent of family medicine has led to a renaissance in medical education involving a reassessment of the traditional medical education environment in a teaching hospital. It is now considered more realistic to train a physician in a community atmosphere, providing exposure to the diseases and problems most closely approximating those that he or she will encounter during practice. The ambulatory care skills and knowledge that most medical graduates will need cannot be taught totally within the tertiary medical center. The specialty of family practice emphasizes training in ambulatory care skills in an appropriately realistic environment, using patients representing a cross-section of a community and incorporating those problems most frequently encountered by physicians practicing primary care.

The lack of relevance in the referral medical center also applies to the hospitalized patient. Figure 1-3 places the health problems of an average community in perspective. In any given month, 800 people will experience at least one symptom. Most of these people will be managed by self-treatment, but 217 will consult a physician. Of these, eight will be hospitalized, but only one will go to an academic medical center. It is obvious that patients seen in the medical center (the majority of cases used for teaching) represent atypical samples of illness occurring within the community. Students exposed to patients in only this manner develop an unrealistic concept

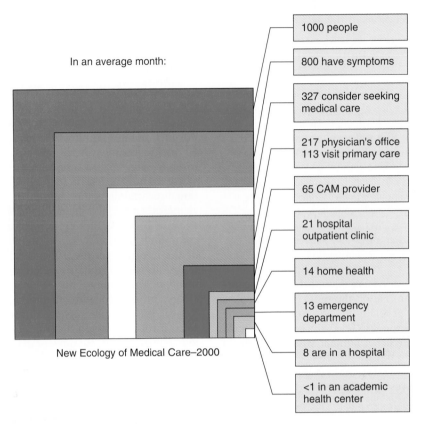

In an average month:

	1000 people
	800 have symptoms
	327 consider seeking medical care
	217 physician's office 113 visit primary care
	65 CAM provider
	21 hospital outpatient clinic
	14 home health
	13 emergency department
	8 are in a hospital
	<1 in an academic health center

New Ecology of Medical Care–2000

Figure 1-3 Number of persons experiencing an illness during an average month, per 1000 population. (From Green LA, Fryer GE Jr, Yawn BP, Lanier D, Dovey SM. The ecology of medical care revisited. N Engl J Med 2001;344:2021–2025.)

of the kinds of medical problems prevalent in society and, particularly, those composing primary care. It focuses their training on knowledge and skills of limited usefulness in later practice. Medical schools should accept the responsibility of providing health care for a defined population, and the dean's office should ensure that the curriculum is congruent with the health needs of that population.

In a typical family physician's practice that cares for 1500 to 3000 individuals, two-thirds will be seen at least once each year. Many practicing family physicians and most family practice residency programs are recording the type and frequency of problems seen. Undergraduate and graduate curricula now are being revised to address more closely the problems that will be encountered in practice.

Practice Content

Family physicians account for a larger proportion of office visits to U.S. physicians than any other specialty. However,

the country's health care (non) system has undergone a major transformation to a market-based system largely dominated by corporate interests and a business ethic. The goal envisioned in the 1960s of rebuilding the U.S. health care system on a generalist base, with all Americans having ready access to comprehensive health care through a personal physician, has not been achieved. Overspecialization was a problem as long as 4000 years ago when Herodotus in 2000 BC noted that "The art of medicine is thus divided: each physician applies himself to one disease only and not more." (Geyman, 2004)

The National Ambulatory Medical Care Survey conducted by the National Center for Health Statistics of the U.S. Department of Health and Human Services has, since 1975, annually reported the problems seen by office-based physicians (in all specialties) in the United States. The 20 most common diagnoses seen by physicians in their offices are shown in Table 1-2. Characteristics of visits to primary care physicians are shown in Table 1-3. Note that diabetes mellitus is the third most common problem and reflects the increasing prevalence of this disease.

Primary care physicians manage an average of 1.65 problems per visit. Of visits to primary care physicians, 61% were for a medical examination compared with 23% for surgical specialists. Although hypertension is the most common problem encountered in offices (see Table 1-2), primary care physicians checked

Table 1-2 Rank Order of Office Visits by Diagnosis
1. Essential hypertension
2. Routine infant or child health check
3. Acute upper respiratory infections, excluding pharyngitis
4. Diabetes mellitus
5. Arthropathies and related disorders
6. General medical examination
7. Spinal disorders
8. Rheumatism, excluding back
9. Normal pregnancy
10. Otitis media and eustachian tube disorders
11. Malignant neoplasms
12. Chronic sinusitis
13. Allergic rhinitis
14. Asthma
15. Gynecologic examination
16. Disorder of lipoid metabolism
17. Heart disease, excluding ischemic
18. Ischemic heart disease
19. Acute pharyngitis
20. Follow-up examination

From National Center for Health Statistics (Woodwell DA, Cherry DK): 2002 Summary: National Ambulatory Medical Care Survey. Advance Data Vital Health Stat no. 346, Aug. 26, 2004.

Table 1-3 Characteristics of Visits to Primary Care Specialists
Accounted for 62.7% of all visits in 2002, with 76% to the patient's designated primary care provider
Major reason for visit to primary care specialists
Acute conditions: 41.5%
Chronic conditions: 29.6%
Preventive care: 23.3%
Top five illness-related diagnoses are
Hypertension: 7.8%
Acute upper respiratory infections (excluding pharyngitis): 5.1%
Diabetes mellitus: 3.1%
Otitis media: 2.4%
Arthropathies: 2.1%
Injury visits accounted for 9.4% of all visits to primary care specialists
Common services ordered or provided
General medical examination: 60.8%
Blood pressure check: 60.1%
Urinalysis: 12.8%
Complete blood count: 10.9%
Diet/nutrition counseling: 19.3%
Exercise counseling: 12.2%
Top therapeutic drug classes were
Vaccines/antisera: 5.7% of drug mentions
Nonsteroidal anti-inflammatory drugs: 5.5% of drug mentions
Antihistamines: 4.8% of drug mentions
Antidepressants: 4.0% of drug mentions
Antihypertensives: 3.9% of drug mentions
Anti-asthmatics: 3.8% of drug mentions
Disposition of visit
Return for an appointment: 53.4%
Return if needed: 33.4%
Referred to another physician: 8.0%
Average face-to-face duration: 17.4 minutes

From National Center for Health Statistics (Woodwell DA, Cherry DK): 2002 Summary: National Ambulatory Medical Care Survey. Advance Data Vital Health Stat no. 346, Aug. 26, 2004.

the blood pressure at 60% of the visits compared with only 20% of surgical specialists and 40% of visits to medical specialists (National Center for Health Statistics [Woodwell DA, Cherry DK], 2004).

Available data concerning primary care indicate that more people use this type of medical service than any other kind and that, contrary to popular opinion, sophisticated medical technology is not normally either required or overused in basic primary care encounters. Indeed, most primary care visits arise from patients requesting care for relatively uncomplicated problems, many of which are self-limiting but cause the patients concern or discomfort. Treatment is often symptomatic, consisting of pain relief or anxiety reduction rather than a "cure." The greatest cost efficiency results when these patients' needs are satisfied while the self-limiting course of the disease is recognized without incurring unnecessary costs for additional tests.

House Calls

Although the number of house calls being made by family physicians has declined significantly, it is now on the increase because of increasing need resulting from shortened hospital stay; increased home care involving intravenous fluids, chemotherapy, and respiratory care previously requiring hospitalization; and the increase in the number of homebound elderly. Adelman et al. (1994) surveyed primary care physicians and found that 63% of family physicians made house calls compared with 47% of general internists and 15% of general pediatricians. Those who made house calls shared the belief that house calls are important for good comprehensive patient care and are satisfying for the physician as well as for the patient.

The house call continues to be a valuable tool used by family physicians to develop a thorough understanding of patients and their environment, and family practice residencies encourage house calls in their training programs. Family physicians who make house calls report an average of 1.6 per week (American Academy of Family Physicians, 1999).

Elderly patients, especially the frail elderly, often have considerable difficulty getting to and from the physician's office. The patient is more comfortable and under less stress at home, and more problems can be identified, leading to improved care. Ramsdell et al. (1989) have shown that home visit assessments reveal, on average, two new problems and as many as eight new treatment recommendations when home visits follow physician office–based assessments. Home visits may be the only way to identify some environmental hazards and to evaluate functional status accurately.

> **Material Available on Student Consult**
>
> Review Questions and Answers about The Family Physician

REFERENCES

Adelman AM, Fredman L, Knight AL. House call practices: A comparison by specialty. J Fam Pract 1994;38:39–44.

Ad Hoc Committee on Education for Family Practice, Council on Medical Education of the American Medical Association (Willard Committee): Meeting the Challenge of Family Practice (Report). Chicago: American Medical Association, 1966.

American Academy of Family Physicians: Congress Reporter, Congress Adopts Revised Definitions Concerning Family Physician, October 5–7, 1993:4–5.

American Academy of Family Physicians. Directors' Newsletter, AAFP Revises Primary Care Definition, and Exhibit 1, February 4, 1994, p 1.

American Academy of Family Physicians. Facts about: Family Practice. Kansas City, MO: American Academy of Family Physicians, 1999.

Anderson GF, Poullier JP. Health spending, access, and outcomes: Trends in industrialized countries. Health Affairs 1999;18:178.

Balint M. The Doctor, His Patient and the Illness. New York: Pitman, 1965.

Beeson PB. Some good features of the British National Health Service. J Med Educ 1974;49:43–49.

Boex JR, Edwards J, Garg M, et al. Generalist and Specialist Practitioner: Analyses of Quality and Costs of Care. Report to the W. K. Kellogg Foundation, Battle Creek, MI, October 7, 1993.

Bulger RJ. The Quest for Mercy: The Forgotten Ingredient in Health Care Reform. Charlottesville, VA: Carden Jennings Publishing, 1998.

Cherkin DC, Rosenblatt RA, Hart LG, et al. The use of medical resources by residency-trained family physicians and general internists: Is there a difference? Med Care 1987;25:455–469.

Citizens' Commission on Graduate Medical Education, American Medical Association (Millis Commission). The Graduate Education of Physicians (Report). Chicago: American Medical Association, 1966.

Cranshaw R, Rogers DE, Pellegrino ED, et al. Patient-physician covenant. JAMA 1995;273:1553.

DeVoe J, Fryer GE, Hargraves L, et al. Does career dissatisfaction affect the ability of family physicians to deliver high-quality patient care? J Fam Pract 2002;51:223–228.

Dunphy JE. Responsibility and authority in American surgery. Bull Am Coll Surg 1964;49:9–12.

Eisenberg L. Whatever happened to the faculty on the way to the agora? Arch Intern Med 1999;159:2251–2256.

Geyman JP. Drawing on the legacy of general practice to build the future of family medicine. Fam Med 2004;36:631–638.

Graduate Medical Education National Advisory Committee. Final Report Vol. 1 (DHHS Publication no. [HRA] 81-651). Hyattsville, MD: Health Resources Administration, 1980.

Hueston WJ, Applegate JA, Mansfield CJ, et al. Practice variations between family physicians and obstetricians in the management of low-risk pregnancies. J Fam Pract 1995;40:345.

Kimball HR, Young PR. A statement on the generalist physician from the American boards of family practice and internal medicine. JAMA 1994;271:315–316.

Landon BE, Reschovsky J, Blumenthal D. Changes in career satisfaction among primary care and specialist physicians, 1997–2001. JAMA 2003;289:442–449.

Leigh JP, Kravitz RL, Schembri M, et al. Physician career satisfaction across specialties. Arch Intern Med 2002;162:1577–1584.

Lown B. The Lost Art of Healing. Boston: Houghton Mifflin, 1996.

Ludmerer KM. Time to heal: American medical education from the turn of the century to the era of managed care. New York: Oxford University Press, 1999.

MacLean DS. Outcome and cost of family physicians' care: Pilot study of three diagnosis-related groups in elderly inpatients. J Am Board Fam Pract 1993;6:588–593.

McGann KP, Bowman MA. A comparison of morbidity and mortality for family physicians' and internists' admissions. J Fam Pract 1990;31:541–545.

National Center for Health Statistics (Woodwell DA, Cherry DK). 2002 Summary: National Ambulatory Medical Care Survey (Advance Data Vital Health Stat no. 346, August 26, 2004). Washington, DC: Government Printing Office, 2004.

Osler W. Aequanimitas, and Other Addresses. Philadelphia: Blakiston, 1904.

Peabody FW. Doctor and Patient. New York: Macmillan, 1930.

Pellegrino ED. The generalist function in medicine. JAMA 1966;198:541–545.

Pellegrino ED. Humanism and the Physician. Knoxville, TN: University of Tennessee Press, 1979.

Ramsdell JW, Swart JA, Jackson JE, et al. The yield of a home visit in the assessment of geriatric patients. J Am Geriatr Soc 1989;37:17–24.

Richards JG. The Nature of General Practice: General Practice in New Zealand, 1997. Wellington, New Zealand: The Royal New Zealand College of General Practitioners, 1997.

Rivo ML, Saultz JW, Wartman SA, et al. Defining the generalist physician's training. JAMA 1994;271:1499–1504.

Robert Graham Center for Policy Studies in Family Practice and Primary Care. The importance of having a usual source of health care. Am Fam Physician 2000;62:477.

Robert Wood Johnson Foundation Annual Report 2002, Princeton, NJ; 2002:1–28.

Smith PC, Westfall JM, Nicholas RA. Primary care family physicians and 2 hospitalist models: Comparison of outcomes, processes, and costs. J Fam Pract 2002;51:1021–1027.

Starfield B. Is primary care essential? Lancet 1994;344:1129–1133.

Starfield B. Is US health really the best in the world? JAMA 2000;284:483–485.

Starfield B. New paradigms for quality in primary care. Br J Gen Pract 2001;51:303–309.

Starfield B, Shi L, Grover A, et al. The effects of specialist supply on populations' health: Assessing the evidence. Health Affairs 2005;0:W5-97–W5-107 (Web Exclusive). Available at http://content.healthaffairs.org/cgi/content/abstract/hlthaff.w5.97v1. Accessed 4/4/06.

Stock Keister MC, Green LA, Kahn NB, Phillips RL, McCann J, Fryer GE. Few people in the United States can identify primary care physicians. Am Fam Physician 2004a;69:2312.

Stock Keister MC, Green LA, Kahn NB, Phillips RL, McCann J, Fryer GE. What people want from their family physician. Am Fam Physician 2004b;69:2310.

Tumulty PA. What is a clinician and what does he do? N Engl J Med 1970;283:20–24.

Weingarten SR, Lloyd L, Chiou CF, Braunstein GD. Do subspecialists working outside of their specialty provide less efficient and lower-quality care to hospitalized patients than do primary care physicians? Arch Intern Med 2002;162:527–532.

World Organization of National Colleges, Academies, and Academic Associations of General Practitioners/Family Physicians. The Role of the General Practitioner/Family Physician in Health Care Systems. Victoria, Australia, World Organization, 1991.

Chapter

2   The Future of Family Medicine

Larry A. Green, Norman B. Kahn, Jr., and James C. Martin

KEY POINTS

1. The American public values the role of a trusted personal physician.
2. The American public views the family physician as a community leader.
3. Characteristics of a family physician include a deep understanding of the dynamics of the "whole" person, a generative impact on patients' lives, a talent for humanizing the health care experience, a natural command of complexity, and a commitment to being available to patients.
4. The key challenges that will affect the success of a family medicine impact on health care include the following:
   a. Promotion of the discipline and its role in the health care system.
   b. A clear public identity and a consistent basket of services.
   c. Respectful enhancement of the role of family medicine in academic centers.
   d. Development of a more attractive career, addressing scope of practice, lifestyle, and compensation.
   e. Incorporation of clinical technology and information into practice.
5. The "New Model" of family medicine is characterized by the following:
   a. Establishment of a personal medical home.
   b. A defined basket of services.
   c. The use of information technology.
   d. The achievement of quality as described in the Institute of Medicine Quality Chasm Report.
   e. Continued assessment of quality patient care improvement and sound business planning and strategies.
6. Future emphasis of family medicine will include the following:
   a. Educational innovation at the residency level.
   b. The incorporation of adult learning techniques in lifelong continuing medical education.
   c. Consideration of a science research agenda for the discipline.
   d. The reassessment of the discipline's role in academic health centers.
   e. Enhanced political and advocacy roles.

Even within the constraints of today's flawed health care system, there are major opportunities for family physicians to realize improvements in both results for patients and economic performance for physicians. A period of active experimentation and redevelopment of family medicine is called for now. The future success of the discipline and its impact on public well-being depend in large measure on family medicine's ability to rearticulate its vision and competencies in a fashion that has greater resonance with the public while substantially revising the organization and processes by which care is delivered. When these goals are accomplished, family physicians will achieve more fully the aspirations articulated by the specialty's core values and contribute to the solution of the nation's serious health care problems (Martin et al., 2004).

HISTORICAL CONTEXT

Historically, the prestige and respect of the medical profession were based on a personal relationship of trust, a respect for the scientifically inquiring mind, and the commitment to place the needs of others above those of the physician. Before World War II, American health care was provided primarily by the general practitioner, a physician who met the characteristics of trust and sacrifice; but, as medical knowledge expanded rapidly, the general practitioner was viewed as less knowledgeable and more limited in the management of complicated disease.

The rapid growth of medical specialties after World War II was accompanied by the decline of general practice, resulting in fragmented health care. By the 1960s, the dominance of medical specialization so highlighted the loss of the generalist function in medicine that society called for the return and prominence of the generalist in medicine, ultimately resulting in the development of the specialty of family medicine in 1969 (Folsom, 1966; Millis, 1966; Willard, 1966). The new specialty of family medicine delivered on its promise to restore what the public needed and wanted as the new family physicians provided frontline medical care to people of all socioeconomic strata and in all regions of the country (Graham et al., 2002). With the establishment of a sufficient family medicine workforce largely addressed after a generation, new challenges emerged.

By the turn of the millennium, a large and growing proportion of the American population lacked health insurance, and almost one fifth of people did not have a usual source of care. Compared with other nations, the United States demonstrated relatively poor health statistics, with persistent disparities in health among population subgroups, while health care expenditures accelerated. Individual health care was recognized once again to be highly fragmented,

error prone, and rarely integrated in a way that satisfied either patients or clinicians. Public health infrastructures were disconnected from primary care. Mental health care, while indivisible from primary care, remained marginalized. There was renewed uncertainty about the adequacy and distribution of the health care workforce, with medical students' interest in primary care careers declining. The public's understanding of both the role of family physicians and the function of primary care was low, and forecasts of collapse of the health care system were frequent fare in the media (Donaldson et al., 1996; Geyman, 2002; Green and Fryer, 2002; Institute of Medicine, 2000, 2001, 2002a,b).

Recognizing the growing frustration among family physicians, confusion among the public about the role of family physicians, and continuing underperformance throughout the U.S. health care system, the leadership of seven U.S. family medicine organizations initiated the Future of Family Medicine (FFM) Project in 2002.

THE FUTURE OF FAMILY MEDICINE PROJECT

The goal articulated for the FFM Project was to "develop a strategy to transform and renew the specialty of family medicine to meet the needs of people and society in a changing environment" (Martin et al., 2004). The work was organized into six national task forces with diverse, interdisciplinary representation. The FFM Project was overseen by a project leadership committee composed of leaders from the sponsoring organizations, staffed by the American Academy of Family Physicians, and financed by the organizations of the discipline and by both public and private organizations.

The project commissioned research conducted by recognized national research organizations not familiar with family medicine. A market research firm performed secondary data analysis of the findings as well as large representative national data sets and literature review and sought opinions of recognized international experts in health care delivery. Through iterative discussions among the task forces, the project leadership committee, panels of reactors from across the country, and the contracted researchers, visions of the future of American health care and family medicine were elaborated, with conclusions and recommendations published in 2004 (Bucholtz et al., 2004; Dickinson et al., 2004; Green et al., 2004; Jones et al., 2004; Martin et al., 2004; Roberts et al., 2004; Spann et al., 2004).

The key findings, conclusions, attributes, and characteristics of family physicians and the major challenges facing family medicine can be summarized as follows.

KEY FINDINGS AND CONCLUSIONS

Family medicine continues to meet both a fundamental public need and the public's demand for integrated, relationship-centered health care. Family physicians currently play a large and critical role in health care throughout the United States while caring for millions of people with the nation's priority health problems (Martin et al., 2004).

Despite their critical role in American health care, family physicians are not well recognized by the public as distinct and differentiated from other physicians. Nonetheless, approximately two thirds of people seeing a family physician correctly identify their physician's specialty (Martin et al., 2004).

Family medicine functions within an overall U.S. health care system that has been characterized by the Institute of Medicine as unsafe, with gaps in quality and disparities in care for population groups. The U.S. health care system is challenged to refocus on the key aims of safety, effectiveness, patient-centeredness, timeliness, efficiency, and equity (Institute of Medicine, 2000, 2001, 2002a,b).

Family medicine's core values of continuing, comprehensive, compassionate, personal care provided in the context of family and community are congruent with the requirements of the 21st century health care system. Equally important, these values are shared by patients (Bucholtz et al., 2004; Green et al., 2004; Jones et al., 2004).

Patients want their doctor to be in their insurance plan, located conveniently, available by appointment quickly, able to communicate with them, and experienced. Beyond these basics, patients value a relationship with their physician above all else, wanting a personal physician who will listen to them, take time to explain things, and integrate their overall care (Green et al, 2004; Stock Keister et al., 2004).

People judge health care quality on relationships, in which they rate family physicians highly. Patients may forgive inadequate service delivered by the system to continue a highly valued relationship with a physician (Green et al., 2004; Stock Keister et al., 2004).

People are skeptical that any one physician can treat people with any condition, believing medicine is too complicated for one doctor to "do it all," yet they define the best physician as someone whom they trust or as a specialist. There is an unresolved tension between the public's desire for a primary physician who treats the patient as a whole person and the desire for access to highly specialized services (Green et al., 2004; Stock Keister et al., 2004).

Family physicians are recognized to have a deep understanding of the dynamics of the whole person, a generative impact on patients' lives, a talent for humanizing the health care experience, a natural command of complexity, and a commitment to being available to their patients in the different ways that different patients require. Family physicians are committed to fostering health and integrating health care for the whole person by humanizing medicine and providing science-based, high-quality care (Martin et al., 2004).

Changes must occur both within the specialty and perhaps more importantly within the broader health care system to ensure the ability of family medicine to fulfill its mission and role. Unless these changes are accomplished, the position of family medicine in a dysfunctional U.S. health system may be untenable in a 10- to 20-year time frame, which would have serious detrimental consequences on the health of the public.

KEY CHALLENGES FACING FAMILY MEDICINE IN THE UNITED STATES

The FFM Project revealed five challenges for family medicine to address to increase its impact in the U.S. health care system.

1. Family medicine should communicate and actively promote a broader, more accurate understanding of the discipline and its role in the U.S. health care system.
2. Family medicine should design its practices so that the discipline attains a clear public identity. As a specialty that admires independence and whose strength is its wide scope and locally adapted practice, the discipline has not clearly communicated to the public who family physicians are, what family physicians do, and what the specialty offers to the public.
3. Despite well-earned respect in practice, winning respect for family medicine in academic circles continues to be a challenge. The academic environment has been recognized as often disparaging of primary care and of family medicine in particular.
4. Successful implementation of the FFM-recommended strategies should make family medicine a more attractive career option. Concerns about the scope of practice, lifestyle, and compensation are integral to the challenges facing the role of family medicine in U.S. health care.
5. Family medicine should address the public's perception that family medicine is less solidly grounded in science and technology than are medical subspecialties. Family medicine has the opportunity to lead medicine in implementing science-based practice. Family medicine should actively incorporate appropriate information and clinical technology into practice.

To address these challenges, changes are needed nearly simultaneously in clinical practice (how family

Table 2-1 Comparison of Traditional versus New Model Practices	
Traditional Model of Practice	**New Model of Practice**
Systems often disrupt the patient-physician relationship	Systems support continuous healing relationships
Care is provided to both genders and all ages and includes all stages of the individual and family life cycles in continuous, healing relationships	Care is provided to both genders and all ages and includes all stages of the individual and family life cycles in continuous, healing relationships
Physician is center stage	Patient is center stage
Unnecessary barriers to access by patients	Open access by patients
Care is mostly reactive	Care is both responsive and prospective
Care is often fragmented	Care is integrated
Paper medical record	Electronic health record
Unpredictable package of services is offered	Commitment to providing directly and/or coordinating a defined basket of services
Individual patient oriented	Individual and community oriented
Communication with practice is synchronous (in person or by telephone)	Communication with the practice is both synchronous and asynchronous (e-mail, Web portal, voice mail)
Quality and safety of care are assumed	Processes are in place for ongoing measurement and improvement of quality and safety
Physician is the main source of care	Multidisciplinary team is the source of care
Individual physician-patient visits	Individual and group visits involving several patients and members of the health care team
Consumes knowledge	Generates new knowledge through practice-based research
Experience based	Evidence based
Haphazard chronic disease management	Purposeful, organized chronic disease management
Struggles financially, undercapitalized	Positive financial margin, adequately capitalized

From Martin JC, Avant RF, Bowman MA, et al. The future of family medicine: A collaborative project of the family medicine community. Ann Fam Med 2004;2(Suppl 1):S3–S32.

physicians organize their practices and how they function), medical education (how family physicians are trained and how they maintain a high level of performance throughout a career), and the health care system of the United States to restore its focus on caring for and meeting the needs of people.

To transform medical care in an unsatisfying health care system, family medicine and the rest of primary care has been swept up in the next period of substantial change in medical practice in the United States. Given the rich interfaces that family medicine has with virtually every other aspect of the health care system, it is not surprising that those in family medicine would feel compelled to respond. It appears to be a time when it is most important to construct not just a rationale for family medicine but the place of family medicine. A substantial revision of the practice setting, supported by a viable business plan, is necessary for future family medicine to achieve top performance (Roberts et al., 2004).

The current shortcomings and dissatisfaction with the U.S. health care system provide family physicians with a compelling opportunity to improve the health of the nation and shape their own destinies by redesigning their model of practice. In

the future, family physicians must not only have the requisite skills in prevention, counseling, diagnosis, prognostication, treatment, and performance of procedures but also competencies in managing relationships, information, and processes of care. The compass headings for the direction of necessary changes in the practice of family medicine were articulated as shown in Table 2-1, contrasting traditional practice with future practice (Green et al., 2004).

Aspects of this New Model have already been implemented on a piecemeal basis by innovative family physicians and are thus known to be practical enough to be achievable now. It is the entire spectrum of characteristics explicitly centered on the needs of patients, incorporating concepts from industrial engineering and customer service, that represents the change in orientation from a traditional model of family medicine to a New Model capable of serving as a personal medical home for any person. The cornerstone of the new model is patient-centered care based on an ongoing patient-physician relationship that is highly satisfying and humanizing to the patient as well as to the physician and practice personnel.

Table 2-2 Basket of Services in the New Model of Family Medicine
Health care is provided to children and adults
Integration of personal health care (coordinate and facilitate care)
Health assessment (evaluate health and risk status)
Disease prevention (early detection of asymptomatic disease)
Health promotion (primary prevention and health behavior/lifestyle modification)
Patient education and support for self-care
Diagnosis and management of acute injuries and illnesses
Diagnosis and management of chronic illness
Supportive care, including end-of-life care
Maternity care, hospital care
Primary mental health care
Consultation and referral services as necessary
Advocacy for the patient within the health care system
Quality improvement and practice-based research

From Martin JC, Avant RF, Bowman MA, et al. The future of family medicine: A collaborative project of the family medicine community. Ann Fam Med 2004;2(Suppl 1):S3–S32.

The future family physician will need to provide care to both genders at all stages of the individual and family life cycle. It is virtually inconceivable to move to the New Model of practice without incorporating an electronic health record (EHR), but adopting an EHR alone will not achieve the new model. Moving toward patient-centeredness and relationship-based care while working in teams is likely to be both rewarding and a challenge. Incorporating discovery and research into routine practice is necessary to complete medicine's knowledge base and ground future family medicine in science-based care.

Achieving sufficient standardization to allow the public to know what they can expect from a family physician while adapting family medicine to the specific requirements of each community will be a critical challenge. In the New Model, every family physician does not need to provide every service at all times, but a New Model practice would guarantee the full basket of services, creating a consistent scope of services, recognizable by the public. A reliable basket of services was identified and is summarized in Table 2-2 (Green et al., 2004).

FINANCIAL IMPLICATIONS OF THE NEW MODEL OF CARE

Scattered across the United States and other countries are practices that exhibit one or more of the characteristics of New Model practice, confirming practical feasibility. However, there is a paucity of practices that have implemented the entire package in the U.S. setting, precluding adequate empirical evaluation of clinical and financial performance of the New Model. This circumstance led to modeling the possible financial effects of implementing the New Model. Based on existing economic policies and management procedures displayed in work patterns from 2001 to 2003 in the United States, expected workloads, revenues, and expenses associated with the New Model were projected. The results found the New Model to be more efficient, resulting in the options for family physicians of working fewer hours with relatively stable income or working the same number of hours with increased earnings, as much as 26% for a prototypical five-physician practice. With revisions in how family physicians are paid, such as payments that blend salary or capitation with fee for service and premium payments for superior results, the financial models could become even more favorable (Spann et al., 2004).

Additional modeling exercises project that the well-documented salutary effects of primary care and the New Model of practice would be expected to result in reduced overall national expenditures for health care, a highly desirable, if unfamiliar, situation. This macrolevel analysis suggested that at least a 5.6% reduction in total health care expenditures (perhaps $67 billion) would be expected if New Model practice could be implemented widely and made available to the entire population (Spann et al., 2004).

In summary, the New Model of family medicine as proposed in the FFM Project appears to be feasible and attractive to patients, family physicians and their professional colleagues, purchasers of health care, and governments. From the perspectives of patients, family physicians, medical students, and residents inclined to be family physicians, the New Model has the potential to achieve unprecedented performance.

RECOMMENDATIONS CONCERNING THE FUTURE OF FAMILY MEDICINE IN THE UNITED STATES

Family physicians are committed to fostering health and integrating health care for the whole person by humanizing medicine and providing science-based, quality care. To remain true to this statement of identity, while continuing to meet the needs of patients and society in a changing health care environment, family medicine must promote active experimentation and innovation in the delivery of clinical services and in the education of clinicians. Family physicians and their organizations must seek out and partner with those who share similar values and a commitment to experimentation, innovation, and transformation of the U.S. health care system.

The following recommendations, which represent a compilation of major recommendations from the FFM task forces, are intended to provide a framework to guide such experimentation and innovation within the discipline (Martin et al., 2004).

New Model of Family Medicine

Family medicine will redesign the work and workplaces of family physicians. This redesign will foster a New Model of care based on the concept of a relationship-centered *personal medical home*, which serves as the focal point through which all individuals, regardless of age, gender, race, ethnicity, or socioeconomic status, participate in health care. In this new medical home, patients receive a basket of acute, chronic, and preventive medical care services that are accessible, accountable, comprehensive, integrated, patient centered, safe, scientifically valid, and satisfying to both patients and their physicians. This New Model will include technologies that enhance diagnosis and treatment for a large portion of problems that patients bring to their family physicians. Business plans and reimbursement will be developed to enable the re-engineered practices of family physicians to thrive as personal medical homes, and resources will be developed to help patients make informed decisions about choosing a personal medical home. A financially self-sustaining national resource will be implemented to provide individual practices with ongoing support in the transition to the New Model of family medicine.

Electronic Health Records

EHRs that meet standards that support the New Model of family medicine will be implemented. The EHR will enhance and integrate communication, diagnosis and treatment, measurement of processes and results, analysis of the effects of comorbidity, recording, and coding elements of whole-person care and promote ongoing, healing relationships between family physicians and their patients.

Family Medicine Education

Family medicine will oversee the training of family physicians who are committed to excellence, steeped in the core values of the discipline, expert in providing family medicine's basket of services within the New Model of family medicine, skilled at adapting to varying patient and community needs, and prepared to embrace new evidence-based technologies. Family medicine education will continue to include training in maternity care, the care of hospitalized patients, community and population health, and culturally effective and proficient care. Innovation in family medicine residency programs will be supported by the Residency Review Committee for Family Practice through 5 to 10 years of curricular flexibility to permit active experimentation and ongoing critical evaluation of competency-based education, expanded training programs, and other strategies to prepare graduates for the New Model. In preparation for this process, every family medicine residency will implement EHRs by 2006.

Lifelong Learning

The discipline of family medicine will develop a comprehensive, lifelong learning program. This program will provide the tools for each family physician to create a continuous personal, professional, and clinical practice assessment and an improvement plan that supports a succession of career stages. This personalized learning and professional development will include self-assessment and learning modules directed at individual physicians and group practices that incorporate science-based knowledge into educational interventions fostering improved patient outcomes. Family medicine residency programs and departments will incorporate continuing professional development into their curricula and will initiate and model the support process for lifelong learning and maintenance of certification.

Enhancing the Science of Family Medicine

Participation in the generation of new knowledge will be integral to the activities of all family physicians and will be incorporated into family medicine training. Practice-based research will be integrated into the values, structures, and processes of family practices. Departments of family medicine will engage in highly collaborative research that produces new knowledge about the origins of disease and illness, how health is gained and lost, and how the provision of care can be improved. A national entity should be established to lead and fund research on the health and health care of whole people. Funding for the Agency for Healthcare Research and Quality should be increased to at least $1 billion per year.

Quality of Care

Close working partnerships will be developed between academic family medicine, community-based family physicians, and other partners to address the quality goals specified in the Institute of Medicine (IOM) Chasm Report. Family physicians and their practice partners will have support systems to measure and report regularly their performance on the six IOM aims of quality health care (safe, timely, effective, equitable, patient centered, and efficient). Family medicine residency programs will track and report regularly the performance of their residents during their training on the six IOM quality measures and will modify their training programs as necessary to improve performance.

Role of Family Medicine in Academic Health Centers

Departments of family medicine will individually and collectively analyze their position within the academic health center setting and will take steps to enhance their contribution to the advancement and rejuvenation of the academic health center to meet the needs of the American people. A summit of policymakers and family medicine leaders in academia and private practice will be convened to review the role of and make recommendations on the future of family medicine in academia.

Promoting a Sufficient Family Medicine Workforce

A comprehensive family medicine career development program and other strategies will be implemented to recruit and train a culturally diverse family physician workforce that meets the needs of the evolving U.S. population for integrated health care for the whole person, families, and communities. Departments of family medicine will continue to develop, implement, disseminate, and evaluate best practices in expanding student interest in the specialty.

Communications

A unified communications strategy will be developed to promote an awareness and understanding of the New Model of family medicine and the concept of the personal medical home. As part of this strategy, a new symbol for family physicians will be created and consistent terminology will be established for the specialty, including use of *family medicine* rather than family practice and *family physician* rather than family practitioner. In addition, a system will be developed to communicate and implement best practices within family medicine.

Leadership and Advocacy

A leadership center for family medicine and primary care will be established that will develop strategies to promote family physicians and other primary care physicians as health policy and research leaders in their communities, in government, and in other influential groups. In their capacity as leaders, family physicians will convene leaders to identify and develop implementation strategies for several major policy initiatives, including ensuring that every American has access to basic health care services. Family physicians will partner with others at the local, state, and national levels to engage patients, clinicians, and payers in advocating for a redesigned system of integrated, personalized, equitable, and sustainable health care.

Much of the work to create this recommended future must be done by the discipline itself. There are opportunities to repair broken linkages, particularly with public health and mental health, while cultivating partnerships necessary to create a supportive environment for family medicine. These actions require collaboration well beyond the discipline and in some instances policy revisions that depend in part on the action of both the private and public sectors.

COMMENTARY

As there is much at stake in this proposed transformation of family medicine, many people have reason to be concerned enough to pay attention to it. Foremost are people in both urban and rural communities who seek health sufficient to live out their hopes and dreams and yearn for enough of the right health care to enable them to do so. Those who have critically examined the evidence of the salutary impact of primary care on health and health care systems will want to facilitate the transformation. Others with much to gain through this transformation include those concerned with the sustainability of health care, the avoidance of waste, health care tailored to each individual, justice in the allocation of resources, over- and undertreatment, and disparities in outcomes.

The next generation of physicians, particularly those who aspire to be the doctors that people in the United States identify as their usual source of care, stand to gain a great deal. Physicians in all specialties have much to gain as the New Model integrates care. Decision makers in and out of health care are likely to have opportunities to support the transformation through their leadership and financing.

A fundamental result of transforming family medicine and the rest of primary care is integrated care. Integration is the pulling together of what often appear to be disparate parts into a coherent whole that has recognized meaning. This integration of health care is the antidote to the frustratingly fragmented care that most Americans now experience. People's problems do not respect the arbitrary boundaries of single disciplines defined by who does what and where for a patient. Consequently, if family physicians are to integrate their patients' care, they must be positioned to work effectively across the health care settings, including hospitals, intermediate care settings, offices, and homes. Integrating health care is, and will remain, high-order intellectual work worthy of the best physicians, of great value to patients, and the crux of the doctoring that family physicians aspire to do and for which patients yearn.

Family medicine may be medicine's largest information management challenge. For the first time, technology exists sufficient to support asynchronous communications, establish an interoperable EHR, and manage the complex information requirements of family medicine. Continuity of care may be achievable as never before possible because of the Internet. When an EHR is united with innovative classifications (Lamberts and Wood, 1987) that capture episodes of care and a robust practice-based research enterprise (Green and Dovey, 2001), New Model practice may be able to achieve family medicine's and primary care's long-standing, ambitious aspirations in the near future.

It is not possible for anyone to state with certainty the future of family medicine. Its future depends on factors not yet known and how family medicine adapts to the challenges and impediments it now faces. These include what the United States does in terms of further commercialization and corporatization of health care and whether relationship-centered care is feasible in the U.S. environment. Whether the United States ever implements universal health care coverage and whether a foundational policy of a medical home for every person is implemented will modulate the degree and rapidity with which family medicine can make the transformation now needed.

A successful business model will be critical in which current inadequacies are corrected such that new model practice is economically sustainable in the market of U.S. medicine. The response of medical students and residents to the ambitious opportunities and daunting challenges facing family medicine and primary care will also be a major determining factor of the future. How general internists, general pediatricians, nurses, and other health care professionals respond to family medicine in the future may help reach critical mass, incite productive competition, or dilute efforts such that no national commitment to primary care and personalized, whole-person, relationship-centered care emerges.

The future of family medicine may depend most on what currently practicing family physicians do next. Overwhelmingly, these family physicians aspire to the opportunity to have a balanced lifestyle while providing personalized care suitable for their patients, patients known by name and with whom they share experiences that are the basis of trust. To make the transformation that is necessary in their practices, those in the discipline have committed to the creation of an assistance organization to help the typical practice of family physicians through consultation and other supporting structures.

CONCLUSION

This is the next moment of adaptive change for family medicine in the United States. Acknowledging the role that the public expects of family medicine, the discipline must effectively address the challenges of transformation. Family medicine must demonstrate the competencies of relationship building, quality care, cost efficiencies, and health outcomes while addressing the macro issues of a research agenda for its science and influencing future health care policy.

If the transformation falters now, it is likely to be a costly failure affecting millions of people. Another rebirth of family medicine in some form would be required in the years ahead. It is time to choose the next adventure and act, from the current position of strength, to respond to immediate opportunities and honor the historic contract between family physicians and the people, who are still waiting for high-performance health care and a personal physician who will stick with them and actually care for them.

Material Available on Student Consult
Review Questions and Answers about The Future of Family Medicine

REFERENCES

Bucholtz JR, Matheny SC, Pugno PA, et al. Task Force 2 Report: Family medicine education and training. Ann Fam Med 2004;2(Suppl 1):S51–S64.

Dickinson JC, Evans KL, Carter J, Burke K. Task Force 4 Report: Communicating the role of family medicine. Ann Fam Med 2004;2(Suppl 1):S75–S87.

Donaldson MS, Yordy KD, Lohr KN, Vanselow NA, eds. Committee on the Future of Primary Care Services. Institute of Medicine. Primary Care. America's Health in a New Era. Washington, DC, National Academy Press, 1996.

Folsom MB. National Commission on Community Health Services. Health Is a Community Affair. Cambridge, MA: Harvard University Press, 1966.

Geyman JP. Health Care in America. Can Our Ailing System Be Healed? Boston: Butterworth-Heinemann, 2002.

Graham R, Roberts RG, Ostergaard DJ, et al. Family practice in the United States. A status report. JAMA 2002;288:1097–1101.

Green LA, Dovey SM. Practice based primary care research networks. They work and are ready for full development and support. BMJ 2001;322:567–568.

Green L, Graham R, Bagley B, et al. Task Force 1 Report: Patient expectations, core values, reintegration and the new model of family medicine. Ann Fam Med 2004;2(Suppl 1):S33–S50.

Green LA, Fryer GE. Family practice in the United States: Position and prospects. Acad Med 2002;77:781–789.

Institute of Medicine. Committee on Quality of Health Care in America. To Err Is Human: Building a Safer Health System. Institute of Medicine. Washington, DC: National Academy Press, 2000.

Institute of Medicine. Committee on Quality of Health Care in America. Crossing the Quality Chasm: A New Health System for the 21st Century. Institute of Medicine. Washington, DC: National Academy Press, 2001.

Institute of Medicine. Committee on Assuring the Health of the Public in the 21st Century. The Future of the Public's Health in the 21st Century. Institute of Medicine. Washington, DC: National Academy Press, 2002a.

Institute of Medicine. Committee on Understanding and Eliminating Racial and Ethnic Disparities in Health Care. Unequal Treatment: What Health Care Providers Need to Know About Racial and Ethnic Disparities in Health Care. Institute of Medicine. Washington, DC: National Academy Press, 2002b.

Jones WA, Avant RF, Davis N, et al. Task Force 3 Report: Continuous Personal, Professional, and Practice Development in Family Medicine. Ann Fam Med 2004;2(Suppl 1):S65–S74.

Lamberts H, Wood M. ICPC: International Classification of Primary Care. New York: Oxford University Press, 1987.

Martin JC, Avant RF, Bowman MA, et al. The future of family medicine: A collaborative project of the family medicine community. Ann Fam Med 2004;2 (Suppl 1):S3–S32.

Millis JS. Citizens Commission on Graduate Medical Education. The Graduate Education of Physicians: The Report of the Citizens Commission on Graduate Medical Education. Chicago: American Medical Association, 1966.

Roberts RG, Snape PS, Burke K. Task Force 5 Report: Family medicine's role in shaping the future health care delivery system. Ann Fam Med 2004;2(Suppl 1): S88–S99.

Spann S, Task Force and the Executive Editorial Team. Report on financing the new model of family medicine. Ann Fam Med 2004;2(Suppl 3):S1–S21.

Stock Keister MC, Green LA, Kahn NB, Phillips RL, McCann J, Fryer GE. What people want from their family physician. Am Fam Physician 2004;69:2310.

Willard WR. American Medical Association. Ad Hoc Committee on Education for Family Practice. Meeting the Challenge of Family Practice: The Report of the Ad Hoc Committee on Education for Family Practice of the Council on Medical Education. Chicago: American Medical Association, 1966.

3 The Relevance of Medical History to Family Medicine

Chester R. Burns, Alice Anne O'Donell, and Barbara Thompson

Imagine that you are Benjamin Rush and that you—along with other congressional delegates assembled in Philadelphia on August 2, 1776—have just signed the American Declaration of Independence.[1] As a very busy general practitioner, you probably need to see a patient in your office, at your home, or at the patient's home. Or you may, in keeping with your unsalaried commitment to impoverished colonials, need to visit a patient in the Pennsylvania Hospital on your way home from the signing ceremony.

What beliefs about health and health care animate your practice? Do you feel responsible for attending to the physical, mental, social, and spiritual maladies of your patients, or is that comprehensive viewpoint too broad? What types of rational information about these maladies are reliable and useful? What types of medical, surgical, psychosocial, and spiritual therapies are available for you to use in caring for a patient? What are the prospects for satisfactory outcomes?

Do you pay any attention to issues of medical ethics and professionalism, and to the realities of the economic and political contexts of your medical practice? In a politically free republic such as the embryonic United States of America, which citizens should monitor the quality of care offered by a variety of medical "professionals" who tout their services as healers? Which citizens are morally and legally responsible for securing the "healths" of their fellow Americans: professionals and/or nonprofessionals (including quacks) who earn income in exchange for remedies and services; nonprofessional volunteers who tout health-promoting advice and gimmicks; and/or governmental agencies that attend to the "public health" needs of all citizens in the specified polity?

Benjamin Rush, probably the most distinguished and influential physician in the colonies and early American Republic, answered these and related questions in numerous articles and books, and historians since then have interpreted his answers in numerous articles and books.[2]

Even though new Latin editions of the writings of Hippocrates and Galen (the most important medical authorities in ancient Greece and Rome) had been prepared by outstanding scholar-physicians and published between 1490 and 1525, Rush (1745–1813) explicitly rejected the theoretical legacies of Hippocrates and Galen, believing them to be irrelevant to his practice in Philadelphia.[3] As a loyal alumnus of the medical school at the University of Edinburgh in Scotland, he accepted the theories of his 18th-century teachers who intentionally rejected the ancient Greco-Roman legacies in favor of the theories of "modern" practitioners: Andreas Vesalius, William Harvey, Thomas Sydenham, Hermann Boerhaave, and William Cullen, to name a few.[4]

How could anyone believe the theories of Hippocrates and Galen after Vesalius, in 1543, and Harvey, in 1628, showed that the revered ancient physicians knew next to nothing about the real structures and functions of the human body? Yet Rush (as did Vesalius, Harvey, Sydenham, Boerhaave, Cullen, and many others) fervently championed the bloodletting and purging legacies of Hippocrates and Galen. During the yellow fever epidemic in Philadelphia in 1799, for example, Rush probably lost some patients because of too much bloodletting. Most formally educated American and European doctors in the late 18th and early 19th centuries subjected their patients to bloodletting and purging. As practical legacies sacrosanct in their teachings, Hippocrates and Galen would have rejoiced![5]

Though an apprentice of Rush who "let blood" from some of their patients in 1799, John Redman Coxe (1773–1864) did not agree with his teacher's rejection of ancient medical theory.[6] Instead, he became an extraordinary disciple of the theories of Hippocrates and Galen. Coxe possessed one of the largest private libraries in Philadelphia (estimated 15,000 volumes). Proudly positioned in this collection was his own synopsis of the medical writings of Hippocrates and Galen. He devoted many hours to the preparation of this "Merck Manual" translation of these ancient writings because he believed that they contained many practical aids that would help him and fellow American doctors make better clinical judgments.[7]

In the same year that Coxe's book was published, about 100 general practitioners assembled in New

York City in May to consider the formation of a national medical society. These physicians established two committees for their new national organization: one on medical education that would identify the theoretical and practical subjects that should be taught in any respectable American medical school, and one on medical ethics that would prepare a code of medical ethics that should be honored by all respectable American physicians. Those general practitioners who attended the first official American Medical Association (AMA) meeting in Philadelphia during the following year unanimously adopted the reports of these two committees.[8]

Some of these doctors may have known John Redman Coxe, but they did not champion the clinical knowledge of Hippocrates and Galen as he did. Like other formally educated American doctors in the mid-19th century, these founders of the AMA had rejected Coxe's viewpoints and the legacies of bloodletting and purging so sacred to their forebears. Instead, they placed their diagnostic and therapeutic trust in (1) their own interpretations of firsthand clinical observations and experiences, (2) "the healing powers of Nature," and (3) a therapeutic approach grounded in a comprehensive view of the physical, mental, social, and spiritual dimensions of health.[9]

Provoked and sanctioned by the same clinical empiricism and experimentalism in France that led to the discrediting of bloodletting and purging, the leading physicians who practiced and taught in the United States between 1830 and 1870 encouraged fellow doctors to embrace the clinical philosophies of their French mentors and marry these philosophies to the Emersonian self-reliance that animated liberally educated Americans at that time.[10] This conceptual marriage resulted in practical maxims that guided every rational physician who made a proper clinical evaluation of a patient: Be a careful observer, take a comprehensive history of the course of the disease, consider the patient's interpretations of symptoms and signs, consult other practitioners who may have treated a patient with similar symptoms and signs, decide on a comprehensive approach to therapy and caregiving, and give "Mother Nature" a chance to show her innate healing powers before and during the course of therapy.[11]

With time and rest and maybe some self-help remedies, "Mother Nature" often healed herself, so to speak. "Bad" colds, vomiting, and diarrhea disappeared regardless of what the patient or healer did. Lacerations and broken bones healed themselves, so to speak. Because of widespread variations in life styles of patients and in therapeutic approaches chosen by a variety of healers, it was very difficult to tell whether a specific remedy or regimen made any real difference in outcomes because it seemed that "Mother Nature" took care of many instances of physical *dis*ease and injury. To be rational, *care*ful,

and ethical, physicians should not choose a remedy or regimen that would interfere with these "healing powers." A professionally conscientious physician "did no harm" better than those who made hasty clinical judgments or resorted to any remedy just to receive a fee.

Yet how did these doctors know whether they were really honoring the revered Hippocratic maxim: "Do no harm"? By the middle of the 19th century, only a few "scientifically" controlled investigations of drugs and surgical techniques had been conducted. Realistically recognizing these conditions, rationally liberal (nonsectarian) physicians and surgeons relinquished their loyalty to bloodletting and purging, embraced an attitude of not aggressively interfering with the healing powers of Nature, and adopted a comprehensive approach to therapy and caregiving. In choosing to assess their professional propriety with these standards of care, these mid-century doctors experienced more than one paradox.

When to use a drug and when to trust the "healing power of Nature" was an ever-present problem of clinical judgment.[12] As John Harley Warner has demonstrated, these mid-century doctors supplemented their trust in Nature not by abandoning the use of drugs but by curtailing excessive drug use and by systematic efforts to correlate the use of specific drugs with specific clinical outcomes.[13]

Feeling simultaneously rejected and idolized by the public was another paradox that suffused the consciences of traditionally educated American doctors. Rejection by the public was probably the most traumatic insult because it affected wallets as well as self-respect. In the eyes of freedom-loving Americans living in a new country with all of its unexplored geographic and cultural frontiers, these strikingly "less-than-heroic" general practitioners who embraced "the healing powers of Nature" and rejected the active therapies of bloodletting and purging were actually behaving as if they did not care, as if they were "un-American" doctors who apparently did not really want to alter the abnormal bodily events of their patients in search of more favorable outcomes.

Not only did many Americans reject these "traditionally" educated physicians, but they employed a host of sectarian practitioners (some formally educated; some not) who rushed into the 19th-century therapeutic vacuum made possible by the abandonment of bloodletting and purging: homeopaths, hydropaths, botanics, eclectics, osteopaths, and others. Even the home remedies of distant relatives and struggling neighbors seemed better than the "do-nothing" behaviors of "regular" physicians. Pragmatic Americans could not accept passive behaviors, especially those of their trusted general practitioners. Hence, they shifted their trust to more aggressive healers who did not reject active therapeutics, even though no one could prove that one therapeutic approach was scientifically better than another.[14]

Dealing with these clinical paradoxes every time they treated patients, the general practitioner founders of the AMA really understood the social, economic, and political realities of mid-19th century America. In responding to these realities, these doctors placed their interpersonal (social) trust in (1) the creation of a national professional association of formally educated physicians who shared the three diagnostic and therapeutic philosophies previously discussed, (2) a code of professional ethics that AMA members would use in self-assessment and in monitoring the behavior of fellow members, (3) the American legal system to administer justice to those physicians who were judged guilty of medical malpractices, and (4) the American system of governance and its local, state, regional, and national agencies that could adopt public health policies and establish appropriate medical institutions to secure the welfare of their political constituents.

Even though this interpersonal trust upheld some of the most important values of medical professionalism in a democratic society, loyal AMA members experienced a fourth paradox that involved their new code of medical ethics. By following the code and participating as an active member of one's local medical society, a physician could be considered ethically acceptable by fellow doctors despite the clinical outcomes for his patients after treatment. If clinical outcomes were so unimportant in assessing professional propriety, how could any group of doctors adopt realistic standards for judging their own as well as their fellow physicians' behaviors at the bedside? To say it another way, the American public could (and did) decide that a non-AMA doctor could be an ethically acceptable American physician, and the same public could (and did) decide that clinical outcomes were highly important criteria for judging professional competence (goodness).

In view of these therapeutic perplexities during the mid-19th century in America, a sick citizen trusted a general practitioner because he was a church-going, formally educated, law-abiding citizen who displayed gentleness toward patients (the cultural meaning of "gentleman"), practiced the philosophy of therapeutics previously discussed, and "swore" allegiance to the AMA code of medical ethics. A traditionally educated doctor was not trusted because he could give no real assurances that his scientific knowledge and clinical remedies would bring about some enduring improvement in the patient's condition.

This scientific uncertainty about therapeutic results was very troubling to patients and their anxious families, who decided to give their money and loyalty to sectarian or quack practitioners who

touted more certainty and charged much less for their advertised remedies. If therapeutic outcomes were so uncertain, why spend a lot of money on clinically unproven drugs? There was no need to waste scarce resources on ignorant doctors who, despite their goodwill, really did not know how to treat most diseases in ways that would "guarantee" good outcomes.

Between 1830 and 1880 especially, Americans confronted many choices among types of "medical practitioners" who offered their wares and services to the sick and injured. These included traditionally educated general practitioners; unlicensed, trial-and-error trained midwives; a variety of sectarians including homeopaths, hydropaths, and botanics; a few who falsely advertised their services as "specialists"; and a host of nostrum vendors, quacks, and charlatans. Political freedom included the freedom to exploit fellow humans who were sick and dying. The sectarians and nostrum vendors attracted many patients. Which healers should sick Americans believe and trust, and why?

Many sick Americans still viewed general practitioners as the traditionally educated healers who could be effective, even comprehensively heroic at times. Popular American novelists captured these sentiments well in some novels that appeared in the late 19th century.

In a novel entitled *Dr. Sevier* (published in 1884), George Washington Cable characterized the motives of a general practitioner as follows: "He waged war—against malady. To fight; to stifle; to cut down; to uproot; to overwhelm,—these were the springs of action." In *A Country Doctor* (1884), Sarah Orne Jewett described Dr. John Leslie as a "self-reliant" commander: "Not only in this farmhouse kitchen, but wherever one might place him, he instinctively took command, while from his great knowledge of human nature he could understand and help many of his patients whose ailments were not wholly physical." In *Dr. Latimer: A Story of Casco Bay* (1893), Clara Burnham celebrated the comprehensive talents of this Boston doctor: "You'd be surprised, Miss Charlotte, to know the things folks'll ask o' Dr. Latimer. Sometimes it's their souls need tinkerin', and then you'd think he was a minister; sometimes it's their bodies, then you'd think he was a doctor; sometimes it's their drains, and then you'd s'pose he was a plumber; then again they've got trouble with their servants or their landlords, and want him to help 'em out, and you'd s'pose he was a lawyer." Sick Americans expected their idealized general practitioners to be all things to all people all the time![15]

As heroic as this may have seemed to imaginative novelists and their readers, the social spectrum of actual doctors more realistically included traditional generalists who were quite habitual in their choice of remedies, opportunists who tended to exploit the sick, caregivers more enthusiastic than knowledgeable, and a steadily growing number of scientifically trained general practitioners who had attended reputable medical schools and gradually realized that they could not, as individuals, really master all of the burgeoning scientific, clinical, and technical knowledge that appeared after 1880.

However, some did try to be comprehensive and professionally responsible, struggling incessantly as they determined acceptable behaviors as persons, professionals, and citizens. Notice the variety of responses in the following glimpses of the careers of five revered general practitioners in Texas between 1889 and 1975.

Born on the family ranch in Travis County in 1867, Uberto Desaix Ezell received a degree from Tulane Medical School in 1889 and became a general practitioner in Kimball, a town in Bosque County where the Chisholm cattle trail crossed the Brazos River. More than once, Ezell almost drowned as he spurred his horse across this raging river to attend patients in Hill and Johnson counties during more than 30 years of practice. In 1918, he moved to Cleburne and became "Uncle Doc" to hundreds of patients for more than 30 years, usually carrying his "black bag" across his right wrist, because four fingers had been amputated after a severe radiation burn from a new x-ray machine.[16]

Born on a family plantation north of Carthage in Rusk County in 1873, Walter D. Biggs worked in a physician-owned drugstore in Sonora as a teenager, graduated from the Fort Worth School of Medicine in 1898, and practiced in Lometa from 1903 to 1945. A Chisholm trail cowtown between 1860 and 1880, Lometa was moved to its present site when the Santa Fe Railroad was built in Lampasas County. "Uncle Walter" was the city's primary doctor and railway surgeon. He delivered more than 3,000 babies, set hundreds of fractures, watched the scars develop on the face of a beautiful girl afflicted with smallpox, prescribed castor oil more than once, broke his right wrist cranking his first Model T Ford, and never lost a patient from snakebite or pneumonia.[17]

Born in Coleman County in 1881, Charles Daniel Cupp was a farm lad in Huron who enjoyed swimming and fishing in the Brazos River. In 1912, he graduated from Tulane Medical School and moved his wife and two boys to Peoria to begin a challenging practice. After a 5-mile horseback ride, for example, Cupp surgically relieved an intestinal obstruction in a 10-year-old boy after placing him on the family's dining room table that had been moved to a "cooler" back porch. During a long peripatetic career as a general practitioner, Cupp followed the oil-driven boom towns, moving to Whitney (1917), Desdemona (1919), Breckenridge (1920), Kilgore (1931), Tyler (1931), and Grand Prairie (1941).

Never sued by a patient and having never purchased malpractice insurance, Cupp celebrated his 94th birthday in 1975 by treating 64 patients and collecting $430 in fees.[18]

Delivered by his grandmother-midwife in Liberty Hill in 1884, J. Gordon Bryson graduated from the University of Texas Medical Branch (UTMB) in 1910 and returned to his home county to serve patients in Pearsall and Bastrop until 1947. Competing with three other doctors when he arrived, Bryson firmly established his reputation when he successfully treated a Mexican laborer with a gunshot wound to the abdomen in June 1911. During his career, Bryson treated many more injuries, delivered many babies, and attended patients with a host of infectious diseases, including one teenager with maggots "completely blocking the passage of one nostril."[19]

Born in Hill County, J.W. Young, Sr., graduated from UTMB in 1907 and moved to the small railroad town of Roscoe (about 1,000 citizens), where he practiced until 1950. When he began, typhoid fever and diphtheria were common diseases. His main medicines then were castor oil, quinine, bismuth, turpentine, and calomel (mercurous chloride). He served patients in the surrounding towns of Blackland, Wastella, Brownlee, Champion, Barnett, Maryneal, Mesquite, and Goode. One night, he rode his horse about 100 miles to attend patients in some of these towns. His office was in the back room of a drugstore that was an "old tin building."[20]

These and other formally educated general practitioners did not ignore the new scientific discoveries about health and disease that emerged from the clinical venues and experimental laboratories of the 19th and 20th centuries. Building on Louis Pasteur's pioneering studies about microorganisms and putrefaction, Joseph Lister, a professor of surgery at the University of Glasgow, discovered ways to save many lives by controlling infection in surgical wounds. Surgeons in Texas and elsewhere used and improved these control techniques during the 1870s, 1880s, and 1890s.[21] Between 1873 and 1889, scientists and clinicians discovered the microorganisms that cause 13 infectious diseases.[22] After it was created in 1891, the antitoxin for diphtheria became an efficacious cure for most children afflicted with this disease.[23] By the turn of the 20th century, humans accurately believed that they were exerting more rational control over infectious diseases than ever before.

As could be gleaned from the previous paragraph about Dr. J.W. Young, Sr., however, American doctors at the turn of the 20th century could prescribe only a few reliable drugs that were scientifically understood and clinically effective. The quickest way to confirm this therapeutic predicament at that time is to read any section about treatment for almost any disease analyzed in William Osler's

Principles and Practice of Medicine, which was published in 1892.[24] Two weeks after its publication, the entire first printing (3,000 copies) had been purchased.[25] By studying this classic text, conscientious and scientifically trained physicians could learn more about the accurate diagnosis of nonsurgical diseases than any cohort of English-speaking physicians had ever understood before.

Yet, during the 1890s and for many years thereafter, these same doctors and their successors would be as perplexed and uncertain about the rationale for most of their prescriptions as their predecessors had been about their prescriptions before 1890. During the late 19th century and throughout the 20th century, a new group of scientifically educated specialist physicians (like Osler) emerged as the new medical heroes. The public often judged these specialists as ethically "better" than general practitioners, because the clinical outcomes for their patients were typically more favorable than the outcomes of those treated by general practitioners.[26]

This did not mean that only specialists were ethical and that all general practitioners were unethical.[27] It did mean that there were significant cultural, scientific, practical, and social distances between the older generations of general practitioners and the younger generations of physicians that included two major types: (1) generalists who, as they aged or encountered the scientific and technical changes of medicine later in their careers, decided to limit their practice to patients with specific diseases, or to patients of certain ages, usually infants and children younger than teens; and (2) specialists who were never generalists but chose to practice one of the evolving specialties when they finished medical school.

Between 1890 and 1970, general practitioners and specialists in the United States struggled for acceptance (some would say prestige, some would say dominance) among the formally educated physicians in the country's medical profession. These doctors were vigorously competing for two cultural and social trophies, so to speak: public acceptance and professional reputation. As Paul Starr documents in *The Social Transformation of American Medicine*, the cultural and social battles involving these doctors and their patrons (sick and potentially sick Americans) were extensive and energetically fought. A sociologist, Starr brilliantly analyzes the competing groups and organizations, and offers numerous provocative interpretations. Starr's book is essential reading for anyone who wants to understand the historical changes in American medicine and health care during the 20th century. As Starr revealed, the vast number of scientific, clinical, therapeutic, institutional, and social changes that occurred between 1882 and 1982 transformed the practice of medicine in so many ways that the contours of practice in late-20th-century America were profoundly different from those of late-19th-century America.[28]

For the historical origins of family medicine as a discrete specialty, three of these changes deserve emphasis: those advances in science and technology that resulted in spectacular improvements in diagnostic and therapeutic techniques; the expansion of clinical specialization with the creation of 24 specialty boards between 1917 and 1980;[29] and the shift of medical care from the homes of patients and the offices of solo practitioners to multiple-specialty private clinics and to multiple-specialty hospitals of varying size and provenance (private, charity, government).

By 1930, the advances in science and technology provided safe blood transfusions, two vitamins (C and D), insulin and other hormones, Pap smears, and iron lungs for polio victims. By 1965, there were electron microscopes, maps of DNA structures, ultrasound and radioactive isotopes, amniocentesis, sulfa drugs, penicillin, streptomycin and tetracyclines, cortisone, tranquilizers, renal dialysis and transplants, heart valves and pacemakers, more vitamins (A, B, E, and K), polio and measles vaccines, the first birth control pills, and laser surgery. By 2000, these advances provided many new drugs including Prozac and Viagra, human babies begun as embryos by artificial insemination, recombinant gene therapies, chemotherapies that destroyed some cancers, AZT for AIDS patients, flexible endoscopes, brain scans, artificial hearts, and other organ transplants (liver, lung, pancreas, cochlea).[30]

With these advances, clinical specialization and subspecialization became entrenched. In Texas before 1940, for example, most doctors were general practitioners. But some became specialists, including some pioneering women physicians. Sofie Herzog established her surgical practice in Brazoria, and she became the chief surgeon for the St. Louis, Brownsville, and Mexico railroad. Claudia Potter was the head of the Anesthesiology Department at Scott and White Hospital in Temple between 1906 and 1947.[31] Specialization proceeded steadily throughout the 20th century, and more women became physicians, especially after mid-century.

The American public was not entirely satisfied with the evolution of these physician specialists and subspecialists. Nevertheless, they sought their services when they needed their specialized knowledge and care. By 1949, only 36% of American doctors were specialists; by 1969 when the American Board of Family Practice was created, the proportion had increased to 77%.[32] As specialization increased, general practice flourished at the local level. Pat Nixon received his medical degree from Johns Hopkins University School of Medicine in 1909 and began a general practice in San Antonio that continued for more than 50 years.[33] Henry Wentz received his medical degree from Jefferson Medical College in 1944, and he was a general practitioner and family physician in the Strasburg, Pennsylvania, area for

40 years (1948–1988).[34] Their reflections and reminiscences provide extraordinary insights into the evolution of medical practice in the United States during the 20th century.

The third major change during this century involved the advent of multiple-specialty care in large clinics and hospitals. When Mavis Kelsey, Sr., began practice as a solo practitioner internist in 1949, the Texas Medical Center was barely beginning. Today it is the largest health care complex in the United States, with 42 institutions situated on more than 900 acres in Houston. As Kelsey notes many times in his autobiography, sharing responsibilities with fellow specialists and generalists became a guiding ethic sustaining the evolution of medical care during the 20th century.[35] From approximately 300 hospitals in the United States in 1882 (about 50 of these mental hospitals), the number of hospitals exceeded 7,000 in 1982. The "hospital standardization" movement was initiated by the American College of Surgeons in 1918; the Joint Commission on the Accreditation of Hospitals was established in 1951; this commission became the Joint Commission on the Accreditation of Healthcare Organizations in 1987.[36] Home care by physicians almost disappeared during these decades. For ethical and practical reasons, solo medical practice was rapidly disappearing into the cultural and social "sunset."

To receive full public acceptance and full respect by all physician specialists, that is, to be professionally ethical in all its cultural meanings, the institutionalized care that was replacing solo medical practice required more cooperation and coordination than ever before in the history of humankind. The new breed of family medicine specialists promised to deliver patient care services grounded in these ultimate values of coordination and cooperation. Moreover, they promised to harness all of the professional and community resources necessary to provide optimum health care to every patient. This was a tall order of premium ideals addressed by many pioneers associated with the advent of family medicine during the 1960s.

Negotiating and renegotiating the new "social contracts" between family medicine pioneers and public institutions occurred repeatedly during this decade that included the intensely challenging events associated with advances in civil rights, women's rights, worker's rights, and rights for hospitalized patients. The advent of Medicare and Medicaid in 1965 also provoked innovative responses from physicians, health care institutions, and community groups participating in these innovative cultural and social negotiations.

Family medicine emerged as a direct response to these public and professional processes of negotiating and renegotiating "social contracts" about the role of physicians and health care institutions in a politically free society. Three path-breaking reports issued in 1966—the Millis Report, the Folsum Report, and the Willard Report—contained the cultural and social "seeds" that generated family medicine and heralded a new day for primary care. Using the contents of these reports, family medicine pioneers transformed the social demands for "rights" and "welfare" and the exhortations for more primary care into an elaborate and extensive set of professional obligations for family medicine specialists.

In 1966, a joint committee of representatives from the American Academy of General Practice (founded in 1947) and the AMA Section on General Practice issued a report titled "The Core Content of Family Medicine." Identifying and emphasizing 26 separate areas of knowledge unique to family medicine, this report is essential reading for anyone who wants to understand the "anatomy and physiology" of the cultural and social values of those physicians who established family medicine as a new specialty.[37]

In February 1969, the AMA officially approved family medicine as a specialty and the American Board of Family Practice was created to certify physicians who chose to become family practitioners. In 1971, the American Academy of General Practice became the American Academy of Family Physicians (AAFP). By the turn of the 21st century more than 500 family practice residencies had been established in the United States, and there were more than 90,000 AAFP members.[38]

In 1999, Robert Taylor, a member of the faculty of the Department of Family Medicine at the Oregon Health Sciences University School of Medicine in Portland, asserted that the new specialty of family medicine had advanced the cultural and professional understanding of medicine in six ways: (1) developed a specialty that emphasized relationship-based health care, (2) utilized comprehensive clinical reasoning, (3) recognized ordinary problems of living as a health care concern, (4) added nuance and richness to the meanings of disease, disability, and pain, (5) advocated a systems approach to primary health care, and (6) analyzed clinical encounters in terms of a definable unit of family practice.[39]

Benjamin Rush, William Osler, and other reflective physicians in America's past would probably celebrate the accomplishments of family physicians and other primary care doctors in the United States during the last 50 years. A sizeable number of previous leaders, such as Rush and Osler, did not ignore the human values contained in the six areas analyzed by Taylor. Lawrence Hirsch, the JAMA reviewer of Robert Rakel's first edition of this book (published in 1977), acknowledged Rakel's "pioneering" efforts to provide a comprehensive look at the "concept of family practice" that, even by then, had "matured into that of family medicine."[40] With the publication of this new edition, the signs of disciplinary maturity for family medicine are even more visible. How these values and behaviors are integrated into future patterns of primary care remain to be negotiated in subsequent decades.[41] Historical information and interpretation can provide valuable insights for family doctors and future negotiations.[42]

Historical inquiry and knowledge can be tools of the human imagination that allow a better understanding of the present and a more deliberate adaptation to its challenges. To be most effective, each individual must pay attention to time and its passage, must construct some evidence-based images about the time-dependent events associated with the individual's interests, and must find some cultural coordinates that help explain and interpret the choices, changes, and causes of the events leading to present conditions. As is evident from the contents of this chapter, the exercise of the historical imagina-

tion requires some focused labor by physicians, residents, students, and others interested in the evolution of family medicine.[43]

Medical history is relevant to family doctors because its study can provide them with a unique perspective about (1) their social identity as members of a healing profession, (2) the multiple influences that have caused cultural and social changes in this identity through time, (3) the moral values expressed in the choices and deeds of past family doctors, and (4) the array of choices and values available for family physicians today as they determine the destinies and legacies that will be remembered as tomorrow's history of family medicine.

Material Available on Student Consult

Review Questions and Answers about The Relevance of Medical History to Family Medicine

---

NOTES

1. Although formally adopted on July 4, 1776, the Declaration was not signed by every member of the new U.S. Congress until August 2, 1776. See "The Declaration of Independence," *The Annals of America*, vol 2, 1755–1783 (Chicago, Encyclopaedia Britannica, 1968, p 447). Family physicians are urged to devote regular attention to the social history of the United States and especially to the histories of family life that have appeared in recent years. For a start, read Steven Mintz and Susan Kellogg, *Domestic Revolutions: A Social History of American Family Life* (New York, Free Press, 1988). To place these stories in the context of our country's general history, spend some time with a recent edition of George Brown Tindall's (with D.E. Shi) *America: A Narrative History* (New York, WW Norton, 1992).

2. For a comprehensive list of these publications, see *Benjamin Rush, M.D. A Bibliographic Guide*, compiled by Claire G. Fox, Gordon L. Miller, and Jacquelyn C. Miller (Westport, CT, Greenwood Press, 1996). Also see Chester R. Burns, "Setting the Stage: Moral Philosophy, Benjamin Rush, and Medical Ethics in the United States before 1846," in Robert B. Baker, Arthur L. Caplan, Linda L. Emmanuel, and Stephen R. Latham (eds), *The American Medical Ethics Revolution: How the AMA's Code of Ethics Has Transformed Physicians' Relationships to Patients, Professionals, and Society* (Baltimore, Johns Hopkins University Press, 1999, pp 3–16). For rich insights about medical practice in the colonies and early American republic, see Richard Harrison Shryock, *Medicine and Society in America: 1660–1860* (Ithaca, NY, Great Seal Books, 1960) and Whitfield J. Bell, Jr., *The Colonial Physician & Other Essays* (New York, Science History Publications, 1975).

3. Reliable evidence about the life of Hippocrates is sparse. He was born on the island of Cos in Greece, probably in 460 BCE and died in 370 BCE. A member of the Asclepiad guild, he practiced and taught medicine. Because he was revered among the ancient Greeks as the "father of rational medicine," those scholars who assembled the anonymous medical writings in Greek from the centuries before 200 BCE titled their collection, *The Writings of Hippocrates*. We do not know if Hippocrates actually wrote any of the treatises in this collection, including the famous Oath. Galen (130 CE –200 CE) was a Greek from Pergamum (in Asia Minor), a city with a popular healing temple to Asclepius, the Greek god of health and healing. Galen taught and practiced in Rome for more than 30 years, serving as physician to some Roman emperors, including Marcus Aurelius. For an introduction to the historical legacies of Hippocrates and Galen, see Owsei Temkin and C. Lilian Temkin (eds), Ancient *Medicine: Selected Papers of Ludwig Edelstein* (Baltimore, Johns Hopkins University Press, 1967); Owsei Temkin, *Galenism: Rise and Decline of a Medical Philosophy* (Ithaca, NY, Cornell University Press, 1973); and Owsei Temkin, *The Double Face of Janus and Other Essays in the History of Medicine* (Baltimore, Johns Hopkins University Press, 1977).

4. Andreas Vesalius (1514–1564), a Belgian physician, was professor of anatomy at the University of Padua and wrote the first textbook of human anatomy based on dissection of a human body.

Published in 1543, this text revolutionized medical science. William Harvey (1578–1657) was a London physician who received his medical degree from the University of Padua. Harvey conducted physiologic experiments on the movement of blood in mammalian bodies and separate experiments on the development of sheep embryos. His theory about the circulation of blood in the human body was published in 1628, and it had a revolutionary impact on medical science similar to that of the anatomic discoveries of Vesalius. Thomas Sydenham (1624–1689) was a British doctor who received his medical degree from the University of Oxford. With his emphasis on detailed observations of patients and their diseases, Sydenham was heralded as the "English Hippocrates." Hermann Boerhaave (1668–1738) was Professor of Botany and Medicine at the University of Leyden. Boerhaave was a superb bedside teacher, and his pupils became the leading medical educators in Edinburgh, Vienna, and other German-speaking academic institutions during the 18th century. William Cullen (1710–1790) was a popular and engaging professor of medicine at Glasgow and Edinburgh. His lectures were given in English, not Latin. Benjamin Rush attended his lectures when he studied in Edinburgh between 1768 and 1769. This is the same Edinburgh cited by Robert E. Rakel in the first chapter of this textbook. For more details about the lives and careers of these and other physicians who practiced before 1930, see the very readable book by Henry Sigerist titled *The Great Doctors* (Garden City, NY, Doubleday Anchor paperback, 1958), and the encyclopedic fourth edition of Fielding Garrison's *An Introduction to the History of Medicine* (Philadelphia, WB Saunders, 1929). The various editions of Garrison's history of medicine were the most accurate and reliable general histories of medicine in English during their time because Garrison had access to the resources of what is now the National Library of Medicine and because he was a meticulous scholar. The fourth edition is still one of the best reference sources for basic facts about much of the world's medical history before the early 20th century.

5. For an introduction to the context of medical therapeutics during the 19th century, see Charles E. Rosenberg, "The Therapeutic Revolution: Medicine, Meaning, and Social Change in Nineteenth-century America" (Persp Biol Med 1977;20:485–506). For a valuable introduction to the evolution of modern medicine from the 17th century to the 1940s, see Richard Harrison Shryock, *The Development of Modern Medicine: An Interpretation of the Social and Scientific Factors Involved* (Madison, University of Wisconsin Press, 1974 paperback reprint of 1947 edition).

6. "Coxe, John Redman," in Howard A. Kelly and Walter L. Burrage, *Dictionary of American Medical Biography* (New York, D. Appleton, 1928, pp 262–263).

7. In his synopsis of the writings of Hippocrates and Galen published in 1846, Coxe gave summaries of 55 separate "treatises" traditionally included in *The Writings of Hippocrates* and summaries of more than 150 "treatises" written by Galen—all eventually transmitted from antiquity to physicians of the "modern" era. The translations published between 1490 and 1525 were the vehicles for this cultural transfer.

8. Morris Fishbein, *A History of the American Medical Association 1847–1947* (Philadelphia, WB Saunders, 1947, pp 19–40).

9. For an analysis of the major cultural legacies about "healths" in Western and American culture, see Chester R. Burns, "Traditions of Healths in Western Culture" (Second Opinion 1986;2:120–136).

10. In the early 19th century in Paris, the clinical studies of Pierre-Charles-Alexandre Louis discredited the tradition of bloodletting in Western medicine; for a crisp summary of the impact of these studies, see Robert P. Hudson, *Disease and Its Control* (Westport, CT, Greenwood Press, 1983, pp 206–207). Ashbel Smith's experiences with bloodletting during a yellow fever epidemic in Galveston in 1839 provide vivid examples of the difficult clinical decisions about bloodletting experienced by those who knew about the clinical studies of Louis. Smith had studied in Paris after graduating from Yale Medical School in 1828. See Smith's report of cases: *An Account of the Yellow Fever Which Appeared in the City of Galveston, Republic of Texas, in the Autumn of 1839; with Cases and Dissections* (Galveston, TX, Cruger & Moore, 1839). When "Self-Reliance" was published in 1841 as the second of 12 essays in his first printed collection of essays, Ralph Waldo Emerson (1803–1882) had abandoned the Unitarian ministry 9 years earlier and was vigorously pursuing his cultural vision of Transcendentalism. For this essay, see *Ralph Waldo Emerson Lectures & Essays* (New York, Library of America, 1983, pp 257–282). For an introduction to Emerson's career, see Peter S. Field, *Ralph Waldo Emerson: The Making of a Democratic Intellectual* (Lanham, MD, Rowman & Littlefield, 2002).

11. From the day of Hippocrates and Galen until the late 19th century, the "healing power of Nature" was a central idea in Western medical therapy.

12. This foremost therapeutic paradox for all doctors, then and now, is that many self-limited diseases do disappear as bodily adaptations occur,

regardless of the therapies used by either professional doctors or loving grandmothers.

13. John Harley Warner, *The Therapeutic Perspective: Medical Practice, Knowledge, and Identity in America, 1820–1885* (Cambridge, MA, Harvard University Press, 1986).

14. The best short introduction to medical self-help and sectarian medicine is *Medicine Without Doctors: Home Health Care in American History*, edited by Guenter Risse, Ronald L. Numbers, and Judith Walzer Leavitt (New York, Science History Publications, 1977).

15. For these and other examples, and their implications for the evolution of general practice in the United States during the last quarter of the 19th century, see Chester R. Burns, "Fictional Doctors and the Evolution of Medical Ethics in the United States, 1875–1900" (Lit Med 1988; 7:39–55).

16. Ray McDearmon, *Without the Shedding of Blood: The Story of Dr. U.D. Ezell and of Pioneer Life at Old Kimball* (San Antonio, TX, Naylor, 1953).

17. Roland Windell, *The Brush of Angels' Wings: The Story of the Country Doctor* (San Antonio, Naylor, 1952).

18. Albert Cupp, *Dad* (Quanah, TX, Nortex Press, 1976) and H. Reginald McDaniel, "Dad Cupp" (Tex Med 1981;77:51–53).

19. J. Gordon Bryson, *One Hundred Dollars & a Horse: The Reminiscences of a Country Doctor* (New York, William Morrow, 1965, p 126).

20. J.W. Young, Sr., *It All Comes Back* (Sweetwater, TX, Watson-Focht, 1962, pp 21, 24).

21. For a short summary of Lister's work, see Robert P. Hudson, *Disease and Its Control* (Westport, CT, Greenwood Press, 1983, pp 156–158). For comments about the expansion of surgical treatment in Texas in the 1880s and 1890s, see Chester R. Burns, "Health and Medicine," in *The New Handbook of Texas*, edited by Ron Tyler, Douglas E. Barnett, Roy R. Barkley, Penelope C. Anderson, and Mark F. Odintz (Austin, Texas State Historical Association, 1996, p 327).

22. See Table 4.1 in Kenneth M. Ludmerer, *Learning to Heal: The Development of American Medical Education* (New York, Basic Books, 1985, p 77).

23. James Bordley, III, and A. McGehee Harvey, *Two Centuries of American Medicine 1776–1976* (Philadelphia, WB Saunders, 1976, pp 604–605) and William Gammon, "The Antitoxine of Diphtheria in Practice" (Trans Tex State Med Assoc 1895, pp 325–334). The John Sealy Hospital was the teaching hospital for University of Texas Medical Branch in Galveston. The hospital opened in 1890, and the first class of medical students matriculated in 1891. See Chester R. Burns, *Saving Lives, Training Caregivers, Making Discoveries: A Centennial History of the University of Texas Medical Branch at Galveston* (Austin, Texas State Historical Association, 2003, pp 9–39).

24. In the mid-1960s, Mac Harvey and Victor McKusick, professors of internal medicine at the Johns Hopkins University School of Medicine in Baltimore, selected portions of chapters about 17 diseases from the 7th edition of Osler's textbook (1909) and invited fellow internists teaching in several U.S. schools to provide commentaries that compared and contrasted the diagnosis and treatment of these diseases during Osler's time and in the mid-1960s. See *Osler's Textbook Revisited*, edited by A. McGeHee Harvey and Victor A. McKusick (New York, Appleton-Century-Crofts, 1967).

25. Michael Bliss, *William Osler: A Life in Medicine* (New York, Oxford University Press, 1999, p 191). Born in Bond Head, Ontario, Canada, on July 12, 1849, to an Anglican evangelist and his wife who had immigrated from England in the spring of 1837, William Osler was the eighth of nine children. Educated in medicine at Toronto Medical College and McGill University's School of Medicine, Osler received his medical degree from McGill in 1872. After studying in London, Berlin, Vienna, and Paris for 2 years, he became a professor at McGill. After 10 years of teaching and writing in Montreal, his career continued in Philadelphia (5 years), Baltimore (16 years), and Oxford (14 years). Osler died in 1919. For a short introduction to Osler's life and career, see Richard L. Golden, "William Osler at 150: An Overview of a Life," in *The Quotable Osler*, edited by Mark E. Silverman, T. Jock Murray, and Charles S. Bryan (Philadelphia, American College of Physicians, 2003, xvii–xxxv).

26. The best introduction to the story of clinical specialization in the United States and the cultural and institutional responses of both physicians and the American public is Rosemary Stevens, *American Medicine and the Public Interest: A History of Specialization* (Berkeley, CA, University of California Press, updated edition, 1998).

27. Chester R. Burns, "Colonial North America and Nineteenth-Century United States," in *Encyclopedia of Bioethics*, revised edition, edited by Warren Reich (New York, Macmillan, 1995, Vol III, pp 1610–1616).

28. Paul Starr, *The Social Transformation of American Medicine* (New York, Basic Books, 1982). Starr divides his book into what he calls Book One and Book Two. After studying his preface and introduction carefully, a first-time reader should then read Book One, and then again read the preface and introduction before reading Book Two. Even another reading of the introduction after digesting Book Two will help a reader better grasp Starr's sociologic jargon.

To fully appreciate the changes described and analyzed by Starr, read the overview of the development of health care in Texas written by Chester R. Burns and published as "Health and Medicine" in *The New Handbook of Texas*, edited by Ron Tyler, Douglas E. Barnett, Roy R. Barkley, Penelope C. Anderson, and Mark F. Odintz (Austin, Texas State Historical Association, 1996, vol 3, pp 524–532) and examine two new books about medical practice in Texas. One describes the incredible changes in a discrete geographic area; see *The History of Medicine in Brazos County (Texas)* by Frank G. Anderson, Jr., and Edith Anderson Wakefield (privately published by Frank G. Anderson, Jr., 2001). The other new book describes fantastic changes in a large academic institution in Dallas; see H. Lawrence Wilsey, *How We Care: The Centennial History of Baylor University Medical Center Baylor Health Care System 1903–2003* (Dallas, TX, Baylor Health Care System, two vols, 2003 and 2004).

29. The following information was compiled from American Board of Medical Specialties, *The Official ABMS Directory of Board Certified Medical Specialists*, 36th edition (St. Louis, Elsevier, 2004).

   1917 American Board of Ophthalmology
   1924 American Board of Otolaryngology
   1930 American Board of Obstetrics and Gynecology
   1932 American Board of Dermatology
   1933 American Board of Pediatrics
   1934 American Board of Radiology
   1934 American Board of Psychiatry and Neurology
   1934 American Board of Orthopedic Surgery
   1934 American Board of Colon and Rectal Surgery
   1935 American Board of Urology
   1936 American Board of Pathology
   1936 American Board of Internal Medicine
   1937 American Board of Anesthesiology
   1937 American Board of Plastic Surgery
   1937 American Board of Surgery
   1940 American Board of Neurological Surgery
   1947 American Board of Physical Medicine and Rehabilitation
   1948 American Board of Thoracic Surgery
   1948 American Board of Preventive Medicine
   1969 American Board of Family Practice
   1971 American Board of Allergy and Immunology
   1971 American Board of Nuclear Medicine
   1979 American Board of Emergency Medicine
   1980 American Board of Medical Genetics

30. For an exceedingly valuable historical overview, see "Looking Back on the Millenium in Medicine" (N Engl J Med 2000;342(1):42–49). Also see Chester R. Burns, *Saving Lives, Training Caregivers, Making Discoveries: A Centennial History of the University of Texas Medical Branch at Galveston* (Austin, Texas State Historical Association, 2003, p 4).

31. For details about these and other pioneering women doctors in Texas, see Elizabeth Silverthorne and Geneva Fulgham, *Women Pioneers in Texas Medicine* (College Station, Texas A&M University Press, 1997). Also see Chester R. Burns, "Health and Medicine," in *The New Handbook of Texas*, edited by Ron Tyler, Douglas E. Barnett, Roy R. Barkley, Penelope C. Anderson, and Mark F. Odintz (Austin, Texas State Historical Association, 1996, vol 3, pp 527–528).

32. Rosemary Stevens, *American Medicine and the Public Interest: A History of Specialization* (Berkeley, University of California Press, updated edition, 1998, p 181).

33. See the biographic sketch of Nixon's life by Chester R. Burns *in The New Handbook of Texas*, edited by Ron Tyler, Douglas E. Barnett, Roy R. Barkley, Penelope C. Anderson, and Mark F. Odintz (Austin, Texas State Historical Association, 1996, vol 4, pp 1021–1022), and *Pat Nixon of Texas: Autobiography of a Doctor*, by Pat Ireland Nixon, edited with an introduction by Herbert H. Lang (College Station, Texas A&M University Press, 1979).

34. Henry S. Wentz, *Patients Are a Virtue: Practicing Medicine in the Pennsylvania Amish Country* (Morgantown, PA, Masthof Press, 1997).

35. Mavis P. Kelsey, Sr., *Twentieth-Century Doctor House Calls to Space Medicine* (College Station, Texas A&M University Press, 1999). Also see Chester R. Burns, "Traditions and Transformations: How Texas Medicine Changed in the 20th Century" (Tex Med 2000;96(1):45–47).

36. The best overviews of these developments are Charles E. Rosenberg, *The Care of Strangers: The Rise of America's Hospital System* (New York, Basic Books, 1987) and Rosemary Stevens, *In Sickness and in Wealth: American Hospitals in the Twentieth Century* (New York, Basic Books, 1989).

37. "The Core Content of Family Medicine" (GP, November 1966;34(5):225–246).

38. The following publications are valuable resources for understanding the historical development of family medicine in the United States: Phillip R. Canfield, "Family Medicine: An Historical Perspective" (J Med Educ 1976;51:904–911); Robert M. Lewy, "The Emergence of the Family Practitioner: An Historical Analysis of a New Specialty" (J Med Educ 1977;52:873–881); P. Curtis, "Three Hundred Years of Family Health Care" (J Fam Pract 1981;12:323–327); William J. Doherty, Charles E. Christianson, and Marvin B. Sussman (eds), *Family Medicine: The Maturing*

of a Discipline (New York, Haworth Press, 1987); David P. Adams, "Evolution of the Specialty of Family Practice" (J Florida Med Assoc 1989;76:325–329); D.P. Adams, *American Board of Family Practice: A History* (Lexington, KY, American Board of Family Practice, 1999); and Robert E. Rakel, "Evolution of Family Medicine in the United States: Sisyphus Revisited," *Proceedings of the 37th International Congress on the History of Medicine*, edited by Chester R. Burns, Ynez Viole O'Neill, Philippe Albou, and Jose Gabriel Rigau-Perez (Galveston, University of Texas Medical Branch, 2002).

39. Robert B. Taylor, "Family Practice and the Advancement of Medical Understanding: The First 50 Years" (J Fam Pract 1999;48:53–57).

40. Lawrence L. Hirsch, "Review of Principles of Family Medicine (1977)" (JAMA 1978;239:2387).

41. Glimpses of this future may be found in Fitzhugh Mullan, *Big Doctoring in America: Profiles in Primary Care* (Berkeley, University of California Press, 2002).

42. In the spring of 2004, Jenny Saurette was one of several seniors at the University of Texas Medical Branch in Galveston who took an elective course in medical history with Dr. Burns. Jenny, now a resident in family medicine in Tyler, Texas, did a superb job of analyzing some of the features about the history of family medicine that were described in this chapter. The authors are most grateful for her insights and wish her all the best in her career as a family physician.

43. Online databases make this labor not as difficult as it was previously. Any reader with access to the Internet can go to the UTMB home page at www.utmb.edu and click on Library. Then click on Internet Resources; then Medical Humanities; then History of Medicine. Under History of Medicine, click on American Association for the History of Medicine (AAHM). More than 30 sites about medical history can be accessed by clicking on Related Sites on the AAHM home page. The most comprehensive of these sites is the one titled History of the Health Sciences World Wide Web Links. These links provide access to more than 300 Internet sites providing information about many topics in the history of medicine and health care.

SUGGESTED READINGS

Burns CR. Fictional doctors and the evolution of medical ethics in the United States, 1875–1900. Lit Med 1988; 7:46–49.

Coxe JR. The Writings of Hippocrates and Galen. Philadelphia, Lindsay and Blakiston, 1846.

Hudson RP. Disease and Its Control. Westport, CT, Greenwood Press, 1983.

Kaufman M, Galishoff S, Savitt TL, eds. Dictionary of American Medical Biography, vols 1 and 2. Westport, CT, Greenwood Press, 1984.

Kelly HA, Burrage WL. Dictionary of American Medical Biography. New York, D. Appleton, 1928.

Powell JH. Bring Out Your Dead: The Great Plague of Yellow Fever in Philadelphia in 1793. Philadelphia, University of Pennsylvania Press, 1949.

Shryock RH. Medicine in America: Historical Essays. Baltimore, Johns Hopkins University Press, 1966.

Silverthorne E. Ashbel Smith of Texas: Pioneer, Patriot, Statesman, 1805–1886. College Station, Texas A&M University Press, 1982.

Tindall GB, with Shi DE. America: A Narrative History. New York, WW Norton, 1992.

Warner JH. The Therapeutic Perspective: Medical Practice, Knowledge, and Professional Identity in America, 1820–1885. Cambridge, MA, Harvard University Press, 1986.

4

Problem Solving in Family Medicine

John C. Rogers and William Y. Huang

KEY POINTS

1. The complete history and physical are not efficient and often not appropriate for handling the brief and varied encounters seen in the ambulatory setting. Students must learn a new way to approach clinical problems in the ambulatory setting that enables them to obtain key information in a focused manner.
2. Different types of ambulatory visits include the new problem visit, chronic illness visit, checkup (prevention) visit, psychosocial visit, and behavior change visit. Family physicians often see "mixed" visits that include two or more of these visit types.
3. Five general tasks to perform in ambulatory visits include assessing the patient's expectations and concerns, acquiring and synthesizing patient information, developing a therapeutic relationship, negotiating a management plan, and learning from the encounter.
4. In performing these general tasks, there is some similarity across different visit types. However, for the acquiring and synthesizing patient information task, different kinds of information must be obtained and processed for each visit type.
5. Selecting the correct visit type(s) and using the general tasks give students an approach to handling different ambulatory generalist encounters in a focused manner.

Medical educators are often concerned about the teaching and assessment of problem-solving skills. Teachers presume that students can learn and use a set of reasoning strategies to solve clinical problems successfully, even novel, complex ones. Research has shown, however, that problem-solving performance varies across different clinical domains, such as nephrology and gastroenterology. Students need more than just a set of generic problem-solving skills; they need specific biomedical knowledge as well. Thus, for effective problem solving in primary care, students need specific knowledge about ambulatory problems (see later chapters about clinical problems) and a foundation of clinical reasoning steps, which this chapter provides.

Introduction to clinical medicine courses present students with one model for approaching clinical problems: the complete history and physical examination (H&P), which is the standard assessment performed when a patient enters the hospital. The H&P consists of the chief complaint, statement of the reliability of the patient as a historian, history of the current illness, medical history, social history, family history, review of systems, complete physical examination, and laboratory test data followed by an impression and initial plans. Students follow this map for physician-patient encounters on internal medicine rotations when doing complete workups on new hospital admissions. Students also follow this map on pediatrics and in an abbreviated form on surgery and obstetrics-gynecology rotations, in which a single problem is more typically the focus of the admission.

In the ambulatory setting, students quickly realize that a complete H&P is not appropriate for most physician-patient encounters. The main issue is the amount of time dedicated to ambulatory visits. The mean time per encounter for the 25 most frequent diagnoses ranges between 9 and 17 minutes, with the bulk of the mean times between 10 and 14 minutes (Rosenblatt et al., 1982 **B**). There is simply not enough time to do an H&P during each ambulatory encounter. The second issue is the wide variety of problems seen in ambulatory care. The top 30 diagnoses seen by office-based family physicians constitute only about two thirds of all problems seen in the outpatient setting (Rosenblatt et al., 1982 **B**). Even the three most common diagnoses (hypertension, general medicine examination, and diabetes mellitus) are seen in only 15% of patient encounters (National Center for Health Statistics, Centers for Disease Control and

---

Evidence levels **A** Randomized, controlled trials (RCTs), meta-analyses, well-designed systematic reviews of RCTs. **B** Case-control or cohort studies, nonrandomized clinical trials, systematic reviews of studies other than RCTs, cross-sectional studies, retrospective studies, certain uncontrolled studies. **C** Consensus statements, expert guidelines, usual practice, opinion.

Prevention, U.S. Department of Health and Human Services, 2002). Parts of an H&P are relevant to the evaluation of new undiagnosed problems (i.e., history of current illness), but care of the other problems (i.e., prevention, chronic illnesses, psychosocial issues, and lifestyle or behavior change) requires information that is not included in a typical H&P.

If the complete workup or H&P model from hospital-based practice does not fit well with office-based, generalist practice, what model does? Unfortunately, a single approach does not work for all types of encounters that family physicians have with patients: new patient visit, new problem visit, follow-up visit, preventive care visit, chronic illness visit, mental health visit, or procedure visit. The H&P map works well for a new patient visit but not for the others. For example, at a chronic illness visit, the physician needs to accomplish several tasks: assess control of the disease, ask about adherence with the treatment plan, check for treatment side effects, seek evidence of end-organ damage, and scan for other risk factors for complications. At a well-person checkup visit, the physician should cover several preventive medicine topics: cancer detection, coronary artery disease risk factors, immunizations and infectious disease risks, trauma prevention strategies, and metabolic disease risk and prevention.

At each of the different types of ambulatory visits, primary care physicians attempt to complete specific tasks in a time-efficient way. This balance is one of the key skills in ambulatory generalist practice: how to efficiently accomplish a number of tasks that synthesize medical knowledge about what constitutes good patient care. The educational challenge for students is to learn which tasks are important in what types of visits and then how to do those tasks. The task-oriented processes in care model (Rogers et al., 2003 ⓑ, 2004) summarizes the different tasks for different visit types and provides students with a framework for organizing their approach to these different visit types.

In the task-oriented processes in care model, the following major processes apply to all visit types and summarize what family physicians do. Together they could be seen as the general model for conducting ambulatory generalist visits. The remainder of this chapter covers these major processes and describes how the student can use them as core problem-solving skills.

1. Assess the patient's expectations and concerns.
2. Acquire and synthesize patient information.
3. Develop a therapeutic relationship.
4. Negotiate a management plan.
5. Learn from the encounter.

Within these major processes, there are specific tasks that are unique to each visit type, especially in the "acquire and synthesize patient information" process.

TASK 1: ASSESS THE PATIENT'S EXPECTATIONS

Assessing a patient's expectations identifies the type of visit and guides patient education and negotiation of the management plan. Four key concepts are involved in this task: goals, requests, explanatory model, and prototypic experiences.

Goals are the ends that patients wish to achieve with regard to health, functional ability, or symptoms. Patients often do not make their goals explicit during the encounter and cannot articulate them easily. Sometimes patients state that they need to be well for an important event, such as a wedding. Others simply want to be rid of the symptoms or be reassured. Still others wish to be able to function for their job. Explicitly identifying a patient's goals can help form an alliance between the physician and the patient.

Requests are patients' notions of the means needed to achieve their goals (Like and Zyzanski, 1986 ⓑ). Patients often want medical information about a problem, such as what it is called, what causes it, how long it is going to last, and which tests may be needed. In addition, patients typically want some biomedical treatment such as medications or surgery for their physical discomfort. At other times, patients want emotional assistance or simply want the physician to listen while they share their own perspective about the problems. Patients also seek advice about general health matters such as diet and exercise. Sometimes patients are explicit about what they expect, but often this opinion is only mentioned indirectly during the visit. By determining a patient's request for the visit, the clinician can address this issue directly with the patient, especially if there seems to be disagreement between the physician's recommendation and the patient's request (Table 4-1).

One source of patients' requests is their explanatory model, which is a concept from the anthropologic literature that refers to the theory about disease (Kleinman, 1980). The Western biomedical model taught in allopathic and osteopathic schools of medicine is one of a number of available models about the causes of diseases, their prognosis, and appropriate treatments. In the community, there are also cultural theories that may use terms from the biomedical model. The beliefs that patients hold often drive their requests and strongly influence what they expect of physicians.

Another determinant of patients' requests is their prototypic experiences, which include personal experience with a problem, experience of a family member or friend, or reading or hearing about the issue through media such as magazines and television (Like and Steiner, 1986 ⓑ). Sometimes these sources of information, particularly significant family members or friends, have great influence in patients' lives.

Gathering information related to each of these four concepts helps focus patient education and nego-

Chapter 4 Problem Solving in Family Medicine

Table 4-1 Examples of Patients' Expectations and Concerns for Different Types of Ambulatory Visits

New problem visit
Diagnose the cause of symptoms
Order diagnostic tests to evaluate symptoms
Concern that symptoms may reflect a severe or life-threatening condition (especially if a family member or friend with similar symptoms turned out to have a severe condition)

Checkup (prevention) visit
Evaluate overall health status
Discuss pros and cons of doing a screening test that the patient wishes to have performed
Desire to be screened for a condition that a family member or friend has

Chronic illness visit
Relieve symptoms or improve control of condition
Discuss lifestyle or medication issues
Avoid target organ damage or other complications from the chronic illness

Psychosocial visit
Diagnose and treat emotional symptoms that may indicate a mental illness or manifestations of a physical illness
Diagnose and treat somatic symptoms that the physician may conclude are related to an emotional condition

Behavior change visit
Relieve current physical symptoms that result from a problem behavior needing change
Discuss how to deal with a problem behavior that the patient knows needs changing
Patient may have no expectations or concerns, but physician may have concerns that a behavior change is causing current symptoms or aggravating the control of a chronic illness

tiation of the management plan. Although collecting this information may seem to be relatively easy, it can be difficult in the busy ambulatory environment to listen to the patient's entire story due to the limited time available for each patient encounter. In one study, physicians interrupted the patient's opening statement of concerns and redirected the interview toward a more specific concern after an average of 18 seconds (Beckman and Frankel, 1984 ⓑ). A later study confirmed that physicians redirected patients after letting them present their opening statement after an average of 23 seconds. However, in this second study, patients allowed to completely express their concerns took only on average six seconds more than those who were interrupted (Marvel et al., 1999 ⓑ). The student must learn to listen to the patient's expectations and concerns and avoid the temptation to take over the interview. In most cases, if the student will allow the patient to completely express his or her concerns, it will not take a significant amount of additional time. This inquiry may reveal that there are no conflicts, no critical gaps in the patient's understanding, and no need for a long-winded discussion by the physician. Alternatively, the physician and patient may discover areas in which brief, focused education and dialogue can be very effective and satisfactory for both parties. This inquiry may even reveal major gaps or conflicts that perhaps can be resolved after serious negotiation or that may lead to the decision that the physician and patient cannot have a successful working relationship. This approach to clinical encounters is sometimes described as patient-centered care in contrast to the focus on diagnostic reasoning or doctor-centered care.

TASK 2: ACQUIRE AND SYNTHESIZE PATIENT INFORMATION

After learning the patient's expectations and concerns, the focus of the visit becomes clearer. Some patients have a new or undiagnosed problem that needs evaluation. Others may desire a checkup or health maintenance examination, have known chronic illnesses that need monitoring, present with psychosocial concerns, or desire help in changing a problem behavior. It is also important to understand that patients in the family physician's office may present with one or more of these concerns at the same time. Indeed, one study demonstrated that 73% of encounters in the family physician's office dealt with more than one problem (Flocke et al., 2001 ⓑ). Understanding the reason for the patient's visit helps the student gather the information necessary for that particular type of visit.

The task-oriented processes in care model describes the different types of patient visits and the information to be gathered and synthesized for each type. The task-oriented processes in care model includes the new problem visit, checkup (prevention) visit, chronic illness visit, psychosocial visit, and behavior change visit (Table 4-2).

New Problem Visit

In this visit, the patient presents with an undifferentiated set of symptoms, and the goal is to diagnose the condition and begin appropriate treatment. This visit is similar to the traditional H&P but more focused. The student elicits the presenting symptom and takes a history of current illness, asks about pertinent history and family and social history, does a brief review of systems, and performs a physical

Table 4-2	**Specific Tasks to Perform in Acquiring and Synthesizing Patient Information**

New problem visit
Assess presenting complaint
Construct a problem list and make a diagnosis

Checkup (prevention) visit
Assess risk factors and previous preventive services for six major areas: cancer, cardiovascular disease, infectious diseases, injury/trauma, metabolic diseases, and emotional health
Recommend preventive services in each area based on risk profile and previous preventive services

Chronic illness visit
Assess severity and control of the condition
Evaluate adherence to and side effects of medications
Scan for target organ damage from the condition
Review status of comorbid conditions

Psychosocial visit
Assess emotional needs of patient and family using the BATHE (see text) model
Evaluate for diagnosable mental illness
Evaluate suicidal risk

Behavior change visit
Get background information on problem behavior
Assess the patient's stage of change

examination focused on systems relevant to the potential diagnoses. While collecting information during the focused H&P, the student develops hypotheses about possible causes and, through an iterative process, tests and revises those hypotheses. With experience, novices become experts in iterative hypothesis testing. The products of this process are a differential diagnosis, a working diagnosis, and eventually a final diagnosis and problem list.

Checkup (Prevention) Visit

In this visit, the patient desires a checkup of current health status and appropriate measures to prevent illnesses and to screen for detectable conditions. Prevention and screening services can be organized into six categories of major causes of death and disability: cardiovascular, cancer, infectious diseases, injury/trauma, metabolic, and emotional health. The student gathers information about the patient's risk factors for particular diseases and about previous preventive and screening services. This information

guides recommendations to the patient about what preventive measures are indicated in each category.

Chronic Illness Visit

In this visit, the patient has a known chronic illness, and the purpose of the visit is to monitor the current status and provide care that will prevent further complications. The student assesses the severity and control of the condition. For patients with diabetes, hemoglobin A1c is one good measure of control. For patients with asthma, the frequency of symptoms, such as wheezing, and peak flow readings are measures of severity and control. Students ask about adherence to the management plan of medication and lifestyle measures and ask whether there are any side effects from the medications. Scanning for target organ damage is an important part of the evaluation of some chronic illnesses. For the patient with diabetes, this includes assessing the patient for retinopathy, coronary artery disease, nephropathy, neuropathy, and peripheral vascular disease. Reviewing comorbid conditions is also an important aspect of the evaluation of some chronic illnesses. For the patient with diabetes, this includes blood pressure, weight, lipids, smoking status, and family history of cardiovascular disease because all these contribute to the patient's risk of developing cardiovascular disease.

Psychosocial Visit

Many patients present to their family physicians with an emotional disorder or psychosocial symptoms. In this visit, the student assesses those needs through use of the BATHE model, which includes understanding the background of the psychosocial situation, the patient's affect or emotional response to the situation, the most troubling aspect of the situation, and how the patient is trying to cope or handle the situation. The student completes the assessment by expressing empathy for the patient's symptoms and situation and pulls the symptoms together to see whether a diagnosable mental illness exists and whether a risk for suicide exists (Stuart and Lieberman, 1986).

Behavior Change Visit

In this visit, the patient presents with a need for behavior change such as starting a diet and/or exercise program or stopping a problem behavior such as smoking or other substance use. The student seeing a patient with this issue first gets background information on the problem to understand why it has been difficult for the patient to change. In asking questions about the patient's motivation and sense of self-efficacy, the student can use the stage of change model to identify the stage of change or readiness of the patient to change (Prochaska and DiClemente,

1992). Patients in the precontemplation or contemplation stage may not be ready for change, and in those cases, it is the goal of the student to educate and help patients consider appropriate information that encourages them to advance to the next stage in the model. Patients in the determination stage are ready to change, and the student can help those patients devise a plan for changing. Patients in the action or maintenance stages, who have already made the change, need encouragement and positive reinforcement on their new behavior and tips on how to avoid relapsing (see Table 4-2).

TASK 3: DEVELOP A THERAPEUTIC RELATIONSHIP

To help solve patients' problems and be healers, physicians foster relationships of mutual trust and respect. In situations with continuity of care over time, there are many opportunities to establish workable therapeutic relationships. When necessary, however, skillful physicians can develop therapeutic relationships in one or two visits.

While physicians' nonverbal cues are a major determinant in establishing an effective relationship, direct questions can foster the desired relationship as well. There are four areas the physician can ask about: (1) the patient's family, work, and sociocultural context; (2) the patient's thoughts about the situation; (3) the patient's feelings in response to the context; and (4) the patient's efforts to cope with the context, thoughts, and feelings (Stuart and Lieberman, 1986).

Gathering contextual information indicates to the patient that the physician is not interested simply in a diseased organ system or pathophysiologic process but is concerned about the person who is experiencing the illness. In addition to listening carefully and maintaining eye contact, asking a patient's context demonstrates the physician's regard for the patient as a person.

By gathering information about the patient's thoughts, feelings, and coping efforts, the physician reinforces the view that the patient's physical complaints cannot be considered in isolation from the rest of the patient's life. This acknowledgment of the interaction of the patient's emotional life and physical well-being also contributes to the development of a personal bond between physician and patient, which is necessary for an optimal healing relationship. Most patients are grateful when a physician takes time to ask and listen. Verbally and nonverbally expressing empathy manifests the unconditional regard necessary in a therapeutic relationship (Stuart and Lieberman, 1986).

In one study, the physician behaviors that were most frequently associated with patient trust included being comforting and caring, demonstrating competency, encouraging and answering questions, explaining, and referring to a specialist if needed (Thom et al., 2001❸). For students to learn to develop a therapeutic relationship, it is important for them to show care, to communicate effectively, and to give the patient confidence in his or her clinical skills (Table 4-3).

TASK 4: NEGOTIATE A MANAGEMENT PLAN

Essential elements of the management plan include medications, diagnostic tests, lifestyle measures, referrals to other specialists or allied health providers, and arranging follow-up.

An important aspect of developing and negotiating the management plan is gaining an understanding of the patient's perspective on the condition. For example, one study demonstrated that physicians focused their attention on managing the laboratory results of patients with diabetes while failing to take into account other psychosocial issues that the patients felt were important (Freeman and Loewe, 2000❸). For successful negotiation of the management plan to occur, it is important for physicians and patients to agree on what needs treatment and then what that treatment will entail. For patients with chronic illnesses, Von Korff et al. (1997) recommend that physicians and patients work together to define what the problems are and then set realistic goals and targets to address the problems. In their suggested model of care, it is important for physicians to help patients know self-management items that can be performed at home and that active, sustained follow-up occur even through telephone contact.

Although it is not fully understood how experienced clinicians make management decisions, there are steps that at least help structure and define the decisions that must be made (Weinstein et al., 1980). One approach is to develop a decision tree that includes the therapeutic options and the outcomes that may result from each option. This structure outlines the treatment alternatives from which the physician and patient can choose as well as the potential outcomes or consequences, both minor and major, of each selection. Describing the options and outcomes to patients involves the patients in their own care.

Obtaining patients' preferences about treatment alternatives and outcomes is helpful.

Physicians do not go through these processes explicitly during every encounter, due to time constraints and variability in patients' desire for direct involvement in medical decisions. Instead, physicians often make decisions informally and quickly in their heads. Patients are grateful, however, if physicians at least list the management options and major outcomes. When patients know why tests or treatments are recommended, they feel more involved and are

Table 4-3 Examples of Strategies to Help Students Develop a Therapeutic Relationship with Patients in Different Types of Encounters

All visit types
Ask about family or social situation; seek to make a connection on a nonmedical topic
Demonstrate interest in the patient
Use facilitating, nonverbal behaviors such as appropriate eye contact, body position, and nods
Hold a genuine, positive regard for the patient

New problem visit
Acknowledge that symptoms are of concern to the patient
Be patient centered by focusing on patient's experiences, thoughts, feelings, and concerns
Include patient preferences in negotiation of the management plan, especially in regard to diagnostic tests and treatment

Checkup (prevention) visit
Acknowledge the patient's concern about a particular condition and desire to have a particular screening test
Patiently work with patients resistant to having a recommended screening

Chronic illness visit
Understand how the chronic illness affects the patient and family
Take a family-focused approach by assessing the needs of patient and family, understanding the relational context in which disease management occurs, and including the family environment in proposing interventions
Encourage continuity of care between physician and patient/family
Work collaboratively with patient and family to manage the illness
Encourage compliance
Demonstrate care and compassion, remembering that "care" may be more important than "cure" in treating many patients who are receiving maximal medical treatment for their chronic illnesses

Psychosocial visit
Recognize that it may be difficult for the patient to share his or her symptoms and situation
Encourage the patient to share his or her symptoms and concerns by being nonjudgmental and empathetic
Include patient preferences in negotiation of the management plan, especially in regard to medication and referrals

Behavior change visit
Demonstrate empathy for the difficulty in changing behavior
Offer partnership, support, and optimism in helping the patient through the change process
Avoid negative labels and terms associated with problem behaviors
Anticipate resistance and be patient in working with the patient
Avoid argumentation but seek to guide the patient in the process of self-discovery

more likely to follow the suggestions or directions. This strategy permits real negotiation between physicians and patients about medical advice and what to do about problems. By providing patients with options and eliciting an idea of patients' preferences, physicians can choose a course of action that is based on the best medical knowledge and patients' values (Table 4-4).

TASK 5: LEARN FROM THE ENCOUNTER

Learning from patient encounters is a principal means by which physicians continue their education. Reflecting on a particular encounter can help the physician determine ways in which the relationship with that patient and the management of that patient's problems can be improved as the care continues. This reflection can also lead to a fuller understanding of the patient's problems in general terms so that the care of other patients is improved.

Reviewing the processes by which a diagnosis was made and the management plan implemented can identify biases or pitfalls that may become habitual and may lead to misdiagnosis or inappropriate management decisions. Errors in problem solving cannot be completely avoided, but by reflecting on encounters and noting when errors occur, clinicians may make these errors less frequently and may avoid the self-deception that all is well with their decision making.

Table 4-4 Examples of Strategies to Negotiate a Management Plan in Different Types of Encounters

All visit types
Management items to discuss
   Diagnostic tests
   Lifestyle measures
   Medications
   Referrals to specialists or allied health providers
   When to return for follow-up

New problem visit
Discussion of possible diagnoses, tests, and prognosis
Negotiation of diagnostic plan by asking the patient about preferences and encouraging the patient to be involved
Support self-care by providing information/patient education material and educating the patient on what he or she can do to care for him- or herself

Checkup (prevention) visit
Recommend preventive or screening services as recommended by accepted guidelines
Negotiation through discussion of options (such as different methods of colorectal cancer screening)
Support the patient's self-care by encouraging healthy lifestyle choices (diet, exercise) that may prevent illnesses, and teach patients to screen themselves where possible (e.g., breast self-examination)

Chronic illness visit
Negotiation of achievable goals and measurable targets and discussion of options such as medication choices, lifestyle measures, and referrals
Support self-care by teaching the patient to mirror what you do in the office: assess severity and control of the condition, monitor compliance with lifestyle measures and medications, scan for target organ damage, observe comorbid conditions

Psychosocial visit
Establish diagnosis by evaluating for appropriate medical and psychosocial conditions
Negotiation through discussion of options such as medications, counseling, and who may be best provider of these services
Support the patient's self-care by encouraging the use of social support networks and counseling services

Behavior change visit
Negotiation of a feasible plan to change the problem behavior that is acceptable and realistic for the patient
Increase the patient's motivation by a discussion of the pros and cons of changing the problem behavior and helping him or her see that the pros outweigh the cons
Increase the patient's self-efficacy by a discussion of the aids and barriers to change and helping him or her see that the aids outweigh the barriers

Individual physician-patient relationships do not remain static but shift over time depending on the clinical setting, clinical problem, and stage of the relationship. Reflecting on the relationship after an encounter may bring insights that will improve future physician-patient encounters (Table 4-5).

It also is useful to identify which decision policies, rules, or protocols are pertinent to the clinical encounter. Each physician develops policies regarding the diagnostic process and therapeutic management. Some of these policies may be related to the goals of diagnosis and therapy. Clinicians also adopt protocol-related policies developed by others, such as diagnostic protocols and algorithms, therapeutic protocols with standard duration and sequencing of interventions, and standard evaluation procedures to monitor the effectiveness of therapy and to detect side effects or complications. A key learning task for all clinicians is to determine which clinical guidelines experts are recommending and how these recommendations are being revised on a continual basis. By reviewing the clinical encounter in these terms, the physician can determine whether his or her practice of medicine is state of the art or behind the times.

SUMMARY: THE AMBULATORY ENCOUNTER CHECKLIST

These five general tasks—assessing the patient's expectations and concerns, acquiring and synthesizing

Table 4-5 Examples of References That Will Help Students Learn from the Encounter

New problem visit
Applicable diagnostic or therapeutic protocols for undifferentiated conditions; many are available at the National Guideline Clearinghouse Web site (www.guideline.gov)

Checkup (prevention) visit
Applicable preventive and screening guidelines; many are available at the U.S. Preventive Services Task Force Web site (www.ahcpr.gov/clinic/uspstfix.htm). The U.S. Preventive Services Task Force provides an excellent summary of the current evidence surrounding each preventive or screening issue and explains how their recommendations were reached through an evaluation of this evidence.

Chronic illness visit
Applicable clinical practice guidelines for chronic illnesses and conditions; many are available at the National Guideline Clearinghouse Web site (www.guideline.gov) or the National Institutes of Health Web site (www.nih.gov)

Psychosocial visit
Diagnostic criteria for mental conditions; many are available from the *Diagnostic and Statistical Manual of Mental Disorders, 4th Edition (DSM-IV)*, American Psychiatric Association, 1994.

Behavior change visit
Applicable guidelines on changing problem behaviors; some guidelines are available at the National Guideline Clearinghouse Web site (www.guideline.gov) and the U.S. Preventive Services Task Force Web site (www.ahcpr.gov/clinic/uspstfix.htm). Students may also learn by reflecting on their own fallibility and need to change.

patient information, developing a therapeutic relationship, negotiating a management plan, and learning from the encounter—provide a checklist to guide young clinicians through ambulatory generalist encounters. Understanding the applicable visit type(s) will help students use these tasks correctly, provide a framework for the visit, treat the patient appropriately, and learn from the encounter.

Material Available on Student Consult

Review Questions and Answers about Problem Solving in Family Medicine

REFERENCES

Beckman HB, Frankel RM. The effect of behavior on the collection of data. Ann Intern Med 1984;101: 692–696. **B**

Flocke SA, Frank SH, Wenger DA. Addressing multiple problems in the family practice office visit. J Fam Pract 2001;50:211–216. **B**

Freeman J, Loewe R. Barriers to communication about diabetes mellitus: Patients' and physicians' different views of the disease. J Fam Pract 2000;49:507–512. **B**

Kleinman A. Patients and Healers in the Context of Culture. Berkeley: University of California Press, 1980:106.

Kleinman A, Eisenberg J, Good B. Culture, illness and care: Clinical lessons from anthropologic and cross-cultural research. Ann Intern Med 1978;88:251–258.

Like R, Zyzanski S. Patient requests in family practice: A focal point for clinical negotiations. Fam Pract 1986;3:216–227. **B**

Marvel MK, Epstein RM, Flowers K, Beckman HB. Soliciting the patient's agenda: Have we improved? JAMA 1999;281:283–287. **B**

National Center for Health Statistics, Centers for Disease Control and Prevention, United States Department of Health and Human Services. National Ambulatory Medical Survey data, 2002. Taken from the American Academy of Family Physicians Web site. Available at www.aafp.org/x25061.xml. Accessed October 14, 2004. **B**

Prochaska JO, DiClemente CC. Stages of change in the modification of problem behaviors. Prog Behav Modif 1992;28:183–218.

Rogers J, Corboy J, Dains J, et al. Task-oriented processes in care (TOPIC): A proven model for teaching ambulatory care. Fam Med 2003;35:337–342. **B**

Rogers JC, Corboy JE, Huang WY, Monteiro FM. Task-Oriented Processes in Care (TOPIC) Model in Ambulatory Care. New York: Springer, 2004.

Rosenblatt RA, Cherkin OC, Schneeweis R, et al. The structure and content of family practice: Current status and future trends. J Fam Pract 1982;15:681–722. **B**

Stuart MR, Lieberman JA. The Fifteen Minute Hour: Applied Psychotherapy for the Primary Care Physician. New York: Praeger, 1986.

Thom DH and the Stanford Trust Study Physicians. Physician behaviors that predict patient trust. J Fam Pract 2001;50:323–328. **B**

Von Korff M, Gruman J, Schaefer J, et al. Collaborative management of chronic illness. Ann Intern Med 1997;127:1097–1102.

Weinstein MC, Fineberg HU, Elstein AS, et al. Clinical Decision Analysis. Philadelphia: WB Saunders, 1980.

Chapter

5 Evidence-Based Medicine

Bernard Ewigman

KEY POINTS

1. Evidence-based medicine (EBM) evolved from the population-based, quantitative, and empirical roots of epidemiology and biostatistics.
2. EBM is a recent approach to clinical decision making and complements rather than supplants pathophysiologic reasoning, clinical experience, and clinical judgment.
3. The key feature that distinguishes EBM from other approaches is the use of explicit and replicable methods to answer clinical questions.
4. InfoRetriever and DynaMed are electronic knowledge resources developed by family physicians that are based on literature surveillance systems.
5. The Family Physicians Inquiries Network is a binational academic consortium of family medicine departments, residency programs, librarians, and other persons and entities dedicated to using information technology to translate research evidence into practice.

WHAT IS EVIDENCE-BASED MEDICINE?

Evidence-based medicine (EBM) is the integration of best research evidence with clinical expertise and patient values (Reilly, 2004; Sackett et al., 2000). The ultimate goal of EBM is to improve patient outcomes by considering the most current, valid, clinical research evidence in patient care decisions. An excellent example of the application of EBM in practice is described in Chapter 6 of this book, "Evaluating the Medical Literature," by Susman and colleagues. They

use the Women's Health Initiative (WHI) randomized trial of hormone replacement therapy (HRT) to make the case that using the best evidence can save lives, to provide concrete examples of using EBM in practice, and to explain some of the methods of EBM (Manson et al., 2003).

EBM is relatively new, roughly a decade old, according to authors writing in a special issue of the *British Medical Journal* (BMJ) published in 2004 (Coomarasamy and Khan, 2004; Gabbay and Le May, 2004; Guyatt et al., 2004; Lockwood, 2004; Reilly, 2004; Strauss and Jones, 2004; Tovey and Godlee, 2004). A MEDLINE search I conducted using the term "evidence-based medicine" resulted in no citations prior to 1992, and only two citations for that year. When the same search term was used for the year 2003, 3,011 citations were generated. A perusal of articles in the 2004 special issue of the BMJ leaves little doubt that EBM has grown exponentially in medical education, clinical training, and clinical practice in the United States, Canada, and Great Britain (Coomarasamy and Khan, 2004; Gabbay and Le May, 2004; Guyatt et al., 2004; Lockwood, 2004; Reilly, 2004; Strauss and Jones, 2004; Tovey and Godlee, 2004).

It remains unclear whether patients have actually benefited from the lofty goals of the EBM philosophy. The EBM model has not yet penetrated the processes of patient care sufficiently to substantively affect patient care outcomes in easily measurable ways, many challenges remain to achieve this objective, and the complex task of proving the effectiveness of EBM will be exceptionally difficult (Strauss and Jones, 2004). Nonetheless, EBM has definitely had an impact on the knowledge, attitudes, and behaviors of practitioners (Coomarasamy and Khan, 2004; Tovey and Godlee,

2004). EBM leaders optimistically predict that the next decade will be as exciting as the last decade, and that the major challenge is to learn how better to use the evidence that is available and how to measure the impact on patient care (Guyatt, 1991; Strauss and Jones, 2004).

EBM has zealous advocates as well as adamant resistors. Its logical objectivity, rooted in the empirical approach to science, is attractive to physicians as scientists. But it clearly complements rather than replaces traditional frameworks for clinical decision making, including pathophysiologic reasoning, clinical experience, and clinical judgment. Doing the systematic searching and rigorous critical appraisal required for EBM is time-consuming and requires specific skills that were not taught in medical school in the past. Even when the evidence is available and has been synthesized into a practice recommendation, there is much more to the practice of medicine than scientific evidence. Any physician who attempted patient care equipped solely with the "current best evidence" would be quickly humbled. EBM appears to be a major advance in the science of medicine, but it is not a medical panacea for the 21st century.

What Are the Distinguishing Characteristics of EBM?

How does EBM differ from more traditional methods of clinical decision making? All physicians are expected to be conscientious and judicious, regardless of their style of practice, so EBM shares those features with other methods. No well-informed EBM adherent would argue with the need to integrate clinical experience and patient values into patient care decisions, nor is that need unique to EBM. The two concepts that distinguish EBM as an innovation are (1) EBM uses systematic methods of identifying and critiquing research evidence, including prespecified hierarchical criteria for identifying "current best evidence," and (2) EBM entails explicit descriptions of the methods and criteria used, which allows others to confirm or refute the findings and recommendations. The teaching case provided here illustrates these concepts and contrasts the findings of an EBM approach and a non-EBM approach to answering a clinical question in a teaching setting.

Teaching Case: A third-year medical student on her first clinical rotation, a family medicine clerkship, saw Mrs. M., a 52-year-old menopausal woman who was making a return visit to her family physician. Mrs. M. had seen Dr. E. twice in the past several weeks for bothersome hot flushes that frequently awakened her at night. Dr. E. had prescribed several remedies, but none had helped, and he had suggested a trial of estrogen. Mrs. M. had read on an Internet site that estrogen causes strokes and heart attacks and wanted to know if that was true.

Dr. E. told her that he would prescribe a low dose of estrogen for only as long as needed for her hot flushes. He said that her risk of a heart attack would not be increased and that if her risk of a stroke were increased at all, the risk would be less than one in a thousand in the next year. Finally, he told her that estrogen would very likely reduce or eliminate the hot flushes altogether.

After the visit was over, Dr. E. suggested to the medical student that she answer a clinical question generated from Mrs. M.'s case as part of fulfilling a clerkship requirement to prepare evidenced-based answers to clinical questions about patients seen with preceptors. The question he suggested was, What is the risk of stroke and coronary heart disease in a postmenopausal woman treated with estrogen only for hot flushes?

The Non-EBM Answer

Our student first looked this up in the most recent edition of a standard textbook on her preceptor's shelf. The book had been published 3 years earlier. She found several statements regarding the benefits of estrogen therapy in postmenopausal women:

> Estrogen replacement therapy (ERT) relieves the symptoms of hot flashes. . . . Postmenopausal women start to experience cardiovascular events at the same rate as their male counterparts. ERT decreases their risk by 50%. . . .

There were no statements about the risk of stroke, and no references were given regarding the decreased risk of cardiovascular events. The student had learned the basic concepts and methods of clinical epidemiology, biostatistics, and literature searching in her preclinical years. She recalled the admonition in *Evidence-Based Medicine: How to Practice and Teach EBM* (Sackett et al., 2000), which was, "Burn your (traditional) textbook." She then proceeded to use her skills in the classic steps of EBM as shown in Box 5-1, knowing that quoting unreferenced statements from a textbook would earn her a failing grade on the assignment.

The EBM Answer

The student searched several databases known to contain the best evidence, including systematic reviews and high-quality original research evidence (Cochrane Library, Clinical Evidence, InfoRetriever, Clinical Inquiries, National Guideline Clearinghouse, U.S. Preventive Services Task Force, UpToDate, DynaMed), and that are updated with current research more or less regularly. In addition, she conducted a search of MEDLINE, the comprehensive research literature database maintained by

<table>
<tr><td>

Box 5-1   **Classic Steps in Evidence-Based Medicine**

1. Formulate a clear, answerable, and specific patient-related clinical question.
2. Conduct a systematic search of the medical literature to identify the relevant research articles.
3. Select the most valid articles based on a priori quality criteria and critically appraise the articles for internal and external validity.
4. Integrate the findings into clinical decision making about the patient.

</td></tr>
</table>

<table>
<tr><td>

Box 5-2   **Methods of Producing Best Evidence**

Clinical Epidemiologic Methods[*]

Randomized trials[†]
Cohort studies[‡]
Case-control studies
Case series

Integrative Methods

Systematic reviews
Meta-analyses
Economic analyses
Decision analyses

</td></tr>
</table>

[*]For establishing cause-and-effect relationships, RCTs are the strongest design, followed by cohort studies, case-control studies, and finally case series, the weakest design for establishing cause and effect.
[†]Study design of choice for questions about diagnosis and prognosis.
[‡]Study design of choice for questions about treatment or preventive interventions.

the National Library of Medicine, and Current Contents, a source of more rapidly indexed citations that captures just recently published research.

Although the student's searches generated a huge number of research articles, reviews, and guidelines, using the principles of EBM, she homed in on one recent (published in April 2004) randomized, controlled trial (RCT). This study clearly stood above numerous older observational studies on estrogen replacement therapy as the strongest study design for determining cause-and-effect relationships (Table 5-1 and Box 5-2) in studies about therapy. This trial was also prominently quoted in UpToDate and DynaMed, and it was the most relevant title found in InfoRetriever. Using the Critical Appraisal Worksheet for Studies of Therapy (reproduced in Appendix 5-1 on the Student Consult), adapted from Sackett et al. (2004), she evaluated the validity and applicability of the Women's Health Initiative study of estrogen versus placebo for the prevention of osteoporosis to her question and the patient case from which the question was generated (Women's Health Initiative Steering Committee, 2004).

Table 5-1 lists the study designs of choice and one of the most important primary criteria for determining the validity of a study according to the

type of questions being asked—diagnosis, prognosis, prevention, or treatment (or harm). A complete listing of the criteria for determining the validity of a study, which are different for each type of question (the RCT is the design of choice only for prevention and treatment questions), is provided in Appendix 5-1. A full description of these criteria (and much more) is available in *Evidence-Based Medicine: How to Practice and Teach EBM* (Sackett et al., 2004), a concise, thorough, and well-written book.

Our student's question was about the harms associated with a treatment. The best study design to answer this question is an RCT. One of the critical criteria for judging validity of an RCT is determining that the random allocation of subjects to treatment and control group was concealed. This helps ensure that the patients in the treatment group are similar to those in the control group in every way except for the intervention. This similarity of groups is what makes RCTs the most powerful design for evaluating treatment (or harm) and determining cause-and-effect relationships. Box 5-2 gives the types of study designs used for generating clinical evidence, and it also gives a list of methods of integrating multiple studies. Integrative methods can be more useful than single studies because they may show consistent findings among studies, or they may have sufficient statistical power when data from several studies are pooled together (meta-analysis).

The estrogen-only WHI study was an RCT that used concealed allocation. It also addressed unopposed estrogen, which is what Dr. E. prescribed for Mrs. M., since she had undergone a hysterectomy

Table 5-1   Primary Criteria for Critical Appraisal of Evidence by Type of Question

Type of Question	Study Design of Choice	Primary Criteria
Diagnosis	Cohort study	Gold standard
Prognosis	Cohort study	Inception cohort
Prevention	RCT	Concealed allocation
Treatment (or harm)	RCT	Concealed allocation

and therefore had no need for the addition of progestin to the estrogen to prevent endometrial cancer. That combination of therapy was evaluated in another WHI trial (WHI combined HRT, August 7, 2003). Although this study was an important RCT, it did not directly address the question that arose in Mrs. M.'s case.

The student's critical appraisal revealed that the WHI estrogen-alone study was a double-blind, randomized trial with concealed allocation of assignment, intention-to-treat analysis, a 98% follow-up of study participants, and equal treatment of the two groups apart from the estrogen therapy in the intervention group. She recognized these factors as the hallmarks of a well-done RCT.

The study showed that there was no increase in the rate of coronary heart disease (hazard ratio [HR] = 0.91; 95% confidence interval [CI] = 0.75–1.12) (note that the 95% confidence interval includes 1.0, or no difference) but that there was an increase in the incidence of stroke (HR = 1.39; 95% CI = 1.10–1.77) (here the 95% confidence interval does not include 1.0, or the possibility of no difference; there is a 95% probability that the true hazard ratio is somewhere between the low of 1.10 or the high of 1.77). However, the rate of stroke was quite low in this population to begin with, so the 39% increase (derived from the HR of 1.39) meant that the actual increase in the rate of strokes amounted to approximately 12 in 10,000 person-years. She also noted that the mean age of the women in the estrogen-alone WHI trial was 63 years. Mrs. M. was only 52, and Dr. E. had prescribed 0.3 mg of estrogen, whereas the estrogen-alone WHI trial used 0.625 mg of estrogen in the treatment group. Dr. E. had told Mrs. M. that he would prescribe the estrogen only as long as she needed it for relief of her hot flushes, which likely would not be nearly as long as the average 6.8 years that women took it in the estrogen-alone WHI study. Mrs. M.'s younger age, the lower dose of estrogen, and the briefer course of therapy all led our student to surmise that Mrs. M.'s risk of a stroke was actually less than the 12 in 10,000 person-years (or 1.2 in 1,000 person-years) reported in the study. In addition, she found a meta-analysis of 26,000 patients in InfoRetriever that showed that mortality was decreased with hormone therapy (combination estrogen and progestin) in women less than 60 years old (Salpeter et al., 2004). Although Mrs. M. was taking estrogen only, the student thought it reasonable to extrapolate these findings to Mrs. M.'s case. Her basic conclusion was that Mrs. M. had no increased risk of heart problems and a maximum increased chance of just over 1 in 1,000 of having a stroke per year while she was being treated, and probably even less.

The student learned several things through this assignment:

1. Sources that are out of date can be misleading. The reference to a 50% reduction in heart disease had likely come from observational case-control studies that, in retrospect, led to erroneous conclusions. An accurate critical appraisal of those studies would have led to a far less enthusiastic endorsement than that given by the textbook author, who did not cite those studies and perhaps did not even read them.

2. In addition to assessing the internal validity of a study, it is important to look closely at the actual population studied, the intervention studied, and the duration of treatment, and think about how the study findings may or may not apply to an individual patient. The combined estrogen plus progestin WHI trial did show an increase in heart disease from HRT; however, that trial did not apply directly to this particular patient, since she was not taking progestins (Manson et al., 2003). On the other hand, since the Salpeter meta-analysis showed decreased mortality in younger patients even though the outcomes in the combination WHI trial were worse than the outcomes in the estrogen-only WHI trial, she found that reassuring. The patient was younger than most women in the estrogen-alone WHI study, the dose of estrogen prescribed was half the dose used in the study, and Mrs. M. was not going to be exposed to estrogen for nearly as long. These nuances significantly affected the student's conclusions and supported the decision made by her family physician preceptor.

3. Some of the so-called best evidence sources actually had not yet updated their information to include this RCT by the end of 2004, when the student conducted her search. Neither the Cochrane Library nor Clinical Evidence, for example, had reviews that included the estrogen-alone WHI trial, even though the student searched these sources 9 months after publication of the study. These collections of rigorous systematic reviews may also be misleading if they are not kept up to date. A quick search of certain databases (Current Contents, PreMEDLINE) will turn up recently published studies to supplement rigorous reviews that are becoming outdated.

4. Sources that do not meet strict criteria for being evidence based may nonetheless reflect the best evidence. UpToDate (www.uptodate.com), for example, included this key trial and others and had incorporated the findings into a clear discussion and a set of recommendations. UpToDate continuously scans several hundred journals and thereby often captures recent evidence. Similarly, DynaMed and InfoRetriever, both of which use the literature surveillance method, also had these critical WHI trials in

their databases. This anecdote suggests that databases employing literature surveillance systems stay abreast of the most important literature more efficiently than the traditional approach of conducting repeated systematic searches on specific topics, and a recent RCT supports this assertion (Alper et al., 2005).

The findings from the WHI trials drew an enormous amount of publicity in the media. There was extensive discussion in the medical literature of the unexpected findings. Nevertheless, many of the sources searched by the student did not include this key evidence. Furthermore, it is uncommon to find a single study, as happened in this case, that definitely answers a clinical question as clearly as the WHI trials did. Most changes in clinical practice occur slowly and over time, based on an accumulation of research studies that, when taken together, make the case for a change in practice. Consequently, most EBM searches must seek out multiple studies and studiously integrate the findings, none of which individually draw much attention at the time of their publication. In other words, practicing EBM using the classic steps is generally more difficult, more time-consuming, and less satisfying than in our example. This points to the value of electronic databases with literature surveillance systems (DynaMed, InfoRetriever) and of collections of brief, evidence-based answers to clinical questions (Clinical Inquiries).

Another fault line that causes a rift between what is known in the literature and what is done in practice is the delay in using evidence that definitely shows a benefit. There is a well-described lag between the publication of research results in journals and the integration of those results into review articles and books written by experts. In the case of treatments for myocardial infarction, for example, many experts were still recommending ineffective or outdated treatments long after definitive evidence showed benefit to new treatments such as thrombolytic therapy (Antman et al., 1992).

Non-evidence-based sources may lead clinicians astray because of the lack of a hierarchical ranking of evidence by prespecified criteria, one of the distinguishing features of EBM. Prior to the WHI studies, the existing evidence on estrogen replacement therapy was not definitive, and the relative benefit versus harm was not clear, although an enormous amount of research had been published on the topic. A strictly EBM approach to this problem prior to the WHS trials would not have graded any recommendations very highly and therefore would not have supported HRT for the prevention of osteoporosis. For example, prior to publication of the WHI trials, the U.S. Preventive Services Task Force (USPSTF) rated information on HRT for the prevention of

osteoporosis as "Insufficient to Recommend For or Against." The EBM model, which the USPSTF uses, generally requires well-done and consistent RCTs before it recommends preventive and therapeutic interventions. Unfortunately, the prevailing non-EBM approach led hundreds of thousands of women to be exposed to this harmful therapy for years, perhaps leading to thousands of excess cases of myocardial infarction, deep vein thrombosis, stroke, or breast cancer.

In summary, this example illustrates some of the distinguishing characteristics of EBM listed in Box 5-3.

What Are the Non-EBM Approaches to Clinical Decision Making?

Our example makes the EBM approach look like the only logical choice for physicians, at least compared with using a standard textbook. One could argue that traditionalists would have eventually incorporated the dramatic findings of such well-publicized research from the WHI trials. Also, most medical knowledge does not change as abruptly as HRT for osteoporosis prevention did, so most of what is in recently published reference books, even several years after publication, is likely to be still valid. But HRT is not an isolated example of the potential for harm to patients that is created by adopting or adhering to practices in the absence of rigorous evidence. The

---

Box 5-3	**Distinguishing Characteristics of EBM**

Explicit methods—Databases searched and search strategies are described.

Systematic searches—The searches are systematic and thorough so that important evidence is not missed.

Standardized critical appraisal—Important sources of potential systematic and random error are assessed in each study.

Hierarchy of study design—More weight is given to stronger study designs.

Designation of levels of evidence—Each study is designated with respect to the strength of the study design and the quality of the evidence in that study.

Grading of recommendations—Each recommendation is graded according to the strength of the accumulated evidence from research studies that support the recommendation.

Verifiable findings—The explicitness of the methods of searching and critical appraisal allows others to verify (or refute) findings or recommendations.

standard (or non-EBM) practices listed in Table 5-2 were adopted with the best of intentions on the basis of one or more traditional models of thinking; definitive evidence has now shown each of these examples to be more harmful, or less beneficial, than the practices based on evidence using an EBM model.

Non-EBM approaches to clinical decision making, or learning how to make clinical decisions, include the apprentice model, deferral to authority, opinion based on experience, the pathophysiologic model, and consensus opinion (Geyman et al., 2000). Each of these has a place in the practice of medicine, despite their deficiencies in comparison with the EBM model.

Apprentice Mode

In the apprentice model, an experienced physician shows or tells a less experienced physician (the apprentice) how the experienced physician practices, and the apprentice learns by emulating the teacher. In the apprentice model, knowledge and skills are passed on with no one questioning the veracity of the knowledge or the usefulness of the skills in improving patient well-being. Both harmful and beneficial practices are passed on to each subsequent generation; evidence from carefully designed studies can help distinguish which are harmful and which are beneficial.

Deferral to Authority

Most physicians appropriately seek out an expert specialist for consultation when necessary and defer to that specialist's opinion. Yet the advice of medical experts has been shown in some cases to be (unknowingly) harmful to patients, as was the case with HRT and the other examples in Table 5-2. The ideal expert specialist not only has extensive training and clinical experience but also incorporates a thorough understanding of the evidence available to guide his or her recommendations.

The definition of an authority is the person who speaks with the greatest confidence.

Opinion Based on Experience

Experience is a powerful teacher and is essential to the development of clinical competence. Incorrect deductions from experience, however, can also mislead the physician. Emotional reactions to dramatic experiences with a bad outcome or an unhappy patient can undermine rational thinking. Clinical experience with single patients or even a large number of patients is best sifted through the net of science so that the valuable lessons are kept and the rest is discarded.

A physician can make the same mistake for 20 years and call it experience.

Pathophysiologic Reasoning

Discoveries about the pathophysiology of disease have revolutionized medical practice over the past 150 years. Basic science and clinical translational research based on an understanding of pathophysiology have led to the development of imaging technology, laboratory methods, laparoscopic surgery, beta-receptor blockers, influenza vaccine, antiretrovirals, and many other powerful diagnostic and therapeutic tools. In addition, understanding the basic pathways and mechanisms of disease is essential for competent management of individual patients, who often have more comorbid conditions than patients enrolled in RCTs, whose disease severity may not fit the spectrum of disease in cohort studies with respect to diagnostic test characteristics, and whose biology may not fit with the biology of the population study; most commonly, there simply is no high-quality evidence to guide the clinician. Nevertheless, the logic of pathophysiologic thinking can lead to harmful, even fatal conclusions.

We did the logical thing, but we killed the patient.

Consensus

Interacting with peers is a powerful and important means of establishing standards and making decisions about how to diagnose and treat patients. This may be the primary way that physicians develop local

---

Table 5-2 Instances in Which Evidence Has Shown That Standard Practices Have Harmed Patients or Resulted in Withholding Effective Therapies

Standard Practice	Evidence-Based Practice
Routine episiotomy performed to prevent complications of vaginal delivery	Episiotomy *avoided* to prevent complications of vaginal delivery
Corneal patching to improve healing of corneal abrasion	Corneal patching shown to delay healing of corneal abrasion
β-blockers contraindicated in: Diabetics Depression Congestive heart failure	β-blockers may be used in: Diabetics Depression Congestive heart failure
HRT used to benefit: Osteoporosis prevention Prevention of heart disease	Harms of HRT overweigh benefit for: Osteoporosis prevention Actually increases rates of heart disease
Narcotics not used in cases of acute abdominal pain for fear of masking diagnoses	Narcotics used to relieve acute acute abdominal pain; do not mask diagnoses

community standards that reflect the conventional wisdom in "communities of practice" (Gabbay and Le May, 2004). The real-world effectiveness of the recommendations made by consensus of a group of physicians is likely to be no greater than that of the authoritative, apprentice, or pathophysiologic approach in the absence of current best evidence. Large groups of intelligent and well-meaning physicians can be wrong and have been wrong on many occasions. Introducing evidence into such communities of practice is a necessary ingredient for success.

There is more convention in the conventional wisdom than there is wisdom.

Each of these non-EBM approaches, and others, have merit and cannot be replaced by a strictly EBM approach. They also have disadvantages, and the EBM model can help rectify those shortcomings when used as one of several ways of problem solving.

The rest of this chapter traces the origins of EBM, describes additional instances in which an EBM approach was clearly superior to a traditional approach, identifies how family medicine has adopted and is shaping EBM, and considers the limitations of EBM.

THE ORIGINS AND EVOLUTION OF EBM

Empiricism: Observation over Theory

The roots of EBM lie deep in medical history, and EBM itself has grown into a distinct species of medical practice style (Feinstein, 1985; Guyatt, 1991; Guyatt and Rennie, 1993; Users' Guides, 2002). As the word *evidence* suggests, EBM is philosophically an empirical approach to clinical decision making. Empiricism in medicine has its roots in the Renaissance. Vesalius made direct and accurate observations of human anatomy and functioning that showed the ignorance of Galen and his anatomical theories. Harvey accurately described the circulation of blood in the 17th century. In the 19th century Jenner developed an inoculation that gave protection against smallpox (in part by inoculating himself!). Jenner's discovery was the first step toward the development of the vaccines now available for protection against many infectious diseases. In 1747 a most interesting clinical trial that included only ten subjects and led to the eventual discovery of vitamin C was undertaken. In this 18th-century experiment, Lind showed that the two British sailors who were given limes to eat while at sea did not develop scurvy, whereas the other eight sailors did. He postulated the existence of an antiscorbutic factor that was later identified as vitamin C. Parenthetically, Lind's work is the origin of *limey,* the sobriquet for British sailors.

Although it was several hundred years before the RCT became the standard by which preventive and therapeutic interventions were evaluated, the seeds of empirical science gradually grew, reproduced, and spread to give life to the tremendous advances of 21st-century scientific medicine. These advances include an emphasis on basic science as the foundation of medicine, as well as an emphasis on epidemiology and biostatistics, the foundational sciences of EBM. By the mid-20th century the dominant mode of medical teaching and research, historically based on theory and experience only, had shifted to empiricism, including direct observation, study of actual human functions, and human experimentation. EBM is one of many expressions of empiricism in medicine in that it uses actual observations in real patient populations using careful and replicable methods. Just as Vesalius rebuffed Galen through direct observation, EBM holds that solid empirical evidence trumps all else, even when the findings are in conflict with prevailing pathophysiologic theory, conventional wisdom, or clinical experience.

Epidemiology: Studying Populations to Care for Individual Patients

The value of studying groups of people or populations to understand human disease was first illustrated when a British general practitioner, John Snow, removed the handle of the pump at the Broad Street well and interrupted the 1854 cholera epidemic in London (Snow, 1936). Based on careful observation of which of his patients did or did not have cholera, he mapped the location of their residences and the well from which they drew their drinking water. He showed that those with cholera were far more likely to use the Broad Street well. This simple intervention, linked to an elegant set of observations, was seminal in the birth of epidemiology, the study of diseases in populations and the evaluation of interventions at a population level as a method of solving the problems of diseases in individuals. John Snow's study was one of many epidemiologic studies that have led to basic science and clinical discoveries, including the discovery of the organism that causes cholera, the human immunodeficiency virus, and the risk factors for coronary artery disease, to name a few of the thousands of examples in which epidemiology has led to major advances in modern medical science.

Biostatistics: Measuring Uncertainty

James Lind had the good fortune of conducting his landmark trial of scurvy prevention in British sailors before statistics was invented, or at least well known, sparing him the embarrassment of having to report that his findings did not achieve statistical significance because of his small sample size and the further embarrassment of seeing his study shunned as a POEM (*patient-oriented evidence that matters*). We now know that all people who lack vitamin C in their diet develop scurvy, and no otherwise healthy person with an adequate intake of vitamin C develops scurvy.

Other conditions have a similar all-or-none cause-and-effect relationship, such as other vitamin deficiencies, antibiotics for bacterial meningitis, and appendectomy for acute appendicitis. Most EBM advocates will concede that the absence of RCTs evaluating all-or-none therapies is not a problem. Those who insist on RCTs for all-or-none therapies can be referred for enrollment in a clinical trial in which EBM zealots who lack clinical judgment are randomly assigned to jump out of an airplane at 5,000 feet with a parachute (intervention group) or without a parachute (control group) (Smith and Pell, 2003). This study, renamed the DUPED study (Does Using Parachutes Eliminate Death) for the purposes of this book, has had severe problems enrolling subjects. According to rumors (admittedly a non-EBM method), the number of hard-headed EBM zealots is steadily decreasing, as they have acknowledged the obvious fact that parachutes do prevent death from jumping out of airplanes, despite the absence of RCTs or POEMs proving this to be the case.

If James Lind were a clinical researcher in the 21st century, he would accept it as axiomatic that the all-or-none therapies are unusual and that most medical interventions are effective in some but not all patients. In other words, there is a theoretical probability that a treatment will be effective in any given patient. He would also know that most diagnostic test results may or may not mean that the patient does or does not have the disease of interest; they only increase or decrease the probability. In the early 1920s Sir Ronald Fisher "fathered" statistical theory and testing as a mathematical method for dealing with such probabilities, although *statistics* as a word dates back several centuries, according to Feinstein, when rulers began collecting information about their subjects (Feinstein, 1985). The people collecting this information were called *statists*. Those who claim Fisher as the father of statistics therefore could have a case of mistaken paternity status. Whoever the father is, all types of analytic clinical research studies now rely heavily on statistical concepts for their design, analysis, and interpretation: case-control studies, cohort studies, and RCTs.

Randomized Controlled Trials

With observers' recognition that agricultural innovations competed with multiple other uncontrollable variables (such as the weather), producing outcomes more or less likely (again, probabilistic), the first modern RCTs were conducted in grain fields in the 1920s. Austin Bradford Hill, another statistician, recognized a similar usefulness of statistics for medicine and called for the formal introduction of statistics into modern medicine in 1937. Ten years later he participated in one of the first true RCTs in medicine, showing that streptomycin was superior to standard therapy for the treatment of pulmonary tuberculosis. The RCT is now the gold standard for the evaluation of preventive and treatment interventions, and thousands of RCTs are completed and published annually (Feinstein, 1985).

Systematic Reviews, Clinical Epidemiology, and EBM

Another general practitioner, Archie Cochrane, from Scotland, in 1972 published a book titled *Effectiveness and Efficiency: Random Reflections on Health Services*, which called attention to the importance of systematic reviews, the importance of high-quality evidence, and the fact that many, if not most, practices lacked solid evidence demonstrating their efficacy or effectiveness (Cochrane, 1999). He made the argument for the routine application of EBM to clinical patient care, emphasizing the need to perform, analyze, and synthesize the findings from RCTs as systematic reviews. The Cochrane Collaboration, named after him, is an international collaborative of physicians and methodologists who perform systematic reviews and meta-analyses of RCTs evaluating medical interventions. The Cochrane Collaboration maintains an electronic library that contains more than 2,000 Cochrane Reviews, a database of abstracts of other systematic reviews, and a worldwide registry of clinical trials. This collaboration set the standard for EBM and remains the single most rigorously evaluated collection of evidence on treatment effectiveness in the world.

Alvin Feinstein, an internist at Yale University, is widely considered the founder of clinical epidemiology, or the epidemiology of medical care. Building on the work of Feinstein and Cochrane, David Sackett, also an internist, and his colleagues at McMaster University in Canada articulated the concept of critical appraisal in the 1970s and began the series of 25 Users' Guides to the Medical Literature, published in *Journal of the American Medical Association*, thereby organizing and articulating the methods that were to form the basis of EBM. Gordon Guyatt coined the term *evidence-based medicine* in 1990 after another term, *scientific medicine*, was roundly rejected by his colleagues, who resisted the new paradigm for teaching residents at McMaster. These individuals and their colleagues in the Evidence-Based Medicine Working Group (from multiple specialties, including family medicine) have been largely responsible for the dissemination of EBM that has occurred in the past 10 years and

Box 5-4 **The Many Descendants of Evidence-Based Medicine**

Evidence-based practice
Evidence-based clinical practice
Evidence-based health care
Evidence-based nursing
Evidence-based dermatology
Evidence-based search engines
Evidence-based otitis media
Evidence-based diabetes
Evidence-based obstetrics
Evidence-based pediatrics
Evidence-based family medicine

deserve the lion's share of credit for laying the foundations and building the primary structures of EBM.

Derivations and Mutations of EBM

If imitation is the most flattering compliment, then EBM has been flattered extensively. Quite a number of variations on the EBM style have developed. A list of examples, not intended to be comprehensive, is shown in Box 5-4. Most of these simply apply traditional EBM or a variation of it to particular disciplines or specialties (nursing, dermatology, obstetrics, pediatrics, family medicine) or to diseases (otitis media, diabetes) or physical diagnosis. Evidence-based literature surveillance employs some of the principles of EBM to systematically select new research, systematic reviews, and guidelines and organize them into electronic databases for easy retrieval as a way to assist physicians with keeping up with new and important research and reviews. DynaMed and InfoRetriever are electronic databases built through evidence-based surveillance systems and are described later in this chapter.

Evidence-based practice, evidence-based clinical practice, and *evidence-based health care* are terms used by authors who want to emphasize the use of EBM in practice, stress the importance of understanding patients', families', and practitioners' beliefs, values, and attitudes as applied to EBM, or more explicitly take evidence into account when considering public health priority setting, resource utilization, and the organization and delivery of health care by doctors and other health care providers. These terms all reflect efforts to apply EBM principles in settings other than those in which individual physicians provide care for individual patients, or developing guidelines for doing so.

MORE ANECDOTES FOR EBM

It is interesting, and not without irony, that the current best evidence supporting the value of EBM is anec-

dotal. Anecdotes are anathema to EBM. By current best evidence in the EBM usage, we refer primarily to original research using the methods of clinical epidemiology (clinical trials, cohort studies, case-control studies, or case series) or systematic syntheses of such research (systematic reviews, meta-analyses, and evidence-based guidelines) as listed in Box 5-2. Yet I am not aware of any such evidence that EBM does what it purports to do, which is good reason for humbleness and for maintaining an open mind about the multiple ways of thinking about best care for patients.

The following anecdotes are examples of situations in which the EBM approach was clearly the winner. In each instance, adherence to a traditional model of thinking or a particular type of methodological error led to incorrect conclusions and, in two of the examples, unfortunate outcomes for patients. No doubt pathologists could give many examples of anecdotes in which pathophysiologic thinking was the clear winner. However, pathology is so well accepted in modern medicine that its value is assumed, and it needs no special chapter to explain or justify its place in medicine.

Patient-Oriented versus Disease-Oriented Evidence

Slawson and Shaughnessy have emphasized the importance of paying particular attention to patient-oriented outcomes (e.g., mortality, morbidity, pain, functional status, quality of life) and of being cautious about research evidence that measures only physiologic or disease-oriented outcomes (e.g., physiologic measures, markers of disease, disease states) (Slawson and Shaughnessy, 2000).

A classic example of the difference between an outcome that matters to patients (a POEM) versus a physiologic outcome is provided by a randomized clinical trial, the CAST study ("Preliminary report," 1989). Published in 1989, the CAST study was designed to determine if a class of anti-arrhythmic drugs that suppressed premature ventricular beats (a physiologic outcome) prevented sudden death (a patient-oriented outcome) as expected. Unfortunately, the trial showed that two of these drugs caused an increase in sudden death among asymptomatic or mildly symptomatic patients. Prior to the findings of the CAST study physicians had prescribed these drugs for thousands of patients based on the findings of improved physiologic outcomes, which likely caused many premature deaths. This is not only an example of disease-oriented evidence, it is also an example of the risks of pathophysiologic thinking and dependence on expert opinion. It certainly is logical that the suppression of premature ventricular beats should reduce sustained ventricular fibrillation or ventricular tachycardia leading to sudden death. Despite the logic, these drugs had pro-arrhythmic effects on the myocardial conduction system that were unrecognized, and patients died as a result.

Selection Bias

Harrison's Principles of Internal Medicine was the textbook used when I was a medical student. *Harrison's* was and remains to this day one of most respected textbooks in internal medicine. But the edition I used in the late 1970s stated that 50% of patients with lymphadenopathy have it because they have cancer. This high risk of such a serious disease should be cause for great concern and would justify an aggressive diagnostic approach, including biopsy. This fact was not well received by my family medicine preceptors in medical school, despite the authoritative stature of the oncologist who wrote it in *Harrison's*.

After its inception as the 19th specialty in 1969, family medicine began to develop its research base, and the evidence from family medicine showed quite a different picture from the one painted by the oncologist in Harrison's textbook. Harold Williamson, an academic family physician in the newly minted specialty, conducted a prospective study to determine the percentage of patients presenting to family physicians with lymphadenopathy who had cancer (or other serious diseases). He identified 249 patients with enlarged lymph nodes. Serious or treatable causes of lymphadenopathy were rare and were always accompanied by clinical conditions that suggested further evaluation. Lymph nodes were biopsied in only 3% of patients. No patient was found to have a prolonged, disabling illness without a prompt diagnosis. He concluded that, in patients without associated signs or symptoms, a period of observation is safe and likely to save unnecessary expense and biopsy.

Why the discrepancy of 50% having cancer versus "rare"? Oncologists see a different population of patients than family physicians do. The patients seen by oncologists (and other specialists and subspecialists whose practice is limited to particular diseases, organs, or procedures) are highly selected, whereas primary care patients are more representative of the general population of patients seeking medical care. Therefore it should come as no surprise that oncologists would come to believe that half of their patients with lymphadenopathy have cancer, an impression borne out by the study quoted in *Harrison's*, which was performed in an oncology clinic. In this case the evidence was valid, but relevant only to patients referred to oncologists and, because of selection bias, was not relevant for primary care. This example also illustrates the point that listing references does not make a statement evidence based, or even necessarily accurate. One must also have discovered all of the studies, critically appraised them for problems such as selection bias, and based conclusions only on the most valid and relevant evidence.

The lymphadenopathy story is not an isolated example of this impact of selection bias. Prior and subsequent research by primary care physicians has documented the pervasive distortion that occurs when clinical experience and research are based on highly selected populations cared for by specialized physicians who limit their practices. Selection bias works in the opposite direction as well. The clinical experience and clinical research conducted by family physicians may be equally irrelevant to other specialists and subspecialists. Williamson's study showing that lymphadenopathy in a patient without suspicious signs and symptoms is rarely due to a serious cause would be equally irrelevant for an oncology practice. Bias in research is not the exclusive domain of any particular specialty.

Pathophysiologic Reasoning and Bad Outcomes

This example illustrates again the hazards of pathophysiologic reasoning put into practice untested in the real-world laboratory of clinical research. It also illustrates the fact that large numbers of expert physicians, and consensus within communities of physicians, can be dead wrong. Again, the book I studied in medical school, *William's Obstetrics,* which was used by every nearly every obstetrician and family physician attending births in the 1970s, recommended that an episiotomy, a surgical cut of the perineum, be performed prior to delivery of the fetal head in every vaginal birth to prevent urinary and fecal incontinence (routine episiotomy). The reasoning was that this cut would provide more space for the fetal head to pass through the vaginal opening and thereby reduce the excess stretching of the tissues presumed responsible for maintaining urinary retention. It was also believed that the risk of extension of a tear into the rectum would be reduced by an episiotomy, and that this in turn would reduce the risk of permanent damage to the anal sphincter and prevent fecal incontinence. Finally, a surgical cut would result in a much better repair than a jagged tear, or so it was reasoned. Although this practice held sway for many decades, there was no empirical evidence demonstrating that routine episiotomy did in fact prevent these complications.

In the 1990s, another academic family physician and his colleagues published a series of RCTs (Klein et al., 1994) showing that routine episiotomy in fact increased the risks for urinary incontinence, increased tears through the rectal sphincter, and interfered with sexual satisfaction. This and other evidence gradually led to a reduction in the routine use of episiotomies, although there are still some who ignore (or are ignorant of) the evidence and adhere faithfully to the dusty pronouncements of their medical school textbooks and medical school professors. Some day the pronouncements of this book and this author will be dusty, and hopefully you will be more insistent on evidence before acting (unless it is an all-or-none phenomenon, like limes for scurvy or parachutes for preventing death from jumping out of airplanes) than your predecessors.

THE FAMILY MEDICINE APPROACH TO EBM

Family medicine has adopted the EBM model in a variety of ways, as much as or perhaps even more so than other specialties. EBM is one of several useful ways to manage the volume of knowledge required for the broad domain of family medicine. All of the major clinical journals in family medicine regularly publish evidence-based systematic review articles. Family physicians routinely participate in national, regional, and local development of evidence-based guidelines. They may represent the American Academy of Family Physicians or other organizations, or they may serve as consultants. All of these activities involve the four steps of EBM and the distinguishing characteristics listed in Box 5-3. Many academic family physicians are engaged in teaching clinical epidemiology or EBM at the medical school, residency, and fellowship levels.

There are also several initiatives by family physicians that are designed with the same goals as EBM in mind but employ more practical strategies in order to make the best available evidence easily accessible to the practicing physician. Three of these initiatives—DynaMed, the Family Physicians' Inquiries Network, and InfoRetriever—are described later in the chapter. The resources developed by these groups do not necessarily adhere strictly to all the criteria listed in Box 5-1 that distinguish EBM in its original formulation, but each of them has advantages that make them useful.

These resources share the goal of helping family physicians meet both recognized and unrecognized information needs. In the next section, the challenge of meeting these two types of information needs is addressed, followed by a description of these resources.

Recognized and Unrecognized Information Needs

The EBM mandate to include current best evidence in decision making generates tremendous information needs for physicians that did not exist 60 years ago. It is estimated that more than 10,000 new research studies per year are published that may reflect current best evidence relevant to the practice of family medicine (Ebell et al., 1999). Obviously, no one practicing physician could possibly stay abreast of all of the relevant original research using the classic EBM approach, and generally speaking, the need to do so is unrecognized in the sense that if a physician does not know about the information, he or she would not recognize the need to access it.

Having easy access to current best evidence for solving patient problems and answering clinical questions during patient care is another unmet information need. In this case, because the physician has a patient problem to solve and needs information to do so, he or she can be said to have a "recognized" information need. Research shows that family physicians have an average of about three questions for every five patients seen, they spend an average of 2 minutes seeking answers to these questions, and the majority (about 71%) of their questions never get answered, much less answered by an EBM process that ensures current best evidence will be used, mainly because answers were never pursued (Ely et al., 1999). Another study showed that physicians do not pursue answers to so many of their questions because of the time required and the difficulty of the steps involved in formulating an adequate answer (Ely et al., 2002).

These observations have led to creative strategies for making best evidence easily integrated into the practice of family medicine by reducing the time required to find answers and doing much of the work for the clinician. These strategies include the development of secondary sources, evidence-based surveillance systems, and evidence-based answers to clinical questions at the point of patient care. All these strategies combine EBM methods with the use of electronic knowledge resources such as Web sites, desktop computers, or portable computers for efficient storage and retrieval of information and the capacity to update frequently.

Literature surveillance systems are designed to assist physicians with meeting unrecognized information needs and to provide easy retrieval of new research to ensure that electronic knowledge resources include current best evidence. Two such systems, InfoRetriever and DynaMed, have been developed by family physicians and are currently available by subscription (www.infopoems.com, www.dynamicmedical.com).

InfoRetriever

Three family physicians—David Slawson, Mark Ebell, and Henry Berry—and a pharmacologist, Allen Shaughnessy, have performed evidence-based literature surveillance for InfoRetriever since 1996. They systematically review more than 1,200 studies from more than 100 journals monthly to identify an average of 30 POEMs each month (Ebell et al., 1999). POEMs stands for *p*atient-*o*riented *e*vidence that *m*atters and is the term used to designate the best evidence identified by the reviewers. A brief structured summary and critique are written and the citation of the study is listed. These reviews are then disseminated on a daily and monthly basis (the entire month of POEMs) by e-mail.

Many family physicians use this system as their primary strategy for keeping up to date with current best evidence (meeting unrecognized information needs). Instead of attempting the impossible, family physicians can read the Daily POEM in just a few minutes with confidence that they are getting the cream of the evidence that has been recently published.

InfoRetriever is the software program used to store and retrieve POEMs on a handheld computer or on the Web. In addition to POEMs, InfoRetriever has Cochrane Systematic Review abstracts, 2,200 diagnostic calculators, more than 200 decision support tools, and more than 700 summaries of evidence-based guidelines. It is updated quarterly and, since the available high-quality evidence that populates InfoRetriever answers only a portion of family physicians' questions, it comes bundled with 5 Minute Medical Consult (5MMC). Although 5MMC is not an evidence-based resource, it does answer most questions (using expert opinion, consensus, and so on). InfoRetriever is therefore useful primarily for recognized information needs, and the Daily POEMs by e-mail are useful mainly for unrecognized information needs (www.infopoems.com).

DynaMed

Brian Alper, a family physician, developed DynaMed in 1993 as a medical student and maintains it based on his surveillance of original research reports, journal review services, systematic review sources (such as Cochrane Reviews and Clinical Evidence), drug information sources, and guidelines. DynaMed has more than 1,800 disease topics, and each disease is organized using a consistent format. DynaMed contains an enormous amount of information, and much of the best evidence is quoted and briefly summarized. However, the evidence is not rated, the methods are not explicit, and it is not peer reviewed. Efforts are under way to peer review the content, and contributors to the database receive a free subscription. Although DynaMed uses a literature surveillance system, it is not useful for unrecognized information needs because users are not alerted to new evidence. However, it is useful for recognized information needs and is the only electronic database besides electronic collections of textbooks that has been shown through research to answer a majority of family physicians' questions (www.dynamic-medical.com) (Alper et al., 2001, 2005).

InfoRetriever and DynaMed both require sorting through a significant volume of material since they are not designed to directly answer specific questions with all of the relevant evidence summarized. InfoRetriever provides a nicely organized list of hits, but knowing which source or combination of sources provides the answer to the clinical question at hand usually requires looking at multiple hits. DynaMed provides an enormous amount of information organized by topic and subtopic, but a fair amount of reading and comparing may be required to find an answer. Nonetheless, expert family physi-

cian searchers were able to find adequate answers in DynaMed in just over 2 minutes (Alper et al., 2001). Young, skilled physicians found their answers in 5 minutes. The quality of the answers was equivalent to other sources (Alper et al., 2005).

Family Physicians Inquiries Network

Members of the Family Physicians Inquiries Network (FPIN) are dedicated to producing concise recommendations based on multiple sources that integrate the best evidence to answer specific clinical questions, provide a pithy summary of the key evidence, and list authoritative recommendations. FPIN is a not-for-profit international academic consortium of 22 family medicine departments, 78 residency programs, 75 academic health sciences librarians, and a network of practice-based research networks (see www.fpin.org). The FPIN vision is to answer 80% of the practicing family physician's questions at the point of patient care within 60 seconds of their time with the best available evidence. The FPIN mission is to translate research into practice at the point of patient care, to teach the clinical scholarship of research translation, and to facilitate the generation of new research from practice. FPIN has two electronic publishing initiatives, Clinical Inquiries and PEPID PCP.

Clinical Inquiries Clinical Inquiries are evidence-based answers to clinical questions developed by FPIN members. Questions are generated from actual patient care problems and selected by Web-based voting by groups of practicing family physicians. A thorough and structured search of the world literature is conducted by one of the trained FPIN librarians. The clinician author or authors who have volunteered to prepare the answer then select and critically appraise the evidence and write the answer in a brief structured format designed for use at the point of care. Each Clinical Inquiry is reviewed by a minimum of four peer reviewers or editors prior to publication in the *Journal of Family Practice* or *American Family Physician*. FPIN makes all Clinical Inquiries available to contributors without charge in the FPIN Electronic Library, a Web-based database maintained by the FPIN consortium. In addition, Clinical Inquiries are included in the Portable Electronic Physicians Information Database (PEPID), Primary Care Plus (PCP), that FPIN members edit, peer review, provide content for, and update regularly. The primary limitation of the Clinical Inquiries database is that the volume of questions and answers is not yet large enough to answer many questions (ca. 300 at the time of this writing), although FPIN is completing 15 to 20 new structured reviews (Clinical Inquiries) per month.

PEPID PCP PEPID PCP is a comprehensive electronic handheld and Web-based resource with

2,100+ disease topics, 5,000+ drugs, a dynamic drug interactions generator, an electronic prescription writing tool, and more than 300 calculators and decision aids. PEPID PCP is available by subscription from the owner, PEPID, Inc. (www.pepid.com), and is free to FPIN contributors. The combination of PEPID PCP content and Clinical Inquiries should answer most questions, and it has the added advantage of a fully integrated drug database. This feature is particularly useful because questions about drug dosages, side effects, indications, and interactions are among the most common questions the family physicians have at the point of care.

Other Useful EBM Resources on the Web

There are many other useful sources for finding current best evidence and for learning more about EBM, and new resources are added frequently. Additional EBM sources are listed in Appendix 5-2 on the Student Consult. These sources include primary sources for searching, search engines designed to prioritize best evidence, secondary sources in which the evidence has already been synthesized and rated, and sites that provide general information about EBM and specific tools for EBM. Appendix 5-1 provides Critical Appraisal Worksheets for each of the four most common question types-diagnosis, prognosis, prevention, and treatment (or harm). It should also be noted that a systematic review addressing a treatment question is evaluated using a different set of questions. In addition, there are also critical appraisal worksheets for economic analysis, studies of differential diagnosis, and many others. Appendix 5-2 lists EBM resources, including general EBM Web sites that provide not only worksheets for critical appraisal but also detailed information about using the worksheets and a lot of other detailed information. A glossary of EBM terms is given in Appendix 5-3 on the Student Consult.

LIMITATIONS OF EBM

EBM has limitations, some of which are inherent to the model and others of which are due to its early stage of development. In addition, EBM has developed a reputation as being synonymous with excellence in medical care. Consequently, in our commercially oriented society, the label is often applied when it is not appropriate, so buyer beware. A simple though not foolproof clue that a resource is evidence based is to look for a grade or strength of recommendation and levels of evidence designations. As of early 2004, there were 40 such systems in use for articles summarizing two or more studies, creating considerable confusion about how to interpret them. The editors of FPIN and the major family medicine journals developed a single system for use in most family medicine publications (Ebell et al., 2004). The Strength of Recommendation Taxonomy (SORT) is a patient outcomes-oriented system for classifying the validity of clinical recommendations based on structured reviews of the literature. Other taxonomies can be converted to SORT to provide a standardized and user-friendly evidence grading system when drawing on numerous other EBM resources.

The types of evidence prized in EBM (clinical trials, prospective cohort studies, systematic reviews, meta-analyses) are all based on population-level data. Yet there is almost always both biological and statistical variation among individuals in clinical populations. In clinical practice, the findings are used for the care of individual patients, not populations. Any particular patient may respond similarly to most patients in a treatment group or may more be like those at the tail end of the distributions and not respond at all, or may respond more dramatically than the patients in the studies. Individual genetic variation between patients or variations in comorbid conditions may result in higher risk, a more aggressive disease, or a different response to therapy. There are also many social, cultural, and economic factors that must be considered, in addition to population-level evidence. EBM proponents recognize the need to consider all of these factors in the care of individual patients, but the primary achievement to date in the EBM movement has been to develop the methods and accumulate valid evidence. Less has been accomplished in the science of how to apply this evidence to individual patient care.

As noted earlier, some publications refer to themselves as evidence based when in fact they are not. Listing references is a time-honored and valuable practice in both journal articles and textbooks, but it does not make an article or a book chapter evidence based. For example, many of the claims in this chapter on EBM do not meet the evidentiary standards of the EBM model, despite the references! Many publications and electronic databases abuse the term evidence based as a marketing tool. Most of these products have excellent qualities and usually emphasize original evidence by extensive referencing, but they do not use the explicit, systematic EBM model. How much this matters is debatable. In my experience the answers and recommendations in well-referenced and reputable sources (such as UpToDate) are often but not always consistent with more explicitly evidence-based sources (and EBM sources are extensively quoted or included frequently in databases such as UpToDate). UpToDate is particularly useful for reviews, and its authors are often leading experts. However, further research is needed to quantify the relative strengths and weaknesses of strictly EBM sources, those that purport to be evidence based or to use variations or shortcuts of the EBM model, and the clearly non-EBM sources.

Also, more creative approaches are needed to fully exploit the combination of EBM principles and electronic technology to close the gap between what we know about best care for patients and getting that care to patients so that they benefit from that knowledge.

CONCLUSION

EBM is a relatively new model for clinical decision making that complements rather than substitutes for traditional models. It is simply another tool to use as appropriate for "doing our best" for patients. EBM has grown enormously in influence in the 10 years since its inception and is likely to continue to develop in importance and usefulness. Mastering the basic concepts and methods of EBM will be necessary to be a competent

physician in the 21st century, as will be learning when evidence is and is not useful in caring for individual patients. Finally, in the spirit of the information mastery model (Slawson et al., 2000), taking advantage of the hard work of others makes practicing medicine with cognizance of the best evidence realistic for all family physicians, as well as for physicians in other specialties.

Material Available on Student Consult

Review Questions and Answers about Evidence-Based Medicine

Appendix 5-1 Critical Appraisal Worksheets

Appendix 5-2 Glossary of EBM Terms

Appendix 5-3 EMB Electronic Resources

REFERENCES

Alper BS, Stevermer JJ, White DS, Ewigman BG. Answering family physicians' clinical questions using electronic medical databases. J Fam Pract 2001;50:960–965.

Alper BS, White DW, Bin G. Physicians answer more clinical questions and change clinical decisions more often with synthesized evidence: A randomized trial in primary care. Ann Fam Med 2005;3:507–513.

Antman EM, Lau J, Kupelnick B, Mosteller F, Chalmers TC. A comparison of results of meta-analyses of randomized control trials and recommendations of clinical experts: Treatments for myocardial infarction. JAMA 1992;268: 240–248.

Cochrane AL. Effectiveness and Efficiency: Random Reflections on Health Services (reprint). London, Royal Society of Medicine, 1999 (London, Nuffield Provincial Hospitals Trust, 1972).

Coomarasamy A, Khan KS. What is the evidence that postgraduate teaching of evidence-based medicine changes anything? A systematic review. BMJ 2004;329: 1017–1019

Ebell MH, Barry HC, Slawson DC, Shaughnessy AF. Finding POEMs in the medical literature. J Fam Pract 1999;48:350–385.

Ely JW, Osheroff JA, Ebell MH, Bergus GR, Levy BT, Chambliss ML, Evans ER. Analysis of questions asked by family doctors regarding patient care. BMJ. 1999; 319:358–361.

Ely JW, Osheroff JA, Ebell MH, Chambliss ML, Vinson DC, Stevermer JJ, Pifer EA. Obstacles to answering doctors' questions about patient care with evidence: Qualitative study. BMJ 2002;324:710.

Feinstein A. Clinical Epidemiology. Philadelphia, WB Saunders, 1985.

Gabbay J, Le May A. Evidence based guidelines or collectively constructed "mindlines"? Ethnographic study of knowledge management in primary care. BMJ 2004;329:1013–1016.

Geyman JP, Deyo RA, Ramsey SD. Evidence-Based Practice: Concepts and Approaches. Butterworth Heinemann, 2000.

Guyatt GH. Evidence-based medicine. ACP Journal Club 1991;114(Suppl 2):A–16.

Guyatt GH, Rennie D. Users' guides to the medical literature. JAMA 1993;270:2096–2097.

Guyatt G, Cook D, Haynes B. Evidence-based medicine has come a long way. BMJ 2004; 329:990–991.

Klein MC, et al. Relationship of episiotomy to perineal trauma and morbidity, sexual dysfunction, and pelvic floor relaxation. Am J Obstet Gynecol 1994;171:591–598.

Lockwood S. "Evidence of me" in evidence-based medicine. BMJ 2004;329:1033–1035.

Manson JE, et al. Estrogen plus progestin and the risk of coronary heart disease. N Engl J Med 2003;349:523–534.

Preliminary report: Effect of encainide and flecainide on mortality in a randomized trial of arrhythmia suppression after myocardial infarction: The Cardiac Arrhythmia Suppression Trial (CAST) Investigators. N Engl J Med 1989;321:406–412.

Reilly BM. The essence of EBM. BMJ 2004;329:991–992.

Sackett DL, Rosenberg WM, Gray JA, et al. Evidence-based medicine: What it is and what it isn't. BMJ 1996;312: 71–72.

Sackett DL, Strauss SE, Richardson WS, Rosenberg W, Haynes RB. Evidence-Based Medicine: How to Practice and Teach EBM, 2nd ed. Edinburgh, Churchill Livingston, 2000.

Salpeter SR, Walsh JME, Greyber E, Ormiston TM, Salpeter EE. Mortality associated with hormone replacement therapy in younger and older women. J Gen Intern Med 2004;19:791–804.

Slawson DC, Shaughnessy AF. Becoming an information master: Using POEMs to change practice with confidence. Patient-Oriented Evidence that Matters. J Fam Pract 2000;49:63–67.

Smith G, Pell J. Parachute use to prevent death and major trauma related to gravitational challenge: A systematic review of randomized trials. BMJ 2003;327:20–27.

Snow J. On the Mode of Communication of Cholera (reprint). New York, Commonwealth Fund, 1936 (London, John Churchill, 1855).

Strauss S, Jones G. What has evidence based medicine done for us? BMJ 2004;329:987–988.

Users' Guides to the Medical Literature. Chicago, American Medical Association, 2002.

Women's Health Initiative Steering Committee. Effects of conjugated equine estrogen in postmenopausal women with hysterectomy: The Women's Health Initiative randomized controlled trial. JAMA 2004;291:1701–712.

SUGGESTED READINGS

Alper BS. Practical evidence based Internet resources. Fam Practice Manage 2003;10:49–52.

Dickinson WP, Stange KC, Ebell MH, Ewigman BG, Green LA. Involving all family physicians and family medicine faculty members in the use and generation of new knowledge. Fam Med 2000;32:480–490.

Ebell MH, Siwek J, Weiss B, Woolf SH, Susman J, Ewigman B, Bowman M. Strength of recommendation taxonomy (SORT): A patient-centered approach to grading evidence in the medical literature. Am Fam Physician 2004;69:548–556.

Evidence-Based Medicine Working Group. Evidence-based medicine: A new approach to the teaching of medicine. JAMA 1992;268:2420–2425.

Grandage KK, Slawson DC, Shaughnessy AF. When less is more: A practical approach to searching for evi-dence-based answers. J Med Library Assoc 2002; 90:298–304.

Herrington DM, Howard TD. From presumed benefit to potential harm: Hormone therapy and heart disease. N Engl J Med 2003;349:519–521.

Kravitz RL, Duan N, Braslow J. Evidence-based medicine, heterogeneity of treatment effects, and the trouble with averages. Milbank Q 2004;82:661–687.

Shaughnessy AF, Slawson DC. What happened to the valid POEMs? A survey of review articles on the treatment of type 2 diabetes. BMJ 2003;327:266.

Tovey D, Godlee F. General practitioners say that evidence based information is changing practice. BMJ 2004; 329:1043.

White B. Making evidence-based medicine doable in everyday practice. Fam Pract Manage 2004;51–55.

Chapter

6 Evaluating the Medical Literature

Jeffrey Susman, Keith B. Holten, and Douglas R. Smucker

KEY POINTS

1. Use the highest quality evidence available to make clinical decisions, prioritizing robust ran-domized controlled trials (RCTs) and systematic reviews, with appropriate patient-oriented out-comes (strength of recommendation [SOR] C).
2. Remember that statistical significance does not always equate to clinical significance (SOR C).
3. Useful sources for clinical evidence include the Cochrane database, the United States Preventive Services Task Force guide to clinical preventive services, and Patient-Oriented Evidence that Matters (POEMs) (SOR C).

Evidence-based medicine (EBM)—asking clear, rele-vant clinical questions; finding appropriate studies; critically appraising the literature; and implementing changes in practice behavior—has become an essen-tial part of medical care. But most busy physicians have neither the time nor the background to answer critically the questions that arise in practice. Primary care physicians identify 2.4 clinical questions for every 10 encounters (Barrie and Ward, 1997) yet spend less than 15 minutes on average with each patient. Furthermore, new evidence about common primary care problems is accumulating at an over-whelming pace, and the broad scope of family medi-cine presents important challenges. Other barriers to the use of EBM include lack of evidence that is per-tinent to an individual patient, quick access to infor-mation at the point of care, and potential negative impacts on the art of medicine (McAllister et al., 1999). How can diligent physicians narrow the gap between their current behaviors and best practices?

This chapter uses hormone replacement therapy (HRT) for postmenopausal women as a case example for understanding the evolution of medical practice vis-à-vis a changing landscape of evidence. Core concepts of EBM and practical tools for family physicians are highlighted.

USING EVIDENCE AT THE POINT OF CARE

Physicians have many sources of clinical information, from "throw-away" or non–peer-reviewed journals to evidence-based searchable databases. Each of these has advantages, disadvantages, and different methods of access (Table 6-1).

One model to help busy physicians stay clinically current, termed *information mastery*, has been advocated by Slawson and Shaugnessy (1999), Ebell (1999), and Geyman (1999). In this model, physicians seek the answer to clinical questions through secondary sources of information that have been created by experts through a review of the medical literature. Secondary sources include evidence-based summaries (Cochrane collaboration reviews, POEMs, and clinical inquiries as published in the *Journal of Family Practice* and elsewhere [Geyman, 1999; Ebell et al., 1999]), systematic reviews (PubMed Clinical Inquiries), guidelines (written by professional societies and accessed through sites such as the National Guideline Clearinghouse on the Web at www.ngc.

gov), and evidence-based databases (InfoPOEMs InfoRetriever) (Table 6-2).

Case Example

A 55-year-old woman sees you because she is experiencing severe vasomotor symptoms (hot flashes). These symptoms are keeping her awake at night. She had a total abdominal hysterectomy and oophorectomy 1 year ago because of uterine fibroids. She is concerned about the dangers of HRT. What is the current evidence? How do you counsel this patient?

A search was performed on PubMed at www.ncbi.nlm.nih.gov/entrez/query/static/clinical.html. Using Clinical Queries and the research methodology, category "therapy" and emphasis "sensitive" were chosen. The search terms were "hormone replacement therapy" and "vasomotor symptoms."

An excellent summary, the position statement from the North American Menopause Society, was found (Neff, 2004). The North American Menopause Society recommends first considering lifestyle changes, alone or combined with a nonprescription remedy (such as dietary isoflavones, vitamin E, or black cohosh), for the relief of mild vasomotor symptoms. For moderate to severe menopause-related hot

---

Table 6-1 Examples of Reference Materials for the Busy Physician: Hormone Replacement Therapy Question

Type of Literature	Advantages	Disadvantages	Availability	Examples
Textbooks	Comprehensive review of topics	Long period from concept to printing; bookshelf space or CD space requirements; cost; reading time	Print, hardcover and paperback; some CD-ROMs and pocket PC	*Novak's Gynecology* ($45.00–$135.00)
Unsolicited medical journals	No cost	Some not peer reviewed; unpredictable topics; large volume of materials	Print; some articles online	*Female Patient* (complimentary)
Subscription peer-reviewed journals	Peer reviewed; pertinent topics	Cost and subscription management; stacks of journals; need to critically appraise	Print and online	*Obstetrics and Gynecology* ($257.00 annually for non-ACOG member)
Evidence-based summaries	Peer reviewed; pertinent topics	Cost; CD management; searches have learning curve	CD ROM and online	Cochrane Reviews: abstracts (complimentary) and full reviews
Searchable evidence databases	Searchable; rapid; focused search possible; point of care access	Learning curve for searches	Pocket PC and online	InfoRetriever ($249.00 annually)

ACOG, American College of Obstetricians and Gynecologists.

Table 6-2 Examples of Evidence Sources

Information Source	Access	Description	Cost
PubMed	www.ncbi.nlm.nih.gov/ entrez/query.fcgi	Service of National Library of Medicine; 15 million citations back to 1950s, includes links to many sites with full text articles	No charge
National Guideline Clearinghouse	www.ngc.gov	Collection of guidelines, regularly updated; joint effort of AHRQ, U.S. Department of Health and Human Services	No charge
U.S. Public Service Task Force Guide to Clinical Preventive Services	www.odphp.osophs. dhhs.gov/pubs/ guidecps	Federal prevention guidelines; public health focus; the AHRQ is the lead agency for the Guide project	No charge
JFP POEMS Database	www.jfponline.com/ display_archives.asp? YEAR=POEMs	Contains all POEMs published in the *Journal of Family Practice* between August 2000 and the present; articles are listed in reverse chronologic order	No charge
Bandolier	www.jr2.ox.ac.uk/ Bandolier	A UK site; monthly, PubMed and Cochrane Library searched for systematic reviews and meta-analyses published; those "both interesting and making sense" appear in Bandolier, first in the print version, then 2 months later on the Web site	No charge
Canadian Task Force on Preventive Care	www.ctfphc.org	Canadian site; Web site; practical guide to health care providers, planners, and consumers for preventive health interventions	No charge
InfoRetriever	www.InfoPoems.com	Database of filtered, synopsized, evidence-based information; quarterly updates; searches a full spectrum of evidence-based resources, including POEMs and Cochrane abstracts, 2200 diagnostic calculators, and >700 summaries of evidence-based practice guidelines	30 days free, then $250/year
Cochrane Database	www.cochrane.org/ reviews/index.htm	An international nonprofit, independent organization that produces and disseminates systematic reviews of health care interventions and promotes the search for evidence in the form of clinical trials and other studies of interventions	$250–$460/year; abstracts free

Continued

Table 6-2   Examples of Evidence Sources (Continued)

Information Source	Access	Description	Cost
TRIP (Turning Research into Practice)	www.tripdatabase.com	UK site; central search engine for high-quality medical literature from a wide range of sources: evidence-based records, clinical guidelines, clinical questions and answers, electronic textbooks, medical images, >13 million peer-reviewed journal articles	5 free searches, then £35 annually
Clinical Inquiries	www.fpin.org	Evolving point of care tool that seeks to answer clinical questions from practice using structured, critical reviews of the literature; evidence graded and explicit; the FPIN bundles access to other products including PEPID, which covers >1800 disease topics and >5000 drugs, and has a drug interactions calculator and multiple other tools	Graduated based on number of subscribers ($100 for single membership to FPIN)

AHRQ, Agency for Healthcare Research and Quality; FPIN, Family Practice Inquiries Network; PEPID, Portable Emergency Physician Database; POEMs, Patient-Oriented Evidence that Matters.

flashes, prescription systemic estrogen-containing products are still the therapeutic standard. Possible treatment options for women with concerns or contraindications to estrogen-containing products include prescription progestogens, venlafaxine, paroxetine, fluoxetine, or gabapentin. The search and review of this article took approximately 3 minutes.

Another PubMed reference from the *New England Journal of Medicine* summarizes the literature and discusses current recommendations on the use of HRT (Timins, 2004). Initially used to treat the vasomotor and vaginal symptoms of menopause, HRT appeared to have many unexpected beneficial effects in early observational trials. It was hailed as a deterrent of atherosclerosis, osteoporosis, cognitive impairment, and Alzheimer's disease. Although its salutary effects on bone mass were substantiated, randomized clinical trials noted an increased risk of breast cancer, coronary artery disease, and thromboembolism and raised doubts about the efficacy of HRT in improving quality of life. This evidence took another 2 minutes to review.

Using the Web-accessed version of the subscription service, InfoRetriever (see Table 6-2), another search was performed. This search tool is convenient and rapid and rates the quality of evidence. The search was performed using keyword search term

"hormone replacement therapy-postmenopausal." The category "treatment by drug" (POEMs/Cochrane only prompted "estrogen" as a choice. One result ("Are low doses of continuous HRT as effective as usual doses for the treatment of vasomotor symptoms and vaginal atrophy in postmenopausal women?") was provided (Utian et al., 2001). This search took approximately 2 minutes. The bottom line was that continuous HRT at less than standard doses was effective in reducing both the number and severity of hot flashes in postmenopausal women. Estrogen alone was a little less effective than estrogen plus progesterone.

Another InfoRetriever reference under category "treatment by drug" (POEMs/Cochrane only) was titled "hormone replacement overall not beneficial." This reference was a review of the Rossouw et al. (2002). This was a large, multiple-site study encompassing several different clinical trials of hormone replacement, calcium supplementation, vitamin D supplementation, and low-fat diet. The trial of conjugated equine estrogen plus progestin (0.625 mg/2.5 mg) in more than 16,000 healthy women with a uterus was stopped early by the study's safety monitoring board because after an average of 5.2 years of follow-up, the HRT group had a higher annual incidence of coronary heart disease (CHD) (0.37% versus 0.30%), invasive breast cancer (0.38% versus 0.30%), stroke (0.29% versus 0.21%,), and venous thromboembolic disease (0.34% versus 0.16%). However, bone fractures were less prevalent in the HRT group (total annual fracture rate, 1.47% versus 1.91%). It is uncertain whether there is the same risk with doses of estrogen and/or progesterone lower than those used in this trial or whether estrogen treatment alone will cause the same outcomes (level of evidence 1b). This search took an additional 2 minutes.

Looking for patient education material was also simple and rapid using InfoRetriever. After choosing search term "hormone replacement therapy-postmenopausal," in the category "education: patient education" was a reference to *AAFP Patient Education Handout: Hormone Replacement Therapy: New Information* (American Academy of Family Physicians, 2004). This source summarized the controversy about HRT, reviewed the Women's Health Initiative (WHI) trial, discussed options for treating vasomotor symptoms of menopause, and referred to two other excellent sites (National Heart Lung and Blood Institute and Mayo Clinic) for patient information. A direct link to the Web page for a printer friendly copy was provided at www.familydoctor.org/x2401.xml (another 1 minute of search time).

This case outlines how a physician with access to searchable databases can quickly review a wide array of clinical evidence and published guidelines. Such resources are based on systematic evaluations of evidence and can provide clinicians with practical guidance at the point of care.

BUILDING CLINICAL EVIDENCE FROM PUBLISHED RESEARCH

Evidence of interventions such as HRT commonly begins with observational studies including unblinded case series and case-control and cohort studies and culminates in RCTs (Fig. 6-1). To better understand how we have arrived at today's clinical understanding of HRT and its effects on heart disease, let us review the progression of research studies and evidence over the past 30 years.

The Story of Hormone Replacement Therapy Research

A series of observational studies in the 1970s and 1980s led to regular prescribing of HRT to prevent a number of significant health conditions in postmenopausal women.

Case-Control Studies

Case-control studies are often the first step in a progression of building clinical evidence because they are relatively inexpensive and rapid studies to complete. Case-control studies always look backward in time (retrospective) to determine a statistical association between an "exposure" and an "outcome." To complete a case-control study of the association of HRT and CHD, a researcher would identify a group of "cases" (women with CHD) and a group of "controls" (women without CHD) and look back in time to determine how many women in each group had been on HRT. The association between exposure (HRT) and outcome (CHD) in a case-control study is commonly summarized by a statistical measure called an odds ratio. An odds ratio is an estimation of the true relative risk (RR) for the outcome in question. A common form of bias in a case-control study is recall bias: errors in accurately determining whether both cases and controls had exposure to HRT in the past.

Cohort Studies

Cohort studies are often the next step in building the strength of evidence regarding an association between an exposure and an outcome. Cohort studies typically are forward looking in their time frame (prospective) and are generally more expensive and take longer to complete than case-control studies. However, they provide a more accurate estimate of

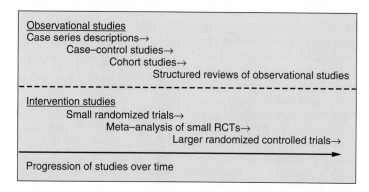

Figure 6-1 Common progression of research in building strength of evidence. RCTs, randomized controlled trials.

the RR between women who are on HRT and those who are not. A cohort study is also an observational study, one that observes outcomes in groups but does not assign participants to a particular exposure or treatment. In a cohort study of HRT and CHD, a researcher would identify a group of women on HRT and a similar group of women who have chosen not to be on HRT, then follow them over time and count the number of CHD events. Because outcome events may be uncommon in each group and may take many months to occur, cohort studies often require large numbers of participants and long follow-up to show significant differences between groups.

The primary statistical measure from a cohort study is the RR. This is a ratio of the rate of CHD events among women who choose to be on HRT divided by the rate among women who choose not to be on HRT. A common form of bias in cohort studies related to prevention is the *healthy user bias*, when participants who choose one preventive measure (such as HRT) also tend to make healthier lifestyle decisions (diet, exercise) that may also prevent the measured outcome (CHD).

Beginning with case-control studies and then larger cohort studies, observational research showed that HRT might reduce the incidence of CHD, fractures, and colorectal cancer. These observational studies also suggested that the same therapy might cause harm with a slightly increased risk of breast cancer, stroke, and venous thromboembolism. On balance, however, even a small positive impact of HRT on preventing CHD was thought to far outweigh the potential adverse effects of HRT

Structured Reviews and Meta-analysis

After a number of studies are completed, whether they are cohort studies or initial small RCTs, they are often reviewed and summarized in publications called structured reviews. Occasionally, data from a series of studies are combined using statistical techniques called meta-analysis, which allows increased statistical power to determine the weight of evidence from a series of studies. The use of HRT was greatly increased during the 1990s based not only on a number of case-control and cohort studies but also on three different meta-analysis studies that further increased the weight of scientific evidence that HRT was protective against CHD (Pettite, 1998).

Indeed, one editorial from 1991 in the *New England Journal of Medicine*, concluded that "a consensus of epidemiologic reports has demonstrated that women who are given postmenopausal estrogen therapy have a reduction of about 40 to 50% in the risk of ischemic heart disease as compared with women who do not receive such therapy" (Goldman and Tosteson, 1991). HRT became a de facto standard for postmenopausal women through the decade of the 1990s.

The Power of Randomized Controlled Trials

In RCTs, participants are randomly assigned to two or more groups and then assigned to either participate in an intervention such as HRT or continue with their usual care. RCTs greatly add to the confidence of measured results because the structure of an RCT helps eliminate many of the inherent biases of observational studies. For example, in cohort studies of HRT and CHD, it is hypothesized that women who choose to go on HRT are generally healthier and have better healthy lifestyle practices than women who do not choose to go on HRT. Because participants in an RCT are randomly assigned to treatment and control groups, they are less likely to have differences in other factors that might prevent or promote heart disease. The decreased likelihood of a "healthy user bias" in an RCT may explain why HRT appeared to be protective in cohort studies but actually proved to be harmful. Because RCTs have this inherent ability to remove many important potential areas of bias, one can have more confidence that they reflect the true association between the HRT and CHD outcomes. Thus, despite decades of work, dozens of observational studies, and structured reviews that strongly suggested a protective effect of HRT for CHD, a single large RCT trumped them all and caused a sudden reversal in physician prescribing behavior.

The release of the major report of a very large RCT of HRT in 2002, the WHI study, sent a shock wave through the medical community (Rossouw et al., 2002). For the first time, a large randomized trial showed that HRT in otherwise fairly healthy postmenopausal women caused a statistically significant increase in CHD events. Within days of the release of the WHI report, hundreds of thousands of women called their physicians to inquire whether they should continue with HRT. Many physicians drastically changed their prescription of HRT based on the WHI study: Within 9 months, prescriptions of the most popular formulation of HRT decreased by as much as 61% (Majumdar et al., 2004). Perhaps more than any other single study in modern medical history, the WHI study dramatically changed a widespread, common medical practice.

UNDERSTANDING THE STATISTICAL SIGNIFICANCE OF STUDY RESULTS

Reports from RCTs such as the WHI study frequently include the RR as a summary measure of differences between the treatment and placebo groups (see Table 6-3). To arrive at the RR, the researcher first measures the incidence rate of an outcome in each of the two study groups (treatment and placebo). The incidence rate for each group is a ratio of the number of new outcome events, such as CHD events, divided by the number of patients at risk of the outcome in that group over a specific period of time. In multiyear studies, the average annual incidence rate is often reported as a summary measure. In a placebo-controlled RCT, the RR is then calculated as simply a ratio of the incidence rate for the treatment group divided by the incidence rate for the placebo group (Table 6-3).

How can one determine whether the reported RR from a study is "significant" enough to influence clinical decisions? The first step is to consider the statistical significance of the summary measure, in this case, the RR. Statistical significance is commonly summarized in published studies by either a P value or a 95% CI for a given summary measure. The P value describes the statistical probability that the observed difference between the groups could have happened simply by chance alone. Thus, a P value less than 0.05, almost universally recognized as the cutoff for statistical significance, means that there is less than a one in 20 chance (5%) that a difference as large as that observed would occur by chance.

When the RR is reported as the summary result of a study, the 95% CI is often used as an alternative to the P value to describe the level of statistical significance of the result. The 95% CI describes the range that will, with 95% certainty, include the stated RR. For the RR, the 95% CI that does not include 1.0 (i.e., no difference between the groups) is a statistically significant result. For example, if a study reported a RR of 1.5 with a 95% CI of 1.2 to 1.8, we could be reasonably certain (95% certain) that the reported difference between the groups was not due to chance. However, if the RR was reported as 1.5 with a 95% CI of 0.90 to 2.1, it would not be considered statistically significant because the CI includes the value of "no difference" (RR = 1.0).

INTERPRETING STUDY RESULTS: STATISTICAL AND CLINICAL SIGNIFICANCE

Although the WHI study showed a statistically significant increase in the RR of CHD events among women who were randomly assigned to take HRT, it is important to consider the absolute difference in CHD events between the two groups to understand the strength of the association and to be able to thoughtfully discuss the risk of HRT with individual patients. Calculating the absolute risk (in addition to the RR) is a helpful way to understand the level of risk that HRT may add for a group of women who are at risk of CHD events (Table 6-4).

In the WHI study, for example, the RR of CHD for participants who were on HRT was 1.29 and was statistically significant with a 95% CI that did not cross 1.0 (95% CI: 1.02 to 1.63). This figure (RR = 1.29) can generally be interpreted as HRT being associated with a 29% increase in CHD events. This summary measure was reported widely in medical journals and the popular press.

When reported in terms of RR, the weight of the association between HRT and CHD sounds ominous (29% increase). However, in terms of the absolute risk attributable to HRT, a less ominous picture emerges (see Table 6-4). In the WHI study, for example, those on HRT had an average rate of CHD events of 0.37% per year (an average of 37 events per 10,000 women each year), whereas those in the placebo group had an annual rate of 0.30% (30 events per 10,000 women each year). Although the adjusted RR of CHD is 1.29 (0.37 ÷ 0.30), the attributable risk or risk difference between the two groups is 0.07% (0.37 − 0.30). In other words, approximately seven additional cases of CHD occurred for 10,000 women using HRT during each year over the course of the study. The attributable risk of the treatment group

---

Table 6-3 Understanding Study Results

Commonly reported summary rates from randomized controlled trials:

$$\text{Incidence rate} = \frac{\text{Number of new cases of disease over a period of time}}{\text{Number of persons at risk during the time period}}$$

$$\text{Relative risk} = \frac{\text{Incidence rate among the treated group}}{\text{Incidence rate among the placebo group}}$$

Summary measures that may be more meaningful for clinicians:

Attributable risk among placebo
= Incidence rate among treated group − Incidence rate among placebo group or risk difference

$$\left(\begin{array}{c}\text{Number needed to treat or}\\\text{number needed to harm}\end{array}\right) = \text{The reciprocal of attributable risk or } \frac{1}{\text{Attributable risk}}$$

Table 6-4 An Example of Summary Rates from the Women's Health Initiative Study

Here is an example of how to take a summary rate commonly reported in published studies (relative risk) and calculate a summary measure (number needed to treat or number needed to harm) that may be more useful in describing the results to clinicians and patients. Let us consider the average annual incidence rates and relative risk of CHD events in the WHI study:

$$\text{Average annual incidence among HRT treated women} = \frac{37 \text{ CHD events per year}}{10,000 \text{ women}}$$

$$\text{Average annual incidence among placebo treated women} = \frac{30 \text{ CHD events per year}}{10,000 \text{ women}}$$

$$\text{Relative risk of CHD} = \frac{\dfrac{37 \text{ CHD events}}{10,000 \text{ women}}}{\dfrac{30 \text{ CHD events}}{10,000 \text{ women}}} = 1.29 \text{ (adjusted)}$$

The relative risk describes a relative 29% increase in CHD events. It may be more useful to consider the absolute difference in incidence rates between the two groups to understand the magnitude of the potential risk for a given patient:

$$\text{Attributable risk} = \frac{37 \text{ CHD events}}{10,000 \text{ women}} - \frac{30 \text{ CHD events}}{10,000 \text{ women}} = \frac{7 \text{ additional CHD events}}{10,000 \text{ women}}$$

The number needed to harm can easily be calculated to describe, on average, how many women must be treated for 1 year to cause one additional CHD event attributable to HRT

$$\text{Number needed to harm} = \frac{1}{\dfrac{7 \text{ CHD events}}{10,000 \text{ women}}} = \frac{10,000}{7} = 1430$$

CHD, coronary heart disease; HRT, hormone replacement therapy; WHI, Women's Health Initiative.
Based on information from Rossouw JE, Anderson GL, Prentice RL, et al. and the Writing Group for the Women's Health Initiative. Risks and benefits of estrogen plus progestin in healthy postmenopausal women. Principal results. From the Women's Health Initiative randomized controlled trial. JAMA 2002;288:321–333.

---

can be summarized as the number needed to harm or, if a study reports a beneficial effect, the number needed to treat. In this case, the number need to harm was approximately 1430 patients per year on average; for every 1430 patients on HRT (the inverse of absolute difference, 0.07 or 10,000 ÷ 7), one additional CHD event occurred (see Table 6-4). The number needed to harm or number needed to treat tends to be much more understandable for both physicians and patients when weighing the risks and benefits of a particular therapy.

OTHER KEYS TO INTERPRETING CLINICAL EVIDENCE

One of the major pitfalls in interpreting the results of a study is to ensure that all relevant patient-oriented outcomes are considered. First, it is important to distinguish among physiologic outcomes (e.g., serum calcium), intermediate outcomes (e.g., bone density), and patient-oriented outcomes (e.g., fractures). Whenever possible, it is more powerful and relevant to see results in terms of outcomes that patients would deem important. Thus, in a trial of HRT for osteoporosis, a decrease in fracture incidence would be much more convincing than a change in a physiologic parameter. Likewise, all important harms (risks) and financial endpoints (costs and savings) should be reported. In a trial of a new antiresorptive agent, the rate of esophagitis, gastritis, and esophageal perforation might be important harms to elaborate, along with such measures as patient satisfaction, costs and savings of care, and global well-being.

When assessing the benefits and harms of such a new treatment, appropriate competing alternatives (including no treatment at all) should be compared. Typically, such a comparison might take the form of a balance sheet, a table comparing each intervention in terms benefits, harms, and, sometimes, economic endpoints. Many studies are randomized, placebo-controlled trials (in which patients either get an active intervention or a placebo or sham intervention). However, the typical question for clinicians is should I change practice to use this intervention instead of an existing one. Thus, an appropriate consideration of patient-oriented outcomes and competing alternatives is of considerable practical importance.

When a study shows no effect, the question of power is raised. Put in simple terms, power is the ability to detect the effect of an intervention; it depends on the number of patients in the study, the magnitude of effect of the intervention, and the variability of the effect from one subject to another. For some interventions, even a small effect may be important. For example, many nonpharmacologic treatments for hypertension (e.g., salt restriction) have relatively modest but important effects. Practically, be skeptical of studies of a small number of patients (<100 to 150) in which statistically insignificant results are found.

Even when a study is positive or shows statistically significant results, it is important to consider whether these findings are clinically significant and applicable to your practice. For example, if a study showed that a drug reduces the risk of heart attack by one in a million patients, we would probably be skeptical of its utility. Likewise, the findings showing that daily borscht reduces fractures in a study done in Russian dockworkers may or may not be transferable to the United States. Moreover, the acceptability of an intervention (e.g., electroconvulsive therapy for depression) may vary. This issue of generalizability or transferability of an intervention is often glossed over. Moreover, the ability to replicate the findings of a study done in a typical research setting is often reduced in real-world practice. Thus, an intervention for osteoporosis requiring daily injections may be demonstrated to be efficacious, but in the average practice setting, its effectiveness might be much more limited.

Finally, we are more frequently relying on the results from not a single study but the synthesis of many studies to change our practices. Such reviews can be systematic, in which very rigorous attempts are made to uncover all studies, published and unpublished, in English and in other relevant languages, or very haphazard, even biased. Some use formal mathematical methods to combine the results of studies (meta-analysis), whereas others are qualitative and synthesize data according to an author's overall judgment. Common biases to look for include the following: were all sources of evidence considered, how were disparate results combined, were relevant patient-oriented outcomes assessed, was there adequate attention to the quality of the studies and their generalizability, and do the authors try to analyze why differences in outcomes may have occurred based on such factors as study design, population, and intervention. As noted, review articles and more elaborate systematic reviews are increasingly important for the busy clinician (see Table 6-1).

For the neophyte clinician, there are many ways to hone your critical appraisal skills including involvement with local journal clubs, work with the Family Practice Inquiries Network, or assisting in the development of POEMs and reading such references as EBM (Sackett et al., 1998). EBM, information mastery, and the application of knowledge at the point of care remain works in progress. By developing a basic understanding of these resources and tools, it is hoped that physicians' care of patients will be effective, safe, and efficient.

Material Available on Student Consult

Review Questions and Answers about Evaluating the Medical Literature

REFERENCES

American Academy of Family Physicians. Hormone Replacement Therapy: New Information. Patient education handout. Leawood, KS: American Academy of Family Physicians, 2004.

Barrie RA, Ward AM. Questioning behavior in general practice: A pragmatic study. BMJ 1997;315:1512–1515.

Ebell M. Evidence-based clinical practice. Information at the point of care: Answering clinical questions. J Am Board Fam Pract 1999;12:225–235.

Ebell MH, Messimer SR, Barry HC. Putting computer-based evidence in the hands of clinicians. JAMA 1999;28:1171–1172.

Geyman JP. POEMs as a paradigm shift in teaching, learning, and clinical practice. J Fam Pract 1999;48:343–344.

Goldman L, Tosteson ANA. Uncertainty about postmenopausal estrogen. N Engl J Med 1991;325:800–802.

Majumdar SR, Amasi EA, Stafford RS. Promotion and prescribing of hormone therapy after report of harm by the women's health initiative. JAMA 2004;292:1983–1988.

McAllister FA, Graham I, Karr GW, et al. Evidence-based medicine and the practicing clinician. J Gen Intern Med 1999;14:236–242.

Neff MJ. NAMS releases position statement on the treatment of vasomotor symptoms associated with menopause. Am Fam Physician 2004;70:393–394,396,399.

Pettite DB. Hormone replacement therapy and heart disease protection. JAMA 1998;280:650–651.

Rossouw JE, Anderson GL, Prentice RL, et al. and the Writing Group for the Women's Health Initiative. Risks and benefits of estrogen plus progestin in healthy postmenopausal women: Principal results. From the Women's Health Initiative randomized controlled trial. JAMA 2002;288:321–333.

Sackett DL, Richardson WS, Rosenberg W, et al. Evidence-based Medicine. Edinburgh: Churchill Livingstone, 1998.

Slawson DC, Shaughnessy AF. Teaching information mastery: Creating informed consumers of medical information. J Am Board Fam Pract 1999;12:444–449.

Timins JK. Current issues in hormone replacement therapy. N J Med 2004;101:21–27.

Utian WF, Shoupe D, Bachman G, et al. Relief of vasomotor symptoms and vaginal atrophy with lower doses of conjugated equine estrogens and medroxyprogesterone acetate. Fertil Steril 2001;75:1065–1075.

7 Ethics in Family Medicine

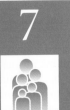

Warren I. Holleman and Baruch A. Brody

KEY POINTS

1. Medicine is a relationship and a profession.
2. When performing evaluations for third-party payers, always clarify the purpose of the evaluation and what information is to be shared and with whom.
3. Respect for confidentiality is essential to an effective doctor-patient relationship.
4. When treating adolescent patients, inform the parents that you will use your professional judgment in determining what information to share with them.
5. Informed consent is not a piece of paper but the verbal agreement between doctor and patient. The purpose of the piece of paper is to document that the conversation occurred and what each party agreed to do.
6. Noncompliance is usually a misnomer. Generally, noncompliance results from poor communication, failures of trust, mental illness, or value differences, each of which can be addressed by a skilled physician.
7. A skilled primary care physician will have the courage to address the medical problems that he or she is qualified to treat and the humility to ask for help when faced with problems beyond his or her expertise.
8. Physicians can avoid burnout if they learn to distinguish between competence and perfectionism, dedication and "workaholism," and compassion and sentimentalism.
9. Physicians have an ethical obligation to help patients live and die with as much dignity, control, and comfort as possible.

Economic, social, legal, and political factors have combined in recent years to effect major changes in medical practice and health care policy. Concern for patient rights and patient autonomy, as well as the demands of third-party payers, have transformed the practice of medicine. The ethical issues discussed in this chapter have taken on new dimensions as a result of this transformation.

MEDICINE AS A RELATIONSHIP AND AS A PROFESSION

At its most fundamental level, the practice of medicine should not be regarded as a science, an art, or a business, even though each of these elements is essential. The practice of medicine—particularly primary care medicine—is rooted, instead, in a relationship between the patient as person and the physician as professional (Jonsen et al., 2002; Smith and Churchill, 1986). Two problems currently threaten the quality of that relationship: a misunderstanding of patient autonomy and inappropriate third-party intervention.

When physicians respect the autonomy of their patients so that patients take control of their health care, the physician is in danger of becoming a hired hand of the patient and the physician-patient relationship is in danger of degenerating into a purely commercial relationship. Patients "own" their bodies, but they should not "own" their physicians. Physicians have an obligation to practice within professional standards of care as well as a right to refrain from doing anything that would violate their own moral and religious convictions (Christie and Hoffmaster, 1986). Yet they should nurture a cooperative relationship with their patients. This is no easy task, but it is through cooperation that the physician and the patient can best work together toward a common goal—to maintain the health of the patient.

The physician-patient relationship also suffers when outside parties interfere inappropriately. When third-party payers set the standard of care, the physician is in danger of becoming a hired hand of the third party. The physician must balance competing loyalties between patients and third parties as well as between professional standards and personal beliefs. In this era of third-party payers, the physician-patient relationship can no longer be exclusive, but it must remain primary. In the remainder of this section, we examine two areas in which these problems are particularly prominent: work-related visits and benefits-related visits.

Work- and School-related Evaluations

Preplacement examinations, work release evaluations, school absence excuses, and athletic physicals constitute a major component of many primary care practices. Inappropriate third-party interventions in these areas challenge the primacy of the physician-patient relationship and the integrity of the medical profession. The following guidelines have been suggested (Holleman and Holleman, 1988; Holleman and Matson, 1991) and should help alleviate some of the problems most commonly associated with these evaluations.

The purpose of the preplacement examination is to determine a person's fitness for work, to protect workers from illnesses and injuries, to protect employers from the costs of preventable job-related illnesses and injuries, and to collect baseline data for the future treatment of such illnesses and injuries. To enable the physician to make such an evaluation, the employer must provide the physician with a detailed job description, including physical requirements, psychological strains, and exposures to toxins. The physician then should tell the employer whether the prospective employee can perform the job without posing a risk to him- or herself or others. As discussed later, the physician should not release medical records to the employer but should keep them on file as baseline data. At the beginning of the evaluation, the physician should advise the patient of the investigative nature of the visit. The physician must warn the prospective employee regarding health risks of the particular occupation (e.g., toxins affecting pregnancies, stresses affecting hypertensive patients) and must tell him or her of any problems detected in the course of the evaluation, regardless of their effect on job performance.

Work release evaluations, school release evaluations, and athletic physical examinations should be performed in accordance with the same guidelines as preplacement physical examinations, but they do present some additional problems. Most work and school release evaluations involve short-term absences for minor problems for which there are few, if any, objective findings. Often workers and students present after their illness or injury has resolved. These absences often reflect personal, family, or job-related problems that are not strictly medical in nature. Investigating such problems for employers and school administrators damages the physician-patient relationship and discredits medi-

cine as a healing profession. Patients will have difficulty trusting a physician who investigates on one occasion but offers therapy on another. We recommend that physicians encourage employers and school administrators to develop nonmedical strategies for policing casual absenteeism. Physicians who do perform these evaluations should minimize the harm to the physician-patient relationship and to the integrity of the profession by evaluating only in the context of treatment and by refusing to release confidential medical information to employers and school administrators.

Many patients present to family physicians seeking to be certified as eligible for worker's compensation, long-term disability, group or individual medical insurance, Medicare, Medicaid, and veteran's benefits. Many others already have been certified and are seeking proper care under the terms of these programs. Physicians must be familiar with the benefits available under these programs as well as the potential abuses. For example, if a patient presents with an on-the-job injury but also requests treatment for some other problem, the physician should file separate bills so that the worker's compensation fund pays for only job-related illnesses and injuries. Long-term abuse of benefits programs can be prevented only if primary care physicians insist that patients receive continuing comprehensive care from one physician or from a small team of physicians who know the patient well.

SPECIAL PROBLEMS IN PRIMARY CARE SETTINGS

Having introduced the concept of medicine as a relationship and as a profession and having seen what this concept means in many primary care contexts, we turn in the next sections to problem areas that challenge our understanding of the physician-patient relationship and of the professional character of medicine.

Confidentiality

The principle of confidentiality is one of the most widely accepted and historically influential principles governing the patient-physician relationship in Western cultures. The Hippocratic Oath mandates that the physician not divulge "whatsoever I shall see or hear in the course of my profession as well as outside my profession in my intercourse with men, if it be what should not be published abroad." The 1980 Principles of Medical Ethics of the American Medical Association mandate that the physician "shall safeguard patient confidences within the constraints of the law."

Confidentiality is important as a way to encourage patients to be frank in their communications with physicians, as a way for physicians to keep an implicit promise to patients that their confidence will be respected, and as a way to emphasize the patient's right to privacy. In all these ways, preserving confidentiality strengthens the relationship between an autonomous patient and a professional physician.

As the delivery of health care has changed from the model of a single physician caring for individual patients to the model of a team of health care workers in an institutional setting providing care to a wide variety of patients, the mandate of confidentiality has changed. The emphasis has switched from physicians' keeping secrets to information about patients being divulged only to those members of the health care team and those institutional employees who have a need for the information, either to provide appropriate care or to meet appropriate institutional needs (e.g., monitoring of quality of care or organizing reimbursement). The underlying theme remains that information should not be provided to anyone else without the patient's consent.

This last point deserves special emphasis because it structures the decision as to when it is appropriate to provide information about the patient to insurance companies and to employers. Providing such information is appropriate if the patient consents; otherwise, it is not. The scope of information supplied and the persons to whom it is supplied are determined by the patient's instructions. If, for example, a patient requests a statement certifying that he or she is fit to return to work, it is not appropriate to give the employer a full account of the patient's illness and treatment, only a statement about the patient's fitness to return to work.

There are circumstances in which our society has judged that the need for information outweighs the principle of confidentiality; these are the circumstances in which the physician is required by law to disclose otherwise confidential information regardless of the wishes of the patient. Laws vary from jurisdiction to jurisdiction, but common circumstances include child custody disputes, suspected abuse of dependent individuals such as children and the frail elderly, venereal and communicable diseases, and gunshot wounds (Bruce, 1996). In recent years, following the *Tarasoff* decision in California (*Tarasoff v Regents of The University of California,* 1976), the concept has emerged that physicians are obligated to warn and/or to take measures to protect third parties threatened by the behavior of their patients, even if doing so involves a breach of confidentiality. The scope of that principle is far from clear; one obvious controversial example is whether physicians should warn the spouses or regular sexual partners of patients who test positive for human immunodeficiency virus about the threat this illness poses.

The principle of confidentiality extends to not providing information to family members of competent adult patients unless the patient wants the information to be shared. An appropriate practice on admitting a patient to a hospital is to ask the patient to identify a particular family member, if any, to whom information should be provided for distribution to the family if the patient is not capable of fulfilling that role (e.g., in the immediate postsurgical period).

Cases involving adolescent patients are particularly troublesome. Information about pediatric patients is, of course, provided directly to the parents of the patients and not to the patients themselves; information about adult patients is, of course, provided directly to the patient and not the patient's parents. What about teenage patients seeking abortions, contraceptive advice, or treatment for venereal diseases, substance abuse, or psychiatric problems? Unless confidentiality can be guaranteed, such patients may not seek out the care they need. If confidentiality is protected, such patients may not get the parental counseling and support from which they also could benefit. Considerable confusion exists about the morally appropriate and legally mandated approach to confidentiality of information involving adolescent patients (Ford et al., 2004; Holder, 1985).

Equally troubling are cases involving elderly patients who are less than fully competent but far from totally demented. Families of such patients often ask physicians to provide them with information about the patient's condition, information that they may not want to share with the patient. Such a request may be perfectly appropriate for the clearly incompetent demented patient, whereas it is obviously inappropriate for normal geriatric patients. How to handle cases that fall between these two extremes is unclear.

Informed Consent

The principle of informed consent is a more recently articulated principle than the principle of confidentiality; the actual phrase *informed consent* first appeared in 1957 in the court case *Salgo v Leland Stanford Jr. University Board of Trustees.* However, it has come to be accepted as a fundamental principle governing the relationship between patients and physicians.

The principle's basic mandate is that a physician must obtain the free and informed consent of a patient if the patient is competent to give that consent or of the patient's surrogate if the patient is not competent before medical treatment is provided. Two exceptions normally are recognized. The first (the *emergency exception*) is invoked when emergency treatment is necessary to protect the patient's life or health and consent cannot be obtained in a timely fashion. The second (the *therapeutic privilege*) is invoked when there is strong reason to believe that the very attempt to obtain consent will be harmful to the patient because of the psychological impact of the information conveyed (Rozovsky, 1990).

Several complementary accounts of the significance of the principle of informed consent are available. One stresses the clinical benefits (in terms of building trust and obtaining compliance) from a therapeutic regimen begun as a result of a joint patient-physician decision rather than as a result of a unilateral physician decision. The other stresses the patient's right to control what happens to his or her body; the resulting obligation of the physician to obtain informed consent is the way in which the physician respects that right.

The standard practice in many institutions is to obtain written documentation of informed consent primarily (if not exclusively) in cases of invasive procedures. This practice should not be understood to mean that the principle of informed consent does not apply to other medical interventions; it applies to all of them. Signed consent forms are merely written evidence of the informed consent already obtained, and the practice reflects the prudent desire to obtain written documentation in cases in which potential liability is highest. Informed consent, as opposed to the written documentation of that consent, should be obtained in all cases, both as a way of obtaining clinical benefits and as a way of respecting patient's rights.

There has been considerable disagreement about the amount and type of information that must be supplied to the patient. Obviously, only a portion of the relevant information known by the physician can be conveyed to the patient. Moreover, any attempt to provide too much information may result in the physician overwhelming and confusing the patient. Some selection of information is required, and the disagreement centers on which principle of selection to adopt.

Two different proposals have been adopted by America's courts (Rozovsky, 1990). The first is the *professional practice standard,* which maintains that a consent is informed if the patient has been provided the information that reasonable medical practitioners would normally provide under similar circumstances. The second is the *reasonable person standard,* which maintains that a consent is informed if the patient has been provided the information that a reasonable person would need to have to make a decision about whether to undergo the therapy in question. The information to be provided would presumably fall under the categories shown in Table 7-1.

Most commentators have argued for the second standard because it best corresponds to the goals of informed consent, but a majority of courts have adopted the usually less demanding professional

Table 7-1	Elements of Informed Consent Under Reasonable Person Standard

Nature of the patient's condition (e.g., hypertension)
Description of the treatment proposed (e.g., particular medication)
Benefits of proposed treatment (e.g., control of hypertension and resulting lowering of risk of disease)
Risks of proposed treatment (e.g., side effects for that medication)
Alternatives (e.g., other medications, diet and exercise, no intervention)
Costs of proposed treatment

From Rakel RE. Textbook of Family Practice, 4th ed. Philadelphia: W.B. Saunders, 1990.

practice standard (Rozovsky, 1990). Clinicians are, we believe, best advised to adopt the reasonable person standard because it provides all the clinical and moral benefits of obtaining informed consent while firmly ensuring that the legal requirement of informed consent is satisfied. Clinicians also must be careful to provide that information using terminology that patients are likely to understand.

A difficult problem arises when one is dealing with patients whose competency is impaired (Freedman, 1996). Informed consent is obtained from the patient when the patient is clearly competent and from the patient's surrogate (a legally appointed guardian, if available, or the closest family member) if the patient is clearly incompetent. What, however, should one do when the patient's mental capacities are impaired but present to some degree? This problem is alleviated partially when one remembers that the assessment of the patient's competency is not an assessment of the patient's total ability to manage all his or her affairs; it is just the assessment of whether at this moment the patient can (1) receive the information relevant to giving or refusing informed consent for this particular treatment, (2) remember that information, (3) appropriately assess and use that information to make a decision, and (4) make a decision (B. A. Brody, 1988). Although no formal test exists to ensure that the patient has the capacity to perform items 1 through 4 in the list, a careful discussion with the patient usually will enable the physician to ascertain whether these criteria are satisfied. If doubt remains, one should obtain consent from both the patient and the surrogate.

A second difficulty involves teenage patients. Informed consent is obtained from parents before one treats children, but from patients once they become adults. How should physicians treat teenage patients? Most states have passed special laws allowing physicians to treat them after obtaining only their consent when (1) the treatment is for venereal disease, pregnancy or contraception, or drug-related problems; (2) they are living away from their parents and are responsible for their own affairs; or (3) they are married. Other cases, such as abortion, are more problematic (Ford et al., 2004; Holder, 1985).

The Noncompliant Patient

Implicit in the principle of informed consent—the principle that medical treatment can be provided only after the patient has freely and knowingly consented to it—is the concept that a patient may choose not to comply with the physician's recommendations and that the choice not to comply must be respected. This concept can be misunderstood, however, leading to a quick, facile, and inappropriate acceptance of a patient's noncompliance before its meaning is properly understood.

Most cases of noncompliance involve failures of communication, lack of trust as a result of previous bad experiences, and psychological and psychopathologic factors. Only a minority of cases involve a true value difference between the physician and the patient. This finding has profound implications for the clinical management of noncompliance. Physicians confronting noncompliant patients need to assess the noncompliance, evaluate its cause, and react appropriately. Table 7-2 indicates how such a noncompliance assessment would proceed. In short, morality does not call on the physician to accept at face value every episode of noncompliance on the part of the patient. Doing so may in fact constitute a form of disrespect for the patient. What morality does call for is a full evaluation of the cause of the noncompliance, appropriate responses where possible to eliminate the cause, and respect for the patient's noncompliance only when it is an informed and competent refusal that is based on a difference between the patient's and the physician's values.

Even in those cases in which noncompliance represents an informed and competent refusal of the physician's recommendations because the patient's values differ, mutually acceptable alternative treatments are often available. Consider a patient who refuses to stay in a hospital for a full evaluation because the patient is concerned about the need to be home to handle personal problems. Such a patient should be scheduled for an outpatient evaluation, even if it is not as satisfactory as a full evaluation in the hospital. Respecting patient values in cases of noncompliance is not a matter of letting the patient win a power struggle; it is, more often, finding a mutually acceptable, although not necessarily optimal, course of action. A failure to seek out such alternatives often may represent a lack of respect for the patient.

A form of noncompliance that deserves special attention is the patient who does not fill the prescription that the doctor writes. This is sometimes the result of the patient's financial condition. The optimal medication from the physician's perspective may cost too much from the patient's perspective. Particularly when dealing with patients who have high medication bills because they need so many drugs or with patients who have very limited means, physicians should raise the question of cost frankly and explore less expensive but satisfactory (even if not optimal) medications.

A similar problem often arises when one considers the question of side effects of various drugs. Different patients with different values and different tolerances may find certain side effects unacceptable. The physician certainly should not assume that a pattern of side effects that is acceptable to the physician will be acceptable to the patient. Taking the patient's values into account in deciding which antihypertensive medication to order is a far clearer example of respecting the patient's values than simply accepting a patient's noncompliance with a particular prescription.

Table 7-2 Evaluation of Noncompliance	
Cause	**Clinical Response**
Problem in communication	Patient should be reinformed about the need for treatment
Failure of trust	Address question of mistrust; involve other health professionals who may be trusted
Psychological factors	Treat anxiety, depression, and so on
Value conflict	Respect patient wishes

From Rakel RE. Textbook of Family Practice, 4th ed. Philadelphia: W.B. Saunders, 1990.

SPECIAL PROBLEMS IN TERTIARY CARE SETTINGS

Quality of care can be improved by careful attention to the components examined thus far: the physician-patient relationship, medicine as a profession, confidentiality, informed consent, and the promotion of patient compliance. When the focus shifts from primary care provided by the family physician to care provided by subspecialists in tertiary care settings, new problems arise and old problems become even more complicated. The next two sections examine ways of resolving some of these problems.

Referrals

Decisions regarding referrals and consultations are often accompanied by great confusion. Referrals to subspecialists practicing in tertiary care institutions can provoke anxiety on the part of patients. The referring physician risks losing a patient and a substantial amount of money and is subject to embarrassment if a mistake is discovered. Referrals sometimes degenerate into power struggles between subspecialists and generalists. Because primary care is a community-based discipline, there is much debate and little consensus as to the primary care physician's role in the tertiary care setting (Christie and Hoffmaster, 1986). The following guidelines about appropriate referrals and about continuity through referrals are intended to help clarify these responsibilities and thus ease the tension and improve the quality of care.

Decisions to use consultants should be based on a realistic assessment of the potentialities and limitations of primary care as a discipline, of oneself as a physician, and of the facilities available in one's geographic region. Unfortunately, a number of other factors (financial and institutional as well as medical) often cloud the decision-making process and disrupt relations between primary and tertiary care physicians.

Many subspecialists in oversubscribed areas have taken it on themselves to enter primary care as a means of bolstering their incomes, despite their inadequate training in this area. Conversely, primary care physicians sometimes feel pressured to go beyond their areas of expertise for financial and professional reasons: They fear losing the patient and the income and fear that their seeking consultation might reinforce the misconception that primary care physicians are inferior.

Knowing when to use consultants requires courage and humility. Courage is the ability to act competently and wisely without being swayed by irrational fears. Some primary care physicians, motivated by unrealistic fears of mistakes and exposure, refer too early. Humility, on the other hand, is the willingness to recognize one's *actual* limitations and to act accordingly. Some primary care physicians, unaware of their limitations, refer too late. A proper combination of courage and humility, along with good working relationships with subspecialists, can prevent most of the problems involved in referring too early or too late.

Even if the primary care physician does decide to refer the patient, he or she remains the patient's primary physician (Christie and Hoffmaster, 1986). Equipped with a strong knowledge of general medicine, the patient's medical history, and the patient's personal traits and committed to treating the disease in the context of the person and the person in the context of the family, the primary care physician is ideally suited to manage the patient throughout the referral.

When initiating a referral, the primary care physician's responsibilities are to educate the patient as to the reasons for referral, to recommend a subspecialist or treatment center best suited to the patient's medical and personal needs, to prepare the patient for what lies ahead, and to provide the specialist with data relevant to the patient's illness. Even after the referral, the primary care physician remains responsible for the quality of the patient's care. This may require translating medical jargon to patients or patient preferences to subspecialists and hospital staff, coordinating the activities of the various consultants, mediating disputes between consultants, ensuring that confidentiality is maintained by the health care team, and counseling patients and their families. The referral process is not complete until the subspecialist and the primary care physician have discussed all findings, treatments, results, and recommendations and the primary care physician has discussed these with the patient (Christie and Hoffmaster, 1986).

Sometimes subspecialists disagree as to how to manage a particular disorder. Consider the different way that surgeons and cardiologists may treat carotid artery disease. Or consider the range of approaches, within particular subspecialties, in treating particular disorders: differences among gynecologists regarding indications for a hysterectomy and differences among neonatologists in managing severely handicapped infants. This makes the referring physician's task a difficult and delicate one. The referring physician must be aware of the differences between subspecialties and between particular physicians within a subspecialty. The referring physician must know the patient and the patient's family well enough to recommend the appropriate subspecialist. In many cases, the principle of informed consent will mandate that the referring physician educate the patient and the family as to the strengths and weaknesses of the available options. Primary care physicians should help their patients find a subspecialist who will be appropriate to both their medical needs and their personal preferences.

Financial Gatekeeping

The soaring costs of health care have led corporations and government agencies to develop prospective payment systems and capitation plans, with primary care physicians often serving as gatekeepers of the health care network. It is hoped that this will save money and streamline the referral process. However, it might drive a bureaucratic wedge into the physician-patient relationship, allow money to compete with quality in determining the standard of care, and inhibit the physician's freedom to practice an individualized style of medicine.

Prospective reimbursement systems (such as the Medicare Diagnosis-Related Group system) save money by limiting the reimbursement available to physicians, thereby encouraging them to do less. Designers of such systems have the legitimate right to require physicians to avoid wasteful procedures and referrals; this prevents unnecessary expenditures and ensures a more just distribution of health care expenditures. Such limitations do not, however, preclude the physician's responsibility to offer the patient the best possible care within the limitations set by those policies. When particular patients require care in excess of the normal level of reimbursement, the primary care physician confronts a major ethical dilemma.

Considerable controversy exists as to whether physicians should do everything that might benefit each patient without regard to costs or other societal considerations or whether physicians must not be allowed to ignore the bottom line (Holleman et al., 1997). Traditionalists tend to ignore the fact that financial considerations always have limited the quality of care available to the poor. The question we are now confronting is whether these considerations may legitimately limit the quality of care available to everyone.

In caring for individual patients, physicians should distinguish between providing what the patient wants and what the patient needs. The controversy concerns whether all procedures and services likely to benefit the patient, as evidenced by outcome data, should be made available to the patient. When patients request unnecessary or marginally beneficial procedures and services, however, physicians must refuse.

THE PHYSICIAN AS HUMAN BEING

The medical profession has, in the past few decades, achieved truly impressive gains in the battle against sickness, suffering, and death. Diseases that killed their victims just a generation ago are now manageable, curable, or even preventable. Yet physicians seem remarkably inept at maintaining their own health and well-being; they have high rates of alcoholism, substance abuse, divorce, burnout, and suicide (Doan-Wiggins et al., 1995; Fields et al., 1995; O'Connor and Spickard, 1997). Why can't the healers heal themselves, and what can they do to get on the road to recovery? To deal with these problems, we recommend that physicians learn to distinguish between competence and perfectionism, dedication and workaholism, and compassion and sentimentalism.

In medical school and residency, young doctors often learn to put their careers ahead of self and family (Gabbard and Menninger, 1988). This dedication is, in some ways, good. Young physicians want to do everything they can to help their patients, but this is often coupled with an unrealistic perception of their capabilities and those of their profession. They allow their egos to become too closely identified with their successes and failures. They become obsessed with insecurity (they are not good enough) and guilt (they do not work hard enough). They worry that they might have missed a diagnosis and fear that their patients will die or suffer unnecessarily. Physicians are not supposed to make mistakes, but they do. Their profession requires staying on top of an ever-expanding field of knowledge; adeptness at a wide range of techniques and skills; making the right decision when fatigued, hassled, or angry; picking up on subtle clues or poorly articulated symptoms; and juggling a plethora of human needs. Mistakes are inevitable, but talking about them is taboo. The only place mistakes are openly discussed, it seems, is the courtroom (Hilfiker, 1985). To be more effective clinicians, physicians must learn to acknowledge their capacity to err and must learn to discuss errors in a constructive manner. Physicians who do not admit their mistakes are doomed to repeat them. Physicians who discuss their mistakes can learn from them and experience healing in the process.

The physician who takes the time to care for personal and family needs is a more effective clinician because he or she is better able to cope with the stresses and strains of a demanding profession. Also, in the case of primary care physicians whose patients know them well, the physician will become a role model for personal health and fitness.

Another area in which physicians must learn to accept their humanity, and the humanity of their patients, is the area of emotions. Clinicians must help patients recognize, express, and interpret their emotions. Clinicians must become aware of their own emotions, recognize their clinical value, and learn how to express and interpret them. The physician who ignores the emotions dehumanizes the physician-patient relationship. The primary care physician who improperly expresses, uses, or interprets emotional factors deprofessionalizes that relationship. Traditionally, physicians have been trained to maintain objectivity, affective neutrality, and clinical detachment. To be scientific, however, does not preclude recognizing the legitimacy of emotions or the necessity of empathy as a legitimate clinical and moral response to suffering. Sometimes a patient's feelings offer a clue to his or her symptoms. Sometimes a physician's feelings in response to a patient offer a clue to the patient's problem. Suffering patients need a physician who will suffer alongside them and who will help them to express and interpret their feelings. When their patients suffer, physicians suffer too. The physician who suffers alongside a suffering patient or family allows the opportunity for healing of self as well as of the patient or family. Many of the physician's feelings, however, cannot be appropriately expressed in the clinical encounter. To maintain personal well-being, therefore, the physician must find appropriate outlets for expression and interpretation.

EUTHANASIA AND ASSISTED SUICIDE

The issues of euthanasia and assisted suicide have provoked considerable public debate and challenged long-standing notions of the physician-patient relationship and the nature of the medical profession. In the coming years, patients may turn increasingly to their family physicians for assistance in dying, and thus it is important for family physicians to be prepared to respond appropriately.

For some time, most Americans have favored legalization of some methods of ending the life of a seriously ill or impaired person. In November 1993, 1254 adult Americans were asked whether they thought that the law should allow doctors to comply with the wishes of a dying patient in severe distress who asks to have his or her life ended. Seventy-three percent responded "yes." Public support of assisted death has increased steadily over the past decade. In 1982, 53 percent responded affirmatively to the same question, and in 1987, 62 percent (Taylor, 1993).

Many fear that aggressive measures to keep them alive, administered against their will, might inflict more suffering and indignity than they wish to bear (Cowart and Burt, 1998). Others worry that the pain and debilitation of the illness itself might become unbearable and want the assurance that escape through euthanasia or assisted suicide is available. These are legitimate concerns: A recent study suggested that terminally ill patients frequently are overtreated against their will and that physicians continue to undertreat pain despite advances in pain and symptom management (Solomon et al., 1993). Another study has shown that most terminal geriatric patients prefer palliative care but that these "patients . . . exert strikingly little influence in the making of the treatment decision" and frequently are misinformed regarding the terminal nature of their condition (Prigerson, 1992). A major factor, according to the study, is physicians' own discomfort with death. Physicians practicing in teaching hospitals were found to be particularly uncomfortable with death, less likely to disclose a terminal diagnosis, and more likely to provide curative treatment in the last months of life (Prigerson, 1992).

Some physicians have urged colleagues to take a more active role in helping patients who request assistance in dying (H. Brody, 1992; Kevorkian, 1991; Quill, 1991). They regard such action as an acknowledgment of medical hubris and an expression of medical compassion and willingness to support the autonomous wishes of patients. The American Medical Association (AMA), however, and a number of prominent physicians and ethicists have opposed efforts to legalize euthanasia and physician-assisted suicide (Gaylin et al., 1988). Physician participation in euthanasia and assisted suicide would, in their view, violate the Hippocratic Oath, confuse patients, erode trust, and tarnish medicine's image as a healing profession.

The most widely publicized model of physician-endorsed euthanasia is found in The Netherlands, where the government does not prosecute physicians who abide by an agreed-on standard of care (de Wachter, 1992). The criteria for euthanasia are that the patient's suffering must be intolerable despite aggressive relief efforts; there must be a low probability of improvement; the patient must be rational and fully informed; the patient's requests for euthanasia must be voluntary and repeated consistently over a reasonable period of time; and two physicians must accede to the request.

Some patient advocacy organizations, most notably the Hemlock Society and Choice in Dying (formerly Society for the Right to Die), urge the adoption of similar standards in the United States, with the government protecting physicians from criminal and civil litigation. These parties believe that aggressive attempts to prolong the lives of terminally ill persons are unnatural and torturous and that euthanasia or assisted suicide is sometimes the most humane alternative. Others, including many of the prolife organizations, hold that the taking of a human life is what is unnatural and immoral and that patients and physicians should always, in the words of the Hebrew scriptures, "choose life." They also express a practical concern that acceptance of this practice will lead to a slippery slope involving involuntary as well as voluntary euthanasia and euthanasia for patients who are not terminally ill or not experiencing unbearable suffering. They point to an apparent erosion of standards in The Netherlands, where, for example, 1000 incompetent patients are euthanized per year (ten Have and Welie, 1992). (Supporters respond that the percentage of life-terminating acts performed without the explicit request of the patient is relatively small, this percentage is stable or shrinking rather than growing, and most of these cases represent patients who requested euthanasia before becoming incompetent [Pijnenborg et al., 1993; van Delden et al., 1993].)

Physician-assisted suicide has been proposed as a way to minimize the role of the physician in the action causing the death of the patient while enabling the physician to provide expertise necessary to make the death as painless as possible. The patient feels a greater sense of control, and the image of the medical profession is not tainted by a stigma of murder attached to the event.

On October 27, 1997, the State of Oregon legalized physician-assisted suicide. The Death with Dignity Act allows physicians to prescribe a lethal dose of barbiturates or other controlled substance to patients who are terminally ill. To qualify, the patient must be an adult resident of Oregon and must make one written and two oral requests; at least 15 days must separate the two oral requests. Primary physician and consultant must confirm the terminal diagnosis and prognosis as well as the patient's competence. If either physician suspects depression or other psychiatric disorder, they must refer for counseling. The primary physician must inform the patient of all reasonable alternatives such as pain and symptom management and hospice care and report all lethal prescriptions to the Oregon Health Division. The physician may not administer the medication (Angell, 1999; Chin et al., 1999).

No significant abuses of the Oregon law have been reported to date. During the first year, only 15 persons chose to end their lives under the terms of the law; all but two had metastatic cancer (Angell, 1999; Chin et al., 1999). Some ethicists have observed that the preference for assisted suicide over euthanasia reflects a cosmetic distinction analogous to the now-obsolete distinction between withholding and withdrawing treatment. Regardless of the methods, the motives and outcome are the same. Preoccupation with taints and stigmas reflects more concern for image than integrity and also may indicate a lack of courage rather than a commitment to principle.

Another concern is that, in this era of cost containment, dying patients will feel unduly pressured to choose suicide rather than spend society's, and perhaps their family's, limited resources. Although such external pressure would be inappropriate, this does raise the question of whether patients have an ethical obligation to limit the costs of their care as they approach the end of life (Hardwig, 1997).

Hospice physicians, who have pioneered in the development of pain and symptom management for terminally ill persons (Ogle et al., 1992; Saunders, 1967), offer help to get beyond the impasse of those physicians who feel torn between wanting to relieve the suffering of the dying but not wanting to serve, directly or indirectly, as the cause of their patient's death. Hospice medicine has shown that the pain of dying persons usually can be palliated by aggressive pharmacologic treatment as well as by attention to "total pain," which includes all the physical, emotional, social, spiritual, and financial sources of the patient's suffering. The existence of this expertise, and the relative ease with which a family physician can master it, implies an obligation to use these methods and, when necessary, to seek consultation from palliative care specialists.

An ethical dilemma persists, however, in the occasional case of a patient whose pain or suffering remains unbearable despite the best care available and who requests assistance in dying (H. Brody, 1992). Patients with severe physical disabilities, such as those with amyotrophic lateral sclerosis, advanced Parkinson's disease, or quadriplegia, also might request assistance in dying. Hospice care offers much less for these patients, and they may turn to their family physician for help. Many family physicians would like to assist such patients but fear legal repercussions. What should those physicians do?

It is disingenuous to deny assistance on the basis of pragmatic considerations, such as slippery slopes, outbreaks of mercy killings, and mistrust of white coats. Withholding and withdrawing treatment also could create slippery slopes and also have been opposed on the basis of inflated fears, but these concerns are now considered insufficient to justify a prohibition against these practices. Most Americans know the difference between the euthanasia as murder and the type of assisted dying currently being discussed, limited to patients suffering unbearably despite aggressive efforts to relieve physical and psychological pain, who request assistance voluntarily and who receive voluntary, compassionate, competent assistance by their physicians. A review process should, of course, be established to ensure that these criteria are met (H. Brody, 1992).

From an ethical perspective, the essential issue is whether the long-standing prohibition against killing, which many regard as absolute, should outweigh all other considerations, such as the patient's autonomy or the degree of pain and suffering. Or does the situation of unbearable pain and suffering pose a special situation that our society ought to regard as an exception to the general prohibition of killing, through granting some types of patients the right to waive their right not to be killed? These two horns of the dilemma embody the crux of the issue, and all other concerns should be regarded as peripheral.

At present, assistance in dying is illegal in most of the United States and much of the world. Whether the legislatures and the courts should stand in the way of physicians who, with compassion and competence, are willing to assist this small category of patients is an issue that our society is in the process of resolving. The ethical obligation for primary care physicians remains to help patients live and die with as much dignity, control, and comfort as possible in light of whatever decision society makes.

CONCLUSION

The ethical questions faced by physicians have been transformed, in ways we have indicated, by changing economic, social, legal, political, and scientific factors. In the end, however, the ethics of medicine remain committed to a view of the patient-physician relationship as a relationship between two autonomous human beings—a patient who is suffering and seeks help and a physician who maintains professionalism, humanity, and a systemic perspective.

REFERENCES

Angell M. Caring for the dying—Congressional mischief. N Engl J Med 1999;341:1923–1925.

Brody BA. Life and Death Decision Making. New York: Oxford University Press, 1988.

Brody H. Assisted death—a compassionate response to a medical failure. N Engl J Med 1992;327:1384–1388.

Bruce JAC. Privacy and Confidentiality of Health Care Information, 3rd ed. Chicago: American Hospital Association, 1996.

Chin AE, Hedberg K, Higginson GK, Fleming DW. Legalized physician-assisted suicide in Oregon—the first year's experience. N Engl J Med 1999;340:577–583.

Christie RJ, Hoffmaster CB. Ethical Issues in Family Medicine. New York: Oxford University Press, 1986.

Cowart D, Burt R. Confronting death: Who chooses, who controls? Hastings Cent Rep 1998;28:14–24.

de Wachter MAM: Euthanasia in the Netherlands. Hastings Cent Rep 1992;22:23–30.

Doan-Wiggins L, Zun L, Cooper MA, et al. Practice satisfaction, occupational stress, and attrition of emergency physicians. Acad Emer Med 1995;2:555–563.

Fields AI, Cuerdon TT, Brasseux CO, et al. Physician burnout in pediatric critical care medicine. Crit Care Med 1995;23:1425–1429.

Ford C, English A, Sigman G. Confidential health care for adolescents: Position paper for the society for adolescent medicine. J Adolesc Health 2004;35:160.

Freedman B. Respectful service and reverent obedience: A Jewish view on making decisions for incompetent parents. Hastings Cent Rep 1996;26:31–37.

Gabbard GO, Menninger RW, eds. Medical Marriages. Washington, DC: American Psychiatric Press, 1988.

Gaylin W, Kass LR, Pellegrino ED, Siegler M. "Doctors must not kill." JAMA 1988;259:2139–2140.

Hardwig J. Is there a duty to die? Hastings Cent Rep 1997;27:34–42.

Hilfiker D. A Physician Looks at His Work. New York: Pantheon Books, 1985.

Holder A. Legal Issues in Pediatrics and Adolescent Medicine. New Haven, CT: Yale University Press, 1985.

Holleman WL, Holleman MC. School and work release evaluations. JAMA 1988;260:3629–3634.

Holleman WL, Holleman MC, Moy JG. Are ethics and managed care strange bedfellows or a marriage made in heaven? Lancet 1997;349:350–351.

Holleman WL, Matson CC. Preemployment evaluations: Dilemmas for the family physician. J Am Board Fam Pract 1991;4:95–101.

Jonsen AR, Siegler M, Winslade WJ. Clinical Ethics: A Practical Approach to Ethical Decisions in Clinical Medicine, 5th ed. New York: McGraw-Hill, 2002.

Kevorkian J. Prescription-Medicine: The Goodness of Planned Death. Buffalo, NY: Prometheus Books, 1991.

O'Connor PG, Spickard A Jr. Physician impairment by substance abuse. Med Clin North Am 1997;81:1037–1052.

Ogle KS, Warren D, Plumb JD. Pain management in advanced cancer. Primary Care 1992;19:793–805.

Pijnenborg L, van der Maas PJ, van Delden JJM, Looman CWN. Life-terminating acts without explicit request of patient. Lancet 1993;341:1196–1199.

Prigerson HG. Socialization to dying: Social determinants of death acknowledgment and treatment among terminally ill geriatric patients. J Health Soc Behav 1992;33:378–395.

Quill TE. Death and dignity: A case of individualized decision making. N Engl J Med 1991;324:691–694.

Rozovsky FA. Consent to Treatment: A Practical Guide, 2nd ed. Boston: Little, Brown, 1990.

Saunders CM. The Management of Terminal Illness. London: Hospital Medicine, 1967.

Smith HL, Churchill LR. Professional Ethics and Primary Care Medicine: Beyond Dilemmas and Decorum. Durham, NC: Duke University Press, 1986.

Tarasoff v Regents of The University of California, 131 Cal Rptr 1976.

Taylor H. Majority support for euthanasia and Dr. Kevorkian increases. The Harris Poll 1993;63.

ten Have HAMJ, Welie JVM. Euthanasia: Normal medical practice? Hastings Cent Rep 1992;22:34–38.

van Delden JJM, Pijnenborg L, van der Mass PJ. The Remmelink study: Two years later. Hastings Cent Rep 1993;23:24–27.

8   Family Dynamics and Health

Therese Zink

KEY POINTS

1. Domestic violence/intimate partner violence/ abuse (IPV) includes physical injury and threats, sexual coercion or threat, and emotional abuse (such as humiliating the victim, controlling what the victim can and cannot do, and isolating the victim from family and friends).
2. The lifetime prevalence of IPV is 7.6% for men and 25% for women.
3. Domestic violence affects the health of the entire family.
4. IPV victims have increased risk of poorer health, depressive symptoms, substance use, developing a chronic disease, chronic mental illness, and injury.
5. Exposure to the abuse between adults is associated with behavioral problems such as acting out, school problems, withdrawal, aggressiveness and disrespect toward the mother, increased involvement in risky behaviors (drugs, sex, alcohol), psychological problems such as depression, anxiety, and posttraumatic stress disorder, eating disorders, and chronic physical complaints.
6. Screening should be done in private without partner or children present. Family members should not be used to translate conversations about abuse.
7. Be nonjudgmental with the victim. Validate that no one deserves to be hurt, share resources, and schedule a follow-up visit at your office.
8. If you are caring for both the victim and perpetrator, maintain strict confidentiality, and always be cognizant of the victim's safety.

INITIAL VISIT

Subjective

Patient Identification and Presenting Illness

Mrs. Mary B. is a 34-year-old woman who is first seen with a headache. The headache gets worse as the day goes on. Sometimes she goes to bed with the headache, and on other days, she wakes up with the headache. No photophobia or nausea is present. Pain is described as throbbing and pounding, involving the entire head, especially the temples.

Her husband and children also are seen at the clinic. Two of the children have been diagnosed with attention-deficit/hyperactivity disorder (ADHD). Her husband has been treated for depression and high blood pressure.

Medical History

Surgical history: appendectomy, tubal ligation. Obstetrics: Gravida 3, Para 3, normal spontaneous vaginal deliveries. Workup for gastric reflux; irritable bowel syndrome. Postpartum depression after last two pregnancies. Many no-show appointments. Once when she accompanied her child to a visit, Mrs. B. had a black eye. She had an emergency department visit for cracked ribs.

Family History

Father: hypertension. Mother: diabetes, migraines.

Health Habits

Occasional glass of wine or bottle of beer, one pack of cigarettes per week, intermittent exercise.

Social History

Mrs. B. lives with her husband and three children.

Review of Systems

Ongoing irritable bowel syndrome, current management plan working.

Evidence levels Ⓐ Randomized, controlled trials (RCTs), meta-analyses, well-designed systematic reviews of RCTs. Ⓑ Case-control or cohort studies, nonrandomized clinical trials, systematic reviews of studies other than RCTs, cross-sectional studies, retrospective studies, certain uncontrolled studies. Ⓒ Consensus statements, expert guidelines, usual practice, opinion.

Objective

Mrs. B is reserved and gives intermittent eye contact. Blood pressure is 120/70, pulse is 72, weight is 140 lb, height is 5 feet 5 inches. Lung and heart examinations are normal. Her neurologic examination is normal.

Assessment

The diagnosis is tension headache, but her poor eye contact, the history of irritable bowel syndrome, postpartum depression, frequent no-shows, and injuries are red flags for intimate partner violence (IPV)/domestic violence (DV). When Mrs. B is asked about her relationship with her husband, she replies curtly that all is fine. You respect her answer but inform her that DV is common and that local resources are available in case she knows anyone who might need them, and you point to the local DV agency's pamphlets in your office.

Plan

Tension headaches are treated with stretching exercises and ibuprofen. Because of the red flags for domestic violence, a follow-up visit is arranged, and the need for further DV assessment is noted.

DISCUSSION

Abusive family dynamics affect the health and well-being of every family member. To date, identification and care of the adult victim of abuse has received the most attention. *Intimate partner violence* and *domestic violence* are often used interchangeably.

Although current evidence does not support or refute the effectiveness of the universal screening for DV in the medical setting, professional organizations recommend identifying patients and sharing resources (American Medical Association, 1992 ⊙; U.S. Preventive Services Task Force, 2004 ⊙). Identifying DV and helping patients understand the impact of this stress on their health and the health of their children are important for quality health care.

This chapter reviews the definition of DV/IPV, prevalence, cost in dollars, health care consequences for all family members, tools for identification, recommended management, and mandatory reporting obligations.

Definition

The Centers for Disease Control defines IPV as physical and sexual abuse or threat of physical or sexual abuse, or emotional/psychological abuse such as humiliating the victim, controlling what the victim can and cannot do, and isolating the victim from family and friends, or a combination of these.

Prevalence

From 11% to 22% of adult women seeking care in primary care practices have experienced physical abuse in the past year. IPV affects one of every four women in the United States. Men also are victims, but the prevalence is 1 in every 14 men, and the degree of injury is much less. The lifetime prevalence is 7.6% for men and 25% for women. The 1-year prevalence of IPV is 0.9% in men and 1.5% in women. IPV occurs in all socioeconomic categories, among all ethnic groups, and in both heterosexual and same-sex relationships. An estimated 3.3 to 10 million children witness IPV annually in the United States (Tjaden and Thoennes, 2000 ⊙).

Health Care Costs

The estimated total cost of IPV (including IPV rape, physical assault, and stalking) against adult U.S. women is $5.9 billion (1995 dollars). Nearly $4.1 billion is for direct medical and mental health care; $0.9 billion is lost productivity from paid work and household chores for victims of nonfatal IPV; and for IPV homicide, $0.9 billion is lost in lifetime earnings. Victims of IPV cost the health care system 50% more than do nonvictims (National Center for Injury Prevention and Control, 2003 ⊙).

Health Effects

Domestic violence affects the health of the entire family. A retrospective cohort survey of adults at Kaiser Permanente found that adverse childhood experiences (emotional, physical, and sexual abuse; a battered mother; parental separation or divorce; growing up with a substance-abusing, mentally ill, or incarcerated household member) were associated with more high-risk behaviors and health conditions than in patients reporting no adverse events in childhood. These conditions include unintended pregnancy, sexually transmitted infections, alcohol abuse, smoking, suicide, depression, and risk factors for heart disease, chronic lung disease, and liver disease (Felitti et al., 1998 ⊙).

Victims

Studies show that both male and female IPV victims have increased risk of poorer health, depressive symptoms, substance abuse, developing a chronic disease, chronic mental illness, and injury (Campbell, 2002 ⊙; Coker et al., 2002 ⊙) (Table 8-1).

Perpetrators

Less is known about the health of IPV perpetrators. Often substance abuse is a problem. Otherwise perpetrators are a heterogeneous group with a wide

Table 8-1	Red-flag Symptoms and Conditions for Victims

- Injuries (Ask about the mechanism of the inquiry; if mechanism does not make sense consider probing further in a nonjudgmental manner.)
- Digestive problems (diarrhea, spastic colon, constipation, nausea, loss of appetite)
- Chronic pain (headache, abdominal pain, pelvic pain, back pain, etc.)
- Genitourinary problems (infections, sexually transmitted diseases, pelvic pain, menstrual problems, sexual dysfunction)
- Vague somatic complaints (fatigue, dizziness)
- Mental health issues (depression, anxiety, post-traumatic stress disorder, substance abuse, suicide)
- Eating disorders
- Pregnancy problems (preterm labor, poor weight gain)

Table 8-2	Red-flag Symptoms and Conditions for Children Exposed

- Symptoms of post-traumatic stress
- Sleep difficulties
- Hypervigilance, poor concentration, and distractibility (ADHD/hyperactivity)
- Behavioral problems, school problems
- Depression
- Anxiety
- Chronic somatic complaints (abdominal pain, headaches, etc.)
- Aggressiveness toward other children
- Teens are more likely to participate in risk-taking behaviors such as smoking, drinking, using illegal drugs, eating disorders, and pregnancy

ADHD, attention-deficit/hyperactivity disorder

variety of needs. Some have depression; others have personality disorders, such as narcissistic or antisocial. Risk factors for perpetrating IPV include witnessing DV in childhood, disrupted attachment patterns, high levels of interpersonal dependency and jealousy, attitudes condoning DV, and lack of empathy (Coben and Friedman, 2002; Holtzworth-Monroe and Meehan, 2004).

Intimate Partner Violence–Exposed Child

Exposure to the abuse between adults is associated with behavioral problems such as acting out; school problems; withdrawal; aggressiveness and disrespect toward the mother; increased involvement in risky behaviors (drug and alcohol use, sex), psychological problems such as depression, anxiety, and posttraumatic stress disorder; eating disorders; and chronic physical complaints. A recent study of 5-year-old twins demonstrated that children exposed to high levels of DV had IQs that were 8 points lower than those of unexposed children, a dose-response relation. (Studies of lead poisoning document a loss of approximately 4 IQ points.) Urban children exposed to DV had higher scores on the Child Behavior Checklist, indicating behavior problems, than did nonexposed children (Kitzmann et al., 2003 ⓑ) (Table 8-2).

Identification of the Intimate Partner Violence Victim

A variety of questions and screening tools have been tested for IPV screening. Some questions are direct, and some are indirect. Both patients and clinicians seem to prefer more-indirect questioning for initial assessment, with more-direct questions for further evaluation. "Do you feel safe in your intimate relationship?" is an example of an indirect screening question. "Have you ever been in a relationship in which your partner has pushed or slapped you?" is a direct screening question. See Table 8-3 for screening tools and questions.

Screening should be done in private without partner or children present. Family members should not be used to translate conversations about abuse. No consensus exists on what method (written vs. verbal) is the best for screening victims about abuse. The most important factor is that the question is asked in a caring, sincere, and nonjudgmental manner. Often victims choose not to disclose the abuse. This should not discourage the clinician from asking the question, and demonstrating that the office is a safe place to discuss IPV is important. Often patients who initially denied the abuse will return to the office at a later date and disclose the abuse when they are ready to ask for assistance. If resources are available to pick up in the office examination rooms and bathrooms, victims have the option of getting assistance without telling anyone (National Advisory Committee, 2002 ⓒ).

Professional organizations recommend routine screening at annual examinations, during prenatal care, and when associated symptoms/conditions, "red flag conditions," are present (see Table 8-1). The American Academy of Pediatrics (AAP) recommends routinely asking mothers about IPV at well-child visits, well-teen visits, and when associated conditions are present (Committee on Child Abuse and Neglect, AAP, 1998 ⓒ) (see Table 8-2). Safety and privacy concerns exist about discussing IPV in front of children. The gravest concern is that the child will report the discussion about the abuse to the perpetrator and that the perpetrator will retaliate with further abuse to the victim. Minimal documentation should be done in the child's chart because the perpetrator, if a guardian, has access to the chart (Groves et al., 2002 ⓒ).

Table 8-3 Intimate Partner Violence Screening Questions and Tools

HITS (Sherin et al., 1998)
Written instrument
How often does your partner
1. Physically hurt you
2. Insult you or talk down to you
3. Threaten you with harm
4. Scream or curse at you

STaT (Paranjape et al., 2003)
1. Have you ever been in a relationship in which your partner has pushed or slapped you?
2. Have you ever been in a relationship in which your partner has thrown, broken, or punched things?
3. Have you ever been in a relationship in which your partner has threatened you with violence?

Woman Abuse Screening Tool (WAST) and WAST-Short (Brown et al., 2000)
1. In general, how would you describe your relationship? (a lot of tension, some tension, no tension)
2. Do you and your partner work out arguments with (great difficulty, some difficulty, no difficulty)?
3. Do arguments ever result in your feeling down or bad about yourself? (often, sometimes, never)
4. Do arguments ever result in hitting, kicking, or punching? (often, sometimes, never)
5. Do you ever feel frightened by what your partner says or does? (often, sometimes, never)
6. Has your partner ever abused you physically? (often, sometimes, never)
7. Has your partner ever abused you emotionally? (often, sometimes, never)

Partner Violence Screen (PVS) (Feldhaus et al., 1997)
1. Have you been hit, punched, or otherwise hurt by someone in the past year? If so, by whom?
2. Do you feel safe in your current relationship?
3. Is a partner from a previous relationship making you feel unsafe now?

Abuse Assessment Screen (AAS) (McFarlane and Parker, 1994)
1. Have you ever been emotionally or physically abused by your partner or someone important to you?
2. Within the last year, have you been hit, slapped, kicked, or otherwise physically hurt by someone?
   If yes, by whom?
   Husband, ex-husband, boyfriend, stranger, other
3. Within the past year, has anyone forced you to have sexual activities?
4. Are you afraid of your partner or anyone listed above?

General questions such as "How is your partner treating you and the kids?" or "Do you feel safe in your relationship with your partner?" are probably okay, but more in-depth questioning or resource sharing should be done in private. If IPV is identified, follow the same procedures as outline later. Helping the mother make decisions about her safety is the best way to assure the safety of the children. Mothers are often afraid that revealing IPV may put them at risk for losing their children (Zink et al., 2003).

Because child abuse occurs in 30% to 60% of homes with DV, the existence of child maltreatment in homes with DV should be assessed and, if suspected, reported according to state laws (Groves et al., 2002⊙).

Management of the Intimate Partner Violence Victim

Thinking of IPV management as requiring the same skills as the management of a chronic illness can help clinicians to be patient with a victim's timing and choices about seeking assistance. Victims weigh a number of issues, such as their financial independ-ence, their attachment to the abuser, their fear of the abuser, the severity of the abuse, their support systems, fear of losing the children, and the children's attachment to the abuser. A victim's awareness of the impact of the abuse on the children often compels the victim to seek help. Seeking a life free of abuse is a process. Some victims must leave the abuser, but some will not. Leaving the abuser is the most dangerous time for the victim. Matching interventions to the patient/victim's stage of coming to terms with his or her abusive relationship may be helpful (Table 8-4).

When a victim discloses abuse, the following steps are critical:

- Create a supportive and nonjudgmental environment
- Assess the impact of IPV on the victim's health
- Assess the victim's safety (Table 8-5)
- Share local DV agency pamphlets and crisis numbers or the names of counselors knowledgeable about IPV
- Respect the victim's choices
- Schedule a follow-up visit

Table 8-4 Stages of Change and Matched Clinician Management
for Patient/Victims of Intimate Partner Violence

Stage of Change: Definition + Substages	Physician Stage-matched Interventions
Precontemplation: patient/victim does not see the relationship as abusive	▪ Ask about IPV when there is an injury; ask how injury occurred. ▪ Ask during pregnancy. ▪ Ask routinely (annual exam and well-child/teen exams) and for red-flag symptoms and illnesses. ▪ Have and make pamphlets available. Do not spend time reviewing them in detail. ▪ Educate about the impact of IPV on the physical and mental health of the victim and her children ▪ Document suspicions about IPV. Assess safety.* If any risk factors are present, share your concern with the patient/victim and/or follow mandated reporting guidelines.
Contemplation: patient/victim sees the relationship as abusive and explores the pros and cons of different options to increase safety Recognition of nondisclosure	▪ Ask about IPV, as above. Despite nondisclosure, women want to be screened. ▪ Listen and watch for clues (hints or evidence of abuse). Victims are seeing if you are willing to discuss the abuse. ▪ Discuss observations about the abuser's controlling behavior: If you observe this, discuss your concern in private with the patient/victim. ▪ Have and make pamphlets available. Do not spend time reviewing them in detail. ▪ Educate about the impact of IPV on the physical and mental health of the victim and her children ▪ Document suspicions about IPV, Assess safety.* If any risk factors are present, share your concern with the patient/victim and/or follow mandated reporting guidelines.
Recognition of disclosure (with disclosure, add the following to other contemplation interventions)	▪ Affirm that abuse is occurring and that no one deserves to be abused. ▪ Review local IPV crisis numbers with the patient/victim. ▪ Offer to have the patient call the crisis number from a private room in your office. ▪ Make referrals for counseling to a counselor knowledgable about IPV for the patient and/or her children. ▪ Document subjective and objective findings. Consider reviewing safety plan* with the patient/victim, or have staff educated about IPV do this, or have the patient do this with the IPV agency.
Action: patient/victim takes steps to create safety	Continue to ask about abuse, affirm that no one deserves to be abused, assess safety, review local resources, and make referrals. Review safety plan.
Maintenance: patient/victim has created ongoing safety	Check on progress, affirm that no one deserves to be abused. Support positive changes, be nonjudgmental if patient returns to abusive/unsafe situation. Share concerns, and repeat steps from contemplation.

IPV, intimate partner violence
*Safety assessment/plan in Table 8-5.

Table 8-5   Safety Assessment and Plan

Safety Assessment
Ask about each of the following:
- Suicide/homicide risk (victim and abuser)
- Abuser's possession of weapons or threat to use weapons
- Drug and alcohol use (victim and abuser)
- Abuse of children
- Abuse of pets
- Escalating severity of abuse
- Increasing fear of abuser

Safety Plan
- Where to go
- Important documents (bank account, birth certificates, insurance records, etc.)
- Health care related: medications, children's immunization records
- Money, keys, clothes, kids' toys, etc.

Proper documentation is critical in case the victim decides to go to court. Include the following in the medical record:

- DV screen completed
- Objective, descriptive documentation on all identified signs of abuse. Record any noted injuries and include location, size, color, shape, and tenderness.
- Documentation of relevant clinical indicators (i.e., laboratory values, radiographs, diagnoses)
- Abuser name, date, time, and place that any injuries were sustained
- Objective descriptions of relevant patient behavior
- Relevant patient, family, and witness quotes
- Photographs to document injury. Consent for photographs must be obtained from adults.
- Referrals made and resources provided

Referrals might include the local DV agency or a counselor familiar with IPV. It may take the victim time to follow up on your referrals. In the meantime, schedule follow-up appointments at your office (National Advisory Committee, 2002 ; Zink et al., 2004a).

Identification and Management of Perpetrators

Research demonstrates that perpetrators will admit perpetration of IPV when questioned in the medical setting. However, perpetrators tend to minimize their violence, and some deny it altogether. Those who do appear for help need support in their decision, encouragement to take responsibility for their actions, and appropriate referrals (Coben and Friedman, 2002).

Be direct, starting with broad questions before becoming more specific. Ask how disagreements or situations of conflict are resolved, before inquiring whether hitting or isolating actions are part of this. For example, "Do you find you want to hit her to make her see sense?" Focus on the abusive conduct, not on the explanations or rationalizations, and make the connection between the perpetrator's behavior and the victim's injuries. For example, "When you hit her on Saturday night, you broke her nose. This is a criminal offence for which consequences follow. You need to make some changes, and we need to consider some things you could do." Help the perpetrator to see DV as a health care issue and to understand that it negatively affects him as well as his partner and children. Ask what effect he thinks his violence has on the victim and children and how it might change his relationship with them. Ask whether he wants the children to learn about violence in relationships from him.

Several approaches to working with perpetrators will help increase the safety of the victim.

- All information from the victim must be kept confidential from the abuser, even though he may be her husband and expect access. Information from third parties also should be kept confidential unless the victim specifically requests that information be shared. Even before sharing information with a perpetrator at the victim's request, the possible dangers and consequences should be reviewed with her.
- Discussion with the perpetrator about DV should never be done in the presence of the victim.
- Ways of discussing DV with perpetrators: Be clear that you are discussing DV as a health care issue. Unless the discussion is specifically covered in a reporting or duty-to-warn situation (fear of danger to self or others), your discussions can remain confidential. You are discussing a health care issue in the same way that it would be discussed with any patient and you are not there to be judgmental or to prosecute a crime.
- Focus on specific descriptions of the abuser's behaviors: "When you threw her to the couch" rather than "when you abused your wife," or "your use of physical force against your partner" rather than "your domestic violence."
- Use a direct, calm approach, and do not continue if the perpetrator becomes angry or objects. He is not ready to go further. You may simply want to let the perpetrator know that you are concerned and ready to discuss it further or make a referral whenever he is ready, and move back to the presenting medical issue. Be prepared that whatever you say may be misquoted back to the victim.

Treatment Options

Referral to accredited behavioral-change programs or to therapists who have expertise in domestic violence counseling may be appropriate for some perpetrators. However, the kinds of referrals that we are accustomed to making in marital disputes such as couples counseling are not useful and can escalate the violence. Couples counseling endangers the victim if she reveals information about the abuse during the sessions. It is unsafe for the victim to discuss the issues that concern her in the abuser's presence.

Anger management and alcoholism or drug-abuse programs deal with one aspect of the perpetrator's problem but do not get to the core. Many communities have batterers' intervention programs. What works and what does not is still unclear. No program approaches have shown themselves to be superior to other approaches. Your local DV agency can refer you to the local program for perpetrators and should have some idea of its quality.

The number of communities that have established and enforce consequences for abuse is steadily growing, as are responses in which law enforcement, courts, and domestic violence agencies form networks of cooperation for this purpose.

Managing the Abusive Couple

In family medicine, it is not unusual to see both the victim and the perpetrator as patients in your office. Confidentiality and safety are critical issues (Table 8-6). If it becomes too difficult to care for both, it

---

Table 8-6   Key Points for Managing the Abusive Couple

- Confidentiality: Maintain confidentiality about your discussions with the victim and abuser. Do not share information.
- Documentation: Document discussions/findings in the patient's chart. Do not document information learned from the abuser in the victim's chart or vice versa.
- Safety assessment of victim: Assess the victim for safety concerns. See safety assessment in Table 8-5. If safety becomes a concern, seek input from domestic violence service agencies.
- Manner of leaving information/messages: Discuss with each patient about how to leave messages about appointments or test results. Home okay, not okay? Cell phone? E-mail? You do not want to compromise the victim's safety by giving the abuser information that the victim does not want the perpetrator to have.
- Discuss abuse with the abuser only with the victim's permission. Before doing so, develop a safety plan with the victim.

From Ferris L, Norton P, Dunn E, Gort E, Degani N. Guidelines for managing domestic abuse when male and female partners are patients of the same physician. JAMA 1997;278:851–857.

---

may be best to refer either the victim or the perpetrator to a partner or another clinician (Ferris et al., 1997).

Managing the Child Exposed to Intimate Partner Violence

Helping the mother create safety for herself is the best way to help the children. Some communities offer programs for children exposed to IPV. These may be helpful. What works and what does not is not clearly understood. Some child-protection agencies are knowledgeable about DV, and some are not.

Mandatory reporting of cases in which children witness IPV as child maltreatment is controversial. Most states do not consider witnessing IPV as child abuse or neglect. Knowing the child maltreatment and reporting statute of one's state is the critical step for understanding reporting obligations. However, county officials and judges may vary in how they interpret the language (Groves et al., 2002 ©; Zink et al., 2002 ©).

Mandatory Reporting for Intimate Partner Violence

Most states (except California, Colorado, and Kentucky) do not require the clinician to report DV unless a weapon is used. In those states with mandatory reporting for DV, the follow-up procedures vary among counties and are dependent on the amount of training about DV provided to local law-enforcement and social-service staff (National Advisory Committee, 2002 ©).

Mandatory Reporting for Child Abuse/Neglect

Clinicians are mandated to report child maltreatment in all 50 states and the District of Columbia. Reports are generally made to a government department of social services, a child welfare agency, or the police. Immunity protection (usually civil and criminal) from prosecution under state and local laws and regulations for individuals making good-faith reports of suspected child abuse or neglect was outlined in the Child Abuse Prevention and Treatment Act of 1974.

Currently all jurisdictions provide immunity to reporters. The most commonly encountered limitation is the "good faith" reporting requirement. Immunity does not extend to reports made maliciously or in bad faith. This means that a clinician is protected from civil or criminal liability for filing a report made in good faith. Although these provisions may not prevent the filing of lawsuits, given the good-faith limitation in some states, they generally prevent negative outcomes for the clinician and other reporters. Clinicians who fail to report suspected child abuse may be held criminally or civilly liable under the state's reporting laws. In most states, it is a misdemeanor and involves a fine or a short time in the local jail (Zink et al., 2004b).

Material Available on Student Consult
Review Questions and Answers about Family Dynamics and Health

RESOURCES

National Domestic Violence Hotline (24-hour). 800-799-SAFE (7233). Translation services available for discussion about domestic violence.
Family Violence Prevention Fund. www.endabuse.org
National Resource Center on Domestic Violence. 800-537-2238 or www.ndvh.org

American Medical Association Domestic Violence Resources, www.ama-assn.org/ama/pub/article/3216-6827.html
American Medical Women's Association online CME course educates physicians about domestic violence. Physicians can earn two CME credits at no charge. www.dvcme.org

REFERENCES

American Medical Association. American Medical Association diagnostic and treatment guidelines for domestic violence. Arch Fam Med 1992;1:39–47.**C**

Brown JB, Lent B, Brett PJ, Sas G, Pederson LL. Development of the woman abuse screening tool for use in the family practice. Fam Med 1996;28:422–428.

Campbell JC. Health consequences of intimate partner violence. Lancet 2002;359:1331–1336.**B**

Coben JH, Friedman DI. Violence: Recognition, management, and prevention: Health care use by perpetrators of domestic violence. J Emerg Med 2002;22:313–317.

Coker AL, Davis KE, Arias I, et al. Physical and mental health effects of intimate partner violence for men and women. Am J Prev Med 2002;23:260–268.**B**

Committee on Child Abuse and Neglect, American Academy of Pediatrics. The role of pediatrician in recognizing and intervening on behalf of abused women. Pediatrics 1998;101:1091–1092.**C**

Feldhaus K, Koziol-McLain J, Amsbury H, Norton I, Lowenstein S, Abbott J. Accuracy of 3 brief screen questions for detecting partner violence in the emergency department. JAMA 1997;277:1357–1361.

Felitti V, Anda R, Nordenberg D, et al. Relationship of childhood abuse and household dysfunction to many of the leading causes of death in adults: The Adverse Childhood Experiences (ACE) Study. Am J Prev Med 1998;14:245–258.**B**

Ferris L, Norton P, Dunn E, Gort E, Degani N. Guidelines for managing domestic abuse when male and female partners are patients of the same physician. JAMA 1997;278:851–857.

Groves B, Augustyn M, Lee D, Sawires P. Identifying and Responding to Domestic Violence Consensus Recommendations for Child and Adolescent Health. San Francisco, Family Violence Prevention Fund, 2002. Available at www.endabuse.org. Accessed 9/27/05.**C**

Holtzworth-Munroe A, Meehan JC. Typologies of men who are maritally violent: Scientific and clinical implications. J Interpers Violence 2004;19:1369–1389.

Kitzmann K, Gaylord N, Holt A, Kenny E. Child witness to domestic violence: A meta-analytic review. J Consult Clin Psychol 2003;71:339–352.**B**

McFarlane J, Parker B. Preventing abuse during pregnancy: An assessment and intervention protocol. MCN Am J Matern Child Nurs 1994;19:321–324.

National Advisory Committee. National Consensus Guidelines: On Identifying and Responding to Domestic Violence Victimization in the Health Care Setting. San Francisco, Family Violence Prevention Fund, 2002. Available at www.endabuse.org. Accessed 9/27/05.**C**

National Center for Injury Prevention and Control. Costs of Intimate Partner Violence Against Women in the United States. Atlanta, Centers for Disease Control and Prevention, 2003.

Paranjape A, Sullivan L, Liebschutz J. STaT: A three question screen for intimate partner violence. J Women's Health 2003;12:233–239.

Sherin K, Sinacore J, Li X, Zitter R, Shakil A. HITS: A short domestic violence screening tool for use in a family practice setting. Fam Med 1998;30:508–512.

Tjaden P, Thoennes N. Extent, Nature, and Consequences of Intimate Partner Violence: Findings from the National Violence Against Women Survey. Washington, DC, National Institute of Justice and the Centers for Disease Control, 2000.**B**

U.S. Preventive Services Task Force. Screening for family and intimate partner violence: Recommendation statement. Ann Intern Med 2004;140:382–386.**C**

Zink T, Jacobson J, Elder N. Screening for domestic violence when the children are present: The victim's perspective. J Interpers Violence 2003;18:872–890.

Zink T, Elder N. Jacobson J, Klostermann B. Medical management of intimate partner violence considering the stages of change: Precontemplation and contemplation. Ann Fam Med 2004a;2:231–239.

Zink T, Kamine D, Musk L, Sill M, Field V, Putnam F. What are physicians' reporting requirements for children who witness domestic violence (DV)? Clin Pediatr 2004b;43:449–460.

Chapter

9

Patient Compliance

Lisa Dolovich, John W. Sellors, and R. Brian Haynes

KEY POINTS

1. Fifty percent is a representative compliance figure for many long-term therapies.
2. Differentiating whether compliance is intentional (e.g., testing out lower doses or discontinuation) or unintentional (e.g., mental deterioration, change in work schedule) can be helpful when developing strategies to improve compliance.
3. Communication with a patient before prescription to discuss the benefits, adverse effects, and use of a medication as well as communication after prescription to verify a patient's medication-taking behavior are important steps to improve medication compliance.
4. Family physicians are unable to detect poor compliers among their patients, because no stereotypic poor complier exists.
5. Dropping out of care is one of the most frequent and most severe forms of noncompliance, and so watching the appointment book and using practice aids such as a manual or

6. computerized ticker system can help identify noncompliance.
7. Provided that the treatment prescribed is known to be efficacious, failure of a patient to respond to treatment can be used as a readily available indicator of noncompliance.
8. Asking the patient directly about compliance can be a very valuable and practical way of determining the pattern of medication consumption.
9. Simple clear instructions are sufficient to improve compliance for short-term treatments.
10. Follow-up of nonattenders by telephone or mailed reminders and multifaceted strategies are needed to improve compliance for longer-term treatments.
11. The physician should be aware that patients often lie when they state that they have taken certain medicines.

[The physician] should keep aware of the fact that patients often lie when they state that they have taken certain medicines.

Hippocrates

Although physicians have dispensed medicines and potions through the centuries in vast quantities, it is only in recent years that there has been systematic examination occurred of whether patients actually take the treatment. It was perhaps to the patient's benefit in the past that little attention was paid to compliance, as poor compliance probably saved the patient's life on many occasions. Some treatments, especially the massive purges and bleeding of the eighteenth century and arsenic and hydrochloric acid of the twentieth century, certainly had lethal

rather than therapeutic potential. Recent incidents of concern with rofecoxib, hormone replacement therapy, nefazodone, and others demonstrate the complexities of balancing benefits and risks of drug interventions to ensure that, on balance, therapies will improve health when they are taken according to the intended management plan. On the whole, our armamentarium of useful treatments is sizable and expanding rapidly; low patient compliance stands squarely in the way of achieving the full benefit of modern therapy.

The extent of poor compliance is distressing. Fifty percent is a representative compliance figure for many long-term therapies. Only 51% to 78% of patients with newly diagnosed hypertension persisted with antihypertensive therapy 1 year after receiving a

---

Evidence levels Ⓐ Randomized, controlled trials (RCTs), meta-analyses, well-designed systematic reviews of RCTs.
Ⓑ Case-control or cohort studies, nonrandomized clinical trials, systematic reviews of studies other than RCTs, cross-sectional studies, retrospective studies, certain uncontrolled studies. Ⓒ Consensus statements, expert guidelines, usual practice, opinion.

new prescription (Caro et al., 1999 **B**; Morgan and Yan, 2004 **B**; Wogen et al., 2003 **B**). Fewer than 40% of patients continued to receive prescriptions for (S)-3-hydroxy-3-methylglutaryl-coenzyme A (HMG-CoA) reductase inhibitors 2 years after their first prescription (Jackevicius et al., 2002 **B**). Only about two thirds of those who continue under care take enough of their prescribed medication to achieve adequate blood pressure control (Haynes et al., 1978). If we look at compliance with lifestyle changes, such as diets and smoking cessation, the figures are considerably more dismal (Best and Block, 1979).

Added to this, physicians—even family physicians—are not good at estimating compliance levels in patients (Gilbert et al., 1980 **B**). Physicians have a strong tendency to overestimate the compliance of their own patients and are usually unable to predict which patients will comply with treatment.

This chapter reviews the practical methods of detecting poor compliance and strategies for improving it.

DEFINITIONS

The trend in medicine, and particularly in family medicine, is toward consumerism and a more democratic approach that involves the patient in medical decisions. The use of the word "compliance" has raised objections because it implies authoritarianism and anything but an equal relationship between physician and patient. Alternative terms such as *adherence* and *concordance* have been proposed to recognize that patients have primary control over the decision to take medications once prescribed and that the use of medications will be improved if patients are seen as partners in the development of treatment plans with their physicians (and other health care providers) (Marinker and Shaw, 2003; World Health Organization, 2003 **C**). Although we agree that the debate over terminology is helpful to gain better insight into how to improve the complex task of taking medications, and we sympathize with the views of those who oppose the term, we use *compliance* throughout this chapter because it is still the most widely used and recognized rubric.

Compliance has been defined as the extent to which a person's behavior (in terms of keeping appointments, taking medications, and executing lifestyle changes) coincides with medical advice (Sackett, 1976). Poor compliance is more difficult to define. What percentage of prescribed medication can a patient forget or omit before being classed as a poor complier? How are patients who take too much medication classified? One way of looking at the problem is to use patient outcomes as a guide. For instance, in hypertension studies, patients taking 80% or more of prescribed medication were consid-

ered compliant because this amount of medication was found to produce systematic blood pressure reduction (Sackett et al., 1975 **A**). Patients taking less than 75% of β-blockers prescribed after an acute myocardial infarction were more than 2.5 to 3 times more likely to die within 1 year (for men) or approximately 2 years (for women) (Gallagher et al., 1993 **B**; Horwitz et al., 1990 **B**).

Compliance also can be thought of in terms of intentionality. The deliberate not starting, stopping, or altering of a drug regimen by the patient has been called intentional noncompliance. Unintentional noncompliance may be due to forgetfulness or may be due to other patient characteristics such as changes in work shifts, mental deterioration, or inability to pay for medications (Royal Pharmaceutical Society of Great Britain, 1997 **C**). The differentiation of compliance behavior by intention can be helpful when trying to identify noncompliance or to develop strategies to improve compliance.

It makes sense that efforts directed at poor compliers should be concentrated on those not achieving therapeutic goals. This obviously leads to more efficient use of resources. However, some patients who respond to treatment may be doing so because of overprescribing rather than because of compliance. Should these patients be hospitalized or placed in some other situation in which compliance may be close to 100%, they may well run into serious effects of overdose.

FACTORS INFLUENCING COMPLIANCE

Many approaches, ranging from complex psychological theories to simplistic or intuitive ideas, have been taken to explain compliance behavior. None is entirely satisfactory, and many address only components of the complex undertaking of compliance; many are lamentably wrong (Leventhal and Cameron, 1987).

In looking at the many factors involved, a natural tendency exists for the physician to feel that poor compliance is the patient's fault; after all, it is the patient who must swallow the pill or keep the appointment. But many other factors leading up to the act of pill taking or returning for an appointment must be considered. For instance, what about the disease or condition being treated: Is it symptomatic or asymptomatic, life threatening or purely a nuisance? Is it an acute or chronic condition? What about the treatment itself: Is it efficacious? Does it have bothersome adverse effects? Is it unpleasant, inconvenient, or expensive? Is the medical environment conducive to regular follow-up? Does the physician inspire confidence in the treatment, or do certain attitudes interfere with compliance? Only some of these factors have an important effect on compliance behavior.

The Patient

General attributes such as age, gender, marital status, education, occupation, intelligence, race, religion, urban versus rural living, and economic status bear no consistent relation to compliance. Two exceptions are the very young and the very old, whose compliance characteristics tend to conform to those of their caregivers. Another exception is the presence of extreme disturbances in functioning and motivation in patients such as those with mental health disorders (DiMatteo et al., 2000🅑; World Health Organization, 2003🅒). Patients will regularly modify their medication regimens or dosing in an attempt to assert control over their health. As Conrad states, "People will change their medication practice, including stopping medication altogether, in order to test the existence or 'progress' of the disorder" (Conrad, 1985). Patients will not usually share the intentional changes they make to their medications unless they are asked about whether they have carried out any medication-taking "tests" within the context of a trusting physician-patient relationship. Numerous theories and models of behavior change have been generated or adapted to explain or better understand compliance. Perhaps the most widely held theory of compliance behavior, probably because of its intuitive appeal, is the communications approach (Leventhal and Zimmersman, 1984). In this model, it is proposed that patients generally do not know enough about their illness or treatment and that this ignorance leads to poor compliance. It follows that adequate instruction or message generation and reception, comprehension, and retention of the message should result in improved compliance. Although it appears that this is true for short-term treatments (<2 weeks in duration), knowledge on its own bears little relation to compliance with chronic disease regimens (Haynes, 1979).

Another popular theory looks at patient motivation and beliefs. By using the health-belief model, Becker (1976) argues that the likelihood of "all individuals undertaking a recommended health action depends on the perception of the level of personal susceptibility to the particular illness or condition; the degree of severity of the consequences of contracting the condition; the potential benefits or efficacy of the treatment in preventing or reducing susceptibility and/or severity; and the physical, psychological, financial, and other barriers or costs involved in initiating or continuing the treatment." The model also requires a stimulus or cue to action to trigger the appropriate behavior (compliance); this cue can be either internal (e.g., a symptom) or external (e.g., screening campaign or physician's advice). This model has been shown to have predictive value for some preventive and short-term therapeutic health actions, such as immunizations and medical regimens for acute disease, but the extent of its predictive value is modest at best (Janz and Becker, 1984).

The information-motivation-behavior skills model (IBM) is a more recently developed model that combines elements from previous literature and models to describe the influences on behavior change (Fisher and Fisher, 1992; Fisher et al., 1996🅑). This model proposes that information and motivation influence behavioral skills (tools and strategies to perform compliance behavior) and that all three of these elements directly influence behavior change. Initial reports evaluating interventions constructed by using this model have shown some promise in influencing behavior change. The model has high face validity; however, more studies are needed to better understand how well the model explains the full extent of behavior change across a variety of conditions.

The transtheoretical stages-of-change model maintains that behavior progresses through five stages—precontemplation, contemplation, preparation, action, and maintenance—and that a decisional balance exists between the pros and cons of the behavior (Prochaska and DiClemente, 1992). It follows that all patients may not be at the same stage of readiness for change in compliance (Keefe et al., 2000🅑; Prochaska et al., 1998), so it is more helpful to identify their highest priority and work on this one behavior. Controlled trials have demonstrated that interventions based on the stages-of-change model can improve health behaviors such as increased exercise in older women (Conn et al., 2003🅐) and smoking cessation (Velicer et al., 1999). Assessment of the stage of change of a noncompliant patient should facilitate counseling that is appropriately tailored to move him or her toward action (Table 9-1) (Willey 1998; Willey et al., 1999).

Other models have been studied, including the behavioral-learning model, which is based on cognitive and social learning theory, and the self-regulating model. As yet, no model adequately explains a person's compliance behavior or gives a clear rationale for modifying it (Haynes et al., 1982).

The behavior models help clinicians understand compliance behavior a bit better, but for helping patients to follow prescribed treatments better the strategies from studies showing successful interventions in the section on prevention and treatment of poor compliance may be of more practical use for helping patients follow prescribed treatment.

The Disease

With few exceptions, disease factors are relatively unimportant as determinants of compliance. Psychiatric patients with schizophrenia, paranoid features, and personality disorders are less compliant

Table 9-1 Behavior-change Strategies for Improving Compliance

Stage	Characteristics
Precontemplation	Resistant to taking medication, fearful, in denial, defensive, misinformed, or demoralized
Contemplation	Ambivalent about taking the medication, concerned about the cons of medication use, lacking commitment to the regimen
Preparation	Understands the pros of taking the medication as directed; planning to improve adherence soon
Action	Recently began taking medication as directed, but this new behavior may still be an effort
Maintenance	Taking medication as directed for ≥6 months, "Now it's easy for me"
Relapse risk	Has been taking the medication as directed for 6 months, but "tests" the degree to which adherence is necessary by taking "drug holidays"

than are other psychiatric patients—a fact that probably reduces the compliance of psychiatric patients as a whole below that of patients with nonpsychiatric disorders.

No relation has been demonstrated between the severity of symptoms and compliance. Surprisingly, the more symptoms a patient reports, the lower his or her compliance is likely to be. Conversely, increasing disability produced by a disease appears to be associated with better compliance. Whether this is a result of increased severity of disease or specifically the result of the *increased supervision* that often accompanies increased disability has not been sorted out.

Chronic diseases requiring long-term treatment have been clearly shown to result in increasingly poor compliance. This fact is of great clinical importance in such potentially serious diseases as tuberculosis and hypertension and is more likely to be a function of the duration of the *treatment* regimen than the duration of the *disease* itself.

The Regimen

Generally speaking, the greater the behavioral demands of a treatment, the poorer the compliance.

Regimens requiring changes in lifestyle, such as dieting, exercising, and stopping harmful habits, result in much poorer compliance than does simply taking pills, because of the substantially greater behavioral changes needed.

Conventional wisdom and common sense suggest that the greater the number of drugs or treatments prescribed for a patient, the greater the probability of poor compliance. However, recent studies have found that patients prescribed (and dispensed) more cardiovascular medications had better medication compliance (based on an examination of their pharmacy records) (Shalansky and Levy, 2002 Ⓑ; Grant et al., 2004 Ⓑ). Likely a set of circumstances exists under which compliance does improve with more medications, and more research is needed to clarify this issue. Despite these recent reports, simplifying the treatment regimen to reduce the number of medications a patient is taking is one of the most important strategies to improve compliance.

Compliance decreases when the frequency of dosing increases. Although no differences in compliance have been identified between once- and twice-daily dosing, compliance decreases with 3- or 4-times daily dosing (Claxton et al., 2001 Ⓑ; Eisen et al., 1990 Ⓑ; Pullar et al., 1988 Ⓑ).

Alternative oral medications for the same condition do not appear to result in substantial differences in compliance, but a difference may be found for different problems. For example, Closson and Kikugawa (1975) found a range from 17% compliance with antacids to 89% with cardiac drugs.

The injection of long-acting preparations, such as benzathine penicillin for acute streptococcal pharyngitis and rheumatic fever prophylaxis, long-acting phenothiazines for schizophrenia, and streptomycin for tuberculosis, has been shown to be acceptable to patients and more effective than oral preparations.

The cost of treatment is an important barrier to compliance for many people (Gregoire et al., 2002 Ⓑ; Tamblyn et al., 2001 Ⓑ; Tseng et al., 2004 Ⓑ). However, a complete understanding of the effect of cost is not as obvious as it might first appear. For instance, one study showed that hospital admissions increased among psychiatric outpatients given drugs at nominal cost compared with admissions for a group paying regular prices (Cody and Robinson, 1977 Ⓑ). Patients without full drug coverage are more likely to use less medication, switch medications, use samples, and report difficulty paying for medications (Tamblyn et al., 2001 Ⓑ; Tseng et al., 2004 Ⓑ).

The Physician

The physician is obviously in a key position to influence compliance. For example, if the frequency of dose affects compliance, then by the very act of prescribing a medication to be taken 4 times a day, the physician is potentially reducing compliance below the level achievable with a single daily dose.

More complex than the mechanics of prescribing, however, is the interaction between physician and patient. Patients are more likely to comply with treatment if their expectations are met by the visit and if they are well satisfied with their care (Francis et al., 1969; Kincey et al., 1975). The concept of a personal physician or the feeling of knowing a physician well also has been associated with increased compliance (Ettlinger and Freeman, 1981❸). Dissecting the physician-patient relationship and measuring the factors that result in increased satisfaction are not easy. This is demonstrated in one study in which some patients felt that they knew their physician well after only one visit, whereas others felt that they still did not know their physicians after as many as 14 visits (Ettlinger and Freeman, 1981❸). Communication with a patient before prescription to discuss the benefits, adverse effects, and use of a medication as well as after prescription to verify a patient's medication-taking behavior are important steps to improve medication compliance (Roberts and Volberding, 1999❸).

DETECTION OF POOR COMPLIANCE

Clinical Judgment

Most of us would like to believe that a good physician can detect poor compliance in patients; surely, this goes along with clinical judgment. Unfortunately, studies have shown that this is not the case: Using clinical judgment has been shown to be no better than flipping a coin as a detection method. The first studies demonstrating this were carried out in specialty settings and with physicians who did not have an ongoing relationship with patients. Unfortunately, the hope that family physicians with their ongoing relationships with their patients might be in a better position to make predictions also has been dispelled. Not only were family physicians unable to detect poor compliers among their patients, but also the length of time that they had known their patients had no effect on their ability to predict (Gilbert et al., 1980❸).

The emphasis on the inaccuracy of clinical judgment is important in that it serves to direct us to alternative approaches to detect poor compliance.

Monitoring Attendance

As mentioned previously, more than 50% of hypertensive patients stop visiting their physicians within a year of starting treatment, and those who do not appear for follow-up appointments are unlikely to be compliers with treatment. Many physicians are unable to detect this type of noncompliance because their appointment systems are inadequate or because the patients do not make follow-up appointments.

It follows, then, that an important method of detecting poor compliance is to watch the appointment book and to use practice aids such as a manual or computerized tickler system. Although no guarantee exists that patients who keep appointments will comply with treatment, no doubt those who do not appear for follow-up will not be in a position to comply with treatment. The importance of monitoring attendance cannot be overstressed: Dropping out of care is one of the most frequent and most severe forms of noncompliance (Stephenson et al., 1993).

Response to Treatment

Provided that the treatment prescribed is known to be efficacious, failure of a patient to respond to treatment can be used as a readily available indicator of compliance levels. For example, high compliance was associated with a 10% lower total A1c in patients on a stable medication regimen for type 2 diabetes relative to patients with low compliance (Krapek et al., 2004❸). However, this method of assessing compliance is not infallible. For example, patients who appear to respond to treatment may do so because they were misdiagnosed and do not have the condition of interest or because their physicians' overprescribing is compensating for their poor compliance. Nevertheless, from the compliance perspective at least, concern is less necessary for patients who have reached the therapeutic goal. Conversely, patients not showing a response to treatment will include those who genuinely do not respond to therapy or who have been prescribed inadequate amounts and will also include a high proportion of poor compliers or noncompliers. If therapeutic response is suboptimal, then noncompliance should be considered and explored as a possible reason for lack of response to treatment before changing management strategies.

Asking the Patient

Although it is not always reliable, asking the patient directly about compliance can be a very valuable and practical way of determining the pattern of medication consumption (see Table 9-2). When asked directly, about half of noncompliant patients will admit to missing at least some medication (Haynes et al., 1980❸; Stephenson et al., 1993). One can be assured that it is highly improbable that a compliant patient will admit to poor compliance, so patients admitting to missing medication have a very high likelihood of being poor compliers. The converse is not true, however, as even under optimal interview conditions about half of noncompliant patients will deny the fact. Patients who admit to missing medication generally overestimate the amount of medication they do take. In one study, the average overestimate was in the region of 20% (Haynes et al., 1980 Ⓑ).

It must be emphasized that the method of questioning is of paramount importance. Asking in a threatening or belligerent manner will result in reflex denial. Approaching the patient with a face-saving, nonthreatening, nonjudgmental question will yield a higher proportion of accurate responses. One way of doing this is to use an approach such as the following: "Many people find it difficult to remember to take medicines: During the past week, have you missed any of your pills?" Taking into account the tendency to overestimate compliance, admission of any noncompliance is associated with an average compliance rate of less than 80% (Haynes et al., 1980 Ⓑ). A similar approach is to ask the four questions based on the simplified Morisky measure of medication adherence (Morisky et al., 1986) (see Table 9-2). If the use of either method of questioning results in the patient answering "yes" to any of the questions asked, then the clinician has the opportunity to engage in further dialogue with the patient to better understand factors associated with noncompliance.

The methods of detecting low compliance described so far can be easily applied in any treatment setting and, if applied with care, will detect the majority of poor compliers. The methods outlined in Table 9-2 may be of help in detecting some of the remainder.

Counting Pills

As a quantitative estimate of compliance over a certain period, pill counts can be relatively reliable so long as they are carried out in the patient's home with strict attention to bookkeeping (Haynes et al., 1980 Ⓑ). Unless the count can be carried out in such a manner that the patient is unaware of what is going on, it becomes a one-time-only procedure. It follows that whereas pill counts are very important research tools, they are not very practical for most clinical situations. It can be reasoned that using pill counts in the office or clinic will result in a bias in the direction of overestimating compliance, in that patients will consciously or unconsciously bring only some of their unused pills with them, giving the appearance that they have taken more of the medication than is actually the case. It is virtually impossible for the bias to go in the opposite direction unless the patient is receiving the same prescriptions from two or more physicians at the same time. In general, pill counts give higher estimates of compliance than do quantitative drug assays and lower (but more accurate) estimates than do patient self-reports or administrative pharmacy claims data (Grymonpre et al., 1998 Ⓑ).

Pharmacy Refill Records

Pharmacy refill records can be used to identify patterns of dispensed medications as a proxy for medication use. These records are especially helpful to detect whether a patient may have stopped taking a long-term medication (Jackevicius et al., 2002 Ⓑ; Morgan and Yan, 2004 Ⓑ; Pilon et al., 2001 Ⓑ; Rijcken et al., 2004 Ⓑ) or did not stop an old medication when a new one was prescribed, especially in cases in which patients cannot remember this information. Pharmacies cannot provide complete medication refill history profiles without the patient's permission; however, pharmacists often provide the date of the previous refill when requesting renewals from the physician's office, and

---

Table 9-2   A Simple Method to Detect Noncompliance

Asking the Patient
The easiest way to detect medication noncompliance is to ask the patient
About 40% of noncompliant patients will admit to missing at least some medications
If patients admit to noncompliance, you can believe them
Patients admitting to poor compliance are most responsive to attempts to improve compliance

How to Ask: One Question
Use a matter-of-fact, nonjudgmental, nonthreatening manner
Use an introduction that allows a patient to save face: "Many people find it difficult to
   remember to take medicines. During the past week, have you missed *any* of your pills?"   Yes ☐   No ☐

How to Ask: Four Questions (Risk Increases with Number of Positive Responses) (Morisky, 1986)

Do you ever forget to take your medicine?	Yes ☐	No ☐
Are you careless at times about taking your medicine?	Yes ☐	No ☐
When you feel better, do you sometimes stop taking your medicine?	Yes ☐	No ☐
Sometimes if you feel worse when you take the medicine, do you stop taking it?	Yes ☐	No ☐

this information can be useful in determining whether the patient appears to be taking his or her medication on schedule. This is an indirect measure, however, and cannot assure whether a patient is actually taking a medication. The patient could, for example, be sharing or hoarding the medications.

Drug Levels

A laboratory test to detect the presence or absence of good compliance is an unrealistic dream in the case of most drugs. For some drugs, however, especially those with long serum half-lives resulting in relatively steady serum levels, the measurement of serum levels can be an extremely useful indicator of compliance. The best examples of this are digoxin and phenytoin, for which plasma levels have been used successfully both to monitor compliance and to improve it through feedback to the patient. Other drugs commonly measured in this way are anticonvulsants, theophylline, tricyclic antidepressants, lithium, and a variety of cardiac drugs. The caution is, however, that a great deal of individual variation is found in drug absorption, metabolism, and excretion. In addition, serum levels of drugs with short half-lives indicate only how recently a dose was taken and give no information on long-term compliance.

Drug levels in urine have also been used as compliance indicators. For instance, the presence or absence of penicillin can be easily detected by observing inhibition of growth of a microorganism, *Sarcina lutea*. Although these methods and others involving inactive markers such as riboflavin and carbon 14 have been used in research, they are not practical methods for the clinician. What is more, as a measure of compliance, single qualitative assessments of urine samples have been shown to be inferior to simply asking the patient (Haynes et al., 1980 **B**).

PREVENTION AND TREATMENT OF POOR COMPLIANCE

Misconceptions

Before discussing prevention and treatment, it is worthwhile to reexamine some popular misconceptions about compliance. The first misconception is that a good clinician can identify poor compliers, as no stereotypic poor complier exists (Vik et al., 2004 **B**). This is very important, because restricting prevention and treatment strategies to patients thought to be potentially poor compliers must result in neglect of a large number of patients who need attention as well as unnecessary attention to some patients who do not.

Another popular and important misconception is that all that stops patients from being near-perfect compliers is their ignorance of either the condition being treated or the treatment being used. Although some evidence indicates that written instructions help improve compliance for short-term regimens, even mastery learning, in which patients were given detailed step-by-step instruction on hypertension, had no beneficial effect on long-term compliance (Sackett et al., 1975 **A**). The belief that it is possible to scare a patient into complying with treatment also has been dispelled (Leventhal et al., 1967; Logan, 1978). A survey of primary care physicians showed that the methods they used to improve compliance were predominantly those that have been found lacking. Methods that have been shown to be effective were not generally applied. The transtheoretical stages-of-change model of readiness to change behavior also can be applied to a physician's own counseling behavior and predicts that unless realistic goals are set for improving monitoring and follow-up of compliance, the physician may become frustrated and slip into inaction (precontemplation) (Prochaska and DiClemente, 1992). Changing the long-term behavior of physicians to manage compliance successfully cannot be done by simply informing or instructing them about efficacious interventions (Evans et al., 1986 **A**; Haynes et al., 1984 **B**).

Prevention

The main thrust in the prevention of poor compliance is to remove barriers to compliance (see Table 9-3). Preventing patients from dropping out of care is of primary importance. Longer waiting times are associated with higher no-show rates (Rockart and Hoffman, 1969), so that one aim is to keep patient waiting time to a minimum. Individual appointments at mutually convenient times help achieve this goal. Ensuring that patients leave the office with a specific time for a future appointment rather than with instructions to call for an appointment in, for example, 3 months, makes detection of those who do drop out much easier.

Simplifying the treatment regimen will remove another barrier to compliance. An essential element of this approach is to eliminate unnecessary medications. In addition, medications should be prescribed that should to be taken as few times daily as possible. The frequency of dosing with many drugs can be reduced below usually prescribed levels with no reduction in efficacy. For example, tricyclic antidepressants can be given as a single bedtime dose, thus reducing dosing frequency and timing side effects so that they occur mainly during sleep. A final strategy is titration to the least amount of medication necessary to achieve the therapeutic goal. Arranging for a comprehensive medication review carried out by a clinical pharmacist or clinical pharmacologist may generate recommendations on how to simplify a patient's medication regimen (Dolovich and Levine, 1997Ⓑ; Hanlon et al., 1996Ⓐ; Sellors et al., 2003Ⓐ).

It has been shown that patients who believe that they are actively involved in their own care are better compliers than are those who do not (Schulman, 1979Ⓑ). Studies also have shown that negotiating care with the patient rather than simply dictating or prescribing it results in better compliance (Eisenthal et al., 1979Ⓑ; Tracy, 1977). Encouraging patients to take greater responsibility for their care by asking more questions of their physicians results in improved attendance (Roter, 1977Ⓐ). It follows that encouraging patients to participate in and take more responsibility for their own care is another strategy for preventing poor compliance, and it not only makes scientific sense but also is consistent with trends in physician-patient relationships.

Treatment

Dropping out of care constitutes a compliance crisis (Table 9-3). Mail and telephone reminders to increase attendance, at least in the short term, can help prevent dropout (Macharia et al., 1992Ⓐ). If the patient does fail to attend, it calls for prompt action by the receptionist or office nurse to reschedule (Takala et al., 1979Ⓐ). A simple method of identifying those patients for whom compliance is important (e.g., the use of chart stickers or special symbols on the written or computerized day sheet) may make the receptionist's task simpler. Personal contact by the physician and the use of outreach services such as public health nurses are other ways of "treating" persistent nonattendance. Most successful compliance interventions have two features in common: increased supervision of, or attention to, the patient; and intentional reinforcement of, reward for, or encouragement of compliance (Haynes et al., 1987).

Low compliance is a chronic condition without a "one-shot" cure, so treatment of poor compliance must continue as long as the regimen of prescribed treatment. To make matters worse, none of the following has improved compliance when tested alone: special learning packages (Rawlings et al., 2003Ⓐ; Sackett et al., 1975Ⓐ) and pamphlets (Swain and Steckel, 1981); special unit-dose reminder pill packaging (Becker et al., 1986Ⓐ); counseling about medication and compliance by a health educator (Levine et al., 1979Ⓐ) or by nurses (Morice and Wrench, 2001Ⓐ; Shepard et al., 1979Ⓑ); visits to patients' homes (Johnson et al., 1978Ⓐ) or pharmacists (Nazareth et al., 2001Ⓐ; Stevens et al., 2002Ⓐ); provision of care at the worksite (Sackett et al., 1975Ⓐ); self-monitoring of blood pressure (Johnson et al., 1978Ⓐ); tangible rewards (Shepard et al., 1979Ⓑ); or group discussions (Shepard et al., 1979Ⓑ). Although these tactics have not worked alone, many have been part of more complex interventions that have been successful; whether they are essential parts of these complex interventions or just along for the ride is difficult to say (McDonald et al., 2002Ⓐ; Von Korff et al., 2003Ⓑ).

A variety of inducements to comply have been used, including feedback of blood-pressure response to hypertensive patients either by the provider (McKenney et al., 1973; Takala et al., 1979Ⓐ) or by patients' taking their own blood pressure (Haynes et al., 1976Ⓐ; Nessman et al., 1980Ⓐ); small tangible rewards for improved compliance or therapeutic response or both (Haynes et al., 1976Ⓐ; Shepard et al., 1979Ⓑ; Swain and Steckel, 1981); medication tailored to daily schedules to decrease forgetting and inconvenience (Haynes et al., 1976Ⓐ; Logan et al., 1979Ⓐ); encouragement of family support (Levine et al., 1979Ⓐ); stimulation of self-help through group support and discussion (Levine et al., 1979Ⓐ; Nessman et al., 1980Ⓐ); negotiation of a brief written contract with the patient to improve health behavior (Swain and Steckel, 1981); and calling back patients who miss appointments (Bass et al., 1986Ⓐ; Peterson et al., 1984Ⓐ; Sellors et al., 1997Ⓐ; Takala et al., 1979Ⓐ).

It is important to note here that many individuals other than physicians have taken an effective part in this process. Nurses, pharmacists, health educators, a psychologist, and even an individual with no formal health training played a key role in successful interventions.

Table 9-3   Keys to Successful Compliance Management

Detection
Monitor attendance and achievement of the therapeutic goal
Ask the patient
Ask the pharmacist

Prevention
Make appointments convenient
Simplify the regimen
Give clear instructions, preferably written
Engage the patient as an active participant
Use telephone or mail reminders

Treatment
Follow up nonattenders
Increase attention and supervision
Use cuing, feedback, and positive reinforcement
Collaborate with pharmacist on strategies and patient follow-up
Schedule frequency of visits to compliance need
Involve spouse or other partner
Maintain compliance interventions as long as compliance is desirable

In summary, the treatment of poor compliance involves many approaches. For short-term treatments, simple clear instructions are sufficient (Al Eidan et al., 2002🅐; McDonald et al., 2002🅐). For longer-term treatments, follow-up of nonattenders by telephone or mailed reminders must occur. In addition, the practitioner must increase the attention paid to poor compliers and provide rewards or positive reinforcement for good compliance that could include simple praise and extending the time between appointments for those responding to treatment. Inui and colleagues (Inui et al., 1976🅐) showed that such maneuvers can be successfully incorporated into regular practice by simply focusing on compliance for a few moments during each encounter, not only to emphasize the importance of following the regimen but also to tailor medication to daily routines. This can be accomplished without necessarily prolonging the visit. It is most important that all compliance interventions applied to noncompliers be maintained for as long as treatment is prescribed.

Ethical Issues

Am I my brother's keeper?

Genesis 4:9

This question highlights the dilemma in which physicians may find themselves when they are pressed to extend their compliance-improving strategies beyond a simple office visit.

The decision to apply tactics deliberately designed to change the compliance of patients should meet several ethical standards that apply to all therapeutic interventions (Levine, 1980). First, the diagnosis must be correct. Second, the therapy to be complied with must be of established efficacy. Third, neither the illness nor the proposed treatment should be trivial. Fourth, the patient must be an informed and willing partner in any attempt to maximize his or her compliance. Finally, the method used to improve compliance must be of demonstrated effectiveness.

After applying these standards and embarking on a course of treatment, it makes no sense, ethically or otherwise, for the physician to abandon a patient at the first sign of poor compliance. Most physicians consider it unethical to withhold efficacious treatment from a patient with a serious physical disease. Why then should it be ethical *to* consider withholding treatment when the condition is noncompliance?

Future Trends

The advent of the personal computer has resulted in increasing use of microcomputers in physicians' offices. Although initial applications have been for business purposes, the computerization of appointment systems and, increasingly, health records affords potential for monitoring patient compliance and assisting in the implementation of reminder systems that allow enhanced management of the poor complier (Hunt et al., 1998🅐).

Computerized appointment systems make it possible to provide patients with appointment times for long periods ahead and can easily be modified to flag nonattenders and produce automatic reminders. The ability to record age, gender, and diagnoses makes it possible to design a system that can improve provider compliance with screening and preventive maneuvers (Bypass et al., 1988🅑). Medication databases that store prescribing information can form the basis of a system that monitors whether patients are at least requesting prescription refill on time (Steiner et al., 1988🅑). Automated telephone messaging technology, Internet-based computer programs, and other new technologies are under development to help improve compliance. The potential is great, but it will require both effort and expenditure by physicians or patients to make it work.

What of other advancements? The technology that brought us the efficacious treatments is also helping with compliance: drugs with long half-lives, long-acting parenteral preparations, conjunctival inserts, and continuous transcutaneous absorption systems. The burgeoning use of high technology could result in an artificial pancreas that will not only dispense insulin but also adjust the dose according to blood levels. What is to stop the development of implanted arterial pressure sensors with automatic dispensing of parenteral antihypertensives? These thoughts make concerns about telephoning nonattenders seem trifling.

CONCLUSION

In dealing with compliance, we have consciously concentrated on compliance with medication, emphasizing long-term medications. This is not because we think that compliance with short-term medications is inconsequential or that no problem of compliance exists with lifestyle or other behavioral changes. On the contrary, both these areas are very important, and noncompliance with lifestyle changes is a monster not to be tamed.

It is our hope that we have raised the level of compliance consciousness in the reader. Awareness of the problem and the difficulties in detecting it is essential before any of these practical treatments can be instituted.

The past two decades have brought the therapist together with the patient, the family, and other members of the health care team in jointly working toward the full effectiveness of potent treatments.

The rewards of this alliance are great: reduction of morbidity, disability, and preventable deaths. The family physician is in an ideal position to help create and share in these rewards.

REFERENCES

Al Eidan FA, McElnay JC, Scott MG, McConnell JB. Management of *Helicobacter pylori* eradication: The influence of structured counselling and follow-up. Br J Clin Pharmacol 2002;53:163–171.🅐

Bass MJ, McWhinney IR, Donner A. Do family physicians need medical assistants to detect and manage hypertension? Can Med Assoc J 1986;134:1247–1255.🅐

Becker LA, Glanz K, Sobel E, et al. A randomized trial of special packaging of antihypertensive medications. J Fam Pract 1986;22:35–36.🅐

Becker MH. Sociobehavioral determinants of compliance. In Sackett DL, Haynes RB, eds. Compliance with Therapeutic Regimens. Baltimore: Johns Hopkins University Press, 1976, pp 40–49.

Best JA, Block M. Compliance in the control of cigarette smoking. In Haynes RB, Taylor DW, Sackett DL, eds. Compliance in Health Care. Baltimore: Johns Hopkins University Press, 1979, pp 202–222.

Bypass P, Hanlon PW, Hanlon LC, Marsh VM, Greenwood BM. Microcomputer management of a vaccine trial. Comput Biol Med 1988;18:179–193.🅑

Caro JJ, Salas M, Speckman JL, Raggio G, Jackson JD. Persistence with treatment for hypertension in actual practice. CMAJ 1999;160:31–37.🅑

Claxton AJ, Cramer J, Pierce C. A systematic review of the associations between dose regimens and medication compliance. Clin Ther 2001;23:1296–1310.🅑

Closson RG, Kikugawa CA. Noncompliance varies with drug class. Hospitals 1975;49:89–93.

Cody J, Robinson AM. The effect of low-cost maintenance medication on the rehospitalization of schizophrenic outpatients. Am J Psychiatry 1977;134:73–76.🅑

Conn VS, Burks KJ, Minor MA, Mehr DR. Randomized trial of 2 interventions to increase older women's exercise. Am J Health Behav 2003;27:380–388.🅐

Conrad P. The meaning of medications: Another look at compliance. Soc Sci Med 1985;20:29–37.

DiMatteo MR, Lepper HS, Croghan TW. Depression is a risk factor for noncompliance with medical treatment: Meta-analysis of the effects of anxiety and depression on patient adherence. Arch Intern Med 2000;160: 2101–2107.🅑

Dolovich L, Levine M. A medication assessment clinic. Can J Hosp Pharm 1997;50:182–184.🅑

Eisen SA, Miller DK, Woodward RS, Spitznagel E, Przybeck TR. The effect of prescribed daily dose frequency on patient medication compliance. Arch Intern Med 1990;150:1881–1884.🅑

Eisenthal S, Emery R, Lazare A, Udin H. "Adherence" and the negotiated approach to patienthood. Arch Gen Psychiatry 1979;36:393–398.🅑

Ettlinger PR, Freeman GK. General practice compliance study: Is it worth being a personal doctor? Br Med J (Clin Res Ed) 1981;282:1192–1194.🅑

Evans CE, Haynes RB, Birkett NJ, et al. Does a mailed continuing education program improve physician performance? Results of a randomized trial in antihypertensive care. JAMA 1986;255:501–504.🅐

Fisher JD, Fisher WA. Changing AIDS-risk behavior. Psychol Bull 1992;111:455–474.

Fisher JD, Fisher WA, Misovich SJ, Kimble DL, Malloy TE. Changing AIDS risk behavior: Effects of an intervention emphasizing AIDS risk reduction information, motivation, and behavioral skills in a college student population. Psychol Bull 1996;15:114–123.🅑

Francis V, Korsch BM, Morris MJ. Gaps in doctor-patient communication: Patients' response to medical advice. N Engl J Med 1969;280:535–540.

Gallagher EJ, Viscoli CM, Horwitz RI. The relationship of treatment adherence to the risk of death after myocardial infarction in women. JAMA 1993;270: 742–744.🅑

Gilbert JR, Evans CE, Haynes RB, Tugwell P. Predicting compliance with a regimen of digoxin therapy in family practice. Can Med Assoc J 1980;123:119–122.🅑

Grant RW, O'Leary KM, Weilburg JB, Singer DE, Meigs JB. Impact of concurrent medication use on statin adherence and refill persistence. Arch Intern Med 2004;164:2343–2348.🅑

Gregoire JP, Moisan J, Guibert R, et al. Determinants of discontinuation of new courses of antihypertensive medications. J Clin Epidemiol 2002;55:728–735.🅑

Grymonpre RE, Didur CD, Montgomery PR, Sitar DS. Pill count, self-report, and pharmacy claims data to measure medication adherence in the elderly. Ann Pharmacother 1998;32:749–754.🅑

Hanlon JT, Weinberger M, Samsa GP, et al. A randomized, controlled trial of a clinical pharmacist intervention to improve inappropriate prescribing in elderly outpatients with polypharmacy. Am J Med 1996;100: 428–437.🅐

Haynes RB. Determinants of compliance: The disease and the mechanics of treatment. In Haynes RB, Taylor DW, Sackett DL, eds. Compliance in Health Care. Baltimore: John Hopkins University Press, 1979, pp 49–62.

Haynes RB, Davis DA, McKibbon A, Tugwell P. A critical appraisal of the efficacy of continuing medical education. JAMA 1984;251:61–64.🅑

Haynes RB, Mattson ME, Chobanian AV, et al. Management of patient compliance in the treatment of hypertension. Hypertension 1982;4:415–423.

Haynes RB, Sackett DL, Gibson ES, et al. Improvement of medication compliance in uncontrolled hypertension. Lancet 1976;1:1265–1268.🅐

Haynes RB, Sackett DL, Taylor DW. Practical management of low compliance with antihypertensive therapy: A guide for the busy practitioner. Clin Invest Med 1978;1:175–180.

Haynes RB, Taylor DW, Sackett DL, Gibson ES, Bernholz CD, Mukherjee J. Can simple clinical measurements detect patient noncompliance? Hypertension 1980;2:757–764.[B]

Haynes RB, Wang E, Gomes MD. A critical review of interventions to improve compliance with prescribed medications. Patient Educ Couns 1987;10:155–166.

Horwitz RI, Viscoli CM, Berkman L, et al. Treatment adherence and risk of death after a myocardial infarction. Lancet 1990;336:542–545.[B]

Hunt DL, Haynes RB, Hanna SE, Smith K. Effects of computer-based clinical decision support systems on physician performance and patient outcomes: A systematic review. JAMA 1998;280:1339–1346.[A]

Inui TS, Yourtee EL, Williamson JW. Improved outcomes in hypertension after physician tutorials: A controlled trial. Ann Intern Med 1976;84:646–651.[A]

Jackevicius CA, Mamdani M, Tu JV. Adherence with statin therapy in elderly patients with and without acute coronary syndromes. JAMA 2002;288:462–467.[B]

Janz NK, Becker MH. The Health Belief Model: A decade later. Health Educ Q 1984;11:1–47.

Johnson AL, Taylor DW, Sackett DL, Dunnett CW, Shimizu AG. Self-recording of blood pressure in the management of hypertension. Can Med Assoc J 1978;119:1034–1039.[A]

Keefe FJ, Lefebvre JC, Kerns RD, et al. Understanding the adoption of arthritis self-management: Stages of change profiles among arthritis patients. Pain 2000;87:303–313.[B]

Kincey J, Bradshaw P, Ley P. Patients' satisfaction and reported acceptance of advice in general practice. J R Coll Gen Pract 1975;25:558–566.

Krapek K, King K, Warren SS, et al. Medication adherence and associated hemoglobin A1c in type 2 diabetes. Ann Pharmacother 2004;38:1357–1362.[B]

Leventhal H, Cameron L. Behavioral theories and the problem of compliance. Patient Educ Couns 1987; 10: 117–138.

Leventhal H, Watts JC, Pagano F. Effects of fear and instructions on how to cope with danger. J Pers Soc Psychol 1967;6:313–321.

Leventhal H, Zimmersman R. Compliance: A self-regulation perspective. In Gentry D, ed. Handbook of Behavioral Medicine. New York: Guilford Press, 1984, pp 369–434.

Levine DM, Green LW, Deeds SG, Chwalow J, Russell RP, Finlay J. Health education for hypertensive patients. JAMA 1979;241:1700–1703.[A]

Levine RJ. Ethical considerations in the development and application of compliance strategies for the treatment of hypertension. In Haynes RB, Matteson ME, Engebretson TOJ, eds. Patient Compliance to Prescribed Antihypertensive Regimens. Washington, DC: U.S. Department of Health and Human Services, H.I.H. Publication No. 81–2102, 1980:229–246.

Logan AG, Milne BJ, Achber C, Campbell WP, Haynes RB. Work-site treatment of hypertension by specially trained nurses: A controlled trial. Lancet 1979;2: 1175–1178.[A]

Logan AS. Investigation of Toronto General Practitioners' Treatment of Patients with Hypertension. Toronto: Canadian Facts, 1978.

Macharia WM, Leon G, Rowe BH, Stephenson BJ, Haynes RB. An overview of interventions to improve compliance with appointment keeping for medical services. JAMA 1992;267:1813–1817.[A]

Marinker M, Shaw J. Not to be taken as directed. BMJ 2003;326:348–349.

McDonald HP, Garg AX, Haynes RB. Interventions to enhance patient adherence to medication prescriptions: Scientific review. JAMA 2002;288:2868–2879.[A]

McKenney JM, Slining JM, Henderson HR, Devins D, Barr M. The effect of clinical pharmacy services on patients with essential hypertension. Circulation 1973;48:1104–1111.

Morgan SG, Yan L. Persistence with hypertension treatment among community-dwelling BC seniors. Can J Clin Pharmacol 2004;11:e267–e273.[B]

Morice AH, Wrench C. The role of the asthma nurse in treatment compliance and self-management following hospital admission. Respir Med 2001;95:851–856.[A]

Morisky DE, Green LW, Levine DM. Concurrent and predictive validity of a self-reported measure of medication adherence. Med Care 1986;24:67–74.

Nazareth I, Burton A, Shulman S, Smith P, Haines A, Timberal H. A pharmacy discharge plan for hospitalized elderly patients: A randomized controlled trial. Age Ageing 2001;30:33–40.[A]

Nessman DG, Carnahan JE, Nugent CA. Increasing compliance: Patient-operated hypertension groups. Arch Intern Med 1980;140:1427–1430.[A]

Peterson GM, McLean S, Millingen KS. A randomised trial of strategies to improve patient compliance with anti-convulsant therapy. Epilepsia 1984;25:412–417.[A]

Pilon D, Castilloux AM, LeLorier J. Estrogen replacement therapy: Determinants of persistence with treatment. Obstet Gynecol 2001;97:97–100.[B]

Prochaska JO, DiClemente CC. Stages of change in the modification of problem behaviors. In Hersen M, Eisler RM, Mille PM, eds. Progress in Behavior Modifications. Sycamore, Ill: Sycamore Press, 1992, pp 188–214.

Prochaska JO, Johnson S, Lee P. The transtheoretical model of behaviour change. In Shumaker SA, Shron EB, Ockene JK, McBee WL, eds. The Handbook of Health Behaviour Change. New York: Springer, 1998, pp 59–84.

Pullar T, Birtwell AJ, Wiles PG, Hay A, Feely MP. Use of a pharmacologic indicator to compare compliance with tablets prescribed to be taken once, twice, or three times daily. Clin Pharmacol Ther 1988;44:540–545.[B]

Rawlings MK, Thompson MA, Farthing CF, et al. NZTA4006 Helping to Enhance Adherence to Antiretroviral Therapy (HEART) study team. Aliment Pharmacol Ther 2003;18:1121–1127.[A]

Rijcken CA, Tobi H, Vergouwen AC, de Jong-van den Berg LT. Refill rate of antipsychotic drugs: An easy and inexpensive method to monitor patients' compliance by using computerised pharmacy data. Pharmacoepidemiol.Drug Saf 2004;13:365–370.[B]

Roberts KJ, Volberding P. Adherence communication: A qualitative analysis of physician-patient dialogue. AIDS 1999;13:1771–1778.[B]

Rockart JF, Hoffman PB. Physician and patient behavior under different scheduling systems in a hospital outpatient department. Med Care 1969;7:463.

Roter DL. Patient participation in the patient-provider interaction: The effects of patient question asking on the quality of interaction, satisfaction and compliance. Health Educ Monogr 1977;5:281–315.[A]

Royal Pharmaceutical Society of Great Britain. From compliance to concordance: Towards shared goals in medicine taking. London: RPS, 1997.**C**

Sackett DL. Introduction. In Sackett DL, Haynes RB, eds. Compliance with Therapeutic Regimens. Baltimore: Johns Hopkins University Press, 1976, p 1.

Sackett DL, Haynes RB, Gibson ES, et al. Randomised clinical trial of strategies for improving medication compliance in primary hypertension. Lancet 1975;1: 1205–1207. **A**

Schulman BA. Active patient orientation and outcomes in hypertensive treatment: Application of a socio-organizational perspective. Med Care 1979;17:267–280.**B**

Sellors J, Kaczorowski J, Sellors C, et al. A randomized controlled trial of a pharmacist consultation program for family physicians and their elderly patients. Can Med Assoc J 2003;169:17–22.**A**

Sellors J, Pickard L, Mahony JB, et al. Understanding and enhancing compliance with the second dose of hepatitis B vaccine: A cohort analysis and a randomized controlled trial. Can Med Assoc J 1997;157:143–148.**A**

Shalansky SJ, Levy AR. Effect of number of medications on cardiovascular therapy adherence. Ann Pharmacother 2002;36:1532–1539.**B**

Shepard DS, Foster SB, Stason WB, et al. Cost-effectiveness of interventions to improve compliance with antihypertensive therapy. Prev Med 1979;8:229.**B**

Steiner JF, Koepsell TD, Fihn SD, Inui TS. A general method of compliance assessment using centralized pharmacy records: Description and validation. Med Care 1988;26:814–823.**B**

Stephenson BJ, Rowe BH, Haynes RB, Macharia WM, Leon G. The rational clinical examination: Is this patient taking the treatment as prescribed? JAMA 1993;269: 2779–2781.

Stevens VJ, Shneidman RJ, Johnson RE, Boles M, Steele PE, Lee NL. *Helicobacter pylori* eradication in dyspeptic primary care patients: A randomized controlled trial of a pharmacy intervention. West J Med 2002; 176:92–96.**A**

Swain MA, Steckel SB. Influencing adherence among hypertensives. Res Nurs Health 1981;4:213–222.

Takala J, Niemela N, Rosti J, Sievers K. Improving compliance with therapeutic regimens in hypertensive patients in a community health center. Circulation 1979;59:540–543.**A**

Tamblyn R, Laprise R, Hanley JA, et al. Adverse events associated with prescription drug cost-sharing among poor and elderly persons. JAMA 2001;285:421–429.**B**

Tracy JJ. Impact of intake procedures upon client attrition in a community mental health center. J Consult Clin Psychol 1977;45:192–195.

Tseng CW, Brook RH, Keeler E, Steers WN, Mangione CM. Cost-lowering strategies used by Medicare beneficiaries who exceed drug benefit caps and have a gap in drug coverage. JAMA 2004;292:952–960.**B**

Velicer WF, Prochaska JO, Fava JL, Laforge RG, Rossi JS. Interactive versus noninteractive interventions and dose-response relationships for stage-matched smoking cessation programs in a managed care setting. Health Psychol 1999;18:21–28.

Vik SA, Maxwell CJ, Hogan DB. Measurement, correlates, and health outcomes of medication adherence among seniors. Ann Pharmacother 2004;38:303–312.**B**

Von Korff M, Katon W, Rutter C, et al. Effect on disability outcomes of a depression relapse prevention program. Psychosom Med 2003;65:938–943.**B**

Willey C. A comparison of two methods of measuring stage of change for adherence with medication. Ann Behav Med 1998;20:S027.

Willey C, Stafford J, Geletko S, et al. Stages of change for adherence with medication. Ann Behav Med 1999;21: S156.

Wogen J, Kreilick CA, Livornese RC, Yokoyama K, Frech F. Patient adherence with amlodipine, lisinopril, or valsartan therapy in a usual-care setting. J Manag Care Pharm 2003;9:424–429.**B**

World Health Organization. Adherence to Long-term Therapies: Evidence for Action: 2003. Geneva: World Health Organization, 2003.**C**

10 Disease Prevention

R. Michael Morse and Charles E. Henley

ROLE OF THE FAMILY PHYSICIAN

The family physician has a special opportunity to be an effective force in disease prevention and health promotion. As the primary care provider for all ages in family units, the family physician has an inherent obligation to screen for a broad range of risk factors associated with preventable diseases and to encourage appropriate preventive measures. Most lifestyle disease-prevention and health-promotion activities are applicable to the entire family unit and should serve as the foundation for more age-specific recommendations and interventions for each individual family member.

Although other medical-surgical problem areas may occasionally require subspecialty consultation, the family physician is the specialist to whom patients and other specialists look for provision of this broad range of health-promotion and disease-prevention activities.

Disease-prevention activities are traditionally classified according to the phase of the disease process in which intervention occurs: tertiary prevention (disease diagnosed and symptoms present); secondary prevention (disease present and diagnosable, but no symptoms present); and primary prevention (no diagnosable disease or symptoms, but risk factors present).

The bulk of medical education focuses on the already ill patient (tertiary prevention), whereas progressively less time is spent on secondary and primary prevention. This may lead medical students and physicians to provide evaluation and treatment primarily in reaction to patient symptoms, rather than in a proactive mode of care—that is, attempting to anticipate problems and to prevent them.

Physicians may encounter a variety of obstacles to providing comprehensive preventive health services. These include heavy demands on the physician's time by patients already ill, lack of financial resources in the patient population, negative third-party attitudes toward reimbursement for preventive health

care, and patients uninformed concerning the benefits of prevention. However, in a capitated environment, family physicians are in a position in which they have the latitude and expectation to provide a full range of preventive health services.

EVALUATING PREVENTIVE HEALTH ACTIVITIES

Where appropriate, recommendations from the U.S. Preventive Services Task Force (USPSTF) are cited. These recommendation categories (Table 10-1) should not be confused with the standard strength-of-evidence categories used elsewhere in this text. Particular attention should be paid to the differences between C and I recommendations. In both cases, USPSTF makes no recommendation, but fair evidence is associated with the C rating (but not enough to weigh benefit vs. harm), and overall insufficient evidence exists to reach any conclusion for an I rating.

Not all diseases lend themselves well to the shift from medical intervention at the tertiary level to prevention at the secondary or primary levels. Several parameters are used to determine the validity of such a shift for each disease and to determine the population group to whom the intervention should be applied. The general criteria are as follows:

1. Is the disease worth screening for? Does it have a significant impact on the quality or length of life, and is it of sufficient prevalence in the population to justify screening?
2. Is sufficient information available to identify accurately, by using risk factors and screening tests, the individual or groups in whom the disease is likely to develop? Or by using diagnostic tests, is it possible to identify those likely already to have the disease at a presymptomatic stage?
3. Are the tests for the screening or early detection satisfactory in terms of accuracy, morbidity, cost, and acceptability to the patient and physician?

Evidence levels Ⓐ Randomized, controlled trials (RCTs), meta-analyses, well-designed systematic reviews of RCTs. Ⓑ Case-control or cohort studies, nonrandomized clinical trials, systematic reviews of studies other than RCTs, cross-sectional studies, retrospective studies, certain uncontrolled studies. Ⓒ Consensus statements, expert guidelines, usual practice, opinion.

Table 10-1 U.S. Preventive Services Task Force Ratings of Recommendations

Recommendation: A
Language: The USPSTF strongly recommends that clinicians routinely provide [the service] to eligible patients. (The USPSTF found good evidence that [the service] improves important health outcomes and concludes that benefits substantially outweigh harms.)

Recommendation: B
Language: The USPSTF recommends that clinicians routinely provide [the service] to eligible patients. (The USPSTF found at least fair evidence that [the service] improves important health outcomes and concludes that benefits outweigh harms.)

Recommendation: C
Language: The USPSTF makes no recommendation for or against routine provision of [the service]. (The USPSTF found at least fair evidence that [the service] can improve health outcomes but concludes that the balance of the benefits and harms is too close to justify a general recommendation.)

Recommendation: D
Language: The USPSTF recommends against routinely providing [the service] to asymptomatic patients. (The USPSTF found at least fair evidence that [the service] is ineffective or that harms outweigh benefits.)

Recommendation: I
Language: The USPSTF concludes that the evidence is insufficient to recommend for or against routinely providing [the service]. (Evidence that [the service] is effective is lacking, of poor quality, or conflicting, and the balance of benefits and harms cannot be determined.)

4. If it is possible to predict the disease or to diagnose it before the onset of symptoms, will a known intervention significantly alter the course of the disease?
5. Is the intervention or treatment satisfactory in terms of proved effectiveness, risk, morbidity, cost, and patient acceptability?

Table 10-2* is a mortality table for the United States. Table 10-3 shows mortality data by sex, Table 10-4 shows mortality by race, and Table 10-5 shows mortality trends over time for each major cause of death. From these tables, one can begin to understand the relative impact of various diseases on death rates. The mortality trends from 1979 to 1998 in Table 10-5 allow assessment of progress in prevention and treatment. In particular, the decreases in mortality from heart disease, stroke, and accidents are highly encouraging and are due primarily to preventive health measures. Conversely, the marked increases in chronic pulmonary disease, pneumonia, influenza, and diabetes are not reassuring when one considers how preventable these deaths are. Finally, careful examination of the consistent patterns of increased risk for male and black subjects highlights a number of lifestyle risks in these groups.

As shown in Table 10-6, nearly 50% of the deaths in the United States are directly attributable to environmental and behavioral issues, most of which are a result of individuals' lifestyle decisions.

*Tables 10-2 through 10-41 appear on the Student Consult.

INTERVENTIONS AND RECOMMENDATIONS

The USPSTF findings form the basis for the evidence-based recommendations in this chapter. Recommendations of other scientific organizations also are presented when appropriate.

CORONARY HEART DISEASE

Epidemiology (American Heart Association, 2003)

Incidence
The yearly national incidence of myocardial infarction is estimated to be 1.2 million. The majority of individuals (50% of men and 64% of women) with coronary heart disease (CHD) have no warning of their disease and are initially seen with either an acute myocardial infarction or sudden death as the initial symptoms.

Prevalence
It is estimated that 13.2 million people alive today have a history of either myocardial infarction or symptomatic CHD, and 1 to 2 million middle-aged men in the United States have asymptomatic but significant CHD. The prevalence of CHD is estimated at 6.4% of the population older than 20 years.

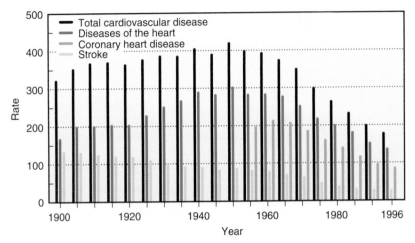

Figure 10-1 Age-adjusted death rates* for total cardiovascular disease, diseases of the heart, coronary heart disease, and stroke,[†] by year, United States, 1900–1996. (Data from Mortality and Morbidity, 1998 Chartbook on Cardiovascular, Lung, and Blood Disease. Rockville, MD, U.S. Department of Health and Human Services, National Institutes of Health, 1998.)
*Per 100,000 population, standardized to the 1940 U.S. population.
[†]Diseases are classified according to International Classification of Diseases (ICD) codes in use when the deaths were reported. ICD classification revisions occurred in 1910, 1921, 1930, 1939, 1949, 1958, 1968, and 1979. Death rates before 1933 do not include all states. Comparability ratios were applied to rates for 1970 and 1975.

CHD is a lifelong process. Pathologic studies of men in their 30s dying of noncardiac causes have shown raised plaque in coronary arteries of up to 50% (Strong et al., 1999). Men older than 50 years have a 20% prevalence of asymptomatic CHD (Strong et al., 1999).

Although difficult, predicting the prevalence in asymptomatic adults is of importance to the physician if early aggressive intervention is to be targeted to the appropriate patients. These high-risk groups are identified by an analysis of the risk factors present for CHD.

Cost of and Impact on Society
It is estimated that the cost of medical treatment and lost productivity for CHD in the United States is $132.2 billion.

Morbidity and Mortality
Mortality rates for cardiovascular diseases and for CHD in male and female subjects and in black and white subjects have been steadily decreasing (Figs. 10-1 and 10-2). Nevertheless, one in every five deaths in the United States is due to CHD: 669,000 per year. In addition, 20% of all persons with a myocardial infarction will die. Of those who survive, about two thirds do not make a complete recovery, although 88% of those younger than 65 years eventually return to work. In the 6 years after myocardial infarction, 7% of men and 6% of women experience sudden death, and 18% of men and 35% of women have another infarction.

Important Facts Relevant to Prevention

1. A major focus for prevention of CHD is encouraging healthy lifestyles for all patients.
2. Risk-factor identification and reduction will reduce the incidence of CHD, particularly when concentrated on blood lipid levels, hypertension, cigarette smoking, and a sedentary lifestyle.
3. Changing the American diet to a low–saturated fat, low–trans-fatty acid, low-cholesterol diet will reduce the levels of serum cholesterol in the population.
5. Regression of coronary lesions is possible with adequate treatment. Even a very low fat diet, combined with exercise and meditation, but without medication, has been shown to be effective.
6. In patients with significantly elevated low-density lipoprotein (LDL) cholesterol, cholesterol-reducing medications have proved effective in reducing the incidence and mortality of myocardial infarction in both symptomatic and asymptomatic adults of all ages.

Screening Test Recommendations for the General Population

1. Screen for lipid disorders in men at 35 years and in women at 45 years (USPSTF, 2001A). Any younger adult with other risk factors also should be screened (USPSTF, 2001B). Measure total and high-density lipoprotein (HDL) cholesterol for screening purposes (USPSTF, 2001A). Patients found to be at high risk based on screening values

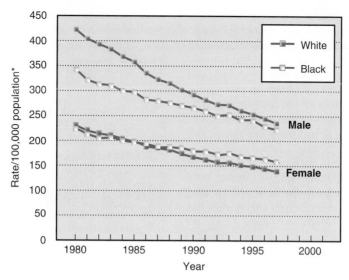

Figure 10-2 Age-adjusted death rates from coronary heart disease by sex and race, United States, 1980–1997. (Data from Cooper R, Cutler J, Desvigne-Nickens P, et al. Trends and disparities in coronary heart disease, stroke, and other cardiovascular diseases in the United States: Findings of the National Conference on Cardiovascular Disease Prevention. Circulation 2000;102:3137–3147.)
*Rates are age-adjusted to 2000 standard.

should obtain a complete fasting lipid panel (total, LDL, and HDL cholesterol plus triglycerides) to determine risk status most accurately. For patients found not to be at risk, a screening interval of every 5 years is recommended by the National Cholesterol Education Program (NCEP), although insufficient evidence is available to determine the optimal interval (USPSTF, 2001I). Generally, children do not need to be screened, but consideration should be made for those who have a parent with high-risk lipid profile or a history of premature heart disease in a first-degree relative (younger than 55 years for men and younger than 65 years for women). A family history of premature heart disease confers a relative risk of 1.5 to 2.0. The Adult Treatment Panel III (ATP III, 2002) recommends beginning screening at age 20 years with a full lipid panel and repetition every 5 years (National Cholesterol Education Program, 2002).

2. Measure blood pressure on all adult patients (USPSTF, 2003A). Insufficient evidence exists to recommend the optimal interval (USPSTF, 2004C). The Seventh Report of the Joint Commission on Prevention, Detection, and Treatment of High Blood Pressure (JNC 7) does not make a specific recommendation for the interval. However, the standard family physician practice of measuring blood pressure at each office visit is reasonable.
3. Update family history at least every 5 years.
4. Update smoking status:
   a. Every 5 years in previous nonsmokers.
   b. Yearly in previous smokers who have quit.

   c. Every visit in current smokers.
5. Monitor activity levels at least every 5 years for every patient for the recommended 30 to 40 minutes of aerobic activity 3 to 4 times weekly.
6. Evaluate for obesity (greater than 20% to 30% more than ideal body weight) yearly.
7. Monitor stress levels yearly (family, occupation). Although this factor is not used to assess risk, it may have a major impact on the physician's approach to risk reduction.
8. Physicians may elect to measure fasting blood sugar every 5 years because the presence of diabetes is a major risk factor, particularly with a family history of diabetes.

Preventive Activities Recommendations

Preventive activities are determined based on calculated risk for CHD by using equations derived from Framingham data. This can be accomplished by using the forms shown in Table 10-7 and Table 10-8. Computerized calculators are available on the website for the National Cholesterol Education Program (NCEP, 2004).

Cholesterol Control
Physicians should prescribe a heart-healthy diet for all patients regardless of age or risk. It is particularly important that children learn healthy eating habits early in life. The American Heart Association provides online and printed nutritional guidelines for healthy adults and children as well as for those needing to reduce their cholesterol to desirable levels. Table 10-9 gives very general guidelines that most

patients can easily implement in a progressive manner. A diet high in soluble fiber (oat bran products, legumes, and some fruits) has been shown in some studies to reduce serum cholesterol, whereas nonsoluble fiber (present primarily in wheat, vegetables, and fruit) has consistently shown no effect on cholesterol.

The presence of risk factors in combination with LDL levels is used to determine the type of intervention. The first step is to determine if the patient has known CHD or its risk equivalent (Table 10-10). If not, then Table 10-11 is used to determine the number of risk factors. Note that HDL may add or subtract from the total, based on its level. Finally, Table 10-12 is used to determine the goal LDL levels. Note that ATP III has created optional, more-aggressive goals based on results from randomized clinical trials using medication to reduce LDL levels (Grundy et al., 2004).

Other methods of altering risk secondary to hypercholesterolemia include weight control, exercise, and drug therapy. The statin family of drugs, in particular, has been shown to significantly reduce the risk of myocardial infarction.

Control of Hypertension

Aggressive treatment of all patients with hypertension is essential, but hypertension is controlled in only 34% of patients (Table 10-13). Risk is doubled for each 20 mm Hg increment in systolic blood pressure and 10 mm Hg increment in diastolic blood pressure. This is true over a blood pressure range of 115/75 to 185/115 (Lewiston et al., 2002). In general, a systolic pressure greater than 140 or a diastolic pressure greater than 90 is used as the cutoff point for hypertension, but this cutoff point, as well as a treatment goal, must be individualized. For instance, the goal for patients with diabetes or renal disease is 130/80.

Before institution of drug therapy for hypertension, nonpharmacologic methods should be considered. These include the "Dietary Approaches to Stopping Hypertension" diet, which is rich in calcium and potassium, salt restriction, weight reduction if obese, and regular aerobic exercise.

Smoking Cessation

Smoking may be the most correctable risk factor for CHD. It presents a serious risk not only for the smokers, but also for all those exposed to secondhand smoke, particularly in the home. Smokers have a 70% increased risk of CHD and will reduce that in half a year after quitting and to the level of nonsmokers after several years. National evidence-based guidelines for clinicians assisting their patients in quitting smoking (Fiore et al., 2000) recommend using the "five As" approach: (1) *ask* patients about smoking, (2) *advise* all smokers to quit, (3) *assess* willingness to make a quit attempt, (4) *assist* those who want to quit, and (5) *arrange* follow-up visits with those trying to quit (Glynn, 1993). These brief clinician interventions can be completed within 2 to 3 minutes at each visit and have been associated with a 30% increase in cessation from 7.9% to 10.2%. In addition, adjunctive use of medication is strongly recommended because of high levels of efficacy in randomized control trials (Table 10-14).

Other Preventive Activities

For patients with CHD or more than 5% 5-year risk of CHD, 75 mg aspirin daily will reduce risk of myocardial infarction by one third (Sanmuganathan, 2001; USPSTF, 2002A). It is recommended that physicians assist all patients to avoid risk-factor development through encouragement of healthy lifestyles (e.g., proper nutrition, avoidance of smoking, regular physical activity, stress management, maintenance of ideal body weight), as well as provision of periodic preventive health care. The exact mechanism of risk reduction for many factors has not been clearly defined. For instance, some dietary factors such as high antioxidant content in the diet (primarily through fruits and vegetables), a high-fiber diet, moderate alcohol consumption, and intake of three or more servings of fish weekly have been associated with a decreased risk of CHD. Yet, in general, trials attempting to test these observations with dietary supplements have failed to show benefit. Recently a strong association has been shown between serum homocysteine levels and the incidence of CHD. Homocysteine is elevated by increased intake of animal protein and reduced by folic acid intake.

Discussion

The mortality of CHD in the United States has been decreasing significantly, as shown in Figure 10-2. More than 50% of this decline is due to lifestyle changes, especially diet modification and smoking cessation. This encouraging information alone provides physicians sufficient reason to pursue further aggressive risk-factor prevention and modification on a population-wide basis.

Although total cholesterol measurement may be appropriate for mass public screening, use of total of LDL plus HDL levels is more appropriate when determining risk for individual patients. Measuring HDL increases the predictive power approximately 6 to 10 times that of measuring total cholesterol alone. A low level of HDL is a strong, independent predictor of CHD (see Table 10-11). Up to 20% of high-risk individuals are not identified by using total cholesterol alone. The USPSTF does not recommend for or against inclusion of triglyceride levels when assessing risk for CHD (USPSTF, 2001I). However, triglycerides are a component in making the diagnosis of metabolic syndrome that conveys a very high risk for CHD.

Whereas national nutritional guidelines continue to emphasize reduction of fat intake, most evidence

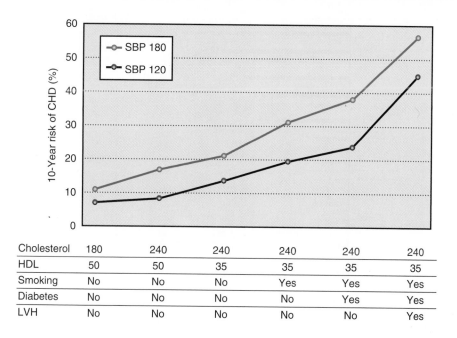

Cholesterol	180	240	240	240	240	240
HDL	50	50	35	35	35	35
Smoking	No	No	No	Yes	Yes	Yes
Diabetes	No	No	No	No	Yes	Yes
LVH	No	No	No	No	No	Yes

CHD, coronary heart disease; HDL, high-density lipoprotein; LVH, left ventricular hypertrophy; SBP, systolic blood pressure

Figure 10-3 Importance of risk factors in determining coronary risk. Estimated 10-year risk of coronary heart disease at age 55 with progressive addition of major risk factors. (Data from Anderson KM, Wilson PWF, Odell PM, Konnel WB. An updated coronary risk profile. A statement for health professionals. Circulation 1991;83:356–362.)

suggests that the type of fat is more important than the amount. In general, many authorities now believe that use of the monounsaturated fats (olive oil, canola oil) and n-3 polyunsaturated fat (found primarily in fish) should be emphasized in the total dietary fat allowance. Although these fats have modest beneficial effects on LDL cholesterol, they are thought also to have antioxidant and antithrombotic actions that reduce CHD risk.

Data suggest that sedentary lifestyle is a potent, independent risk factor that has an effect equal to that of the other major risk factors. Exercise can have beneficial effects on insulin resistance, HDL, triglycerides, obesity, and blood pressure. The American Heart Association considers sedentary lifestyle to be a major risk for CHD.

Assessing total risk for individual patients may be complicated by the presence of more than one risk factor. Figure 10-3 shows the progressive increase in risk as major risk factors are added. However, it must be recognized that most major risk factors vary in impact as their values change.

The authors also recommend structured long-term follow-up with maximal support and encouragement from physician and office staff.

Impact on the Family Unit

The lifestyles that are important for prevention of CHD cannot be easily implemented by an individual without due consideration of the person's family and environment. The chances of abstinence from smoking are dimmed considerably when other smokers are in the home. Diet changes are especially difficult to implement for only one individual in a family unit. Major changes in knowledge, attitudes, and habits in the entire family are often required so that the desirable foods can be purchased, properly prepared, and consumed with an agreed-on common family goal of improved health. Anything less can lead to resentments, confusion, and outright rebellion.

STROKE

Epidemiology

Incidence

Incidence of new and recurrent strokes is 700,000 people per year, of which 88% are ischemic. Five hundred thousand of these are new strokes. The yearly incidence increases dramatically with age. Overall incidence in men is 25% greater than women, and blacks have twice the incidence of first-ever strokes compared with whites. Figure 10-4 shows the increased relative risk of first ischemic stroke in the most at-risk ethnic and racial populations. Significant decreases have occurred in the last 30 years because of recognition and management of risk factors and lifestyle modification.

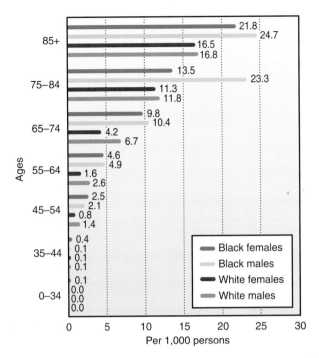

Figure 10-4 Annual rates of first cerebral infarction by age, sex, and race, Greater Cincinnati/Northern Kentucky Stroke Study, 1993–1994. (Data from American Heart Association. Heart Disease and Stroke Statistics, 2004 update. Dallas, TX, American Heart Association, 2003.)

Prevalence

There are 4.8 million living stroke victims in the United States. Prevalence increases markedly after age 74 years (Fig. 10-5). These data do not include the millions of individuals with significant asymptomatic atherosclerotic cerebrovascular disease who are at high risk for stroke.

Cost of and Impact on Society The yearly cost of stroke to society is estimated at $53.6 billion for medical costs and indirect costs, such as lost productivity.

Morbidity and Mortality

Stroke is the cause of 1 in 15 deaths or 282,000 deaths per year and is the third leading cause of death in the United States after CHD and cancer. Acute stroke mortality is 20%. Twenty-two percent of male and 25% of female stroke victims die within 1 year, and 50% are dead within 5 years. In addition to the high mortality, stroke is the leading cause of long-term disability. Fifteen percent to 30% of stroke survivors are permanently disabled and require special services. Two percent require institutional care at 3 months after onset.

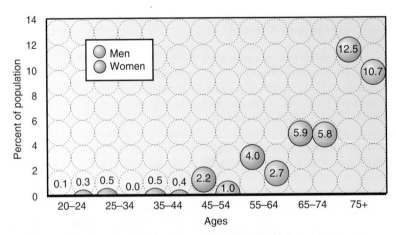

Figure 10-5 Prevalence of stroke by age and sex. (From Third National Health and Nutrition, Examination Survey, 1988–1994.)

Important Facts Relevant to Prevention

Physical activity is strongly and inversely related to stroke incidence. A major risk factor for stroke is hypertension, and risk increases disproportionately at all ages as either systolic or diastolic pressures increase (Figs. 10-6 and 10-7). The other major risk factors for atherosclerosis, with the exception of dyslipidemia, also are predictive for stroke risk. The known presence of heart disease (CHD or atrial fibrillation) carries a high risk for emboli to the brain. Atrial fibrillation increases stroke risk 5 times and is responsible for 15% of cerebral infarcts. Diabetes mellitus, even if mild, carries a significant increased risk for stroke and this risk increases disproportionately if diabetes also is present or if criteria are met for metabolic syndrome (Table 10-15).

In a large cohort study, a transient ischemic attack (TIA) conferred a 10.5% risk of subsequent stroke in the following 90 days (Johnston et al., 2000). One of five stroke victims has had at least one of four major symptoms suggestive of TIA in the prior year: (1) temporary loss of vision (especially if in one eye), (2) unilateral numbness, (3) aphasia, and (4) focal weakness.

Patients with carotid bruits have a 1% to 3% incidence of stroke per year. Although aspirin, anticoagulants, and surgery are commonly prescribed, the current data are not sufficient to show that these treatments effectively reduce the risk of stroke in patients with asymptomatic carotid bruits. Such studies are in progress and will provide further guidance in the future. Other risk factors for stroke include family history of stroke, cigarette smoking, oral contraceptive use, hyperlipidemia, and elevated hematocrit.

Screening Test Recommendations

Blood pressure and smoking status are the two major modifiable risk factors and should be determined. The optimal interval for this screening is not known, but it is often done each office visit. Other risk factors (similar to those for CHD) for atherosclerosis should be sought, as previously recommended in the discussion on CHD. The USPSTF has concluded that insufficient evidence exists to recommend for or against screening asymptomatic persons for carotid artery stenosis by using physical examination or carotid ultrasound. (USPSTF, 1996I).

Preventive Activities Recommendations

Prevention of stroke is aimed primarily at prevention and treatment of sustained, even mild, hypertension and other known risk factors for atherosclerosis.

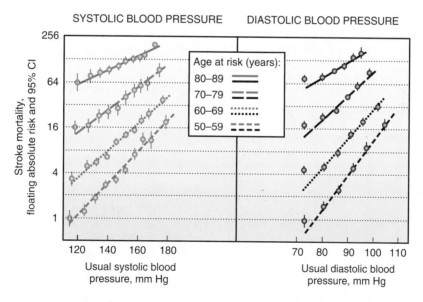

Stroke mortality rate, pictured on a log scale with 95 percent confidence intervals, in each decade of age in relation to the estimated usual systolic and diastolic blood pressure at the start of that decade. Stroke mortality increases with both higher pressures and older ages. For diastolic pressure, each age-specific regression line ignores the left-hand point (i.e., at slightly less than 75 mm Hg), for which the risk lies significantly above the fitted regression line (as indicated by the broken line below 75 mm Hg).

Figure 10-6 Stroke mortality related to blood pressure and age. Note that mortality is on a log scale. (Data from Prospective Studies Collaboration. Age-specific relevance of usual blood pressure to vascular mortality: A meta-analysis of individual data for one million adults in 61 prospective studies. Lancet 2002;360:1903–1913.)

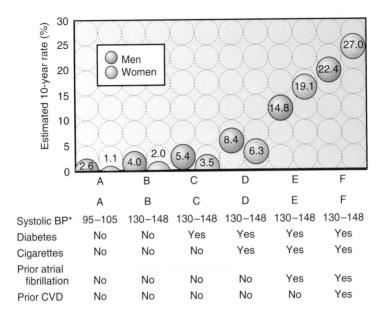

Systolic BP*	95–105	130–148	130–148	130–148	130–148	130–148
	A	B	C	D	E	F
Diabetes	No	No	Yes	Yes	Yes	Yes
Cigarettes	No	No	No	Yes	Yes	Yes
Prior atrial fibrillation	No	No	No	No	Yes	Yes
Prior CVD	No	No	No	No	No	Yes

Figure 10-7   Estimated 10-year stroke risk in 55-year-old adults according to levels of various risk factors, Framingham Heart Study. (Data from Wolf PA, D'Agostino RB, Belanger AJ, Kannel WB. Probability of stroke: A risk profile from the Framingham Study. Stroke 1991;22:312–318.)
*Blood pressures are in millimeters of mercury (mm Hg)

Smokers, in particular, should be strongly advised to stop and should be offered assistance in that effort. Aspirin has not been shown to be effective in primary prevention of stroke. Anticoagulation with warfarin is proven to be effective primary prevention in patients with atrial fibrillation and average-to-high risk of stroke (Segal et al., 2000 Ⓐ). Secondary prevention in patients with TIAs includes prophylaxis with aspirin or other antiplatelet agents (unless otherwise contraindicated), anticoagulation in certain circumstances, and carotid endarterectomy, depending on the degree of stenosis. In the acute phase of an ischemic stroke, thrombolytic therapy has been shown to be effective. However, few patients can be treated within the recommended 3-hour time frame.

Discussion

Despite the lack of evidence that dyslipidemia increases stroke risk, treatment with statin drugs has been shown to lower risk by 24% to 29% (Corvol et al., 2003 Ⓐ). The most important reason to consider screening for carotid bruits is to document the existence of significant atherosclerosis in high-risk individuals and thus alert the physician to the need to modify risk factors more aggressively. However, a theoretical risk with this approach is that it may initiate a process that includes angiography and endarterectomy, procedures that have no clear consensus as to their proper use in asymptomatic individuals.

SUBSTANCE ABUSE, ALCOHOLISM, AND OTHER DRUG DEPENDENCY

Epidemiology

Incidence

Inability to identify a specific time that an individual meets criteria for alcohol, or drug abuse or dependence makes incidence rates very difficult to determine reliably. Centers for Disease Control and Prevention (CDC) studies have shown an incidence of fetal alcohol syndrome (FAS) of 0.2 to 1.5 per 1000 live births. The incidence of less severe variants is approximately 3 times that of FAS.

Prevalence

More than 17 million, or 17%, of U. S. individuals 12 years of age or older abused or were dependent on alcohol or illicit drugs in 2001 (Substance Abuse and Mental Health Administration, 2002). Figure 10-8 shows the proportions for users of alcohol and drugs. The male-to-female ratio is 2:1. The highest rate of abuse of or dependence on alcohol or illicit drugs was among 18- to 25-year-olds and American Indians/Alaska natives. One study of primary care practices showed that 16.5% of patients were "problem drinkers" (Fleming et al., 1997 Ⓐ).

Cost of and Impact on Society

The estimated yearly cost of alcohol abuse and dependence in the United States is $184.6 billion, including $134.2 billion from lost employment and

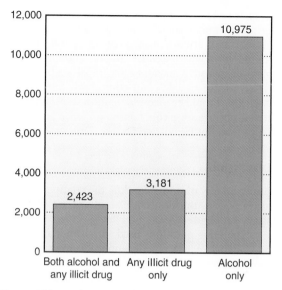

Figure 10-8 Estimated numbers (in thousands) of persons aged 12 or older reporting past year abuse or dependence for any illicit drug or alcohol, 2001.

reduced productivity and $26.3 billion in health care costs (Harwood, 2000). The estimated total cost of illicit drug use is $160.7 billion of which $14.9 billion is for health care (Office of Drug Control Policy, 2001). The social consequences of problem drinking, although not quantifiable, may be as great as the costs of the medical consequences. Abusers have a higher rate of injury, divorce, domestic violence, unemployment, and poverty.

Morbidity and Mortality The contribution of alcohol misuse to overall mortality is 3.5% of all deaths, and that of illicit drugs is 0.7% (see Table 10-6). Patients with alcoholism have 2.5 times the normal overall risk of mortality. Overall mortality is 30% to 38% higher among men and more than doubled in women who drink more than six drinks per day. More than 100,000 deaths per year are related to alcohol abuse, and half of these are related to accidental deaths.

The morbidity for chemical dependency (alcohol and drug abuse) is substantial, ranging from the extremely high association with crime to cirrhosis, psychosis, depression, cardiomyopathy, peptic ulcer disease, overdose, cancer of directly exposed organs (lips, mouth, larynx, pharynx, esophagus, stomach, liver), pancreatitis, suicide, various infections (hepatitis, acquired immunodeficiency syndrome [HIV], endocarditis, pneumonia), fetal alcohol syndrome, violence, and accidents of all types.

However, it should be kept in mind that regular alcohol consumption has a beneficial association with a 30% to 40% reduction of risk of death from cardiovascular diseases (Thun et al., 1997). This benefit is evident at low to moderate levels of intake and does not increase with additional alcohol intake. Overall, low point of a J-shaped mortality curve is associated

with small volumes (one drink or less per day) of alcohol consumption because of the cardiovascular benefits, but as volume increases, the many adverse effects overcome these benefits (Enlish, 1995).

Important Facts Relevant to Prevention

A wide variety of serious individual social, psychological, and physical health problems are strongly associated with misuse of alcohol. FAS is a permanent, severe syndrome of mental retardation and birth defects that is 100% preventable. Society bears a large burden of social, legal, and economic problems as a result of alcohol and drug abuse.

The USPSTF recommends "screening and behavioral counseling interventions to reduce alcohol misuse by adults, including pregnant women, in the primary care setting" (USPSTF, 2004B). Insufficient evidence exists to recommend for or against this approach for adolescents (USPSTF, 2004I).

Measures to increase enforcement of drinking and driving laws, to increase prices for alcoholic beverages, and to increase the legal drinking age have been successful in reducing either alcohol consumption or the frequency of the legal consequences of drinking. Whether education can reduce the rate of alcoholism is not known. Strong cultural biases (e.g., Orthodox Jews) against drunkenness substantially reduce the prevalence of abuse and dependence.

Children of alcoholics are at 3 to 4 times greater risk of alcoholism, whether or not their biologic parents raise them.

Although spontaneous recovery from alcoholism is reported in more than 20% of patients (American Psychiatric Association, 1994), psychosocial treatment has been reported to result in a 30% to 60% 1-year abstinence rate (Finney et al., 1996). Even brief interventions in the outpatient setting have shown significant reduction in high-risk drinking behavior for up to 48 months (Fleming et al., 2002Ⓐ). Increasing evidence shows that the use of adjunctive pharmacotherapy agents such as naltrexone and acamprosate provides added benefit. One must remember that studies use a variety of definitions of both alcoholism and recovery.

Screening Test Recommendations

All patients older than 12 years should be screened regularly for alcohol and substance abuse. A yearly frequency of screening can deliver a strong educational message to the patient, although the optimal screening interval has not been determined.

The first step in screening individuals who consume alcohol is evaluating volume and frequency of drinking. Risky drinking is defined for female subjects as more than three drinks any day during the prior month or more than seven drinks average per week, and for male subjects, as four drinks any day or more than 14 drinks average per week. Adverse consequences with continued drinking are the major common criteria for abuse and dependence in the *Diagnostic and Statistical Manual of Mental Diseases* (DSM-IV), with additional elements, including physiologic effects (tolerance, with-drawal) and further loss of control, necessary for dependence (Tables 10-16 and 10-17).

The ultimate goal of screening questions is to ascertain whether the patient is having or has ever had a health, legal, or personal problem as a result of drinking alcohol. The CAGE questionnaire is the most widely used screening tool (Table 10-18). Any positive response should be explored. Two or more positive responses to the CAGE questions in the past year are highly suggestive of alcohol abuse or dependence and require further investigation. The T-ACE questions have been validated for use in pregnancy (Table 10-19). The increased sensitivity of the T-ACE compared with the CAGE during pregnancy is shown in Table 10-20. Guidelines published by the U.S. Department of Health and Human Services are a very useful evidence-based resource for effective strategies for dealing with alcohol problems in the outpatient medical setting (U.S. Department of Health and Human Services, 2003).

The Two-Item Conjoint Screen (TICS), a two-question screen for detection of either alcohol or drug use disorder, has shown a likelihood ratio of 1.93 for one positive response and 8.77 for two. The two questions are as follows: (1) "In the last year, have you ever drunk or used drugs more than you meant to?" and (2) "Have you ever felt you wanted or needed to cut down on your drinking or drug use the last year?" (Brown et al., 2001⊜).

Preventive Activities Recommendations

The presence or absence of alcoholism in first-degree relatives should be a part of the family history. A positive answer identifies a high risk for alcohol problems and affords an opportunity to inquire about the patient's drinking history and current status. Any patient with a family history of alcoholism should be counseled concerning his or her high-risk status and encouraged to become a member of Al-Anon or the Children of Alcoholics Foundation.

All patients, including children, should be asked yearly if any problems within the family involve alcohol.

Those caring for female patients during the childbearing years should assure that these patients are aware of the risk of FAS and its less severe variants. If they might become pregnant, they must not consume alcohol.

Literature concerning the warning signs of alcoholism and sources of help should be freely available in every medical office. If the subject of chemical dependency is dealt with openly, an increased likelihood exists of their seeking help through the family physician. All pregnant women should be advised against the use of alcohol and drugs during pregnancy, and all users should be advised against driving and performing other dangerous behaviors while intoxicated.

Evidence-based counseling and intervention guidelines should be followed for those individuals who screen positive for alcohol abuse or dependence (U.S. Department of Health and Human Services, 2003).

Discussion

A helpful way of understanding the relation between alcohol consumption and resultant problems is shown in Figure 10-9.

The same questions used for alcohol abuse and dependence may be equally applicable to drug abuse. Certain cues found in alcoholics, and often in other drug-dependent patients, help lead to the correct diagnosis: problems with children, separation, divorce, job changes, depression, anxiety, hypertension, macrocytosis of red blood cells, low resistance to infections, recurrent accidents, arrests and other legal problems, upper gastrointestinal complaints, and abnormal liver enzymes.

Impact on the Family Unit

The family is at the epicenter of the alcoholic earthquake. As the rumblings of the disease progress, so does pathology within the family. One in four American children is exposed to alcohol abuse or dependence in the family (Grant et al., 2000) and is at significant risk of serious physical and psychological consequences. Most prominent is the role of the "co-alcoholic" or "enabler," who assumes the abnegated responsibilities of the alcoholic, covers for the alcoholic, and makes possible his or her continued drinking. This person is often the major focus of the alcoholic's hostility. Treatment should include healing of the entire family.

CANCER

General Information

About 1,368,030 new cancer cases are expected to be diagnosed in 2004 (Fig. 10-10). Since 1990, more than 18 million new cases of cancer have been diagnosed. However, the National Cancer Institute (NCI) estimates that approximately 9.6 million Americans with a history of cancer were alive in January 2000. Death rates from all cancers combined have been decreasing since the 1990s. Death rates decreased for 11 of the top 15 cancers in men and 8 of the top 15 cancers in women (NCI, 2004). The mortality trends since 1930 for all major cancers are shown in Figures 10-11 and 10-12.

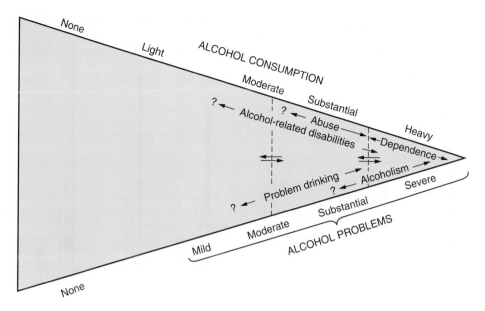

Figure 10-9 A terminological map of alcohol use.

LEADING SITES OF NEW CANCER CASES AND DEATHS—2004 ESTIMATES*

Estimated New Cases*		Estimated Deaths	
Male	**Female**	**Male**	**Female**
Prostate 230,110 (33%)	Breast 215,990 (32%)	Lung and bronchus 91,930 (32%)	Lung and bronchus 68,510 (25%)
Lung and bronchus 93,110 (13%)	Lung and bronchus 80,660 (13%)	Prostate 29,500 (10%)	Breast 40,110 (15%)
Colon and rectum 73,620 (11%)	Colon and rectum 73,320 (11%)	Colon and rectum 28,320 (10%)	Colon and rectum 28,410 (10%)
Urinary bladder 44,640 (6%)	Urinary corpus 40,320 (6%)	Pancreas 15,440 (5%)	Ovary 16,090 (6%)
Melanoma of the skin 29,900 (4%)	Ovary 25,580 (4%)	Leukemia 12,990 (5%)	Pancreas 15,830 (6%)
Non-Hodgkin's lymphoma 28,850 (4%)	Non-Hodgkin's lymphoma 25,520 (4%)	Non-Hodgkin's lymphoma 10,390 (4%)	Leukemia 10,310 (4%)
Kidney 22,080 (3%)	Melanoma of the skin 25,200 (4%)	Esophagus 10,250 (4%)	Non-Hodgkin's lymphoma 9,020 (3%)
Leukemia 19,020 (3%)	Thyroid 17,640 (3%)	Liver 9,450 (3%)	Urinary corpus 7,090 (3%)
Oral cavity 18,550 (3%)	Pancreas 16,120 (2%)	Urinary bladder 8,780 (3%)	Multiple myeloma 5,640 (2%)
Pancreas 15,740 (2%)	Urinary bladder 15,600 (2%)	Kidney 7,870 (3%)	Brain 5,490 (2%)
All sites 699,560 (100%)	All sites 668,470 (100%)	All sites 290,890 (100%)	All sites 272,810 (100%)

Figure 10-10 Leading sites of new cancer cases and deaths, 2004 estimates. (Data from The American Cancer Society. *Cancer Facts and Figures 2004.* Atlanta, American Cancer Society, 2004.)
*Excludes basal and squamous cell skin cancers and in situ carcinoma except urinary bladder.
Note: Percentages may not total 100% due to rounding.

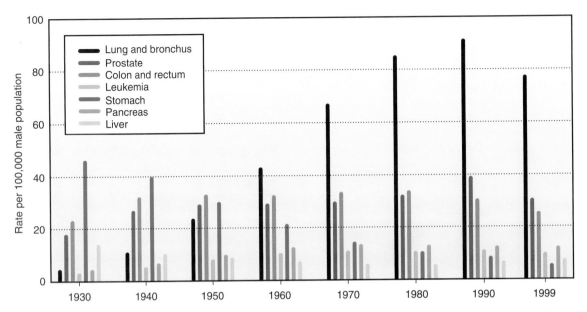

Figure 10-11   Age-adjusted death rates, males* by site, United States, 1930–1999. (Data from U.S. Mortality Public Use Data Tapes, 1960–1999, U.S. Mortality Volumes, 1930–1959. National Center for Health Statistics, Centers for Disease Control and Prevention, 2002. American Cancer Society, Surveillance Research, 2003)
*Per 100,000, age-adjusted to the 2000 U.S. standard population.
Note: Due to changes in ICD coding, numerator information has changed over time. Rates for cancers of the liver, lung and bronchus, and colon and rectum are affected by these coding changes.

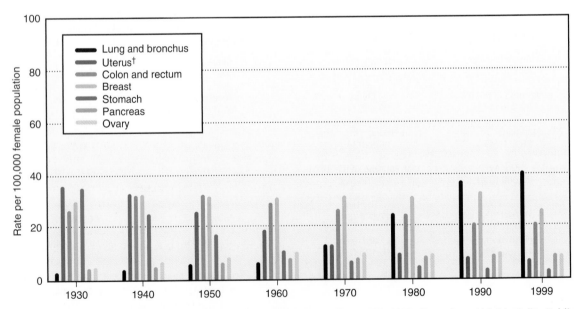

Figure 10-12   Age-adjusted death rates, females* by site, United States, 1930–1999. (Data from U.S. Mortality Public Use Data Tapes, 1960–1999, U.S. Mortality Volumes, 1930–1959. National Center for Health Statistics, Centers for Disease Control and Prevention, 2002. American Cancer Society, Surveillance Research, 2003.)
*Per 100,000, age-adjusted to the 2000 U.S. standard population.
†Uterus cancer death rates are for uterine cervix and uterine corpus combined.
Note: Due to changes in ICD coding, numerator information has changed over time. Rates for cancers of the liver, lung and bronchus, colon and rectum, and ovary are affected by these coding changes.

Definition of Cancer

Cancer is a group of diseases characterized by uncontrolled growth and spread of abnormal cells. Cancer is caused by both external factors such as tobacco, ionizing radiation, chemicals, and infectious organisms, and internal factors such as inherited mutations, hormones, immune conditions, and mutations that occur from metabolism. All cancers involve some form of gene malfunction that controls cell growth and division. Often a long latent phase occurs between exposure and development of detectable cancers.

General Cancer Prevention

All cancers related to cigarette smoking and heavy alcohol consumption are completely preventable. Evidence suggests that about one third of the 563,700 cancer deaths expected to occur in 2004 will be related to nutrition, physical inactivity, obesity, and other lifestyle factors, and thus also could be prevented. Infectious agents such as hepatitis B virus, human papilloma virus, and HIV also are implicated in the etiology of certain cancers, and the risk for acquiring these infections could be reduced significantly through behavioral change. Regular screening can result in the detection of cancers of the breast, cervix, colon, prostate, oral cavity, and skin at a stage at which treatment is more likely to be beneficial.

Who Is at Risk?

About 76% of all cancers are diagnosed at age 55 or older. Lifetime risk in the United States is less than one in two for men, and a little more than one in three for women. Relative risk is a measure of the strength of the relation between risk factors and a particular cancer compared with that in those individuals who do not have the exposure. For example, in male smokers, lung cancer is 20 times more likely to develop than in nonsmokers, so the relative risk is 20. However, women who have a first-degree relative with breast cancer have a twofold increased risk of breast cancer developing compared with women who do not have a family history, so their relative risk is only 2. The actual probability of cancer developing, by age and sex in the general population, is shown in Table 10-21.

Lung Cancer

Epidemiology

Incidence The NCI reports the 2004 incidence for both small cell and non–small cell lung cancer in the United States at 173,770 new cases. This makes it the second highest cancer incidence for both males and females in the United States (see Fig. 10-10). However, in the 2004 NCI *Annual Report to the Nation*, lung cancer incidence rates among women have leveled off for the first time, after increasing for many decades.

Morbidity and Mortality Lung cancer is the leading cause of cancer death in the United States, with 160,440 resulting deaths in 2004, and it remains one of the leading causes of preventable death worldwide. Because of the high case-fatality rate for the disease, the incidence and mortality rates are nearly identical. The age-adjusted lung cancer death rate in the United States is 56.9 per 100,000 population in 1988. Small cell carcinoma is the most aggressive type and carries the worst prognosis, with a median survival from diagnosis of only 2 to 4 months without treatment. Although the prognosis for the heterogeneous group of cancers classified as non–small cell (epidermoid, large cell, and adenocarcinoma) cancers is better, the overall survival rate for all types is just 5% to 10%.

Important Facts Relevant to Prevention

A single etiologic agent, cigarette smoking, is the leading cause of lung cancer. This causal relation between cigarette smoking and lung cancer is unequivocal and represents one of the most intensely studied relations in medical research. Approximately 90% of all new cases of lung cancer are attributed to cigarette smoking, and smokers are at a 20-fold increased risk for developing lung cancer compared with people who never smoked. Even with the strong causal association with smoking, a few other etiologies also have been associated with lung cancer, such as occupational exposures to arsenic, asbestos, chromate, hydrocarbons, chloromethyl ethers, nickel, and radon. Emerging evidence also exists for a genetic susceptibility factors such as polymorphism in the cytochrome *p450* enzymes and mutations in the *k-ras* oncogene and the *p53* gene. Environmental tobacco smoke continues to be an important source of risk and a significant public health issue. The only evidence-based advice for reducing cancer risk is not to smoke or to stop smoking; however, 50% of all new lung cancers are diagnosed in former smokers.

Screening Test Recommendations

Even though lung cancer is one of the most preventable of cancers, no major professional organization currently recommends screening for lung cancer, including the USPSTF. Studies on the use of chest radiographs and 3-day pooled sputum cytology showed an insufficient efficacy in detecting lung cancer compared with low-dose helical computed tomography (CT). Although still no evidence exists that screening tests reduce the rate of cancer-specific mortality, a growing interest is found in the potential of low-dose helical CT for improving screening efficacy.

Preventive Activities Recommendation

Smoking cessation is a key component of any prevention strategy. Patients at all ages should receive a strong health message concerning smoking, including an offer of assistance for current smokers from their physicians (USPSTF, 2003A): "It's addicting. Don't start. If you have started, stop." The risk for lung cancer decreases among those who quit smoking compared with those who continue to smoke. Diet as a preventive of lung cancer has been studied by various groups (Wright, 2000), and foods such as flax seeds, fruits and vegetables, and foods rich in sulforophane, such as broccoli sprouts, and selenium, folic acid, vitamin B_{12}, vitamin D, and antioxidants have all been implicated in a cancer-prevention diet. β-Carotene has been especially touted as being effective in preventing lung cancer, although randomized placebo-controlled trials have not shown a significant protective effect. The β-carotene and retinol efficacy trial (CARET) conducted in the United States and the Alpha Tocopherol Beta-Carotene (ATBC) trial conducted in Finland showed an actual increased risk associated with β-carotene supplementation.

Discussion

The prevention of lung cancer is dependent on the identification of exposures to known carcinogens such as cigarette smoking. The epidemiology of lung cancer shows irrefutable correlation with the onset of lung cancer and the introduction of the first manufactured cigarette by R.J. Reynolds in 1913. Lung cancer was a rare disease before the turn of the century, but the incidence of lung cancer increased along with the increase in smoking, which peaked at around 1965. Even though smoking has been in decline, the rates of lung cancer will continue to increase until the peak incidence rate for past smokers has been reached. The populations at greatest risk for lung cancer based on smoking prevalence are 18- to 24-year-olds, American Indians and Alaskan Natives, and those who have not completed high school (Table 10-22, Figs. 10-13 and 10-14). Physicians can continue to have a major impact on the risk of this disease through community and patient intervention and education. Targeting certain cohorts at higher risk, such as young women and certain ethnic groups, also makes sense as part of an overall prevention strategy. Excellent support materials are available from the American Academy of Family Physicians, the American Cancer Society (ACS), and the American Heart Association. Physician recommendation has a great potential impact on patients' decisions to stop smoking.

Impact on Family Unit

A single smoker in a family can be a source of secondary smoke exposure for the rest of the family. Angina, respiratory symptoms, and increased risk of lung cancer can result in those exposed. A relatively high number of lung cancer cases from never-smokers have been attributed to exposure to passive smoking. Children from households with smokers have a higher school absence rate as a result of increased incidence of respiratory illnesses, infections, and middle-ear

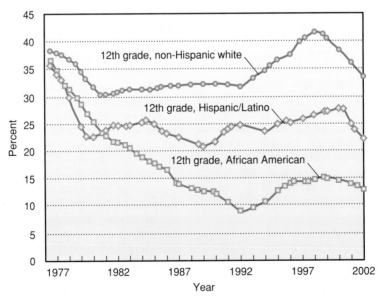

*Used cigarettes in the last 30 days.

Figure 10-13 Current* cigarette smoking among 12th graders, by race and ethnicity, 1977–2002. (Data from American Cancer Society. Cancer Prevention and Early Detection Facts and Figures, 2004. Atlanta, American Cancer Society, 2004.) * Used cigarettes in the last 30 days.

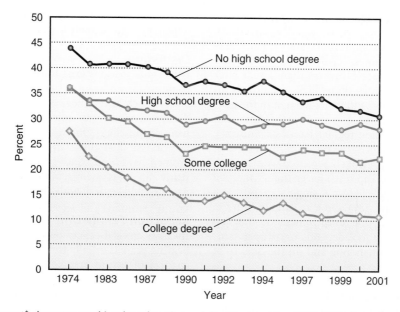

Figure 10-14 Current* cigarette smoking by education, adults 25 and older, 1974–2001. (Data from National Health Interview Survey, 1974–2001, National Center for Health Statistics, Centers for Disease Control and Prevention, American Cancer Society. American Cancer Society, Surveillance Research.)
*Adults 25 and older who have smoked 100 cigarettes in their lifetime and who are current smokers (regular and irregular).

infections. Infants born to mothers who smoked during pregnancy are more likely to die of sudden infant death syndrome. Couples who smoke create a special problem for the physician who wishes to help. It is difficult to persuade one smoker to quit while the other continues, and it is equally problematic to bring two smokers to the point of wishing to stop at the same time. The withdrawal period is one of great stress and requires family education and support.

Cervical Cancer

Epidemiology
Incidence In 2004, the incidence of invasive cervical carcinoma (new cases) was 10,520, although declining. The overall incidence rates in the United States have decreased from 14.2 per 100,000 women in 1973, to 7.8 cases per 100,000 women in 1994. The NCI Surveillance, Epidemiology, and End Results (SEER) program reports the incidence of invasive cervical cancer from in the United States, from 1995 to 1999, in women age 20 to 24 years, to be 1.7/100,000 per year. Worldwide, cervical carcinoma is the most common malignancy in women, whereas in the United States it is the 10th most common form of malignancy among woman.

Morbidity and Mortality The mortality for invasive carcinoma of the cervix in 2002 was 4100 women, although the mortality has declined 70% from the mid-1920s since the introduction of the Papani-

colaou (Pap) test to screen for preinvasive cancer. Cervical cancer that is detected in the preinvasive stages, such as carcinoma in situ, has a 100% cure rate with proper treatment, whereas localized cancer has a 91% 5-year survival rate. The Healthy People 2010 target for cervical cancer is a reduction in mortality to 2.0 deaths per 100,000 women. Since 1998, the rate has been approximately 3.0 deaths per 100,000.

Important Facts Relevant to Prevention
Squamous cell carcinoma of the cervix occurs almost exclusively in women who are sexually active, with the risk for developing a precancerous lesion increasing with increasing numbers of sexual partners. The American Cancer Society guidelines on early detection of cervical neoplasia describe the mean time for progression from mild dysplasia (CIN I-1) carcinoma in situ (CIN III) or cancer as 70 to 80 months in women older than 50 years, 41 to 42 months for women aged 26 to 50 years, and 54 to 60 months in women younger than 25 years. The mean time for further progression to invasive carcinoma is an additional 10 years. The rate of progression for any one individual is unpredictable, with some intraepithelial lesions regressing spontaneously in 30% to 50% of cases, depending on age. In adolescent women, aged 13 to 21 years, 70% of high-grade and 90% of low-grade lesions have been shown to regress within 3 years, whereas 30% of older patients with CIN III have progression to invasive carcinoma.

Major risk factors are early age for first intercourse, multiple sexual partners, HIV infection, herpes simplex virus infection, history of condylomas (human papilloma virus, or HPV infection), smoking, and low socioeconomic status. Early sexual intercourse has an especially dramatic effect on risk. Women who had coitus less than 1 year after menarche are 26 times more likely eventually to have cervical carcinoma than are women in the general population. From 15% to 20% of American women do not undergo regular Pap tests, and they account for the majority of cases of carcinoma of the cervix. Among previously screened women with a history of normal Pap tests, fewer than 1 in 1000 will have a high-grade lesion. A single Pap test has a sensitivity of around 58% and a specificity of 99%. Major variability in the effectiveness of the Pap smear as a screening tool depends on proper sampling and specimen handling and on the quality of the laboratory.

Screening Test Recommendations

The USPSTF recommendations for screening for cervical cancer include beginning Pap smears approximately 3 years after sexual activity begins, but no later than age 21 years, and continued screening at 3-year intervals (USPSTF, 2005A). Most organizations recommend having a Pap test at least once yearly for 3 years and then, after at least three negative annual Pap tests, the frequency may be reduced to as little as every 3 years, at the discretion of the physician. The USPSTF advises against Pap tests in women older than 65 years who have had consistently negative examination and in women who have had a total hysterectomy for benign disease (USPSTF). Suggestive Pap tests should be evaluated by direct observation with colposcopy. Although the Food and Drug Administration (FDA) has approved hybrid capture II technology for screening for HPV, and a clear association is shown with HPV as the etiology of cervical cancer, the USPSTF does not yet recommend testing for HPV with polymerase chain reaction or hybrid capture II as an alternative or an adjunct to primary Pap screening (USPSTF). HPV testing may be worthwhile if it can be shown to distinguish reliably between women who would benefit from more intensive Pap testing or colposcopy. In women who do have HPV DNA testing done, and are positive for one of the high-risk HPV types such as 16, 18, 31, or 45, colposcopy examination would be warranted, even if they have normal Pap tests.

Preventive Activities Recommendations

Risk status should be re-evaluated at each preventive health visit, especially in groups who may have an increased likelihood of multiple sexual partners. Women should be advised of their risk status, with emphasis on the importance of regular re-evaluation. Although barrier contraception has only theoretical benefits, it also can be strongly recommended to help prevent sexually transmitted diseases (STDs).

Discussion

Other good reasons exist to request many women to come in for an examination more often than every 3 years, such as monitoring use of birth control pills, dietary advice, contraceptive counseling, and prepregnancy counseling. Only a minority of women may need to visit their physician less often than once yearly. Women have been educated for many years that the yearly Pap test is essential but not that other important issues should be dealt with during these visits.

Impact on Family Unit

Invasive cervical cancer occurring during the childbearing years is usually treated surgically, ending the chances of future pregnancy. This has a profound effect on a single woman's approach to possible marriage and on a married couple's plans and relationship. The family physician's role only begins with referral for appropriate treatment. Preventive counseling is necessary in these situations. Women past the childbearing years may still have a loss of identity similar to, but not as intense as, that of the breast cancer victim.

Skin Cancer

Epidemiology

Incidence There are 800,000 cases of basal and squamous skin cell cancer yearly plus an additional 38,300 malignant melanomas. This is more than twice the cancer incidence of that in any other organ system. Since the 1960s, the incidence of cutaneous squamous cell carcinoma has been increasing dramatically at 4% to 8% per year.

Morbidity and Mortality Of the 9430 deaths each year, 7300 are from malignant melanoma. Mortality is rare with nonmelanoma cancers, but substantial morbidity can be prevented with effective screening.

Important Facts Relevant to Prevention

The most important risk factor for all skin cancer is exposure to ultraviolet (UV) light. Major risk factors include severe sunburns as a child, fair complexion, multiple or atypical moles, a family or personal history of skin cancer, poor tanning ability, freckles, history of local treatment with ionizing radiation, and immunosuppression (Table 10-23). Occupational exposures to coal tar, pitch, arsenic, radium, and creosote all increase risk.

Screening Test Recommendations

The most efficient screening programs target individuals at higher risk for the development of skin cancers (Wolfe, 1999). For melanoma, that means light-skinned people a history of excessive skin exposure, a family history of melanoma, multiple nevi, or dysplastic nevi. During regular preventive health examinations, the skin should be thoroughly examined for suggestive lesions. All lesions suggestive of malignancy should be sampled by biopsy or prophylactically excised and submitted for pathologic interpretation. Randomized trials have not proven the efficacy of either melanoma or nonmelanoma skin cancer screening, yet physicians discover approximately 20% of melanomas when the patient did not notice anything unusual. Unfortunately, many primary care physicians do not take the opportunity to examine the skin when patients are seen for other problems. This routine screening of the skin for cancerous lesions within the usual context of care should become more commonplace, especially for higher-risk patients.

Preventive Activities Recommendation

For primary prevention, all patients at risk should be counseled in measures for UV-wave avoidance (sun or artificial tanning), protection with higher sun protection factor (SPF) number sunscreens (15 or greater), and use of protective clothing (see Table 10-23) (USPSTF, 2003A). Secondary prevention includes regular self-examination. This is a logical activity, especially for patients with already existing melanotic nevi.

The physician also should be alert to actinic keratoses and treat these as appropriate with 5-fluorouracil or retinoic acid topical application when generalized or with local means such as cryocautery.

Prostate Cancer

Epidemiology

Incidence Prostate cancer is the second leading cause of cancer death in American men age 50 years or older. Approximately 230,000 new cases and 30,000 deaths occur each year in the United States. A dramatic, transient 20% increase in incidence was found for several years after 1986 when the FDA approved the prostate-specific antigen (PSA) test for screening for prostate cancer. It continues to increase 6% per year, probably secondary to increased detection efforts. African-American men tend to have a higher incidence of prostate cancer, 37% higher than that of white men.

Prevalence Prevalence increases with age. Some studies have found microscopic evidence of prostate cancer in 30% of autopsies of men age 30 to 49 years. Estimates of the prevalence in men older than 80 years range up to 100%.

Morbidity and Mortality According to the SEER program, the mortality rates for prostate cancer declined after 1991 in white men and in 1992 in black men. These declines were due to declines in distant disease mortality, which in turn was due to a decrease in distant disease incidence and not to improved survival of patients with distant disease. Because of the potential for morbidity associated with progression of prostate cancer to widespread metastases, many experts believe that the increased detection of prostate cancer with PSA before it becomes metastatic is responsible for the reduced morbidity in both white and black men.

Important Facts Relevant to Prevention

Only a small minority of men with microscopic evidence of prostate cancer ever has clinical evidence of the disease. Population studies have suggested that dietary fat may be related to increased risk of prostate cancer.

Screening Recommendations

The principal screening tests are digital rectal examination, serum tumor markers such as the PSA, and transrectal ultrasound. The sensitivity and specificity of these tests are difficult to calculate. Although these tests have been shown to increase the diagnosis of disease, it remains to be seen whether these screening tests will lead to interventions that will prolong life. A recommendation for routine screening is controversial. It is possible that a screening program sensitive to the risk factors and targeting patients with curable disease could decrease the rates of mortality and morbidity. Conversely, routine screening for prostate cancer also can result in patients being offered curative treatments when their disease does not require extensive treatment. Physicians are advised to counsel all men older than 50 years of the availability, risks, and benefits of PSA testing. Insufficient evidence exists to recommend for or against screening (USPSTF, 2002).

Endometrial Cancer

Epidemiology

Incidence and Mortality See Figures 10-10, 10-11, and 10-12.

Important Facts Relevant to Prevention

Endometrial cancer is the most common cancer of the genital tract and represents 10% of all cancers diagnosed in women. It is primarily a postmenopausal disease, with 97% of endometrial cancers being adenocarcinoma. Endometrial cancer can arise from malignant transformation of atrophic endometrium, but the major causative factor appears to be unopposed estrogen, whether physiologic or iatrogenic, with estrogen excess giving rise to atypical hyperplasia of the endometrium. The most important early-warning sign is abnormal vaginal bleeding. Risk factors are obesity, prolonged treatment with estrogen alone, age, chronic anovulation, and increased number of years of menstruation (early menarche, late menopause, or no pregnancies). Hypertension and diabetes are associated with risk, probably because of the prevalence of obesity in these patients. An association is found between the use of tamoxifen as an adjuvant treatment for breast cancer and the development of endometrial cancer (Crabbe, 1996). Tamoxifen works as an antiestrogen in breast tissue, but it also has estrogenic properties that can affect the endometrium as well as other tissues, such as bones and the cardiovascular system. It is estimated that 2 of 1000 women who are taking tamoxifen for breast cancer are at higher risk for developing endometrial cancer. However, the benefits may outweigh the risks.

Screening Test Recommendations
Insufficient evidence exists to recommend for or against routine screening (NCI, 2005). Most cases of endometrial cancer are diagnosed by symptoms, and high proportions are diagnosed at an early stage and have high rates of survival. Endometrial cells are occasionally found on Pap smear, but this is not an adequate screen. Any endometrial cells found on a postmenopausal Pap smear should be considered abnormal. All postmenopausal women with abnormal bleeding of any amount must have endometrial sampling performed.

Preventive Activities Recommendation
Risk factors should be established at menopause and modified when possible. All women with an intact uterus who are treated with estrogen replacement therapy also should be prescribed a progestational agent, although the use of hormone replacement therapy (HRT) is recommended against routine use (USPSTF, 2005D) for the prevention of osteoporosis or other postmenopausal conditions, because of the potential for serious complications of heart disease and a higher breast cancer risk.

Breast Cancer

Epidemiology
Incidence, Morbidity, and Mortality Breast cancer is the leading cause of death in women worldwide. In the United States, 192,000 new cases of invasive breast cancer occurred in 2001, with 40,200 deaths, and 1500 cases of breast cancer in men, with 400 deaths.

Important Facts Relevant to Prevention
The etiology of breast cancer in men is poorly understood, but in women, several associations should be considered. The risk factors for breast cancer are shown in Table 10-24. Women who delay childbirth until after age 30 years have a twofold increase in the risk of breast cancer developing. The excessive use of alcohol also may play a role. A small increase in risk appears to occur in women with a family history of breast cancer who take estrogen birth control pills, with an association between the prolonged use (>10 years) of HRT and breast cancer risk. The risk seems to be 6% increase in breast cancer risk for every 5 years of estrogen replacement and a 9% increase in risk for every 5 years of estrogen plus progestin therapy. However, the major association seems to be in the cancer-susceptibility genes *BRCA1* and *BRCA2*, which account for 45% of the hereditary forms of breast cancer (Brewster, 2001). The cumulative risk of breast cancer developing in a woman with a mutation in *BRCA1* and *BRCA2* is 84% by age 70 years. The use of selective estrogen-receptor modulators such as tamoxifen has been advocated as a primary prevention of breast cancer in high-risk women such those with a strong family history of first-degree relatives having breast cancer or carrying the *BRCA1* or *BRCA2* genes. Certainly, evidence exists that hormonal manipulation will play an important role in reducing cancer risks, because prophylactic oophorectomy in *BRCA1* and *BRCA2* carriers has been shown to reduce the risk of breast cancer developing by 50% to 70%. One of the potential side effects of using tamoxifen is its association with endometrial cancer. Raloxifene, another selective estrogen-receptor modulator, has not been shown to have the same association with endometrial cancer. Clinicians should consider both the risks of breast cancer and the risks of adverse effects when recommending chemoprophylaxis. USPSTF (2005D) recommends against routine use of tamoxifen or roloxifene in low or average risk women.

Screening Test Recommendations
Although the evidence is inconclusive concerning the added value of clinical breast examination, most clinicians believe that the clinical breast examination is an important part of the detection of breast cancer. Mammography alone has a sensitivity of 30% in women with very dense breast tissue and 80% in women with fatty breast tissue. The ACS recommends that all women should start having annual mammograms at age 40 years, or earlier if they have strong risk factors for breast cancer. The USPSTF now also recommends starting at age 40 years for routine screening and no longer recommends that screening with mammograms cease after age 70 years (USPSTF, 2002B). The prevalence of mammography screening varies by population, with the uninsured having rates of less than 40% (Table 10-25). The clinical breast examination has an I rating from the USPSTF, whereas the ACS strongly recommends it.

Preventive Activities Recommendation
It is important for family physicians to understand the risk factors and associations with HRT, family history, age of pregnancy, and *BRCA* carrier state to

advise women on their options for screening and primary prevention.

Ovarian Cancer

Epidemiology

Incidence In the United States, 23,000 women are diagnosed with ovarian cancer every year, representing a 1.7% lifetime risk for developing the disease. Two genes, *BRCA1* and *BRCA2,* are linked with both hereditary breast and ovarian cancer (Modugno, 2003). Testing positive for the genetic marker does not mean that cancer will develop, but it does increase the lifetime risk to between 16% and 60%. The incidence of ovarian cancer also increases with age, with the majority of cases occurring between the ages of 55 and 74 years, with the average being 61 years.

Morbidity and Mortality Every year, 14,000 women die of ovarian cancer, accounting for 52% of all gynecologic cancer deaths. Seventy-five percent of ovarian cancers are not diagnosed until the cancer has advanced to stage III or IV, giving the patient a 5-year survival rate of only 20%.

Important Facts Related to Prevention

A documented decreased risk for ovarian cancer is found in women who use birth control pills. This is probably because of the prolonged suppression of ovarian function. The risk for ovarian cancer in women who are positive for the *BRCA* genes also goes down with each live birth, although increased risk is associated with the use of HRT for longer than 10 years. The use of estrogen replacement for less than 10 years does not seem to be associated with an increased risk. Other risk factors for ovarian cancer include a documented first-degree relative (mother, daughter, sister) with ovarian cancer, a high-fat diet, nulliparity, infertility, age older than 30 years at time of first pregnancy, use of talcum powder in feminine hygiene, and living in North America or Northern Europe. Having two or more first-degree relatives with ovarian cancer increases the lifetime risk of the disease developing to almost 50%.

Screening Test Recommendations

The mortality data for ovarian cancer have not improved in three decades because a reliable screening mechanism for ovarian cancer still does not exist. The tumor marker CA-125 is too nonspecific, and pelvic examinations are operator dependent. It is estimated that 10,000 pelvic examinations would have to be done to identify one ovarian cancer. Today three main approaches to screening exist: transvaginal ultrasound, C-125 tumor marker, and pelvic examinations. Only 80% of ovarian cancers produce C-125, and the C-125 antigen has a low specificity, especially in premenopausal women.

Because of its low specificity, no recommendation exists to use C-125 in premenopausal women as a screening device. C-125 can be used in postmenopausal women with an adnexal mass, or in detecting relapse of a known ovarian cancer. Other conditions, such as pancreatitis, chronic hepatitis, endometriosis, alcoholic hepatitis, adenomyosis, renal failure, pelvic inflammatory disease, and pregnancy, also can release small amounts of CA-125, which may confuse the screening process. The difficulty is in differentiating between ovarian cancer and benign ovarian masses. The risk for ovarian cancer increases with increasing size of any ovarian cyst, to the point at which a cyst on ultrasound that is larger than 10 cm has a 60% chance of being malignant. The FDA and the NCI have jointly published data using artificial intelligence computer programs to identify correctly patterns of serum proteins from a finger-stick blood sample in patients with ovarian cancer. This had a sensitivity of 100% and a specificity of 95%, with a positive predictive value of 94%, compared with 35% for C-125. This may prove to be a worthwhile screening tool in the future, especially for women who are *BRCA1* positive or have a strong family history of ovarian cancer. Currently, a negative C-125 test cannot rule out the presence of ovarian cancer. Fair evidence indicates that screening may lead to important harms (USPSTF, 2004D).

Preventive Activities Recommendation

No proven primary prevention therapies are known for ovarian cancer, although a case could be made for treating high-risk women desiring birth control with oral contraceptive pills. Knowing and advising women about their personal risk factors is presently one of the most useful tasks for the primary care physician.

Colorectal Cancer

Epidemiology

Incidence, Morbidity, and Mortality According to the ACS, colorectal cancer is the third leading cause of cancer-related death in the United States in both men and women, with 148,000 new cases and 56,600 deaths estimated in 2002.

Important Facts Related to Prevention

An individual's lifetime risk for developing colorectal cancer is 6%, with 90% of all cases occurring after age 50 years. The risk factors for colorectal cancer are shown in Table 10-26. Colorectal cancer is considered a preventable disease. It is the result of accumulated genetic mutations over many years, leading to the formation of adenoma and ultimately to carcinoma. The disease can be prevented if this adenoma-to-carcinoma sequence is not initiated or can be interrupted. A strong association between high dietary fiber and low incidence of colorectal cancer can play a role in reducing the incidence of colorectal cancer. The epidemiologic strength for such a statement is overwhelming, even though it now appears that the major reason for this association is that, in general, populations with low fiber intake consume higher levels of saturated fat. Evidence also indicates that nonsteroidal anti-inflammatory drugs (NSAIDs), either aspirin or nonaspirin cyclo-oxygenase (COX)-1 and COX-2 inhibitors, can have a beneficial effect in preventing the development of adenomatous polyps. Case reports exist of adenomatous regression in patients with familial polyposis using NSAIDs. The risk reduction for colorectal cancer with the use of NSAIDs may be as much as 40% to 50%. However, no long-term clinical trials looked at the effect of NSAIDs on the actual reduction of colorectal cancer, and the evidence for such an association is inferential from other studies. A study sponsored by the NCI was begun in 2000 to study the effectiveness of the COX-2 inhibitor celecoxib (Celebrex) in preventing adenomatous polyps, a precursor of colon cancer. The study (the Adenoma Prevention with Celecoxib, or APC trial) was to run until 2005 but was halted when analysis by an independent data safety board showed a 2.5-fold increase in risk of fatal and nonfatal cardiovascular events compared with placebo. This follows another report in September 2004 that the COX-2 inhibitor rofecoxib (Vioxx) also caused a twofold increase in cardiovascular toxicities in a trial to prevent adenomas. Because of these findings, we cannot recommend this class of drugs for prevention of adenomatous polyps.

Screening Test Recommendations

Because primary prevention and lifestyle changes are difficult to initiate and take many years to accomplish, it is important that effective screening programs also be in place. Some controversy exists over the relative value of screening with flexible sigmoidoscopy versus colonoscopy. Conclusive evidence indicates that fecal occult blood testing alone can decrease the mortality of colorectal cancer by identifying patients who then undergo colonoscopy to identify their cancers. However, the false positives encountered with this test create a large burden of resulting colonoscopies on patients with no disease, with a huge cost to the health care system. The addition of flexible sigmoidoscopy to fecal occult blood testing means that many more actual polyps will be detected and removed, without the need for conscious sedation. However, several proximal cancers or adenomatous polyps may be missed by not visualizing the right and transverse colon. Colonoscopy has several advantages in detecting colorectal cancer. The entire colon is visualized, and suggestive lesions can be sampled or removed. Part of the success of the fecal occult blood screening is that it results in colonoscopies. However, it may be difficult to recommend the use of colonoscopy as a screening tool based

on cost and limited access. A recent Veterans Administration cooperative study showed the majority of cancers detected by colonoscopy were identified in an early stage, suggesting that colonoscopy screening may be able to identify potentially curable cancers. The current recommendations for screening are to determine the risk status of the individual in terms of family history and personal medical history. Individuals with a history of ulcerative colitis, acromegaly, or a first-degree relative with colorectal cancer or familial polyposis should undergo colonoscopy examination every 1 to 3 years. The average-risk person should begin annual fecal occult blood and flexible sigmoidoscopy screening or full colonoscopy by age 50 years, with periodic re-examination every 3 to 5 years (USPSTF, 2002A) (Dove, 2001). Compliance with screening guidelines is low (Table 10-27). The use of CT colonography also may show promise in detecting adenomatous polyps and cancers without the effects of conscious sedation. With colonoscopy as the standard, this technique has been shown to have a 60% to 90% sensitivity in detecting large polyps.

Preventive Activities Recommendation

Although some evidence exists for the use of aspirin or other NSAIDs along with diet in the primary prevention of colorectal cancer, this cannot be considered a substitute for colorectal cancer screening. Adherence to screening protocols should be the overriding effort of primary care physicians. Trials of population screening with fecal occult blood tests have shown a significant decrease in mortality, whereas trials of once-only flexible sigmoidoscopy and colonoscopy are still under way. Patients should also be instructed on the long-term health benefits of a high-fiber and low-fat diet. Other possibly effective chemoprevention therapies include the use of oral folate and calcium. Folate intake should be at the level of 400 µg/day. Calcium supplements also have been associated with lower colorectal cancer risk, possibly by binding bile and fatty acids in the bowel lumen or by directly inhibiting the colonic epithelial cell proliferation. The recommended dosage is 1800 mg of calcium daily.

In Brief: Screening for Other Cancers

Testicular Cancer

Testicular cancer is relatively rare. Physician examination and self-examination of the testes have not been demonstrated to be effective enough to recommend mass screening. However, it is appropriate to examine the testes as part of an examination for other reasons.

Pancreatic Cancer

Cancer of the pancreas is the fourth leading cause of cancer death in American men and women.

However, because of a lack of evidence of effectiveness, screening in asymptomatic persons by palpation, ultrasonography, or serologic markers is not recommended.

Oral Cancer

Primary care physicians are advised to include an oral examination in routine preventive health screening, particularly in high-risk persons, such as smokers and people using snuff or chewing tobacco. Patients should be advised against the use of all tobacco products, and the heavy use of alcohol.

Bladder Cancer

Routine screening for bladder cancer is not advised. However, patients who smoke tobacco double their risk of bladder cancer and should be advised to stop.

Thyroid Cancer

Thyroid cancer is rare. Screening of asymptomatic patients is not recommended, but examination at intervals may be advised for patients with an increased risk, such as those with a childhood history of head or neck irradiation.

Childhood Cancer

Although an estimated 9300 new cases of childhood cancers are expected in children aged 0 to 14 years in 2004, childhood cancers showed some of the largest improvements in cancer survival, with an absolute survival-rate increase of 20% in boys and 13% in girls. An estimated 1510 deaths are expected in 2004, about one third from leukemia. In spite of these figures, childhood cancer remains a relatively rare disease.

OSTEOPOROSIS

Epidemiology

Incidence

Although it is difficult to determine the yearly incidence of osteoporosis, the major complication of fractures secondary to osteoporosis is estimated to be 1.5 million per year. Osteoporosis causes a fracture in more than half of all women after menopause, most commonly in the vertebral column, with the remainder in the hip, distal forearm, and other sites.

Prevalence

It is estimated that 5 million women older than 50 years have osteoporosis and are therefore at increased risk for fractures. Another 14 million have osteopenia. Seventy percent of women older than 70 years have osteoporosis at one or more sites. Black women have rates approximately half those of white women (Fig. 10-15).

Cost of and Impact on Society

The National Osteoporosis Foundation estimates the medically related costs of caring for patients with fractures secondary to osteoporosis are $17 billion each year.

Morbidity and Mortality

Hip fractures are associated with an increased mortality of 10% to 20% in the following year. Hip and vertebral fractures lead to significant morbidity. Chronic pain, loss of mobility and independence, as well as the serious medical consequences of multiple vertebral fractures (restrictive lung disease, gastrointestinal

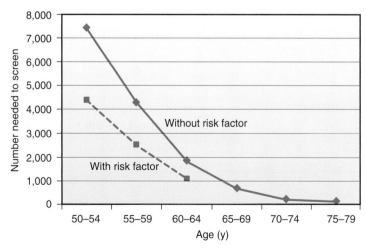

Figure 10-15 Number needed to screen to prevent one hip fracture in 5 years with advancing age and for women younger than 65 with at least one risk factor. (Data from Nelson HD, Helfand M, Woolf SH, Allan JD. Screening for postmenopausal osteoperosis: A review of the evidence for the U.S. Preventative Services Task Force. Available at www.preventiveservices.ahrq.gov. Accessed 1/24/2006.)

problems from altered abdominal anatomy) all have adverse effects on well-being.

Important Facts Relevant to Prevention

Ultimately, the degree of osteoporosis is dependent on two major factors: the peak bone density at age 20 to 30 years and the rate of bone loss thereafter. The risk of osteoporosis and resultant fractures increases with age. Compared with age 50 to 54 years, women age 65 to 69 years have 5.9 times the risk of osteoporosis, and those age 75 to 79 years have 14.3 times the risk (Siris et al., 2001). In women, bone loss abruptly increases to 2% to 3% per year at menopause and then gradually returns to premenopausal rates. Men follow a similar sequence, but without the accelerated phase. Total loss of bone mass in men is about two thirds that of women.

Before age 30 years, adequacy of calcium intake affects the peak bone mass, and after age 30 years, slows the rate of loss of bone mass slightly. All women and men need 1.0 g of elemental calcium daily to maintain a zero calcium balance. In postmenopausal women not prescribed estrogen replacement therapy, increasing this amount to 1.5 g still does not maintain zero calcium balance. An 80% prevalence of inadequate calcium intake is found among female patients of all ages.

Bone mineral density measurements using dual energy x-ray absorptiometry accurately predict risk for osteoporotic fractures.

Available treatments for osteoporosis in asymptomatic women reduce fracture risk. Effective medications include bisphosphonates, selective estrogen-receptor modulators, and calcitonin. Although no longer recommended because of other associated risks, estrogen replacement therapy is an effective method of preventing the accelerated phase of bone-mass loss after menopause and reducing fracture risk.

Other methods of maximizing peak bone mass and slowing bone-mass loss include regular weight-bearing exercise. Actual gains in lumbar bone mass have been demonstrated in postmenopausal women placed on a weight-bearing exercise regimen. This effect was sustained as long as the exercise was continued.

Many risk factors exist for osteoporosis plus multiple additional medical conditions that may place an individual at higher risk (Table 10-28).

Obesity, because of increased endogenous estrogen levels, and thiazide diuretics, because of decreased calcium excretion, have a protective effect.

Screening Test Recommendations

The USPSTF recommends screening all women beginning at age 65 years and all high-risk women beginning at age 60 years by using dual energy x-ray absorptiometry (USPSTF, 2002B). The optimal screening interval for repeated testing has not been determined.

Preventive Activities Recommendations

All patients, especially women, should be educated regarding the recommended intake of 1000 mg of dietary calcium. Postmenopausal women not receiving estrogen should increase calcium intake to 1500 mg. Major nutritional sources of calcium are listed in Table 10-29. Dairy products should be low fat as part of the overall prudent diet. Women unable to meet minimal calcium needs through diet should be advised to use supplemental calcium plus vitamin D, 400 to 800 IU daily.

Risk status should be reviewed for all females, preferably at menarche, and re-evaluated at the time of routine preventive health visits. Additional counseling concerning osteoporosis prevention should be given to those at higher risk.

All patients should be counseled to maintain regular aerobic weight-bearing activities as part of the overall program for general preventive health care. Although 50 to 60 minutes of exercise 3 times weekly has been shown to increase bone mass, the minimal levels necessary have not been determined.

Discussion

Falls are one of the major reasons for the increase in morbidity and mortality in individuals with osteoporosis. Thus evaluating elderly individuals for fall risk and instituting preventive measures are particularly important for those with osteoporosis.

Contributing factors may be easily overlooked when an illness that may increase risk of osteoporosis consumes the focus of attention. A good example might be the elderly white woman in otherwise good health in whom polymyalgia rheumatica develops. The attention required to make the diagnosis and the resulting treatment with corticosteroids become the major focus. It is easy to forget that such a person, 2 years later, may be free of polymyalgia symptoms but debilitated by vertebral fractures.

Impact on the Family Unit

Family eating patterns primarily determine the peak bone mass achieved. Therefore counseling of women in the childbearing years should include recommendations for the entire family.

Elderly patients who are already at high risk create a dilemma for the family physician. The resulting impact of severe fractures is sudden loss of independence. In an elderly family member, this has great impact in both emotional and financial terms. The resulting major decisions that must be made often reverse the parent and child roles. Intimate knowledge of the elderly patient, his or her functional capacities, and the living situation place the family physician in a pivotal role in fracture prevention.

SEXUALLY TRANSMITTED DISEASES

Epidemiology

Incidence

More than 25 diseases are transmitted primarily through sexual activity. Hepatitis A, B, and C, in addition to their primary modes of infection, also can be sexually transmitted. More than 834,000 cases of chlamydia infection, more than 350,000 cases of gonorrhea, and more than 6,800 cases of syphilis are reported each year in the United States. The rates of chlamydia and syphilis are slowly increasing, whereas gonorrhea incidence is decreasing slightly. The actual incidence of these diseases beyond reported cases is not known, but more than 3 million actual new infections with chlamydia each year and more than 650,000 new cases of gonorrhea are estimated. The CDC reports that one fourth of these infections are in teenagers, with the overall incidence of these being highest in women age 15 to 19 years, in men age 20 to 24 years, and in blacks. The estimated incidence and prevalence of the most common STDs (excluding HIV) is shown in Table 10-30. The estimated annual incidence of new HIV infections is 40,000. Forty-two percent of these are in men who have sex with men, and 54% are in blacks.

Prevalence

Chlamydia infection is particularly insidious because 70% to 90% of women and a high percentage of men with infections are asymptomatic. At least 45 million people in the United States are estimated to have genital herpes simplex virus infection and 20 million to have HPV (see Table 10-30). An estimated 850,000 to 950,000 persons in the United States are living with HIV, including 180,000 to 280,000 who do not know they are infected.

Cost of and Impact on Society

The total estimated cost of STDs in the United States, including sexually transmitted HIV, is more than $16.6 billion. Table 10-31 shows the breakdown by disease.

Morbidity and Mortality

Of the estimated 15 million individuals in the United States who contract one or more STDs each year, half will have a lifelong infection. This leads to an estimated prevalence of 65 million persons with an incurable STD (Cates et al, 1999). HIV is the leading cause of death in black men, age 25 to 44 years.

Each disease has it own short-term and long-term consequences. These include chronic or recurring pain, infertility, disseminated disease with multiorgan damage, transmission to newborn children and sexual contacts, cancer of the cervix, death, and others.

Important Facts Relevant to Prevention

The fact that many of these infections are incurable and have a high prevalence of asymptomatic carriers has led to STDs being categorized as the "hidden epidemic."

The risk factors for STDs are sexual behaviors in individuals or groups of individuals that predispose to sexual transmission of disease (Table 10-32). Only abstinence and properly used condoms are effective in reducing the risk of disease transmission through sexual contact.

The presence of chlamydia or herpes infection has been shown to enhance significantly the likelihood of sexually transmitted infection when the individual is exposed to HIV.

Screening Test Recommendations

The USPSTF recommends routine screening for chlamydia infection in all sexually active women younger than 25 years and in all other high-risk non-pregnant women (USPSTF, 2001A) as well as in these groups during pregnancy (USPSTF, 2001B). The evidence is not strong enough to recommend for or against screening other women whether pregnant or not (USPSTF, 2001C). The evidence for and against screening men for chlamydia infection is too close to justify a general recommendation (USPSTF, 2001C). The optimal screening interval or timing of screening during pregnancy for chlamydia is not known (USPSTF, 2001). In its 1996 Second Report, the USPSTF made recommendations for gonorrhea screening similar to those for chlamydia. The USPSTF has not made recommendations concerning screening for HPV infection, but the Canadian Task Force on Preventive Health Care (2003D) has determined that fair evidence exists to recommend against routine screening.

The USPSTF recommended that all at-risk individuals including pregnant women and those who live in higher-prevalence areas be periodically screened (USPSTF, 1996A).

Preventive Activities Recommendations

Areas of the country with the largest declines of STDs have been those that have active public health education and screening programs. High schools have the highest-risk population and present the best opportunity for systematic prevention efforts. The prevalence of sexually active high school students engaging in early intercourse at younger than 13 years and with four or more sexual partners is shown in Table 10-33. Family physicians should support and, when possible, actively participate in public health efforts to reduce STDs.

The advent of reasonably accurate, noninvasive screening tests for chlamydia by using urine specimens makes the process and acceptability of broader screening more achievable for both male and female subjects. Clinicians should consider routine use of these tests for their high-risk patients.

Discussion

An example of the epidemiology of the consequences of STDs follows. From 75% to 90% of women with chlamydia infection have no symptoms, yet in 40% of women with untreated chlamydia infections, pelvic inflammatory disease will develop, and one in five of these women will become infertile. The usual source of infection is from the 50% of infected men who have no symptoms.

Impact on the Family Unit

The incrimination that can result when a husband or wife is diagnosed with an STD may lead to major family disruption. The physician plays the key role in interpreting the meaning of such an episode and bringing the couple to a mutual understanding. It is therefore critical that the physician know the natural course of the disease. Because of the high percentage of asymptomatic infected individuals with many of these infections, it is often impossible to know accurately when the patient was initially infected.

The high prevalence of STDs among teens creates some very challenging issues for both the teens and the parents. Assuring that children are educated concerning their risk is paramount, and creating an environment that fosters open and honest communication will help assure appropriate evaluation and treatment, should infection be suspected.

VACCINE-PREVENTABLE INFECTIONS

Epidemiology

Incidence
One of the greatest public health achievements of the 20th century has been the dramatic effect of immunization on the incidence of infectious disease, particularly in children. Table 10-34 shows the nearly 100% decrease in the morbidity of diseases for which immunizations are universally recommended in children. Poliomyelitis has been virtually eliminated from the Western Hemisphere, and smallpox has been eliminated worldwide.

Prevalence
Vaccines such as childhood immunizations may be recommended universally or specifically for at-risk groups such as those traveling to areas in which the disease is endemic. The prevalence of coverage for recommended immunizations for children has met or continues to increase toward meeting the Healthy People 2010 goal of 90% coverage. The rates for the elderly have been less successful, with only 66% coverage for influenza and 56% for streptococcal pneumonia disease.

Cost of and Impact on Society
Immunization is highly cost-effective. For instance, influenza and streptococcal pneumonia immunization in the elderly produce $30 to $60 of savings for every dollar spent. Measles, mumps, rubella immunization in children saves $16.34 for each dollar spent (CDC, 1999).

Important Facts Relevant to Prevention

Many of the historically most severe, often epidemic, infectious diseases are now well controlled by safe, effective immunizations that have an excellent cost-to-benefit ratio.

Preventive Activities Recommendations

Family physicians should regularly update recommended schedules for pediatric (Fig. 10-16) and adult immunizations (Fig. 10-17). Documentation and reminder systems are important strategies in assuring optimal protection of patients from vaccine-preventable illness.

A variety of vaccines also are recommended for individuals with special medical conditions (Fig. 10-18), as well as those undertaking international travel. Up-to-date information is available at www.cdc.gov/nip/default.htm.

INJURY PREVENTION

Epidemiology

Incidence
The medical system cares for 24.6 million injury and poisoning episodes per year: 104 million by office-based physicians, 10.8 million by hospital outpatient departments, and 39.2 million by emergency departments. The estimated number of total injuries per year exceeds 57 million.

Morbidity and Mortality
More than 160,000 injury deaths occur each year. The major causes of those deaths are shown in Table 10-35. Unintentional injury is the leading cause of death for all age groups from age 1 to 34 years (Table 10-36). Motor vehicle traffic is the leading cause of unintentional injury death for all age groups except those younger than 1 year and older than 65 years, for whom it is second (Table 10-37). For intentional

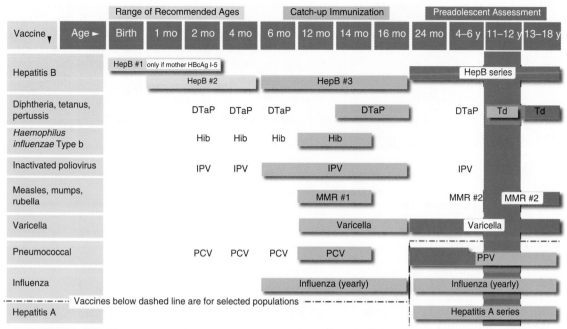

Figure 10-16 Recommended childhood and adolescent immunization schedule, United States, July through December 2004. (Data from Advisory Committee in Immunization Practices. Recommended Childhood and Adolescent Immunization Schedule, United States, July through December 2004. MMWR Morb Mortal Wkly Rep. 2004;53:Q1–Q3.)

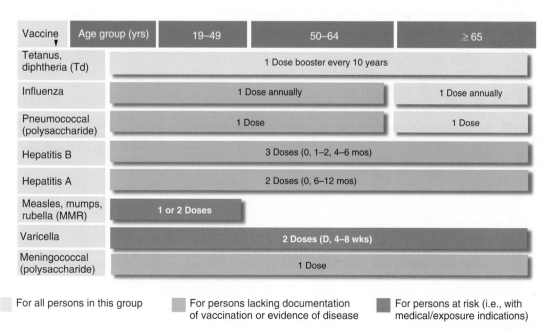

Figure 10-17 Recommended adult immunization schedule, by vaccine and age group, United States, October 2004 through September 2005. (Data from Centers for Disease Control and Prevention. Recommended Adult Immunization Schedule, United States, October 2004 through September 2005. MMWR Morb Mortal Wkly Rep 2004;53:Q1–Q4.)

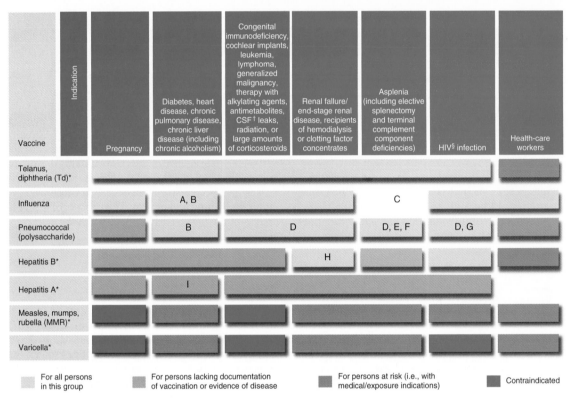

Vaccine	Pregnancy	Diabetes, heart disease, chronic pulmonary disease, chronic liver disease (including chronic alcoholism)	Congenital immunodeficiency, cochlear implants, leukemia, lymphoma, generalized malignancy, therapy with alkylating agents, antimetabolites, CSF† leaks, radiation, or large amounts of corticosteroids	Renal failure/end-stage renal disease, recipients of hemodialysis or clotting factor concentrates	Asplenia (including elective splenectomy and terminal complement component deficiencies)	HIV§ infection	Health-care workers
Tetanus, diphtheria (Td)*							
Influenza		A, B			C		
Pneumococcal (polysaccharide)		B	D	D, E, F	D, G		
Hepatitis B*				H			
Hepatitis A*		I					
Measles, mumps, rubella (MMR)*							
Varicella*							

For all persons in this group

For persons lacking documentation of vaccination or evidence of disease

For persons at risk (i.e., with medical/exposure indications)

Contraindicated

*Covered by the Vaccine Injury Compensation Program.
†Cerebrospinal fluid.
§Human immunodeficiency virus.

Special Notes for Medical and Other Indications

A. Although chronic liver disease and alcoholism are not indications for influenza vaccination, administer one dose annually if the patient is aged ≥50 years, has other indications for influenza vaccine, or requests vaccination.
B. Asthma is an indication for influenza vaccination but not for pneumococcal vaccination.
C. No data exist specifically on the risk for severe or complicated influenza infections among persons with asplenia. However, influenza is a risk factor for secondary bacterial infections that can cause severe disease among persons with asplenia.
D. For persons aged <65 years, revaccinate once after ≥5 years have elapsed since initial vaccination.
E. Administer meningococcal vaccine and consider *Haemophilus influenzae* type b vaccine.
F. For persons undergoing elective splenectomy, vaccinate ≥2 weeks before surgery.
G. Vaccinate as soon after diagnosis as possible.
H. For hemodialysis patients, use special formulation of vaccine (40 μg/mL) or two 20 μg/mL doses administered at one body site. Vaccinate early in the course of renal disease. Assess antibody titers to hepatitis B surface antigen (anti-HB) levels annually. Administer additional doses if anti-HB levels decline to <10 mIU/mL.
I. For all persons with chronic liver disease.
J. Withhold MMR or other measles-containing vaccines from HIV-infected persons with evidence of severe immunosuppression (see *MMWR* 1998;47 [No. RR-8]:21-2 and *MMWR* 2002; 51[No. RR-2]:22–4).
K. Persons with impaired humoral immunity but intact cellular immunity may be vaccinated (see *MMWR* 1999; 48[No. RR-6]).

Figure 10-18 Recommended adult immunization schedule, by vaccine and medical and other indications, United States, October 2004 through September 2005. (Data from Centers for Disease Control and Prevention. Recommended Adult Immunization Schedule, United States, October 2004 through September 2005. MMWR Morb Mortal Wkly Rep 2004;53:Q1–Q4.)

injury deaths, homicide is one of the top five causes of death for groups age 1 to 34 years, and suicide is one of the top five for groups from ages 10 to 54 years (Table 10-38).

Based on emergency department treatment records, the large preponderance of more serious nonfatal injuries is unintentional. Of these nonfatal injuries, the leading cause in all age groups except 15 to 24 years is falls (Table 10-39).

Important Facts Relevant to Prevention

Alcohol use is a major factor in multiple types of intentional and unintentional injuries. The most effective interventions have been those that are legislated or require no action on the part of the individual or family (or both). Examples are safer vehicles and child-proof safety caps.

Specific measures that have been shown to reduce injury include seat belts, children's car seats, vehicle air bags, helmets for cyclists, smoke detectors, and absence of firearms in the home. Office-based interventions increase compliance with preventive recommendations such as seat-belt use.

Screening Test Recommendations

Physicians should consider screening patients for injury risk factors such as use of safety restraints when driving, fire alarms in the home, firearms in the home, violence in the home or community, and alcohol abuse. Additional risk-assessment questions are age specific, such as safety measures in the home for young children and the elderly. The USPSTF has one screening recommendation related to injury prevention, which cites insufficient evidence to recommend for or against screening for family and intimate partner violence (USPSTF, 2004I).

Preventive Activities Recommendations

The guidelines for prevention listed under alcohol abuse and osteoporosis should be followed. The USPSTF recommends counseling all patients and parents of patients concerning use of occupant restraints in vehicles, use of helmets when riding motorcycles, refraining from driving or participating in other dangerous activities when under the influence of alcohol or drugs, and reduction of unintentional injury risk for children, adolescents, and adults. Parents should be encouraged to ensure that all children are taught to swim. Homes should be safety-proofed. All homes should have working fire alarms. Medications, poisons, toxins, and firearms should all be inaccessible when small children are in the home. When elderly persons are within the home, specific measures should be taken to reduce the risk of falls. Families should be counseled to place sleeping infants on their backs to decrease the incidence of sudden infant death syndrome. The USPSTF evidence ratings for injury prevention are shown in Table 10-40.

Discussion

Whereas the incidence of many types of injuries is declining, many others are worsening. These include nonfatal head injuries. Overall, emergency department visits for injury, nonfatal poisonings, overall unintentional injury deaths, motor vehicle crash deaths, nonfatal pedestrian injury, motorcycle helmet use, child-maltreatment fatalities, and homicides show a worsening trend.

The facts that the leading cause of death for ages 1 to 34 years is unintentional injury and that the most frequent source of these fatal injuries is motor vehicle accidents create an important opportunity for screening and counseling this age group. This should include screening for alcohol abuse, because 40% of fatal motor vehicle accidents are alcohol related.

Impact on the Family Unit

In addition to the immediate trauma, nonfatal accidents affect the individual and the family directly. An issue that must be confronted is the injured person's and the other family members' own mortality. Although some families grow closer at these times, others may distance themselves as a defense mechanism. Fatal accidents present a special problem. The loss is unexpected and often occurs in those who are otherwise young and healthy. The process of grieving may become particularly difficult or pathologic.

DIABETES MELLITUS

Recommendations

Despite the high morbidity, mortality, and cost associated with diabetes, the long presymptomatic stage, the high prevalence, and the ease of diagnosis, the USPSTF is unable to find sufficient evidence to recommend for or against routine screening for type 2 diabetes (USPSTF, 2003I). It is known that aggressive management of diabetes can reduce microvascular complications, but no evidence indicates that earlier diagnosis and treatment will affect the outcomes. However, the USPSTF (2003B) has recommended screening for type 2 diabetes in adults with hypertension or hyperlipidemia. This recommendation is supported by evidence of improved cardiovascular outcomes in patients with hypertension or hyperlipidemia if the target goals for treatment are adjusted when diabetes also is present.

Discussion

As the target levels for blood pressure and LDL now have been reduced significantly, one could make the case that any patient with higher levels should be screened for diabetes as part of determining what each individual's blood pressure and lipid goals should be.

GLAUCOMA

Prevalence

The prevalence of glaucoma increases from 0.5% of persons younger than 65 years to 2% to 4% of those older than 75 years. Glaucoma is 4 to 6 times more prevalent in blacks than in whites.

Important Facts Relevant to Prevention

The ultimate result of untreated glaucoma is blindness. Primary open-angle glaucoma is the most common type of glaucoma and is asymptomatic until severe, often irreversible damage has occurred. The benefits of treatment have not been conclusively demonstrated.

The two major criteria for diagnosis are visual field defects and optic disc pallor and cupping. In glaucoma, the optic cup diameter is 30% greater than that of the disc. The funduscopic changes on direct ophthalmoscopy are best seen with the red filter. Patients with upper-normal intraocular pressure can have glaucoma and secondary blindness, yet only in a minority of patients with elevated intraocular pressure does glaucoma develop.

The risk factors for glaucoma are elevated intraocular pressure, family history, black race, diabetes mellitus, and age.

Screening Test Recommendations

The value of screening for elevated intraocular pressure with the Schiotz tonometer is controversial. If the family physician elects to use this method, patients should be screened starting at age 40 years and every 5 years thereafter until age 60 years, at which time the screening interval should be reduced to 2 to 3 years. Funduscopic evaluation by a well-trained physician at the time of tonometry increases the sensitivity of screening. The USPSTF (2005I) states that insufficient evidence exists to recommend for or against screening.

Preventive Activities Recommendations

Although the treatment of elevated intraocular pressure is the standard of care, no proven primary or secondary preventive measures are available once elevated pressure is found.

Discussion

Elevated intraocular pressure has a less than 30% positive predictive value for glaucoma developing. In addition, up to 50% of patients with glaucoma have normal intraocular pressure on a single random measurement. These facts make it important that high-risk patients have more extensive screening by an ophthalmologist, and that patients who are screened only with tonometry be advised that they are still at risk.

OTHER SCREENING RECOMMENDATIONS

Routine screening for thyroid disease with thyroid-stimulating hormone level is effective for detecting subclinical thyroid disease in asymptomatic children and adults. However, the USPSTF (2004I) found insufficient evidence to recommend for or against screening. Routine screening of newborns is recommended and is done routinely by all hospitals (USPSTF, 1996A).

The USPSTF (1996B) recommends screening high-risk children and pregnant women for iron-deficiency anemia. Insufficient evidence exists for general screening for iron-deficiency anemia.

Obesity is an increasingly prevalent disease in the United States (Fig. 10-19). Obesity increases the risk for cardiovascular disease, diabetes, and other chronic illness. The USPSTF (2003) makes a B recommendation for screening patients for obesity (body mass index ≥ 30) and providing access to intensive behavioral counseling.

All children at increased risk should be screened for lead levels at least once at age 1 year (USPSTF, 1996B). Very high-risk children and children living in communities with a high prevalence of lead levels should be considered for subsequent testing.

ADDITIONAL PREVENTIVE ACTIVITIES

The family physician provides a large amount of general medical care and, in the course of this care, may easily identify patients who can benefit from individualized screening tests not recommended for the general population. These screening activities also include the discovery of patients who can benefit from lifestyle and other health-related counseling. These can include counseling to prevent tobacco use, to optimize physical activity, to achieve and maintain ideal weight, and to consume a healthy diet. Other helpful services include providing information about safe sexual practices and identifying potential occupational hazards. Older adults should be screened for hearing impairment at least by questioning about a deficit. Examples in the behavioral science area include screening for dementia, depression, suicide risk, family and youth violence, as well as drug and alcohol abuse in persons at risk.

Prevention of unwanted pregnancies is another important role for the family physician. Each year an estimated 1 million pregnancies occur in teenagers age 15 to 19 years. Of these, 78% are unplanned. Although rates are declining, the U.S. rate remains the highest for developed countries. Family physicians are in a position to identify teenagers at risk for sexual activity and to provide counseling for contraception and prevention of STDs for those who are sexually active.

Yet another area of disease prevention is the preconception obstetric risk assessment. Health promotion, patient education, and therapeutic intervention can reduce risk and improve outcome. Risk is associated with systemic disease, family history, genetics, demography, environment, and lifestyle. Regular supplementation of 0.4 mg of folic acid daily is recommended for all women who could become pregnant and of 1.0 mg daily once pregnancy has occurred. Identifying risks and providing appropriate counseling before conception may help formulate important health-promotional aspects of optimal health care.

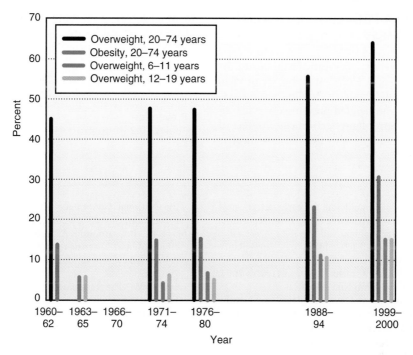

Figure 10-19   Percentage of overweight and obese individuals by age, United States, 1960–2000. (Data from National Center for Health Statistics. Health, United States, 2003. Hyattsville, MD, 2003; Freid VM, Prager K, MacKay AP, Xia H. Chartbook on Trends in the Health of Americans. Health. United States, 2003. Hyattsville, MD, National Center for Health Statistics. 2003.)

LIFESTYLES FOR HEALTH

Of the diseases discussed in this chapter, a strikingly common theme is seen in their etiology and prevention: An individual's lifestyle is the major modifiable determinant of health.

Proper diet is of paramount importance to prevent the nation's number one killer: CHD; it is estimated that one third of cancers, the nation's number two killer, are secondary to diet and physical activity habits (Byers et al., 2002). Fortunately, the specific dietary recommendations for prevention of one disease also are beneficial in general. Therefore it is possible to make broad, prudent nutritional recommendations as a basis on which all physicians and patients can build: Dietary guidelines are outlined in Table 10-9, on the Internet (American Heart Association, Dietary Guidelines for Healthy Adults), and in booklets that can be made available in the physician's office (American Heart Association, 2000).

Cohort studies have shown a significant protective effect for all-cause mortality in both men and women engaging in even modest levels of exercise (Blair et al., 1996). Sedentary lifestyle imparts the same 1.5- to 2-times degree of increased risk for CHD as do smoking and other major risk factors. Weight-bearing exercises substantially reduce the risk of osteoporosis and its associated fractures. Anxiety and depression both appear to have lower incidence in those who exercise, as well as benefiting individuals already suffering from these disorders. Hypertension, obesity, and type 2 diabetes are all benefited by regular exercise. It is recommended that all patients be counseled as to the most appropriate types, amount, and intensity of exercise for their current health and risk status. General guidelines for all healthy adults are to engage in at least 30 minutes of moderate aerobic physical activity most days of each week. These 30 minutes may be accumulated over the day. Adding additional exercise to increase muscle strength and joint flexibility also is recommended. Parents should ensure that their children engage in regular activities that involve vigorous exercise.

Another common prevention theme is the critical importance of avoiding toxins, especially the addictive substances nicotine and alcohol. Smoking accounts for 18% of all deaths and 30% of all cancer deaths, as well as being a major factor in CHD. Each year, 435,000 deaths can be directly attributed to cigarette smoking. It is estimated that each pack of cigarettes sold results in a cost of $7.18 for medical care and lost productivity (American Cancer Society, 2003). Alcohol is a risk factor for colon and breast cancer, obesity, liver disease, suicide, homicide, and accidents of all kinds.

Table 10-41 shows the major diseases discussed and the lifestyle issues and genetics implicated as risk factors for each one.

DEVELOPING A PREVENTIVE HEALTH CARE FLOWSHEET

Electronic health records can greatly facilitate health-maintenance tracking, with automatic reminders increasing the family physician's ability to offer systematically the recommended preventive services in a cost-efficient manner. If an electronic health record is not available, a simple and flexible flowsheet is essential for the continuity and comprehensiveness of preventive health care.

> ### Material Available on Student Consult
>
> Review Questions and Answers about Disease Prevention
> Tables 10-2 through 10-41.

REFERENCES

American Cancer Society guideline for early detection of cervical neoplasia. Available at http://caonline.amcancersoc.org/cgi/content/full/52/6/342. Accessed

American Cancer Society. Facts and Figures, Surveillance and Research, 2004.

American Cancer Society. Cancer Facts and Figures 2004. Am Cancer Soc 2003;Pub No. 5008.04.

American Heart Association. Dietary guidelines for healthy adults. Available at www.americanheart.org/presenter.jhtml?identifier=1330. Accessed 9/11/2004.

American Heart Association. An eating plan for healthy Americans: Our American Heart Association Diet. Channing Bete Company (Product Code 50–1481), 2000.

American Heart Association. Heart Disease and Stroke Statistics, 2004 update. Dallas, TX, American Heart Association, 2003.

American Psychiatric Association. Diagnostic and Statistical Manual of Mental Disorders, 4th ed. Washington, DC, American Psychiatric Association, 1994:195–204.

Anderson KM, Wilson PWF, Odell PM, Konnel WB. An updated coronary risk profile. A statement for health professionals. Circulation 1991;83:356–362.

Blair SN, Kampert JB, Kohl HW III, et al. Influences of cardio-respiratory fitness and precursors on cardiovascular disease and all-cause mortality in men and women. JAMA 1996;276:205–210.

Brewster A. Breast cancer epidemiology, prevention, and early detection [Review]. Curr Opin Oncol 2001;13:420–425.

Brown RL, Leonard T, Saunders LA, Papasouliotis. A two-item conjoint screen for alcohol and other drug problems. J Am Bd Fam Pract 2001;14;95–106. ⓑ

Byers T, Nestle M, McTiernan A, et al. American Cancer Society guidelines on nutrition and physical activity for cancer prevention: Reducing the risk of cancer with healthy food choices and physical activity. CA Cancer J Clin 2002;52:92–119.

Cates W, et al. Estimates of the incidence and prevalence of sexually transmitted diseases in the United States. Sex Transm Dis 1999;26(Suppl):S2–S7.

Centers for Disease Control and Prevention. An Ounce of Prevention: What Are the Returns? 2nd ed. Atlanta, U.S. Department of Health and Human Services, 1999.

Centers for Disease Control and Prevention. Recommended Adult Immunization Schedule, United States, October 2004 through September 2005. MMWR Morb Mortal Wkly Rep, 2004;53:Q1–Q4.

Cooper R, Cutter J, Desvigne-Nickens P, et al. Trends and disparities in coronary heart disease, stroke, and other cardiovascular diseases in the United Staes: Findings of the National Conference on Cardiovascular Disease Prevention. Circulation 2000;102:3137–3147.

Corvol JC, Bouzamondo A, Sirol M, et al. Differential effects of lipid-lowering therapies on stroke prevention: A meta-analysis of randomized trials. Arch Intern Med 2003;163:669. ⓐ

Crabbe WW. The tamoxifen controversy. Oncol Nurs Forum 1996;23:761–766.

Dove-Edwin I, Thomas HJW. Review article: The prevention of colorectal cancer. Aliment Pharmacol Ther 2001;15:323–336.

Enlish DR, Holman CDJ, Milne E, et al. The Quantification of Drug Caused Morbidity and Mortality in Australia, 1992. Canberra, Australia, Canberra Commonwealth Department of Human Services and Health, 1995.

Finney JW, Hahn AC, Moos RH. The effectiveness of inpatient and outpatient alcohol abuse; the need to focus on mediators and moderators of setting effects. Addiction 1996;91:1773–1796.

Fiore MC, Bailey WC, Cohen SJ, et al. Treating Tobacco Use and Dependence: Clinical Practice Guideline. Rockville, MD, U.S. Department of Health and Human Services, Public Health Service, June 2000.

Fleming MF, Barry KL, Manwell LB, Johnson K, London R. Brief physician advice for problem alcohol drinkers: A randomized controlled trial in community-based primary care practices. JAMA 1997;277:1039–1045. ⓐ

Fleming MF, Mundt MP, French MT, Manwell LB, Staauffacher EA, Barry KL. Brief physician advice for problem drinkers: Long-term efficacy and cost-benefit analysis. Alcohol Clin Exp Res 2002;26:36–43. ⓐ

Glynn TJ, Manley MW, How to Help Your Patients Stop Smoking: A National Cancer Institute Manual for Physicians. Bethesda, MD, U.S. Department of Health and Human Services, Public Health Service, National Institutes of Health, National Cancer Institute, 1993. NIH Publication No. 93–3064.

Grant BF. Estimates of U.S. children exposed to alcohol abuse and dependence in the family. Am J Public Health 2000;90:112–115.

Grundy SM, Cleeman JI, Merz NB, et al. Implications of recent clinical trials for the National Cholesterol Education Program Adult Treatment Panel III Guidelines. Circulation 2004;110:227–239.

Harwood H. Updating estimates of the economic costs of alcohol abuse in the United States: Estimates, update methods, and data. Lewin Group for the National Institute on Alcohol Abuse and Alcoholism, 2000.

Available at http://pubs.niaaa.nih.gov/publications/economic-2000/alcoholcost.pdf. Accessed 12/27/2005.

Johnston SC, Gress DR, Browner WS, Sidney S. Short-term prognosis after emergency department diagnosis of TIA. JAMA 2000;284:2901–2906.

Lewiston S, Clarke R, Qizilbash N, et al. Age-specific relevance of usual blood pressure to vascular mortality: A meta-analysis of individual data for one million adults in 61 prospective studies. Lancet. 2002;360:1903–1913.

Modugno F. Ovarian cancer and high risk women: Implications for prevention, screening and early detection. Gynecol Oncol 2003;91:15–31.

National Cancer Institute, U.S. National Institutes of Health. Endometrial cancer (PDQ): Screening health professional version, summary of evidence, 2005. Available at www.cancer.gov. Accessed 5/1/2005.

National Cholesterol Education Program Expert Panel of Detection, Evaluation, and Treatment of High Blood Cholesterol in Adults (Adult Treatment Panel III): Third report of the National Cholesterol Education Program (NCEP) on detection, evaluation, and treatment of high blood cholesterol in adults (Adult Treatment Panel III) final report. Circulation 2002;106:3143–51.

National Cholesterol Education Program. Risk assessment tool for estimating 10-year risk of developing hard CHD (myocardial infarction and coronary death). Available at hin.nhlbi.nih.gov/atpiii/calculator.asp Accessed 9/11/2004.

NCI, U.S. National Institutes of Health, Annual Report to the Nation. 2004. Available at www.Cancer.org. Accessed 12/20/2005.

NCI, U.S. National Institutes of Health Surveillance: Epidemiology and End Results, SEER cancer statistics. 2004. Available at www.Cancer.gov. Accessed 12/20/2005.

Nelson HD, Helfand M, Woolf SH, Allan JD. Screening for postmenopausal Osteoperosis: A review of the evidence for the U.S. Preventative Services Task Force. Available at www.preventiveservices.ahrq.gov. Accessed 1/24/2006.

Office of National Drug Control Policy. The economic costs of drug abuse in the United States, 1992–1998. Washington, DC, Executive Office of the President, 2001. Pub no. NCJ 190636.

Prospective Studies Colloboration. Age-specific relevance of usual blood pressure to vascular mortality: A meta-analysis of individual data for one million adults in 61 prospective studies. Lancet 2002;360:1903–1913.

Sanmuganathan PS, Ghahramani P, Jackson PR, et al. Aspirin for primary prevention of coronary heart disease: Safety and absolute benefit related to coronary risk derived from meta-analysis of randomized trials. Heart 2001;85:2. Ⓐ

Segal JB, McNamara RL, Miller MR, et al. Prevention of thromboembolism in atrial fibrillation: A meta-analysis of trials of anticoagulants and antiplatelet drugs. J Gen Intern Med 2000;15:56–67. Ⓐ

Siris ES, Miller PD, Barrett-Connor E, et. al. Identification and fracture outcomes of undiagnosed low bone mineral density in postmenopausal women: Results from the National Osteoporosis Risk Assessment. JAMA 2001;286:2815–2822.

Strong JP, Malcom GT, McMahon CA, et al. Prevalence and extent of atherosclerosis in adolescents and young adults. JAMA 1999;281:727–735.

Substance Abuse and Mental Health Administration. Substance abuse or dependence. The NHSDA Report, October 11, 2002.

Thun MJ, Peto R, Lopez AD, et al. Alcohol and consumption and mortality among middle-aged and elderly U.S. adults. N Engl J Med 1997;337:1705–1714. Ⓑ

U.S. Preventive Services Task Force. Screening for cervical cancer, recommendations and rationale. Available at ARHQ.gov/clinic/3rduspstf/cercanrr.htm. Accessed 12/20/2005.

U.S. Preventive Services Task Force. Screening for chlamydia infections: Recommendations and rationale. Am J Prev Med 2001;20:90–94.

U.S. Preventive Services Task Force. Screening for Osteoporosis in Postmenopausal Women: Recommendations and Rationale. Rockville, MD, Agency for Health Care Research and Quality, 2002. Available at www.ahrq.gove/clinic/3rduspstf/osteoporosis/osteoorr.htm. Accessed 9/25/2005.

U.S. Department of Health and Human Services, National Institutes of Health, National Institute on Alcohol Abuse and Alcoholism: Helping Patients with Alcohol Problems: A Health Practitioners Guide. Bethesda, MD, NIH Publication No. 03–3769, 2003.

Wolf PA, D'Agostino RB, Belanger AJ, Kannel WB. Probability of stroke: A risk profile from the Framingham Study. Stroke 1991;22:312–318.

Wolfe JT. The role of screening in the management of skin cancer. Curr Opin Oncol 1999;11:123.

Wright GS, Gruidl ME. Early detection and prevention of lung cancer. Curr Opin Oncol 2000;12:143–148.

SUGGESTED READINGS

Abenaa B, Helzisouer K. Breast cancer epidemiology, prevention, and early detection. Curr Opin Oncol 2001;13:420–425

Gandelman G, Bodenheimer MM. Screening coronary arteriography in the primary prevention of coronary artery disease. Heart Dis 2003;5:335–344.

Humphrey LL, Tensch S, Johnson M. U.S. Preventive Services Task Force, lung cancer screening with sputum cytological examination, chest radiography, and computed tomography: An update for the preventive services task force. Ann Intern Med 2004;140:740–753.

Institute of Medicine. The Hidden Epidemic: Confronting Sexually Transmitted Diseases. Washington, DC, National Academy Press, 1997.

Ladabaum U, Chopra CL, Huang G, et al. Aspirin as an adjunct to screening for prevention of sporadic colorectal cancer, Ann Intern Med 2001;135:769–781.

Office of Applied Studies, Substance Abuse and Mental Health Administration. Results from the National Osteoporosis Risk Assessment. JAMA 2001;286:2815–2822.

11

Integrative Medicine

David P. Rakel and Adam Rindfleisch

KEY POINTS

1. Integrative medicine takes an individualized, health-oriented approach to healing, emphasizing a strong provider-patient relationship. It incorporates evidence-based medicine as much as possible while also taking into account the patient's personal beliefs and cultural background. The patient has an active role in the healing process.

2. Integrative medicine makes use of therapies commonly referred to as "complementary" or "alternative," provided they are safe, potentially effective, and likely to benefit the individual patient. Evidence of risk and benefit must always be carefully weighed for all interventions.

3. Patients commonly use a wide array of complementary and alternative therapies. Health care providers must be able to advise them regarding the safety and efficacy of these approaches.

4. In developing a treatment plan for a given patient, care of the patient might be improved through incorporating any or all of the following into the care plan: nutrition, herbs and other supplements, physical activity, manipulative therapies, energy medicine, mind-body techniques, spirituality, and other healing systems, such as traditional Chinese medicine, Ayurveda, and homeopathy.

5. Primary care providers should understand how to make reasonable and appropriate referrals to practitioners of complementary and alternative therapies.

6. No therapy is without associated risks. Be familiar with supplement side effects, potential dangers of exercise and manipulative techniques, and how various treatments may interact with standard medical care. Urgently needed biomedical care should not be delayed to try unvalidated therapeutic techniques.

INTEGRATIVE MEDICINE IS FAMILY MEDICINE

Integrative medicine is healing-oriented medicine that takes account of the whole person (body, mind, and spirit), including all aspects of lifestyle. It emphasizes the therapeutic relationship and makes use of all appropriate therapies, both conventional and alternative.

The field emerged in response to a need to bring a better balance to health care delivery, combining the advances made by disease-oriented care with those that help facilitate health and healing.

In the 1990s, a significant increase was found in public interest in complementary and alternative medicine (CAM). This was related in part to the deterioration of the physician-patient relationship, the overutilization of technology, and the inability of the medical system to treat chronic disease adequately. At that time, more visits to CAM providers occurred than those to all primary care medical physicians, and the public paid an estimated $13 billion out of pocket for such visits (Eisenberg et al., 1993). This trend continued throughout the 1990s, with 42% of the public using CAM therapies and CAM expenditures increasing to $27 billion from 1990 to 1997 (Eisenberg et al., 1998).

Integrative medicine reflects an attempt to shift our focus back toward the enhancement of health as part of health care delivery. The foundation of this approach is based in relationship-centered care, in which a caring physician takes time to listen to a patient's story and gain insight into the person who has the disease. Developing this relationship allows a physician to more easily create a health plan that outlines what actions are needed to improve health. Box 11-1 highlights key components of an integrative approach.

Facilitating health and healing is a dynamic process, as illustrated in Figure 11-1. It involves four steps:

1. When individuals are in poor health and in need of medical attention, they will seek care from

---

Evidence levels Ⓐ Randomized, controlled trials (RCTs), meta-analyses, well-designed systematic reviews of RCTs. Ⓑ Case-control or cohort studies, nonrandomized clinical trials, systematic reviews of studies other than RCTs, cross-sectional studies, retrospective studies, certain uncontrolled studies. Ⓒ Consensus statements, expert guidelines, usual practice, opinion.

Box 11-1	Defining Integrative Medicine

Provides relationship-centered care
Integrates conventional and complementary methods for treatment and prevention
Involves removing barriers to activate the body's healing response
Uses natural, less invasive interventions before costly, invasive ones when possible
Engages mind, body, spirit, and community to facilitate healing
Contends that healing is always possible, even when curing is not.

someone they trust. Ideally, the relationship that results leads to rapport and empathy, and insight develops. Insight generates the ideas the physician uses to develop an efficient treatment plan that will facilitate positive changes in individual health.

2. What a physician suggests to optimize individual health will be influenced by a number of factors. The patient's belief system and culture must be considered. In addition, research findings and science must guide the choice of which therapeutic modalities to use. Individual uniqueness also must be taken into account.

3. Once the foundation of relationship-centered care is established and insight into the patient's unique situation is developed, the physician and the patient must agree on a plan of action that both believe will lead to improved health. This often includes a collaborative approach that may involve both conventional and complementary treatment. For example, a patient with cancer may have a team that includes the primary care physician, an oncologist, a nutritionist, a traditional Chinese medicine practitioner, and a spiritual advisor or chaplain. The primary practitioner is in the best position to organize the team that will best suit the patient's needs. Most important, this approach requires that the patient be an active participant in the healing process. This includes participating in decisions regarding behaviors and positive lifestyle changes. Patients are empowered to make positive changes themselves instead of simply being passive recipients of care.

4. The healing process is a dynamic, continuous process that constantly needs re-evaluation if the balance that best facilitates health is to be maintained. What works at one time may require modification and adaptation in the future. These changes will best occur with the involvement of a primary care practitioner who knows how the patient's unique situation is influenced by biopsychosocial and spiritual influences on health.

As this process continues to unfold, the physician and patient constantly learn from past experiences and develop new insights into how to maintain the balance of health. In so doing, they often develop a deeper understanding of the patient's core health needs. This inward journey leads to an understanding of why symptoms exist and what can be done to resolve them within a continuously changing environment.

If this inner exploration does not occur, the body-mind will continue to rely on external influences to reduce the severity of symptoms. The learning that could arise from the illness experience may be lost. Symptoms can often be red flags that exist to

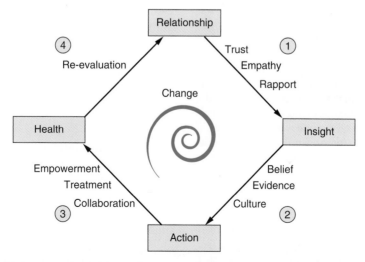

Figure 11-1 Steps in facilitating healing. (Reprinted with permission from Rakel D. The healing power of relationship-centered care. In Rakel D, Faass N, eds. Complementary Medicine in Clinical Practice. Sudbury, MA: Jones and Bartlett Publishers, 2005.)

alert us to lifestyle habits or situations that are not conducive to health and well-being. If we simply suppress a symptom without learning what it is trying to teach us, we may never understand what is needed to permanently resolve it. An example would be the suppression of dyspepsia with a proton-pump inhibitor. Whereas some medications act on the underlying cause of a disease, others are strictly for symptom control. Both are important, but if the question of why the problem exists in the first place is not explored, lasting attempts to improve health are less likely to occur. Why does the patient have symptoms of dyspepsia in the first place? If the main focus becomes what is needed for healing, fewer symptom-suppressing therapies will be required, resulting in lower health care costs and improved quality of life for patients. This is health-oriented, as opposed to disease-oriented, care.

In this chapter, we use a case study to illustrate how integrative medicine can be used to stimulate the body's self-healing mechanisms. We also look at some key studies illustrating how integrating complementary therapies into family medicine can improve health. We also review common CAM therapies.

AN INTEGRATIVE MEDICINE CASE STUDY

History and Present Illness

Joan is a 53-year-old woman who tells you, "Doc, I'm a mess. My bowels are giving me trouble again, and I'm always tired. What else can I do to feel like myself again?"

Joan has a long history of multiple chronic medical problems. She was diagnosed with irritable bowel syndrome (IBS) 4 years ago while she was going through a divorce, and for the past 3 months, she has been having two episodes of diarrhea daily. She refuses IBS medications because they led to dizziness and nausea in the past. In addition, she notes feeling "tired all the time," even though she sleeps at least 8 hours per night. Joan has poor libido, anhedonia, and increased appetite. She denies suicidal thoughts, but states, "No one would really care if I was gone. My ex and my son would probably throw a going-away party." A sleep study and thyroid tests were normal 2 months ago.

Medical History

Joan's medical history also includes seasonal allergies, morbid obesity, weekly migraine headaches, and, according to another provider she saw, fibromyalgia. She injured her lower back 20 years ago and still has intermittent pain. She refuses narcotics because they make her "loopy," and her son "would just steal them anyway." A chiropractic visit several years ago helped her back pain for several months. Joan has hypertension and was told recently that her lipids are borderline. Past surgeries include an appendectomy and a cholecystectomy.

Medications, Supplements, and Botanicals

Medications include aspirin and lisinopril. She lists multiple drug allergies, many symptoms of which are not commonly associated with the drugs in question. She is not taking any herbals or other supplements, but her sister has suggested that she try some. She wants your opinion first.

Patient Profile

Joan is divorced and lives alone. Her 19-year-old son was arrested a few months ago for possession of marijuana. Her father died at 67 years of a heart attack, and her 82-year-old mother lives nearby with Joan's sister. Joan's mother and sister both have type 2 diabetes. Joan's father was an alcoholic who was often physically abusive. Her son has depression. Joan has smoked a half pack of cigarettes daily for 35 years and is a social drinker, but she does not use illicit drugs. She is employed as an administrative assistant in a busy real estate firm but dreams of becoming a professional artist. She enjoys painting, reading mystery books, movies, and going to the park. When asked about stress, she states, "My whole life is a stressor." Joan was brought up Catholic but attends mass only on holidays. She states that her sister and friends at work are her main social contacts.

Joan eats a typical American diet, with significant diet soda and coffee consumption. She averages fewer than four servings of fruits and vegetables daily and eats red meat and dairy products frequently. She craves cookies and chocolate. She used to enjoy swimming and walking but is currently not exercising.

Review of Systems

Review of systems is positive for almost every system reviewed.

Physical Examination

Notable examination findings include abdominal obesity, and a blood pressure of 142/94. She has diffuse abdominal tenderness with no rebound or guarding, and pain on palpation of the paralumbar muscles.

Note that an integrative approach incorporates elements not always covered in a standard history and physical, including relationships, life stressors, nutrition, and spirituality. Such topics provide useful additional insights to guide the creation of an individualized care plan. Please refer to the boxes labeled "Suggestions for Joan" after each section of this chapter for examples of how integrative medicine providers might approach Joan's case.

INTEGRATIVE MEDICINE: EIGHT PERSPECTIVES

Integrative medicine makes use of a wide array of healing modalities, each with different philosophical, diagnostic, and therapeutic underpinnings. Eight perspectives that can be used to assess a person's health needs are outlined. All of them can be relevant to a patient encounter, but areas of focus will differ from one person to the next.

1. Nutrition

Good nutrition is central to health, but it is given only minimal attention in most medical training programs. A growing body of research indicates that diet can play a key role in preventing and treating a number of disorders, including hypertension, dyslipidemias, and diabetes. Dietary modification also may improve illnesses associated with chronic inflammation, such as rheumatoid arthritis, inflammatory bowel disease, and eczema. Nutritional recommendations are frequently incorporated into integrative treatment plans for various cancers, dementia, multiple sclerosis, chronic fatigue, and any number of other diseases (Mahan and Escott-Stump, 2004).

Integrative medicine makes use of several nutritional tools. These include the glycemic index and load, the anti-inflammatory diet, elimination diets, and supplementation with vitamins, minerals, and other nutrients.

Glycemic Index and Glycemic Load

Glycemic index is an indicator of the immediate effect a food has on postprandial blood glucose levels. White bread and glucose, which cause the fastest and sharpest increase, are assigned a value of 100. All other foods are then assigned a value relative to this reference, based on how they affect test subjects' glucose levels over time. Foods with a higher glycemic index cause the pancreas to release more insulin, leading to a decrease in blood glucose to below the fasting level approximately 2 hours after eating. This rebound hypoglycemia can be characterized by fatigue, which decreases substantially when foods with a higher glycemic index are removed from the diet (Johnson, 2003 Ⓑ). Interestingly, a low-glycemic-index meal will result in a lower glycemic response for the next meal eaten as well (Wolever, 1990). Overall, meal size tends to be smaller as well.

Glycemic load takes the concept of glycemic index a step further, accounting not only for how rapidly a food's carbohydrates are converted to glucose, but also for the relative amounts of carbohydrate the food contains. Glycemic load is generally held to be a more accurate measure of a food's overall effect on pancreatic insulin release and serum glucose levels.

The Anti-inflammatory Diet

Inflammation is a major contributor to many illness states, from autoimmune disorders and Alzheimer's disease to cancer and inflammatory bowel disease. Certain fats (the omega-6 fatty acids in partially hydrogenated oils) lead to the formation of arachadonic acid and other inflammatory precursors. Conversely, omega-3 fatty acids, found in foods such as fish oil and flaxseed, have been found to reduce inflammation. If omega-3 fatty acid intake is increased and omega-6 intake decreased, inflammation and its associated symptoms may diminish over time.

Elimination Diets

Elimination diets are used to determine if a specific food or group of foods is contributing to a person's symptoms. Food allergies tend to arise relatively rapidly after foods are consumed and can be evaluated by standard allergy testing. Food intolerances, in contrast, can be quite challenging to diagnose. Symptoms of food intolerance may arise up to 3 days after exposure. The causes and manifestations of food intolerance are still hotly debated, but one theory is that foods cause problems in patients who have increased intestinal permeability, or a "leaky gut." Increased intestinal permeability permits the absorption of larger, potentially harmful molecules into the bloodstream; these subsequently trigger an immune response (Joneja, 1998 Ⓑ).

In elimination diets, specific foods or groups of foods are removed entirely from the diet for a set period, usually 10 to 14 days. After that time, if symptoms have improved, eliminated foods are reintroduced into the diet in 3-day increments. If symptoms return or worsen after the food is eaten, that food is considered one to which the subject is intolerant.

Vitamins, Minerals, and Other Nutrients

In a review of vitamin use in chronic disease, Fairfield and Fletcher (2002 Ⓐ) concluded: "We recommend that all adults take one multivitamin daily. This practice is justified mainly by the known and suspected benefits of supplemental folate and vitamins B_{12}, B_6, and D in preventing cardiovascular disease, cancer, and osteoporosis and because multivitamins at that dose are safe and inexpensive." At least 30% of U.S. residents use vitamin supplements regularly (Balluz et al., 2000), and many more need them. A survey conducted in 2000 found that only 20% to 30% of the American population met the goal of at least five servings of fruits and vegetables daily (Flood and Schatzkin, 2000).

Dose recommendations for vitamins and minerals are now referred to as reference daily intakes. For a full list of reference daily intakes and food sources of various nutrients, see Mahan and Escott-Stump, 2004 (Box 11-2).

2. Herbal Medicine

Herbal remedies have been used by cultures worldwide for thousands of years, and an estimated 25% of modern pharmaceuticals are based on compounds found in plants (Schulz et al., 2001). In the late 1990s, the consumption of herbal remedies increased dramatically. Astin (1998) concluded that 12% of American adults used herbs over the course of a 1-year period. Other studies have placed this number as high as 49% (Johnston, 2000).

For physicians, providing advice regarding the use of herbal remedies is fraught with challenges. Many people who use herbal remedies do not tell their primary care physicians, largely because the doctor "never asked" or because they "did not feel it was important for him/her to know" (Eisenberg et al., 2001❸). However, given the popularity of herbal remedies, the potential for herb-drug interactions, and a growing body of evidence indicating that

many herbs have beneficial therapeutic effects, it is important for health care providers to have a working knowledge of herbal medicine.

Information about herb-drug interactions is derived from a number of sources. Some randomized trials exist, but most information is based on case reports, animal studies, in vitro studies, or theoretical assumptions made based on known chemical components of the herb. A 2001 review collected information from a wide array of sources and scored them on a 10-point scale based several factors, including whether a clear causal relation occurred between herb consumption and untoward effects and whether patients' comorbidities were taken into account. In total, 108 herb-drug interaction reports were found worldwide. Of these, 74 interactions were classed as unevaluable, 20 as possible, and 14 as likely (Fugh-Berman and Ernst, 2001❸) (Box 11-3).

3. Exercise and Movement Therapies

Only 25% of American adults meet recommended levels of physical activity, and 29% report no regular leisure-time physical activity whatsoever (Centers for Disease Control and Prevention, 2001). Obesity has reached epidemic proportions, contributing to an

---

Box 11-2	**Suggestions for Joan: Nutrition**

Evidence-based dietary advice is useful for practically all patients, and Joan is no exception. Given her obesity (and her abdominal body fat distribution), elevated lipids, hypertension, and family history of type 2 diabetes, she is at high risk for vascular disease. An anti-inflammatory diet can decrease this risk and may help both decrease her chronic pain symptoms and improve her mood. Following a diet of foods with a low glycemic load can help prevent insulin resistance. Since she mentioned that certain foods seem to worsen her irritable bowel symptoms, an elimination diet trial (especially removing dairy products) might prove helpful. Joan's homocysteine level should be checked, and if it is elevated, she can add folate, Vitamin B_6, and B_{12} for heart disease prevention. Calcium and vitamin D intake should be assessed. Magnesium supplementation may be beneficial for her periodic migraines.

Box 11-3	**Suggestions for Joan: Herbal Remedies**

Joan is interested in trying herbal remedies. Some useful suggestions would include:

Enteric-coated peppermint oil capsules, which are often effective for diarrhea-predominant irritable bowel symptoms. Recommending enteric-coated capsules prevents release in the stomach, which can relax the lower esophageal sphincter resulting in gastro-esophageal reflux.

Herbal anti-inflammatories. Boswellia, turmeric, and ginger all have anti-inflammatory properties and may serve as useful adjuncts or alternatives to nonsteroidal anti-inflammatory drugs.

A treatment for depression is probably indicated in Joan's case. St. John's wort or S-adenosyl methionine (SAMe) are alternatives that have shown promise in the treatment of mild to moderate depression.

Probiotics would be suggested. Probiotic supplements contain bacteria that are normally present as part of healthy intestinal flora. They are often useful in decreasing diarrhea associated with antibiotics; they also may help normalize Joan's intestinal motility and alleviate symptoms related to food intolerance.

estimated 300,000 deaths in the United States yearly (Allison et al., 1999), and pediatric obesity rates are soaring. All-cause mortality rates are doubled for those with low activity levels (Blair et al., 1996).

Given these sobering statistics, encouraging physical activity is of key importance. Physical activity can lead to improvements in any number of physical and emotional symptoms in addition to improving overall well-being.

A number of therapeutic modalities are based on movement. These therapies, including hatha yoga, tai chi, qigong, and Feldenkrais, can be used for both prevention and treatment of various disorders (Box 11-4).

4. Manipulative Therapies

Manipulative therapies use direct physical contact to facilitate healing. Practitioners focus on the relation between structure and function; parts of the body are moved in various ways to alleviate pain and other symptoms. Examples include chiropractic, osteopathic manipulative treatment (OMT), and therapeutic bodywork. Although these techniques are used most commonly to treat musculoskeletal disorders, they may be used to treat "visceral" problems (e.g., asthma, gastrointestinal problems, or otitis) as well (Erickson et al., 2004 **B**).

Chiropractic

Chiropractic was founded in Iowa in 1895 by D. D. Palmer. Palmer believed that manipulation of the spine could be used to remove subluxations, or misalignments of the vertebrae, which he believed were the underlying causes of many symptoms. The definition of subluxation has broadened over the years, and chiropractic focuses on restoring proper alignment to joints and their related structures. Decreased range of motion, inflammation, alterations in motor

Box 11-4	Suggestions for Joan: Exercise and Movement Therapies

Exercise counseling should be tailored to Joan's individual needs, recognizing the limitations imposed by her chronic pain. Extremely small amounts of exercise (even 5 minutes at a time, increasing only a minute or two every few weeks) may be all she can handle with her symptoms of fatigue and her fibromyalgia. Water-based activities or tai chi are less likely to exacerbate her back pain. Exercise will likely reduce her depressive symptoms. A visit with a skilled bodyworker may be beneficial, provided this person has experience working with fibromyalgia patients' extremely low pain thresholds.

function, and pain are all potentially treatable. Many people associate chiropractic with high-velocity, low-amplitude adjustments, in which a joint is forcibly moved until a pop or "release sound" is heard. This is but one of many methods used. Techniques are modified based on a patient's individual situation. Different techniques may be used on pregnant women, infants, and people with bleeding disorders or bone disease.

Now more than 65,000 chiropractors practice in the United States (Chapman-Smith, 2004). Chiropractors train for 4 or 5 academic years, with intense basic science experiences, in 16 training institutions in the United States. Accreditation is regulated through state licensing boards.

A 2005 Cochrane review concluded, based on the results of 39 randomized controlled trials, "There is no evidence that spinal manipulative therapy is superior to other standard treatments for patients with acute or chronic low-back pain" (Assendelft et al., 2005). However, other reviews and individual studies show a consistent overall trend suggesting chiropractic decreases low back pain (Erickson et al., 2004 **B**). A 2001 systematic review concluded that spinal manipulation was comparable to medical prophylaxis for treating tension and migraine headaches (Bronfort et al., 2001 **A**). Neck-pain data are mixed in terms of showing a benefit or not (Rindfleisch and Rakel, 2003 **B**) Evidence is thus far limited to randomized or prospective trials that are relatively small. More methodologically rigorous chiropractic investigations are currently under way. It is worth noting that patient-satisfaction ratings tend to be consistently higher for chiropractic than for conventional medical care (Erickson et al., 2004 **B**).

Osteopathic Medicine

Osteopathic medicine was developed by Andrew Taylor Still, MD, who became disillusioned with biomedicine when three of his children died of meningitis in 1864. In 1874, he developed OMT, and in 1892, he founded the first medical school to grant the degree of doctor of osteopathy (DO). Now 20 osteopathic training schools exist in the United States. Training overlaps significantly with medical doctorate (MD) training, and osteopaths compose 6% of practicing physicians in the United States. Currently, only a small percentage of osteopaths practice manipulation on a routine basis. Overall, research relating to the efficacy of OMT remains limited in part because of challenges of double-blinding and in part because of a historical lack of research funding support. However, it has shown promise for many of the indications.

Therapeutic Bodywork

Therapeutic bodywork is a general term used to describe any of a number of techniques in which the practitioner uses a hands-on approach. Many techniques bodyworkers use overlap with those used in osteopathy and chiropractic. Massage, one of the most common forms of bodywork, has a higher rate of physician referral in the United States than does any other complementary modality (Astin et al., 1998). A recent Cochrane review concluded, "Massage might be beneficial for patients with sub-acute and chronic non-specific low-back pain, especially when combined with exercises and education" (Furlan et al., 2004Ⓑ). Physical and occupational therapists often make use of such techniques in their practices (Box 11-5).

5. Energy Medicine

We are continually surrounded by energy in various forms. Heat, light, sound, electromagnetic radiation—all of these can affect our physical state. Modern medicine frequently makes use of various energy fields for diagnostic purposes (e.g., electrocardiograms, ultrasounds, and electroencephalograms), but it remains controversial whether an energy field exists around the human body, the pattern of which can be altered to affect a person's health (Benor, 2002).

Throughout history, the concept of energy (also referred to as vital force, bioelectric field, chi, and many other names) has played a significant part in most cultures' healing systems.

Research into the scientific basis of energy medicine is ongoing but far from definitive (Oschman, 2002). Hundreds of energy medicine studies are now listed in various medical databases. In 2000, Astin and colleagues performed a systematic review of 23 trials that met inclusion criteria (primarily randomized controlled trials) involving prayer, therapeutic touch, or "other distant healing methods." Thirteen of the 23 trials, which involved a total of 2774 patients, showed a positive treatment effect. Only one trial showed a negative effect, in that wounds treated with energy healing seemed to heal more slowly (Astin et al., 2000Ⓑ). A 2003 update to this review, published in Germany, concluded that subsequent studies call some of these likely benefits into question (Ernst, 2003Ⓑ).

A 2000 review focused on 37 randomized trials in which energy therapy was given to human subjects with a variety of conditions. Only 22 of the studies were accessible as published reports, and 10 reported a significant effect. Studies measured an array of outcomes, and a variety of energy modalities were used. Methodologic shortcomings were noted to be significant, and the author ultimately concluded that no firm conclusions could be drawn (Abbot, 2000 Ⓑ).

The challenge facing health care providers is to determine how such information could guide clinical practice. It is reasonable to inform patients that energy medicine modalities are, in general, quite safe but that evidence is inconclusive (Box 11-6).

6. Mind-Body Influences

The mind-body influence goes in both directions, from the mind to the body and vice versa. If we are more depressed and anxious, pain is exacerbated. If we have more pain, we are more likely to become depressed and anxious. Such topics are the subjects of a field of study called psycho-neuro-endo immunology, which explores how our body's systems are uniquely interrelated. What happens in one system affects others. For example, nerve endings have been found in the tissues of the immune system such as the spleen, lymph nodes, and bone marrow (Felten and Felten, 1991). Cells in the immune system have been found to produce chemicals previously thought to be confined to the neurologic and endocrine systems. Lymphocytes have been found not only to secrete neuropeptides and hormones, but also to have receptors for them on their surfaces (Ackerman et al.,

---

Box 11-5	Suggestions for Joan: Manipulative Therapies

Joan had a positive interaction with a chiropractor previously, and some form of manipulation could be tried. Her low back pain is likely to respond well. Given that much of her pain seems to be muscular, a strain-counterstrain or trigger point release could be attempted.

Box 11-6	Suggestions for Joan: Energy Medicine

Successful referrals to an energy medicine practitioner rely in part on the openness of the patient to the therapy. If Joan were willing, information about local energy healers could be provided. Often these modalities will address deep-seated emotional issues, such as those related to abuse experienced as a child. Choosing an appropriately discrete and competent provider is important. The type of energy medicine recommended would depend in part on Joan's past experience and what is available in the community. Energy practitioners often note that when someone suffers from a myriad of complaints or describes his or her problems as being related to "low energy levels," energy modalities may prove helpful when other approaches fail.

1991). Just as chemicals of the neuroendocrine system have been found in our immune cells, those of the immune system have been found in the neuroendocrine system. Several immunoregulatory cytokines, including interleukin (IL)-1, IL-2, IL-6, interferon-gamma, and tumor necrosis factor, have been found on the brain side of the blood-brain barrier, especially in the region of the hypothalamic-pituitary axis (Ferencik and Stvrtinova, 1997). Clearly, the body's systems are set up to communicate through multidirectional pathways.

From a clinical standpoint, how do we positively influence this intricate system? Many different ways exist. It is important to seek out what lies at the root of a problem so as to cause a fundamental change that can start a cascade of positive effects on health and well-being. Examples of such changes could include making a career transition, forgiving someone for a past traumatic experience, altering overall outlook so that events do not seem as stressful as they might once have, and disclosing suppressed emotions. Helping patients make conscious choices that result in a greater sense of peace enhances their bodies' self-healing so that fewer medications are needed to suppress symptoms.

One important aspect of defining mind-body influences when taking a medical history is to listen to metaphor. For example, someone with neck pain may say, "My boss is a pain in the neck." Someone with irritable bowel may say, "This divorce is eating me up inside." When people understand how these stressors can influence their physical health, symptoms may resolve.

A pathologist named William Boyd said at the turn of the 20th century, "The Sorrow that hath no vent in tears, may make other organs weep." Expressing emotions through talking or writing can be very helpful. For example, simply writing about past stressful life experiences has been found to result in symptom reduction in patients with asthma and rheumatoid arthritis. One hundred and seven patients with these diseases were assigned to write about either the most stressful event of their lives (study group) or daily events (control group) for just 20 minutes over a consecutive 3-day period. Four months after journaling, the asthma patients in the treatment group showed a 20% improvement in lung function versus no improvement in the control group. The patients with rheumatoid arthritis who wrote about stressful events showed a 28% reduction in disease severity, whereas the control group showed no change (Smyth et al., 1999🅐).

Other tools also use the mind-body connection to improve symptoms. Examples include hypnosis, guided imagery, biofeedback, and specific relaxation exercises. In the treatment of IBS, hypnosis has been found to have lasting positive effects up to 5 years after therapy. Of more than 200 patients with IBS studied,

---

Box 11-7	Suggestions for Joan: Mind-Body Therapies

Joan has a significant amount of stress in her life. Sources of this include her divorce and dealing with her teenage son. She reports that her "whole life is a stressor." It is no surprise that she suffers from stress-related conditions such as irritable bowel syndrome, fatigue, and depression. One way to help Joan escape stressful thoughts is to encourage her to participate in a mindfulness-based stress reduction program. As she learns how to control her stress, you can teach her a relaxation technique to help reduce the severity of her pain and emotional distress. Examples of such techniques include breathing exercises, progressive muscle relaxation, and self-hypnosis techniques. Joan may also benefit from expressing her emotions through writing (keeping a journal). She may also benefit from seeing a therapist for hypnosis for her irritable bowel syndrome.

71% of patients initially responded to therapy. Of these, 81% maintained their improvement over time, whereas the majority of the remaining 19% claimed that worsening of symptoms had only been slight (Gonsalkorale et al., 2003 🅑) (Box 11-7).

7. Other Medical Systems

Other medical systems, based on entirely different philosophical underpinnings from those of biomedicine, can play a key role in providing integrative care. Traditional Chinese medicine, Ayurveda, naturopathy, and homeopathy are systems commonly found in the United States (Box 11-8).

8. Spiritual Connection

Spirituality is difficult to conceptualize. It is similar to the wind. It is invisible, but you can feel its effects. It is defined as a journey toward, or experience of, connection with the source of ultimate meaning. Edgar Cayce said, "Spirit is the life, mind is the builder, physical is the result." When we set our goals according to those things in life that have great meaning and purpose for us, our health often improves as a side effect.

It is easier to understand how to discuss spirituality with our patients if we realize that religion and spirituality are not synonymous. Think of religion as a poem and spirituality as the flower it describes. Our job is to understand with which poem the individual resonates the most. We can then know how best to facilitate the connections that give life mean-

Box 11-8	Suggestions for Joan: Other Medical Systems

Recommendations for Joan will depend on what is available in her community, but several nonbiomedical systems could be considered. Traditional Chinese medicine would characterize Joan's symptoms in terms of yin and yang and the effects of organ systems on one another. Ayurveda would do the same using the three doshas. The Chinese, Ayurvedic, or homeopathic systems can potentially link Joan's multiple symptoms into an overall explanatory model that can allow for a simplification of treatment. For example, acupuncture along one of the energy channels, or meridians, may simultaneously affect her bowels, her back, and her emotional status.

healing. A body can be cured but not healed and vice versa. Although curing can occur without spiritual exploration, it is very difficult to facilitate healing without it. This is how a disease such as metastatic cancer can stimulate spiritual growth. Healing occurs because the disease encourages an individual to reconnect with what gives life meaning and purpose. These influences cannot be directly defined with medical imaging or serum analysis. Often the only clue we have to see whether this takes place is by looking into someone's eyes or hearing them tell their story. Seeing and experiencing this is one of the greatest joys in the practice of medicine.

There is no "right" answer to how we can explore spirituality with patients. Each individual defines spirituality in a unique way. Our task is to encourage this exploration to help patients draw from this powerful and mysterious influence that results in healing and well-being.

ing and purpose. Spirituality may or may not involve formal religion. A person's poem may be defined through nature or human relationships.

In exploring how spirituality influences health, we can also understand how curing differs from

Material Available on Student Consult
Review Questions and Answers about Integrative Medicine
Tables 11-1 through 11-21

REFERENCES

Abbot N. Healing as a therapy for human disease: A systematic review. J Altern Complement Med 2000;6:159–169.B

Ackerman KD, Bellinger DL, Felton SY, et al. Ontogeny and senescence of noradrenergic innervation of the rodent thymus and spleen. In Ader R, Cohen N, Felton DL (eds): Psychoneuroimmunology, 2nd ed. New York, Academic, 1991, pp 71–125.

Allison DB, Fontaine KR, Manson JE, et al. Annual deaths attributable to obesity in the United States. JAMA 1999;282:1530–1538.

Assendelft WJJ, Morton SC, Yu EI, Suttorp MJ, Shekelle PG. Spinal manipulative therapy for low back pain. Cochrane Database Syst Rev 2005;3:CD00047.

Astin J, Marie A, Pelletier K, et al. A review of the incorporation of complementary and alternative medicine by mainstream physicians. Arch Intern Med 1998;79:1440–1447.

Astin JA. Why patients use alternative medicine: Results of a national study. JAMA 1998;279:1548–1553.

Astin JA, Harkness E, Ernst E. The efficacy of "distant healing": A systematic review of randomized trials. AIM 2000;132:903–910.B

Balluz LS, Kieszak SM, Philen RM, Mulinare J. Vitamin and mineral supplement use in the United States: Results from the third National Health and Nutrition Examination Survey. Arch Fam Med 2000;9:258–262.

Benor DJ. Energy medicine for the internist. Med Clin North Am 2002;86:105–125.

Blair SN, Kampert JB, Kohl HW, et al. Influences of cardiorespiratory fitness and other precursors on cardiovascular disease and all-cause mortality in men and women. JAMA 1996;276:205–210.

Bronfort G, Assendelft WJJ, Evans R, et al. Effects of spinal manipulation for chronic headache: A systematic review. J Manipul Physiol Ther 2001;24:457–466.A

Centers for Disease Control and Prevention. Physical activity trends: United States, 1990–98. MMWR 2001;50:166–169.

Chapman-Smith D. Chiropractic report: Origin and professional organization. Available at www.chiropracticreport.com/chiropractic.htm. Accessed on 12/5/2004.

Eisenberg DM, Davis RB, Ettner SL, et al. Trends in alternative medicine use in the United States, 1990–1997: Results of a follow-up national survey. JAMA 1998;280:1569–1575.

Eisenberg DM, Kessler RC, Foster C, Norlock FE, Calkins DR, Delbanco TL. Unconventional medicine in the United States: Prevalence, costs and patterns of use. N Engl J Med 1993;328:246–252.

Eisenberg DM, Kessler RC, Van Rompay MI, et al. Perceptions about complementary therapies relative to conventional therapies among adults who use both: Results from a national survey. Ann Intern Med 2001;135:344–351.B

Erickson K, Rosier A, Rainone F. Chiropractic and osteopathic care. In Kligler B, Lee R (eds): Integrative

Medicine: Principles for Practice. New York, McGraw Hill, 2004, pp 153–176.🅑

Ernst E. Distant healing: An "update" of a systematic review. Wien Klin Wochenschr 2003;115:241–245.🅑

Fairfield KM, Fletcher RH. Vitamins for chronic disease prevention in adults: Clinical applications. JAMA 2002; 287:3127–3129.🅐

Felten SY, Felten DL. The innervation of lymphoid tissue. In Ader R, Cohen N, Felton DL (eds): Psycho-neuroimmunology, 2nd ed. New York, Academic, 1991, pp 27–70.

Ferencik M, Stvrtinova V. Is the immune system our sixth sense? Relation between the immune and neuroen-docrine systems. Brisl Lek Listy 1997;98:187–198.

Flood A, Schatzkin A. Colorectal cancer: Does it matter if you eat your fruits and vegetables? J Natl Cancer Inst 2000;92:1706–1707.

Fugh-Berman A, Ernst E. Herb-drug interactions: Review and assessment of report reliability. Br J Clin Pharmacol 2001;52:587–595.🅑

Furlan AD, Brosseau L, Imamura M, Irvin E. Massage for low-back pain. Cochrane Database Syst Rev 2004; 2:CD001929.🅑

Gonsalkorale WM, Miller V, Afzel A, Whorwell PJ. Long term benefits of hypnotherapy for irritable bowel syn-drome. Gut 2003;52: 1623–1629.🅑

Johnson K. The glycemic index. In Rakel D (ed): Integrative Medicine. Philadelphia, WB Saunders, 2003, pp 661–666.🅑

Johnston BA. Prevention Magazine assesses use of dietary supplements. HerbalGram 2000;48:65–72.

Joneja JV. Dietary Management of Food Allergies and Intolerances: A Comprehensive Guide, 2nd ed. Vancouver, BC, Hall Publications, 1998.🅑

Mahan LK, Escott-Stump S (eds). Krause's Food, Nutrition and Diet Therapy, 11th ed. Philadelphia, Elsevier, 2004.

Oschman JL. Energy Medicine: The Scientific Basis. New York, Churchill Livingstone, 2002.

Rindfleisch JA, Rakel D. Neck pain. In Rakel D (ed): Integrative Medicine. Philadelphia, WB Saunders, 2003, pp 433–445.🅑

Schulz V, Hansel R, Tyler VE. Rational Phytotherapy: A Physician's Guide to Herbal Medicine. New York, Springer Verlag, 2001.

Smyth JM, Stone AA, Hurewitz A, Kaell A. Effects of writ-ing about stressful experiences on symptom reduction in patients with asthma and rheumatoid arthritis. JAMA 1999;281:1304–1309.🅐

Wolever TM. The glycemic index: Aspects of some vita-mins, minerals, and enzymes in health and disease. World Rev Nutr Diet 1990;62:120–185.

Chapter

12   The Electronic Medical Record

Bruce Bagley and David Kibbe

KEY POINTS

1. The goal of incorporating information technology into health care practices is to improve patient care and outcomes through efficient management of time, resources, and data.
2. The electronic medical record (EMR) provides a comprehensive mechanism for integrating and subsequently accessing patient data.
3. The EMR facilitates exchange of information with referring physicians, consultants, nurses, and other care providers.

4. The EMR is especially useful as a tool in practice management for large physician groups with multiple practice sites.
5. To realize the full advantages of the EMR, standards related to data exchange and interoperability will need to be in place.
6. Appropriate electronic platforms and solutions to implementation issues are expected to evolve over time.

The contemporary practice of medicine requires a high level of information management. Electronic applications can be used to achieve high-quality, consistent health care outcomes through an integrated, logical approach to patient data management. The electronic medical record (EMR) is the principal tool for efficiently managing, accessing, and sharing patient data. This tool represents an advance over existing knowledge retrieval and sharing capabilities already available through Internet databases and PDA messaging and lookup functions by aggregating patient data in one electronic location with common access.

THE ELECTRONIC MEDICAL RECORD

The EMR provides clear and concise information about the patient and so improves patient care and outcomes. Information is organized in a way that is easy to use and to access. Chart notes, laboratory test results, and X-ray reports can all be entered into the EMR, accessed, and reviewed in an efficient and logical manner (Box 12-1). Problem lists, immunization records, and medication lists are all automatically updated during the process of caring for the patient, and the updated information can be immediately shared with nurses and physicians. Because the EMR makes use of relational database concepts and technology, it is no longer necessary to enter the same information in multiple places in the chart. Some of the most important patient safety

and data management areas in which the EMR is proving its worth are discussed in this chapter.

Applications and Functionalities

Medication Prescription

A provider need only enter the information for a new prescription in the EMR, and that information is put on the patient's medication list. The computer keeps track of when the prescription was written, the amount ordered (and later dispensed by the pharmacy), and the number of refills. This capability saves time and improves communication with the patient, the pharmacist, and subsequent care providers. Most systems can check to see if medications are on a specific formulary and can even advise the physician of the probable cost to the patient for the drug.

Medication Reconciliation

Managing multiple medications has increased the complexity of everyday patient care, especially care of the elderly. The computer automatically checks for allergies and drug-drug interactions whenever a new drug is entered. Although not all of the drug interaction alerts generated by the computer are clinically significant, the physician is prompted to consider the severity of the conflict and act accordingly. If the physician is not knowledgeable about the type or cause of the interaction, a full explanation is available at the touch of a screen or with a single keystroke. Pharmacy computers can keep track of prescription

142

<table>
<tr><td>**Box 12-1**</td><td>**Electronic Medical Record Functionalities**</td></tr>
</table>

Intra-office messaging, phone calls, and prescription refills

Prescription writing; allergy and interaction warnings

Laboratory tests: order entry, review and tracking of abnormal results

Referral letters and health plan notification

Reimbursement: billing, coding, and documentation for payment

Patient education

Office visit documentation

Comprehensive problem list management

Efficient filing of clinical information from outside the office

Enhanced e-mail communication with patients

Clinical data tracking for quality improvement purposes

refills and alert the physician if the patient appears not to be taking a medication regularly. Other physicians can access the patient's medication profile in the EMR before prescribing a new drug.

Laboratory Test Results

Ordering laboratory tests and reviewing the results on a timely basis is an important component of patient care. When laboratory tests are ordered electronically, the information is entered into a log, so that tracking the return and review of results is reliable and efficient. For laboratory work that is performed in the office, such as blood tests, electrocardiograms, or radiographs, the computer automatically captures the proper information for billing purposes. When results are returned to the physician, they are reviewed, and the patient can be notified of normal results or of the need for further testing. At the time blood is drawn or other test is performed, the nurse determines the patient's preferred method of notification about results. An electronic method of tracking and obtaining results reduces delays in patient care provision and eliminates periods of concern for both patient and physician.

Record of Office Visit

An accurate record of the office visit is essential to the provision of good patient care. Various members of the clinical team enter information using templates. The nurse or medical assistant may enter a portion of the note, such as the reason for the current visit, any concerns expressed by the patient, vital signs, and a review of current medications. Physicians usually enter information about the patient's history and physical findings, along with diagnostic impressions or conclusions.

The traditional written narrative in the office visit note may easily obscure both normal and abnormal findings by embedding them in the middle of a paragraph or page, requiring the reader to scan the entire page to find the one piece of information the reader is looking for. It would be far more efficient if normal and abnormal items were highlighted in some way for easy recognition. A wad of text may not be the best way to record and communicate important information.

Structured data entry allows information to be entered into the computer in a way that is easy to search and retrieve. Pick-lists allow clinicians to choose from standard complaints, history items, and physical findings in the course of constructing the final note. There is also the option of displaying the note either in tabular form or in narrative form. With structured data entry, the necessary elements for coding and billing can be determined more readily. However, the pick-lists do limit some of the richness of the history (which often helps to substantiate the diagnosis or conclusion), and the time required to construct the note is longer than the time needed to dictate a traditional narrative note. A plan of action or follow-up recommendations complete the office visit note.

Physicians often use a combination of structured data entry, keyboard entry, dictation, and voice recognition software to enter the visit record. Because of the drawbacks of voice recognition systems and editing, some combination of structured data entry and traditional dictation, with the transcribed note later entered into the record, is likely to be most widely used for the near future.

Managing the Practice

Physicians have used computerized practice management systems for years to help with scheduling, billing, and collections. The addition of the EMR allows clinical and billing information generated during the process of care to be integrated with business information in the practice management software. The result is improved accuracy and timely submission of bills to appropriate payers.

From this basic union of patient care and reimbursement data, additional useful information can also be gathered from the EMR. Inventory control is a fairly obvious application of EMR data. The cost of care can be tracked, as can provider efficiency, productivity, and time required for specific tasks. This information is crucial to analyzing and managing office systems and process. Tracking supply and demand for services enables office managers to reduce waiting time for a provider's services.

Office Workflow

One of the greatest benefits of the EMR is to facilitate office workflow. Intra-office messaging, responding to patient phone calls or e-mail messages, and providing medication refills are all part of the daily office workload. Even though the average family physician may see 25 to 30 patients face-to-face in the office each day, an additional 75 to 100 interact with the office through some other means—phone, fax, or e-mail. They may call for advice about minor problems, prescription refills, or referrals to other providers. In a paper-only system, each of these 100+ interactions requires a clerk to manually access the chart folder, attach a note, and deliver the chart to the location. The EMR allows any member of the care team to access the medical record at any time, regardless of location. Most systems allow multiple users to access the same patient's chart at the same time. This capability is essential for efficient time management and to reduce waiting times and delays. The ability to access patient records from remote sites is especially important for physican groups with multiple practice sites and for physicians who are on call while at home or at the hospital.

STANDARDS

Most office-based health information technology in use today, including the EMR, cannot be used to exchange much information with laboratories, pharmacies, or patients and family members. Connectivity between the practice EMR and these important sources of information within and outside the office practice environment is necessary to prevent computerized systems from becoming data islands. The acceptance and promulgation of IT standards can increase low-cost connectivity and data exchange solutions at the level of the medical practice. A growing number of data content, format, vocabulary, and messaging standards play an important role in health IT adoption. Perhaps the most significant to family physicians is the new interoperability standard called the Continuity of Care Record (CCR).

A quarter of a century ago, a uniform ambulatory medical care minimum basic data set was designed and reported to the U.S. National Committee on Vital and Health Statistics. In the early 2000s, the Institute of Medicine (IOM) articulated yet again the enormous potential for IT to improve health care quality by enabling safe, effective, patient-centered, timely, efficient, and equitable care. The IOM recognized that the health care system will move away from the current medical record (an arti-fact of the focus on visit-based care) to health care information that is interactive, real time, and prospective. The potential for this technology, however, has remained an unfulfilled promise.

The CCR is a document standard for basic health information that uses XML (extensible markup language). A number of groups, among them ASTM International, the Massachusetts Medical Society, the Health Information Management and Systems Society, the American Academy of Pediatrics, and the American Academy of Family Physicians, are developing it jointly (Box 12-2). The CCR is intended to foster continuity of patient care, to reduce medical errors, and to increase patients' role in managing their own health care. It will also enable epidemic monitoring, public health research, and ensure at least a minimum standard of secure health information transportability. The CCR is not an electronic health record but rather a snapshot of the information the medical record contains at a given point in time. The CCR is compatible with other efforts to standardize health information systems and can work in conjunction with these efforts.

The nationwide transmittal of data as important as health care information should be as easy as using an ATM card. The number of health information system vendors is increasing, however, and most offer only their own proprietary software. A survey of nearly 1,300 family physicians who used electronic health records in their practices found

---

Box 12-2	**Continuity of Care Record**

- Provides a snapshot of the individual patient's medical history at a given point in time.
- Contains most of the relevant clinical information needed for a variety of clinicians, in various settings, to provide safe, efficient and informed care to the patient.
- Can be updated anytime changes are made.
- Data are formatted in XML language, which allows any operating system or electronic health record to "read" the data and populate its own data structure.
- Can be stored and transferred as a digital file that can be opened and converted to readable text or read by an EMR system.
- Will serve as the "universal interface" for clinical information among disparate electronic health record systems.
- Can serve as a vehicle to collect and report clinical data for quality improvement or accountability efforts.

264 different software vendors were represented, but even the largest was used by only 148 physicians. None of the 264 systems used currently can share data with any of the other systems. The software being developed for the CCR addresses this lack of compatibility by allowing disparate information technologies and software programs to read, interpret, and transmit a core summary of personal health information. A growing number of clinical information systems companies have agreed to implement the CCR. The prospects are good that widespread adoption of this first interoperability standard can be achieved by 2006.

The CCR is also portable, allowing patients to carry with them a summary of their most important personal medical information. It can be printed out, carried on a USB flash drive or smart card, e-mailed directly to a physician, or uploaded to a secure Web site, where it can be accessed with consent. Wherever a patient carries or sends the CCR, the data in it, such as recent blood pressure readings, a current list of medications, medication allergies, and laboratory test results, can be accessed for immediate use.

QUALITY SYSTEMS EMBEDDED

Calls for better quality of care and more consistent care have come from many different groups. Improved patient safety standards and the reduction of medical errors will be at the top of the health care policy agenda for the next decade. The EMR allows quality improvement and patient safety to be built into systems of care.

Quality improvement focuses on reducing waste and variability in process and systems. The goal is to have office systems that deliver reliable health care outcomes and enjoy the support of excellent customer service. Well-designed EMR systems will include functions that help physicians manage health maintenance and chronic illness. A registry is a system to identify and track patients with a specific condition. It helps to ensure that patients get what they need, when they need it, to optimally manage their chronic illness such as diabetes or hypertension. Common office tasks, such as tracking and reporting laboratory results, can be seamlessly integrated into the flow of patient care processes.

There is great interest in monitoring and collecting data on the quality of care delivered to patients. Performance measures have been developed to monitor and improve office systems. The EMR should be designed to collect data for these quality improvement measures during the process of care. This step would eliminate costly and time-consuming retrospective chart audits.

CHALLENGES

Computer Hardware

Computer hardware is constantly evolving, so it is not possible to make lasting recommendations about what configurations are best. Most EMR vendors offer software that can serve the office needs on a completely self-contained system. The *enterprise system*, as it is called, usually has all the computer equipment installed and maintained in the office. Many vendors now offer the *application service provider* (ASP) version of software, which can provide the same functions from remote computers that are accessed via high-speed Internet connections. There are pros and cons to both approaches. The cost advantage of ASP systems has diminished as hardware prices have continued to fall. Maintenance and downtime are considerations with both approaches. Other useful office technology includes local area networks (linked intra-office network of computers), handheld devices on which the EMR can be accessed at the bedside or in the physician's off-site location, and portable printers available in each examination room for printing out results for patients to take with them (Box 12-3).

Box 12-3	The ACID Test for EMR Systems

Electronic medical records systems must pass the ACID test.

A Affordability—Office-based IT should be affordable to family physicians and other office-based clinicians who face challenging economic environments and decreasing reimbursement.

C Compatibility—Physicians should not have to replace entire systems when purchasing a component or be locked into a single vendor's products due to proprietary interfaces or predatory pricing tactics. Systems should be "plug and play" with regard to interfacing.

I Interoperability—Data exchange schemas should facilitate data transfer, import, and export among different vendors' systems and in different settings, such as interoffice exchange or office to hospital, to nursing home, and to patient/patient home.

D Data stewardship—Physicians reserve the right to choose the keepers and guardians of their data and should have some control over how the data are used.

The Paperless Office

Most physicians still work in a world of paper, and making the transition to a paperless office environment can be fraught with problems, not least the need to gain the endorsement of all users. The Electronic Health Record Readiness Assessment tool from the AAFP Center for Health Information Technology provides information and guidance on switching over to a paperless environment in stages, addressing both educational and office-culture needs and technology product evaluation needs. A list of useful Internet sites for obtaining further information about EMRs, standards, and transitioning to a paperless office is provided in Box 12-4.

The EMR and electronic practice management system must support the core business needs of the office. It is tempting to wanst to have all the extra features up and running right away, but it is more important to stabilize and refine the basics first. The computer will serve as a platform for office system redesign, and simply computerizing the same "mess" that is currently in place is a missed opportunity. The benefits of improved efficiency and improved patient care will not be realized. Leadership and change management are important skills for physicians who are going through the transformation to a paperless office. Forming a project team, providing good individualized training, and developing and implementing strategies that minimize lost productivity are essential leadership skills.

In summary, the ability to deliver high-quality health care in the 21st century requires that patient care teams be supported by IT. Knowledge management, clinical information management, and communication with patients and other providers all benefit from the assistance of computers. IT comes in many forms and can be implemented slowly, with software and knowledge training integrated into new skills. The EMR is expected to be the prime patient data management tool in the very near future, with support from the CCR and similar standards.

Box 12-4	Internet Resources

Institute for Healthcare Improvement (www. ihi.org)

Institute of Medicine (www.iom.edu)

American Academy of Family Physicians Center for Health Information Technology (www. centerforhit.org)

Continuity of Care Record (www.centerforhit.org)

National Committee on Vital and Health Statistics (www.cdc.gov/nchs/products/pubs/pubd/other/ncvhs/ncvhs.htm)

Electronic Health Records Readiness Assessment (www.centerforhit.org)

American Academy of Family Physicians Quality Initiative (www.aafp.org/x3843.xml)

Agency for Healthcare Quality and Research. Healthcare Informatics (www.ahrq.gov/data/infoix.htm)

American Medical Association Physicians Consortium on Performance Measurement (www.ama-assn.org/ama/pub/category/4837.html)

Material Available on Student Consult

Review Questions and Answers about The Electronic Medical Record

SUGGESTED READING

Martin JC, et al. The future of family medicine: A collaborative project of the family medicine community. Ann Fam Med 2004;2(Suppl 1):S3–S32.

13 Interpreting Laboratory Tests

Stephen Scott

KEY POINTS

1. Test results are often ambiguous.
2. Always consider the clinical context when interpreting a laboratory test result.
3. The more tests ordered, the more likely that a result will fall outside the reference range, despite being a "normal" result.
4. Reference ranges may require adjustment based on the patient's age and other factors.

INTERPRETING LABORATORY TESTS

Laboratory tests are very useful tools to aid in the diagnosis and treatment of illness. However, it is important to understand the inherent limitations of tests. Whereas it might seem that many tests give clear "yes" or "no" results, the reality often is not so, and test results may be ambiguous or difficult to interpret. A temptation always exists to order and interpret tests without adequately considering the patient and the clinical context. Falling prey to any of these pitfalls can lead to unnecessary testing, expensive workup, and even misdiagnosis.

Some of the reasons for test ambiguity are covered in Chapter 6, including test characteristics of sensitivity and specificity. Some additional important areas to consider include reference range, predictive value, patients with multiple illnesses, and treatment assumptions.

Reference Ranges

Although clinicians and patients often refer to test results as "normal" or "abnormal," it is more accurate to define a reference interval for normal individuals in an "average" population. For statistical reasons, the reference range for a particular test generally includes 95% of healthy or normal results. This means that 5% of normal results will fall outside the reference range. This is particularly important to consider when faced with a large panel of tests. Based on probability alone, the chance of having a result fall outside the reference range will increase simply on the basis of an increasing number of tests. At 20 tests, the probability that all of the results will be within the reference range in a normal individual is only 36%. (Stated differently, this means that a 64% chance exists that at least one result will be outside the reference range, despite being a normal result.) Most clinical laboratories report both the result of a test and the reference range for their laboratory; these ranges usually do not vary considerably from laboratory to laboratory, but they may take into consideration testing methods or local populations.

Many factors can influence a test result, which often necessitates adjusting a reference range or interpreting a result with caution. For example, reference intervals for adults are often not appropriate for children, and separate reference ranges must be considered. Other states that affect test results and corresponding reference ranges include gender, pregnancy, exercise, ethnicity, lean body mass, some drugs (including hormones, ethanol), physiologic fluctuations, posture, diet, sampling problems, and specimen handling.

Reference ranges also may be hard to define. For example, some controversy occurs about the appropriate upper limit of normal for serum thyroid-stimulating hormone (TSH). Most laboratories have for some time used values of 4.5 to 5.0 mU/L. However, a recent report indicated that 95% of rigorously screened euthyroid volunteers have serum values between 0.4 and 2.5 mU/L, and that the reference range should be adjusted appropriately (Baloch et al., 2003Ⓒ). However, if this change in reference range is implemented, the number of patients in the United States diagnosed with subclinical hypothyroidism (asymptomatic persons with TSH > 2.5 mU/L) would increase. Given the accompanying uncertainty about whether asymptomatic

Evidence levels Ⓐ Randomized, controlled trials (RCTs), meta-analyses, well-designed systematic reviews of RCTs. Ⓑ Case-control or cohort studies, nonrandomized clinical trials, systematic reviews of studies other than RCTs, cross-sectional studies, retrospective studies, certain uncontrolled studies. Ⓒ Consensus statements, expert guidelines, usual practice, opinion.

hypothyroidism should be treated, it is unclear whether changing the reference range would provide any meaningful clinical benefit.

Predictive Value of a Test

In conjunction with the sensitivity and specificity of a test, it is important to consider the predictive value of the test. The predictive value answers the question, "What is the frequency of disease among all persons with an abnormal test result?" To calculate the predictive value for a particular disease, the prevalence of the disease in the population under study must be known. If the disease prevalence in a population is high, then more of the patients who test "positive" will actually have the disease. However, if the disease prevalence is low, then the proportion of patients who both test positive and have disease will be lower (i.e., more false-positive results will be found relative to true-positive results).

These important considerations apply in several ways. First, for many diseases, the prevalence is often 1% or less. To be a good screening test in healthy individuals, a test must have a sensitivity that approaches 100%; even in such cases, false positives may outnumber true positives by a factor of 100 or more, resulting in many "abnormal" results in healthy individuals. Second, predictive value is important to consider before ordering a test. The more likely a patient is to have a disease state, the more predictive an abnormal result will be; if a patient is unlikely to have a disease, then an abnormal result is more likely to be a false-positive result.

Multiple Concurrent Illnesses

Some test results may be within reference range despite the presence of underlying disease. For example, a patient with iron deficiency and folate deficiency (as can be seen in alcoholism) may have a normal mean corpuscular volume despite a mixed population of microcytic and macrocytic red cells. The same can occur in early treatment of iron deficiency, in which new reticulocytes, which are larger than iron-deficient red cells, may obscure the population of microcytic cells.

Treatment Assumptions

Even when a reference range is well defined and a result is more clearly outside the range, differences can still occur in interpretation. This can happen when potentially competing treatment goals exist or when the proper follow-up or treatment of an abnormal result is controversial. In these cases, the clinicians' view of which priorities are most important (e.g., minimizing test cost, minimizing adverse outcomes, or minimizing cost of treatment) will

shape interpretation as much as or more than the characteristics of a given test.

Summary

The sources of variation are numerous, and the proper interpretation of test results demands consideration of the entire clinical picture. Even with guidelines and decision-support analyses, the interpretation of a particular result can be a complex process. Rational and judicious use of testing is always warranted.

The following sections consider a number of common tests that are used in everyday clinical practice. For each test, the physiologic basis, common indications, causes of abnormal results, potential pitfalls in interpretation, and clinical guidelines are reviewed, and related tests are grouped. The discussions and tables are intended to serve as a clinically useful, introductory guide. In keeping with this goal, specialized testing as well as tests in development are not covered here, and for these as well as more in-depth consideration of individual tests, the reader is referred to more exhaustive references.

Each section includes "normal" values for the tests. Although it is more accurate to refer to reference ranges, in practice, clinicians and patients more often refer to tests as normal or abnormal. It should be understood that determination of normal or abnormal requires consideration of numerous factors, as discussed. Where appropriate, units are given both in conventional and système international (SI) units along with conversion factors; in the United States, conventional units are commonly used.

BLOOD CELL TESTS

Hemoglobin and Hematocrit

Most modern hematology instruments directly measure the hemoglobin (Hgb) and calculate the hematocrit (Hct) from the measured red blood cell (RBC) and mean corpuscular volume (MCV). The hematocrit also can be measured by centrifugation of a microcapillary tube filled with whole blood. The hematocrit is defined as the percentage volume of RBCs after maximal packing has occurred. For most purposes, the hemoglobin and hematocrit are related by a factor of three, where Hct = 3 × Hgb.

It is reasonable to use the hemoglobin and hematocrit interchangeably except for patients with abnormally shaped RBCs (i.e., sickle cell disease). In such patients, the measured hematocrit is artificially high because the RBCs fail to pack maximally. In such individuals, the hemoglobin is a better test to follow.

Little evidence indicates any benefit from screening the general population with routine hemoglobin or hematocrit measurements. However, screening may be indicated in groups at high risk for anemia, such as infants, pregnant women, the institutionalized elderly, or menstruating women. It also may be used to screen individuals undergoing a procedure associated with blood loss and to screen hospitalized patients on admission. In addition to screening, the hemoglobin or hematocrit is an essential test for any patient suspected to have anemia, blood loss, or polycythemia (Table 13-1).

The most common abnormal finding is a mild, unsuspected anemia that is often asymptomatic. When it is found, it is important to uncover the cause of the anemia, as it is often a clinically important diagnosis (e.g., poor nutrition, menorrhagia, pernicious anemia, or colon cancer).

A common error when interpreting hemoglobin or hematocrit is to rely on it as an indicator of acute blood loss. Unfortunately, about 12 to 24 hours is needed before equilibration of hemoglobin and hematocrit occurs. It is only then that these values can be used to indicate the extent of blood loss.

White Blood Cell Count

Changes in the white blood cell (WBC) count are seen with many infectious, hematologic, inflammatory, and neoplastic diseases (Table 13-2). This variety of influences makes the WBC count a nonspecific test. It can, however, be a sensitive indicator of disease in some clinical situations. Its degree of increase or decrease often correlates with the severity of the disease process. Monitoring changes in WBC count over time can provide useful information about the course of an illness.

Five types of WBCs are commonly counted in the WBC differential: neutrophils, lymphocytes, monocytes, eosinophils, and basophils. Changes in the relative percentages of these cells may correlate with some types of illness (e.g., prominence of neutrophils is often seen in acute infections [sometimes called a *left shift*] lymphocytes are often predominant in viral illnesses, leukemia, and pertussis).

Leukopenia, which usually indicates neutropenia, may occur with severe infections, autoimmune disorders, collagen vascular diseases (including lupus), human immunodeficiency virus (HIV), or chemotherapy. In patients with congenital neutropenia, levels may be low with or without evidence of infection.

Lymphopenia is frequently seen in association with physiologic stress and is often of no clinical significance. Elevation of eosinophils (eosinophilia) may be seen in parasitic infections.

An increased WBC count can be seen in a wide variety of illnesses, although it is most used as an indicator of acute infection. Of note, WBC counts

Table 13-1 Hemoglobin		
Diagnostic units, g/dL (g/L) SI conversion factor, 10.0 Normal (adult): males, 13.9–16.3; females, 12.0–15.0 Normal values are higher in the first few months of life and are approximately 18.5–21.5 at birth		
Hemoglobin (g/dL)	**Diagnoses to Consider**	**Actions to Consider**
Increased		
>16.5	Dehydration	Smoking history
	Diuretic use	Check volume status
	Polycythemia vera	Check for splenomegaly
	Secondary polycythemia	Urinalysis
	High altitude	CBC
	Pulmonary disease	Platelet count
	Cardiac disease	Alkaline phosphatase
	Renal tumor	
>22	Severe polycythemia	Consider phlebotomy
Decreased		
<11	Blood loss	History of chronic disease
	Menstrual history	Stool for occult blood
	Decreased blood cell survival	Check for splenomegaly
	Decreased marrow production	RBC indices
	RBC sequestration	Reticulocyte count
		Iron studies
		Folate, B_{12} studies
<8	Severe anemia	Transfusion if patient is symptomatic

CBC, complete blood count; RBC, red blood cell.

Table 13-2 White Blood Cell (WBC) Count

Diagnostic units, cells/mm³ (cells × 10⁹/L)
SI conversion factor, 0.001
Normal (adult), 3200–9800
Varies by age, 9000–30,000 at birth;~5000–18,000 from age 1 wk to 2 yr

WBC Count (cells/mm³)	Diagnoses to Consider	Actions to Consider
Decreased 500–3200	Infections	Complete drug history
	Severe bacterial infection	Peripheral smear
	Influenza	Platelet count
	Infectious mononucleosis	CBC
	Typhoid fever	Mononucleosis test
	Drugs	ANA
	Cytotoxicity	HIV
	Idiosyncratic drug reaction	Folate, vitamin B₁₂ level
	Congestive splenomegaly	Bone marrow biopsy
	Felty syndrome	
	SLE	If very low (<500), consider frequent exam,
	Aplastic anemia	antibiotics for fever, given risk of serious
	Congenital neutropenia	bacterial infections
Increased 9800–30,000	Physiologic reaction to stress	Physical exam (looking for sites of infection,
	Infection	organomegaly)
	Tissue destruction	Peripheral blood smear
	Leukemia	
	Cancer	
	Hemorrhage	
	Splenectomy	
>30,000	Leukemia	
	Leukemoid reaction	

ANA, antinuclear antibody; CBC, complete blood count; HIV, human immunodeficiency virus; SLE, systemic lupus erythematosus.

vary with age and generally are higher in neonates and children. They also increase during pregnancy. Counts greater than 30,000/mm³ often are associated with leukemia or other blood disorders.

Platelet Count

The platelet count is often routinely performed as a part of a complete blood count, because most automated cell counters do an automated platelet count as a part of the test. As a result, the most common platelet abnormality is a small increase or decrease from normal in an otherwise asymptomatic individual (Table 13-3). Usually no benefit is found from further testing or repeating the platelet count in such cases.

Preoperative screening platelet counts are indicated for patients when blood loss is expected. They also are useful for evaluating patients with abnormal bleeding, bruising, purpura, petechiae, or splenomegaly.

A low platelet count can be caused by a reduction in the marrow's production of platelets (due to marrow suppression or infiltration), increased destruction of platelets, or sequestration of platelets in the spleen. A platelet count also is a useful indicator of marrow sensitivity to cytotoxic medications in the treatment of cancer.

It is important to note that platelets may be adequate in number but defective in function. Medications, including aspirin, other nonsteroidal antiinflammatory drugs, alcohol, and penicillins are the most common reason for abnormal platelet function.

Mean Corpuscular Volume

The MCV is an indication of the size of the RBCs. It is used primarily to differentiate the anemias into macrocytic, normocytic, or microcytic types, which often correlate with specific differential diagnoses (Table 13-4). However, it is important to note several potentially confusing scenarios. First, reticulocytes and other young RBCs are larger than mature RBCs, and a rapid release of RBCs may produce an increase in MCV. It is possible to confuse this with other causes of macrocytosis. Mixed populations of microcytic and macrocytic cells may produce an average MCV in the normal range, despite underlying abnormalities. This may occur in early treatment of iron

Table 13-3　Platelet Count

Diagnostic units, platelets $\times 10^9$/L
Normal, first week of life, 84–478; after first week of life, 140–400

Platelets (10^9/L)	Diagnoses to Consider	Actions to Consider
Decreased		
100–140	Response to viral or bacterial illness	Repeat test
50–100 (may have bleeding with major surgery)	Thrombocytopenic purpura After transfusion Splenic sequestration Marrow infiltration (i.e., leukemia) Response to cytotoxic drugs Marrow infiltration DIC	Drug history Alcohol history Examine for splenomegaly CBC Trial off all medications Bone marrow biopsy
20–50 (may have bleeding with minor procedure)		Platelet transfusion with procedure
<20 (may have spontaneous GI or CNS bleeding)		Platelet transfusion
Increased		
400–600	Splenectomy Infection Blood loss Inflammatory bowel disease Collagen vascular disease	
600–1000	Malignancy Polycythemia vera	Evaluate for malignancy
>1000		Administer antiplatelet drugs

CBC, complete blood count; CNS, central nervous system; DIC, disseminated intravascular coagulation; GI, gastrointestinal.

Table 13-4　Mean Corpuscular Volume

Diagnostic units, cubic micrometers (fL)
SI conversion factor, 1
Normal, 76–100 fL

MCV (fL)	Diagnoses to Consider	Actions to Consider
Increased		
100–120	Reticulocytosis Folate deficiency Vitamin B_{12} deficiency Hypothyroidism Response to chemotherapy	Reticulocyte count Peripheral smear Serum vitamin B_{12}, folate TSH
>120	Folate deficiency Vitamin B_{12} deficiency	
Decreased		
70–76	Iron deficiency Thalassemia Anemia of chronic disease Hereditary sideroblastic anemia Lead poisoning RBC fragmentation (burns, sickle disease)	Reticulocyte count Peripheral smear Serum iron, TIBC, ferritin Hgb electrophoresis
<70	Severe iron deficiency Thalassemia	

Hgb, hemoglobin; RBC, red blood cell; TIBC, total iron-binding capacity; TSH, thyroid-stimulating hormon.

deficiency (i.e., microcytic cells plus macrocytic reticulocytes) and in alcoholic patients who may be both iron and folate deficient.

ELECTROLYTES

Sodium

Sodium is the major cation in extracellular fluid. It is most useful to interpret sodium values as a measure of total body water and effective circulatory volume, and not simply as a measure of total body sodium. In the normal state, the body maintains a constant serum osmolality, or overall concentration of solutes in the blood plasma. When the osmolality increases, the body compensates by increasing thirst (increasing free water) and by secreting antidiuretic hor-

mone (ADH), which acts to reduce water excretion by the kidneys. When osmolality decreases, thirst disappears, and ADH secretion is reduced, allowing free water to be excreted. When the body is adjusting water levels appropriately, serum sodium concentration remains about the same.

However, in situations in which the effective circulatory volume is reduced, the body may sacrifice a normal osmolality in an effort to maintain the circulatory volume. In this setting, the sodium concentration may decrease as fluid is retained or ingested in an effort to maintain circulation. The most common causes of hyponatremia result from this effective depletion of circulating volume and include volume losses from sweating, vomiting, diarrhea, or urinary losses, heart failure, cirrhosis, and medications including thiazide diuretics (Table 13-5). Another

Table 13-5 Sodium

Diagnostic units, mEq/L (mmol/L)
SI conversion factor, 1
Normal, 135–147

Sodium (mEq/L)	Diagnoses to Consider	Actions to Consider

Increased
>147
	Fluid loss in excess of salt
	  Sweating
	  Diarrhea
	  Diabetes mellitus (osmotic diuresis)
	  Diabetes insipidus
	  Hyperaldosteronism
	Reduced fluid intake
	  Altered mental status (unable to drink)
	  Vomiting
		Assess fluid status
		Serum electrolytes
		BUN/Creatinine
		Serum glucose
		Urine specific gravity
		Oral fluids
		For symptomatic or very elevated sodium (>160), slow hydration with isotonic saline to reduce serum sodium no faster than 10 mEq/L/day; rapid changes in sodium can induce CNS changes and serious injury

	Excessive salt intake
	  Infant formula
	  Hypertonic nasogastric feeding
	  Salt poisoning	

Decreased
<135
	Excess water
	  Psychogenic polydipsia
	  Excessive IV hydration
	Decreased circulatory volume
	  Diuretic therapy
	  Congestive heart failure
	  Cirrhosis
	  Nephrotic syndrome
	  Dehydration with free water access
	Inability to excrete water
	  Renal failure (CrCl <15)
	  SIADH
	Sodium depletion
	  Gastrointestinal loss
	  Excessive sweating
	  Adrenal insufficiency
	Pseudohyponatremia
		Assess fluid status
		Serum albumin
		Serum electrolytes
		BUN/Creatinine
		Urine and serum osmolality
		Urine protein
		Urine specific gravity
		Water restriction

BUN, blood urea nitrogen; CNS, central nervous system; CrCl, creatinine clearance; IV, intravenous; SIADH, syndrome of inappropriate antidiuretic hormone.

important cause is the syndrome of inappropriate ADH secretion (SIADH), which often results in a stable reduction of serum sodium to 125 to 135 mEq/L. In advanced renal failure, ADH may be secreted appropriately, but the diseased kidney is simply unable to dilute the urine sufficiently to prevent solute and water loss. Dilution of serum sodium also may occur in the presence of excess water intake, as occurs in primary polydipsia.

Pseudohyponatremia results when marked elevations of other solutes in the plasma occur, effectively reducing the measured serum sodium concentration, and may be seen with hyperglycemia, severe hyperlipidemia, or hyperproteinemia.

Hypernatremia generally occurs in states in which free water losses exceed sodium loss, fluid intake is reduced, or excessive salt is ingested (including intravenous administration of hypertonic sodium solutions). As noted, the body very effectively regulates plasma osmolality. When the serum osmolality increases, ADH is secreted, and thirst increases. As a result, one of the most common reasons for hypernatremia is the inability of patients to express thirst normally. This occurs frequently in impaired elderly patients, who may already be prone to volume depletion due to reduced intake, medicines, or illness.

Potassium

Potassium is the major intracellular cation, and 98% of total body potassium is contained within cells. The kidneys regulate the concentration of extracellular potassium, and hyperkalemia and hypokalemia occur primarily as a result of renal disorders, medications, or abnormalities in the intake of potassium.

Measuring potassium is useful for patients with renal disease, for patients taking diuretics, and in patients who complain of weakness (Table 13-6). It is

Table 13-6 Potassium

Diagnostic units, mEq/L (mmol/L)
SI conversion factor, 1
Normal, 3.5–5.0

Potassium (mEq/L)	Diagnoses to Consider	Actions to Consider
Decreased		
2.5–3.5	Renal loss	Drug and diet history
	Thiazide or loop diuretics	Serum electrolytes
	Renal tubular acidosis	Urine electrolytes
	Hyperaldosteronism	ECG (ST and T depression, presence of U waves)
	Gastrointestinal loss	
	Vomiting	Oral potassium replacement
	Diarrhea	
	Inadequate dietary potassium	
<2.5	Hypokalemia arrhythmias	ECG, close monitoring
		Neurologic exam
		IV and/or oral potassium
Increased		
5.0–7.5	Hemolyzed specimen	Repeated K on new specimen
	Drugs	Drug and diet history
	Potassium-sparing diuretics	ECG (peaked T waves)
	NSAIDs	Creatinine
	ACE inhibitors	Serum electrolytes
	Decreased renal excretion	Urine electrolytes
	Acute renal failure	
	Chronic renal failure	
	Addison's disease	
	Acidosis	
	Tissue destruction	
>7.5	Hyperkalemic arrhythmias	ECG (peaked T waves, wide QRS, absent P waves)
		Calcium gluconate
		Kayexalate (absorbs potassium from GI tract)
		Bicarbonate
		Dialysis

ACE, angiotensin-converting enzyme; ECG, electrocardiogram; GI, gastrointestinal; IV, intravenous; NSAID, nonsteroidal anti-inflammatory drug.

frequently included in a basic metabolic panel, which is often performed in acutely ill hospitalized patients because of the frequent use of intravenous infusions, nasogastric tubes, or other interventions that potentially alter the body's usual homeostatic mechanisms.

The most common potassium disorder is a mild hypokalemia in patients taking thiazide or loop diuretics. These patients are often asymptomatic, but low potassium levels are usually monitored, and oral potassium replacement is given as needed to prevent clinically significant hypokalemia. Mild hypokalemia can be associated with vague complaints such as weakness, muscle cramps, and paresthesias. Severe hypokalemia may cause cardiac arrhythmias, paralytic ileus, or paralysis.

Hyperkalemia is most commonly seen with hemolysis of red blood cells during blood collection or processing. If in doubt, serum potassium should be retested before having the patient undergo an extensive workup for unknown causes of hyperkalemia. Other common causes include some medications, such as potassium-sparing diuretics, and renal disease. Severe hyperkalemia may be associated with bradycardia, hypotension, ventricular fibrillation, and cardiac arrest. Clinically significant hyperkalemia is usually associated with electrocardiogram (ECG) findings, as noted in Table 13-6.

Chloride

Chloride is the major extracellular anion in the body, but it is clinically useful only in selected circumstances.

Most dietary chloride is absorbed, and the level is controlled by renal excretion. Chloride levels change primarily in relation to shifts in the serum carbon dioxide (CO_2) content. CO_2 content decreases in metabolic acidosis or with metabolic compensation for respiratory alkalosis (where excess CO_2 is blown off by the lungs). In these situations, chloride levels increase in response to the decrease in CO_2 content. In settings in which CO_2 content is increased (metabolic alkalosis or respiratory acidosis), the chloride is reduced to compensate for the increased CO_2 content.

Chloride can be depleted by either gastrointestinal losses (vomiting) or renal losses (salt-losing renal diseases) (Table 13-7). In these circumstances, chloride depletion results in a persistent metabolic alkalosis.

The most frequent use of the chloride test is in determining the anion gap, which is calculated by subtracting the total measured anions (chloride + CO_2) from the total cations (sodium + potassium). The normal range for anion gap is 16 ± 4 mEq/L. Increases in the anion gap indicate the presence of unmeasured anions such as ketoacids, methanol, or salicylates.

Carbon Dioxide

The CO_2 content of blood is made up of bicarbonate, carbonic acid, and dissolved CO_2. Of the total CO_2 content, 95% is bicarbonate (HCO_3^-). Bicarbonate is the second most important anion in serum and is the most available base that is capable of buffering a metabolic acid load. As a result, CO_2 has a primary role in the body's acid-base balance. The two mechanisms for control of CO_2 are respiratory elimination of CO_2 and renal reabsorption of filtered bicarbonate. Bicarbonate also can be lost pathologically from the gastrointestinal tract.

The most common CO_2 content abnormality is a decrease due to metabolic acidosis. In this setting, it is useful to calculate the anion gap (discussed

Table 13-7 Chloride

Diagnostic units, mEq/L (mmol/L)
SI conversion factor, 1
Normal, 95–105

Chloride (mEq/L)	Diagnoses to Consider	Actions to Consider

Increased >105	Metabolic acidosis
	    Loss of bicarbonate
	    Production of metabolic acids
	Respiratory alkalosis with metabolic compensation
	Dehydration
		HCO_3^-, Na, K, pH, BUN
		Calculate anion gap

Decreased <95	Metabolic alkalosis
	    Hydrogen ion loss
	    HCO_3^- retention
	Respiratory acidosis with metabolic compensation
	Salt-losing renal disease
	Thiazide diuretics
		Urinalysis
		HCO_3^-, Na, K, pH, BUN

BUN, blood urea nitrogen; HCO_3^-, bicarbonate; K, potassium; Na, sodium.

under Chloride), which may provide a clue to the cause of the acidosis (Table 13-8).

Metabolic alkalosis may be initiated by the loss of hydrogen ion, as is seen with nasogastric suction. Maintenance of metabolic alkalosis requires greater than normal reabsorption of bicarbonate by the kidneys. Therefore in patients with an elevated CO_2 content, also consider diseases that affect the handling of bicarbonate by the kidneys.

Calcium

Calcium is an essential component of the skeleton and also plays a key role in neuromuscular function. The ionized form is the physiologically active form and represents about 43% of the total serum calcium; the remainder is bound to plasma proteins, primarily albumin. Diseases that result in elevated total calcium levels also result in elevated ionized calcium levels. For simplicity, both tests can be viewed as a measure of serum calcium levels.

The serum level of calcium is under the complex control of parathyroid hormone (PTH) and calcitonin. These hormones and others control the rate at which calcium is absorbed from the gastrointestinal tract, excreted in the urine, and gained or lost to bone (Table 13-9).

The most common abnormality is a low total calcium level in patients with a low serum albumin. In this case, the disorder is primarily of albumin, not serum calcium, and the ionized calcium remains unchanged. In this setting, it is possible to correct mathematically the total calcium in light of the decreased albumin (1-g/dL reduction in albumin leads to a 1-mg/dL reduction in calcium).

Hypocalcemia produces symptoms that result from neuromuscular excitability: carpopedal spasm, seizures, tetany, stiffness, fatigue, memory loss, and confusion. It can be seen with vitamin D deficiency, renal insufficiency (mediated by elevated phosphorus, which binds calcium), and gastrointestinal malabsorptive disorders.

Table 13-8 Carbon Dioxide (CO_2)

Diagnostic units, mEq/L (mmol/L)
SI conversion factor, 1
Normal, 22–28

CO_2 (mEq/L)	Diagnoses to Consider	Actions to Consider

Decreased <22	Metabolic acidosis
	Bicarbonate loss
	  Diarrhea
	  Renal tubular acidosis
	  Primary hyperparathyroidism
	Failure to reabsorb bicarbonate
	  Triamterene, spironolactone
	  Renal tubular acidosis
	Production of metabolic acids
	  Renal failure
	  Diabetic ketoacidosis
	  Lactic acidosis
	  Methanol
	  Ethylene glycol
	  Salicylates
	  Alcoholic ketoacidosis
	Respiratory alkalosis with compensation
	  Anxiety
	  Sepsis
	  Salicylates
	  CNS injury
		Drug history
		Serum electrolytes
		Blood gas
		Calculate anion gap

Increased >28	Metabolic alkalosis
	  Volume contraction
	  Nasogastric suction
	  Vomiting
	  Postassium depletion
	  Furosemide
	  Cushing syndrome
	Chronic respiratory acidosis with compensation
		Serum electrolytes
		Blood gas
		Urine electrolytes

CNS, central nervous system.

Table 13-9 Total Calcium

Diagnostic units, mg/dL (mmol/L)
SI conversion factor, 0.2495
Normal, 8.8–10.3 (2.20–2.45)

Calcium (mg/dL)	Diagnoses to Consider	Actions to Consider
Increased 10.3–13.0	Hyperparathyroidism Cancer Thiazide diuretics Immobilization Vitamin D intoxication Milk-alkali syndrome Multiple myeloma Sarcoidosis Thyrotoxicosis	Repeated serum calcium Drug history Diet history Ionized calcium, albumin, phosphorus, PTH, TSH Chest radiograph Hand radiographs Evaluation for malignancy
>13.0	Hypercalcemic coma	Hydration Furosemide Close monitoring
Decreased 7.0–8.8	Hypoalbuminemia Chronic renal failure Hypoparathyroidism (neck surgery) Malnutrition Vitamin D deficiency Nutritional Anticonvulsants Malabsorption Liver disease Hypomagnasemia Pancreatitis	Serum albumin Drug history Alcohol history Serum creatinine, phosphate, magnesium, PTH
<7.0	Hypocalcemic seizures Hypocalcemic arrhythmia	Calcium gluconate IV Ionized calcium Magnesium level

IV, intravenous; PTH, parathyroid hormone; TSH, thyroid-stimulating hormone.

Hypercalcemia is associated with fatigue, depression, constipation, polydipsia, ulcers, and hypertension. In the outpatient setting, the most common cause of hypercalcemia is hyperparathyroidism. Many of these patients are asymptomatic. Ionized calcium may be more sensitive in detecting hypercalcemia in these patients. Malignancy is the second most common cause and is often seen in the inpatient setting. The mechanism involves secretion of a PTH-related protein by the tumor. The most common cancers that produce hypercalcemia are in the lung (particularly primary squamous cell cancer), breast, kidney, liver, and ovary.

Calcium has frequently been included in routine screening chemistry panels, with the rationale that many cases of hyperparathyroidism are asymptomatic. However, it is unclear whether asymptomatic hyperparathyroidism requires treatment. Hence, the use of calcium as a screening test in healthy individuals is of questionable value.

GLUCOSE

Glucose levels are commonly ordered to diagnose diabetes, follow up the course of diabetes treatment, or diagnose hypoglycemia. It is important to distinguish between random and fasting glucose levels, which are interpreted differently. A random specimen taken 2 hours after lunch should not be treated in the same way as a fasting specimen. Fasting glucose levels are a key feature of screening and diagnostic tests for diabetes.

Causes of elevated glucose levels other than diabetes include specimens taken after eating, specimens that are taken from a vein just above an intravenous glucose infusion site, stress states, steroid therapy, Cushing's syndrome, and other metabolic disorders.

Many causes of hypoglycemia are noted, and before embarking on a detailed workup, it is important to consider whether a patient's symptoms correlate with a low blood sugar. If a low blood sugar value does not produce symptoms, it may not be clinically significant. The lower limit of the reference range for normal glucose usually is between 40 and 55 mg/dL; hypoglycemia is then defined as a blood sugar below this level at the same time symptoms are present.

Fasting hypoglycemia is seen primarily in those with diabetes and alcoholism, and it usually occurs only after a long period of fasting or with excess insulin administration. Symptoms include confusion, jitteriness, unusual behaviors, or seizures, and may be more gradual in onset in alcoholics. Other causes of hypoglycemia include insulin-secreting tumors, adrenal insufficiency, hypopituitarism, and drugs (including insulin, sulfonylureas, and salicylates).

Various standards for interpreting glucose levels have been established. Glucose values vary slightly by the type of specimen, and venous specimens are used as the reference standard. When used as a screening test, a fasting glucose greater than or equal to 126 mg/dL or any random glucose level greater than 200 mg/dL is diagnostic of diabetes. The upper limit of a normal glucose level may vary by laboratory but usually is about 110. If a fasting glucose is in the intermediate range between about 110 mg/dL and 126 mg/dL, repeated testing or glucose tolerance testing may serve as an aid to diagnosis.

Additional testing is most commonly used to confirm diabetes in pregnancy. If an initial glucose level is greater than or equal to 140 mEq/dL 1 hour after ingestion of a 50-g glucose load, a 3-hour confirmatory test is performed. In this test, the fasting level is obtained, a 100-g glucose load is ingested, and glucose values are measured at 1, 2, and 3 hours. If more than two of the four values exceed the accepted reference value (≥95, 180, 155, and 145 for fasting, 1-, 2-, and 3-hour values), the woman is considered to have gestational diabetes.

GLYCOSYLATED HEMOGLOBIN

The glycosylation of hemoglobin occurs continuously during the life of an RBC and is directly related to the average glucose concentration. The measurement of glycosylated hemoglobin (HbA_{1c}) has therefore become a useful clinical test to assess the "average" glucose control in patients with diabetes. Increased percentages of glycosylated hemoglobin reflect increased hyperglycemia. Glycosylation of the RBC is irreversible, and because the life of the average RBC is about 3 to 4 months, the HbA_{1c} value can be viewed as a measure of diabetes control for the previous few months.

The HbA_{1c} value does not change with rapid hour-to-hour or day-to-day variations in serum glucose. As a result, it is inappropriate to use HbA_{1c} values when making decisions about insulin or drug therapy in acutely ill patients. Although it may influence treatment decisions in the outpatient who is not acutely ill, the best source for data, especially for altering insulin regimens, is regular, premeal home glucose monitoring.

Reference values for HbA_{1c} vary by laboratory; a representative range is given in Table 13-10. The HbA_{1c} may be falsely elevated with uremia, alcoholism, and aspirin use; it may be falsely reduced in patients with anemia, hemoglobinopathies, or pregnancy.

HUMAN CHORIONIC GONADOTROPIN

Human chorionic gonadotropin (hCG), a glycoprotein secreted by placental trophoblastic tissues, is essential for support of the corpus luteum during early pregnancy. With sensitive tests, hCG can be found in the maternal serum within 24 hours of implantation. The levels then increase rapidly and peak at 10 weeks of gestation. For the remainder of the pregnancy, levels continue at approximately one tenth of the peak level.

Qualitative and quantitative hCG tests are available. The most common are qualitative tests that are used on urine specimens to diagnose pregnancy. The sensitivity and specificity of these tests have steadily improved since they were first introduced in the 1970s. Most, including over-the-counter

---

Table 13-10   Glycosylated Hemoglobin

Diagnostic units, % of total hemoglobin
Normal, 4–6 (varies by laboratory)

HbA_{1c} (%)	Diagnoses to Consider	Actions to Consider
Increased		
<7*	Good diabetic control	No change in therapy
7–9	Average diabetic control	Home glucose monitoring; initiate or change medications
>9	Poor diabetic control	Evaluate for causes of poor diabetic control

*Achieving a more stringent glycemic goal (i.e., to a normal HbA_{1c} of <6.0%) reduces the risk of complications of diabetes (i.e., cardiovascular disease, retinopathy, and nephropathy) at the cost of an increased risk of hypoglycemia (particularly in those with type 1 diabetes).
From Diabetes Care 2004;27(Suppl 1):S91–S93.

Table 13-11   Human Chorionic Gonadotropin (hCG)

Diagnostic units, mIU/L
Normal, <5 (women of childbearing age); <0.8 (postmenopausal women); <0.7 (men)

Normal Pregnancy:

Gestational week	hCG (mIU/L)
1	<30
2	50–500
3	100–10,000
10	50,000–300,000
2nd trimester	10,000–25,000
3rd trimester	5,000–15,000

hCG (mIU/L)	Diagnoses to Consider	Actions to Consider
Increased >5	Pregnancy Ectopic pregnancy Gestational trophoblastic disease After abortion (≤2 wk) Choriocarcinoma Ovarian cancer Testicular cancer	Correlate with ultrasound Repeated hCG to document trend

commercially available kits, are now sensitive enough to detect pregnancy several days before the time of missed menses.

If a patient is possibly pregnant but the hCG test is negative, a repeated test in 1 to 2 days on a concentrated first-morning specimen can be performed. A quantitative serum test is not needed in these cases, as serum tests are not more sensitive than current urine tests.

Quantitative serum hCG tests are commonly used to evaluate the viability of an "at risk" pregnancy, such as a pregnant woman with bleeding. Quantitative hCG tests may be ordered serially every few days. On average, a 66% increase in hCG should be found between values, although significant variability in doubling times may be seen in normal pregnancies (ranging from 1.4 to 5.0 days). hCG doubling times are most useful up until the sixth gestational week. By week 9, cardiac activity detected by ultrasonography can be used reliably to determine fetal viability. Unfortunately, no definitive test determines viability in women who have bleeding between 6 and 9 weeks of gestation.

If serum hCG values are higher than expected or increase more rapidly than expected, diagnoses to consider include gestational trophoblastic disease, multiple pregnancy, and cancer. Abnormally low rate of increase of hCG values may be associated with ectopic pregnancies (Table 13-11).

IRON STUDIES

Multiple studies are used to differentiate among the various disorders of iron metabolism; of these, the most frequently used are iron (Fe), iron-binding capacity (TIBC), and ferritin. In brief, iron is a direct measure of the serum iron. TIBC is a measure of the saturation of the serum with iron (and approximates the transferrin saturation, which may be used instead of TIBC); it will be increased in simple iron deficiency because of the increased "binding capacity" available from reduced iron levels. Ferritin is a protein produced by the reticuloendothelial system, and it serves as the primary iron-storage protein in the body. In general, the ferritin level is proportional to the total body iron-storage level.

Iron deficiency is a frequent cause of anemia, and iron studies are frequently indicated when microcytosis is seen in patients with anemia. In patients with uncomplicated iron deficiency, such as occurs from chronic blood loss or inadequate intake of iron, the serum iron level will be decreased, the TIBC (or transferrin) level will be increased, and the ferritin will be normal or decreased. In iron-deficiency states, ferritin often decreases before anemia, microcytosis, a low iron, or an elevated TIBC appears. Therefore it is more sensitive than either iron or TIBC in detecting iron deficiency. Iron, TIBC, and ferritin levels quickly respond to iron therapy, even though total body iron stores may take months of therapy to restore.

Ferritin is most commonly used to differentiate iron-deficiency anemia from anemia of chronic disease in patients with a normal or low MCV (Table 13-12). It can also be used to determine a patient's response to iron therapy, or to evaluate for iron-overload states, particularly in patients with hemolytic anemia. It is less sensitive as a marker of overload

Table 13-12 Ferritin

Diagnostic units, ng/mL (mg/L)
SI conversion factor, 1
Normal: 20–300 (males); 20–120 (females)

Ferritin (ng/mL)	Diagnoses to Consider	Actions to Consider
Decreased <20	Iron deficiency Hypothyroidism	Evaluate for GI blood loss CBC Dietary history TSH
Increased >300	Iron overload Hemochromatosis Transfusion Hemolytic anemia Liver disease Chronic inflammation Malignancies Hyperthyroidism	Iron, TIBC CBC ESR Thyroid studies Liver tests

CBC, complete blood count; ESR, erythrocyte sedimentation rate; GI, gastrointestinal; TIBC, total iron-binding capacity; TSH, thyroid-stimulating hormone.

Table 13-13 Interpreting Iron Studies

Disease	Ferritin	TIBC (or Transferrin)	Serum Iron
Iron deficiency	↓	↑	N or ↓
Anemia of chronic disease	N or ↑	N or ↓	↓
Hemolytic anemia	↑	N or ↓	N or ↑
Hemochromatosis	↑	↓	↑↑
Acute liver disease	↑	Varies	↑

N, normal; TIBC, total iron-binding capacity.

than it is of iron deficiency; if iron overload is suspected, iron and TIBC assays are the preferred tests.

A cause for iron deficiency should always be sought, as it may lead to diagnosis of an occult gastrointestinal tract cancer.

Some common causes of iron overload include hemochromatosis, hemolytic anemias, hepatitis, and inappropriate iron therapy.

A brief summary of iron studies is found in Table 13-13.

LIVER TESTS

These tests are commonly ordered as a group, although often the investigator is interested in just one or two of the individual tests. Although commonly called liver-function tests, some tests are a measure of function (such as manufacture of albumin and clotting factors), and others more clearly indicate whether injury is present (such as the aminotransferase enzymes, levels of which are elevated in settings of hepatic injury).

Albumin

Albumin is produced by the liver and is the most abundant plasma protein, accounting for 90% of the plasma oncotic pressure. It is unclear how albumin is processed and degraded, but the half-life is about 20 days. The concentration of plasma albumin depends on the rate of synthesis, degradation, loss, and overall plasma volume.

Serum albumin testing is not recommended for general screening of healthy individuals, but it can be useful for evaluating patients with liver disease, edema, or suspected malnutrition (Table 13-14). An elevated albumin value is not thought to be of any clinical significance, although it may occur with dehydration.

Protein (Total)

Total protein measured by laboratory instruments includes albumin plus the various globulins. Decreased levels of total protein are seen in a wide variety of illnesses. In most cases, these diseases are better monitored by measurement of albumin.

Table 13-14 Albumin

Diagnostic units, g/dL (g/L)
SI conversion factor, 10
Normal: 4.0–6.0 (40–60)

Albumin (g/dL)	Diagnoses to Consider	Actions to Consider

Decreased
<4.0
	Decreased synthesis
	  Liver insufficiency
	  Malnutrition
	  Malignancy
	Increased loss
	  Nephrotic syndrome
	  Extensive burns
	  Protein-losing enteropathy
	Pregnancy
	Inflammatory illness
		Dietary history
		Urinalysis
		24-hr urine protein
		Creatinine
		Other liver-function tests
		Complete blood count

Increased levels of total protein are occasionally seen and may lead to an evaluation for multiple myeloma, which may be associated with increased (and sometimes decreased or normal) protein levels (Table 13-15). When a question occurs about the interpretation of any abnormal total protein, a protein electrophoresis may be considered. This test separates the albumin from the various globulins, and the electrophoretic pattern that results may be diag-nostically useful. Further immunologic typing can be performed to test for multiple myeloma.

Alkaline Phosphatase

Alkaline phosphatase (ALP) is produced by a large number of tissues, primarily liver and bone (accounting for about 80% of total activity) but also including intestine, kidney, and placenta. When elevated, it pro-

Table 13-15 Protein (Total)

Diagnostic units, g/dL (g/L)
SI conversion factor, 10
Normal: 6.0–8.0 (60–80)

Protein (g/dL)	Diagnoses to Consider	Actions to Consider

Decreased
<6.0
	Decreased synthesis
	  Liver insufficiency
	  Malnutrition
	  Malignancy
	Increased loss
	  Nephrotic syndrome
	  Extensive burns
	  Protein-losing enteropathy
	Pregnancy
	Inflammatory illness
	Myeloma
	Increased intravascular volume
		Dietary history
		Urinalysis
		24-hr urine protein
		Creatinine
		Other liver-function tests
		Complete blood count

Increased >8.0	Dehydration Chronic inflammation Monoclonal gammopathy Sarcoidosis Multiple myeloma	BUN Creatinine Protein electrophoresis Chest radiograph

BUN, blood urea nitrogen.

Table 13-16   Alkaline Phosphatase

Diagnostic units, units/L (g/L)
SI conversion factor, 10
Normal: 50–120*

Alkaline Phosphatase (units/L)	Diagnoses to Consider	Actions to Consider
Increased >120	Related to the liver	Recheck in 6 mo (if <2× normal and patient is asymptomatic)
	Cirrhosis	Other liver tests, including GGT and bilirubin
	Hepatitis	Alkaline phosphatase isoenzymes
	Infiltrative liver disease (sarcoid, TB, amyloidosis, tumor, abscess)	Liver ultrasound
	Autoimmune cholangiopathy	
	Gilbert's syndrome	
	Related to bone	
	Bone growth	
	Healing fracture	
	Acromegaly	
	Osteogenic sarcoma	
	Liver or bone metastases	
	Leukemia	
	Myelofibrosis	
	Other	
	Sepsis	
	Drugs	
	Nonfasting specimen	

*Normal values are higher in pediatric, pregnant, and menopausal patients.
GGT, γ-glutamyl transferase; TB, tuberculosis.

vides a useful, but not very specific, indication of possible liver or bone disease (Table 13-16). In the liver, ALP is produced by the biliary epithelium and excreted in the bile. When the biliary tract becomes obstructed, ALP may increase in the serum and usually corresponds with elevated bilirubin levels. When in doubt about the source of ALP, serum γ-glutamyl transferase (GGT), an enzyme found in liver and biliary epithelium, can be measured. GGT is elevated in most diseases that cause acute damage to the liver or bile ducts. ALP isoenzyme determinations also can be made by electrophoresis and may help to distinguish the source of ALP. A low ALP is not commonly encountered but may be seen with hypothyroidism, drug side effects, pernicious anemia, or Wilson's disease.

Aminotransferases

Alanine aminotransferase (ALT) and aspartate aminotransferase (AST; ALT was formerly referred to as serum glutamate pyruvate transaminase [SGPT], and AST was formerly referred to as serum glutamic-oxaloacetic transaminase [SGOT]) are enzymes that occur primarily in liver cells and appear in the serum as a result of tissue injury. Of the two enzymes, ALT is more specific for detection of hepatocyte injury than

is AST, which may be elevated with muscle (skeletal or cardiac) injury as well as hemolysis. In most circumstances, both will be elevated in the presence of liver injury, and ALT is usually elevated more than AST. A useful exception occurs in the case of alcoholic hepatitis, in which AST is often several-fold greater than ALT. When the ratio is more than 3:1, 96% of patients will have alcoholic liver disease (Table 13-17).

Aminotransferase tests are very useful for diagnosing and monitoring liver disease. They are not useful for screening healthy individuals; however, they are frequently ordered as a precursor to or for monitoring of potentially hepatotoxic drugs, such as isoniazid (for treatment of latent or active tuberculosis), or statin-type medications (for treatment of hypercholesterolemia).

Low aminotransferase levels are not usually of any clinical significance. They may be seen in advanced cirrhosis or fulminant hepatitis, in which a normal or low level can indicate that the disease has progressed so far that few hepatocytes remain.

Bilirubin

Bilirubin is an integral component of the heme ring, the oxygen-carrying molecule within RBCs. When

Table 13-17 Aminotransferases

Diagnostic units, units/L (0.17–0.68 μkat/L)
SI conversion factor, 1.0
Normal: males, 10–40; females, 8–35

Aminotransferase (units/L)	Diagnoses to Consider	Actions to Consider
Increased >40	AST and ALT increased	Repeated testing
	Steatohepatitis (fatty liver)	Hepatitis exposure history (drugs, travel, transfusion, blood-borne illness risks)
	Hepatitis	
	Alcoholic hepatitis (AST often > ALT)	Alcohol history
	Biliary obstruction	Other liver function tests, including bilirubin and alkaline phosphatase
	Drugs (prescription, over-the-counter, and illicit)	Hepatitis virus testing
	Hemochromatosis	CBC, peripheral smear (for hemolysis)
	Wilson's disease	If initial serologic tests negative, or persistent elevation, consider
	α-Antitrypsin deficiency	Ultrasound
	Only AST elevated	ANA
	Myocardial infarction	Smooth muscle antibody
	Hemolysis	Ceruloplasmin
	Skeletal disorders	α-Antitrypsin
		Liver biopsy

ALT, alanine aminotransferase; ANA, antinuclear antibody; AST, aspartate aminotransferase; CBC, complete blood count.

RBCs are degraded, the bilirubin attaches to albumin and is transported to the liver. There, it is processed into its water-soluble, or *conjugated*, form and is then excreted in the bile, where it later passes into the intestine to be reabsorbed and reprocessed.

Laboratories measure the total bilirubin and conjugated (or *direct*) bilirubin; the unconjugated (or *indirect*) bilirubin fraction is then obtained by subtraction. In normal serum, less than 15% of the total bilirubin is conjugated.

Common causes of elevated bilirubin are increased RBC destruction, liver disease, and biliary tract obstruction (Table 13-18). Interpretation of elevated bilirubin levels is often aided by considering other liver test results in conjunction with the clinical picture. For example, most cases of elevated bilirubin caused by infectious hepatitis will be associated with marked elevations in aminotransferases; only modest elevation of aminotransferases and marked elevation in ALP levels or GGT (or both) with hyperbilirubinemia suggests an obstructive process, and isolated elevations of bilirubin occur in neonatal jaundice and with inborn errors of bilirubin metabolism such as Gilbert and Dubin-Johnson syndromes.

Hyperbilirubinemia and jaundice are common in newborns, and, in most cases, physiologic. Physiologic jaundice and bilirubin levels usually peak by the third or fourth day of life in term neonates, and acceptable upper reference limits vary appropriately. A bilirubin level should be obtained in all infants with suspected jaundice, and in some centers, routine testing of all infants may be performed.

When bilirubin increases above acceptable levels, treatment with phototherapy or, in severe cases, exchange transfusions, is warranted. Of primary concern is the prevention of kernicterus, a devastating injury caused by deposition of unconjugated bilirubin in the brain. Transcutaneous bilirubin testing is becoming more widely available, but after 10 days of life, endogenous carotenoids interfere with transcutaneous measurements.

Prothrombin Time

The prothrombin time (PT) is the only coagulation test commonly used in the outpatient setting. It is defined as the time required to initiate clotting when tissue thromboplastin is mixed with blood. The PT is a measure of both the extrinsic clotting system (i.e., factor VII) and factors common to the intrinsic and extrinsic systems (i.e., factor X, factor V, prothrombin, and fibrinogen).

The thromboplastin reagents used as a part of the test may vary considerably in their clotting activity; as a result, PT values are converted to a normalized value by every laboratory to an international normalized ratio (INR), which is standardized to the World Health Organization's reference thromboplastin. In practice, the INR is what is actually used when interpreting PT results.

PT is most commonly used to monitor the anticoagulation effects of warfarin (Coumadin) (Table 13-19). Acceptable therapeutic ranges for PT are often defined for specific diagnoses. For example,

Table 13-18   Bilirubin (Total)

Diagnostic units, mg/dL (μmol/L)
SI conversion factor, 17.1
Normal: adults, 0.3–1.0 (5–17); newborns, varies by age and gestation of newborn; for term infants, upper
limit is approximately <6.0 at 24 hr, <10.0 at 24–48 hr, and <12–15 at >48 hr

Bilirubin (mg/dL)	Diagnoses to Consider	Actions to Consider
Increased: neonates (see note above for ranges)	Physiologic Breast-feeding ABO or Rh incompatibility Hemorrhage, hematomas Sepsis Infections (toxoplasmosis, cytomegalovirus, rubella, syphilis) Maternal diabetes Inborn errors of metabolism (galactosemia, G6PD, pyruvate kinase deficiency)	Maternal, prenatal, and birth history Maternal and infant blood type Direct Coombs' test Hematocrit Phototherapy Exchange transfusion

Adults: >1.0 mg/dL	Hepatobiliary disease
	  Hepatitis
	  Cholangitis
	  Cholecystitis
	  Cirrhosis
	Hemolytic anemia
	  Transfusion reaction
	  Hematoma
	  Pulmonary embolus
	  Congestive heart failure
	Drugs
	Isolated bilirubin elevation
	  Dubin-Johnson or Gilbert's syndrome
	  Wilson's disease (often in conjunction with decreased alkaline phosphatase)
		Alcohol history
		Drug history
		Travel, dietary, blood exposure history
		ALT, AST, GGT, conjugated bilirubin
		Complete blood count
		Reticulocyte count
		Direct Coombs' test
		Viral hepatitis tests
		Ultrasound

ALT, alanine aminotransferase; AST, aspartate aminotransferase; G6PD, glucose 6-phosphate dehydrogenase deficiency; GGT, γ-glutamyl transferase.

Table 13-19   Prothrombin Time (PT) and International Normalized Ratio (INR)

Units, PT in seconds; INR is a ratio and has no units
Normal, PT varies; INR, 0.8–1.3

INR	Diagnoses to Consider	Actions to Consider
Increased >1.3	Liver disease Malabsorption DIC Warfarin therapy Factor II, V, VII, X deficiency Vitamin K deficiency	Liver tests PTT Clotting factor assays Serum carotene 72-hr stool fat Administer vitamin K

DIC, disseminated intravascular coagulation; PTT, partial thromboplastin time.

patients with atrial fibrillation commonly have INR values maintained between 2.0 and 3.0; for patients with prosthetic heart valves, the range is usually slightly higher at 3.0 to 4.5.

PT also is a useful test for evaluating any patient with abnormal bleeding. However, it is important to note that PT is normal in people with classic hemophilia (i.e., factor VIII deficiency) and in those with von Willebrand's disease. Clotting factors are generally produced by the liver; hence PT also can be used to evaluate the liver's synthetic function.

PANCREATIC ENZYMES

Amylase

Amylase is an enzyme that breaks down dietary starches into smaller polysaccharides and is produced by the pancreas and the salivary glands. Most of the amylase produced goes directly into the gut, but a small amount is absorbed into the circulation. Usually, about one third of the serum amylase is of pancreatic origin, and two-thirds is from the salivary glands. Amylase is excreted primarily by the kidneys.

The most common cause of an elevated serum amylase is pancreatitis, and a serum amylase is often ordered to evaluate patients with acute unexplained abdominal pain (Table 13-20). When the source of amylase is in doubt, it is sometimes useful to distinguish the P (pancreatic) and S (salivary) forms of the enzyme, a test that can be performed in most hospital laboratories. Given its renal excretion, modest elevations of 2 to 3 times normal can be seen in patients with chronic renal failure.

However, pancreatitis can occur without elevation in amylase levels in up to 10% of patients, especially in those with recurrent disease or long duration of symptoms before testing. In such cases, serum lipase testing (often ordered at the same time as amylase testing) may be useful.

In some individuals, amylase can become bound to other large serum polysaccharides, which can lead to macroamylasemia, and these individuals can have persistently elevated, fluctuating amylase levels. This condition is sometimes associated with chronic illnesses such as celiac disease, HIV infection, lymphoma, ulcerative colitis, rheumatoid arthritis, and monoclonal gammopathy.

Low serum amylase levels are rarely of clinical significance.

Lipase

Pancreatic lipase breaks down triglycerides into glycerol and free fatty acids. Similar to amylase, lipase is produced by several body tissues including the tongue, pancreas, intestine, and liver. It is excreted by the kidney. Bile acids inhibit the activity of lipases, but the activity of pancreatic lipase is preserved in the intestine because of the presence of another enzyme, colipase. A commonly used test for lipase combines bile acids and colipase to the assay to

Table 13-20 Amylase		
Diagnostic units, Somogyi units/dL (units/L) Normal, 50–150 (0–130)		
Amylase (Somogyi units/dL)	Diagnoses to Consider	Actions to Consider

Increased >150	Gastrointestinal
	 Pancreatitis
	  Alcohol
	  Gallstones
	  Trauma
	  Hyperlipidemia
	  Infectious
	  Drug-induced (thiazide
	   diuretics, aspirin,
	   some antibiotics)
	  Familial
	  After ERCP
	 Perforating ulcer
	 Bowel obstruction
	  or infarction
	 Salivary gland disease
	Renal
	 Chronic renal failure
	Neoplastic
	 Cancer that secretes amylase
	 Macroamylasemia
		Complete drug history
		Lipase
		Amylase isoenzymes
		Ultrasonography
		CT scan abdomen
		Amylase-to-creatinine clearance ratio (ratio
		  of <1% in a 24-hr collection supports
		  diagnosis of macroamylasemia; ratio is
		  increased in acute pancreatitis, severe
		  burns, and diabetic ketoacidosis)

CT, computed tomography; ERCP, endoscopic retrograde cholangiopancreatography.

Table 13-21   Lipase

Diagnostic units, units/dL (units/L)
SI conversion factor, 10
Normal, 0–160

Lipase (units/dL)	Diagnoses to Consider	Actions to Consider

Increased >160	Gastrointestinal
	  Pancreatitis (see under amylase)
	  Cholecystitis
	  Bowel obstruction or infarction
	  Salivary gland disease
	Renal
	  Chronic renal failure
	Neoplastic
	  Cancer that secretes amylase
	  Pancreatic cancer
	Iatrogenic
	  Drugs
	    Furosemide
	    Thiazide diuretics
	    Cholinergics
	    Narcotics
	    Oral contraceptives
		Complete drug history
		Ultrasonography
		CT scan abdomen
		MRI or EUS

Decreased	Drugs
	  Salicylates
	  Calcium
	  Hydroxyurea
	  Protamine
	  Somatostatin
		Drug history

CT, Computed tomography; EUS, endoscopic ultrasound; MRI, magnetic resonance imaging.

inhibit other forms of lipase, providing a specific assay for pancreatic lipase.

Elevation of lipase levels is most commonly associated with pancreatitis, and markedly elevated levels of lipase are very specific for pancreatitis (Table 13-21). Because of its longer half-life (7 to 13 hours), lipase remains elevated longer than amylase, and hence may remain elevated after the amylase has returned to normal. Low lipase levels may be associated with some medications.

RENAL TESTS

Blood Urea Nitrogen and Creatinine

Urea is the end product of protein metabolism, synthesized by the liver, and freely excreted by the renal glomeruli. It is commonly used to indicate renal function but may be altered by the nitrogen load, water intake, and urine flow. Creatinine is released from skeletal muscle and is excreted unchanged in the urine. Few factors affect its excretion, and it is the best common test for monitoring renal function. An increase in creatinine represents a decrease in the renal glomerular filtration rate (GFR).

Because creatinine is released by skeletal muscle, it is affected by total muscle mass. Small or elderly people may have a normal creatinine even with reduced renal function. Hence it is often more useful to estimate creatinine clearance. The following is a commonly used formula:

$$\text{Cr clearance} = \frac{(140 - \text{age})(\text{weight in kg})}{72 \times \text{Cr in mg/dL}}$$

As a rough guideline, a creatinine level of 2 mg/dL is equivalent to a creatinine clearance of 50 mL/min; a creatinine level of 4 mg/dL is equal to a creatinine clearance of 20 mL/min; and a creatinine level of 6 mg/dL is equivalent to a creatinine clearance of 10 mL/min. When necessary, creatinine clearance can be more accurately measured through collection of a 24-hour urine specimen.

Serum creatinine increases exponentially in response to a decrease in the GFR, and small increases in creatinine can represent a significant decline in GFR. This is especially important in early decline, because a 50% reduction in GFR leads to an increase of creatinine from only 1.0 to 2.0 mg/dL. It also is important to note that creatine increases slowly in response to changes in renal function. In sudden, severe renal failure (e.g., tubular necrosis after shock), the creatinine may increase as little as 1 mg/dL daily, despite a creatinine clearance of zero.

The blood urea nitrogen (BUN)/creatinine ratio can be useful in assessing abnormalities of nitrogen load, water intake, or urine flow (Table 13-22). A high ratio (>20:1) suggests overproduction or impaired excretion and is commonly associated with prerenal failure (decreased renal blood flow or decreased perfusion); examples include congestive heart failure, shock, volume loss, dehydration, and, when extreme (>36:1), upper gastrointestinal bleeding. Low ratios may be found with low-protein diet, malnutrition, pregnancy, severe liver disease, or rhabdomyolysis.

Chronic renal insufficiency is generally defined as a creatinine level of 1.5 to 3.0 and chronic renal failure, as Cr > 3.0. The dosages of most renally excreted drugs must be adjusted appropriately or avoided altogether in patients with reduced renal function.

THYROID TESTS

Thyroid-stimulating Hormone

Thyroid-stimulating hormone (TSH), also known as pituitary thyrotropin, is produced by the anterior pituitary gland in response to levels of thyroid hormone in the plasma. Very small changes in the circulating thyroid hormone T_4 produce large changes in TSH; hence thyroid function is usually best assessed by measurement of TSH. It is often used to screen patients at risk for hypothyroidism (as in patients with diabetes or who have a family history of hypothyroidism) (Table 13-23). More often, it is used to monitor therapy in patients taking thyroid replacement. If the serum TSH is high (representing a hypothyroid state), the dose should to be increased; if it is low, the dose should be decreased.

In hyperthyroid patients, TSH is suppressed. First-generation tests for TSH were not sensitive in the low range, but second- and third-generation tests are sensitive below 0.5 µIU/mL and can be

Table 13-22 Creatinine

Diagnostic units, mg/dL (µmol/L)
SI conversion factor, 88.4
Normal, 0.6–1.2 (50–110)

Creatinine (mg/dL)	Diagnoses to Consider	Actions to Consider
Increased		
1.2–1.6	Mild renal impairment	Repeated test
	Muscle injury	Urinalysis
		Creatinine clearance
>1.6	Prerenal cause	Urinalysis
	Dehydration	Creatinine clearance
	Blood loss	Bladder catheterization
	Heart failure	Renal imaging
	Liver failure	
	Intrinsic renal failure	
	Diabetes mellitus	
	Hypertension	
	SLE	
	Nephrotoxins	
	Glomerulonephritis	
	Acute tubular necrosis	
	Postrenal failure	
	Urethral obstruction	
	Upper tract obstruction	
>6.0	Severe renal failure	Electrolyte measurements
		Correction of potassium (hyperkalemia), acidosis
Decreased		
<0.6	Decreased muscle mass	Observation
	Small stature	Treatment of underlying disorder
	Muscle diseases	
	Advanced liver disease	
	Long-term steroids	

SLE, systemic lupus erythematosus.

Table 13-23 Thyroid-stimulating Hormone

Diagnostic units, μIU/mL (mU/L)
SI conversion factor, 1
Normal, 0.5–6.0 (Variations in reference values will depend on laboratory and method used)

TSH (μIU/mL)	Diagnoses to Consider	Actions to Consider
Increased >6.0	Primary hypothyroidism (gland failure) Thyroiditis Inadequate levothyroxine therapy	Drug history Physician examination T_4, T_3 uptake TRH stimulation test
Decreased <0.5	Hyperthyroidism Excessive levothyroxine intake Secondary hypothyroidism (pituitary failure) Tertiary hypothyroidism (hypothalamic failure)	Physical examination Drug history T_4, T_3 uptake TRH stimulation test

TRH, thyroid-releasing hormone.

useful as an aid to diagnosis of hyperthyroidism. However, in early stages of treatment, TSH may be suppressed and remain subnormal for several months. T_3 and T_4 levels change more rapidly, and because T_3 concentrations are typically higher than T_4, serum T_3 measurements can be valuable in assessing and monitoring patients with hyperthyroidism.

Thyroxine and Triiodothyronine

Thyroxine (T_4) is the principal hormone secreted by the thyroid gland and is virtually all bound to serum proteins, including thyroxine-binding globulin (TBG), transthyretin, or thyroxine-binding prealbumin (TBPA). T_3, another form of thyroid hormone, is less tightly bound to TBG and TBPA, but more

Table 13-24 Thyroxine (T_4)

Diagnostic units, μg/dL (nmol/L)
SI conversion factor, 13
Normal, 5.5–12.5 (72–163)

Thyroxine (μg/dL)	Diagnoses to Consider	Actions to Consider
Increased >12.5	Hyperthyroidism Elevated TBG Birth control pills Pregnancy Estrogen therapy Liver disease Drugs Propranolol Amphetamines Cocaine Amiodarone Heparin	TSH Free T_4 T_3 uptake Thyroid scan Complete drug history
Decreased <5.5	Hypothyroidism Decreased TBG Malnutrition Liver diseases Nephrotic syndrome Androgens Glucocorticoids Sick thyroid syndrome	TSH Free T_4 Albumin Liver tests Urinary protein

T_3, triiodothyronine; T_4, thyroxine; TBG, thyroxine-binding globulin; TSH, thyroid-stimulating hormone.

Table 13-25   Interpreting Thyroid Function Tests

	Total T_4	T_3-resin uptake or THBI	Free T_4
Hyperthyroidism	↑	↑	↑
TBG excess	↑	↓	Normal
Hypothyroidism	↓	↓	↑
TBG deficiency	↓	↑	Normal

TBG, thyroid-binding globulin; THBI, thyroid hormone binding index.
From Kamath PS. Clinical approach to the patient with abnormal liver test results. Mayo Clin Proc 1996;71:1089–1095.

tightly bound to albumin than is T_4; measurements of T_3 also are used in the assessment of thyroid function (Table 13-24). It is generally held that the active form of the thyroid hormones is the unbound or free form, which is available for uptake into cells and interaction with nuclear receptors. The bound hormone represents a circulating storage pool.

Drugs and illness can alter the concentration of binding proteins, which may cause elevated total T_4 and T_3 measurements even though the free, physiologically active form remains in the normal range. Estrogen may induce production of TBG, which may then increase TBG-bound hormone levels, elevating total T_4 measurements. Normal ranges for free T_4 and T_3 measurements depend on the method used; most methods use a formula to estimate the actual free hormone level.

T_3-Resin Uptake and Thyroid Hormone Binding Ratio

Other tests have been developed to try to measure the effect of binding protein on hormone levels; among these, T_3-resin uptake has been traditionally most used. The patient's serum is incubated with a radiolabeled T_3 tracer, and then an insoluble resin (often dextran-coated charcoal) is added that traps the remaining unbound radiolabeled T_3. The percentage of tracer that is bound to the resin is reported as the T_3 uptake, and it varies inversely with the number of available free binding sites for T_3. For example, if a large percentage of available T_3 is bound to the resin, it indicates either excess T_3 or a low-ratio TBG-bound hormone. Using this value in conjunction with other thyroid tests helps distinguish between these two scenarios (Table 13-25). Many laboratories convert the T_3-resin uptake to a ratio value called the thyroid hormone uptake ratio or index (THBR or THBI):

$$THBI = \frac{\text{patient's } T_3 \text{ resin}}{\text{normal pool } T_3 \text{ resin}}$$

A typical reference range for THBI is 0.83 to 1.16.

Antithyroid antibody tests also are available to help in the evaluation of other abnormal thyroid states, such as Graves' disease and other autoimmune disorders.

Material Available on Student Consult

Review Questions and Answers about Interpreting Laboratory Tests

REFERENCES

Baloch Z, Carayon P, Conte-Devolx B, et al. Laboratory medicine practice guidelines: Laboratory support for the diagnosis and monitoring of thyroid disease. Thyroid 2003;13:3–126.

Kamath PS. Clinical approach to the patient with abnormal liver test results. Mayo Clinic Proc 1996;71:1089–1095.

Management of hyperbilirubinemia in the newborn infant at 35 or more weeks of gestation. Pediatrics 2004;114: 297–316.

14

Selecting Radiographic Tests: Radiographs, Computed Tomography, Magnetic Resonance Imaging, Ultrasound, and Nuclear Imaging

J. Mark Beard and David P. Losh

KEY POINTS

1. Regular x-ray is best for detecting changes in bone, air, soft tissue, and fat densities but is limited by its two-dimensional representation of structures.

2. Compared tomography, with or without contrast, allows digital reconstruction of cross-sectional images of body without the super imposition of other structures that frequently occurs on standard x-ray films.

3. Standard contrast agents can significantly improve the accuracy of imaging modalities but can also increase the cost of the study and, in some instances, cause mild or serious reactions and renal failure.

4. Renal failure complications can be prevented with the use of other imaging modalities that do not require nephrotoxic contrast or can be reduced with the use of nonionic contrast, good hydration, and prophylactic acetylcysteine.

5. MRI uses a strong magnetic field for imaging, allowing for better visualization of **soft tissues** surrounded by bone structures without radiation exposure. MRI should not be used in patients with ferrous metallic structures or fragments in their body. MRI contrast is nontoxic to the kidney.

6. Ultrasound utilizes sound waves for imaging and is preferred for abdominal and cardiac imaging, gynecologic or pregnant patients, and children because of its lack of radiation risks. It can be combined with color flow to assess vascular integrity of structures.

7. For most **head trauma**, head CT scanning without contrast provides the best method for assessment of fractures and hemorrhagic complications.

8. CT scanning is used to acutely evaluate a patient suffering an evolving or a completed **stroke** to assess for a hemorrhagic component that would preclude systemic anticoagulation.

9. The occurrence of **TIA** requires no acute imaging, but a carotid Doppler and ultrasound and echocardiogram are used to determine the cause and source of the ischemic or embolic phenomenon.

10. Most **acute low back pain** occurring in minimally traumatic cases does not require radiographic imaging. When imaging is required, CT is preferred for suspected bone injury. MRI is the preferred modality for soft tissue injury as it is superior in visualizing tissue within surrounding bone.

11. Most causes for **headache** can be diagnosed with an accurate history and physical. In **severe headaches of sudden onset,** a non-contrast CT is obtained. When imaging is required otherwise, a CT with contrast is preferred.

12. Plain x-rays are used in the initial assessment of **spinal trauma** to assess for fracture or stability of the bone structures and followed by CT when needed. MRI is preferred to assess the spinal cord and exiting nerve roots.

13. CT with contrast and MRI are both used to assess **cerebral tumors and metastases.**

14. Echocardiography is the best method for evaluation of **heart failure** once ischemic causes are resolved.

Continued

Evidence levels Ⓐ Randomized, controlled trials (RCTs), meta-analyses, well-designed systematic reviews of RCTs. Ⓑ Case-control or cohort studies, nonrandomized clinical trials, systematic reviews of studies other than RCTs, cross-sectional studies, retrospective studies, certain uncontrolled studies. Ⓒ Consensus statements, expert guidelines, usual practice, opinion.

KEY POINTS (Continued)

15. A chest x-ray and D-dimer test followed by a ventilation/perfusion scan is the initial choice in evaluating patients with suspected **pulmonary embolism.**

16. Chest x-ray followed by CT with contrast is used for **thoracic aneurysms.** Ultrasound is used for the initial evaluation of **abdominal aneurysms.**

17. Cholelithiasis is best diagnosed and evaluated with abdominal ultrasound due to ease, availability, and cost.

18. Cholecystitis is best evaluated with abdominal ultrasound followed by radionuclide scanning, if needed.

19. Ultrasound is the easiest and most cost-effective method for evaluating causes of biliary **tract obstruction.** Other modalities of imaging can be used in special circumstances.

20. Plain x-rays of the abdomen remain the standard to evaluate **small bowel obstruction** in its initial phases. Contrast studies can follow for further identification of the cause or location.

21. Direct endoscopy of the affected site is preferred in the evaluation of **gastrointestinal bleeding** as treatment of the causative site can occur simultaneously.

22. Ultrasound is the imaging modality of choice if the biliary tree is compromised by a **pancreatic mass** although CT scans have better resolution in most other cases.

23. Radionuclide scanning is the most commonly used approach in evaluating **hepatosplenomegaly.**

24. Although ultrasound is used for most hepatic masses, CT scanning with contrast is best for **hepatic metastases.**

25. Fine-needle aspiration biopsy is the best method for evaluation of a single **thyroid nodule.** A radionuclide thyroid scan can assess function of a nodule when needed.

26. A radionuclide thyroid scan is recommended in the initial evaluation of an **enlarged thyroid without obvious nodule.**

27. Enlarged or hypersecretory **parathyroid glands** as well as adrenal masses are assessed with the use of radionuclide scans to assess areas of increased or decreased function. Plain lateral skull x-rays followed by MRI may be used to assess **hyperprolactinemia.**

28. Standard x-rays are most often used to evaluate possible **fractures.** CT scan or radionuclide bone scan can be performed if the diagnosis remains in question following x-ray films.

29. DEXA scans are the favored form of evaluation for **osteoporosis** both for initial diagnosis and subsequent exams to follow treatment response.

30. Standard x-ray can detect 80% of **urinary stones.** If not successful, a noncontrast spiral CT is done to further evaluate the urinary tract and has generally supplanted the intravenous pyelogram as the study of preference.

31. **Renal failure** is best evaluated radiographically with the ultrasound to assess size and structure of the kidneys. A Duplex study can be done to assess renovascular disease.

32. Ultrasound is the preferred imaging method for **renal mass** appraisal. CT can be obtained to evaluate a mass further, as indicated.

33. **Testicular torsion** is best assessed acutely with color flow Doppler ultrasound. Standard ultrasound is recommended for the initial evaluation of other scrotal masses.

34. **Breast mass** evaluation begins with a clinical exam and is frequently followed by a mammogram or ultrasound to further define the cause of any irregularities. In most cases, a biopsy of the palpable mass is clinically indicated even if the imaging modalities are otherwise normal.

Exponential advances in medical imaging have occurred with the advent of progressively more sophisticated equipment and more complex computer technology. As computers have become more powerful, they have allowed digitalization of images, integration of numerous pictures in multiple planes, and improvement in image clarity. Computerized tomography (CT), magnetic resonance imaging (MRI), ultrasound (US), and nuclear medicine studies have revolutionized the type and quality of information obtained from medical imaging. This technology has provided the family physician with many new and sometimes expensive choices for diagnostic testing. It is therefore important for the family physician to judge the cost-benefit ratio of a particular test and to select the most effective imaging strategy for a particular clinical problem. Medical imaging should be used as a diagnostic tool only after a provider performs an appropriate history and physical examination. Individual patient characteristics and circumstances must be considered and a differential diagnosis developed before the most appropriate imaging study can be selected. The imaging results from the consulting radiologist can be fully interpreted only by a physician seeing the findings in the specific context of an individual patient (Mettler et al., 2000). Because the field of diagnostic imaging is quite technical and has so many new and expensive techniques, the family physician is encouraged to discuss cases and diagnostic dilemmas regularly in consultation with radiologists. This chapter provides background information on the most commonly available imaging studies and provides an imaging strategy for many common diagnostic problems encountered in family medicine.

BASIC IMAGING TESTS AVAILABLE TO THE CLINICIAN

Standard Radiographic X-Rays and Contrast Material

An electric tube generating electrons from a heated filament and accelerating them toward a rotating anode produces traditional x-rays. The x-rays generated by this process are passed through the body and are differentially absorbed by various densities of tissue. A detector such as x-ray film, a fluoroscope, or an analog-to-digital converter records the x-rays remaining after they pass through tissues. Variations in the types of x-ray tubes, films, and patient positioning allow different special images such as mammograms and soft tissue views (Figs. 14-1 and 14-2). Tomograms are an application of standard x-rays in which the x-ray source and the detector are rotated to blur tissue above and below the desired level of examination. This allows better visualization of a specific structure on one plane when overlying tissues or items on a different plane in standard radiographs obscures it. Fluoroscopy is performed by using continuous x-rays to evaluate a moving process, such as in tube placement or in evaluation of peristalsis. Standard radi-

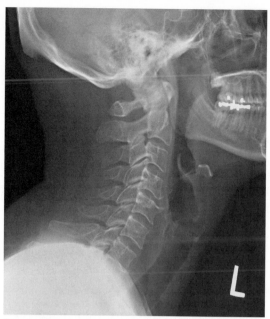

Figure 14-2   Soft tissue radiograph of neck with lateral view. Note good visibility of hyoid bone, thyroid cartilage, and trachea.

ographs have the advantage of being relatively inexpensive and portable and are used occasionally for applications at the bedside. The cost of standard radiographs varies according to the study requested. Examinations such as an upper gastrointestinal series, a barium enema, or an intravenous pyelogram cost about 2.5 to 3 times that of a standard chest radiograph. Standard radiographs are best for detection of bone (Figs. 14-3 and 14-4), air, soft tissue, and fat densities, with more-dense tissues appearing lighter (bone) and less-dense tissues darker (air) (Fig. 14-5). Radiographs are limited by their two-dimensional representation of a three-dimensional structure and in their ability to detect small differences in tissue density with superimposition of surrounding structures. Table 14-1 outlines further details on cost of specific standard diagnostic radiology imaging.

The Selection of Contrast Material

Contrast agents are used to define structures that frequently are inadequately visualized on standard imaging. They can be introduced intravascularly or intraluminally to define fully the structure in question (Fig. 14-6). When ordering imaging studies, the family physician is required to weigh the value and risk of an examination requiring contrast and may even need to decide what type of contrast material to recommend. High-osmolarity ionic contrast material is a water-soluble material containing iodine. It is frequently used in imaging of the urinary tract and in angiography. Contrast material also is used in enhanced CT applications, such as

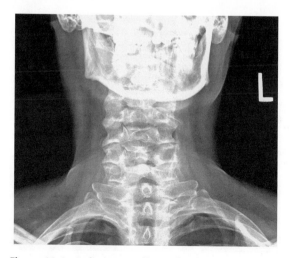

Figure 14-1   Soft tissue radiograph of neck from anterior to posterior view.

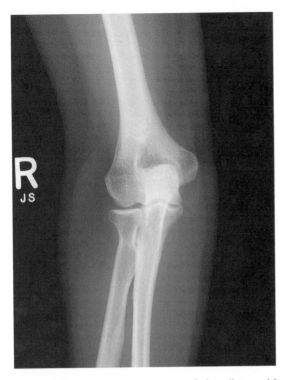

Figure 14-3 Anteroposterior view of the elbow with standard radiograph.

examinations of the head, chest, and abdomen. When used with CT, contrast material can determine the vascularity of a region and the outline of a hollow viscus. When receiving ionic contrast material, up to 5% of patients may experience a mild reaction and feel a sense of altered taste, heat, nausea, tachycardia, or flushing. Hives and wheezing are not uncommon side effects. Although fatal reactions occur in fewer than one per 100,000 doses (Eisenberg and Margulis, 1996), serious adverse reactions such as anaphylaxis, cardiovascular collapse, laryngospasm, or bronchospasm can occur in about one patient in 500 to 1000 doses (American College of Radiology [ACR], 1991 Ⓑ). The cause of adverse reactions is unknown but may be related to the high osmolarity of the solution or to true anaphylactic reactions. Many of the adverse reactions may be avoided by the use of low-osmolarity, non-ionic contrast materials. However, these newer non-ionic contrast agents are expensive and in some cases may double the cost of a procedure. In addition, traditional contrast material must be used with great caution in patients with reduced renal perfusion caused by hypovolemia, advanced congestive heart failure or vascular disease, and baseline preexisting renal disease (serum creatinine >1.5 mg). Contrast agents can cause potentially irreversible kidney

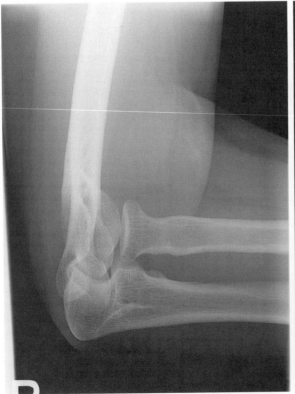
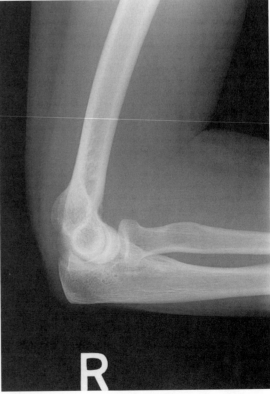

Figure 14-4 Two lateral views of the elbow with standard radiographs.

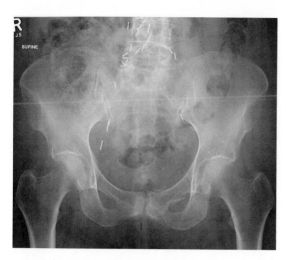

Figure 14-5 Radiograph of pelvis showing fracture of left pubic ramus and bowel gas, stool, and surgical clips overlying the lumbar spine.

failure in these high-risk patients. The following approaches have been advocated to manage potential adverse reactions to contrast material.

Acute renal failure can be a serious complication with the use of radiographic contrast agents, particularly for those with impaired renal function before the examination. A serum creatinine greater than 1.5 or a creatinine clearance less than 60 mL/min identifies a patient at higher risk for radiocontrast-induced nephropathy. The best prevention for renal dysfunction is use of an alternate noncontrast imaging modality such as MRI. If a contrast test is still required, the provider should order use of lower-dose non-ionic contrast (Rudnik et al., 1995Ⓐ), should adequately

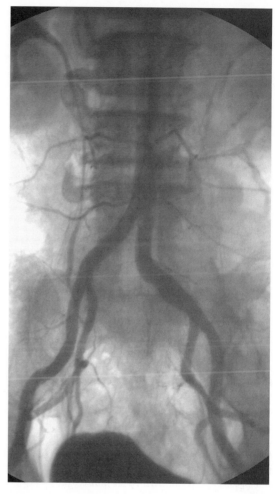

Figure 14-6 Angiogram of aorta with visible aorta and branching vessels.

Table 14-1 Approximate Costs of Diagnostic Radiology Imaging

Diagnostic Radiology Imaging	CPT Code	Cost*	Medicare MPFS†
Chest radiography, 2v.	71020	$90	$38.09
Abdomen, 1v.	74000	$75	$31.48
Lumbar spine, 2v.	72100	$125	$40.45
Pelvis, 1v.	72170	$85	$31.10
Hand, 2v.	73120	$70	$29.08
Ankle, 2v.	73600	$70	$29.08
Barium enema	74270	$250	$110.27
Enteroclysis	74251	$225	$107.30
Intravenous pyelogram	74400	$250	$98.27
Mammogram	76091	$180	$101.66
Dexascan	76075	$200	$148.49
Coronary angiogram	93508	$1700	$785.44
Cerebral angiogram	75671	$1400	$626.50
Pulmonary angiogram	75743	$1400	$625.49

V, views

*Approximate relative charge based on average of survey of current charges at two hospital systems in Seattle, Washington, 2004.

†2004 maximum payment for Healthcare Common Procedure Code for locality 0083602, King County, Washington, Medicare Physician Fee Schedule. Available at www.cms.hhs.gov/physicians/mpfsapp/display.asp. Accessed 10/8/2004.

hydrate the patient before the imaging study (Solomon et al., 1994🅐), and should consider use of acetylcysteine prophylactically (Alonso et al., 2004🅐). One successful method to reduce the risk of radiocontrast nephropathy is to hydrate the patient by using 0.45% saline at 1 mL/kg/hr for 12 hours before the procedure and to give 600 mg of acetylcysteine twice a day on the day before and day of the imaging procedure (Tepel et al., 2000🅐). Care also should be taken with patients taking medications that can lead to metabolic acidosis, such as metformin or topiramate. Ideally, metformin should be withheld for 48 hours before and after an intravascular contrast procedure (ACR, 1997🅒).

Prophylactic medication has provided good protection from anaphylaxis when a possibility of an allergic reaction to ionic contrast material exists. The following prophylactic regimen may be used to reduce a reaction: 50 mg prednisone orally, 13, 7, and 1 hour before the study, and 50 mg diphenhydramine 1 hour before the study. This regimen does not, however, protect against direct radiocontrast toxicity to the kidney. The American College of Radiology (2001a🅒) recommends the use of non-ionic contrast material in patients with a history of a previous adverse reaction to contrast material, asthma or prior serious allergic reaction, renal insufficiency, known cardiac dysfunction, generalized debilitation, or on recommendation by the radiologist. In addition, others have recommended that the following patients also be considered for non-ionic contrast material: children age 2 years or younger; patients with sickle cell disease; patients with renal failure; patients with major trauma including hypotension, shock, neurotrauma, or spinal precautions; and patients requiring angiography.

Computed Tomography

In CT, x-ray beams are aimed through the patient from many different angles. Instead of striking film, radiation detectors identify the x-rays, and the results are recorded as digital information in a computer. The computer produces images that may be manipulated in many ways and recorded on film. Standard CT images are axial cross sections through the body and are viewed as if oriented at the foot of the patient looking toward the head (Fig. 14-7). For standard studies, axial images are generated every 5 to 10 mm throughout the body. However, images may be obtained every 1 to 3 mm for some specialized studies. The main advantage of CT scans is the ability to obtain cross-sectional images through the body without the visual superimposition of other structures. They also are able to detect much smaller differences in tissue density than are standard radiographs. Disadvantages are the frequent need to use ionic or non-ionic con-

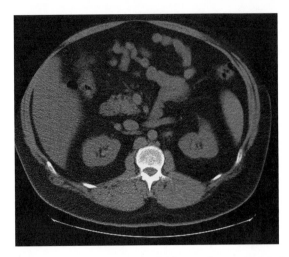

Figure 14-7 Transverse or axial image from computed tomography of abdomen. Note liver is to the left, and spleen is to the right, as if viewed from patient's feet. Note kidneys without contrast toward spine at bottom and small and large intestine in center. Aorta without contrast is just anterior to spine.

trast, the image artifacts occurring with patient movement, and the increased exposure to radiation in generating the multiple images. Although CT scans offer much more detail, because of the complexity of the examination and the cost of the equipment, CT scans are more expensive than standard radiographs, and they are not portable. CT scans are generally in the cost range of 7 to 10 times that of a standard chest radiograph.

CT scans may be obtained with or without contrast and performed with or without angiography. Over the past decade, CT has been modified to improve image quality and usefulness. A standard CT moves the patient on its table through the scanner in a stepwise fashion. Helical (spiral) CT allows the patient to move through the scanner continuously and rapidly, in one patient breath. This allows near elimination of movement artifact, identification of much smaller lesions, less scan time, and use of lower doses of contrast material. Multidetector CT (MDCT) provides multiple rows of x-ray detectors, allowing even shorter scan times, increased resolution, and thinner slices for more specific detail, particularly with angiography (Chen et al., 2004). These CT scanners can obtain images in less than 1 second and allow visualization of the vascular system with injection of intravenous contrast material without catheterization. They also provide a large number of scan planes that can be used to recreate three-dimensional images. The ability to obtain three-dimensional images has revolutionized CT angiography and allowed visualization of arterial, capillary, and venous vascular phases in an organ. Its use also has been expanded to provide CT colonography (virtual colonoscopy) that allows a patient to forgo the need for sedation for a colonoscopy but, obviously, does not allow directed tissue biopsy. Table 14-2 defines costs associated with CT scanning.

Magnetic Resonance Imaging

MRI produces images by subjecting the body to a very strong magnetic field and then exposing the body to pulses of radiofrequency energy. These radiofrequency pulses cause randomly oriented hydrogen nuclei to realign in the body and then return to their original neutral position, releasing energy sensed by the scanner. The MRI computer is able to recreate a picture in any sagittal, coronal, or axial plane. Because the magnetic field of an MRI scanner is so strong, it can potentially dislodge traditional nerve stimulators, pacemakers, internal defibrillators, and some very specific mechanical heart valves, making these devices absolute contraindications to MRI scan. Patients with any ferrous metal in their body, such as intraorbital metallic fragments, should not receive MRI scans. In patients with surgical clips, such as cerebral aneurysm clips, MRIs are contraindicated as well. Titanium wires, most mechanical heart valves, and most orthopedic hardware are made from nonferrous metals, allowing MRI scanning to proceed. A plane radiograph can be used before MRI to assess for any ferrous metal object as needed. Although MRI is expensive, it is particularly useful in evaluating soft tissue around bony structures that normally interfere with image clarity on a CT scan. MRI is especially helpful in imaging the central nervous system for masses and other abnormalities of the brain, spinal cord, and nerve roots (Figs. 14-8 and 14-9). MRI also is useful for evaluating the musculoskeletal system, including the joints and spine, and is being used to evaluate the pelvis, retroperitoneum, mediastinum, and large vessels. Two types of weighted images are available on MRI to assist in better visualization of tissue densities. The T_1-weighted images show fluids as a dark image on the film and fatty tissue as a white or bright image, whereas the T_2-weighted images show fluids as a light color and fats as dark (Figs. 14-10 and 14-11). Bones are not well visualized on MRI, and what is actually imaged is the fat present in the marrow. These weighted images allow better image definition and evaluation of tissue density (i.e., solid, cystic, or fatty lesions). Advantages of MRI are its increased contrast resolution and lack of radiation exposure for the scan. The cost of an MRI study may be in the range of 8 to 12 times that of a standard chest radiograph.

Contrast agents are available with MRI as well. The most frequently used contrast agent is gadolinium dimeglumine. Significantly fewer adverse reactions to gadolinium are found in comparison with

Table 14-2 Approximate Costs of Computed Tomography and Magnetic Resonance Imaging

	CPT Code	Cost*	Medicare MPFS†
Computed Tomography			
Head without contrast	70450	$550	$247.07
With contrast	70460	$650	$301.27
Chest without contrast	71250	$800	$313.78
With contrast	71260	$950	$367.46
Abdomen without contrast	74150	$750	$304.34
With contrast	74160	$850	$359.55
Magnetic Resonance Imaging			
Head, without contrast	70551	$1150	$557.39
With contrast	70552	$1350	$669.06
With and without	70553	$1950	$1189.42
Knee	73721	$1200	$543.56
Lumbosacral spine	72158	$2200	$1189.72
MRA head, without contrast	70544	$1300	$542.17
With contrast	70545	$1400	$542.17
With and without	70546	$2000	$1036.15

MRA, magnetic resonance angiography.
*Approximate relative charge based on average of survey of current charges at two hospital systems in Seattle, Washington.
†2004 maximum payment for HCPC for locality 0083602, King County, Washington, Medicare Physician Fee Schedule. Available at www.cms.hhs.gov/physicians/mpfsapp/display.asp. Accessed 10/8/2004.

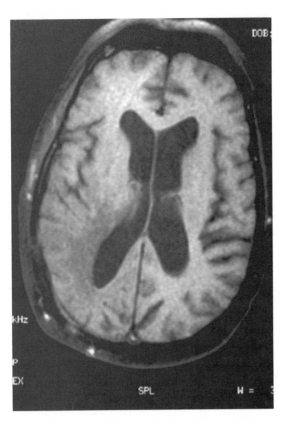

Figure 14-8 Magnetic resonance imaging of brain in axial view. Note right posterior horn of lateral ventricle (on the reader's left in picture) has an abnormality in the surrounding brain parenchyma.

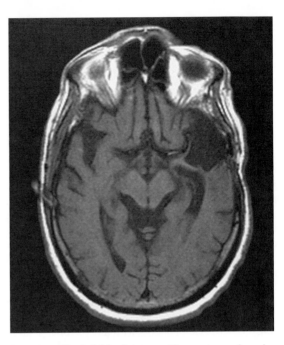

Figure 14-10 Axial brain magnetic resonance imaging with T$_1$-weighted image, with fluids appearing dark on the film. Note patient's left temporal lobe (to reader's right) with prior craniotomy and cerebral defect.

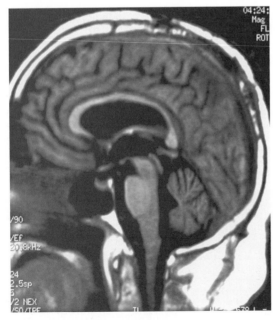

Figure 14-9 Magnetic resonance imaging of brain in sagittal view.

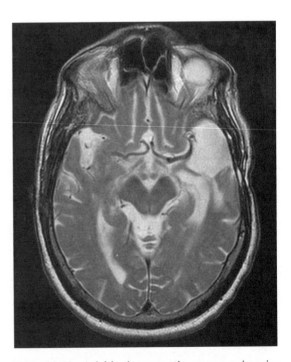

Figure 14-11 Axial brain magnetic resonance imaging with T$_2$-weighted image, with fluids now appearing lighter on the film. Note enhancement of left temporal lobe region with cerebrospinal fluid after recovery from craniotomy.

those to standard radiographic contrast, but these include dizziness, nausea, vomiting, headache, and paresthesias. The gadolinium may add $200 to $300 to the cost of the imaging study.

MR angiography (MRA) is a technique of studying the blood vessels with or without the need for intravenous contrast. Short scan times, as quick as one breath hold, have allowed this technique to replace various types of traditional angiography. Imaging techniques such as fast spin echo, fast gradient echo, diffusion imaging, perfusion imaging, and echo planar imaging with MRI have provided many new uses for these scanners. These techniques are now being used in the evaluation and treatment of strokes. Another application is magnetic resonance cholangiopancreatography (MRCP), which allows noncontrast evaluation of the biliary system in patients unable to tolerate standard or endoscopic contrast evaluations (ACR, 2001a©).

Most MRI machines are designed as long tubes open at both ends. Standard scans take several minutes to complete and require the patient to remain motionless. Newer open MRI machines are now available for patients prone to claustrophobia or who may have problems with traditional MRI machines. Recently introduced echo planar machines have reduced the imaging time to less than 1 second, thus reducing the artifacts of breathing movement and allowing imaging of the heart, lungs, and abdomen. Costs of some selected MRI and MRA scans are outlined in Table 14-2.

Ultrasound

US creates images by using high-frequency sound waves generated by a hand-held transducer. When the transducer is passed over a thin layer of gel on the surface of the body, it captures the returning sound waves or echoes that reflect off of the structures being imaged. The waves returning are transformed into a picture by a computer. To improve images, gel is used between the transducer and patient's skin to eliminate any air pocket that would normally reflect nearly all of the sound waves. Once produced by the transducer, US waves spread out from the transducer into the body and are reflected back at different frequencies by varying tissue planes. The returning signals diminish as they pass through tissue, making US a difficult imaging modality for deeper structures.

Because US delivers no ionizing radiation, it is thought to be comparatively safe and has been widely used in applications related to pregnancy, such as imaging of the fetus and pelvic structures. However, US has limitations, especially because it cannot penetrate bone and gas. Bowel gas can interfere with the examination. The technique works poorly when imaging structures in the lung, brain, and, frequently, the central retroperitoneum and pancreas. Because US is very portable, many applications may be done at the bedside.

US has been found to be particularly useful in evaluation of structures such as the heart in echocardiography or the gallbladder in an abdominal study. Doppler US is a technique used to assess organ perfusion and blood flow. Color flow Doppler assigns a different color for faster- or slower-flowing fluids that permits evaluation of arterial and venous blood flow to specific sites. This can be used in obstetric US of umbilical cord blood flow or to assess vascularity of some abdominal or pelvic masses. It is particularly useful in cardiac applications with echocardiography and in identifying ischemic processes, such as testicular torsion.

Transluminal US or sonography has been recently refined to provide methods for evaluation of structures around any hollow lumen. This technique can evaluate the heart with transesophageal echocardiography, the prostate with a transrectal ultrasound probe, pelvic structures with transvaginal ultrasound and hysterosonography, and masses or tumors of the gastrointestinal tract with endoluminal probes. Intravascular catheters have recently been developed to assess vascular stenoses and plaque formation in vessels. Three-dimensional US has improved with computer digitalization. This process is used to define structures and volumes in abdominal US and, more important, in definition of fetal congenital anomalies in obstetric ultrasound. The cost of a standard US examination is in the range of 2 to 3 times that of a standard chest radiograph, although some examinations such as echocardiography may cost nearly twice that. Selected US costs are outlined in Table 14-3.

Nuclear Imaging

Nuclear imaging uses gamma rays emitted from isotopes that are administered to the patient by the oral or intravenous route. The isotopes, such as ^{99m}technetium, are bound to different metabolically active chemicals that determine the biodistribution of the compound in different tissues. The gamma rays are then counted and displayed as a picture by a gamma camera and computer. Nuclear imaging is particularly useful in determining the functional physiologic status of certain organs or tissues instead of giving a simple pictorial representation. Applications that assess the function of the heart, thyroid, lung, gallbladder, kidneys, and skeleton are particularly common. Although the function can be assessed, the detail of structures is less defined than with other techniques.

Improved definition of specific tissues is possible with single-photon emission CT (SPECT) scans. SPECT scans use a rotating gamma camera to improve images by focusing on a thin slice of tissue

Table 14-3 Approximate Costs of Nuclear Medicine and Ultrasound Imaging

	CPT Code	Cost*	Medicare MPFS†
Nuclear Medicine			
Bone scan, total body	78306	$550	$228.47
Myocardial perfusion	78460	$475	$147.03
Pulmonary, ventilation/perfusion	78596	$600	$369.40
HIDA scan	78223	$450	$201.36
MUGA scan	78473	$850	$430.98
Ultrasound			
Abdomen, total	76700	$300	$127.60
Obstetrical, <14 wk	76801	$150	$142.87
>14 wk	76805	$285	$142.87
Echocardiogram, TTE	93307	$450	$216.35
TEE	93312	$575	$282.35
Stress echocardiogram	93350	$370	$156.14

HIDA, hepatobiliary iminodiacetic acid; MUGA, multigated acquisition; TEE, transesophageal echocardiography; TTE, transthoracic echocardiography; CPT, current procedural terminology.
*Approximate relative charge based on average of survey of current charges at two hospital systems in Seattle, Washington.
†2004 maximum payment for HCPC for locality 0083602, King County, Washington, Medicare Physician Fee Schedule. Available at www.cms.hhs.gov/physicians/mpfsapp/display.asp. Accessed 10/8/2004.

and blurring the surrounding tissues in a way similar to standard tomograms. This technique has increased the resolution and sensitivity of the examination but is nearly double the cost of the standard nuclear imaging technique.

Positron emission tomography (PET) scans take advantage of binding positron-emitting isotopes to metabolically active compounds (such as nitrogen, oxygen, carbon, or glucose) to assess their uptake in specific tissues. This technique can been used to identify more metabolically active tumors and the uptake or release of specific compounds during activities in the brain. Because the radionuclides are produced by a cyclotron and are short lived, PET is extremely expensive and is available at relatively few large medical centers only. The cost may be reduced with the recent development of upgraded gamma camera-based scanners. Most nuclear imaging techniques deliver less radiation to the patient than do standard x-ray techniques because multiple pictures can be taken with a single isotope injection. The cost of most nuclear imaging studies is in the range of 5 to 9 times that of a standard chest radiograph. Some particular nuclear medicine testing costs are listed in Table 14-3.

SELECTED DIAGNOSTIC STRATEGIES FOR COMMON CLINICAL PROBLEMS

For a family physician, diagnostic imaging strategies are complex and rapidly changing. An outline of suggested imaging options is helpful to a busy provider to allow rapid reference to recommended studies. Alternative choices are given in cases in which certain tests may not be widely available or are particularly expensive. It should be understood that as the cost of certain procedures change and certain studies become more widely available, these recommended approaches would change. In some cases, a more expensive test is recommended first, because the test is so sensitive or specific that it may save the added expense of doing less-focused tests first. Because of the limited scope of this chapter, only selected problems that either represent diagnostic controversy or are thought to be most common in family medicine are addressed. Many resources are available to the reader for other disease entities or symptom complexes, some of which are outlined in the references. The tables in this article give an approximate comparison of the charges for various imaging studies and procedures as a reference. Also given is the Medicare Physician Fee Schedule for payment on these procedures in one locale.

Neurologic System

With a few exceptions, as noted later, MR and CT are the most useful examinations with which to study the central nervous system.

Cranial Trauma

Skull trauma can be easily assessed with standard radiographs, although CT scan may be helpful in delineating an acute fracture from cranial suture lines or defining a small intranasal or intraorbital fracture. In head trauma and in suspected intracranial or subarachnoid hemorrhage, head CT without contrast is the best imaging method. MRI is generally inappropriate for the initial examination in head trauma. MRI is practical when symptoms remain unexplained. It may be useful in subacute or chronic conditions or in brainstem contusions in which posterior fossa bone structures preclude clear CT imaging.

Transient Ischemic Attack

Frequently, no acute imaging is necessary with a transient ischemic attack (TIA), which is defined as neurologic changes lasting less than 24 hours. US and Doppler are primarily used to evaluate the carotid arterial system and, frequently, the vertebral and intracranial arterial system if adequate views can be obtained either around or through bone. If a significant arterial plaque or occlusion is identified with US that may require carotid endarterectomy, angiography is frequently requested for preoperative conformation of anatomy (Fig. 14-12). New procedures performed by some interventional radiologists include cranial arterial stenting with the aid of direct angiography. For those patients found with a carotid bruit on examination, US Doppler offers the only cost-effective method to screen for significant stenosis. Patients who have contraindications for an angiography, such as renal disease, can undergo an MRA on either the carotid or vertebral arterial systems, as indicated.

Stroke

CT without contrast is used immediately to identify hemorrhagic strokes and can distinguish ischemic strokes after 12 to 24 hours. CT also can exclude several problems that appear similar to a stroke, such as a tumor or an abscess. MRI may be useful if CT does not fully explain the clinical findings, or when a posterior fossa or brainstem infarction is suspected. Fast imaging MRI is now being implemented in the evaluation of evolving stroke symptoms and is able to detect smaller regional blood-flow changes. In initial evaluation, MRI has had significant difficulty successfully identifying hemorrhage accurately, so usually it is maintained as a secondary imaging modality. If an aneurysm is suspected, one must keep in mind that MRA or CT angiography is less precise if lesions are smaller than 5 mm. Standard angiography is much more exact and may be performed when surgery is being considered for carotid or vertebral artery disease or when other vascular abnormalities are suspected or noted on CT or MRI (ACR, 2000©). Standard angiography is vital at some medical centers in the initial evaluation of a patient within the first 2 to 4 hours of an evolving acute stroke. An interventional radiologist places an angiographic catheter for the immediate identification of the vascular supply. This allows the infusion of thrombolytics for reversal of an acute infarction, placement of a vascular stent, or introduction of a coil for embolization of an aneurysm.

Back Pain and Suspected Lumbosacral Disk Herniation with Nerve Root Compression

More than 80% of patients with acute back pain respond to conservative therapy and do not require radiologic imaging initially. If conservative therapy is not successful within 4 to 6 weeks or an initial risk is present of nonmuscular causes for the back pain, imaging is appropriate. Initial images should be considered in significant traumatic injuries, immunosuppression, unexplained weight loss, unexplained fever, use of intravenous drugs, prolonged use of corticosteroids, osteoporosis, and in those older than 70 years. Plain lumbosacral spine films have low sensitivity and specificity but may provide a rational starting point to rule out such abnormalities as fracture or metastases and can provide a correlation with further studies when they are needed (Figs. 14-13 and 14-14). If clinically indicated, more extensive five-view radiographic imaging can be obtained to assess neuroforamina, facet structure, and pedicle stability. If a fracture is not clearly seen but is clinically suspected, CT may be helpful in evaluating the bony structures. SPECT scanning may be rarely needed in specific instances to visualize small fractures that are then seen as metabolically active or to identify an inflamed facet joint before injection. SPECT also is used to assess localized vertebral pain after a spinal fusion because of anatomic changes interfering with other modalities. Total-body nuclear medicine bone scans are completed when distant bone metastases in cancer are suspected. When disk herniation, nerve root compression, or both are suspected, MRI is the preferred imaging modality

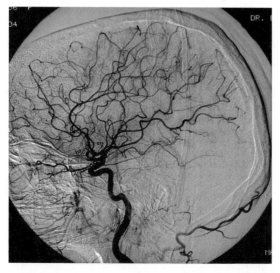

Figure 14-12   Brain angiogram of middle cerebral artery.

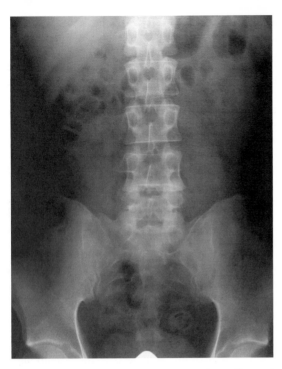

Figure 14-13 Standard anterior to posterior radiograph of lumbosacral spine. Note abdominal bowel gas overlying spine.

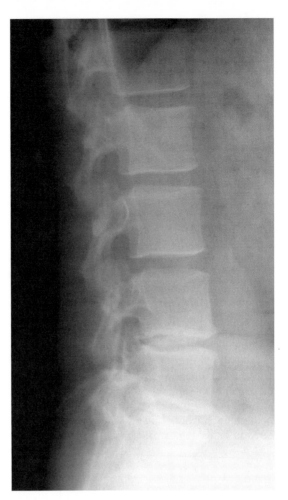

Figure 14-14 Standard lateral radiograph of lumbosacral spine. Note loss of normal lordotic curve.

(Fig. 14-15). Random use of MRI or CT in back-pain patients is discouraged, as it may identify lumbosacral spine abnormalities that are frequently present in asymptomatic individuals and may be unrelated to the current medical concern (ACR, 1999c ©). Controversy exists over whether CT or MRI is the study of choice for suspected disk herniation and nerve compression. MRI is preferred by many because of its ability to obtain views in multiple planes and because it shows excellent anatomic detail and avoids ionizing radiation. CT also is useful for detecting herniated disks, but it is limited to certain views by its one-plane imaging abilities. Its imaging is improved with use of a myelogram (placement of contrast in the spinal fluid space) to differentiate tissue planes and nerve root outlets. Myelography also is used preoperatively, in occasional cases, to define further a herniated intervertebral disk or nerve root compression. CT is the study of choice for bone abnormalities such as suspected spinal stenosis, osteophyte impingement, degenerative disease of the facets, and spondylolysis in adults. Nuclear bone scans with SPECT are now being used in children suspected of having spondylolysis because of its lower dose of radiation and its relatively high specificity in children.

Headache

The majority of headaches seen by the family physician may be diagnosed with reasonable accuracy by a careful history and physical examination. A CT with contrast should be considered when focal disease is suspected from the history or physical examination, when the pattern of the headaches changes significantly, or if further screening history or tests suggest the presence of an intracranial process such as cancer. Concerns for focal disease include aphasia, memory impairment, or focal sensory, motor, or coordination deficits. Headaches of sudden onset and described as the worst headache of a patient's life suggest a potential aneurysmal bleed that is best evaluated initially with noncontrast CT. Lumbar puncture for red blood cell detection is used in some suspected cases only after a normal CT is obtained. Angiography can be used if an aneurysm or hemorrhage is identified to define the anatomy clearly for surgery or even for direct embolization (ACR, 1999i ©).

Infections

The diagnosis of meningitis is determined with a lumbar puncture examination. Generally before the

ularly useful in evaluating for bone changes. If plain views reveal no fracture, and focal pain is present, flexion and extension views may be considered or a CT may be done to clarify the diagnosis. If no focal pain or bone injury is seen, yet suspicions remain regarding cord trauma or a myelopathy, then MR should be considered as the next step to evaluate clearly the soft tissue structures and spinal cord.

Cerebral Tumors or Metastases

CT with contrast will visualize most cerebral metastases. MRI with contrast is even more sensitive and is used to diagnose or monitor primary brain tumors (Figs. 14-16 and 14-17). If symptoms or findings suggest a posterior fossa mass or small anterior cerebral mass, MRI can be particularly helpful. As neurosurgical techniques have improved, so have some imaging techniques that map the exact extent of neoplastic lesions. Functional MRI scans that track regional blood flow with specific motor activity and standard angiography are sometimes used to assist in specific surgical and radiologic procedures. Although quite expensive and of limited availability, PET scan can be used to identify tumor recurrence in patients who have complex structural anatomic changes after initial surgical resection.

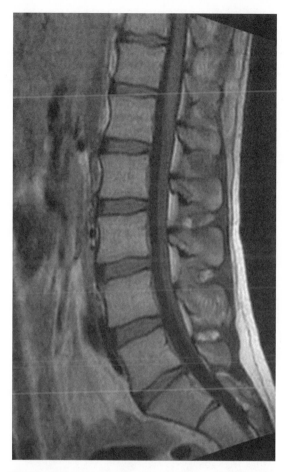

Figure 14-15 Normal sagittal magnetic resonance imaging view of lumbosacral spine in T_1-weighted image.

lumbar puncture, a CT scan is performed to evaluate for space-occupying lesions or midline shift. These findings indicate increased risk of high intracranial pressure that can potentially result in brainstem herniation with a lumbar puncture. CT must be done within the first 30 minutes and should not delay the start of antibiotics when bacterial meningitis is suspected (Losh, 2004). MRI is the imaging method of choice for other intracranial infections. Its enhanced visualization of soft tissues allows identification of abscesses, cerebritis, subdural infections, and human immunodeficiency virus–related changes or secondary infections.

Spinal Injuries

A plain lateral film should be taken during the initial assessment to assess spinal stability at any level. If no fracture is seen, then further plain film views (oblique, anteroposterior [AP], open-mouth views) are obtained. If a fracture is suspected but not definitely seen, CT may be obtained because it is partic-

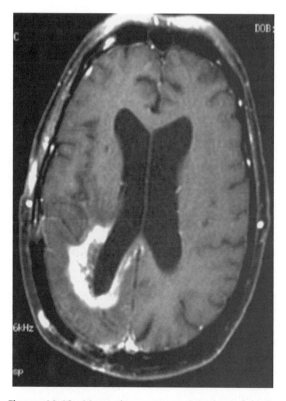

Figure 14-16 Magnetic resonance imaging of brain with T_1-weighted image of film in Figure 14-8. Note contrast enhancement of right posterior lateral ventricle.

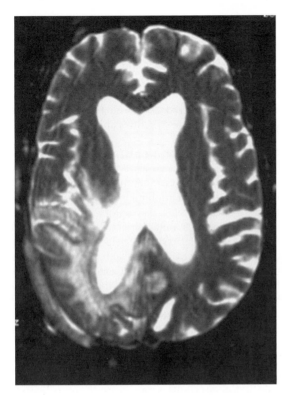

Figure 14-17 Magnetic resonance imaging of brain with T$_2$-weighted image of film in Figure 14-8. Note contrast enhancement of right posterior lateral ventricle.

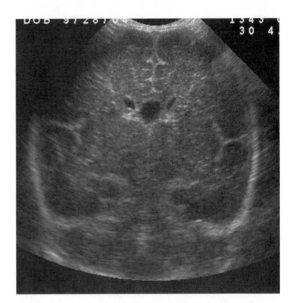

Figure 14-18 Coronal view of fetal brain from an echoencephalogram through one of the fontanelles.

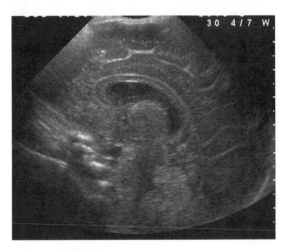

Figure 14-19 Sagittal view of fetal brain from an echoencephalogram.

Specific Pediatric Applications

Because of the noncalcified anterior and posterior fontanelles in newborns and young infants, US is an imaging modality used to assess intracranial structures and not available to older children or adults (Figs. 14-18 and 14-19). This modality can be used to assess for intracranial hemorrhage, hydrocephalus, or mass in the first 4 to 8 months of life with no radiation exposure. It may be done at the bedside and rarely requires sedation.

Cardiovascular System and Respiratory System

Angina Pectoris and Suspected Coronary Artery Disease

In a nonemergency situation, a resting electrocardiogram (ECG) should be obtained as the first step in the evaluation of chest pain of suspected cardiac origin, along with serologic cardiac markers, such as CK-MB and troponin. A chest radiograph may be beneficial to rule out other causes of chest pain, such as pneumothorax, pulmonary embolism, rib fracture, ascending aortic aneurysm, aortic dissection, or congestive heart failure with pulmonary edema. Transthoracic echocardiogram can be used to evaluate for causes of other chest pains, such as pericarditis or pericardial effusion, which can mimic myocardial ischemic pain. If the initial resting ECG shows no abnormalities that preclude valid exercise stress testing, such as a left bundle branch block or ST-segment changes, exercise stress testing is appropriate. For approximate costs of stress testing, see Table 14-4. Controversy exists over whether to do an exercise stress test or to proceed directly to noninvasive imaging studies. Most patients with good exercise capacity and a normal exercise ECG may avoid further more-expensive testing. An abnormal or equivocal exercise stress test is more likely to be a true reflection of disease in those patients at highest risk for coronary artery disease. However, these high-risk patients are the ones most likely to require further

Table 14-4	Approximate Costs of Selected Nonradiology Tests		
	CPT Code	**Cost***	**Medicare MPFS†**
Cardiac			
stress test	93015	$225	$1000
ERCP, alone	43260	$113.36	$328.04

ERCP, endoscopic retrograde cholangiopancreatography.
*Approximate relative charge based on average of
survey of current charges at two hospital systems
in Seattle, Washington.
†2004 maximum payment for HCPC for locality
0083602, King County, Washington, Medicare
Physician Fee Schedule. Available at www.cms.hhs.
gov/physicians/mpfsapp/display.asp. Accessed
10/8/2004.

diagnostic studies, and it can be argued that with them, the most effective approach is to proceed directly to noninvasive diagnostic studies.

Noninvasive imaging studies include stress echocardiography as the first choice. Poorly perfused myocardial tissue does not contract effectively when exercised. Wall-motion abnormalities can be detected by echocardiography done within a minute of exercise completion. The test requires the patient to be free of advanced chronic obstructive pulmonary disease (COPD) or massive obesity and to be able to achieve 85% to 90% of the maximal heart rate during exercise. In patients who cannot exercise, the heart may be stressed to obtain similar results by administering one of the vasodilators, dipyridamole or adenosine, or the sympathomimetic agent, dobutamine. If stress echocardiography is unavailable or the patient has significant COPD, nuclear medicine myocardial imaging studies should be considered. The thallium stress test is based on the failure of areas of ischemic myocardium to take up the thallium radiopharmaceutical during exercise. [201]Thallium has been largely replaced by another radiopharmaceutical, [99m]technetium sestimibi. SPECT imaging is used to yield highly sophisticated images. The sensitivities of SPECT nuclear imaging and stress echocardiography are about the same. Stress echocardiography is generally less expensive (about $400) than nuclear imaging (about $650).

When intervention is planned, it is necessary to proceed to coronary angiography. Coronary angiography yields the most information about the coronary artery anatomy and the exact location and degree of stenosis. This can guide either acute or subacute angioplasty of vessels, coronary artery stenting, and coronary artery bypass graft surgery. Contrast injected into the ventricle allows study of the contractility of the heart and, in addition, direct measurements of the cardiac chamber and ejection fraction. The cost of coronary angiography is in the range of $2000 to $4000 when all costs are totaled.

A form of CT termed electron beam tomography (EBT) is being used at some centers to assess calcium deposition around coronary arteries as an indirect and noninvasive method of assessing risk of coronary events (ACR, 1999b●). Ultrafast cine CT scanners are now able to produce images of the coronary arteries after a peripheral injection of contrast material. It is thought that these technologies may begin to supplant some of the currently available imaging techniques in the evaluation of coronary artery disease.

Congestive Heart Failure

Certainly if ischemia is the primary cause of congestive heart failure (CHF), the evaluations outlined earlier for ischemic heart disease should be the initial evaluation. If, conversely, CHF is caused by nonischemic disease, echocardiography (ECHO) becomes the most dependable mode of assessment after a standard chest radiograph. ECHO provides assessment of valvular function and dysfunction, pericardial effusion, chamber size, myocardial muscle mass and function, and an estimate of ejection fraction and pulmonary artery pressures. It also appraises both systolic and diastolic function of the heart, guiding the selection of appropriate medications or treatments. Systolic failure is characterized by a decrease in contractility, with the heart usually dilated and the ejection fraction less than 40%. Diastolic failure, conversely, is associated with a normal or slightly hypertrophic heart and a normal ejection fraction. ECHO assesses chamber size and thickness to guide therapy for either a hypertrophic or dilated cardiomyopathy, if present. Echocardiography is usually sufficient to estimate the cardiac ejection fraction. If a more precise measurement of ejection fraction is needed, consideration should be given to a nuclear ventriculogram displayed as a multigated acquisition (MUGA) study. A MUGA study is a series of images created by a computer as ^{99m}Tc]-labeled red blood cells flow through the heart after their intravenous injection.

Echocardiography is useful in cases of cardiomyopathy, cardiac tumors, congenital heart disease, cor pulmonale, endocarditis, valvular heart disease, cardiac tamponade, and pericardial effusion. In general, most standard ECHO examinations are done through the anterior chest, or transthoracically. For more accurate visualization of the posterior heart and left atrium, a transesophageal ECHO (TEE) is performed. A TEE is frequently used to assess for an atrial appendage thrombosis in the setting of an embolic stroke or peripheral vascular occlusion with atrial fibrillation. TEE also can be used for identification of other left atrial pathology, such as a myxoma or tumor, or for the assessment of a mediastinal mass. Echocardiography generally costs more than $400.

Pulmonary Embolus

Chest pain, dyspnea, tachypnea, or hemoptysis raises the clinical suspicion for pulmonary embolus and, therefore, the question of whether anticoagulation is necessary. The physician is often faced with the dilemma of determining whether a ventilation/perfusion (V/Q) scan should be done on an emergency basis. If the symptoms are suggestive of pulmonary embolus, or the patient has risk factors such as prolonged bed rest, recent surgery, myocardial infarction or heart failure, an indwelling venous catheter, or venous thrombosis of the pelvis or proximal lower extremities, then the first step should be a plain chest radiograph (Figs. 14-20 and 14-21). The chest radiograph will usually be nonspecific or normal but is important in excluding other chest pathology and is helpful in interpreting the V/Q scan if baseline radiologic abnormalities exist. A nuclear V/Q scan consists of two parts. The perfusion portion is accomplished by intravenously administering technetium-labeled macroaggregated albumin, which lodges in the vascular bed of the lungs and is then scanned. In the ventilation portion of the study, the patient breathes radioactive-labeled xenon gas for a scan that determines the portion of the lung being ventilated. If the V/Q scan is normal, showing good perfusion, it virtually eliminates pulmonary embolus from the diagnosis. Areas of lung with poor alveolar ventilation also have resultant vasospasm. Therefore the two areas of decreased ventilation and perfusion uptake should "match." When perfusion and ventilation

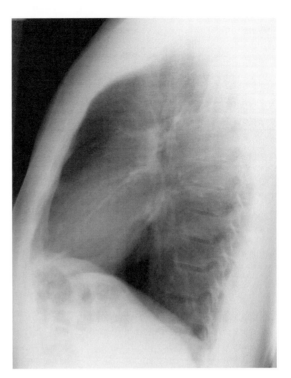

Figure 14-21 Standard lateral radiograph of chest. Note curvature of diaphragm and heart in anterior chest.

defects match, in the absence of other parenchymal disease, the scan will be read as "low probability." Clinical judgment will be required regarding anticoagulation, because about an 80% chance exists that no embolus is present. "Indeterminant" scans are reported with multiple areas of poor perfusion and ventilation, making interpretation difficult, or when the V/Q deficit is associated with a lung lesion of undetermined etiology. The risk of embolus in indeterminant scans may range between 30% and 70%. If the scan shows normal ventilation of a segment, but with a perfusion deficit, then the scan is read as "highly probable," with enough certainty that, in the absence of other contraindications, the patient should be given anticoagulation. A V/Q scan costs about $600.

With the advent of rapid-scan CT machines, CT of the chest with contrast is frequently used in patients with baseline chest radiograph abnormalities, as seen in pulmonary fibrosis, sarcoidosis, mass lesions, and other cardiopulmonary disease. These patients have a high likelihood of an abnormal ventilation scan, which frequently leads to indeterminant V/Q scans. Even with rapid-scan techniques, some patients with pulmonary decompensation are unable to hold their breath for the needed 20 to 30 seconds. In these cases, pulmonary angiography is an option if clinical suspicion remains.

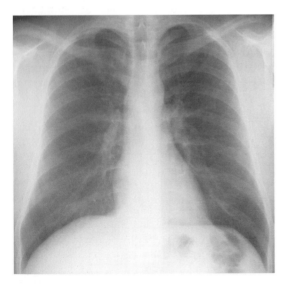

Figure 14-20 Standard radiograph of chest in posteroanterior view.

Pulmonary angiography is reserved for those cases in which a high clinical suspicion of pulmonary embolus is present in the setting of a nondiagnostic or indeterminant V/Q scan or CT scan. Pulmonary angiography is very sensitive and specific. It costs about $1500 and is associated with a mortality rate of between 0.5% and 1% (Grossman et al., 1995b ●). Duplex Doppler compression examination of the lower extremities is used as an adjunct in the evaluation of the patient with suspected pulmonary embolus to determine the location of the embolism source, but it is not used to diagnose the lung component. If further definition of a suspected lower-extremity deep venous thrombosis is need or the US is equivocal, contrast venography with standard radiographs may be used (ACR, 1999h ●).

Other Chest Pathology

Aortic dissection is best diagnosed by first obtaining a chest radiograph and then proceeding to CT with and without contrast (ACR, 1999a ●). If the patient cannot be given contrast, MRI should be considered. In general, an initial plain radiograph and rarely following it with CT, when needed, is appropriate for the first two steps in many diagnoses related to the chest (Fig. 14-22). This approach has been used with diseases such as lung abscesses, persistent atelectasis, asbestosis, blunt chest trauma, bronchiectasis, bronchogenic carcinoma, bronchopleural fistula, emphysema with recurrent pneumothoraces, empyema, pulmonary metastases, anterior and middle mediastinal masses, some cases of pneumonia, sarcoidosis, Wegener's granulomatosis, pneumothorax, and solitary lung nodules. US can be used to evaluate pleural effusions, particularly for thoracentesis when needed, and any soft tissue abnormality of the chest wall. Fiberoptic bronchoscopy may be useful after the chest radiograph in selected cases of hemoptysis or suspected bronchogenic carcinoma. CT may be needed if symptoms persist despite negative findings on bronchoscopy. MRI is acquired only to help stage some lung cancers and mediastinal masses that are suspected of central vascular involvement. A barium swallow may be indicated if esophageal pathology is suspected in the posterior mediastinum, and a thyroid nuclear scan may be indicated in the evaluation of a superior mediastinal mass.

Aneurysms

US is the first choice when evaluating for a suspected abdominal aortic aneurysm. CT with contrast should be considered with suspicion of a retroperitoneal hematoma secondary to a leaking aneurysm. Ultrasound with color Doppler is the initial assessment for peripheral aneurysms, although CT or MRI with contrast may be required for subclavian artery aneurysms.

Sinusitis

Acute sinusitis requires no form of imaging study in its regular clinical presentation. If sinusitis persists after initial clinical treatment, or if mechanical obstruction of the sinus passages is suspected, imaging becomes appropriate. Traditionally, sinus radiographs have been used to evaluate causes of obstructive sinusitis with a Waters' view (frontal view angled upward) and a lateral view. These can show a solid mass or an air/fluid level indicating obstruction. Any life-threatening complication of acute sinusitis or chronic sinusitis lasting longer than 3 months warrants further evaluation, and CT is the preferred method (Fig. 14-23). Imaging with CT defines the nasal bone structure, sinus ostia, fluid accumulation, mucosal reaction, and any obstructing polyp, tumor, or cyst. Frequently, a CT is ordered before endoscopic sinus surgery to define anatomic structures. If intracranial complications of sinusitis are suspected, MRI best defines the areas and their extent.

Gastrointestinal System

Cholelithiasis

US has replaced the oral cholecystogram as the study of choice for the detection of gallstones in the presence of appropriate symptoms. Gallstones appear as very echogenic foci with an intense acoustic shadow and are easily seen within the gallbladder or biliary system. The sensitivity of this test approaches 100% when the examination is done by an experienced technician. CT of the abdomen can visualize stones, but not optimally. When the US is indeterminant and stones are suspected in the biliary tree with elevated appropriate liver-function tests, cholangiography should be performed with endoscopic retrograde cholangiopancreatography (ERCP) or MRI (MRCP).

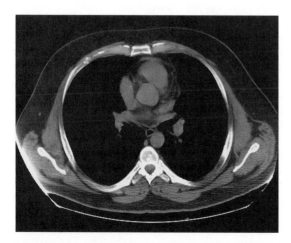

Figure 14-22 Transverse or axial view of computed tomography of the chest. Note the lungs laterally and heart and great vessels centrally. Aorta is just anterior to spine.

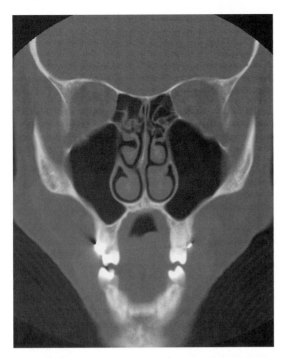

Figure 14-23 Coronal view of sinus computed tomography scan visualizing the maxillary and ethmoid sinuses.

Acute Cholecystitis

An abdominal US examination is particularly useful for confirmation of the diagnosis of acute cholecystitis or if the diagnosis is even somewhat uncertain. An US study can localize the gallbladder and allow the ultrasonographer to confirm the area of pain (a sonographic Murphy's sign). It will identify stones, gallbladder wall thickening, and edematous fluid around the gallbladder. The finding of gallstones plus either a positive Murphy's sign or gallbladder wall thickening is highly suggestive of acute cholecystitis. If only one of these findings is present, and the diagnosis is uncertain, a nuclear [^{99m}Tc]-hepatobiliary iminodiacetic acid (HIDA) scan may be done. This radioactive-labeled substance is rapidly excreted from the liver into the biliary system. An injection of intravenous morphine is used to constrict the sphincter of Oddi and aid in the concentration of the HIDA in the gallbladder. HIDA is useful to determine whether the gallbladder is functional and whether the cystic duct is obstructed. If the gallbladder does not fill with HIDA, acute obstructive cholecystitis is highly likely. If the cystic duct is open, the likelihood of obstructive cholecystitis is virtually eliminated. Rare cases of acalculous cholecystitis are possible, especially after cardiopulmonary bypass surgery; however, the combination of HIDA and ultrasound is usually sufficient to make an appropriate clinical diagnosis. US has a variable accuracy of 64% to 88% in acute cholecystitis. Conversely, HIDA scintigraphy

has a more consistent accuracy of 85%, but with a higher cost for the scan, and frequently it takes up to 4 hours to complete the test (ACR, 1999e ⓒ). Abdominal US costs about $250, and HIDA is slightly more expensive at $400.

Biliary Tract Obstruction

An approach similar to that in cholecystitis is used in these cases. US will reveal dilated biliary and hepatic ducts with a specificity of 71% to 96% and sensitivity of 55% to 95%, depending on technique, although occasionally they can be normal early in the course of the obstruction. HIDA scan is useful if obstruction is highly suspected but the ducts appear normal on US. CT may be necessary when the cause of the obstruction and ductile dilatation is not apparent or is revealed by US and has a specificity of 90% to 94% and sensitivity of 74% to 96% (ACR, 1999f ⓒ). CT can be helpful in locating tumors in the head of the pancreas, as US cannot frequently visualize this area with accuracy. MRI has no advantage over CT in this indication. ERCP may be necessary to define further the anatomy or location of the obstruction. For approximate costs of ERCP, see Table 14-4. This procedure involves cannulation of the duct with the use of an endoscope. Contrast material may be injected into the common bile duct, and sometimes an obstructing stone can be removed with a balloon catheter or sphincterotomy of the sphincter of Oddi. MRCP depicts three-dimensional anatomy of the biliary system and is used primarily for a patient who cannot tolerate ERCP or for whom it fails. Occasionally, percutaneous transhepatic cholangiography (PTC) is necessary as well. This procedure involves a US-guided injection of an intrahepatic biliary duct with contrast material through a thin needle to outline the biliary tree distal to the injection site. With this technique, a stent can be placed simultaneously to bypass the obstruction.

Appendicitis

Most of the time, the diagnosis of appendicitis is made with reasonable certainty on clinical and laboratory examination and without imaging studies. However, when the diagnosis remains clinically uncertain, imaging studies are of assistance in establishing the diagnosis. Groups of people that may have atypical abdominal pain or uncertain findings include the elderly, infants and young children, women in pregnancy or of childbearing age, and cases of suspected appendiceal rupture. Abdominal plain radiographic films are helpful in ruling out other pathology, such as small bowel obstruction, a mass effect, or perforation of a viscus with intra-abdominal air. However, an appendicolith can be seen only about 10% of the time. The next step is to decide between US and CT. CT is the best choice in patients other than pregnant women, infants, and young children. It is especially useful when appendiceal rupture is suspected. CT is often able to detect an abnormal appendix or an appendicolith with surrounding inflammatory changes. US should be ordered as an alternative in pregnant women or in infants or young children (ACR, 1999d ☉). US is less sensitive than CT at detecting a perforated appendix, and technical problems with loops of bowel, obesity, and retrocecal appendix location may hamper the examination.

Esophageal Dysfunction

A barium swallow with fluoroscopy is a reasonable first step in the management of most cases of dysphagia (Fig. 14-24). It costs about one-fourth the cost of endoscopy. This examination can be tailored to the specific type of dysphagia symptoms by giving various thicknesses of barium or barium-coated solids. This is especially important if the patient has dysphagia or suspected aspiration from a stroke or other neurologic problem. Endoscopy is usually required next with evidence of any strictures, ulcerations, tumors, or webs to allow direct visualization, biopsy, or treatment (ACR, 2001d ☉).

Small Bowel Obstruction

Plain films of the abdomen (supine, upright, and decubitus) looking for air/fluid levels or evidence of air-filled small bowel loops with decreased colonic gas are the initial evaluation for small bowel obstruction (SBO). Barium studies are considered next. They are contraindicated with evidence of free air in the abdomen. If an obstruction is suspected in the distal small bowel or colon, one should proceed to a barium enema before an upper gastrointestinal (UGI) barium series (Fig. 14-25). This order is important because barium may be difficult to evacuate when it is proximal to the obstructing lesion. Partial and intermittent small bowel obstructions can sometimes be better detected by a technique called enteroclysis. With this technique, a bolus of barium and methylcellulose is injected directly into the jejunum via an oral tube placed under fluoroscopic guidance. CT may have a role in the diagnosis of small bowel obstruction, but it should probably be reserved for those cases in which the barium studies are inconclusive or an extraintestinal mass is suspected (ACR, 1999g ☉).

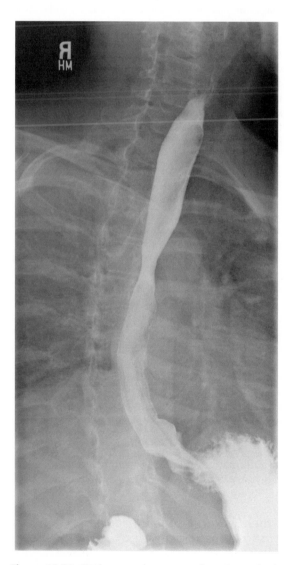

Figure 14-24 Barium esophagogram done to evaluate the swallowing mechanisms.

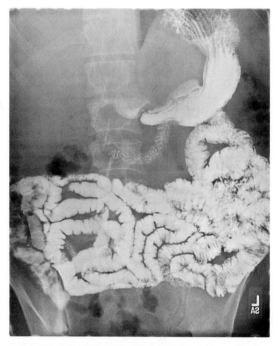

Figure 14-25 Upper gastrointestinal series with small bowel follow-through (UGI/SBFT). Note stomach and small bowel with barium contrast agent.

Acute Gastrointestinal Bleeding

Endoscopy is indicated for the evaluation of acute gastrointestinal bleeding, as both visualization and treatment can occur simultaneously in 95% of cases (ACR, 2002 ⊙). However, if endoscopy cannot locate the bleeding source, a [^{99m}Tc]-red blood cell study may serve to document active bleeding, if 0.05 to 0.1 mL/min or more of blood flow is present, before considering an angiogram. If active bleeding of more than 0.5 to 1 mL/min is present, the angiogram is very good at localizing duodenal or stomach bleeding but is rarely helpful in detecting bleeding from esophageal varices (Grossman et al., 1995a ⊙). Angiography also can be used therapeutically by allowing embolization of a vessel or injection of vasoconstrictive agents.

Pancreatic Lesions

A radiograph of the acute abdomen in acute pancreatitis can show a paralytic ileus of the small bowel overlying the pancreas and can be misinterpreted as an SBO. US is the initial choice in the evaluation of the jaundiced patient with an unknown cause. However, CT may be the initial study in the nonjaundiced patient. CT has better resolution of the retroperitoneal structures and can define pancreatic edema, mass, tumor, abscess, or bleeding.

Hepatomegaly or Hepatosplenomegaly

A nuclear liver and spleen scan can document enlargement of the liver or spleen. However, CT may be needed if the etiology of the enlargement is in question. US is more cost effective with documentation of splenomegaly alone.

Hepatic Metastases

CT with contrast is generally the study of choice for hepatic metastases. If contrast material is contraindicated, or clinical suspicion continues despite a normal CT, an MRI is indicated. If the MRI is unavailable, an alternative is a nuclear liver and spleen scan with SPECT. Extrahepatic metastases may be best defined with either CT or MRI with contrast.

Endocrine System

Thyroid Nodule

The dilemma for the practitioner when a central lower neck nodule is identified is determining whether the nodule actually arises from the thyroid gland. US of the thyroid gland region may be helpful in locating the nodule to confirm its location. If the nodule arises from the thyroid, the question becomes whether the nodule is benign or malignant. The best test in euthyroid patients is fine-needle aspiration biopsy (FNAB) of the thyroid nodule. This test may be done without a radiologic imaging study. It yields usable material about 85% of the time and has 95% accuracy.

A minority of nodules not yielding diagnostic material on a biopsy may have repeated FNAB with US guidance as necessary. A nuclear thyroid scan is reserved for situations in which an FNAB is unavailable, the FNAB yields inconclusive results, or the patient is hyperthyroid. If a nuclear medicine thyroid scan is necessary, it will yield one of several results (Fig. 14-26). If the scan reveals a solitary nonfunctioning "cold" nodule, the risk of malignancy is between 15% and 40%. Although a US examination may be able to differentiate between cystic and solid lesions, some malignant lesions may have cystic components, and US cannot rule out malignancy with certainty. A functioning or "hot" nodule or nodules, conversely, can generally be assumed to be benign. Although multiple cold nodules are usually benign adenomas or cysts, malignancy cannot be ruled out, and a tissue diagnosis should be obtained. A tissue diagnosis also must be obtained for irregular cold areas. They may represent a malignancy or may represent benign lesions such as scars or an atypical adenoma. If thyroid cancer is diagnosed, CT or MRI is obtained to assess for cervical or thoracic metastasis as well as for preoperative surgical planning. If papillary thyroid cancer is diagnosed, [^{131}I]-radionuclide scanning is performed to assess for metastases, as it is the only thyroid tumor that actively incorporates iodine (Grossman et al., 1995c ⊙).

Thyroid Gland Enlargement

The recommended approach to a diffusely enlarged thyroid gland is a nuclear medicine thyroid scan with [^{99m}Tc]-pertechnetate. When the results reveal an enlarged gland with multiple increased- and decreased-function areas, the diagnosis is usually a *multinodular goiter*. A gland with partial replacement by multiple cysts, poorly functioning normal tissue, and fibrosis characterizes this condition. If a hard, growing, or dominant cold nodule is found in a thyroid gland with multinodular goiter, it should be diagnosed by tissue biopsy to rule out cancer. A diffusely enlarged homogeneous gland with increased uptake is suggestive of Graves' disease, although it may rarely represent an organification defect in which iodine is trapped in the gland but not converted to thyroid hormone. An enlarged homogeneous gland with normal uptake may represent early Graves' disease, a stage of Hashimoto's or subacute thyroiditis, a multinodular goiter of fine consistency, or a normal variant. A large gland with poor uptake probably represents subacute thyroiditis and does not require further imaging.

Other Endocrine Abnormalities

Parathyroid adenomas may be visualized by using a technetium sestamibi scan (MIBI) with SPECT. CT is the most common approach to adrenal masses. The CT must be done with very thin slices because most

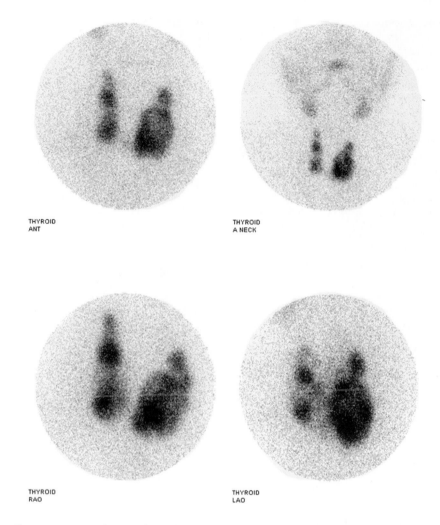

THYROID
ANT

THYROID
A NECK

THYROID
RAO

THYROID
LAO

Figure 14-26 Nuclear medicine thyroid scan showing uptake of the radioactive tracer.

adrenal tumors are smaller than 2 cm in diameter. CT is usually the first step for adrenal adenomas, aldosteronomas, and pheochromocytomas. However, [^{131}I]iodocholesterol scans, [^{131}I]metaiodobenzyl-guanidine (MIBG) scans, and adrenal vein sampling are available if the CT results are incongruous with the clinical findings or if further characterization of a nodule is necessary.

Skeletal System

Fractures

Plain radiographic films can detect the majority of fractures adequately. Because fractures can occur in different planes of the bone, it is vitally important to obtain at least two views of the area suspected of fracture (Figs. 14-27 through 14-30). In a few exceptions, plain films are not diagnostic. When initial radiographs are negative, and a high clinical suspicion remains of a long-bone fracture or fracture of a bone such as the navicular (scaphoid) bone in the hand, a

repeated radiographic film done 10 to 14 days later may show resorption along the fracture line or a periosteal reaction at the site of a fracture. In cases that cannot wait for this approach, either CT or MRI should be ordered. CT can be used in most cases and is less expensive; however, MRI is preferred in elderly patients with a clinically suspected fracture of the femoral neck despite normal plain films. When the clinical diagnosis remains unclear, a nuclear bone scan detecting more metabolically active bone repair may be helpful in confirming the diagnosis of a fracture. Bone scans may be used to detect a stress fracture because the plain radiographic films are often normal. Common areas for stress fractures include the tibia, fibula, and feet in runners or other athletes. Although the uptake of radionuclide can result from a number of conditions such as inflammation, trauma, neoplasm, or arthritis, these conditions are rarely confused when searching for a stress fracture of high clinical suspicion. A stress fracture is essentially ruled out by a negative bone scan.

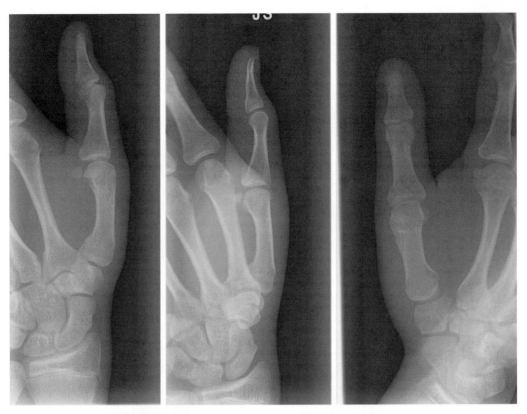

Figure 14-27 Standard three-view series of films to evaluate for fractures. Note fracture of proximal radial aspect of first proximal phalanx.

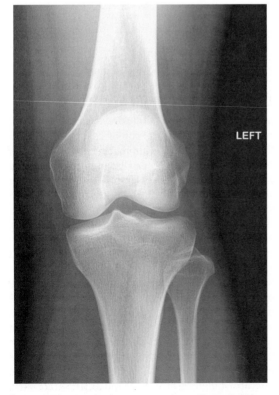

Figure 14-28 Standard anteroposterior radiograph of knee.

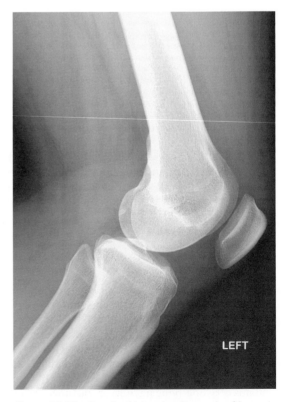

Figure 14-29 Standard lateral radiograph of knee.

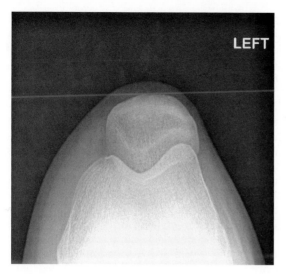

Figure 14-30 Standard sunrise-view radiograph of patella on top of distal femur at the knee.

Osteoporosis

Plain radiographic films are useful only late in the course of osteoporosis because at least 30% of the bone density must be lost before the loss is apparent on the standard radiograph. Therefore x-ray absorptiometry techniques were developed to detect this problem in its earlier stages and to follow up the progress of therapy. Among the more widely available techniques are both dual-photon absorptiometry (DPA) and the faster and more reliable dual x-ray absorptiometry (DEXA). DEXA is generally preferred because of its low precision error, its low radiation, and its ability to measure at multiple skeletal sites. These techniques measure the absorption of x-rays or gamma rays through selected bones of the body, such as the hip or lumber spine. All pre- and postmenopausal women, men with testosterone deficiency, persons with primary hyperparathyroidism, persons with long-term use of corticosteroids, and those with vertebral or other suggestive bone fractures should discuss ways to prevent osteoporosis with their family physician. For the majority of patients, the decision on how and whether to treat is a clinical decision based on the patient's risk factors. Bone-density measurement should be obtained when the results would influence the physician's therapeutic recommendations or the patient's compliance, or when it is necessary to monitor a patient's therapeutic progress. If a DEXA scanner is not available, a quantitative CT scan can be done by any CT scanner, but it is much more expensive, has a higher radiation dose, and is not mobile for easy screening of patients. Newer quantitative US is available for osteoporosis screening because of its low cost, portability, and lack of radiation. Unfortunately, the US technique is not sufficient to monitor treatment success (ACR, 2001e ⓒ). The cost

of absorptiometry imaging is in the range of $150 to $250.

Knee Injury with Meniscal Tear

When the diagnosis of a meniscal injury is supported by history and physical findings after a knee injury, it is reasonable to first consider plain radiographic films of the knee. Although the plain knee radiographs do not show the knee cartilage directly, they are useful as a first step to evaluate for joint effusion and other potential knee pathology such as an associated fracture. If a meniscal tear is suspected, and it is not responding to conservative therapy or is interfering significantly with the patient's activity, arthroscopic surgery is considered. The family physician should discuss the approach to this problem with the intended arthroscopic surgeon to determine whether MRI would be indicated in the particular patient. If the symptoms are suggestive enough that surgery is likely, it may be most cost effective to proceed directly to arthroscopic surgery, costing around $3000. An MRI is useful to determine the exact location and severity of meniscal and ligamentous injuries to the knee if further definition of the injury is needed. It can be done at less cost (about $1000) than arthroscopy and is noninvasive. MRI may be useful in identifying meniscal tears or cruciate ligament tears that are in locations difficult to visualize with the arthroscope, as well as injuries to the articular cartilage or underlying bone associated with these knee injuries (Figs. 14-31 and 14-32). However, if arthroscopic surgery is ultimately required, MRI can add significantly to the total expense. MRI has largely replaced arthrography as the imaging study for the evaluation of meniscal tears.

Urinary and Reproductive Systems

Obstructive Uropathy including Renal and Ureteral Stones

A plain radiographic kidney, ureter, and bladder (KUB) film of the abdomen should be the first imaging study when evaluating for renal or ureteral stones or other causes of obstructive uropathy. Nearly 80% of stones incorporate calcium into their structure at some point and are, therefore, radiopaque and easily seen. When it is available, a noncontrast spiral (helical) CT may used to locate the stone because it is faster and requires no contrast agent, when compared with an intravenous pyelogram (IVP). An IVP may be considered next, in place of a CT or when CT is not available, in patients who are producing adequate amounts of urine and are free of significant renal disease or impairment. A renal US examination should take the place of the IVP if the patient is anuric, has severe renal disease, or is suspected to have obstruction from outside the urinary tract itself. The US examination is useful to define renal pelvis

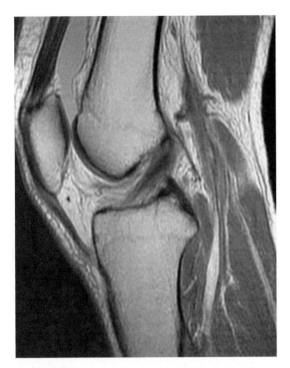

Figure 14-31 Normal magnetic resonance imaging of knee. Note anterior cruciate ligament traversing from superior tibia anteriorly to posterior femur superiorly.

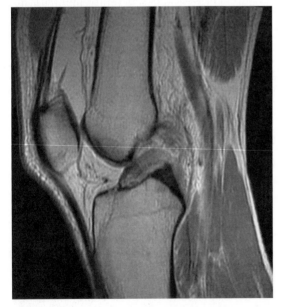

Figure 14-32 Magnetic resonance imaging of knee with anterior cruciate ligament tear noted in center of knee beginning at tibia and not attaching to posterior aspect of femur. Area of tear shows moderate to severe edema of ligament.

and calyceal enlargement, often reveals both radiopaque and radiolucent stones if larger than 5 mm, and examines the kidney structures, regardless of their function. Antegrade and retrograde pyelo-

grams or a voiding cystourethrogram may be needed if the cause and location of the obstruction remain obscure (ACR, 2001b ◉).

Renal Failure

The renal US examination is the best initial imaging method and has several other applications in addition to the detection of stones and obstructive uropathy. It is the main imaging method in the evaluation of renal failure, especially when obstruction is a possible cause (ACR, 2001f ◉). It also can assess renal atrophy resulting from various causes. Duplex US is frequently used to assess the renal vasculature as a cause of secondary hypertension, which occurs in fewer than 5% of patients. A nuclear medicine captopril renal study also can be used to assess for renovascular causes of hypertension. The captopril causes temporary restriction of the affected renal artery and, therefore, a decrease in perfusion and deposition of the radionuclide (ACR, 2003 ◉).

Renal Mass

US is one of the first imaging studies to consider when evaluating a renal mass. If the mass is cystic, the workup often ends at that point, as frequently this represents a benign cyst. CT may be necessary when the mass is indeterminant or of solid character. CT or MRI is used to assess a renal mass preoperatively to evaluate for renal capsule extension and metastasis. When percutaneous image-guided needle aspiration or biopsy is needed, renal US is used for needle guidance.

Testicular Torsion and Other Scrotal Lesions

When it is available on an emergency basis, color Doppler US examination of the scrotum is the preferred method to evaluate a patient for possible torsion of the testicle in acute-onset scrotal pain (Fig. 14-33). Because it is important to operate within

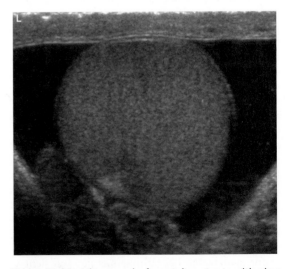

Figure 14-33 Ultrasound of scrotal contents with view of testicle.

hours of an acute testicular torsion, and because the clinical examination is frequently inconclusive, emergency imaging is necessary. An acceptable alternative method of imaging when Doppler is unavailable is a testicular nuclear medicine scan. The scan does an excellent job of differentiating between decreased flow found in testicular torsion and increased flow found in epididymitis (ACR, 2001c ⓒ). US imaging also is useful in the diagnosis of painful swelling arising from trauma and in differentiating mass lesions of the scrotum. US can be used to identify or locate a testicle in cryptorchidism. Staging of any testicular tumors can be done with abdominal and pelvic CT with contrast.

Prostate Carcinoma

If a nodule is palpated on examination, or if an unexplained high prostate-specific antigen (PSA) is obtained, biopsy is necessary and is usually done under US guidance. Transrectal US is the approach of choice to evaluate the prostate and guide transrectal biopsy. MRI is beginning to have an important role in the evaluation of prostate cancer staging, because it evaluates local pelvic nodes or local spread more effectively than CT or US. Nuclear bone scan can be used to assess for distant bone metastases.

Gynecology

Breast

The diagnostic approach to a breast lump is addressed in Chapter 10. Screening for breast cancer is an important issue related to diagnostic imaging and the role of family physicians in health maintenance. The incidence of breast cancer increased to 115 in 100,000 women in 1997, and justifiable public concern exists over this health problem. Breast cancer is the most common cancer diagnosed in women and accounts for approximately one third of all newly diagnosed cancers in women. The risk of developing breast cancer is age dependent. For example, the probability of acquiring breast cancer is about 1:72 for a woman in her 40s, about 1:36 for a woman in her 50s, and about 1:29 for a woman in her 70s. Screening mammography (Fig. 14-34) has been shown to reduce the breast cancer (Fig. 14-35) mortality rate about 30% for women older than 50 years, although less evidence is found for a benefit at younger than 50 years. For this reason, a lack of consensus exists over when mammography screening should begin for the average-risk woman. The risk of radiation exposure with screening mammography has been judged to be negligible for women older than 40 years when mammographers use low-dose equipment and adhere to high quality-control standards. One of the problems with screening mammography is its relatively low positive predictive value of 2% to 22% and the need for further diagnostic evaluation, meaning that it results in a large number of

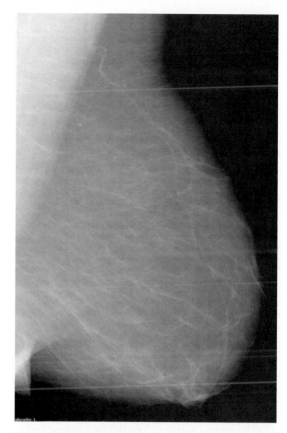

Figure 14-34 Mammogram of breast.

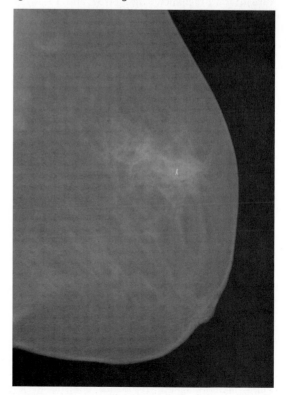

Figure 14-35 Mammogram of breast showing density in upper central aspect evident by small marker placed.

biopsies for benign findings. Specificity of a single mammogram is 94% to 97%, whereas sensitivity is 77% to 95%. For this reason, the physician must never be falsely assured about a palpable breast lump that is followed by a negative mammogram. A tissue diagnosis of a breast lump must be obtained regardless of the result of the mammogram. All women between ages 50 and 70 years should have an annual breast examination and mammography at least every 2 years. For average-risk women between ages 40 and 50 years, who desire mammography, it should be made available yearly despite lack of strong evidence of its clinical efficacy and should be available every 1 to 2 years for those older than 70 years who desire it. High-risk women should have annual mammography starting at age 35 years, or 5 years before the age at which their first-degree relative acquired cancer. US is routinely used in younger women with denser breasts or in those with probable cystic disease, as it is able to discern fluid phases in a cyst better than does mammography. US should not be used to assess a solid mass. Recent advances have begun to use MRI as an imaging modality for breast evaluation when an abnormal potential cancerous mass is found on routine mammography screening (U.S. Preventive Services Task Force, 2002 Ⓒ) (Fig. 14-36).

Ectopic Pregnancy and Adnexal Masses

US examination is the preferred imaging study when evaluating a pregnancy (Figs. 14-37 and 14-38) or

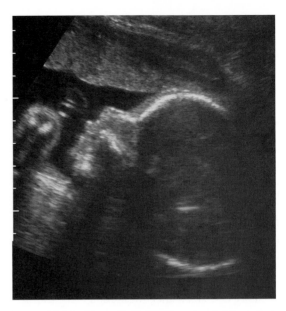

Figure 14-37 Obstetrical ultrasound of fetus. Note transverse view of fetal face.

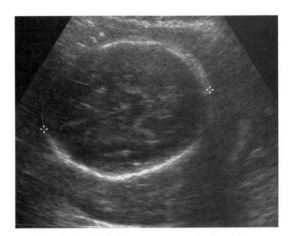

Figure 14-38 Obstetrical ultrasound of fetus. Note axial view of fetal head and measurement of cranial diameter.

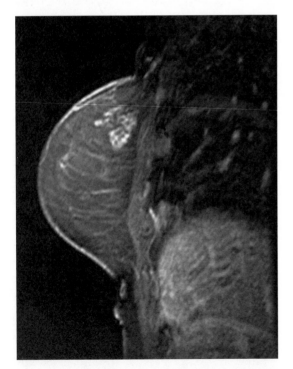

Figure 14-36 Magnetic resonance imaging of left breast. Note enhancing lesion of upper outer quadrant, consistent with breast cancer.

adnexal mass. Imaging studies must always be preceded by a clinical physical examination to determine that the patient is in a stable condition and is able to proceed with the diagnostic evaluation. In most cases, enough time is found to obtain a serum β-human chorionic gonadotropin (β-hCG), which will help determine whether an ectopic or intrauterine pregnancy needs to be considered. When the β-hCG is more than 1800 IU/L, either abdominal US or transvaginal US may be used to confirm an intrauterine pregnancy. Transvaginal US is superior to the abdominal US in detecting an ectopic pregnancy and is usually able to diagnose an intrauterine pregnancy when the β-hCG is more than 1000 IU/L. β-hCG levels less than 1000 will warrant careful serial monitoring if the transvaginal US fails to

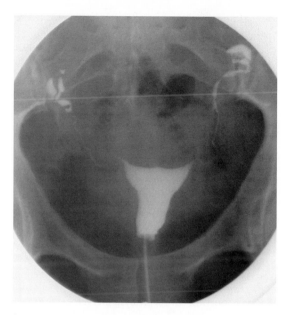

Figure 14-39 Hysterosalpingogram. Note exiting dye at ends of patent fallopian tubes.

detect an intrauterine pregnancy and detects no other explainable pathology. Transvaginal US also may be useful when evaluating a suspected adnexal mass if equivocal findings or technical problems with the abdominal US occur (Tulandi, 2004 **C**). A color flow Doppler US of the ovarian vessels is used to evaluate an acute ovarian pain suggestive of ovarian torsion. Obstruction of fallopian tubes can be assessed with a hysterosalpingogram when needed to assess infertility or chronic salpingitis (Fig. 14-39). Many adnexal masses are nonspecific in their appearance on US and appear to have both cystic and solid components. When this is the case in postmenopausal women, or in premenopausal women without evidence for infection, a biopsy should be obtained to rule out malignancy. CT may be helpful in the staging process of ovarian cancer.

Material Available on Student Consult

Review Questions and Answers about Selecting Radiographic Tests

REFERENCES

Alonso A, Lau J, Bertrand L, Weintraub A, et al. Prevention of radiocontrast nephropathy with *N*-acetylcysteine in patients with chronic kidney disease: A meta-analysis of randomized, controlled trials. Am J Kidney Dis 2004; 43:1–9.**A**

American College of Radiology (ACR). Manual on Iodinated Contrast Media. Reston, VA, ACR, 1991.**B**

American College of Radiology (ACR). Metformin (Glucophage) Therapy and the Risk of Lactic Acidosis [Bulletin]. Reston, VA, ACR, 1997.**C**

American College of Radiology (ACR). Acute Chest Pain: Suspected Aortic Dissection, ACR Appropriateness Criteria, 1999a. Available at www.acr.org/dyna/?doc=departments/appropriateness_criteria/text.html. Accessed 9/23/2004.**C**

American College of Radiology (ACR). Acute Chest Pain: Suspected Myocardial Infarction, ACR Appropriateness Criteria, 1999b. Available at www.acr.org/dyna/?doc=departments/appropriateness_criteria/text.html. Accessed 9/23/2004.**C**

American College of Radiology (ACR). Acute Low Back Pain: Radiculopathy. ACR Appropriateness Criteria, 1999c. Available at www.acr.org/dyna/?doc=departments/appropriateness_criteria/text.html. Accessed 9/23/2004.**C**

American College of Radiology (ACR). Evaluation of Acute Right Lower Quadrant Pain, ACR Appropriateness Criteria, 1999d. Available at www.acr.org/dyna/?doc=departments/appropriateness_criteria/text.html. Accessed 9/23/2004.**C**

American College of Radiology (ACR). Evaluation of Patients with Acute Right Upper Quadrant Pain, ACR Appropriateness Criteria, 1999e. Available at www.acr.org/dyna/?doc=departments/appropriateness_criteria/text.html. Accessed 9/23/2004.**C**

American College of Radiology (ACR). Imaging Strategies in the Initial Evaluation of the Jaundiced Patient, ACR Appropriateness Criteria, 1999f. Available at www.acr.org/dyna/?doc=departments/appropriateness_criteria/text.html. Accessed 9/23/2004.**C**

American College of Radiology (ACR). The Patient with Suspected Small Bowel Obstruction: Imaging Strategies, ACR Appropriateness Criteria, 1999g. Available at www.acr.org/dyna/?doc=departments/appropriateness_criteria/text.html. Accessed 9/23/2004.**C**

American College of Radiology (ACR). Suspected Lower Extremity Deep Venous Thrombosis, ACR Appropriateness Criteria, 1999h. Available at www.acr.org/dyna/?doc=departments/appropriateness_criteria/text.html. Accessed 9/23/2004.**C**

American College of Radiology (ACR). Atraumatic Isolated Headache: When to Image? ACR Appropriateness Criteria, 1999i. Available at www.acr.org/dyna/?doc=departments/appropriateness_criteria/text.html. Accessed 9/23/2004.**C**

American College of Radiology (ACR). Cerebrovascular Disease, ACR Appropriateness Criteria, 2000. Available at www.acr.org/dyna/?doc=departments/appropriateness_criteria/text.html. Accessed 9/23/2004.**C**

American College of Radiology (ACR). ACR Practice Guideline for the Use of Intravascular Contrast Material. Reston, VA, ACR, 2001a.**C**

American College of Radiology (ACR). Acute Onset Flank Pain, Suspicion of Stone Disease, ACR Appropriateness Criteria, 2001b. Available at www.acr.org/dyna/?doc=departments/appropriateness_criteria/text.html. Accessed 9/23/2004.**C**

American College of Radiology (ACR). Acute Onset of Scrotal Pain: ACR Appropriateness Criteria, 2001c.

Available at www.acr.org/dyna/?doc=departments/appr opriateness_criteria/text.html. Accessed 9/23/2004.©

American College of Radiology (ACR). Imaging Recommendations for Patients with Dysphagia, ACR Appropriateness Criteria, 2001d. Available at www. acr.org/dyna/?doc=departments/appropriateness_ criteria/text.html. Accessed 9/23/2004.©

American College of Radiology (ACR). Osteoporosis and Bone Mineral Density, ACR Appropriateness Criteria, 2001e. Available at www.acr.org/dyna/?doc=departments/ appropriateness_criteria/text.html. Accessed 9/23/2004.©

American College of Radiology (ACR). Radiologic Investigation of Causes of Renal Failure, ACR Appropriateness Criteria, 2001f. Available at www.acr.org/ dyna/?doc=departments/appropriateness_criteria/text. html. Accessed 9/23/2004.©

American College of Radiology (ACR). Hematemesis, ACR Appropriateness Criteria, 2002. Available at www.acr.org/ac_pda. Accessed 9/23/2004.©

American College of Radiology (ACR). Radiologic Investigation of Patients with Renovascular Hypertension, ACR Appropriateness Criteria, 2003. Available at www.acr. org/dyna/?doc=departments/appropriateness_criteria/ text.html. Accessed 9/23/2004.©

Chen MYM, Pope TL, Ott DJ. Basic Radiology. New York, Lange Medical Books/McGraw-Hill, 2004, pp 6–7.

Eisenberg, RL, Margulis, AR. Radiology Pocket Reference: What to Order When. Philadelphia, Lippincott-Raven, 1996, p 441.

Grossman ZD, Katz DS, Santelli ED, et al. Acute gastrointestinal bleeding in the adult. In: Cost-Effective Diagnostic Imaging: The Clinician's Guide, 3rd ed. St. Louis, CV Mosby, 1995a, pp 63–69.©

Grossman ZD, Katz DS, Santelli ED, et al. Pulmonary embolism. In: Cost-Effective Diagnostic Imaging: The Clinician's Guide, 3rd ed. St. Louis, CV Mosby, 1995b, pp 179–187.©

Grossman ZD, Katz DS, Santelli ED, et al. Thyroid nodule/thyroid enlargement. In: Cost-Effective Diagnostic Imaging: The Clinician's Guide, 3rd ed. St. Louis, CV Mosby, 1995c, pp 394–403.©

Losh DP. Central nervous system infections. Infect Dis Clin Fam Pract 2004;61:41.

Mettler FA, Guiberteau MJ, Voss CM, Urbina CE. Primary Care Radiology. Philadelphia, WB Saunders, 2000.

Rudnick MR, Goldfarb S, Wexler L, et al. Nephrotoxicity of ionic and nonionic contrast media in 1196 patients: A randomized trial. Kidney Int 1995;47:254.©

Solomon R, Werner C, Mann D, et al. Effects of saline, mannitol, and furosemide on acute decreases in renal function induced by radiocontrast agents. N Engl J Med 1994;331:1416.©

Tepel M, Van der Giet M, Schwarzfeld C, et al. Prevention of radiographic-contrast-agent-induced reductions in renal function by acetylcysteine. N Engl J Med 2000;343:180–184.©

Tulandi T. Clinical Manifestations and Diagnosis of Ectopic Pregnancy, Up To Date, 2004. Available at www.upto dateonline.com. Accessed 10/10/2004.©

U.S. Preventive Services Task Force. Screening for Breast Cancer: Recommendations and Rationale. Rockville, Md: Agency for Healthcare Research and Quality, 2002. Available at www.ahrq.gov/clinic/3rduspstf/ breastcancer/brcanrr.htm.©

Part II

Case Studies

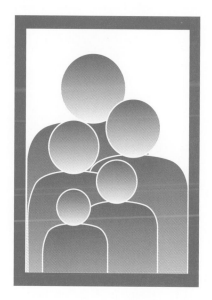

15 Nasal Congestion in a 15-Month-Old Girl (Immunizations)

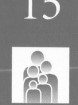

Richard D. Clover

KEY POINTS

1. Simultaneously administer as many indicated vaccines as possible.
2. Remind parents when vaccinations are due, and send recall notices to parents whose children are overdue for vaccinations.
3. Influenza vaccine is now recommended for all children at 6 to 23 months of age.
4. Children with mild, acute illnesses with or without fever can be vaccinated.
5. Low-grade fever by itself is not a contraindication to immunization.
6. Children with HIV infection should receive all routine inactivated vaccines.
7. Current antimicrobial therapy is not a contraindication to immunization.
8. Recent exposure to infectious disease is not a contraindication to immunization.

INITIAL VISIT

Subjective

Patient Identification and Presenting Problem

Kristin C. is a 15-month-old girl who presents in October with a runny nose. Her mother states that Kristin was in her usual good health until approximately 3 days ago, when she developed a runny nose, nasal congestion, and a low-grade fever. Yesterday Kristin's fever resolved, but her nasal congestion has persisted. Because Kristin has a history of ear infections, Mrs. C. is concerned that she may have another ear infection. Mrs. C. states that Kristin has not had a cough, difficulty breathing, vomiting or diarrhea.

Medical History

Kristin was born after a term gestation to a 27-year-old white woman. The pregnancy and delivery were uneventful. Kristin has been treated successfully with amoxicillin three times previously for otitis media. Her growth and development have been normal. Her

immunization record is as follows: hepatitis B vaccine (Hep B) at 2 days of age; diphtheria and tetanus toxoids and acellular pertussis vaccine (DTaP), *Haemophilus influenzae* type b vaccine (Hib), Hep B, pneumococcal conjugate vaccine (PCV), and inactivated poliovirus vaccine (IPV) at 8 weeks of age; DaTP, Hib, PCV, and IPV at 4 months of age; and DTaP, Hib, PCV, IPV, and Hep B at 6 months of age.

Family History

Kristin's father, a physician, is in good health at age 28. Her mother, a teacher, is in good health. Her maternal grandmother died at age 32 from lymphoma. Her other grandparents are in their fifties with no major medical problems.

Objective

Physical Examination

Kristin's vital signs include a temperature of 37.3°C (99.1°F), a respiratory rate of 20, a heart rate of 100, and a weight of 25 pounds. She is generally alert and active, although obviously nasally congested. Her tympanic membranes are normal. She has clear rhinorrhea, and her throat is mildly injected but without exudate. Her neck is supple, with no cervical lymphadenopathy. Lung, heart, and abdominal examinations are within normal limits. Findings on the neurologic examination are appropriate for her age. Her skin is without rashes.

Assessment

Working Diagnosis

The working diagnosis is an upper respiratory tract infection, probably viral in origin. This visit is also an opportune time to check on her immunization status, which needs updating. Kristin has had DTaP × 3, Hib × 3, Hep B × 3, PCV × 3, and IPV × 3; she therefore needs measles-mumps-rubella vaccine (MMR), varicella vaccine, and her fourth dose of DTaP, Hib, and PCV vaccines. In addition, since it is October, she will need her first influenza vaccine.

Differential Diagnosis

The differential diagnosis includes allergic rhinitis and a nonviral respiratory tract infection. *Allergic rhinitis* is usually associated with clear rhinorrhea, a more chronic history, and no fever. In this case, the acute onset and initial fever make an infectious etiology more likely.

A *nonviral respiratory infection,* although possible, is also unlikely. Although multiple organisms may produce a respiratory infection, the improving course of this illness (i.e., resolved fever) makes a self-limited viral infection the most probable etiology.

Plan

Diagnostic
No diagnostic tests are appropriate at this time.

Therapeutic
Kristin is administered the following vaccines: DTaP, Hib, PCV, MMR, varicella, and influenza. She also receives symptomatic treatment for rhinorrhea (a saline nasal spray).

Patient Education
Mrs. C. is advised that Kristin's symptoms should continue to improve. She is also informed of the potential side effects and adverse reactions to each of the vaccines and is given the appropriate vaccine information handouts. Acetaminophen may be given to Kristin for the fever and discomfort that accompany immunizations.

Disposition
Mrs. C. is asked to bring Kristin back in 4 weeks for the child's second influenza vaccine if her condition deteriorates.

DISCUSSION

Immunization programs have reduced the incidence of many childhood infections. Through these initiatives, global eradication of smallpox has been accomplished, and polio has been eliminated from the Western hemisphere. Significant reductions in the incidence of other vaccine-preventable diseases have been accomplished. Varicella, hepatitis B, and hepatitis A have recently been added to the list of vaccine-preventable diseases. The reemergence of measles in the years 1989 to 1992 reminds us of the importance of these programs.

Several factors are involved in children and adults not receiving age-appropriate vaccines. These factors include patient, provider, and system issues. Although this discussion addresses certain indications, contraindications, and compliance issues as they exist at the time of this book's publication, providers should refer to the published recommendations of the Advisory Committee on Immunization Practices (ACIP) for a more detailed discussion and up-to-date recommendations.

The leading reasons for delayed or missing immunizations are failure of simultaneous administration, invalid contraindications, missed opportunities, missed appointments, and parental concerns including vaccine safety and religious beliefs. In order to raise the vaccination levels, Standards for Pediatric Immunization Practice were recommended by the National Vaccine Advisory Committee and approved by the U.S. Public Health Service. These standards address many of the factors that have been identified as contributing to underimmunization of children. Following are some of the standards:

Vaccination services are readily available.

Vaccinations are coordinated with other health care services and provided in a medical home when possible.

Barriers to vaccination are identified and minimized.

Patient costs are minimized.

Health care professionals review the vaccination and health status of patients at every encounter to determine which vaccines are indicated.

Health care professionals assess for and follow only medically accepted contraindications.

Parents or guardians and patients are educated about the benefits and risks of vaccination in a culturally appropriate manner and in easy-to-understand language.

Health care professionals follow appropriate procedures for vaccine storage and handling.

Up-to-date, written vaccination protocols are accessible at all locations where vaccines are administered.

People who administer vaccines and staff who manage or support vaccine administration are knowledgeable and receive ongoing education.

Health care professionals simultaneously administer as many indicated vaccine doses as possible.

Vaccination records for patients are accurate, complete, and easily accessible.

Health care professionals report adverse events after vaccination promptly and accurately to the Vaccine Adverse Events Reporting System (VAERS) and are aware of a separate program, the Vaccine Injury Compensation Program (VICP).

All personnel who have contact with patients are appropriately vaccinated.

Systems are used to remind parents or guardians, patients, and health care professionals when vaccinations are due and to recall those who are overdue.

Office- or clinic-based patient record reviews and vaccination coverage assessments are performed annually.

Health care professionals practice community-based approaches.

The frequent changes in the immunization schedules have produced uncertainties in providers.

Figure 15-1 summarizes the recommendations and schedules as published for July through December, 2004 (recommendations may change, and providers should seek current recommendations from appropriate agencies). This schedule includes a recent change in the recommendations. Influenza vaccine is now recommended for all children aged 6 to 23 months. If this year's administration of trivalent inactivated influenza vaccine is the child's first vaccination, a second dose is administered at least 4 weeks later. In addition, family members of children aged 0 to 6 months old should be vaccinated.

In special circumstances, the provider will need to alter the recommended schedule. In immunocompromised individuals, killed or inactivated vaccines do not represent a danger and generally should be administered as recommended for healthy children. Steroid therapy usually does not contraindicate administration of live virus vaccines (MMR, varicella vaccine) when such therapy is short term (<2 weeks), of low to moderate dose, provided in maintenance physiologic doses, or administered topically, by aerosol, or by intra-articular, bursal, or tendon injection. A dose of prednisone equal to or greater than 2 mg/kg of body weight or 20 mg/day should raise concern about the safety of immunization with live virus vaccines. Physicians should wait at least 3 months after discontinuation of therapy before administering a live virus vaccine to patients who have received high-dose, systemic steroids for 2 weeks or longer.

Children with HIV infection should receive all routine inactivated vaccines. In general, live vaccines should be avoided, with the following exceptions: MMR can be given to children with HIV infection with no to moderate immunosuppression, and varicella can be administered to HIV-infected children with no immunosuppression. Children with severe, non-HIV-related immunocompromise should receive all routine inactivated vaccinations as scheduled. It is recommended that children with HIV or who are severely immunocompromised receive both pneumococcal and influenza vaccines. Varicella virus vaccine should not be given to individuals who may be immunocompromised from cancer except for children with acute lymphocytic leukemia in remission.

Contraindications

Providers' knowledge of relative and absolute contraindications is variable. Some of the most common invalid contraindications are mild illness, such as a low-grade fever, upper respiratory infection, colds, otitis media, or mild diarrhea. Children with mild acute illnesses can and should be vaccinated. Several large studies have shown that young children with upper respiratory tract infection, otitis media, diarrhea, and/or fever respond as well to measles vaccine as those without these conditions. Low-grade fever by itself is not a contraindication to immunization. Other invalid contraindications to vaccination include concurrent antibiotic therapy, disease exposure or convalescence, pregnancy in the household, and breast-feeding of an infant.

Nonspecific allergies and nonsevere allergies are frequent invalid contraindications. Infants and children with nonspecific allergies, duck or feather allergy, allergy to penicillin, relatives with allergies, and children taking allergy shots can be immunized. Children with egg allergies can be vaccinated with MMR vaccine. Table 15-1 summarizes the true and invalid contraindications.

Accelerated Schedules

A common problem for providers is determining what vaccinations a child needs when the child is behind schedule. Table 15-2 is the recommended accelerated immunization schedule for infants at least 4 months of age and children younger than 7 years of age who start the series late or who are more than 1 month behind in the immunization schedule (i.e., children for whom compliance with scheduled return visits cannot be assured). Table 15-3 is the recommended immunization schedule for children older than 7 years who were not vaccinated at the recommended time in early infancy.

Material Available on Student Consult
Review Questions and Answers about Immunizations

RECOMMENDED CHILDHOOD AND ADOLESCENT IMMUNIZATION SCHEDULE[1]
UNITED STATES, JULY-DECEMBER 2004

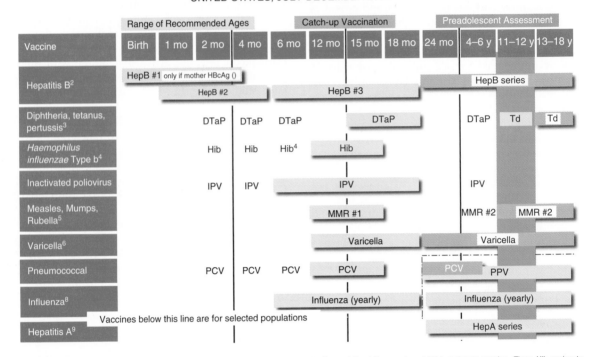

1. Indicates the recommended ages for routine administration of currently licensed childhood vaccines, as of April 1, 2004, for children through age 18 years. Any dose not given at the recommended age should be given at any subsequent visit when indicated and feasible. ▨ Indicates age groups that warrant special effort to adminster those vaccines not given previously. Additional vaccines may be licensed and recommended during the year. Licensed combination vaccines may be used whenever any components of the combination are indicated and the vaccine's other components are not contraindicated. Providers should consult the manufacturer's package inserts for detailed recommendations. Clinically significant adverse events that follow vaccination should be reported to the Vaccine Adverse Event Reporting System (VAERS). Guidance about how to obtain and complete a VAERS form is available at http://www.vaers.org/ or by telephone, 800-822-7967.
2. Hepatitis B vaccine (HepB). All infants should recive the first dose of HepB vaccine soon after birth and before hospital discharge: the first dose also may be given by age 2 months if the infant's mother is HBsAg-negative. Only monovalent HeB vaccine can be used for the birth dose. Monovalent of combination vaccine containing HepB may be used to complete the series; 4 doses of vaccine may be administered when a birth dose is given. The second dose should be given at least 4 weeks after the first dose except for combination vaccines, which cannot be administered before age 6 weeks. The third dose should be given at least 16 weeks after the first dose and at least 8 weeks after the second dose. The last dose in the vaccination series (third or fourth dose) should not be administered before age 24 weeks. Infants born to HBsAg-positive mothers should receive HepB vaccine and 0.5 mL hepatitis B immune globulin (HBIG) within 12 hours of birth at separate sites. The second dose is recommended at age 1-2 months. The last dose in the vaccination series should not be administered before age 24 weeks. These infants should be tested for HBsAg and anti-HBs at age 9-15 months. Infants born to mothers whose HBsAg status is unknown should receive the first dose of the HepB vaccine series within 12 hours of birth. Maternal blood should be drawn as soon as possible to determine the mother's HBsAg status; if the HBsAg test is positive, the infant should receive HBIG as soon as possible (no later than age 1 week). The second dose is recommended at age 1–2 months. The last dose in the vaccination series should not be administered before age 24 weeks.
3. Diphtheria and tetanus toxoids and acellular pertussis vaccine (DTaP). The fourth dose of DTaP may be administered at age 12 months provided that 6 months have elapsed since the third dose and the child is unlikely to return at age 15-18 months. The final dose in the series should be given at age ≥4 years. Tetanus and diphtheria toxoids (Td) are recommended at age 11-12 years if at least 5 years have elapsed since the last dose of tetanus and diphtheria toxoid-containing vaccine. Subsequent routine Td boosters are recommended every 10 years.

4. *Haemophilus influenzae* type b(Hib) conjugate vaccine. Three Hib conjugate vaccines are licensed for infant use. If PRP-OMP (PedvaxHIB© or ComVax© [Merck]) is administered at ages 2 and 4 months, a dose at age 6 months is not required. DTaP/Hib combination products should not be used for primary vaccination in infants at ages 2,4, or 6 months but can be used as boosters after any Hib vaccine. The final dose in the series should be given at age ≥12 months.
5. Measles, mumps, and rubella vaccine (MMR). The second dose of MMR is recommended routinely at age 4-6 years but may be administered during any visit, provided at least 4 weeks have elapsed since the first dose and both doses are administered beginning at or after age 12 months. Those who have not received the second dose previously should complete the schedule by the visit at age 11-12 years.
6. Varicella vaccine (VAR). Varicella vaccine is recommended at any visit at or after age 12 months for susceptible children (i.e., those who lack a reliable history of chickenpox). Susceptible persons aged ≥13 years should receive 2 doses given at least 4 weeks apart.
7. Pneumococcal vaccine. The heptavalent pneumococcal conjugate vaccine (PCV) is recommended for all children aged 2–23 months and for certain children aged 24-59 months. The final dose in the series should be given at age ≥12 months. Pneumococcal polysaccharide vaccine (PPV) is recommended in addition to PCV for certain high-risk groups. See MMWR 2000;49(No. RR-9):1-35.
8. Influenza vaccine. Influenza vaccine is recommended annually for children aged ≥5 months with certain risk factors (including but not limited to asthma, cardiac disease, sickle cell disease, HIV, and diabetes), health care workers, and other persons (including household members) in dose contact with persons at high risk (see MMWR 2004;53;[RR][in press]) and can be administered to all others wishing to obtain immunity. In addition, healthy children aged 6-23 months and close contacts of healthy children aged 0-23 months are recommended to receive influenza vaccine, because children in this age group are at substantially increased risk for influenza related hospitalizations. For healthy persons aged 5–49 years, the intranasally administered live, attenuated influenza vaccine (LAIV) is an acceptable alternative to the intramuscular trivalent inactivated influenza vaccine (TIV). See MMWR 2003;52(No.RR-13):1-8. Children receiving TIV should be administered a dosage appropriate for their age (0.25 mL if 6-35 months or 0.5 mL if ≥3 years). Children aged ≤8 years who are receiving influenza vaccine for the first time should receive 2 doses (separated by at least 4 weeks for TIV and at least 6 weeks for LAIV).
9. Hepatitis A vaccine. Hapatitis A vaccine is recommended for children and adolescents in selected states and regions and for certain high-risk groups. Consult your local public health authority and MMWR 1 999;48(No.RR-12):1–37. Children and adolescents in these states, regions, and high-risk groups who have not been immunized against hepatitis A can begin the hepatitis A vaccination series during any visit. The 2 doses in the series should be administered at least 6 months apart.

Additional information about vaccines, including precautions and contraindications for vaccination and vaccine shortages is available at http://www.cdc.gov/nip or from the National Immunization Information Hotline, 800-232-2522 (English) or 800-232-0233 (Spanish). Approved by the Advisory Committee on Immunization Practices (http://www.cdc.gov/nip/acip), the American Academy of Pediatrics (http:www.aap.org), and the American Academy of Family Physicians (http://www.aafp.org).

Figure 15-1 Recommended childhood and adolescent immunization schedule—United States, July–December, 2004. (From Advisory Committee in Immunization Practices (ACIP). Recommended Childhood and Adolescent Immunization Schedule—United States, July–December 2004. MMWR Morb Mortal Wkly Rep 2004;53:Q1–Q3.)

Table 15-1 Guide to Contraindications* and Precautions† to Commonly Used Vaccines, *by Vaccine*

Vaccine	True Contraindications and Precautions#	Untrue (Vaccines Can Be Administered)
General for all vaccines, including diphtheria and tetanus toxoids and acellular pertussis vaccine (DTaP); pediatric diphtheria-tetanus toxoid (DT); adult tetanus-diphtheria toxoid (Td); inactivated poliovirus vaccine (IPV); measles-mumps-rubella vaccine (MMR); Haemophilus influenzae type b vaccine (Hib); hepatitis A vaccine, hepatitis B vaccine; varicella vaccine; pneumococcal conjugate vaccine (PCV); influenza vaccine; and pneumococcal polysaccharie vaccine (PPV)	**Contraindications** Serious allergic reaction (e.g., anaphylaxis) after a previous vaccine dose Serious allergic reaction (e.g., anaphylaxis) to a vaccine component **Precautions** Moderate or severe acute illness with or without fever	Mild acute illness with or without fever Mild to moderate local reaction (i.e., swelling, redness, soreness); low-grade or moderate fever after previous dose Lack of previous physical examination in well-appearing person Current antimicrobial therapy Convalescent phase of illness Premature birth (hepatitis B vaccine is an exception in certain circumstances)+ Recent exposure to an infectious disease History of penicillin allergy, other nonvaccine allergies, relative with allergies, receiving allergen extract immunotherapy
DTaP	**Contraindications** Severe allergic reaction after a previous dose or to a vaccine component Encephalopathy (e.g., coma, decreased level of consciousness; prolonged seizures) within 7 days of administration of previous dose of DTP or DTaP Progressive neurologic disorder, including infantile spasms, uncontrolled epilepsy, progressive encephalopathy; defer DTaP until neurologic status clarified and stabilized. **Precautions** Fever of >40.5°C ≤48 hours after vaccination with a previous dose of DTP or DTaP Collapse or shock-like state (i.e., hypotonic hyporesponsive episode) ≤48 hours after receiving a previous dose of DTP or DTaP Seizure ≤3 days of receiving a previous dose of DTP/DTaP^ Persistent, inconsolable crying lasting ≥3 hours ≤48 hours after receiving a previous dose of DTP or DTaP Moderate or severe acute illness with or without fever	Temperature of <40.5°C, fussiness or mild drowsiness after a previous dose of diphtheria toxoid-tetanus toxoid-pertussis vaccine DTP or DTaP Family history of seizures^ Family history of sudden infant death syndrome Family history of an adverse event after DTP or DTaP administration Stable neurologic conditions (e.g., cerebral palsy, well-controlled convulsions, developmental delay)

Continued

Table 15-1 Guide to Contraindications* and Precautions† to Commonly Used Vaccines, *by Vaccine* (Continued)

Vaccine	True Contraindications and Precautions#	Untrue (Vaccines Can Be Administered)
DT, Td	**Contraindications** Severe allergic reaction after a previous dose or to a vaccine component **Precautions** Guillain-Barré syndrome ≤6 weeks after previous dose of tetanus toxoid-containing vaccine Moderate or severe acute illness with or without a fever	
IPV	**Contraindications** Severe allergic reaction to previous dose or vaccine component **Precautions** Pregnancy Moderate or severe acute illness with or without fever	
MMR@	**Contraindications** Severe allergic reaction to previous dose or vaccine component Pregnancy Known severe immunodeficiency (e.g., hematologic and solid tumors; congenital immuno-deficiency; long-term immunosuppressive therapy## or severely symptomatic human immunodeficiency virus [HIV] infection) **Precautions** Recent (≤11 months) receipt of antibody-containing blood product (specific interval depends on product)$$ History of thrombocytopenia or thrombocytopenic purpura Moderate or severe acute illness with or without fever	Positive tuberculin skin test Simultaneous TB skin testing++ Breast-feeding Pregnancy of recipient's mother or other close or household contact Recipient is child-bearing-age female Immunodeficient family member or household contact Asymptomatic or mildly symptomatic HIV infection Allergy to eggs
Hib	**Contraindications** Severe allergic reaction to previous dose or vaccine component Age <6 weeks **Precautions** Moderate or severe acute illness with or without fever	
Hepatitis B	**Contraindications** Severe allergic reaction to previous dose or vaccine component **Precautions** Infant weighing < 2000 g Moderate or severe acute illness with or without fever	Pregnancy Autoimmune disease (e.g., systemic lupus erythematosus or rheumatoid arthritis)

Table 15-1 Guide to Contraindications* and Precautions† to Commonly Used Vaccines, *by Vaccine* (Continued)

Vaccine	True Contraindications and Precautions#	Untrue (Vaccines Can Be Administered)
Hepatitis A	**Contraindications** Severe allergic reaction to previous dose or vaccine component **Precautions** Pregnancy Moderate or severe acute illness with or without fever	
Varicella@	**Contraindications** Severe allergic reaction to previous dose or vaccine component Substantial supression of cellular immunity Pregnancy **Precautions** Recent (≤11 months) receipt of antibody-containing blood product (specific interval depends on product)$$ Moderate or severe acute illness with or without fever	Pregnancy of recipient's mother or other close or household contact Immunodeficient family member or household contact Asymptomatic or mildly symptomatic HIV infection Humoral immunodeficiency (e.g., agammaglobulinema)
PCV	**Contraindications** Severe allergic reaction to previous dose or vaccine component **Precautions** Moderate or severe acute illness with or without fever	
Influenza	**Contraindications** Severe allergic reaction to previous dose or vaccine component, including egg protein **Precautions** Moderate or severe acute illness with or without fever	Nonsevere (e.g., contact) allergy to latex or thimerosal Concurrent administration of coumadin or aminophyaline
PPV	**Contraindications** Severe allergic reaction to previous dose or vaccine component **Precautions** Moderate or severe acute illness with or without fever	

*Contraindications: A contraindication is a condition in a recipient that increases the risk for a serious adverse reaction. A vaccine will not be administered when a contraindication is present. Consult the MMWR article, "General Recommendations on Immunizations" for a full definition including examples.

†Precautions: A precaution is a condition in a recipient that might increase the risk for a serious adverse reaction or that might compromise the ability of the vaccine to produce immunity. Injury could result, or a person might experience a more severe reaction to the vaccine than would have otherwise been expected; however, the risk for this happening is less than expected with a contraindication. Under normal circumstances, vaccinations should be deferred when a precaution is present. However, a vaccination might be indicated in the presence of a precaution because the benefit of protection from the vaccine outweighs the risk for an adverse reaction. Consult the MMWR article, "General Recommendations on Immunizations" for a full definition including examples.

Continued

#Events or conditions listed as precautions should be reviewed carefully. Benefits and risks of administering a specific vaccine to a person under these circumstances should be considered. If the risk from the vaccine is believed to outweigh the benefit, the vaccine should not be administered. If the benefit of vaccination is believed to outweigh the risk, vaccine should be administered. Whether and when to administer DTaP to children with proven or suspected underlying neurologic disorders should be decided on a case-by-case basis.

+Hepatitis B vaccination should be deferred for infants weighing <2000 grams if the mother is documented to be hepatitis B surface antigen (HbsAg)-negative at the time of infant's birth. Vaccination can commence at chronological age 1 month. For infants born to HbsAg-positive women, hepatitis B immunoglobulin and hepatitis B vaccine should be administered at or soon after birth regardless of weight. See MMWR article, "General Recommendations on Immunizations" text for details.

^Acetaminophen or other appropriate antipyretic can be administered to children with a personal or family history of seizures at the time of DTaP vaccination and every 4–6 hours for 24 hours thereafter to reduce the possibility of postvaccination fever (Source: American Academy of Pediatrics. Active immunization. In Pickering LK, ed: 2000 Red Book: Report of the Committee on Infectious Diseases. 25th ed. Elk Grove Villege, IL, American Academy of Pediatrics, 2000).

@MMR and varicella vaccines can be administered on the same day. If not administered on the same day, these vaccines should be separated by ≥28 days.

##Substantially immunosuppressive steroid dose is considered to be >2 weeks of daily receipt of 20 mg or 2 mg/kg body weight of prednisone or equivalent.

++Measles vaccination can suppress tuberculin reactivity temporarily. Measles-containing vaccine can be administered on the same day as tuberculin skin testing. If testing cannot be performed until after the day of MMR vaccination, the test should be postponed for >4 weeks after the vaccination. If an urgent need exists to skin test, do so with the understanding that reactivity might be reduced by the vaccine.

$$See text for details.

^^ If a vaccinee experiences a presumed vaccine-related rash 7–25 days after vaccination, avoid direct contact with immunocompromised persons for the duration of the rash.

From General Recommendations on Immunizations of the Advisory Committee on Immunization Practices (ACIP). MMWR Morb Mortal Wkly Rep 2002;51(RR02):1–36.

Table 15-2 Schedule of Accelerated Immunizations for Children under Age 7

Dose 1 (Minimum Age)	Minimum Interval between Doses			
	Dose 1 to Dose 2	Dose 2 to Dose 3	Dose 3 to Dose 4	Dose 4 to Dose 5
DTaP (6 wk)	4 wk	4 wk	6 mo	6 mo[1]
IPV (6 wk)	4 wk	4 wk	4 wk[2]	
Hep B[3] (birth)	4 wk	8 wk (and 16 wk after 1st dose)		
MMR (12 mo)	4 wk[4]			
Var (12 mo)	4 wk: if 1st dose given at age < 12 mo	4 wk[6]: if current age < 12 mo		
Hib[5] (6 wk)	8 wk (as final dose): if 1st dose given at age 12–14 mo No further doses needed: if 1st dose given at age ≥ 15 mo 4 wk: if 1st dose given at age < 12 mo and current age ≤ 24 mo	8 wk (as final dose)[6]: if current age ≥ 12 mo and 2nd dose given at age <15 mo No further doses needed: if previous dose given at age ≥ 15 mo 4 wk: if current age < 12 mo	8 wk (as final dose): this dose only necessary for children age 12 mo–5 y who received 3 doses before age 12 mo	
PCV[7] (6 wk)	8 wk (as final dose): if 1st dose given at age ≥ 12 mo or current age 24–59 mo No further doses needed: for healthy children if 1st dose given at age ≥ 24 mo	8 wk (as final dose): if current age ≥ 12 mo No further doses needed: for healthy children if previous dose given at age ≥ 24 mo	8 wk (as final dose): this dose only necessary for children age 12 mo–5 y who received 3 does before age 12 mo	

Notes

1 DTaP: The fifth dose is not necessary if the fourth dose was given after the fourth birthday.

2 IPV: For children who received an all-IPV or all-oral poliovirus (OPV) series, a fourth dose is not necessary if third dose was given at age ≥ 4 years. If both OPV and IPV were given as part of a series, a total of 4 doses should be given, regardless of the child's current age.

3 HepB: All children and adolescents who have not been immunized against hepatitis B should begin the HepB immunization series during any visit. Providers should make special efforts to immunize children who were born in, or whose parents were born in, areas of the world where hepatitis B virus infection is moderately or highly endemic.

4 MMR: The second dose of MMR is recommended routinely at age 4–6 years but may be given earlier if desired.

5 Hib: Vaccine is not generally recommended for children age ≥ 5 years.

6 Hib: If current age of child is < 12 months and the first 2 doses were PRP-OMP (PedvaxHIB or ComVax [Merck]), the third (and final) dose should be given at age 12–15 months and at least 8 weeks after the second dose.

7 PCV: Vaccine is not generally recommended for children age ≥ 5 years.

From Advisory Committee on Immunization Practices (ACIP). Recommended Childhood and Adolescent Immunization Schedule—United States, July–December 2004. MMWR Morb Mortal Wkly Rep 2004;53(16);Q1–Q3.

Table 15-3 Schedule of Accelerated Immunizations for Children over Age 7

Minimum Interval between Doses		
Dose 1 to Dose 2	*Dose 2 to Dose 3*	*Dose 3 to Booster Dose*
Td: 4 wk	Td: 6 mo	Td[1]: 6 mo: if 1st dose given at age < 12 mo and current age < 11 y 5 y: if 1st dose given at age ≥ 12 mo and 3rd dose given at age < 7 y and current age ≥ 11 y 10 y: if 3rd dose given at age ≥ 7 y
IPV[2]: 4 wk Hep B: 4 wk	IPV[2]: 4 wk Hep B: 8 wk (and 16 wk after 1st dose)	IPV[2,4]
MMR: 4 wk VAR[3]: 4 wk		

Notes

[1] Td: For children age 7–10 years, the interval between the third and booster dose is determined by the age when the first dose was given. For adolescents age 11–18 years, the interval is determined by the age when the third dose was given.

[2] IPV: Vaccine is not generally recommended for persons age ≥ 18 years.

[3] Varicella: Give 2-dose series to all susceptible adolescents age ≥ 13 years.

[4] IPV: For children who received an all-IPV or all-oral poliovirus (OPV) series, a fourth dose is not necessary if third dose was given at age ≥ 4 years. If both OPV and IPV were given as part of a series, a total of 4 doses should be given, regardless of the child's current age

Reporting Adverse Reactions: report adverse reactions to vaccines through the federal Vaccine Adverse Event Reporting System. For information on reporting reactions following immunization, please visit www.vaers.org or call the 24-hour national toll-free information line 800–822–7967.

Disease Reporting: report suspected cases of vaccine-preventable diseases to your state or local health department. For additional information about vaccines, including precautions and contraindications for immunization and vaccine shortages, please visit the National Immunization Program Web site at www.cdc.gov/nip or call the National Immunization Information Hotline at 800–232–2522 (English) or 800–232–0233 (Spanish).

From Advisory Committee on Immunization Practices (ACIP). Recommended Childhood and Adolescent Immunization Schedule—United States, July–December 2004. MMWR Morb Mortal Wkly Rep 2004;53(16);Q1–Q3.

SUGGESTED READINGS

Advisory Committee on Immunization Practices (ACIP). General Recommendations on Immunization. Recommendations of the Advisory Committee on Immunization Practices. MMWR Morb Mortal Wkly Rep 2002;51(RR02):1–36.

Advisory Committee on Immunization Practices (ACIP). Recommended Childhood and Adolescent Immunization Schedule—United States, July–December 2004. MMWR Morb Mortal Wkly Rep 2004;53:Q1–Q3.

Advisory Committee on Immunization Practices (ACIP). Standards for Child and Adolescent Immunization Practices. Pediatrics 2003;112:958–963.

Advisory Committee on Immunization Practices (ACIP). Standards for Adult Immunization Practices. Am J Prev Med 2003;25:144–150.

16

Worsening Low Back Pain (Metastatic Cancer Pain Management)

Frederick Lambert

KEY POINTS

1. Attempt to characterize chronic pain as nociceptive or neuropathic based on clinical history.
2. Believe the patient, as he is or she is the best source of how much pain he or she is currently experiencing.
3. Use the World Health Organization three-step analgesic ladder to help guide therapy.
4. Nonopioid medications all have a ceiling to their analgesic effects, and they have potentially serious adverse effects.
5. Opioids do not have a ceiling effect to their analgesia, and short-acting oral opioid agents can be titrated rapidly to achieve pain control.
6. Side effects from opioids are usually manageable. Constipation from opioids must be treated aggressively, and the risk of respiratory depression from opioids is overestimated.
7. Opioids do not cause the psychological dependence involved in addiction, and addiction is rare when opioids are used appropriately for pain management.
8. Tricyclic antidepressants and anticonvulsant medications such as gabapentin (Neurontin) are indicated for neuropathic pain.

CLINICAL SCENARIO

M.W. is a 61-year-old woman who is on disability as a result of chronic low back pain secondary to osteoarthritis of her lumbar spine. Her pain is usually well controlled with naproxen (Naprosyn). Two years earlier, she was diagnosed with colon cancer, which was treated with surgical resection followed by 1 year of adjuvant chemotherapy with 5-fluorouracil.

She has had worsening low back pain for the last 3 weeks. Her pain consists of severe throbbing, pressure-like pain that radiates around her hip to her left groin (10 of 10 on a numeric analog scale). Initially, she is prescribed a higher dose of naprosyn in combination with a mild opioid agent, hydrocodone with acetaminophen (Vicodin). Her pain does not respond to this regimen, and a magnetic resonance imaging (MRI) scan is ordered, which reveals multiple metastatic lesions in her lower thoracic and lumbar spine. She is admitted to the hospital for further pain management, and her pain is quickly controlled with intravenous morphine administered by means of patient-controlled analgesia (a PCA pump).

On discharge, she is prescribed a strong opioid, sustained-release oxycodone (Oxycontin), 40 mg orally twice daily, in addition to her naproxen, and short-acting oxycodone with acetaminophen (Percocet) for breakthrough pain. She also begins radiation therapy for her spinal metastases. After 3 weeks, her pain remains uncontrolled on this regimen, and a second strong opioid, transdermal fentanyl (Duragesic patch) is added. After titration of the fentanyl, her pain is finally well controlled. Five months later, herpes zoster (shingles) of her left L3 and L4 dermatomes develops, resulting in burning left groin pain. Sciatica of her left leg also develops, with shooting electrical pains down to her left foot as well as numbness and tingling of her left leg. Both of these conditions respond to the addition of amitriptyline and gabapentin (Neurontin).

DISCUSSION

Each year, approximately 25 million Americans experience acute pain due to injury or surgery, and another 50 million have chronic pain. About one of every three Americans will seek medical attention for severe chronic pain at some point during their lifetimes. Cancer is one cause of chronic pain, but there are several other nonmalignant causes of chronic pain. Such painful conditions include osteoarthritis,

Evidence levels Ⓐ Randomized, controlled trials (RCTs), meta-analyses, well-designed systematic reviews of RCTs. Ⓑ Case-control or cohort studies, nonrandomized clinical trials, systematic reviews of studies other than RCTs, cross-sectional studies, retrospective studies, certain uncontrolled studies. Ⓒ Consensus statements, expert guidelines, usual practice, opinion.

chronic low back pain, fibromylagia, spinal cord injury, peripheral neuropathy, neuralgia, and chronic regional pain syndromes. Furthermore, the Joint Commission of Accreditation of Healthcare Organizations (JCAHO) equates pain to "the fifth vital sign" and mandates that physicians and hospitals screen for the presence and assess the nature and intensity of pain in all patients.

Despite such mandates, despite the prevalence of chronic pain, and despite the availability of effective treatments and medications for pain, many patients with chronic pain remain undertreated. This is in part due to fears and misconceptions related to the prescribing of opioid medications for pain. For instance, many physicians, as well as patients, fear that using medications such as morphine for chronic pain will cause addiction. Addiction is characterized by a psychological dependence on drugs and usually includes behaviors such as compulsive drug use (even when patients are pain free) and continued drug use despite harm. If prudent dosing guidelines are followed, addiction is quite rare in patients who are receiving opioid medicines for pain control.

Like any other chronic symptom, pain requires adequate assessment in every patient. This includes the usual historic parameters of location, severity, quality, associated symptoms, and aggravating or mitigating factors. Proper assessment of pain also includes the impact of the pain on the patient's activities of daily living and his or her quality of life, as well as evaluating the impact of the patient's pain in the personal context of psychological, social, and spiritual issues. Several instruments are available to help patients quantify the location and severity of pain as well as its impact on their lives. Pain scales are available for children or patients who cannot communicate verbally: scales such as the Wong-Baker Faces Scale can be used with patients as young as 3 years of age (Fig. 16-1).

Based on history, chronic pain can generally be classified as either nociceptive or neuropathic in origin. Nociceptive pain is presumed to involve direct stimulation of intact pain fibers (nociceptors) with transmission of electrical signals along normally functioning nerves. Nociceptive pain is usually sharp, aching, or throbbing. Somatic pain (i.e., from skin, soft tissue, muscle, and bone) is usually easy for patients to localize, whereas visceral nociceptive pain (for example, from the gastrointestinal tract, genitourinary tract, or lungs) is more achy and harder to localize. Neuropathic pain, conversely, is caused by aberrant signal processing either in the peripheral or central nervous system, sometimes as a result of previous nerve injury. Such pain is usually burning, shooting, stabbing, tingling, or electrical and may be accompanied by paresthesias. Although both types of pain usually respond to opioids, adjuvant analgesics (such as tricyclic antidepressants and gabapentin) are often required to achieve adequate relief of neuropathic pain.

When treating chronic pain, whether from cancer or from nonmalignant illness, it is important to prescribe effective medication and to achieve adequate pain control as quickly as possible. To this end, in 1986 the World Health Organization developed the three-step analgesic ladder (Fig. 16-2). It provides a simple and well-tested approach to the rational selection, administration, and titration of many analgesics.

Management can begin at the corresponding step depending on the severity of the patient's pain. For instance, patients with mild pain (1 to 3 of 10 on a numeric analog scale) can usually be started with medications from step 1. Patients with moderate pain (4 to 6 of 10) usually enter the ladder at step 2, whereas those with severe pain (7 to 10 of 10) usually require medications from step 3. Adjuvant analgesics that are used to enhance the effects of pain medication, such as tricyclic antidepressants, can be used at any stage.

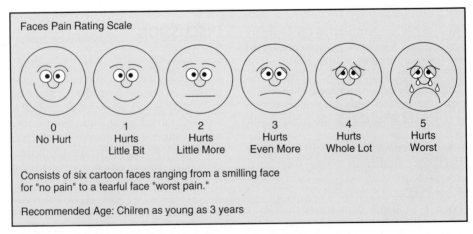

Figure 16-1 The Wong-Baker Faces Scale. (From Wong D, Baker C. Pain in children: Comparison of assessment scales. Pediatr Nurs 14(1): 9–17, 1988.)

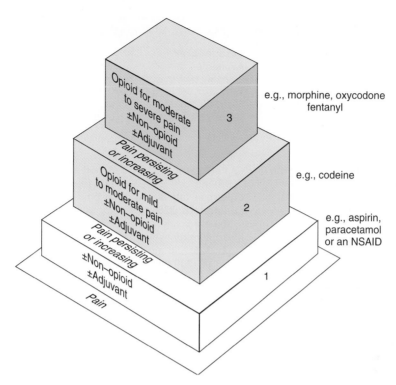

Figure 16-2 The World Health Organization analgesic ladder.

It is important to note that every patient's response to pain is different, so medication regimens must be individualized based on specific patient complaints and individual pain scores. Remember, the patient is his or her own best judge of how much pain he or she is currently experiencing—not the doctor, and not the family. It is not necessary for patients to traverse each step of the pain ladder sequentially; for example, a patient with severe pain may need to be prescribed step 3 opioids right away.

Step 1 analgesics (Table 16-1) include medications such as aspirin, acetaminophen, and nonsteroidal anti-inflammatory drugs (NSAIDs). All of these medications have ceiling effects to their analgesia: a maximal dose above which no further analgesia can be expected or obtained. These medications are good for mild pain, such as the well-controlled osteoarthritis that the patient in our clinical scenario initially has. Acetaminophen use is limited primarily by hepatotoxicity, with the maximum safe dose being 4 g (4000 mg) in 24 hours. Alcohol use and preexisting liver disease can magnify this risk, even with lower doses. NSAIDs also are limited by side effects, most notably gastric ulceration, renal insufficiency, hemorrhage, elevations in blood pressure, and fluid retention. Although selective cyclo-oxygenase (COX)-2 inhibitors may offer theoretical advantages in preventing gastric ulcers, they otherwise have the same serious side-effect profile as do nonselective NSAIDS, and they are no more efficacious than tra-

ditional NSAIDs in relieving pain. In addition, questions are emerging about the cardiovascular safety of COX-2 inhibitors, prompted by the recent withdrawal of rofecoxib (Vioxx) from the global drug market.

Step 2 analgesics generally include lower-potency opioids such as codeine, hydrocodone, oxycodone, and tramadol (Table 16-2). In the United States, these medications are usually available in combination with a step 1 analgesic. Examples include acetaminophen with codeine (Tylenol 3), acetaminophen with hydrocodone (Vicodin), acetaminophen with tramadol (Ultracet), and hydrocodone with ibuprofen (Vicoprofen). Acetaminophen with short-acting oxycodone (Percocet) is generally the most potent of the step 2 analgesics. These medications are a natural second step in the treatment of pain that is not responding to nonopioid analgesics. They also are a good first choice in patients who are having mild to moderate acute pain after injuries or surgery. These medications are usually dosed every 4 to 6 hours, and although they do have opioid-related side effects such as constipation and sedation, the maximal dose is usually limited by side effects of the nonopioid component.

When patients have severe pain or pain that does not respond completely to step 1 or 2 analgesics, high-potency opioids (step 3 medications) are generally indicated. This group of medications includes morphine, hydromorphone (Dilaudid), fentanyl, and methadone (see Table 16-2). Oxycodone in

Table 16-1 Step 1 Analgesics Commonly Used in the United States

Generic Name	Trade Name(s)	Dosage Forms Available	Usual Dosing	Recommended Maximum Dosing
Acetaminophen	Various, Tylenol Plain and Extra Strength are examples	Tabs: 325, 500 mg Elixir: 80 mg/mL Supp: 325, 650 mg	325–650 mg po, pr q4h routinely or prn	650 mg po, pr q4h (4 g/24 h)
NSAIDs and ASA				
Acetylsalicylic acid (ASA) (salicylic acid derivative)	Various, Aspirin is an example	Caplets, tabs: 325, 500 mg Children's tab: 80 mg Coated tabs: 325, 500 mg Elixir: 80 mg/mls Supp: 325, 650 mg	325–650 mg po, pr q4h routinely or pm	650 mg po, pr q4h (5 g/24 h)
Celecoxib (CO-2 selective)	Celebrex	Cap: 100, 200 mg	100–200 mg po bid	200 mg po bid
Choline magnesium trisalicylate (salicylic acid derivative)	Trilisate	Tabs: 500, 750, 1000 mg Salicylate Elixir: 500 mg/5 mL	1–1.5 g po q12h or 0.5–1.0 g po q8h	1.5 g po q8h (4.5 g/24 h)
Diclofenac (acetic acid derivative)	Various, Cataflam, Voltaren are examples	IR tabs: 50 mg SR tabs: 25, 50, 75, 100 mg (with 200 µg misoprostol: Arthrotec 50, 75 mg)	IR: 50–75 mg po, pr q6–8h or SR 75–100 mg po q8–12h	50 mg IR po q6h or 75 mg SR po q8h (225 mg/24 h)
Diflunisal (salicylic acid derivative)	Various, Dolobid is an example	Tabs: 250, 500 mg	250–500 mg po q8–12h	500 mg po q8h (1.5 g/24 h)
Etodolac (acetic acid derivative)	Various, Lodine is an example	IR tabs: 200, 300, 400, 500 mg SR tabs: 400, 500, 600 mg	200–500 mg po q6–12h	400 mg po q8h SR: 1200 mg q d
Flurbiprofen (propionic acid derivative)	Various, Ansaid is an example	Tabs: 50, 100 mg	50–100 mg po q12h	200–300 mg/24 h
Ibuprofen (propionic acid derivative)	Various, Motrin is an example	Tabs: 200, 400, 600, 800 mg Elixir: 100 mg/5 mL	200–800 mg po q6–8h	800 mg po q6h (3.2 g/24 h)
Indomethacin (indole)	Various, Indocin is an example	IR tabs: 25, 50 mg SR tabs: 75 mg Supp: 50 mg elixir, 25 mg/5 mL	25–75 mg po q8–12h or 75 mg SR po q12–24h	50 mg po q6h (200 mg/24 h)
Ketoprofen (propionic acid derivative)	Various, Orudis is an example	Cap: 25, 50, 75 mg SR tabs: 100, 150, 200 mg	150–200 mg po/24 h IR: q6–8h or SR: q12–24h	75 mg po q6h (300 mg/24 h)
Ketorolac (acetic acid derivative)	Various, Toradol is an example	Tab: 10 mg Inj: 15, 30 mg/mL	10 mg po qid or 60 mg IM, IV loading dose, then 10–30 mg IM, IV q6h	40 mg po/24 h or 120 mg IM, IV/24 h for ≤5 days
Nabumetone	Various, Relafen is an example	Tabs: 500, 750 mg	1–2 g po q12–24h	1 g po q12h (2 g/24 h)
Naproxen (propionic acid derivative)	Various, Naprosyn is an example	IR tabs: 250, 375, 500 mg SR tabs: 375, 500 mg	250–500 mg po q8–12h	500 mg po q8h (1.5 g/24 h)
Piroxicam (oxicam)	Various, Feldene is an example	Caps: 10, 20 mg	10–20 mg po q12–24h	20 mg po q12h (40 mg/24 h)

Table 16-1 Step 1 Analgesics Commonly Used in the United States (Continued)

Generic Name	Trade Name(s)	Dosage Forms Available	Usual Dosing	Recommended Maximum Dosing
Salsalate (salicylic acid derivative)	Various, Disalcid is an example	Tabs: 500, 750 mg	1000–1500 mg po bid	3000 mg/d
Sulindac (indole)	Various, Clinoril is an example	Tabs: 150, 200 mg	150 mg po q12h	200 mg po q12h (400 mg/24 h)

See individual opioids for combination medications.
IR, Immediate release; SR, sustained release; $\uparrow$, upper dose limited only by need and adverse effects. NSAID, nonsteroidal anti-inflammatory drug; ASA, acetylsalicylic acid.
From Emmanuel LL, von Gunten CF, Ferris FD, eds. Module 4: "Pain Management," the Education for Physicians on End-of-Life Care (EPEC) Curriculum. The Robert Wood Johnson Foundation, 1999.

Table 16-2 Step 2 and 3 Analgesics Commonly Used in the United States

Generic Name	Trade Name(s)	Dosage Forms Available	Usual Dosing	Recommended Maximum Dosing
Codeine (alone) (methylmorphine, naturally occurring opioid metabolized into morphine)	Various	IR tabs: 15, 30, 60 mg Elixir: 15 mg/5 mL Inj: 30, 60 mg/mL	15–60 mg po, SC, IM q4h routinely/ q1h pm	600 mg/24 hr
Codeine + acetaminophen combinations	Various, Tylenol 3, 4 are examples	Tabs: 30, 60 mg codeine + 325 mg acetaminophen (may include caffeine, butalbital)	1–2 tabs po q4h routinely or prn	Limited to 12 tabs/24 h by acetaminophen
Fentanyl	Various, Duragesic, Actiq, Sublimaze are examples	Patch: 25, 50, 75, 100 μg/hr Lozenge: 200, 400, 600, 800, 1200, 1600 μg Inj: 50 μg/mL	Patch: 25–$\uparrow$ μg/h q72h Lozenge:200 μg q1h prn	Limited only by need and adverse effects
Hydrocodone + acetaminophen	Various, Vicoden, Lortab, Norco are examples	Tabs: 2.5/500, 5/500, 7.5/500, 7.5/750, 10/325, 10/500, 10/660 Elixir: 7.5/500 in 15 mL	1–2 tabs po q4–6h routinely or prn	Limited to 4 g acetaminophen in 24 hr
Hydrocodone + ibuprofen	Vicoprofen	Tab: 7.5/200	1–2 tabs po q4–6h routinely or prn	Limited to 2400 mg ibuprofen in 24 hr
Hydromorphone	Various, Dilaudid is an example	Tabs: 1, 2, 4, 8 mg Elixir: 1 mg/mL Inj: 2, 10 mg/mL Powder: 250 mg/vial	1–$\uparrow$ mg: po q4h routinely/q1h prn, SC, IM q3h routinely/q 30 min pm, or SC, IV q1h via infusion + breakthrough q 30 min pm	Limited only by need and adverse effects
Levorphanol	Levo-Dromeran	Tab: 2 mg inj: 2 mg/mL	2–$\uparrow$ mg po q6–8h	Limited only by need and adverse effects
Meperidine (pethidine, synthetic opioid not related to morphine, useful for rigors)	Various, Demerol is an example	Tabs: 50, 100 mg Inj:50, 75, 100 mg/mL Syrup: 50 mg/5 mL	50–150 mg po, IM, SC, IV q4h pm NOT RECOM-MENDED FOR CHRONIC DOSING Active metabolite normeperidine may produce adverse effects	150 mg q3–4h, 900–1200 mg/ 24 hr

Continued

Table 16-2 Step 2 and 3 Analgesics Commonly Used in the United States (Continued)

Generic Name	Trade Name(s)	Dosage Forms Available	Usual Dosing	Recommended Maximum Dosing
Methadone	Various Dolophine is an example	Tabs: 5, 10, 40 mg Elixir: 10 mg/mL	5 mg po q8h Titrate dose q 3–5 days due to delayed clearance	Limited only by need and adverse effects
Morphine, IR	Various	IR tabs: 5, 15 mg Elixir: 1, 2, 20 mg/mL Supps: 5, 10, 20, 30 mg Inj: 1, 2, 10, 15, 25, 50 mg/mL	1–↑ mg: po, pr q4h routinely/q1h prn, SC, IM q3h routinely/q 30 min prn, or SC, IV q1h via infusion + break through q 30 min prn	Limited only by need and adverse effects
Morphine, SR	Capsule: Kadian Tabs: Ora-Morph-SR, MS-Contin	Kadian capsules: 20, 50, 100 mg (q12–24h) MS-Contin tabs: 15, 30, 60, 100, 200 mg (q8–12h) Ora-Morph-SR tabs: 15, 30, 60, 100 mg (q8–12h) (Kadian capsules may be opened and pellets mixed with fluids or soft food)	10–↑ mg: po, pr q8–24h routinely only (depending on product). Provide break-through doses using IR morphine q1h prn	Limited only by need and adverse effects
Oxycodone (alone)	IR: Various SR: Oxycontin	IR tabs: 5, 10 mg SR tabs: 10, 20, 40, 80 mg Elixir: 20 mg/mL	5–↑ mg IR po, pr q4h routinely, q1h pm or 10–↑ mg SR po q12h	Limited only by need and adverse effects
Oxycodone + Acetaminophen combinations	Various, Percocet is an example	5 mg oxycodone + 325 mg acetaminophen (may include caffeine)	1–2 tabs po q4h routinely or prn	Limited to 12 tabs/24 hr by acetaminophen
Oxycodone + ASA combinations	Various Percodan is an example	5 mg oxycodone + 325 mg ASA (may include caffeine)	1–2 tabs po q4h routinely or prn	Limited to 12 tabs/24 hr by ASA
Tramadol	Ultram	Tab: 50 mg	1–2 tabs po q6h	2 tabs po q6h

IR, Immediate release; SR, sustained release; ↑, upper dose limited only by need and adverse effects.

From Emmanuel LL, von Gunten CF, Ferris FD, eds. Step 2 and 3: "Pain Management," the Education for Physicians on End-of-Life Care (EPEC) Curriculum. The Robert Wood Johnson Foundation, 1999.

doses greater than 5 to 10 mg also is used for severe pain. Many opioid medications have similar pharmacologic properties and follow first-order kinetics. This means that they are eliminated from the body in a direct and predictable way, irrespective of dose. These medications are first conjugated in the liver, and then the metabolites are almost exclusively eliminated in the urine by the kidneys. As a result, these medications (especially morphine) can quickly accumulate in patients with oliguria and renal failure, and such patients must be watched very carefully for signs of toxicity such as delirium, excessive sedation, and seizures. All of these medications (with the exception of methadone and fentanyl) have effective half-lives of approximately 3 to 4 hours, and therefore steady-state concentrations are usually attained within a day. This allows relatively rapid titration of opioids on a daily basis to achieve pain control, especially in the inpatient setting.

In general, patients who are in severe pain are started with a moderate dose of a short-acting step 2 or step 3 opioid every 4 hours. If pain is not controlled within 24 hours, then the dose of the opioid can be increased by 25% to 50% (or even more for severe pain). Unlike NSAIDs, no ceiling effect is found in opioid analgesia, and the dose can be raised until either adequate analgesia is achieved or side effects become limiting. Frequently, titration of pain medications in the inpatient setting requires use of parenteral narcotics (intravenous or intramuscular); but once adequate pain relief is achieved, one can easily convert to oral narcotics by using an equianalgesic dosing table. Table 16-3 provides an example.

If a patient continues to require frequent dosing of short-acting opioids, or if a patient has chronic pain that is stable, consideration should be given to administering oral sustained-release formulations of opioids such as morphine (MS Contin) and oxycodone (Oxycontin). These formulations generally provide a baseline level of analgesia for 8 to 12 hours and may result in improved patient compliance and decreased dosing of short-acting or breakthrough medications. However, they should not be used for initial dose titration in patients with severe pain. Patients should be informed that sustained-release medications such as MS Contin and Oxycontin must be swallowed whole and cannot be broken, crushed, or chewed. Oxycontin in particular can be lethal if it is not taken properly, and it has a very high abuse potential, so proper patient selection is important.

Another option in patients with severe pain is transdermal fentanyl (Duragesic). Because of the unique pharmacokinetics of the fentanyl patch, patients need to be counseled that when starting the patch or increasing the dose of fentanyl, the full effect of the medicine will not peak until 24 hours later. Once a steady state is reached, the duration of pain relief from the fentanyl patch is approximately 72 hours in most patients.

Several currently available opioids should not be used as pain medications. Meperidine (Demerol) has significant adverse effects, such as tremors, dysphoria, myoclonus, and seizures, especially when given in repeated doses. An active effort is under way in many hospitals to remove meperidine from their formularies. Propoxyphene (Darvocet), when compared with other available step 2 analgesics, produces relatively little analgesia, and its use is generally not recommended by most pain-management specialists. Mixed opioid agonists-antagonists, such as pentazocine (Talwin), butorphanol (Stadol), and nalbuphine (Nubain) also should not be used for the management of chronic pain. Not only do these medications have side effects, but they also have ceiling effects to their analgesia, and they can produce acute withdrawal in patients who are already taking other opioids for pain.

Opioid medications do have many common side effects, including constipation, dry mouth, sedation, sweats, and nausea and vomiting. Patients must be educated that such side effects are not allergic reactions, and true allergies to opioids are uncommon. Patients sometimes do experience urticaria or pruritis with opioids, which can usually be treated with either sedating or nonsedating antihistamines. Pharmacologic tolerance to side effects (except constipation) develops in most patients within a relatively short period. Constipation due to opioids is almost universal and should be anticipated and treated aggressively. Usually stool softeners such as docusate (Colace) are ineffective by themselves, and often they must be combined with either stimulant laxatives such as senna (Senokot) or bisacodyl (Dulcolax) to produce regular bowel movements. Prokinetic medications, such as metoclopromide (Reglan), and osmotic agents, such as prune juice and lactulose, also may be required.

Sedation from opioids can be troublesome for some patients and their families, but it usually disappears within several days when tolerance develops. If sedation persists, a different opioid can be tried. Other serious side effects from opioids are actually rare. Delirium, with hallucinations, agitation, myoclonic jerks, and seizures, rarely occurs in patients with normal renal function if opioids are administered in a prudent fashion. However, delirium should be a concern in patients who have renal failure, oliguria, sepsis, and dehydration, and in patients who may be near the end of life.

The risk of respiratory depression from opioids when they are used for pain management is grossly exaggerated. In patients who are receiving opioids

Table 16-3	Equianalgesic Doses of Opioid Analgesics	
Oral/Rectal Dose (mg)	Analgesic	Parenteral Dose (mg)
100	Codeine	60
—	Fentanyl	0.1
15	Hydrocodone	—
4	Hydromorphone	1.5
2	Levorphanol	1
150	Meperidine	50
10	Methadone	5
15	Morphine	5
10	Oxycodone	—

When converting to or from transdermal fentanyl patches, published data suggest that a 25-μg patch is equivalent to 45 to 135 mg of oral morphine/24 hr. However, clinical experience suggests that most patients will use the lower end of the range of morphine doses (i.e., for most patients, 25 μg is about equivalent to 45 to 60 mg of oral morphine/24 hr).
Adapted from Emanuel LL, von Gunten CF, Ferris FD, eds. The EPEC Curriculum. Available at www.epeconline.net. Accessed 1/24/2006;Levy MH. Pharmacologic treatment of cancer pain. N Engl J Med 1996;335:1124–1132.

for pain, respiratory depression does not occur suddenly in the absence of overdose, and somnolence always precedes respiratory depression. Thus PCA and even continuous morphine intravenous drips can be safely used in most patients, provided they are closely monitored for sedation.

Both patients with cancer and those with non-malignant chronic pain may require escalating doses of opioids as their pain or disease progresses. If opioids must be discontinued because of side effects, they should be tapered slowly to prevent withdrawal symptoms such as tachycardia, diaphoresis, nausea, vomiting, diarrhea, abdominal pain, and hallucinations. If withdrawal symptoms do occur, they can usually be managed with clonidine or low doses of benzodiazepines. Once again, patients and families should be educated that tolerance and signs of physiologic dependence (as evidenced by withdrawal symptoms) are *not* evidence of addiction to opioids. They should be reassured that opioids by themselves do not cause psychological dependence or craving, and that addiction is an extremely rare outcome of pain management without a history of substance abuse. Even most patients with prior substance abuse can be given opioids safely for chronic pain, but they may need to adhere to strict dosing protocols, and contracting may be required.

Several medications can be used as adjuvant medications to enhance analgesia and as primary treatments for neuropathic pain. Low-dose tricyclic antidepressants, in doses of 10 to 25 mg at night, are a good first choice. Amitriptyline (Elavil) is the most extensively studied of the tricyclics and can be especially useful in patients with insomnia. It also has more anticholinergic and cardiac toxicity than other medications in its class, and desipramine (Norpramin) and nortriptyline (Pamelor) may be safer and better tolerated, especially in elderly patients. Gabapentin (Neurontin) has become a potent treatment for many types of neuropathic pain, including postherpetic neuralgia and pain that is shooting or stabbing. Sometimes a combination of a tricyclic and gabapentin must be used for complex neuropathic pain, as illustrated by the patient in our scenario. If gabapentin is not successful, other anticonvulsant medications such as carbamazepine (Tegretol) and valproic acid can be tried.

Finally, many nonpharmacologic modalities can be useful for patients whose pain is not entirely responsive to traditional medications. Such modalities include physical therapy, acupuncture, transcutaneous electrical nerve stimulation (TENS units), relaxation therapy, guided imagery, art and music therapy, and biofeedback, among others. Like medical therapy, such interventions must be tailored according to the individual patient's plan of care.

In conclusion, as family doctors begin to encounter increasing numbers of patients with chronic pain, we as a specialty will need to feel more comfortable prescribing medications to relieve pain and suffering. This chapter has illustrated that potent pain medications are in our armamentarium, and the World Health Organization analgesic ladder is a useful tool in helping us guide our therapy. If physicians prescribe opioids in a prudent and rational manner, and patients are monitored carefully for side effects, then we can begin to make a profound impact on patients who are currently not receiving adequate treatment for their chronic pain.

Material Available on Student Consult

Review Questions and Answers about Metastatic Cancer Pain Management

SUGGESTED READINGS

Berry PH, Chapman CR, Covington RC, et al., eds. Pain: Current Understanding of Assessment, Management, and Treatments. Monograph produced jointly by the National Pharmaceutical Corporation, and by the Joint Commission on Accreditation of Healthcare Organizations, 2001. Available at www.jcaho.org and www.npcnow.org. Accessed 1/18/2006.Ⓒ

Emanuel LL, von Gunten CF, Ferris FD, eds. Pain management. In The Education for Physicians on End-of-life Care (EPEC) Curriculum. The EPEC Project, The Robert Wood Johnson Foundation, 1999. Available at www.epeconline.net Accessed 1/18/2006.Ⓒ

Levy MH. Pharmacologic treatment of cancer pain. N Engl J Med 1996;335:1124–1132. Ⓑ

Chapter

17

Sore Throat
(Acute Pharyngitis)

Roberto Cardarelli

KEY POINTS

1. The most common etiologic agent of acute pharyngitis is a virus.
2. The drug of choice for treating group A β-hemolytic streptococcus is penicillin V.
3. The most important parts of the diagnostic workup for pharyngitis are a thorough history and an accurate physical examination.
4. The heterophil antibody test misses a third of infectious mononucleosis cases in the first week of the disease.
5. All patients first seen with pharyngitis should receive appropriate analgesics, antipyretics, and supportive care.

OFFICE VISIT

Subjective

Patient Identification and Presenting Problem

Leanne, a 13-year-old girl, complains of a sore throat and fever, which started abruptly while at her family's lake house yesterday. She admits to a decreased appetite due to feeling mildly nauseated without vomiting or diarrhea. Leanne states that she feels "worn out" with a slight headache. Her throat is what bothers her the most, even swallowing her own saliva. She also admits that her ears ache. She denies being around anyone who is sick but privately admits that she kissed a boy in her class for the first time last week.

Medical History

Allergies No known drug allergies.

Medical Leanne is the youngest and the only girl of three children. Her mother had no complications

during the prenatal and delivery course. She is up to date with all her immunizations. She has been in the 60th percentile for weight and height all her life. She takes no medications. She has had two episodes of streptococcal pharyngitis in the last 4 years, the last episode being 1.5 years ago. She did require tympanostomy tubes when she was 2 years old because of recurrent middle ear infections.

Surgical Tympanostomy tubes at age 2.

Family History

Both of Leanne's parents are in good health. Her maternal grandmother died at age 62 of breast cancer. The rest of her relatives are alive and well.

Social History

Leanne is in 8th grade and is on the honor roll. She plays volleyball and is a member of a traveling soccer team. She has never attempted cigarettes or illicit drugs. She tasted a wine cooler once at her friend's house but never tried any other alcoholic beverage since. Her father smokes outside the house, and he avoids smoking in the car. She gets along well with her two older brothers, who are 15 and 17 years old.

Review of Systems

Aside from that mentioned earlier, she denies abdominal pain, discolored urine, dizziness, nasal congestion, sinus pressure, or skin rashes. A dry cough developed since this morning.

Objective

Vital Signs

Height, 59 in
Weight, 104 pounds
Temperature, 101.3°F
Blood pressure, 98/68
Pulse, 96 (regular) beats per minute
Respiratory rate, 14 respirations per minute

Evidence levels Ⓐ Randomized, controlled trials (RCTs), meta-analyses, well-designed systematic reviews of RCTs. Ⓑ Case-control or cohort studies, nonrandomized clinical trials, systematic reviews of studies other than RCTs, cross-sectional studies, retrospective studies, certain uncontrolled studies. Ⓒ Consensus statements, expert guidelines, usual practice, opinion.

Physical Examination

General Leanne is a slightly tired-appearing young girl in no acute distress and appropriately dressed.

Skin Normal skin turgor and pigmentation. No rashes are appreciated.

Head, Eyes, Ears, Nose, and Throat Normocephalic. Eyes are anicteric, and the conjunctivae are clear. Her tympanic membranes are without erythema or fluid levels. Nasal mucosa is slightly swollen, and the oropharynx shows swollen and erythematous tonsils with exudates. Several petechiae are appreciated on the upper palate and uvula. No sinus tenderness is present.

Neck The thyroid is not palpable. Bilateral prominent and tender anterior cervical lymph nodes are palpated. No posterior cervical, pre- or postauricular lymph nodes are appreciated.

Chest Lungs are clear to auscultation bilaterally.

Heart Regular rate and rhythm. No murmurs are appreciated. Pulses are +2 throughout.

Abdomen Flat, normal bowel sounds, soft and nontender. No masses are appreciated. No hepatosplenomegaly is noted.

Assessment

Working Diagnosis

The working diagnosis is acute pharyngitis. Differential etiology includes group A β-hemolytic streptococcus, viral not otherwise specified (NOS), infectious mononucleosis.

Plan

Diagnostic

A rapid streptococcal antigen test is ordered and returns positive. No other tests are ordered.

Treatment

1. Leanne is given penicillin V, 500 mg, to take by mouth every 8 hours for 10 days, because she refused the intramuscular injection.
2. Over-the-counter analgesics are recommended for fever and pain. Analgesic throat spray also is mentioned for her consideration.
3. She is instructed to drink plenty of fluids and to gargle with warm salt water for symptomatic relief.
4. She is given a school absence note and instructed to avoid sharing utensils and cups with others. She should take the antibiotic for at least 24 hours before coming into contact with others.
5. She is instructed to return to clinic if she does not improve, if a rash develops, if dark urine is noticed, or if symptoms worsen.

DISCUSSION

Pharyngitis is one of the most common medical conditions encountered in ambulatory care offices. It accounts for little more than 1% of all office visits in primary care offices (Cherry et al., 2003). The ultimate decision that must be made by physicians is whether antibiotics are indicated. A delicate balance exists between overprescribing antibiotics, appropriately ordering diagnostic tests, and preventing complications from untreated pharyngitis. This is accomplished by a taking a good history, completing an accurate physical examination, and appropriately ordering diagnostic tests.

Differential Diagnosis

The numerous causes of pharyngitis are listed in Table 17-1 (Bisno et al., 2002 Ⓒ; Kazzi, 2005 Ⓑ; Vincent et al., 2004 Ⓑ). Most cases are seen in the late fall/early winter and early spring (Gerber, 1998 Ⓑ). Our discussion focuses on the infectious causes of pharyngitis, primarily viral and bacterial agents, with an emphasis on group A β-hemolytic streptococcus (GABHS).

Viral pharyngitis is the most common type of pharyngitis (Bisno et al., 2002 Ⓒ; Gerber, 1998 Ⓑ), with adenovirus and Epstein-Barr virus being two of the more common viral agents. The latter is known to cause infectious mononucleosis (Mono), with signs and symptoms of fever, fatigue and malaise, tonsillar exudates, pharyngitis, posterior cervical lymphadenopathy, and occasionally hepatosplenomegaly. If patients with Mono are given an antibiotic, in 90% of them, a classic maculopapular rash will develop (Peter and Ray, 1998 Ⓑ). Patients who are diagnosed with Mono should be instructed to rest and to avoid any vigorous activities that may place them at increased risk for splenic rupture. Other viral causes of pharyngitis, such as adenovirus, are commonly accompanied by typical symptoms such as rhinorrhea, conjunctivitis, low-grade fever, and malaise (Bisno et al., 2002 Ⓒ). Atypical symptoms can include abdominal pain, nausea with or without vomiting, and diarrhea (Middleton, 1996 Ⓑ).

Approximately 15% to 30% of pharyngitis cases in children are attributable to GABHS, whereas only 5% to 15% of adult cases are caused by the bacterium (Bisno, 2001 Ⓒ; Bisno et al., 2002 Ⓒ; Snow et al., 2001 Ⓒ). The objective in treating GABHS infection is to improve symptoms, decrease the spread of disease, and prevent, although rare, life-threatening complications, such as rheumatic fever, acute glomerulonephritis, and peritonsillar abscesses (Bisno et al.,

Table 17-1 Causes of Sore Throat

Infectious	Noninfectious
Viruses	Gastroesophageal reflux
Adenovirus	Neoplasm
Epstein-Barr virus	Foreign body
Rhinovirus	Dry air
Influenza A and B virus	Chemical injury
Coxsackievirus A/B	Postnasal drip/allergies
Herpes simplex	Smoking
Cytomegalovirus	Recent endotracheal intubation
Human immunodeficiency virus	Ludwig angina
Bacteria	Thyroiditis
Group A β-hemolytic streptococci	Retropharyngeal abscess
Group C, G, and F streptococci	
Neisseria gonorrhoeae	
Corynebacterium diphtheriae	
Mycoplasma pneumoniae	
Chlamydia pneumoniae	
Arcanobacterium haemolyticus	
Candidiasis	
Epiglottitis	
Croup	
Peritonsillar abscess/cellulitis	

Data from Bisno AL, Gerber MA, Gwaltney JM, et al. Practice guidelines for the diagnosis and management of group A streptococcal pharyngitis. Clin Infect Dis 2002;35:113–125; Cooper RJ, Hoffman JR, Bartlett JG, et al. Principles of appropriate antibiotic use for acute pharyngitis in adults: Background. Ann Interm Med 2001; 134:509–517; Kazzi AA, Wills J. Pharyngitis. eMed J. Available at www.emedicine.com/emerg/topic419.htm. Accessed 8/28/2005.

2002 Ⓒ). The most common signs and symptoms of GABHS infection include severe pharyngitis with tonsillar exudates, anterior cervical lymphadenopathy, fever, and palatine petechiae. If untreated, GABHS pharyngitis can last for about 7 to 10 days and individuals can be infectious for up to 1 week after the acute phase (Ebell et al., 2000 Ⓑ; Gerber, 1998 Ⓑ). With treatment, symptoms are shortened by 1 to 2 days, and the infectious period is reduced to 24 hours (Ebell et al., 2000 Ⓑ; Snow et al., 2001 Ⓒ; Vincent et al., 2004 Ⓑ). Treatment also prevents most complications, although this is unclear for peritonsillar abscesses (Bisno et al., 2002 Ⓒ; Snow et al., 2001 Ⓒ; Vincent et al., 2004 Ⓑ).

Diagnostic Workup

A thorough history and accurate physical examination will allow the practitioner to refine his or her differential diagnosis in a matter of minutes. Refractory cases of sore throat with negative cultures may lead the practitioner to consider noninfectious causes, such as gastroesophageal reflux disease or neoplasm.

Infectious Mononucleosis

As already discussed, the presenting signs and symptoms will help make the diagnosis of Mono. Many times, the typical presentation of Mono requires no further testing (Brigden et al., 1999 Ⓐ). A blood count

with more than 10% lymphocytes helps support the diagnosis (Brigden et al., 1999 Ⓐ). The heterophil antibody test (Monospot test) misses one third of the cases in the first week of the disease, but the sensitivity increases to 80% by the second week (Brigden et al., 1999 Ⓐ). Testing for immunoglobulin M (IgM) antibodies against the Epstein-Barr virus can be used in uncertain circumstances.

Group A β-Hemolytic Streptococcus

Clinical decision rules have been developed to help in accurately diagnosing GABHS pharyngitis because no single element in the history or examination is sensitive or specific enough to diagnose or rule out streptococcal pharyngitis (Gerber, 1998 Ⓑ). Others have supported such an approach (Cooper et al., 2001 Ⓒ. McIsaac and colleagues (2000 Ⓑ) developed a scored approach by using five criteria: age, tonsillar swelling or exudate, anterior cervical lymphadenopathy, absence of cough, and fever higher than 100.4°F (Table 17-2). Based on the score, patients are placed in the low-, intermediate-, or high-risk group. Patients in the low-risk group should not receive treatment and should have no further testing. Those in the high-risk group should be given empiric antibiotics, and a throat culture or rapid streptococcal antigen test or both may be considered. Patients in the intermediate group should have further testing with the rapid streptococcal

Table 17-2 Sore Throat Score

Give 1 point for each:
    The patient is younger than 15 years
    Tonsillar swelling or exudates
    Tender anterior cervical lymphadenopathy
    Temperature >100.4°F
    Absence of cough
Subtract 1 point if:
    The patient is older than 45 years

Scoring

−1 to 0	Low risk: Antibiotic therapy, rapid strep test, and throat culture are not indicated.
1 to 3	Intermediate risk: Perform rapid strep test and treat accordingly. If rapid strep test is negative, consider throat culture for children.
4 to 5	High risk: Empiric antibiotics. Rapid strep test and/or culture is optional.

Data from Bisno AL, Gerber MA, Gwaltney JM, et al. Practice guidelines for the diagnosis and management of group A streptococcal pharyngitis. Clin Infect Dis 2002;35:113–125; Ebell MH, Smith MA, Barry HC, et al. The rational clinical examination: Does this patient have strep throat? JAMA 2000;284:2912–2918; Snow V, Mottur-Pilson C, Cooper RJ, Hoffman JR. Principles of appropriate antibiotic use for acute pharyngitis in adults. Ann Intern Med 2001;134:506–508; and Vincent MT, Celestin N, Hussain AN. Pharyngitis. Am Fam Physician 2004;69:1465–1470; McIssac WJ, Goel V, To T, Low DE. The validity of a sore throat score in family practice. CMAJ 2000;163:811–815.

antigen test or throat culture or both. All refractory cases should have a throat culture performed. It is advocated that children with a negative rapid streptococcal antigen test should have the result confirmed by a throat culture (Bisno et al., 2002❻). A negative rapid streptococcal antigen test does not require confirmation by a throat culture in adults (Bisno et al., 2002 ❻). The rapid streptococcal antigen test has an approximate sensitivity of 95% and specificity of 97% (Vincent et al., 2004❸). The throat culture has an approximate sensitivity of 97% and specificity of 99%, depending on the technique and medium used (Vincent et al., 2004❸).

Therapy

All patients initially seen with pharyngitis should receive appropriate analgesics, antipyretics, and supportive care, such as gargling with warm salt water (Snow et al., 2001❻). Precautions should be discussed with all patients, especially those with infectious mononucleosis, about the risk of splenic rupture. Duration of symptoms should be discussed to give patients a realistic expectation of when the symptoms will improve.

Appropriate antibiotic choices for treating GABHS should have a narrow spectrum of action that includes GABHS. Options for treatment are shown in Table 17-3 (Bisno at al., 2002❻; Cooper et al., 2001❻; Hayes and Williamson, 2001❸; Kazzi, 2005❸). Penicillin is the preferred antibiotic when it

Table 17-3 Antibiotic Choices for Group A β-Hemolytic Streptococcus

Antibiotic	Pediatric Dose	Adult Dose	Frequency	Duration
Penicillin V	250 mg	500 mg	Three times daily	10 days
Benzathine penicillin	600,000 units	1,200,000 units	One IM injection	—
Amoxicillin	13.3 mg/kg/dose	500 mg	Three times daily	10 days
Ampicillin	12.5 mg/kg/dose	500 mg	Four times daily	10 days
Amoxicillin-clavulanate potassium	20 mg/kg/dose	875 mg	Two times daily	10 days
Erythromycin ethylsuccinate	10 mg/kg/dose	400 mg	Four times daily	10 days
Azithromycin	12 mg/kg/dose	500 mg on day 1 and 250 mg on days 2–5	Once daily	5 days
Cephalexin	6.25–12.5 mg/kg/dose	250 mg	Four times daily	10 days

IM, intramuscular.

Data from Bisno AL, Gerber MA, Gwaltney JM, et al. Practice guidelines for the diagnosis and management of group A streptococcal pharyngitis. Clin Infect Dis 2002;35:113–125; Cooper RJ, Hoffman JR, Bartlett JG, et al. Principles of appropriate antibiotic use for acute pharyngitis in adults: Background. Ann Intern Med 2001;134:509–517; Hayes CS, Williamson H. Management of group A beta-hemolytic streptococcal pharyngitis. Am Fam Physician 2001;63:1557–1564; and Kazzi AA, Wills J. Pharyngitis. eMed J. Available at www.emedicine.com/emerg/topic419.htm. Accessed 8/28/2005.

is indicated (Cooper et al., 2001©). Erythromycin should be considered in someone with a penicillin allergy (Cooper et al., 2001©). Penicillin can be given in two ways; orally with penicillin V, 250 to 500 mg, three or four times per day for 10 days, or intramuscularly with benzathine penicillin, 1.2 million units (adults) in one dose.

Patients can follow-up as necessary and should be instructed to return immediately to the clinic if symptoms worsen or are not improving. It is impor-tant to remember that avoiding the indiscriminate use of antibiotics will help avoid antimicrobial resist-ance and limit the risks of allergic reactions.

Material Available on Student Consult

Review Questions and Answers about Acute Pharyngitis.

REFERENCES

Bisno AL. Acute pharyngitis. N Engl J Med 2001;344: 205–211.❸

Bisno AL, Gerber MA, Gwaltney JM, et al. Practice guidelines for the diagnosis and management of group A strepto-coccal pharyngitis. Clin Infect Dis 2002;35:113–125.❹

Brigden ML, Au S, Thompson S, et al. Infectious mononu-cleosis in an outpatient population: Diagnostic utility of 2 automated hematology analyzers and the sensitiv-ity and specificity of Hoagland's criteria in heterophile-positive patients. Arch Pathol Lab Med 1999;123: 875–881.❹

Cherry DK, Burt CW, Woodwell DA. National Ambulatory Medical Care Survey: 2001 Summary. Adv Data 2003; 337:1–44.

Cooper RJ, Hoffman JR, Bartlett JG, et al. Principles of appropriate antibiotic use for acute pharyngitis in adults: Background. Ann Intern Med 2001;134: 509–517.❹

Ebell MH, Smith MA, Barry HC, et al. The rational clinical examination: Does this patient have strep throat? JAMA 2000;284:2912–2918.❸

Gerber MA. Diagnosis of group A streptococcal pharyngi-tis. Pediatr Ann 1998;27:269–273.❸

Hayes CS, Williamson H. Management of group A beta-hemolytic streptococcal pharyngitis. Am Fam Physician 2001;63:1557–1564.❸

Kazzi AA, Wills J. Pharyngitis. eMed J. Available at www.emedicine.com/emerg/topic419.htm. Accessed 8/28/2005.

McIsaac WJ, Goel V, To T, Low DE. The validity of a sore throat score in family practice. CMAJ 2000;163: 811–815.❸

Middleton DB. Pharyngitis. Prim Care 1996;23:719–739.❸

Peter J, Ray CG. Infectious mononucleosis. Pediatr Rev 1998;19:276–279.❸

Snow V, Mottur-Pilson C, Cooper RJ, Hoffman JR. Principles of appropriate antibiotic use for acute pharyngitis in adults. Ann Intern Med 2001;134: 506–508.❹

Vincent MT, Celestin N, Hussain AN. Pharyngitis. Am Fam Physician 2004;69:1465–1470.❸

18

Nasal Congestion (Allergic Rhinitis)

David Q. Hutcheson-Tipton

KEY POINTS

1. Allergic rhinitis is common. It exacts a heavy toll in lost work and school days.
2. Diagnosis is usually based on clinical picture but, if in doubt, can be clarified by radioallergosorbent test or skin testing.
3. The cornerstone of treatment is avoidance (at least minimization) of allergens.
4. Medicinal treatment may involve intranasal steroids, oral antihistamines, and decongestants, among others.

INITIAL VISIT

Subjective

Patient Identification and Presenting Problem

Alice is a 36-year-old woman with complaints of nasal congestion and a frequent need to blow her nose.

Present Illness

Alice relates that her rhinorrhea and nasal congestion had a gradual onset 3 weeks ago. At the time, she thought she was catching a cold, but the symptoms lasted longer than her usual cold. They have neither improved nor worsened during that time. She has had no fever, malaise, or general achiness. Neither has she had a sore throat, more than rare cough, or headache. She denies using an over-the-counter intranasal decongestant. She tried diphenhydramine (Benadryl), and although it relieved her symptoms some, she found herself too drowsy when taking it, even if she took it only once a day before bedtime.

Medical History

Alice was diagnosed with eczema as a baby but has had no further skin problems. She had a tonsillectomy at age 5 years and an extraction of her wisdom teeth as a teenager but no other surgeries. She had a normal spontaneous vaginal delivery of one child.

Family History

Her brother, 25 years old, had asthma as a child. In a maternal aunt, breast cancer developed at age 60 years. She is not aware of any family history of allergies or eczema. Besides her brother, no other family members have had asthma.

Social History

Alice works as a local convenience store manager. She lives in a two-bedroom apartment with her 12-year-old daughter and a kitten given to them about a month ago by a co-worker. She does not use tobacco in any form, drinks one to two alcoholic beverages weekly, and denies use of recreational drugs. She runs several miles most evenings with a friend.

Review of Systems

Alice denies fever, chills, night sweats, unintended weight loss, nausea, vomiting, diarrhea, and constipation. She denies a change in her senses of smell and taste or any dyspnea, wheezing, chest pain, or chest tightness. She denies sore throat and heartburn. She also denies feelings of increased or decreased energy, hair or skin changes, or changes in bowel habits. On questioning, she admits that her nose has been rather itchy lately. She denies that her eyes have been either itchy or watery.

Objective

Physical Examination

General Alice is a pleasant, well-developed, well-nourished woman who appears her stated age. She

Evidence levels Ⓐ Randomized, controlled trials (RCTs), meta-analyses, well-designed systematic reviews of RCTs. Ⓑ Case-control or cohort studies, nonrandomized clinical trials, systematic reviews of studies other than RCTs, cross-sectional studies, retrospective studies, certain uncontrolled studies. Ⓒ Consensus statements, expert guidelines, usual practice, opinion.

often rubs her nose with the side of her hand and occasionally clears her throat during the office visit.

Vital Signs Blood pressure, 122/84; heart rate, 75; respirations, 14 per minute; temperature, 98.4°F; height, 5 feet 8 inches; weight, 130 pounds; peak expiratory flow rate, 540.

Head, Eyes, Ears, Nose, and Throat Her external auditory canals are clear. Both tympanic membranes are slightly retracted but without erythema: They move easily to pneumatic otoscopy. Her oropharynx is cobblestoned without visible exudate. Her nasal turbinates are boggy and somewhat pale. Some watery discharge is visible on the walls of her nares. No sinus tenderness to palpation is noted. Her neck is supple and without palpable lymphadenopathy or thyromegaly.

Lungs Both lungs are clear to auscultation, with good air movement.

Heart Her heart has a regular rate and rhythm without adventitious sounds.

Skin Her skin appears and feels normal except for some mild dryness in the antecubital areas of her arms.

Assessment

Working Diagnosis
Allergic rhinitis.

Differential Diagnosis
1. *Infectious rhinitis* is generally viral in origin, from an upper respiratory tract infection. It is often accompanied by rhinorrhea and nasal congestion. Many people—patients, even some physicians—believe that yellow nasal discharge (so-called purulent rhinitis) is invariably a sign of a sinus infection. Many people during the course of the common cold have at least one day of this symptom; should a computed tomography (CT) scan of their sinuses be obtained at that time, it might even show radiologic sinusitis (i.e., opacification of one or more of the paranasal sinuses). This does not mean they need antibiotics: The vast majority will pass quickly through this phase and get better. Should the purulence last more than several days, however, the diagnosis of rhinosinusitis likely to be responsive to antibiotic therapy should be strongly considered (American Academy of Allergy, Asthma, and Immunology, 2005©).
2. *Eosinophilic nonallergic rhinitis* is a year-round (perennial) rhinitis; congestion is the predominant symptom. A nasal smear shows numerous eosinophils (as it does with allergic rhinitis [AR]), but skin testing for allergies is negative. Intranasal steroids are quite helpful.
3. *Acute rhinosinusitis* often is first seen with rhinorrhea and nasal congestion as prominent symptoms. Most often, sinusitis is a complication of allergic rhinitis or a viral respiratory infection (or both) and has as cardinal symptoms headache, sore throat, and cough. The latter two symptoms are often worse at night, as the sinuses drain best when the body is in a supine position. Antibiotics are the cornerstone of therapy.
4. *Vasomotor or idiopathic rhinitis* occurs without any eosinophilia. Allergic skin testing is negative. Ipratropium bromide (Atrovent), the 0.03% solution, is helpful, as at times are intranasal steroids, oral decongestants, regular nasal saline washes, or a combination of these.
5. *Hormonal rhinitis.* Hypothyroidism can cause rhinorrhea: This etiology should always be considered with an atypical presentation. Rhinitis also is quite common in late pregnancy and, if particularly bothersome, can be treated with oral decongestants (these should generally be avoided in the first trimester). Some women, at certain times in the menstrual or life cycles (or both), have hormonal rhinitis (Howarth, 2003©).
6. *Rhinitis medicamentosa* is a problem that occurs with overuse of over-the-counter intranasal decongestants, the most popular being oxymetazoline. Such agents are extremely effective and can have a place in the treatment of various forms of rhinitis. Patients should be warned against using them for more than 3 days at a time, however, as rebound congestion can be worse than the original.
7. *Other etiologies* include sinus polyps, other anatomic problems such as septal deviation, and complications of certain head and neck surgeries (American Academy of Allergy, Asthma and Immunology, 2005©).

Plan

Diagnostic
No laboratory, radiologic, or other diagnostic evaluation is needed at this time. A medication trial with good response will be helpful. Alice should also notice any increase in symptoms on exposure to suspected offending allergens—in her case, her cat.

Therapeutic
Several options are discussed with her, and the patient chooses a trial of an intranasal steroid once daily. Adverse effects are discussed.

Patient Education
Alice is encouraged to try to identify and avoid, as much as possible, triggers for her symptoms. The

temporal relation of having a cat in her residence with subsequent onset of her symptoms cannot be overlooked: It strongly suggests that her leading (or sole) allergen is cat dander. Animal dander contains many allergenic proteins in and on the skin of the animal, which is sloughed off on a continual basis. In the case of cats, who groom themselves so fastidiously, a protein in their saliva adheres to their skin and becomes airborne. The protein is among the most allergenic known.

Because a good chance exists that Alice is allergic to her new kitten, she is advised to bathe it weekly, a measure that reduces the quantity of dander that becomes airborne. She should also keep the animal out of her bedroom.

Disposition

The patient is instructed to return to or phone the clinic should her symptoms worsen or fail to improve within the next week to 10 days. An appointment in a month is made to review the effectiveness of the steroid.

DISCUSSION

Allergic rhinitis (AR) is an inflammation of the nasal mucosa and is caused by several chemicals, including leukotrienes and histamine, the latter mediated by immunoglobulin E (IgE) released from the degranulation of mast cells (Howarth, 2003 ©). It is basically the body trying to reject harmless airborne substances (e.g., pollen, mold, animal dander) that it should ignore.

AR is extremely common, affecting approximately 40 million people in the United States. Its importance is often underestimated by the general public as well as by physicians. It has significant morbidity, yearly causing millions of days of school and work to be lost (American Academy of Allergy, Asthma and Immunology, 2005©).

Alone or with allergic conjunctivitis—a dual presentation is common—AR is one of the three common atopic (allergic) disorders, the other two being atopic dermatitis (eczema) and asthma. The tendency to atopy is strongly heritable, making a family (or personal) history of any one or a combination of these problems extremely relevant (such a history is not by any means essential to diagnosing this problem). An atopic diathesis can evolve into actual symptoms at any time in the life cycle, although it is usually before adulthood. Symptoms also can vanish for a while—the patient "grows out of" the disease or moves to an area with different allergens—only to return.

Traditionally, AR has been categorized into two types: seasonal and perennial. In the seasonal variety, popularly called "hay fever," symptoms appear at particular times of year when specific airborne allergens (aero-allergens) are present (such as tree pollen in the spring, grass pollen in midsummer, and weeds in autumn). In perennial AR, the patient is allergic to one or more stimuli that are always present (airborne particles from dust mites, decomposed cockroaches, animal dander). Both types can coexist. Allergic rhinitis of either variety also results in a hypersensitivity of the nasal mucosa to many nonspecific stimuli such as smoke, smells, and changes in temperature or humidity. Symptoms then occur on exposure to these stimuli.

Details of the history are exceedingly important in diagnosing AR (American Academy of Allergy, Asthma and Immunology, 2005©). Rhinorrhea, sneezing fits, pruritus of the nose and eyes, nasal congestion, and a sensation of "sinus pressure" are common. It is a strong clue if symptoms worsen on the patient's encounter with specific allergens—when she or he is around a dog, for instance—or at certain times of the year.

The physician begins the physical examination the moment he or she walks into the room. The patient with AR may sniffle, rub or blow the nose frequently, and clear the throat or sneeze or both. Specific examination of the head, eyes, ears, nose, and throat, of course, yields the most information. When AR is active, tympanic membranes are often retracted (from swelling of pharyngeal tissues where the eustachian tubes drain). Eyes can be injected or watery or both if allergic conjunctivitis is present. Sometimes periorbital edema with a bluish hue is seen, causing the so-called allergic shiners. Nasal mucosa may be swollen. Turbinates may be pale and boggy, with clear drainage. The oropharynx is often injected and sometimes "cobblestoned" from postnasal drip. The neck is supple but may have some (reactive) shotty lymphadenopathy. Lungs should be evaluated for signs of possible asthma (e.g., wheezing). Skin can be observed by vision and palpation for dryness or lichenification, which can occur with atopic dermatitis.

Most frequently for the family physician, the diagnosis of AR is a clinical one, based on presentation and examination. If the symptom cluster responds to appropriate treatment for allergies, no need exists for further assessment (American Academy of Allergy, Asthma and Immunology, 2005©). An argument can be made (and is at times by allergists) for universal testing of patients with AR signs and symptoms. This is usually not necessary, though, for a family physician. If doubt remains about the etiology of rhinitis, allergic testing can be done. A simple, rapid test is to obtain a specimen of nasal secretions and apply Hansel's stain. If eosinophils are present, the differential diagnosis is narrowed to either AR or nonallergic eosinophilic rhinitis. Polymorphonuclear lymphocytes point to an infectious etiology.

A more frequently used and still quite expedient and relatively inexpensive form of testing is the radio-allergosorbent test (RAST), in which circulating antibodies to substances are detected. Although RASTs will often demonstrate reactivity to, say, certain pollens or molds, if the tests are negative, allergies are not ruled out. Allergists usually perform skin testing, which is more accurate. Here the clinician applies solutions containing small amounts of substances that represent classes of allergens (e.g., pollen, mold, trees) to small breaks in the skin created by small needle pricks. When a patient is allergic to a substance, the skin at the application site swells and develops an area of surrounding redness (the so-called wheal and flare effect).

Minimizing, preferably eliminating, exposure to identified or suspected allergens is the cornerstone of AR treatment. Washing a pet weekly and keeping it out of the bedroom will help reduce exposure. Many people with perennial AR are allergic to decomposing dust mites that live in bedding. Covering pillow and mattress with plastic or tightly woven cloth, as well as washing all bedding and bed clothes at least weekly in hot water, will reduce exposure to this common allergen. If pollens are offenders, keeping windows closed and using a HEPA filter can help. Likewise with mold from the outside; indoor mold can be reduced by dehumidification and minimization of carpeting.

Several medicinal options exist. Intranasal steroids are recommended as first-line medication by the International Board for the Treatment of Allergic Rhinitis (Ledgerwood and Johnson, 2002). Several versions are available. They are all used once or twice daily. Although many patients will have some relief sooner, it is important to warn that the maximal effectiveness is usually not reached for 2 to 3 weeks. Most common side effects are local: sneezing, epistaxis, or bad taste. Pretreatment with nasal saline may help attenuate these.

The most popular type of medications are oral antihistamines. The "first-generation" antihistamines—those like hydroxyzine (Atarax) and diphenhydramine (Benadryl)—are not used nearly as frequently as before. Although they are inexpensive in comparison to their successors, their side-effect profile is high. Sedation is a particularly bothersome effect, with growing evidence that even when these medications are taken at bedtime, daytime attention may be impaired, leading to decreased performance in school or work or both, as well as more serious

consequences, including motor vehicle collisions (Casale et al., 2003 ⓒ).

"Second-generation" antihistamines are much preferred now. Both fexofenadine (Allegra), either 60 mg twice daily or 180 mg daily for adults, and loratadine (Claritin)—10 mg daily for adults and children 6 years old and older—are nonsedating (the only antihistamines approved by the Federal Aviation Administration for pilots). Cetirizine (Zyrtec) is sedating to some. Its usual dose is 5 to 10 mg daily for adults and children 6 and older; 2.5 mg daily for children age 2 to 5 years.

Decongestants are often used to treat the congestion that often accompanies AR (American Academy of Allergy, Asthma and Immunology, 2005 ⓒ). The most common one is pseudoephedrine (Sudafed), the adult dose of which is 60 mg every 6 hours. It also comes in a slow-release 12-hour version (120 mg) that often causes less-pronounced sympathomimetic effects such as restlessness, dry mouth, and palpitations. Pseudoephedrine is available in numerous preparations in combination with various antihistamines.

Another decongestant used is topical: oxymetazoline (Afrin). The usual dose is two sprays in each nostril, twice daily. As mentioned earlier, patients should not use these for more than 3 to at most 5 days, or they risk rebound congestion.

Other treatments are available but much less frequently used. They include intranasal antihistamines, cromolyn sodium and ipratropium; nasal saline; and montelukast (Singulair) (can be particularly useful when congestion is a targeted symptom). A short course of oral corticosteroids is rarely given (prednisome 50 mg daily for 5 to 10 days) to relieve severe symptoms rapidly.

Finally, for selected patients, allergic immunotherapy (AIT)—so-called allergy shots—may be appropriate. AIT requires quite a time commitment (usually 3 to 5 years). It works approximately two thirds of the time. Although a few family physicians do this (along with prior diagnostic skin testing) in their offices, this therapy is usually considered in consultation with and administered by an allergy specialist.

Material Available on Student Consult

Review Questions and Answers about Allergic Rhinitis

REFERENCES

American Academy of Allergy, Asthma and Immunology. The Allergy Report: Science-Based Findings on the Diagnosis and Treatment of Allergic Disorders. Available at www.theallergyreport.org. Accessed 9/9/2005.ⓒ

Casale TB, Blaiss MP, Gelfand E, et al. First do no harm: Managing antihistamine impairment in patients with allergic rhinitis. J Allergy Clin Immunol 2003; 111:S835–S842. ⓒ

Howarth PH. Allergic and nonallergic rhinitis. In Adkinson NF, Yunginger JW, Busse WW, et al. (eds): Middleton's Allergy: Principles and Practice, 6th ed. Philadelphia, Mosby, 2003, pp 1391–1393. Ⓒ

Ledgerwood GL, Johnson RL. Allergy. In Rakel R (ed): Textbook of Family Practice, 6th ed. Philadelphia, WB Saunders, 2002, pp 473–493.

Scadding GK. Corticosteroids in the treatment of pediatric allergic rhinitis. J Clin Allergy Immunol 2001;108 (1 Suppl):S59–S64. Ⓒ

Chapter

19 Fever and Fussiness in a 22-Month-Old Child (Acute Otitis Media)

John G. O'Handley

KEY POINTS

1. Ear pain has many causes.
2. A definite diagnosis of acute otitis media (AOM) requires (1) a history of sudden onset, (2) evidence of inflammation, and (3) evidence of middle ear effusion (MEE).
3. The age of the patient and the severity of the disease dictate the use of antimicrobials and length of treatment of AOM.
4. It can take as long as 3 months for MEE to gradually resolve.
5. MEE may be monitored without treatment in patients not at risk for speech or hearing problems.
6. Antibiotics, decongestants, and antihistamines do not accelerate MEE resolution.
7. Referral to an otolaryngologist for pressure-equalization tubes should be accompanied by documentation of hearing loss and length of time MEE has persisted.

INITIAL VISIT

Subjective

Patient Identification and Presenting Problem

Hannah R. is a 22-month-old child with a 2-day history of fever, fussiness, crying, and decreased appetite. The child has also been pulling at her left ear, and when asked by her mother if it hurt, Hannah nodded in the affirmative. Three days previously, Hannah had a runny nose.

Present Illness

Hannah's mother phoned the office this morning after a night of very little sleep for both mother and daughter. She has been giving the child liquid acetaminophen every 4 hours, but the fever and fussiness returned before the medication was due again. Hannah has eaten some juice and milk but has not eaten solid food for 2 days. The family had been at a family reunion 6 days earlier, and some of the children there had been sick with colds.

Evidence levels Ⓐ Randomized, controlled trials (RCTs), meta-analyses, well-designed systematic reviews of RCTs. Ⓑ Case-control or cohort studies, nonrandomized clinical trials, systematic reviews of studies other than RCTs, cross-sectional studies, retrospective studies, certain uncontrolled studies. Ⓒ Consensus statements, expert guidelines, usual practice, opinion.

Medical History

Hannah is the product of a term vaginal delivery and has received all her appropriate immunizations. She has had colds in the past but has never been given any antibiotics. Developmental milestones are normal.

Social History

Hannah is the only child of her parents, Katie and Brendan R. Neither parent smokes. The child does not attend day care.

Review of Systems

Respiratory, gastrointestinal, genitourinary, and integumentary system reviews are noncontributory.

Objective

Physical Examination

Hannah appears to be alert and well nourished. She clings to her mother in the examination room and cries when put on the examination table. Her height is 34 inches, and her weight is 28 pounds, which puts her in the 75th percentile. Her temperature is 102.2°F. Her cheeks are flushed, but no rash is observed on any part of her body. The right ear canal is impacted with cerumen, but the left tympanic membrane (TM) is erythematous and bulging into the canal. The nose is illed with yellowish-white mucus, but the mouth is moist and the throat is clear. The neck is supple with some shotty jugulodigastric nodes present. The lungs are clear to auscultation, and the heart is regular in rate and rhythm. The abdomen is soft except when the child cries, and no masses are palpated.

Assessment

Working Diagnosis

The working diagnosis is acute otitis media (AOM) following an upper respiratory infection. Three criteria are needed to make a diagnosis of AOM: (1) signs and symptoms with an abrupt onset, (2) the presence of a middle ear effusion (MEE), and (3) signs or symptoms of middle ear inflammation (American Academy of Pediatrics/American Academy of Family Practice [AAP/AAFP], 2004 ⓒ). MEE is present with decreased mobility of the TM, bulging of the TM, an air/fluid level visible behind the TM, or pus draining from the middle ear space. Middle ear inflammation is noted by erythema of the TM or ear pain that disrupts sleep or normal activities. The erythema of AOM must be distinguished from the erythema caused by crying. The latter does not cause bulging of the TM. Tympanometry can be used to detect MEE when the physician is unsure of the presence of MEE. Pneumatic otoscopy can also aid in the diagnosis of MEE. Often the diagnosis in infants and young children remains unconfirmed, even after all

available tools have been used. In one study the prevalence of true AOM by AAP/AAFP criteria was only 70% among clinicians in a variety of settings (Rosenfeld, 2002 ⓐ). In the presence of an uncertain diagnosis, the physician must base his decision for treatment on knowledge of the patient and the reliability of the patient's family to return for follow-up.

Differential Diagnosis

Because middle ear inflammation and effusion cause pressure in a closed space, ear pain is invariably present (Table 19-1). It is not always easy to distinguish different types of ear pain, especially when the patient does not speak. Therefore, the clinician must separate the possible sources of ear pain. Sources of pain from the external ear include otitis externa or swimmer's ear. These are identified by pulling back on the external ear or applying pressure over the tragus. A foreign body in the external ear can also cause pain, and this is diagnosed by direct visualization of the canal. Ear pain can also be caused by furunculosis of the external canal, which is diagnosed by direct visualization. Inflammation of the TM itself without MEE can be the cause of pain and is referred to as myringitis or tympanitis. In addition, a cholesteatoma, although slow growing, can eventually lead to ear pain.

Pain arising from the middle ear is not always AOM. Barotrauma can be diagnosed from a recent history of deep-sea diving or airplane travel. Acute eustachian tube obstruction also can lead to pain and will eventually result in MEE. Acute mastoiditis and extradural abscess, although rare in the antibiotic era, must be considered when the origin of the ear pain remains uncertain. Table 19-1 also lists the

Table 19-1	Differential Diagnosis of Ear Pain	
External Ear	**Middle Ear**	**Referred from Elsewhere**
Otitis externa (OE)	Acute otitis media	Sinusitis
Foreign body	Barotrauma	Pharyngitis/tonsillitis
Trauma	Acute eustachian tube obstruction	TMJ syndrome
Furunculosis		Tonsillar cancer
Impacted cerumen		Trigeminal neuralgia
Tympanitis/myringitis	Acute mastoiditis	Elongated styloid process (Eagle's syndrome)
Cholesteatoma	Extradural abscess	Dental abscess
		Cervical disk disease

TMJ, temporomandibular joint.

causes of ear pain referred from other areas of the head and neck; these sources of pain must be included in the differential diagnosis when faced with ear pain in the presence of a normal ear exam.

Plan

Diagnostic

Direct visualization of the left ear reveals a bulging erythematous TM. The condition of the TM, the history of acute onset after an upper viral infection, and a fever of 102.2°F fulfill the three criteria necessary to make a diagnosis of AOM: (1) history of sudden onset, (2) MEE (bulging TM), and (3) signs or symptoms of middle ear inflammation (redness and fever) (Table 19-2). There is no need for tympanometry or pneumatic otoscopy in this case. There is no need to remove the cerumen in the right canal to observe the right TM because it would not alter the therapy.

Therapeutic

The management of pain in a patient, although often looked on as peripheral, must be addressed. The parents must be instructed to give acetaminophen or ibuprofen for mild to moderate pain because this is strongly recommended and evidence based (AAP/AAFP, 2004ⓒ). Topical benzocaine (Auralgan, Americaine Otic) can provide additional, but brief, relief and can be administered to the affected ear, 2–4 drops three or four times daily as needed. With a certain diagnosis of AOM in a child 6 months to 2 years, use of an antibacterial agent is recommended. In a child who is not penicillin allergic, the first-line choice of antimicrobial is amoxicillin in a dose of 80 to 90 mg/kg/day divided two or three times daily. The higher dose of amoxicillin improves the cure rate, especially in light of increasing *Streptococcus pneumoniae* resistance to penicillin in younger age groups.

Patient Education

It is important to inform the patient's caregiver to report any pain or fever that continues after 2 to 3 days. Persistent pain and fever could indicate that the organism is resistant to the chosen antibiotic, which must then be changed. In the case of uncertain diagnosis when the patient is being observed without antimicrobial therapy, continuation of symptoms or fever would necessitate adding antimicrobial therapy. It is important to determine whether the patient's caregiver is reliable and can afford the prescribed medication. Instructing the caregiver to call the office in 2 to 3 days, regardless of initial treatment or subsequent outcome, will improve the likelihood of proper follow-up. Resolution of MEE can take up to 3 months, so scheduling a return visit sooner than 4 weeks is not cost effective.

Disposition

Hannah's parents are asked to call back in 2 days to assess the therapy and to make an appointment in 6 weeks to have Hannah evaluated for MEE.

DISCUSSION

Diagnosis

Each patient is different in presentation of illness and response to therapy and must be treated individually. However, a subcommittee on management of otitis media of the American Academies of Pediatrics and Family Practice (AAP/AAFP, 2004ⓒ) examined an extensive body of literature and recommended guidelines that can assist clinicians in their decision-making process. The first recommendation is to establish the diagnosis of AOM. Acute onset, presence of MEE either by visualizing a bulging TM, otorrhea, or an air/fluid level behind the TM or using tympanometry or pneumatic otoscopy; and signs and symptoms of middle ear inflammation by redness of the TM or distinct otalgia are the requirements for a certain diagnosis.

Treatment

In an effort to decrease the cost and side effects of medicine and to diminish the emergence of resistant bacteria, a 2- to 3-day period of observation is recommended in children older than 2 years if the three criteria are not satisfied. In that same age group, antimicrobial treatment may be withheld if the child has a temperature less than 102.2°F and only mild pain (Table 19-3). The choice of antimicrobial is based on many factors including the severity of the illness, the age of the patient, penicillin allergy, and local experience with resistant organisms. The three main organisms at which antimicrobial therapy is aimed are *Streptococcus pneumoniae, Haemophilus influenzae,* and *Moraxella catarrhalis.* The incidence of these pathogens in AOM is 25% to 50% for *S. pneumoniae,* 15% to 30% for nontypeable *H. influenzae,* 3% to 20% for *M. catarrhalis,* and 5% to 22% for viruses. By age 12 months, 70% of children are colonized by at least

---

Table 19-2 Definition of Acute Otitis Media

1. Acute onset of signs and symptoms
2. The presence of middle ear effusion
3. Signs or symptoms of middle ear inflammation

Adapted from American Academy of Pediatrics, American Acedemy of Family Physicians. Subcommittee on Management of Acute Otitis Media. Diagnosis and management of acute otitis media. Pediatrics 2004;113:1451–1465.

Table 19-3	Criteria for Initial Treatment or Observation of Acute Otitis Media in Children	
Age	**Certain Dx**	**Uncertain Dx**
<6 mo	Antibiotics	Antiobiotics
6 mo to 2 yr	Antibiotics	Antibiotics if severe illness; otherwise, observe
>2 yr	Antibiotics if severe; otherwise, observe	Observe

From American Academy of Pediatrics, American Acedemy of Family Physicians. Subcommittee on Management of Acute Otitis Media. Diagnosis and management of acute otitis media. Pediatrics 2004;113:1451–1465.

one of these three pathogens. During viral upper respiratory infections, colonization with these organisms increases dramatically (Sinus and Allergy Health Partnership, 2000©). Amoxicillin is still the first choice to treat these pathogens, with a dose of 80 to 90 mg/kg/day in two or three doses per day. With severe AOM (temperature greater than 102.2°F or moderate to severe otalgia), amoxicillin/clavulanate (Augmentin ES-600) in a dose of 90 mg/kg/day of the amoxicillin component in two divided doses is recommended. About 29% of *S. pneumoniae* are not susceptible to penicillin because of alteration of penicillin-binding proteins. The mechanism of resistance in *H. influenzae* and *M. catarrhalis* is β-lactamase production, and currently resistance rates are running 40% and 98% for

H. influenzae and *M. catarrhalis*, respectively (Sinus and Allergy Health Partnership, 2000©). Risk factors affecting the resistance of bacteria to antimicrobials are attending day care, receiving antimicrobials within the previous 30 days, and age younger than 2 years.

When the child is penicillin allergic, other therapies must be used, depending on whether the reaction was type 1 (urticaria or anaphylaxis) or non-type 1 (Table 19-4). If the child is vomiting, ceftriaxone can be given in a dose of 50 mg/kg/day (up to 1 g IM), for 3 consecutive days.

When symptoms and signs persist after an initial treatment with amoxicillin, amoxicillin/clavulanate (Augmentin ES-600) in a dose of 90 mg/kg/day of the amoxicillin component divided every 12 hours (Table 19-5). If the child had severe AOM and was first treated with amoxicillin/clavulanate but that therapy failed, then either ceftriaxone in the previously mentioned dose or clindamycin in a dose of 8 to 25 mg/kg/day in three or four doses for 5 to 10 days may be given orally.

The duration of treatment also has been studied from an evidence-based perspective, and for children 6 years and older with mild to moderate disease, a 5- to 7-day course is appropriate. For children 5 years or younger or for any child with severe disease, as defined earlier, a 10-day course is advised.

There is no evidence supporting the use of complementary or alternative medicine for treatment of AOM (AAP/AAFP, 2004©).

Risk Factors

A number of risk factors in the etiology of AOM can be altered, reducing the chance of illness (Table 19-6). Breastfeeding children during the first 6 months of

Table 19-4	Antimicrobial Therapy in Pediatric Penicillin-allergic Patients
Drug	**Dosage**
Non–type 1 Reaction	
Cefdinir (Omnicef)	14 mg/kg/day (to a maximum of 600 mg/day) in one or two doses
Cefpodoxime (Vantin)	10 mg/kg/day (to a maximum of 400 mg/day) every 12 hr
Cefuroxime (Ceftin)	30 mg/kg/day (to a maximum of 100 mg/day) in two doses
Type 1 Reaction (Urticaria or Anaphylaxis)	
Azithromycin (Zithromax)	10 mg/kg/day on day 1 and then 5 mg/kg/day for 4 days in a single dose or 10 mg/kg/day every 24 hr for 3 days
Clarithromycin (Biaxin)	15 mg/kg/day in two doses for 5 to 10 days
Erythromycin/sulfasoxazole (Pediazole)	50 mg/kg/day in three to four doses for 5 to 10 days
Sulfamethoxazole/trimethoprim (Bactrim)	5 ml susp./10kg (up to 20 mL) per dose po bid for 5 to 10 days
Ceftriaxone (Rocephin)	50 mg/kg/day (up to 1 g) for 3 consecutive days, IM or, if vomiting, IV
Clindamycin (Cleocin)	8–25 mg/kg/day in three or four doses for 5 to 10 days

Table 19-5   Treatment after Initial Failure

Treatment after Initial Failure on Amoxicillin
Amoxicillin/ clavulanate (Augmentin ES-600):
    90 mg/kg/day of amoxicillin in two doses for
    5 to 10 days

**Treatment after Failure on Amoxicillin/
Clavulanate**
Ceftriaxone (Rocephin): 50 mg/kg/day up to 1 g IM
    in a single dose for 3 consecutive days
Clindamycin (Cleocin): 8–25 mg/kg/day in three or
    four doses for 5 to 10 days

**Table 19-6   Preventable Risk Factors for
Acute Otitis Media**

Day care attendance
Bottle feeding for the first 6 mo of life
Supine bottle feeding ("bottle propping")
Pacifier use in the second 6 mo of life
Passive tobacco smoke

**Table 19-7   Non preventable Risk Factors
for AOM**

Premature birth
Native American/Inuit ethnicity
Genetic predisposition
Male gender
Siblings in the household
Low socioeconomic status

life helps prevent early episodes of AOM. Altering day-care attendance patterns in infancy and early childhood can decrease the number of respiratory infections and significantly reduce the incidence of recurrent AOM. It is not as clear whether avoiding pacifier use, "bottle propping," and passive tobacco smoke also decrease the incidence of AOM, but some evidence supports these measures. The benefit of pneumococcal conjugate vaccines in preventing AOM is small, but some studies have shown a 6% reduction in the incidence of AOM. Risk factors that cannot be altered are listed in Table 19-7.

Natural History of MEE

MEE resolves slowly after the middle ear fluid becomes sterile. Antimicrobials will eliminate bacteria in the middle ear in 2 to 3 days. By 2 weeks, 30% to 40% of MEE will be resolved, and by 1 month, 60% of MEE will be cleared. Even at 3 months, it is possible to have 10% to 25% of patients with MEE (AAFP/AAO-HNS/AAP, 2004◉). It is important for the clinician to identify children at risk for speech,

language, or learning problems and to intervene even before 3 months. Such children include those with Down syndrome, autism, visual impairment, cleft palate, developmental delays, and permanent hearing loss independent of MEE. Management of these at-risk children includes speech and language evaluation and hearing tests. Interventions include hearing aids, tympanostomy tube insertion, and repeated hearing testing after the resolution of MEE. Little harm occurs in watchful waiting for children not at risk for speech, language, or learning problems. In the past, physicians have used antihistamines and decongestants, antimicrobials, and corticosteroids. But current evidence strongly suggests that these treatments are not efficacious in the long run and are certainly not recommended for routine management (Williamson, 2002◉). The tendency to "do something" must be avoided in healthy children with persistent MEE. Despite modest short-term benefits from antimicrobials in persistent MEE, long-term benefits have not been proven (Williamson, 2002◉). The side effects of antimicrobials also warrant avoidance of this therapy in healthy children with persistent MEE. Children not at risk may be monitored at 3-month intervals with hearing tests to determine the effect of MEE (AAFP/AAO-HNS/AAP, 2004◉). If the hearing test shows 40 dB or more loss in the affected ear, immediate referral to an otolaryngologist is recommended. If the decibel loss is between 21 and 39 (mild hearing loss), the physician has the option of surgery referral or continuing to monitor the patient at 3- to 6-month intervals. The choice is determined on an individual basis and in concert with a full discussion of the options with the patient's parents. A hearing loss of 20 dB or less may require repeated hearing evaluation and assessment for MEE in 3 to 6 months. If the clinician believes the child needs a referral to an otolaryngologist, he or she should document the episode of AOM and the length of time that the MEE has persisted. The results of hearing tests also must be communicated to the referral physician. Explaining to the parents that many alternatives exist for the management of persistent MEE and that surgery is not necessarily the desired outcome will help facilitate the referral from the parents' perspective as well. Persistent MEE in children younger than 3 years without risk factors does not require immediate insertion of PE tubes because developmental outcomes do not differ when the procedure is postponed for 6 months (Paradise, 2001◓). For children at risk (Table 19-8), surgical intervention may occur earlier to prevent the sequelae of persistent MEE. When PE tubes become the recommended procedure, adenoidectomy should not be performed unless nasal obstruction from the adenoids or chronic adenoiditis is seen. Twenty percent to 50% of children will have recurrence of MEE after the PE tubes come out, and in those cases

Table 19-8	Risk Factors for Developmental Difficulties in Children with Persistent Middle Ear Effusion

Permanent hearing loss independent of OME
Suspected or diagnosed speech and language delay or disorder
Autism–spectrum disorder and other pervasive developmental disorders
Syndromes (e.g., Down) or craniofacial disorders that include cognitive, speech, and language delays
Blindness or uncorrectable visual impairment
Cleft palate with or without associated syndrome
Developmental delay

OME, Otitis media with effusion.
Adapted from American Academy of Family Physicians, American Academy of Otolaryngology-Head and Neck Surgery, American Academy of Pediatrics. Subcommittee on Otitis Media with Effusion. Otitis media with effusion. Pediatrics 2004;113:1412–1429.

adenoidectomy plus myringotomy with or without PE tube placement should be used. In the case of a child with cleft palate and recurrent MEE, adenoidectomy is not recommended. On average, the PE tubes remain in position for 12 to 14 months and provide ventilation to the middle ear during that time.

Conclusion

In addition to the decreased incidence of AOM from the use of pneumococcal conjugate vaccines, in recent years the killed and live-attenuated intranasal influenza vaccines in children older than 2 years have been shown to reduce the incidence of AOM by 30% during the cold season. With further research the diagnosis and treatment of AOM will continue to evolve.

More antimicrobials are prescribed for AOM than for any other childhood infection in the United States. In 2000 the total number of office visits for otitis media was 16 million, and for these visits 13 million prescriptions were written. In the United States, infants in the first year of life average 1.2 episodes of AOM and 1.1 episodes in the second year of life (Baumer, 2004). The direct and indirect costs of this infection approach $3 billion per year. A large percentage of these visits are to family physicians, so it is important that physicians feel confident diagnosing and treating this common problem. The guidelines given here are meant to help the practitioner choose a course of action when he or she is unsure of how to proceed. Part of the impetus for these guidelines has been the emergence of resistant strains of organisms causing AOM, making judicious and proper use of antimicrobials important for society in general. As practitioners benefiting from experience in our own practice and information provided to us, we can continue to offer medical care that is grounded in evidence-based knowledge and affords our patients the latest in medical advances.

Material Available on Student Consult

Review Questions and Answers about Acute Otitis Media

REFERENCES

American Academy of Family Physicians, American Academy of Otolaryngology-Head and Neck Surgery, American Academy of Pediatrics (AAFP/AAO-HNS/AAP). Subcommittee on Otitis Media with Effusion. Otitis media with effusion. Pediatrics 2004;113:1412–1429.🅒

American Academy of Pediatrics, American Academy of Family Physicians. Subcommittee on Management of Acute Otitis Media. Diagnosis and management of acute otitis media. Pediatrics 2004;113:1451–1465.🅒

Baumer JH. Comparison of two otitis media guidelines. Arch Dis Child Educ Pract Ed. 2004;89:ep76–ep78.

Dowell SF, Marcy SM, Phillips WR, Gerber MA, Schwartz B. Otitis media: Principles of judicious use of antimicrobial agents. Pediatrics 1998;101:165–171.🅐

Paradise JL, Feldman HM, Campbell TF, et al. Effect of early or delayed insertion of tympanostomy tubes for persistent otitis media on developmental outcomes at the age of three years. N Engl J Med 2001;344:1179–1187.🅐

Rosenfeld RM. Diagnostic certainty for acute otitis media. Int J Pediatr Otorhinolaryngol 2002;64:89–95.🅐

Sinus and Allergy Health Partnership. Antibacterial treatment guidelines for acute bacterial rhinosinusitis. Otolaryngol Head Neck Surg 2000;123:525–531.🅒

Williamson I. Otitis media with effusion. Clin Evid 2002;7:469–476.🅒

20 Hiccups

Stephen G. Cook

INITIAL VISIT

Subjective

Patient Identification and Presenting Problem

Alice B. is a 56-year-old African-American woman who complains of continuous hiccups for the past 6 weeks. She states they have been unremitting, making it difficult for her to sleep at night and interrupting meals as well because of their frequency. She has ried a number of home remedies suggested by friends and family, including drinking water with her head upside down, holding her breath, and having friends surprise her by popping a paper bag loudly, but none of these have been successful.

Medical History

Alice has mild hypertension, for which she takes atenolol daily. She has been a two-pack-per-day smoker since age 15, although she states that she is trying to cut back. Chronic obstructive pulmonary disease was diagnosed 5 years ago, and she uses a steroid inhaler daily as well as ipratropium and albuterol inhalers when breathing difficulties worsen. She had a negative treadmill test 1 year ago after an episode of chest pain and has never had a heart attack.

Surgical History

Alice had two children by cesarean section. She also had a laparoscopic cholecystectomy 3 years before presentation.

Family History

Her father died of myocardial infarction at age 54. Her mother is alive at 81 but has diabetes and hypertension. Two brothers also have hypertension but are in otherwise good health.

Social History

She smokes two packs of cigarettes per day. She drinks a few glasses of wine several times a week. She lives with her husband of 31 years, who is also a smoker.

Review of Systems

She reports a chronic cough that is the worst in the morning and seems to have worsened in the past year. She says she has lost 10 pounds in the past 2 months. She has had no recent acute illnesses and feels generally well.

Objective

Physical Examination

Alice is a very pleasant woman who appears somewhat older than her stated age.

Vital Signs Her temperature is 36.9°C (98.5°F), blood pressure is 142/86, pulse is 100 and regular, respiratory rate is 16, weight is 135 pounds, and height is 67 inches.

Skin Leathery skin with deep creases and wrinkles around her eyes and mouth but warm and well perfused.

Head, Eyes, Ears, Nose, and Throat Tympanic membranes are unremarkable. Teeth are yellow stained but without significant caries; tongue is mildly

---

Evidence levels Ⓐ Randomized, controlled trials (RCTs), meta-analyses, well-designed systematic reviews of RCTs. Ⓑ Case-control or cohort studies, nonrandomized clinical trials, systematic reviews of studies other than RCTs, cross-sectional studies, retrospective studies, certain uncontrolled studies. Ⓒ Consensus statements, expert guidelines, usual practice, opinion.

yellow stained as well. No other abnormalities of oropharynx or nares.

Neck No thyromegaly; shotty nontender adenopathy in posterior and anterior cervical chains.

Lungs Hiccups noted with a frequency of one per 5 to 10 seconds. Distant breath sounds with faint end-expiratory wheezes but no rales or rhonchi. The expiratory phase is notably prolonged, with an inspiratory:expiratory ratio of 1:3.

Heart Regular rate and rhythm; no murmurs, gallops or rubs.

Abdomen Nondistended abdomen with minimal amount of subcutaneous fat. Normal bowel sounds. No masses or hepatosplenomegaly. No tenderness to palpation or percussion.

Neurologic Alert, pleasant female in no apparent distress. Speaks in full sentences except as interrupted by her hiccups.

Extremities Yellow-stained fingers; thinly muscled arms and legs with normal distal pulses.

Assessment

Working Diagnosis

Hiccups are an extremely common malady, affecting all ages from newborns to the very elderly. The medical term for hiccups is singultus, although it is probably best to refer to this common disorder by its common name. While quite annoying, they most often are a benign and self-limited problem. Patients normally do not present for medical attention for hiccups unless the occurrence is quite prolonged.

"Acute hiccups" are episodes up to 48 hours in duration. "Persistent hiccups" are defined as those lasting longer than 2 days. Episodes lasting longer than 1 month are termed "intractable hiccups" (Viera and Sullivan, 2001❸). Although hiccups themselves are benign, prolonged cases of hiccups have been associated with other morbidity including weight loss, exhaustion, insomnia, anxiety, and even suicide (Schiff et al., 2002); cases of aspiration pneumonia and respiratory arrest have been described (Moretti et al., 2004 ❸). Because intractable hiccups can be an indication of severe underlying disease, patients presenting with this complaint should be evaluated thoroughly.

Despite their prevalence, understanding of both the cause and purpose of hiccups remains limited.

Technically, hiccups are an involuntary spasmodic contraction of the diaphragm followed by sudden closure of the glottis, which causes the characteristic hiccup sound. The hiccup reflex arc consists of the vagus and phrenic nerves, as well as the sympathetic chain arising from T6-12. Irritation of the phrenic or vagus nerves anywhere along their course is thought to result in spasm of the diaphragm and external intercostal muscles (Schiff et al., 2002). However, central nervous system abnormalities, toxins, drugs, and metabolic disorders can lead to hiccups as well, possibly by removing inhibitory control of an inspiratory nucleus in the brain (Moretti et al., 2004❸).

More than 100 causes of hiccups have been identified, most of which are gastrointestinal (Box 20-1). Gastroesophageal reflux disease is perhaps the most frequently identifiable cause. A full medication list is essential in working up this problem. In fact, many of the same drugs used to treat hiccups can also cause them. Hiccups have also been described as a complication following surgery, including laparoscopic procedures such as Nissen fundoplication. Of the more sinister possible causes, head/neck and chest or mediastinal masses may impinge on the phrenic or vagus nerves. Appropriate imaging studies to look for these should be used (Smith and Busracamwongs, 2003❸).

Plan

Diagnostic

Alice is classified as having intractable hiccups. Her medications (atenolol, inhaled steroids, ipratropium, and albuterol) are unlikely to be causal. She has a history of laparoscopic abdominal surgery, but Alice's hiccups arose long after surgery. While her physical examination does not immediately reveal a cause, she has a number of physical signs consistent with her long-term tobacco use; therefore, further evaluation of her chest and lungs is indicated.

A complete metabolic panel is normal. A chest radiograph reveals that Alice has a mass obscuring the right hilum. She is referred for bronchoscopy and biopsy, which reveals squamous cell carcinoma arising from the right mainstem bronchus.

Therapeutic

As hiccups are predominantly a symptom rather than an illness in themselves, therapy is first directed toward treating an underlying cause if one can be identified. Due to the size of the tumor at the time of presentation, Alice is referred to oncology, where she is scheduled to begin chemotherapy and radiation treatment to shrink the tumor.

Treatment options for the hiccups themselves are numerous, but it should be noted that no treatment

---

Box 20-1	**Partial List of Causes of Hiccups**

Gastrointestinal Causes

Gastroesophageal reflux disease
Gastric distention or insufflation
Esophageal or small bowel obstruction
Excessive food or alcohol intake
Sudden change in gastric temperature
Aerophagia

Tumor Masses, Benign or Malignant

Head/neck tumors, including goiter
Mediastinal masses
Lung/chest masses

Metabolic Causes

Diabetes mellitus
Hyponatremia
Hypocalcemia
Addison's disease
Uremia

Medications/Toxins

Neuroleptics
Corticosteroids
Benzodiazepines
Alcohol
Tobacco use

Central Nervous System Diseases

Stroke
Arteriovenous malformation
Cerebral contusion or hematoma
Temporal arteritis
Encephalitis or meningitis
Neurosyphilis
Multiple sclerosis
Hydrocephalus

Infectious Diseases

Psychogenic Causes

Other Causes

Laparoscopic surgery
Laryngeal mask airway insertion
Foreign body in external ear canal
Epidural steroid injection

Idiopathic Causes

---

method has been proven effective by evidence-based criteria, and no one treatment has been shown to be better than another. The literature is rife with therapies ranging from drug treatments to acupuncture (Schiff et al., 2002). One case report even indicates sexual intercourse may be a treatment for chronic intractable hiccups (Peleg and Peleg, 2000).

Most patients have tried a wide range of home remedies before presentation. Most home remedies seem to work by either stimulating the nasopharynx or by disrupting the normal respiratory cycle: Drinking ice water, breath holding, and being spooked all are part of the popular repertoire, as are a variety of Valsalva maneuvers. Others, like breathing in and out of a paper bag, seem to work in part because hiccups decrease as CO_2 rises. Still others, like drinking out of the far side of a glass, are based on little but folklore (Viera and Sullivan, 2001Ⓑ).

Once the patient presents for assistance, some simple in-office efforts, such as elevating the uvula with a cotton-tipped applicator or stimulating the nasopharynx with a rubber catheter, may be successful. If these fail, numerous medications have been used to treat hiccups, all with varying degrees of

success (Viera and Sullivan, 2001Ⓑ). These include a wide range of drug classes:

1. Neuroleptics such as haloperidol (Haldol) or chlorpromazine (Thorazine)
2. Anticonvulsants including phenytoin (Dilantin), gabapentin (Neurontin), and valproate (Depakote)
3. Gastrointestinal motility drugs like metoclopramide (Reglan)
4. Antihypertensives, especially nifedipine (Procardia)
5. Muscle relaxants such as baclofen (Lioresal)

Case reports of other medications being used include lidocaine by IV infusion or nebulizer, atropine, and methylphenidate (Ritalin) (Moretti et al., 2004Ⓑ). In the most severe cases, surgical management such as phrenic nerve interruption or the placement of diaphragmatic pacemakers has been used. (Viera and Sullivan, 2001Ⓑ).

Patient Education

Again, information should primarily attend to the underlying cause if one is identified. If medications are used to treat hiccups, patients should be aware of the potential side effects of the agent being employed. For instance, if neuroleptic drugs are used, patients should be aware of normal concerns for extrapyramidal side effects.

FOLLOW-UP VISIT

Subjective

Alice returns to clinic after her first week of chemotherapy. She continues to report persistent hiccups. She has lost an additional 5 pounds and still is unable to sleep through the night. She says that she thinks the hiccups are worse than the effects of chemotherapy.

Objective

Alice appears visibly more fatigued, with dark circles under her eyes. Aside from her weight decreasing to 130 pounds, her examination is unchanged.

Assessment

Alice's hiccups are most likely caused by direct irritation of the phrenic and vagus nerves by the tumor surrounding her bronchus. Thus, treatment options are limited while the tumor continues to affect the nerves. It is possible that if chemotherapy and radiation are successful in shrinking her tumor, her hiccups might be alleviated. If they persist, surgical ligation of the phrenic nerve may be considered.

Plan

Alice says she is desperate to get rid of her hiccups. She is started on gabapentin (Neurontin), 400 mg orally three times per day for 3 days, then reduced to 400 mg orally once daily, based on case reports of success with this in neurologic patients (Moretti et al., 2004Ⓑ). She understands that this treatment is not based on proven efficacy by normal standards and is informed of possible side effects.

Material Available on Student Consult
Review Questions and Answers about Hiccups

REFERENCES

Moretti R, Torre P, Antonello RM, Ukmar M, Cazzato G, Bava A. Gabapentin as a drug therapy of intractable hiccup because of vascular lesion: A three-year follow up. Neurologist 2004;10:102–106.Ⓑ

Peleg R, Peleg A. Case report: Sexual intercourse as potential treatment for intractable hiccups. Can Fam Physician 2000;46:1631–1632.

Schiff E, River Y, Oliven A, Odeh M. Acupuncture therapy for persistent hiccups. Am J Med Sci 2002;323:166–168.

Smith HS, Busracamwongs A. Management of hiccups in the palliative care population. Am J Hospice Palliative Care 2003;20:149–154.Ⓑ

Viera A, Sullivan SA. Remedies for prolonged hiccups. Am Fam Physician 2001;63:1684–1685.Ⓑ

21 Fever without Source in Children (Fever)

Jennifer E. Lochner

INITIAL VISIT

Subjective

Patient Identification and Presenting Problem

Zoe W. is a 5-week-old infant brought in by her father for evaluation of fever. He first noted that she felt "warm" a few hours ago. He took her temperature with a tympanic thermometer and found it to be 38.2°C (100.7°F). Dad reports that she seems somewhat more fussy than usual but otherwise is acting normally (eating well with the usual number of wet and dirty diapers per day). He has noted no cough, nasal congestion, or rash.

Medical History

Zoe was the product of an uncomplicated pregnancy and spontaneous vaginal delivery at 39 weeks. She went home from the hospital on day 2 of life. This is the first health problem that she has encountered in her life. She has not yet had any vaccinations and is exclusively breast-fed.

Family History

Zoe has no siblings. Her father has hypothyroidism, and her mother has no medical problems.

Social Hstory

Zoe lives at home with her parents and two pet cats. No one in the home smokes. She is cared for by her parents and is not in day care. There are no ill contacts.

Review of Systems

Zoe's father has not noted any apparent difficulties with breathing. Zoe frequently spits up a small amount of breast milk after eating; this is unchanged from usual. There is no bilious vomiting or diarrhea.

Objective

Physical Examination

General Zoe is an alert and interactive infant who is fussy with examination but easily consolable by her father.

Vital Signs Her blood pressure is 86/42, pulse is 110, respiratory rate is 32, rectal temperature is 38.6°C (101.5°F), and weight is 5.1 kg (11.2 pounds).

Head, Eyes, Ears, Nose, and Throat Her anterior fontanelle is soft and open, and her pupils are equal, round, and reactive to light; there is no nasal discharge. Her posterior pharynx has no redness or exudate.

Neck There is no cervical lymphadenopathy.

Heart The heart has a regular rate and rhythm without murmur.

Lungs The lungs are clear to auscultation bilaterally.

Abdomen Soft; bowel sounds are present. The abdomen is nontender and nondistended with no mass.

Extremities Extremities are warm, with capillary refill less than 2 seconds at the fingers and toes.

Neurology Zoe moves all four extremities.

Skin No rash is noted.

Assessment

Working Diagnosis
Fever without source in a 5-week-old infant.

DISCUSSION

Evaluation of Infants and Children Younger than 36 Months of Age with Fever without Source

Fever is defined as a rectal temperature of 38°C (100.4°F) or higher. Other methods of measuring temperature (oral, axillary, tympanic) are not accurate measures of core body temperature and therefore are considered not to be sufficiently reliable to assess for fever in infants and children. Fever without source refers to an acute febrile illness in which the etiology of the fever is not apparent after a careful history and physical examination.

With an SBI constituting a low percentage of the causes of fever in infants and children, many other causes are more likely. Viruses are by far the most likely culprit. Some viruses are easily identified by their clinical syndrome (e.g., varicella), but most have nonspecific syndromes and some appear only to cause fever. Self-limited febrile illnesses that have no source identified are presumed to have been viral in nature.

The main goal of evaluation of infants and young children with fever is to distinguish those with mild self-limiting illness from those with SBIs (meningitis, sepsis, bone and joint infection, urinary tract infection, pneumonia, enteritis). This is more difficult than in older children and adults due to the failure of clinical signs and symptoms alone in reliably differentiating these two groups (Baker et al., 1990[B]). Younger children also have a higher incidence of SBI than their older counterparts. It is these two principles that form the underlying basis for the guidelines that follow.

The youngest classification of febrile infants includes those age 28 days and younger. They appear to be at highest risk of SBI with studies showing that 7% to 16% of febrile infants in this age category to have an SBI (Baker and Bell, 1999[B]; Chiu et al., 1994[B]; Ferrera et al., 1997[B]; Kadish et al., 2000[B]).

These studies showed variable utility of guidelines such as the Rochester criteria (Table 21-1) in identifying which febrile young infants are at lowest risk of SBI. The percentage of infants classified in the lowest risk group who were eventually found to have an SBI varied from 0.4% to 6.4% (Baker and Bell, 1999[B]; Chiu et al., 1994[B]; Ferrera et al., 1997[B]; Kadish et al., 2000[B]). Because of this variability and the potentially serious risk in missing an SBI, there is general agreement that all febrile infants age 28 days and younger should have a full evaluation for SBI including admission to the hospital for cerebrospinal fluid, blood, and urine cultures, with coverage with parenteral antibiotics while awaiting culture results (Baraff et al., 1993[C]). This is true regardless of how well the infant may appear, whether the infant meets all the low-risk criteria, and whether the infant has signs and symptoms of a less serious source of infection (e.g., upper respiratory infection, otitis media). A slight variation in this recommendation comes from Jaskiewicz et al. (1994[B]) who, based on the results of their study, propose this evaluation, but with careful inpatient observation without parenteral antibiotics while awaiting culture results for infants age 28 days and younger who meet all the Rochester criteria for low risk of SBI. These options are included in Figure 21-1.

Older infants (28 to 90 days old) are the next group considered. In this age group, the Rochester criteria discussed previously have also been used to identify infants at low risk of SBI. With fewer reports of infants meeting low-risk criteria being found to have an SBI (and those eventually found to have an SBI subsequently doing well after an initial delay in treatment), options exist as to the management of this group of patients (Baraff et al., 1993[C]). Parent and physician level of concern and acceptability of risk guide the approach to evaluation rather than a strict set of guidelines. An aggressive strategy identical to that described for infants 28 days and younger (admission to the hospital for cerebrospinal fluid, blood, and urine cultures, with coverage with parenteral antibiotics while awaiting culture results) can also reasonably be used in infants 28 to 90 days old. Alternatively, if a patient meets all the Rochester criteria described in Table 21-1, less aggressive strategies may be used. The first option is blood, urine, and cerebrospinal fluid cultures with parenteral antibiotics but with outpatient rather than inpatient follow-up. A second option is urine culture only with no empirical antibiotics, also with close outpatient follow-up. The physician must feel comfortable with the parent's ability to adhere to the close monitoring and follow-up needed before a less aggressive strategy for management is chosen. Infants who do not meet low-risk criteria should be evaluated aggressively with hospital admission, cultures, and empirical antibiotics while awaiting culture results.

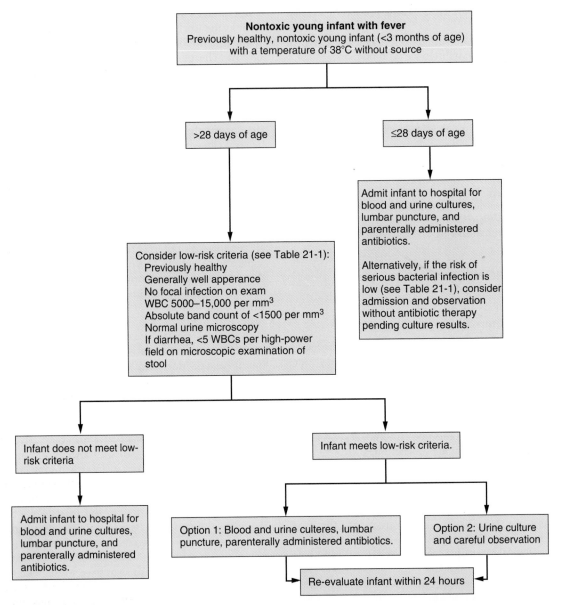

Nontoxic young infant with fever
Previously healthy, nontoxic young infant (<3 months of age) with a temperature of 38°C without source

>28 days of age

≤28 days of age

Admit infant to hospital for blood and urine cultures, lumbar puncture, and parenterally administered antibiotics.

Alternatively, if the risk of serious bacterial infection is low (see Table 21-1), consider admission and observation without antibiotic therapy pending culture results.

Consider low-risk criteria (see Table 21-1):
Previously healthy
Generally well apperance
No focal infection on exam
WBC 5000–15,000 per mm³
Absolute band count of <1500 per mm³
Normal urine microscopy
If diarrhea, <5 WBCs per high-power field on microscopic examination of stool

Infant does not meet low-risk criteria

Infant meets low-risk criteria.

Admit infant to hospital for blood and urine cultures, lumbar puncture, and parenterally administered antibiotics.

Option 1: Blood and urine culteres, lumbar puncture, parenterally administered antibiotics.

Option 2: Urine culture and careful observation

Re-evaluate infant within 24 hours

Figure 21-1 Algorithm for the management of nontoxic young infants with a temperature of 38°C (100.4°F) without source. (Modified with permission from Baraff LJ, Bass JW, Fleisher GR, et al. Practice guideline for the management of infants and children 0 to 36 months of age with fever without source. Pediatrics 1993;92:1–12.)

Remember also that included in the Rochester criteria are the results of evaluations including white blood cell count (WBC) and urinalysis, so none of these recommendations include decision making based on clinical appearance alone. See Figure 21-1 for an algorithm of the above.

Evaluation of Children Age 3 Months to 3 Years with Fever without Source

Children age 3 months to 3 years with fever without source are at lower risk than their younger counter-

parts of developing significant sequelae including sepsis and meningitis. Children with higher fevers and higher WBCs are at higher risk. Although these facts help guide decision making, controversy exists over the optimal management of these children. In evaluating fever without source in this age group, temperature is the first factor used in deciding further evaluation. In children with a temperature lower than 39°C (102.2°F) and no focus of infection identified on a careful physical examination, no initial tests or antibiotics are indicated if the child appears well. If fever persists or the child has

Table 21-1 Rochester Criteria for Identifying Febrile Infants at Low Risk of Serious Bacterial Infection

Infant appears generally well
Infant has been previously healthy
    Born at term (≥37 weeks' gestation)
    No perinatal antimicrobial therapy
    No treatment for unexplained hyperbilirubinemia
    No previous antimicrobial therapy
    No previous hospitalization
    No chronic or underlying illness
    Not hospitalized longer than mother
Infant has no evidence of skin, soft-tissue, bone, joint, or ear infection
Infant has these laboratory values
    White blood cell count 5000–15,000/mm³
    Absolute band count ≤1500/mm³
    ≤10 white blood cells per high-power field on microscopic examination of the urine
    ≤5 white blood cells per high-power field on microscopic examination of stool in infant with diarrhea

worsening symptoms, re-evaluation is necessary. With temperatures higher than 39°C (102.2°F), options for evaluation are more complicated and are outlined in Figure 21-2 (Luszczak, 2001). Urinary tract infections are a significant cause of fever without source in this age group, and urine culture is recommended in male infants younger than 6 months old and female infants younger than 2 years old because these are the highest risk groups for urinary tract infections. In making the decision as to whether blood cultures and/or empirical antibiotics are indicated, the WBC count may be of assistance. It remains an option to obtain blood cultures and empirically treat all children aged 3 months to 3 years with fever higher than 39°C (102.2°F) with parenteral antibiotics. Another option is to use the cutoff of a WBC of less than 15,000 to identify children at lower risk of SBI in whom it is reasonable to not obtain these studies. Both groups of children require close follow-up (within 24 to 48 hours) to identify any localizing signs of infection or clinical deterioration (Baraff et al., 1993©).

Issues in Diagnostic Evaluation of Children with Fever

Method of Obtaining Urine

Urethral catheterization and suprapubic aspiration are the best methods for obtaining urine for use in evaluation of the infant or child with fever. Bag collection of urine results in an unacceptably high false-positive rate on urine culture. If, however, a bag urine

sample results in a negative culture, this is considered adequate in ruling out a urinary tract infection (American College of Emergency Physicians Clinical Policies Committee: American College of Emergency Physicians Clinical Policies Subcommittee on Pediatric Fever, 2003⑧).

Urinalysis Versus Urine Culture

For children younger than 2 years old, urinalysis has not been shown to be sensitive enough to rule out urinary tract infection. As many as 10% to 50% of patients eventually shown to have a urinary tract infection (by urine culture) had a negative urinalysis. Urine microscopy also has inadequate sensitivity in ruling out urinary tract infection (American College of Emergency Physicians Clinical Policies Committee: American College of Emergency Physicians Clinical Policies Subcommittee on Pediatric Fever, 2003 ⑧). For this reason urine culture is necessary to determine whether a child younger than age 2 years has a urinary tract infection.

Utility of a Chest Radiograph

In the absence of signs or symptoms of respiratory infection, it is highly unlikely that a chest radiograph will be abnormal in children younger than 3 months of age (Bramson et al., 1993⑧). It has been reported in children older than 3 months, however, that a small but significant percentage of children without respiratory signs or symptoms but with temperatures higher than 39°C (102.2°F) and a WBC count of more than 20,000 have occult pneumonia as the source of their illness (Bachur et al., 1999⑧). A chest radiograph should be considered in this group of patients but is not necessary in the evaluation of children younger than 3 months who do not have signs or symptoms of respiratory illness.

Other Issues

Toxic Appearance Toxic-appearing infants and children are those who appear lethargic and have signs of poor perfusion, hypoventilation, hyperventilation, or cyanosis. They constitute a separate category and warrant immediate and intensive evaluation and either treatment aimed at an identifiable cause of illness or empirical antibiotic therapy while awaiting culture results.

Children with Chronic Illnesses Another category of children not addressed thus far are those with known chronic illnesses (e.g., congenital heart disease, cystic fibrosis, human immunodeficiency virus disease). Such children are at much higher risk of SBI and complications from infections and therefore warrant aggressive evaluation and treatment of febrile illnesses.

Persistent Fever In some cases, a fever may persist without a source being identified. Fever of unknown

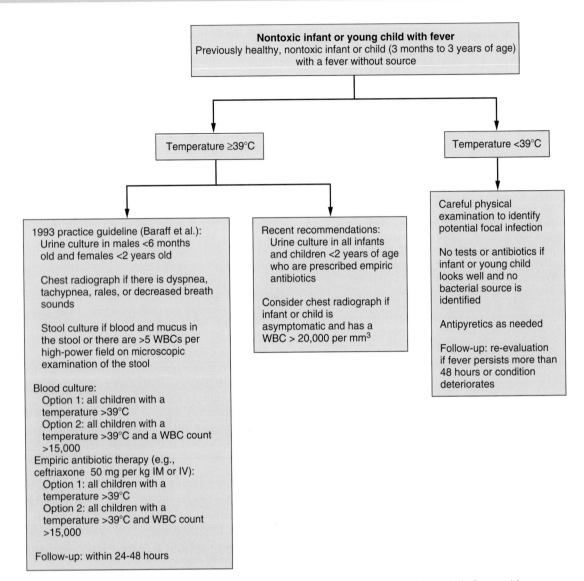

Figure 21-2 Algorithm for the management of nontoxic infants and young children with fever without source. (Modified with permission from Baraff LJ, Bass JW, Fleisher GR, et al. Practice guideline for the management of infants and children 0 to 36 months of age with fever without source. Pediatrics 1993;92:1–12.)

origin is a specific term referring to a fever whose source has not been identified after 3 weeks of evaluation in the outpatient setting or 1 week of evaluation in the inpatient setting. Although infections remain high on the list of possible diagnoses in these patients, it is important to remember that fever can be caused by illnesses other than infections. Rheumatologic diseases, neoplasms, inflammatory disease, and diseases of hypersensitivity such as drug fevers are important considerations. The evaluation for such diseases may appropriately include serum biochemical analysis, imaging such as computed tomography or magnetic resonance imaging, and biopsy of any potentially abnormal areas identified.

Effect of Newer Vaccines on the Risk of Serious Bacterial Infection in Children Until recently, the types of bacteria most commonly identified in children with SBI included *Streptococcus pneumoniae* and *Haemophilus influenzae* type B (Hib). It has already been demonstrated that since the introduction of the vaccine against *H. influenzae* type B, the rates of SBI cause by this pathogen have significantly declined (Black and Shinefield, 1992❸). It remains to be seen the extent to which the same may be true of invasive pneumococcal disease as more and more children are vaccinated with the conjugated pneumococcal vaccine active against seven of the most pathogenic serotypes of *S. pneumoniae*. If the overall rates of SBI decline as expected in response to this vaccine, the preceding recommendations for the evaluation of children with fever could significantly change.

Plan

Based on historical and clinical information, Zoe appeared to be at low risk of an SBI. To complete the assessment as to whether she met the low-risk Rochester criteria, a WBC count and urinalysis were performed. Results included a WBC count of 11,300, an absolute band count of 300, and a normal urinalysis with fewer than five white blood cells per high-power field. With this information, Zoe's father and physician came to the decision that her risk of serious infection was low, and both preferred to avoid further invasive testing with lumbar puncture. Zoe's father agreed to carefully observe her for any further signs of illness and to bring her back for evaluation the next day. Zoe's urine was sent for culture in the meantime.

Follow-up

In the clinic the next day, Zoe's father reported that she had continued to look well, and that she was eating, urinating, defecating, and breathing normally. Her temperature taken at the clinic was 38.1°C (100.6°F) rectally; the rest of her examination remained unremarkable. Urine culture returned showing no growth. Again, close parental monitoring was discussed, and she returned home with instructions for the father to call the clinic the next day to report how she was doing. By the next day, she remained well and axillary temperature had come down to 37.2°C (99.0°F). She continued to remain well and afebrile thereafter with no source for her fever having been identified.

Material Available on Student Consult

Review Questions and Answers about Fever

REFERENCES

American College of Emergency Physicians Clinical Policies Committee: American College of Emergency Physicians Clinical Policies Subcommittee on Pediatric Fever. Clinical policy for children younger than three years presenting to the emergency department with fever. Ann Emerg Med 2003;42:530–545.**C**

Bachur R, Perry H, Harper MB. Occult pneumonias: Empiric chest radiographs in febrile children with leukocytosis. Ann Emerg Med 1999;33:166–173.**B**

Baker MD, Anver JR, Bell LM. Failure of infant observation scales in detecting serious illness in 4- to 8-week-old infants. Pediatrics 1990;85:1040–1043.**B**

Baker MD, Bell LM. Unpredictability of serious bacterial illness in febrile infants from birth to 1 month of age. Arch Pediatr Adolesc Med 1999;153:508–511.**B**

Baraff LJ, Bass JW, Fleisher GR, et al. Practice guideline for the management of infants and children 0 to 36 months of age with fever without source. Pediatrics 1993;92:1–12.**C**

Black SB, Shinefield HR. Immunization with oligosaccharide conjugate Haemophilus influenzae type B (HbOC) vaccine on a large health maintenance organization population: Extended follow-up and impact on *Haemophilus influenzae* disease epidemiology. The Kaiser Permanente Pediatric Vaccine Study Group. Pediatr Infect Dis J 1992;11:610–613.**B**

Bramson RT, Meyer TL, Silbiger ML, et al. The futility of the chest radiograph in the febrile infant without respiratory symptoms. Pediatrics 1993;92:524–526.**B**

Chiu CH, Lin TY, Bullard MJ. Application of criteria identifying febrile outpatient neonates at low risk for bacterial infections. Pediatr Infect Dis J 1994;13:946–949.**B**

Ferrera PC, Bartfield JM, Snyder HS. Neonatal fever: Utility of the Rochester criteria in determining low risk for serious bacterial infection. Am J Emerg Med 1997;15:299–302.**B**

Jaskiewicz JA, McCarthy CA, Richardson AC, et al. Febrile infants at low risk for serious bacterial infection—an appraisal of the Rochester criteria and implications for management. Febrile Infant Collaborative Study Group. Pediatrics 1994;94:390–396.**B**

Kadish HA, Loveridge B, Tobey J, et al. Applying outpatient protocols in infants 1–28 days of age: Can the threshold be lowered? Clin Pediatr 2000;39:81–88.**B**

Luszczak M. Evaluation and management of infants and young children with fever. Am Fam Physician 2001;64:1219–1226.**C**

22 Cough (Possible Asthma)

Frank J. Domino and Robert A. Baldor

KEY POINTS

1. Chronic cough (cough lasting longer than 4 weeks) is common.
2. Cough in the first hour after eating or that is worse while supine may reflect gastro-esophageal reflux.
3. A single wheeze pitch with discrete starting and stopping points and cough should encourage evaluation for foreign body aspiration or tracheomalacia.
4. For some asthmatics, cough is the most prominent symptom of their illness.
5. Tuberculosis may be subtle in children; tuberculin skin testing should be considered if the child is at high risk of exposure.

INITIAL VISIT

Subjective

Patient Identification and Presenting Problem

K.M. is a 9-year-old boy who presents to your office for follow-up of a cough.

Present Illness

Three weeks ago K.M. came to your office for a cough that had persisted for over a month. Your associate examined him but could not make a definitive diagnosis. He treated him with erythromycin empirically for "bronchitis." K.M.'s mom now reports that he continues to cough intermittently, especially at night.

Medical and Surgical History

K.M. has been very healthy in general. He has not had any hospitalizations or surgery. His immuniza-

tions are up to date. He takes no medications except for a daily multivitamin. He has no known drug allergies.

Family History

His mother and father are healthy, although his father smokes cigarettes. K.M. has a 15-year-old sister who is healthy and without any medical problems.

Personal and Social History

K.M. lives with his parents, his sister, and a cat. He plays soccer and does well in school (getting As and Bs).

Review of Systems

General: healthy male, born by spontaneous vaginal delivery at 39 weeks without complications; has made all developmental and growth milestones without difficulty. Head, eyes, ears, nose, and throat: 2 to 3 months of slight "itchy" eyes and sneezing in the mornings and at night but less so at school. Respiratory: cough is dry and nonproductive; no shortness of breath recognized. Dermatologic: last winter had "blotches" after showers and sporting activities. Other systems benign.

Objective

Physical Examination

General K.M. is a well-appearing male in no acute distress.

Vital Signs Temperature is 37.2°C (99.0°F), respiratory rate is 12, blood pressure is 96/55, and pulse is 88.

Head, Eyes, Ears, Nose, and Throat Tympanic membranes are clear; nasal turbinates are bulging and erythematous. Oropharynx is slightly reddened and injected; no postnasal drip.

Neck No lymphadenopathy.

Evidence levels Ⓐ Randomized, controlled trials (RCTs), meta-analyses, well-designed systematic reviews of RCTs. Ⓑ Case-control or cohort studies, nonrandomized clinical trials, systematic reviews of studies other than RCTs, cross-sectional studies, retrospective studies, certain uncontrolled studies. Ⓒ Consensus statements, expert guidelines, usual practice, opinion.

Lungs Positive breath sounds in all fields; no rales or rhonchi.

Abdomen Positive bowel sounds, soft, nontender, no hepatosplenomegaly.

Extremities No clubbing, cyanosis, or edema.

Assessment

Working Diagnosis

Chronic cough. Cough lasting longer than 4 weeks is common, with an estimated prevalence of 5% to 7% in preschoolers and 12% to 15% in older children. It is more common in boys than in girls up to 11 years of age and may be less common in developing countries than in affluent countries (Bush, 2002©; Chang and Powell, 1998©; Chung and Chang, 2002©).

Differential Diagnosis

The differential diganosis for a chronic cough includes cough-variant asthma, gastroesophageal reflux disease (GERD), allergic rhinitis, chronic sinusitis, cough receptor hypersensitivity, chronic pulmonary infection, cardiac disease, cystic fibrosis, functional disorders, and some combination of these diagnoses (Bush, 2002©).

1. *Cough-variant asthma.* For some asthmatics, cough is the most prominent symptom of their illness. Individuals with cough-variant asthma typically have atopy and reversible obstruction. Initial empirical treatment of these children includes bronchodilators with appropriate holding chamber (spacer) or oral theophylline (National Institutes of Health et al., 2004 ©). Some literature exists that the use of oral steroids in combination with inhaled beta agonists does not provide benefit in relieving cough (Chung and Chang, 2002 ©).
2. *GERD.* Little is known about the prevalence and natural history of GERD in children and adolescents. Children at increased risk of GERD include those with neuromuscular disorders such as muscular dystrophy, cerebral palsy, cystic fibrosis, and Down syndrome. Children with GERD may be at increased risk of developing respiratory complications, including aspiration pneumonia.
3. *Allergic rhinitis.* This syndrome is characterized by paroxysms of sneezing, rhinorrhea, nasal obstruction, and itching of the eyes, nose, and palate. It is frequently associated with postnasal drip, cough, irritability, and fatigue. It can be further classified as seasonal if symptoms typically occur at a particular time of the year or perennial if they occur year round.
4. *Chronic sinusitis.* This is typically uncommon in pediatric populations. Its presence should alert the physician to consider cystic fibrosis or nasal polyps. Rarely, fungal elements may play a role.

5. *Increased cough receptor sensitivity.* Some children appear to have increased cough receptor sensitivity. The etiology of this hypersensitivity may be viral illness or other exposures.
6. *Habit cough.* Psychogenic (habit) cough is a common type of chronic cough in children and adolescents. The cough is a barking or honking sound after a short inhalation. It may develop following an upper respiratory infection. It is typically absent at night and when the child is otherwise engaged. Its presence can result in significant secondary gain for the child, as it often results in multiple physician visits and disrupts the school classroom. The cough may worsen when attention is paid to it in the doctor's office. Habit cough is a diagnosis of exclusion and can be related to Tourette's syndrome or tic disorders (Tan et al., 2004 ©).

When history and physical examination do not provide a single diagnosis, then two or more of the listed causes in combination may be the etiology. Alternatively, functional disorders (including habit cough and tic) should be considered.

Plan

Diagnostic

The diagnosis is often made on the basis of history and examination. Additional testing may be of value, but sensitivities are low in pediatric populations, and if the cough does not appear to be of serious etiology, further testing may lead to unnecessary exposures and false securities. Pulmonary function tests can be considered. When performed optimally, spirometry may show signs of obstruction when obstructive disorders and restriction in interstitial or chest wall restrictive processes are present. This test measures FEV_1 (forced expiratory volume in 1 second) and forced vital capacity and, when the result is positive, can help make the diagnosis (Faniran et al., 1999 ©). False results may occur if the child exerts a suboptimal effort; this will result in a restrictive picture.

FEV_1 less than 80% implies an obstructive pattern. Following a positive test or when a test is normal but asthma is suspected, a bronchodilator can be given. Should the patient have a greater than 12% improvement in FEV_1, reversible obstructive disorders like asthma can be diagnosed. However, a lack of a response to a bronchodilator does not rule out an obstructive disorder.

Bronchoprovocation is the most sensitive method for determining reactive obstruction. It can be accomplished by using methacholine, cold air, or exercise, as these may induce acute bronchospasm; bronchoprovocation may be contraindicated in some age groups.

Peak expiratory flow rate is easy to measure but is very dependent on the patient's abilities. Thus its role is to monitor an asthmatic's status over time rather than to make the diagnosis of asthma.

In younger children with chronic cough, aspiration of a foreign body should be considered. In such cases a chest radiograph should be ordered. If a history of aspiration is likely, a computed tomography scan may be needed. Finally, because the presentation of tuberculosis may be subtle in children, tuberculin skin testing should be considered if the child is at high risk of exposure.

Therapeutic
Empirical therapy for asthma (albuterol inhaler), allergic rhinitis (steroid inhaler), sinusitis (antibiotic, steroid inhaler), or GERD (raising head of bed, not eating 2 hours before bedtime) can be implemented when history and/or physical examination suggest that these will be helpful.

When no clear diagnosis is discerned, a trial of over-the-counter cough or cold medicine can be considered, but there are no data supporting the effectiveness of these medicines for cough. Often the physician can do little other than reassure the patient and provide close follow-up. If secondary gain or psychological stress plays a role, cognitive-behavioral therapy may be tried. For psychogenic cough, successful therapies include hypnosis, suggestion, and biofeedback.

Patient Education
In the case of a chronic cough without other worrisome signs, the patient should be reassured that the condition is not serious but may improve with careful attention to potentially aggravating environmental factors (Schwartz, 2004; Smith et al., 2000). In this case, K.M. is exhibiting allergic symptomatology, and his father is advised to quit smoking or at least to smoke outside the home. In addition, K.M. is advised to limit his exposure to cats, and the cat should not be allowed to sleep in his room. If medication is prescribed, correct instructions in its use must be given, and the patient must be encouraged to have patience with medications (inhaled nasal steroids, for example) that may take several doses to take effect.

Disposition
K.M. is started on a steroid nasal inhaler, beclomethasone (42 μg/spray), one spray in each nostril twice daily. He is advised to use the inhaler faithfully over the next 10 days and to return to the office for reassessment in 2 weeks. Depending on his response to this empirical therapy, further testing/treatment will be considered at that time.

DISCUSSION

Chronic cough in children can have many etiologies, but the diagnosis can often be made with attention to a careful history and physical examination. The medical history should include an account of the pregnancy, labor, and delivery, as well as the neonatal course. Low-birth-weight and/or premature neonates are at risk of developing atopic sensitization and asthma. Neonates who are small for gestational age may have congenital infection. In addition, prematurity and neonatal respiratory distress syndromes are precursors for bronchopulmonary dysplasia, which in turn may predispose to chronic lung disease.

Additional historical features may help lead to a diagnosis. Chronic paroxysmal cough triggered by exercise, cold air, sleep, or allergens is often seen in patients with asthma. Cough due to asthma typically occurs following exposure to characteristic asthma triggers (i.e., allergens, smoke, exercise, cold air), and typically worsens during sleep (Bush, 2002; Stein et al., 1999; National Institutes of Health et al., 2004).

A chronic productive (or wet) cough suggests a suppurative process and may require further investigation to exclude bronchiectasis, cystic fibrosis, active infection, immune deficiency, or congenital malformation.

Cough that appears in the first hour after eating or that is worse when the patient is supine may reflect GERD. Although cough due to postnasal drip is also typically worse during changes of position, in this case the patient is more likely to complain of a tickle in the back of the throat, and this maybe accompanied by a nasal discharge.

Barking or a brassy cough suggests a process in the trachea or more proximal airways, such as airway malacia, laryngotracheobronchitis, and foreign body.

Psychogenic cough is present during the day, disappears at night, and is typically the worst and most disruptive during school classes. Cough that is honking ("Canada goose–like") and disappears at night suggests a psychogenic or habitual cough.

A careful history should be obtained for current illness in family members or close contacts; such individuals with cough, weight loss, and night sweats should arouse suspicion of tuberculosis. Family history of atopy or asthma increases the risk in offspring and suggests a diagnosis of either allergic rhinitis or asthma in the child with chronic cough.

It is also important to obtain a information on who lives in the home with the child and the travel histories of these people. Indoor exposures also play a role. Wood-burning and gas stoves can cause respiratory symptoms. Second-hand or active exposure to smoke from tobacco, marijuana, cocaine, or other substances can result in chronic cough. Contact with pets can lead to allergy or asthma-induced cough.

Ascertaining whether there has been a response to previous treatments may discern the cause of chronic cough. Response to antihistamines suggests rhinitis and postnasal drip, whereas response to an empirical trial of inhaled bronchodilators may suggest asthma. Previous response to medications, and in particular antibiotics, must be interpreted with special caution, as many causes of cough are self-limiting, and cessation of symptoms may have been coincidental (Schroeder and Fahey, 2002Ⓐ).

Finally, when performing the physical examination, close attention should be paid to the following signs:

- Delayed growth or developmental milestone attainment
- Extremes of weight (wasting or obesity)
- "Shiners" (bluish discolorations under the eyes), swollen nasal turbinates, nasal polyps, allergic nasal crease, scarred tympanic membranes, halitosis, tonsillar hypertrophy, pharyngeal cobblestoning, high arched or cleft palate, hoarseness
- Respiratory rate, retractions, accessory muscle use, abnormal breath sounds (reduced intensity, wheezing, stridor, crackles)

- Murmurs, abnormal heart sounds, abnormal pulses
- Hepato- and/or splenomegaly, abdominal masses
- Edema, cyanosis, and/or clubbing of the digits

The character of a wheeze may give some clue to its etiology. Wheezing with different pitches, associated with cough, is typical of asthma. In children with this type of wheeze and atopic symptoms (rhinitis, conjunctivitis, and/or eczema), asthma is the likely cause of the cough (Bush, 2002Ⓒ; National Institutes of Health et al., 2004Ⓒ).

A single wheeze pitch with discrete starting and stopping points and cough should encourage evaluation for foreign body aspiration or tracheomalacia.

Material Available on Student Consult

Review Questions and Answers about Possible Asthma

REFERENCES

Bush A. Paediatric problems of cough. Pulm Pharmacol Ther 2002;15:309–315.Ⓒ

Chang AB, Powell CV. Non-specific cough in children: Diagnosis and treatment. Hosp Med 1998;59:680–684.Ⓒ

Chung KF, Chang AB. Therapy for cough: Active agents. Pulm Pharmacol Ther 2002;15:335–338.Ⓒ

Faniran AO, Peat JK, Woolcock AJ. Measuring persistent cough in children in epidemiological studies: Development of a questionnaire and assessment of prevalence in two countries. Chest 1999;115:434–439.Ⓐ

Schroeder K, Fahey T. Should we advise parents to administer over the counter cough medicines for acute cough? Systematic review of randomised controlled trials. Arch Dis Child 2002;86:170–179.Ⓐ

Schwartz J. Air pollution and children's health. Pediatrics 2004;113:1037–1043.Ⓒ

Smith KR, Samet JM, Romieu I, Bruce N. Indoor air pollution in developing countries and acute lower respiratory infections in children. Thorax 2000;55:518–532.Ⓒ

Stein RT, Holberg CJ, Sherrill D, et al. Influence of parental smoking on respiratory symptoms during the first decade of life: The Tucson Children's Respiratory Study. Am J Epidemiol 1999;149:1030–1037.Ⓑ

Tan H, Buyukavci M, Arik A. Tourette's syndrome manifests as chronic persistent cough. Yonsei Med J 2004;45:145–149.Ⓒ

National Institutes of Health, National Heart, Lung and Blood Institute. National Asthma Education and Prevention Program. Guidelines for the Diagnosis and Management of Asthma—Update on Selected Topics 2002 and Expert Panel Report 2 (1997). Available at www.nhlbi.nih.gov/guidelines/asthma/index.htm. Accessed 9/15/2004.Ⓒ

23 Insomnia

Venita W. Morell

KEY POINTS

1. Insomnia is a symptom that can be caused by many disease states or environmental conditions. To best treat the insomnia complaint, find the cause and target treatment to that specific cause.
2. The evaluation of a patient complaining of insomnia relies primarily on the excellent history and physical examination. Laboratory testing and other evaluation are often unnecessary.
3. Polysomnography should be reserved for patients refractory to treatment, patients suspected of having a sleep-related breathing or limb movement disorder, or those with chronic insomnia without a diagnosable medical, neurologic, or psychiatric cause.

INITIAL VISIT

Subjective

Present Illness

Janet B., a 30-year-old white woman with asymptomatic human immunodeficiency virus infection on highly active antiretroviral therapy, is in the clinic for her 3-month checkup. She recently had a change of social situation and is now living in her parents' home and working during the day. She complains of insomnia and requests sleeping pills. Before this change, she slept 5 hours during the day, worked at night, and was not bothered by sleep-related issues. Now, she tries to go to bed with the rest of the household at about 9 PM but remains awake until after midnight. Once she falls asleep, she does not wake until 6 AM. She has always experienced episodes at work when she feels sleepy but denies falling asleep easily during the day or while performing activities

such as driving. She does occasionally nap. She denies restless leg sensation or any discomfort or distraction that seems to interfere with her ability to fall asleep. She has a history of depression but denies any exacerbation of her depressive symptoms at present. She snores occasionally.

Medical History

Janet contracted human immunodeficiency virus 8 years ago through sexual contact. She elected to take highly active antiretroviral therapy 2 years ago when testing of her viral load showed an increase in the amount of virus in her blood and showed that her CD4 counts had begun to decline. She has been on the same highly active antiretroviral therapy regimen for 2 years.

She has chronic depression, which has been well controlled with medication. No other medical or surgical history is noted.

Family History

Janet is an only child. Both parents smoke cigarettes and are suspected alcohol abusers.

Social History

Janet is single and sexually abstinent. She works full time as a clerk in a convenience store. She smokes one pack of cigarettes per day and occasionally marijuana. She drinks two to four beers per day. Caffeine is consumed in soda and iced tea in as many as six drinks per day. She has no known allergies to medicine.

Her current medications are efavirenz (Sustiva) 600 mg at bedtime, a lamivudine/zidovudine combination (Combivir) twice daily, fluoxetine (Prozac) 20 mg once daily, and a multiple vitamin daily.

Objective

Physical Examination

Janet is a well-developed, well-nourished, alert, white woman in no distress. She smells strongly of tobacco smoke. Her vital signs are all within normal limits.

Her head and neck examination shows no abnormality of the airway or thyroid, and no lymphadenopathy is noted. Her lungs are clear. Her cardiac examination is unremarkable. Her extremities show no edema. Her abdomen is benign. A detailed neurologic examination is unremarkable. Her mood is normal and her affect is normally reactive. Her thought is normal.

Assessment

Differential Diagnosis

Insomnia is a symptom, not a disease. Insomnia can be caused by many different disease states or can be the perception of impaired sleep in the absence of any disease state or true sleep problem (Mahowald et al., 1997◉). The patient with insomnia may describe inadequate quantity or quality of sleep. Like Janet, patients complaining of insomnia may have difficulty initiating sleep. They may also have difficulty maintaining the sleep state, or they may wake frequently or early. Patients may complain of daytime sleepiness or may wake feeling unrefreshed.

Documenting the specifics of the sleep problem and the duration of the problem helps generate the differential diagnosis of insomnia. For example, acute insomnia of less than 3 weeks' duration may have different causes than more chronic symptoms. Common causes of transient insomnia include the following (Graeber, 1994):

- Uncomfortable sleep environment (noise, light, temperature, unfamiliar surroundings)
- Change in sleep/wake cycle (shift change)
- Mental stress (worry about work, school, or family dysfunction)
- Acute illness
- Central nervous system stimulants (caffeine or decongestants)
- Jet lag

Janet's symptoms have been present for longer than 3 weeks, and thus the differential diagnosis must consider causes of chronic insomnia (Chokroverty, 2004◉). These include the following:

- Medical disorders (the nocturnal dyspnea associated with congestive cardiomyopathy)
- Medications (efavirenz for human immunodeficiency virus treatment or theophylline for asthma)
- Chronic illicit drug or alcohol use
- Psychiatric disorders (anxiety may cause delayed or disrupted sleep, psychosis may cause extreme sleep disruption, and depression typically causes early morning awakening but sometimes may cause delayed sleep)
- Primary sleep disorders (idiopathic/childhood-onset insomnia or psychophysiologic insomnia as a developed response after stress)

- Sleep state misperception (normal sleep pattern in a patient who perceives insomnia)
- Inadequate sleep hygiene (poor habits to promote sleep)
- Insufficient sleep syndrome (chronic accumulated lack of enough time in sleep)
- Altitude insomnia (accompanying other symptoms at altitudes of more than 4000 m)
- Restless legs syndrome (urge to move legs often accompanied by uncomfortable sensations that worsen at rest) (Consensus Recommendation from an Expert Panel, 2004◉)
- Periodic limb movement disorder (intermittent limb flexion)
- Central sleep apnea syndrome (usually associated with daytime sleepiness)
- Circadian rhythm disorders (normal function during waking hours and normal sleep but shifting of the normal sleep period)

Janet's insomnia may have multiple causes. She is noted to snore, but without excessive daytime sleepiness, sleep apnea is unlikely. She suffers from depression, but this problem seems to be well controlled and does not seem to be a contributor to her insomnia complaint. Her normal physical examination and history do not indicate any uncontrolled medical illness that would interfere with her sleep. She does take a prescription medication, efavirenz, which is known to interfere with sleep, but she has taken this medication since long before her insomnia complaint arose. She does ingest alcohol on a daily basis; chronic alcohol ingestion may be interfering with her sleep patterns. Her sleep hygiene, especially related to the use of stimulants such as tobacco and caffeine, can be improved. Janet may also have some degree of sleep state misrepresentation. She does not complain of daytime sleepiness or seem impaired by the lack of restorative sleep. The insomnia complaint did not occur until she needed to adjust her routine to fit the patterns of a new household and define her sleep to new norms.

Plan

Testing and Consultation

Patients presenting with insomnia complaints should have a complete history and physical examination performed. The history should include specifics of any drug use that may affect sleep, any chronic alcohol use, psychiatric problems, family history of sleep problems, and any medical or neurologic problems. Because insomnia is primarily a clinical diagnosis, there are no laboratory evaluations that are routinely recommended for evaluation of patients with this complaint. However, there are several studies that may be helpful.

Completion of a sleep log is often helpful in obtaining detailed information about the time a patient attempts to sleep and the time he or she actually spends asleep. The patient should also record comments about any related issues, such as perceived impediments to sleep, changes in daily routine, or daytime naps. The sleep log helps clarify the history for the clinician and can also clarify insomnia issues for the patient.

Multiple sleep latency testing can also be helpful. This informal assessment of daytime sleepiness can be accomplished by asking the patient to attempt to nap in a dark room four or five times during the day for as long as 20 minutes. If sleep occurs within that time, especially if it occurs within only minutes and on all occasions, pathologic daytime sleepiness is suspected and diagnoses that lead to insufficient restorative sleep are highly suspect. Without excessive daytime sleepiness, the diagnosis of sleep apnea syndrome or insufficient sleep syndrome, for example, is unlikely.

Actigraphy and polysomnography are also available for evaluation of insomnia complaints. In actigraphy, sensors are used to detect movement, and patients are assumed to be in a sleep state when movement is absent and awake when movement is documented. When used in correlation with a sleep log, actigraphy can be useful in diagnosing causes of insomnia or in helping patients identify sleep state misperception.

Polysomnography is generally done in a sleep laboratory, although there are home tests available with less elaborate sensor readings. A combination of sensors records respiratory air flow, heart rate, muscle activity, brain wave activity, and other activity. In sleep laboratories, the patient is also observed or videotaped. The electroencephalographic recording of waves associated with the sleep state can be correlated with other sensor readings and used to diagnose the cause of sleep disruption. The American Sleep Disorders Association Standards of Practice Committee Guidelines do not suggest polysomnographic testing for the routine evaluation of insomnia. These guidelines suggest polysomnography may be helpful when (1) a sleep-related breathing or limb movement disorder is suspected; (2) chronic insomnia without medical, neurologic, or psychiatric cause is present; or (3) a treatment-refractory insomnia exists (Committee of the American Sleep Disorders Association, 1995🅐, 1997🅐).

In some areas, expert consultation with a physician specializing in sleep disorders may also be available.

Treatment

All patients should be asked to pay attention to their sleep hygiene. Here are commonsense sleep hygiene measures to discuss:

- Avoid the use of stimulants in pre-bedtime hours (including caffeine, nicotine, and over-the-counter medications such as decongestants).
- Get regular exercise, but do not perform vigorous exercise in the hours before bedtime.
- Provide a comfortable sleep environment (temperature, lighting, bedding, noise, lack of hunger, empty bladder, use of minor analgesics for pain).
- Avoid alcohol near bedtime.
- Reduce stress and worry overall, and deal with distracting worries before bedtime.
- Maintain a regular schedule for sleep and waking, even on weekends.
- Create a bedtime routine.
- Do not nap during the day.

In addition to these generally recognized sleep hygiene principles, Bootzin's stimulus control technique discusses the use of the bedroom for sleep and sex exclusively. If the patient cannot sleep within a reasonable amount of time, he or she is instructed to leave the bedroom and to return when sleepy. Eventually, the bed comes to be associated with sleep in the patient's mind.

Various forms of relaxation therapies have helped patients with insomnia fall asleep. Techniques such as progressive muscle relaxation, biofeedback, and deep breathing can be quickly taught by the office practitioner. Additionally, sleep restriction therapy, which involves the time allotted for sleep each progressive day, has been successfully used to help address insomnia (Lacks and Morin, 1993).

The main treatment of insomnia is nonpharmacologic, but careful use of hypnotic medication may also be indicated. Pharmacologic treatment of insomnia should be used only after nonpharmacologic treatment options have been instituted. Although hypnotic medications are very effective short-term treatments for insomnia, they do not work well for the treatment of chronic insomnia. In addition, hypnotic medications may be contraindicated in pregnant patients because of concerns about their effects on the developing fetus and in some patients with compromised renal, hepatic, or pulmonary function.

Benzodiazepines are among the most commonly used hypnotic medications. These may cause amnesia, rebound insomnia, daytime somnolence, and exacerbation of anxiety disorders. When used long term, dependence on and tolerance to the medications develop. As a result, dosage must be increased to maintain hypnotic effects in the patient, and withdrawal symptoms occur when the medication is discontinued. Benzodiazepines should be used with caution when used to treat chronic insomnia.

Zolpidem (Ambien) and zaleplon (Sonata) do not have a benzodiazepine structure but act through the benzodiazepine receptor. Other nonbenzodiazepine hypnotics that have been used for insomnia include antidepressants with sedative side effects, such as the tricyclics, and sedating antihistamines. These medications may cause daytime sleepiness as well as other side effect problems. Their effect as hypnotic agents is transient, as tolerance to the side effect develops, making them ineffective for use in treating chronic insomnia.

It is best to identify and treat a specific disease state that may be the cause of insomnia symptoms, while avoiding the use of general hypnotic medication. For example, patients with restless legs syndrome benefit greatly from targeted treatment for that illness. Patients with sleep apnea will show improvement in their daytime sleepiness if their nighttime ventilation is improved. Likewise, the sleep of patients with depression improves with treatment of underlying psychiatric disease.

FOLLOW-UP

Janet completes a sleep log and participates in a multiple sleep latency test. This demonstrates she is sleeping about 7 hours a night and napping 30 minutes to an hour during the evening. She does not fall asleep during most of her nap opportunities, con-firming the absence of excessive daytime sleepiness. These results reassure her that she does not have a serious insomnia problem and support the diagnosis of sleep state misrepresentation. We discuss sleep hygiene relevant to her case. She succeeds in eliminating her evening naps, cutting down her alcohol intake, and avoiding caffeine after lunchtime. She also is told to get up from the bed if unable to sleep within 20 minutes, to go to the family room to read, and to return to bed when sleepy. She is encouraged to stop smoking and increase aerobic exercise, but she is not receptive to these changes. We instruct Janet in the technique of progressive muscle relaxation while lying in bed attempting to sleep. Finally, she is given a small quantity of zolpidem to use as often as twice weekly when all conservative measures fail to help her fall asleep by midnight. After a month, she reports using the zolpidem only once, and states she is rarely troubled by difficulty falling asleep. We will continue to address tobacco cessation and exercise with her in the future.

Material Available on Student Consult

Review Questions and Answers about Insomina

REFERENCES

Chokroverty S. Epidemiology and causes of insomnia. Available at www.uptodate.com, 2004. Ⓐ

Consensus Recommendation from an Expert Panel. Restless legs syndrome: Diagnosis and treatment strategies for the primary care provider. 2004;5.Ⓐ

Graeber RC. Jet lag and sleep disruption. In Kryger MH, Roth T, Dement WC, eds. Principles and Practice of Sleep Medicine. Philadelphia, WB Saunders, 1994, p 463.

Mahowald MW, Chokroverty S, Kader G, Schenck CH. Sleep disorders. Continuum. A Program of the American Academy of Neurology, 1997, p 48.Ⓒ

Lacks P, Morin CM. Recent advances in the assessment and treatment of insomnia. J Consult Clin Psychol 1993;60:586–594.

Practice parameters for the use of polysomnography in the evaluation of insomnia. Standards of Practice Committee of the American Sleep Disorders Association. Sleep 1995;18:55–57.Ⓐ

Practice parameters for the indications for polysomnography and related procedures. Polysomnography Task Force, American Sleep Disorders Association Standards of Practice Committee. Sleep 1997;20:406–422.Ⓐ

24 Pruritus (Atopic Dermatitis)

Jennifer E. Lochner

KEY POINTS

1. Itch is a nociceptive sensation with some similarities to pain.
2. Dermatologic conditions commonly cause itch, but systemic illness may cause itch as well.
3. Treatment of itch may be general in nature or specific to the source condition.

INITIAL VISIT

Subjective

Patient Identification and Presenting Problem

Steven J. is a 17-year-old young man who presents to the clinic with intractable itching. He states that he has had "eczema" since childhood and that his current symptoms seem to be related to a flare of his eczema. He reports red, dry patches over various parts of his body with intense itching. It seems to get worse the more he scratches it, but the itching is so intense that he simply cannot avoid scratching. He has tried moisturizing creams, which he thinks help relieve some of the dryness, but the itching persists. He has also tried over-the-counter hydrocortisone 1% cream (which has worked for his eczema in the past) with minimal relief.

Medical History

In addition to the eczema reported, Steven has seasonal allergies that are controlled with over-the-counter antihistamines. He reports no other medical illnesses or surgeries.

Family History

Steven's mother has a similar history of seasonal allergies. His father and two siblings are alive and well.

Social History

Steven lives with his parents and siblings. He is a junior in high school and denies using tobacco, alcohol, and illicit drugs.

Review of Systems

Steven reports feeling otherwise well and specifically denies headache, shortness of breath, chest discomfort, abdominal pain, and bladder or bowel symptoms.

Objective

Physical Examination

Steven is an alert male who is actively scratching his arms but is otherwise in no apparent distress. His blood pressure is 126/68, pulse is 62, temperature is 37.1°C (98.8°F), respiration is 16, height is 5 feet 10 inches, and weight is 180 pounds. Skin examination shows thick, red, dry patches over the flexor surfaces of his wrists, elbows, knees, and ankles. No pustules or papules are noted.

Assessment

Working Diagnosis

Itch caused by atopic dermatitis.

DISCUSSION

Itch, also called pruritus, is most easily defined as an unpleasant sensation that evokes the desire to scratch. It is similar to pain in that it is a modality of nociception with a reflex response. With pain, the reflex is to withdraw from the source, whereas with itch, the reflex is to scratch the source.

Itch has been found to be mediated by C fibers that transmit signals via the spinothalamic tract to the cerebral cortex. No single mechanism exists to trigger these signals, and in fact several different

---

Evidence levels Ⓐ Randomized, controlled trials (RCTs), meta-analyses, well-designed systematic reviews of RCTs. Ⓑ Case-control or cohort studies, nonrandomized clinical trials, systematic reviews of studies other than RCTs, cross-sectional studies, retrospective studies, certain uncontrolled studies. Ⓒ Consensus statements, expert guidelines, usual practice, opinion.

neurotransmitters have been implicated in the generation of itch. Histamine is well known for its involvement in allergy-associated pruritus. Other substances that appear to be involved in various types of itch include serotonin, substance P, and opioids.

Categories of itch have been proposed based on their differing origins. It is possible for itch in a single clinical entity to be explained by more than one type of itch. The classic example of this is atopic dermatitis in which it appears that both prurioceptive and neurogenic itch are involved.

Prurioceptive Itch

Prurioceptive itch originates in the skin. Inflammation or other skin damage is the source; C nerve fibers transmit the itch message. Common examples of this type of itch include the itch of dry skin and insect bites.

Neuropathic Itch

Neuropathic itch originates in the afferent nerve pathway of itch. Diseases that can affect this pathway and induce itch include postherpetic neuralgia and multiple sclerosis.

Neurogenic Itch

Neurogenic itch originates centrally but without evidence of damage in the nervous system pathway. Chemicals such as opioids, whether endogenous or exogenous, induce itch via this mechanism.

Psychogenic Itch

Psychogenic itch is associated with psychologic abnormalities such as delusional states and obsessive compulsive disorders (Yosipovitch et al., 2003).

Differential Diagnosis of Itch

In most cases of itch, a clinically apparent dermatologic condition is the source.

Common Dermatologic Conditions Associated with Itch

Atopic Dermatitis
It is still not clear whether the itch precedes or follows the rash seen in atopic dermatitis (also known as atopic eczema or simply eczema). It is clear that no matter what the initial inciting event is, a vicious cycle of itch and scratch follows in which the damage induced by scratching makes the itch worse and induces further scratching. Atopic dermatitis often has its onset in childhood and may persist into adulthood. It is often associated with other atopic

diseases including asthma and allergic rhinitis. Common locations of the rash in atopic dermatitis include the flexor surfaces of the elbows, wrists, knees, and ankles. Acutely, skin appears swollen and red in poorly defined areas. When present more chronically, skin tends to thicken from the persistent scratching. Dryness can lead to painful fissures.

Xerosis
Xerosis refers to dry skin. As a source of itch, it is most common in older adults and affects the lower legs, back, flank, abdomen, and waist. Scratching the dry skin results in red plaques with fissures.

Allergic Contact Dermatitis
An itchy rash can develop in response to contact with particular substances in susceptible people. Poison ivy is a common cause of such a rash. The rash is typically erythematous with overlying vesicles and sharply demarcated borders.

Scabies
Scabies can be easily diagnosed when it presents with the typical burrows in web spaces of the fingers. Other times it presents less specifically with red pruritic papules. Itch can be intense both before treatment and as long as a week afterward due to the continued presence of organisms in the skin.

Psoriasis
Skin findings in psoriasis include papules and plaques covered with a silvery scale. Some types of psoriasis include pustules as well. Distribution can be isolated to a particular body part or generalized. Commonly affected areas include the elbows, knees, scalp, and intertriginous areas.

A more complete list of dermatologic causes of pruritus can be found in Table 24-1.

Systemic Causes of Itch

When no clear dermatologic source of itch is apparent, systemic sources of itch should be considered. Additionally, when appropriate treatment for a dermatologic source of itch (such as xerosis) does not result in abatement of symptoms, systemic disease should be considered as an additional source of itch.

Cholestasis and Liver Disease
The specific details of the pathogenesis of itch in cholestasis are not understood; there may be more than one contributing factor. It has been suggested that impaired secretion of bile leads to an accumulation of some pruritogenic substance. Levels of bile salts themselves, however, appear not to be correlated with the level of itch. Significant evidence exists that endogenous opioids play a role in pruritus in cholestasis, and many treatments aimed at

Table 24-1 Dermatologic Causes of Pruritus

Diagnosis	Features
Allergic contact	Sharply demarcated erythematous lesion with dermatitis overlying vesicles; reaction within 2–7 days of exposure
Atopic dermatitis	"Itch that rashes (when scratched)" in patients with atopic conditions (e.g., allergic rhinitis, asthma); involvement of flexor wrists and ankles as well as antecubital and popliteal fossae
Bullous pemphigoid	Initially pruritic urticarial lesions, often in intertriginous areas; formation of tense blisters after urticaria
Cutaneous T-cell lymphoma (mycosis fungoides)	Oval eczematous patch on skin with no sun exposure (e.g., buttocks); possible presentation as new eczematous dermatitis in older adults; possible presentation as erythroderma (exfoliative dermatitis)
Dermatitis herpetiformis	Rare vesicular dermatitis affecting lumbosacral spine, elbows, or knees
Folliculitis	Pruritus out of proportion to appearance of dermatitis; papules and pustules at follicular sites on chest, back, or thigh
Lichen planus	Lesions often located on the flexor wrists, the "6 Ps": pruritus, polygonal, planar, purple papules, and plaques
Pediculosis (lice infestation)	Occiput of school-age children; genitalia in adults (sexually transmitted disease)
Psoriasis	Plaques on extensor extremities, low back, palms, soles, and scalp
Scabies	Burrows in hand web spaces, axillae, and genitalia; hyperkeratotic plaques, pruritic papules, or scales; face and scalp affected in children but not in adults
Sunburn	Possible photosensitizing cause (e.g., nonsteroidal anti-inflammatory drugs, cosmetics)
Xerotic eczema	Intense itching in elderly patients (often during winter months in northern climates); involvement of back, flank, abdomen, waist, and distal extremities

Reprinted with permission from Moses S. Pruritus. Am Fam Physician 2003;68:1135–1142, 1145–1146.

antagonizing the opioid receptor appear to have some benefit. Diseases that involve cholestasis include primary biliary sclerosis, primary sclerosing cholangitis, and cholestasis of pregnancy.

Some liver diseases classified as primarily non-holestatic have been associated with itch as well. Patients with alcoholic cirrhosis, viral hepatitis, and autoimmune hepatitis have been found to have pruritus with varying frequency. Again, the pathogenesis is not well understood in these cases, and management should be the same as in cholestasis.

Uremia

Itch has been reported in 25% to 85% of patients with renal failure but appears to be becoming less prevalent due to improved dialysis techniques. The exact reason for itch in uremia is not completely understood, but accumulation of endogenous opioids has been proposed as a contributing factor.

Human Immunodeficiency Virus Disease

Many diseases associated with itch, both dermatologic (e.g., scabies, xerosis) and nondermatologic (chronic renal or liver disease), are associated with human immunodeficiency virus disease. It also appears that

human immunodeficiency virus itself can cause itch because itch has been found in patients with human immunodeficiency virus but no other infection or condition known to be associated with itch.

Medication Effect

Opioids are the medications most clearly known to induce itch. Epidural and spinal anesthesia have the highest incidence of associated itch with an incidence of 30% to 100% (Szarvas et al., 2003), but itch is also a well-known side effect of intravenous and intramuscular administration. The exact route by which opioids exert this pruritogenic effect is not known. Evidence of the involvement of serotonin in the pathway includes the fact that ondansetron, a 5-HT3 antagonist, has been shown to relieve itch after intrathecal morphine (Yeh et al., 2000 Ⓐ).

Other systemic causes of itch are described in Table 24-2.

Pregnancy-Related Causes

Pruritus has been reported in 3% to 14% of all pregnancies (Sherard and Atkinson, 2001). The causes unique to pregnancy are discussed in the following sections.

Table 24-2 Systemic Causes of Pruritus

Cause	Features
Cholestasis	Intense itching (hands, feet, pressure sites) that becomes worse at night; reactive hyperpigmentation that spares the middle of the back (butterfly-shaped dermatitis)
Chronic renal failure	Severe paroxysms of generalized itching, worse in summer
Delusions of parasitosis	Focal erosions on exposed areas of arms and legs
Hodgkin's lymphoma	Prolonged generalized pruritus often preceding diagnosis
Human immunodeficiency virus infection	A common presenting symptom resulting from secondary causes (eczema, drug reaction, eosinophilic folliculitis, seborrhea)
Hyperthyroidism	Warm, moist skin; possibly pretibial edema; associated conditions: onycholysis, hyperpigmentation, vitiligo
Iron deficiency anemia	Signs in addition to pruritus: glossitis, angular cheilitis
Malignant carcinoid	Intermittent head and neck flushing with explosive diarrhea
Multiple myeloma	In elderly patients: bone pain, headache, cachexia, anemia, renal failure
Neurodermatitis or neurotic excoriations	Bouts of intense itching that may awaken patients from sound sleep; involvement of scalp, neck, wrist, extensor elbow, outer leg, ankle, and perineum
Parasitic infections	Usually in returning travelers or immigrants
Filariasis	Tropical parasite responsible for lymphedema
Schistosomiasis	Freshwater exposure in Africa, the Mediterranean area, or South America
Onchocerciasis	Transmitted by black fly in Africa or Latin America
Trichinosis	Ingestion of undercooked pork, bear, wild bear, or walrus meat
Parvovirus B19 infection	"Slapped cheek" appearance in children; arthritis in some adults
Peripheral neuropathy	
Brachioradial pruritus	Involvement of lateral arm in white patients who have traveled to the tropics
Herpes zoster	Pruritus accompanying painful prodrome 2 days before appearance of rash
Notalgia paresthetica	Pruritus in middle of back with hyperpigmented patch
Polycythemia rubra vera	Pricking-type itch persisting for hours after hot shower or bath
Scleroderma	Nonpitting extremity edema, erythema, and intense pruritus; edema phase with pruritus occurring before fibrosis of skin
Urticaria	Response to allergen, cold, heat, exercise, sunlight, or direct pressure
Weight loss (rapid) in eating disorders	Signs in addition to pruritus: hair loss, fine lanugo hair on back and cheeks, yellow skin discoloration, petechiae

Reprinted with permission from Moses S. Pruritus. Am Fam Physician 2003;68:1135–1142, 1145–1146.

Pruritic Urticarial Papules and Plaques of Pregnancy Most commonly, this disorder presents with erythematous urticarial plaques and papules. Other variations have been observed, however, including vesicles and target lesions. Lesions tend to first appear within abdominal striae and then spread to the rest of the trunk and extremities. Pruritic urticarial papules and plaques of pregnancy are most common in primigravidas, with most cases beginning in the third trimester and resolving after delivery, although it is possible for this condition to first appear in the immediate postpartum period. The increased incidence in twin pregnancies and increased maternal weight gain suggest that the physical stretching of the skin plays an etiologic role. Treatment involves topical steroids and antihistamines. Prognosis is excellent with no fetal risks identified. The condition is unlikely to recur with subsequent pregnancies.

Herpes Gestationis Occurring in approximately one in 50,000 pregnancies, herpes gestationis is uncommon. It presents with an intensely pruritic urticarial lesion on the trunk in the second or third trimester. It then spreads to the rest of the body, sparing only the face, palms, soles, and mucous membranes. Most cases spontaneously remit in the late third trimester, although it may flare at delivery or in the postpartum period. Flares have also been reported with the use of oral contraceptives postpartum and with menses. Diagnosis can be confirmed with skin biopsy showing C3 complement in a linear band along the basement membrane. Treatment is with systemic corticosteroids. Controversy exists as to whether the fetus is at risk with this disease. Initial reports showed no fetal risks, but subsequent studies have shown an increased risk of stillbirth, prematurity, and low birth weight (Sherard and Atkinson, 2001). With these data, third trimester fetal monitoring is recommended, including non-stress tests and amniotic fluid volume evaluations. Herpes gestationis is likely to recur in subsequent pregnancies.

Intrahepatic Cholestasis of Pregnancy The dermatitis in this disorder is from scratching. Pruritus may or may not be accompanied by jaundice. It most typically develops in the third trimester with the itch most

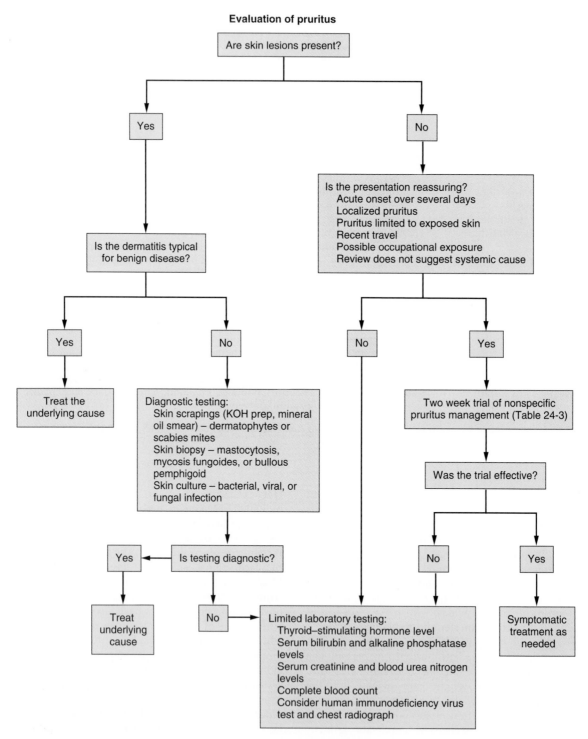

Figure 24-1 Algorithm for the evaluation of pruritus. (Adapted from Moses S. Pruritus. Am Fam Physician 2003;68: 1135–1142, 1145–1146.)

prominent on the palms, soles, and trunk. In cholestasis of pregnancy, laboratory studies rather than skin biopsy findings are diagnostic. Bile acids (cholic acid, deoxycholic acid, and chenodeoxycholic acid), direct bilirubin, and aspartate aminotransferase are all elevated. As with many other disorders related to pregnancy, the signs and symptoms disappear within 1 to 2 weeks of delivery. Cholestasis of pregnancy commonly recurs with subsequent pregnancies. Most worrisome with cholestasis of pregnancy is the increase in perinatal morbidity including prematurity and stillbirth. For this reason, fetal surveillance is warranted with delivery as soon as fetal lung maturity is established.

Evaluation of Itch

Because the majority of causes of itch are due to dermatologic disease, a thorough history and physical examination will yield a diagnosis in most cases. Exposure history is important in suspected contact dermatitis or itch due to infectious agents such as scabies. Skin examination is often diagnostic and may need to include microscopic examination of scrapings or skin biopsy if clinical appearance cannot rule out more serious skin disease such as cutaneous T-cell lymphoma. The physical examination should not be limited to the skin, however, especially if the skin examination is found to be normal. Systemic causes of itch may have physical findings involving the liver (in cholestasis) or lymph nodes (in human immunodeficiency virus disease), for example.

Some historical features of pruritus are more associated with a nonsystemic source of itch and are therefore more benign in nature. Acute onset, localized symptoms, limitation of itch to exposed skin, presence of itch in family members, occupational exposure, and recent travel are all reassuring findings and may allow a trial of nonspecific treatment rather than an exhaustive search for systemic illness. Figure 24-1 is an algorithm for a systematic approach to evaluating pruritus.

Treatment of Itch

Treatment of itch may be specifically directed toward the etiology of itch or it may be nonspecific in nature. Nonspecific treatment includes many therapies that have not been evaluated in clinical trials but have been around for decades and have stood the test of time (Table 24-3). Treatment aimed at prurioceptive itch includes capsaicin cream, topical doxepin, and topical aspirin. Neurogenic itch tends to respond more to treatments aimed at blocking the opioid pathways including naltrexone, naloxone, and nalmefene. Neuropathic itch is difficult to treat; anecdotal evidence supports the use of lidocaine and gabapentin, medications more commonly known in their treatment of neuropathic pain. In inflammatory conditions, topical steroids are often a mainstay of therapy. It

---

Table 24-3   Nonspecific Management of Pruritus

Use skin lubricants liberally: petrolatum or lubricant cream at bedtime; alcohol-free, hypoallergenic lotions frequently during the day.
Decrease frequency of bathing and limit bathing to brief exposure to tepid water; after bathing, briefly pat skin dry and immediately apply skin lubricant.
Use mild, unscented, hypo-allergenic soap two to three times per week; limit daily use of soap to groin and axillae (spare legs, arms, and torso).
Humidify dry indoor environment, especially in winter.
Choose clothing that does not irritate the skin (preferably made of doubly rinsed cotton or silk); avoid clothing made of wool, smooth-textured cotton, or heat-retaining material (synthetic fabrics); when washing sheets, add bath oil (e.g., Alpha Keri) to rinse cycle.
Avoid use of vasodilators (caffeine, alcohol, spices, hot water) and excessive sweating.
Avoid use of provocative topical medications, such as corticosteroids, for prolonged periods (risk of skin atrophy) and topical anesthetics and antihistamines (may sensitize exposed skin and increase risk of allergic contact dermatitis).
Prevent complications of scratching by keeping fingernails short and clean and by rubbing skin with the palms of the hands if urge to scratch is irresistible.

Treatments
  Standard topical antipruritic agents: menthol and camphor (e.g., Sarna lotion), oatmeal baths (e.g., Aveeno), pramoxine (e.g., PrameGel), calamine lotion (Caladryl; use only on weeping lesions, not on dry skin), doxepin 5% cream (Zonalon).
  Topical antipruritic agents for refractory pruritus (e.g., severe atopic dermatitis): Burrow's solution (wet dressings), Unna's boot, tar emulsion.
  Systemic antipruritic agents (used in allergic and urticarial disease): doxepin (Sinequan), 10–25 mg at bedtime; hydroxyzine (Atarax), 25–100 mg at bedtime; nonsedating antihistamines (e.g., fexofenadine [Allegra]).

Reprinted with permission from Moses S. Pruritus. Am Fam Physician 2003;68:1135–1142, 1145–1146.

Table 24-4 Specific Management of Pruritic Conditions

Condition	Management
Cholestasis	Cholestyramine (Questran), 4–6 g orally 30 min before meals Ursodiol acid (Actigall), 13–15 mg/kg/day orally Ondansetron (Zofran), 4–8 mg IV, then 4 mg orally every 8 hr Opiate receptor antagonist such as nalmefene (Revex), 20 mg orally twice daily Rifampin (Rifadin), 300 mg orally twice daily Bile duct stenting for extrahepatic cholestasis Bright-light therapy
Neurotic excoriation	Pimozide (Orap) orally for delusions of parasitosis Selective serotonin reuptake inhibitor (e.g., fluvoxamine [Luvox], fluoxetine [Prozac], paroxetine [Paxil])
Notalgia paresthetica	Capsaicin 0.025% cream (Zostrix) applied to localized areas four to six times daily for several weeks
Polycythemia vera	Aspirin, 500 mg orally every 8–24 hr Paroxetine (Paxil), 10–20 mg/day orally Interferon alfa, 3–35 million IU/wk
Spinal opioid-induced pruritus	Ondansetron, 8 mg IV, concurrent with opioid Nalbuphine (Nubain), 5 mg IV, concurrent with opioid
Uremia	Ultraviolet B phototherapy twice weekly for 1 mo Activated charcoal, 6 g/day orally Capsaicin 0.025% cream applied to localized areas four to six times daily for several weeks

IV, intravenously.
Reprinted with permission from Moses S. Pruritis. Am Fam Physician 2003;68:1135–1142, 1145–1146.

is important to remember that corticosteroids do not directly relieve itch and should not be used in pruritic conditions that are not inflammatory in nature. In systemic illness, treatment of the underlying condition often relieves itch. Options for the management of specific pruritic conditions are listed in Table 24-4.

Plan

Diagnostic

Based on the typical history and physical examination findings, atopic dermatitis is likely to be the cause of Steven's itching, and therefore no further diagnostic tests are indicated at this time. If symptoms persist despite appropriate treatment, skin biopsy could be performed to provide additional diagnostic information.

Therapeutic

Before initiating drug treatment for atopic dermatitis, less intensive management strategies may be tried. Moisturizing is extremely important because dry skin is a significant contributor to itch in atopic dermatitis. Nonspecific therapies for itch such as avoiding skin irritants and heat may aid in the prevention of flares of

the disease. If these basic measures fail to control the disease, topical corticosteroids are a good choice for treatment because of the inflammatory nature of atopic dermatitis. It is important to use the lowest effective potency and dose to minimize the chances of side effects such as thinned skin. Alternatives to corticosteroids are the topical immunosuppressant medications tacrolimus and pimecrolimus. Again, these medications are aimed at treating the inflammatory cause of atopic dermatitis and have no direct antipruritic effect. Steven was instructed in the importance of moisturizing his skin and avoiding irritants. He was prescribed triamcinolone 0.1% ointment, a moderate potency topical corticosteroid.

Disposition

Steven was advised to follow up in 2 to 3 weeks if his symptoms were not controlled with these treatment recommendations or if he had any concerning side effects or new symptoms.

Material Available on Student Consult

Review Questions and Answers about Atopic Dermatitis

REFERENCES

Moses S. Pruritus. Am Fam Physician 2003;68:1135–1142, 1145–1146.

Sherard GB, Atkinson SM. Pruritic dermatological conditions in pregnancy. Obstet Gynecol Surv 2001;56: 427–432.

Szarvas S, Harmon D, Murphy D. Neuraxial opioid-induced pruritus: A review. J Clin Anesth 2003;15:234–239.

Yeh HM, Chen LK, Lin CJ, et al. Prophylactic intravenous ondansetron reduces the incidence of intrathecal morphine-induced pruritus in patients undergoing cesarean delivery. Anesth Analg 2000;91:172–175.Ⓐ

Yosipovitch G, Greaves MW, Schmelz M. Itch. Lancet 2003;361:690–694.

Chapter

25 Dizziness (Vestibular Neuritis)

Jeanne M. Ferrante

KEY POINTS

1. The majority of dizziness cases are self-limited and benign.
2. The history and physical examination are most important in the workup of dizziness.
3. Dizziness can be classified into vertigo, presyncope, dysequilibrium, and nonspecific lightheadedness.
4. Laboratory tests are of little value in most patients complaining of dizziness.
5. Patients with cerebrovascular risk factors or neurologic deficits should undergo magnetic resonance imaging of the posterior fossa.
6. Holter monitoring and echocardiogram may be indicated in patients with palpitations, underlying heart disease, or an abnormal cardiac examination.

INITIAL VISIT

Subjective

Patient Identification and Presenting Problem

Tom W. is a 41-year-old white man who presents for the first time with a complaint of dizziness. Tom states that he began to feel ill 1 week ago with fatigue, slight sore throat, nasal congestion, and dry cough. This morning he awoke with severe dizziness, described as "the room spinning" associated with nausea, vomiting, and generalized weakness. Any movement of his head makes his symptoms worse. He has been feeling dizzy and nauseated all day and has not been able to keep anything down. This is the first time that he has experienced these symptoms. He denies recent head or neck trauma, barotrauma, headache, hearing loss, discharge from the ears, tinnitus, or fullness in his ears. There is no blurry vision, double vision, difficulty swallowing, changes in his speech, or weakness or numbness in his face, arms, or legs.

Medical History

Tom has had no major medical illnesses or surgery. He has no history of recurrent ear infections. He does not take any medications and has not been on antibiotics recently.

Family History

Tom has no siblings. His parents are alive and well.

Social History

Tom is married and works as a mechanic. He has smoked one pack of cigarettes per day for 25 years.

Evidence levels Ⓐ Randomized, controlled trials (RCTs), meta-analyses, well-designed systematic reviews of RCTs. Ⓑ Case-control or cohort studies, nonrandomized clinical trials, systematic reviews of studies other than RCTs, cross-sectional studies, retrospective studies, certain uncontrolled studies. Ⓒ Consensus statements, expert guidelines, usual practice, opinion.

He drinks alcohol rarely on weekends. He denies illicit drug use.

Review of Systems

The patient denies headache, neck pain, shortness of breath, chest pains, palpitations, depression, anxiety, fainting, and falling.

Objective

Physical Examination

General Tom is a well-developed, well-nourished alert white man lying on the table in mild to moderate distress.

Vital Signs His height is 5 feet 10 inches, weight is 165 pounds, temperature is 37.3°C (99.1°F), respiratory rate is 20, blood pressure is 138/88, and pulse is 90. There is no orthostatic change in blood pressure or pulse.

Head, Eyes, Ears, Nose, and Throat His head is without lesions or signs of trauma. His external ear canals and tympanic membranes are clear bilaterally; hearing is intact by testing with tuning forks. His conjunctivae are pink; pupils are equal, round, and reactive to light and accommodation; extraocular muscles intact with horizontal nystagmus with a rotational component (fast phase) toward the left. His nose is clear; the maxillary and frontal sinuses are nontender to percussion. He has poor dentition. His oropharynx is clear.

Neck It is supple, with no bruits and no lymphadenopathy. The thyroid is normal.

Lungs The lungs are clear to auscultation.

Heart He has normal sinus rhythm without murmurs, rubs, or gallops.

Neurologic He is oriented to person, place, and time. He has a normal but slowed gait. Cranial nerves II through XII are intact. Deep tendon reflexes are 2+ in upper and lower extremities bilaterally. Strength is 5 of 5 in all extremities. Sensorium is intact to light touch and pinprick. Cerebellum is intact to finger-to-nose pointing and rapid alternating movements. Romberg test shows falling toward the right. Dix-Hallpike maneuver is positive on the right for nystagmus and vertigo after a latency of approximately 3 seconds. This lasted for less than 1 minute.

Assessment

Working Diagnosis

The working diagnosis is peripheral vertigo caused by acute vestibular neuritis. Vertigo can be caused by peripheral or central disorders. Peripheral causes of vertigo include lesions of the vestibular nerve, labyrinth, or both (Froehling et al., 1994 Ⓑ). Central vertigo is caused by disorders of the lower brain stem or cerebellum. Patients with brain stem disease have symptoms typical of vertebrobasilar insufficiency, such as diplopia, dysarthria, dysphagia, paresthesia, and changes in sensory and motor function. Patients with cerebellar disease may have truncal ataxia and difficulty with rapid alternating movements and finger-to-nose testing. Tom had none of the history or physical findings of central vertigo. The result of the Dix-Hallpike maneuver also helps to point to a peripheral cause of the vertigo. The Dix-Hallpike maneuver (also referred to as the Nylen-Barany maneuver) is a head hanging maneuver that helps to distinguish peripheral vertigo from central causes of vertigo (Hoffman et al., 1999 Ⓑ). The Dix-Hallpike maneuver is performed with the patient initially sitting on the examination table. Quickly the patient is brought into the lying position by the examiner with the patient's head turned approximately 30 degrees to one side and slightly hyperextended over the end of the table (Fig. 25-1). The patient should be given clear instructions to keep his or her eyes open. The patient is then observed for symptoms of nausea and vertigo and signs of nystagmus. This maneuver is then repeated with the head turned to the opposite side. If the symptoms are reproduced and nystagmus occurs after a brief latency period (3 to 20 seconds) but resolves in less than 1 minute, then the dizziness is more likely to have a periphera cause. If there are mild or no symptoms, and nystagmus is present immediately and persists for longer than 1 minute, then a central cause of vertigo should be suspected.

Vestibular neuritis, the most common cause of vertigo seen in primary care offices (Sloane et al., 2001 Ⓑ), is thought to be due to inflammation of the vestibular nerve from either an acute viral infection or reactivation of dormant herpes simplex virus type 1. It is characterized by the acute onset of severe persistent vertigo (made worse by head movement), nausea, and vomiting, in the absence of hearing loss or tinnitus. When there is cochlear involvement (tinnitus, hearing loss), then the disorder is termed labyrinthitis (Hoffman et al., 1999 Ⓑ). An upper respiratory tract infection precedes 50% of cases. Tom developed acute persistent symptoms, and he had a recent upper respiratory tract infection. He has no hearing loss or tinnitus and no signs of a central cause of the vertigo. Tom's history and physical findings make vestibular neuritis the most likely diagnosis.

Differential Diagnoses

Other common causes of peripheral vertigo include benign paroxysmal positional vertigo and Meniere's

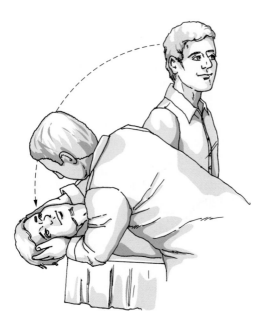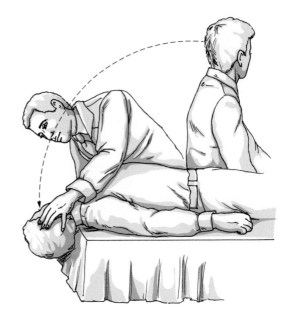

Figure 25-1 The Dix-Hallpike maneuver. (From Reilly BM. Practical Strategies in Outpatient Medicine, 2nd ed. Philadelphia, WB Saunders, 1991.)

disease. Benign paroxysmal positional vertigo is the most common cause of vertigo in referral settings (Sloane et al., 2001🅑). Patients usually have sudden intermittent episodes of vertigo initiated by position change or head turning only. The episodes last less than 1 minute, and there is no hearing loss. In most cases, it is idiopathic and results from accumulation of free-floating debris in the endolymph of the posterior semicircular canal. A precipitating factor may be a recent middle ear infection, vestibular neuritis, head trauma, or ear surgery. Peak occurrence is between ages 50 and 70. Ménière's disease is caused by an abnormal collection of endolymphatic fluid in the inner ear. It is defined by a classic triad of episodic vertigo, low-frequency sensorineural hearing loss, and tinnitus (Froehling et al., 1994🅑). Ear fullness may also be present. Patients are usually between the ages of 30 and 60 years at the onset. These patients have clusters of vertiginous exacerbations coinciding with increased hearing loss and intensity of tinnitus. During periods of remission, episodes of vestibular dysfunction and even hearing loss and tinnitus may significantly resolve for weeks or months. Other rare causes of peripheral vertigo are associated with hearing loss and include perilymphatic fistula (history of pressure changes such as diving or air flight, worsened with straining), cholesteatoma (complication of chronic otitis media with conductive hearing loss and ear drainage), temporal bone trauma, ototoxicity (from aminoglycoside antibiotics), and Ramsay Hunt syndrome (from herpes zoster infection with ear pain, facial palsy, and vesicles in the ear canal) (Froehling et al., 1994 🅑).

Plan

Diagnostic

Because Tom does not have symptoms and signs of a more severe cause of vertigo, no tests are indicated at this time. If the symptoms do not resolve after 6 weeks or if hearing loss or tinnitus develops, then audiometry and vestibular assessment (including calorics with or without electronystagmography) may be indicated.

Therapeutic

The patient was given meclizine 25 mg three to four times daily for the dizziness and nausea.

Patient Education

The patient is educated on the benign course of vestibular neuritis and that it gradually resolves over 2 days to 6 weeks. He is instructed to move slowly initially and to take the meclizine as needed for symptoms. Once the nausea and vomiting subside, habituation exercises (deliberately repeating the head maneuvers that elicit the vertigo) may lessen the duration and severity. He is also advised to stop smoking.

Disposition

The patient is instructed to make a second appointment in 6 weeks or sooner if his symptoms are not relieved by the meclizine or if he develops hearing loss, tinnitus, or other neurologic symptoms.

DISCUSSION

Dizziness is prevalent in the community, ranging from 1.8% in young adults to more than 30% in the elderly (Sloane et al., 2001⑬). Dizziness can be caused by a disturbance in any of a number of balance control systems, including the visual pathways, the vestibular apparatus, the cardiovascular system, and the proprioceptive tracts of the central nervous system. Dizziness is a general and vague term that means different things to different people. History taking is most important to clarify what the patient means by dizziness. Dizziness can be classified into four main categories: vertigo, presyncope, dysequilibrium, and nonspecific lightheadedness (Table 25-1). Vertigo is an illusion of movement, as if the patient or the room is spinning. Vertigo can be peripheral (discussed previously) or central in origin. Central vertigo is rare and can be caused by neoplastic, vascular, or neurologic disorders of the lower brain stem or cerebellum (Froehling et al., 1994⑬). In patients with posterior fossa tumors, vestibular dysfunction is usually slow in onset due to the slow growth of typical neoplasms. These patients usually have imbalance and coordination difficulties. Acoustic neuroma is a benign tumor that usually causes progressive unilateral high-frequency hearing loss, tinnitus, and imbalance (particularly in the dark). Vertigo occurs in less than 20% of patients. The lesion is in the cerebellopontine angle and will also affect, when advanced, other cranial nerves (i.e., fifth and seventh). Vascular diseases include vertebrobasilar transient ischemic attacks, cerebellar or brain stem strokes, and vertebrobasilar migraines. Neurologic disorders include complex partial seizures and multiple sclerosis. Complex partial seizures may present with an aura of dizziness, vertigo, or unsteadiness. In multiple sclerosis, vertigo can present initially in 5% of patients and ultimately in as many as 50% of patients. Symptoms are usually episodic and associated with a wide variety of other neurologic symptoms.

In presyncope, patients describe the feeling of almost fainting or the world going gray and out of focus, especially when they stand. This can be caused by orthostatic hypotension due to decreased

---

Table 25-1 Classification of Dizziness

Vertigo	**Presyncope**
Peripheral	Postural symptoms with or without orthostatic hypotension
Vestibular neuritis	Medications
Labyrinthitis	Anemia
Benign paroxysmal positional vertigo	Infections
Ménière's disease	Dehydration
Perilymphatic fistula	Metabolic diseases (electrolyte disturbance, diabetes, thyroid)
Cholesteatoma	Cardiac disease
Temporal bone trauma	Aortic stenosis
Ototoxicity from medications	Mitral regurgitation
Ramsay Hunt syndrome	Hypertrophic cardiomyopathy
Central	Arrhythmias
Posterior fossa tumors	Heart blocks
Acoustic neuroma	
Vertebrobasilar transient ischemic attack	**Nonspecific Lightheadedness**
Brain stem or cerebellar strokes	Depression
Vertebrobasilar migraines	Anxiety
Complex partial seizures	Panic attacks
Multiple sclerosis	Somatization disorder
	Substance abuse
Dysequilibrium	
Multiple sensory deficits	
Decreased vision	
Peripheral neuropathy	
Diabetes mellitus	
Alcoholism	
Medications	
Anticonvulsants	
Benzodiazepines	
Neuroleptics	
Antidepressants	
Neurologic disorders	

baroreceptor responsiveness, medications (antihypertensives, antidepressants), anemia, dehydration, metabolic diseases (e.g., diabetes mellitus, thyroid diseases), or cardiovascular disorders. Structural cardiac disease (e.g., aortic stenosis, mitral regurgitation, and hypertrophic cardiomyopathy), arrhythmias, and heart blocks may also cause dizziness associated with near-syncope or syncope.

Dysequilibrium is a sensation of unsteadiness and imbalance when standing or walking and resolves at rest. The patient feels a lack of coordination and a sense of impending falls. This is commonly seen in the elderly. The cause is usually multifactorial including multiple sensory deficits (e.g., decreased visual acuity and peripheral neuropathy with impaired proprioception), medications affecting the central nervous system (e.g., anticonvulsants, benzodiazepines, neuroleptics, and antidepressants), or other neurologic disorders (Sloane et al., 2001❸).

Patients with nonspecific lightheadedness are usually vague in their description, sometimes feeling sensations of floating, feeling apart or far away from the environment, fatigue, or tightness or fullness in the head. Patients may also complain of headache, numbness or tingling around the mouth or in the hands, or abdominal pain. These patients tend to have psychiatric disorders including depression, anxiety, panic attacks, somatization disorder, and substance abuse.

Once the character of the dizziness is determined, it is helpful to find out how long it has persisted and whether it occurs in attacks. In addition, the physician should ask about what provokes or worsens the dizziness (standing up, head turning or rolling over in bed, coughing or straining, stress or emotional upset), and what was happening when the dizziness began (e.g., loud noise, blow to the head, flulike symptoms, or a cold beforehand). Inquiring about general health problems such as high blood pressure, diabetes, heart disease, thyroid disease, migraine headaches, seizure disorder, anxiety, and depression is also helpful. Medications and drug use should always be noted. A system review is important to identify symptoms that are related to the dizziness including generalized weakness; loss of consciousness; headaches; nausea; vomiting; diplopia; blurry vision; dysarthria; dysphagia; hearing loss; discharge from the ears; tinnitus or fullness in the ears; numbness or tingling in the face, around the mouth, or in the hands or feet; chest pain; and a pounding or rapid heartbeat.

The physical examination can help to narrow the differential diagnosis. Vital signs, especially postural changes in blood pressure, should be obtained to check for orthostatic hypotension. A head, eyes, ears, nose, and throat examination should focus on the ears, eyes, and sinuses. Spontaneous nystagmus can usually be observed in vertiginous patients. However, in peripheral vestibular disorders, visual fixation can suppress spontaneous nystagmus. Visual acuity should be tested in patients with dysequilibrium. The neck examination includes checking for bruits and thyroid abnormalities. The cardiovascular examination is important to check for size of the heart, murmurs, and arrhythmias. The neurologic examination should focus on the cranial nerves (eye movements, facial strength and sensation, hearing), strength, gait observation, Romberg testing, and cerebellar functions. If the dizziness is described as vertigo, then the Dix-Hallpike maneuver should be performed. If a psychogenic cause is suspected, an often recommended test is to have the patient hyperventilate for 3 minutes in an attempt to reproduce symptoms. This test, however, has poor specificity (Kroenke et al., 1992❸). Laboratory tests are of little value in most patients complaining of dizziness (Hoffman et al., 1999❸). Patients who appear to have fatigue or metabolic abnormalities can be screened with a standard biochemical profile and complete blood count. Thyroid function tests may be indicated if thyroid disease is suspected. A rapid plasma reagin or Venereal Disease Research Laboratories (VDRL) test may be useful in patients suspected of Ménière's disease because secondary or early tertiary syphilis may present with symptoms identical to those seen in Ménière's disease. An electrocardiogram can document cardiac abnormalities if they are suspected based on the history and physical examination. When the history, physical examination, and laboratory studies rule out organic disease, psychogenic factors should be addressed.

Advanced diagnostic tests are helpful if more severe causes of dizziness are suspected based on the history and physical examination. In patients with chronic peripheral vertigo or vertigo associated with hearing loss, audiometric testing and vestibular assessment by the audiologist are indicated. Patients with cerebrovascular risk factors or neurologic deficits such as dysarthria or numbness should undergo magnetic resonance imaging of the posterior fossa. Tests such as Holter monitoring and echocardiogram may be indicated in patients with palpitations, underlying heart disease, or an abnormal cardiac examination. Treatment of dizziness depends on the suspected underlying cause. Acute vertigo and associated vegetative symptoms can be treated symptomatically with the antihistamines meclizine or dimenhydrinate in doses of 25 to 50 mg three or four times daily. In severe cases, diazepam, which decreases brain stem response to vestibular stimuli, in doses of 2.5 to 5.0 mg three times daily can be used. Methylprednisolone, starting at 100 mg/day and tapering to 10 mg over 3 weeks was shown in a recent randomized controlled trial to reduce long-term vestibular dysfunction in vestibular neuritis (Strupp et al., 2004❹). Benign paroxysmal positional vertigo can be effectively treated by a canalith repositioning

1. Have the patient lie down quickly onto her back.

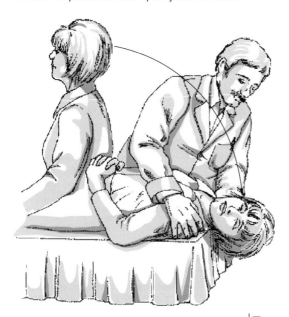

2. First, turn the patient's head to the symptomatic side at a 45° angle for 30–60 seconds.

3. Then turn the head to the opposite side for 30–60 seconds.

4. Finally, roll the head facing 45° downward on the same side. Return the patient to a sitting position.

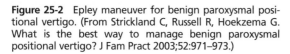

Figure 25-2 Epley maneuver for benign paroxysmal positional vertigo. (From Strickland C, Russell R, Hoekzema G. What is the best way to manage benign paroxysmal positional vertigo? J Fam Pract 2003;52:971–973.)

procedure, such as the Epley maneuver, which takes the patient through a series of head positions (Hilton and Pinder, 2004Ⓐ) (Fig. 25-2). This returns debris from the semicircular canal into the utricle, where its movement does not cause vertigo. Ménière's disease is treated with salt restriction, diuretics, or both. The more serious causes of peripheral vertigo are best handled by otolaryngologic specialists. Corrective surgical procedures may sometimes be helpful. Patients with dysequilibrium are usually managed supportively. Adjustment of medications may be necessary, and steps to improve function in the elderly (e.g., treatment of cataracts, physical therapy for gait and balance training, use of walkers) can help to prevent secondary disability, isolation, depression, and falls. Cardiovascular and neurologic disorders are treated accordingly. Nonspecific lightheadedness can be managed by reassurance and addressing the specific psychiatric disorder.

In summary, dizziness can be caused by a disturbance in any of a number of balance control systems. The history and physical examination are most important in the workup for dizziness. Dizziness in primary care very rarely represents a life-threatening problem. Because the majority of cases are self-limited and benign, conservative management strategies, including observation and supportive treatment, are often appropriate.

Material Available on Student Consult

Review Questions and Answers about Vestibular Neuritis

REFERENCES

Froehling DA, Silverstein, MD, Mohr DN, Beatty CW. Does this dizzy patient have a serious form of vertigo? JAMA 1994;271:385–388.Ⓑ

Hilton M, Pinder D. The Epley (canalith repositioning) manoeuvre for benign paroxysmal positional vertigo (Cochrane Review). The Cochrane Library. Vol. 3. Chichester, UK, John Wiley & Sons, 2004.Ⓐ

Hoffman RM, Einstadter D, Kroenke K. Evaluating dizziness. Am J Med 1999;107:468–478.Ⓑ

Kroenke K, Lucas CA, Rosenberg ML, et al. Causes of persistent dizziness. A prospective study of 100 patients in ambulatory care. Arch Intern Med 1992;117: 898–904.Ⓑ

Reilly BM. Practical Strategies in Outpatient Medicine, 2nd ed. Philadelphia, WB Saunders, 1991.

Sloane PD, Coeytaux RR, Beck RS, Dallara J. Dizziness: State of the science. Ann Intern Med 2001;134: 823–832.Ⓑ

Strickland C, Russell R, Hoekzema G. What is the best way to manage benign paroxysmal positional vertigo? J Fam Pract 2003;52:971–973.

Strupp M, Zingler VC, Arbusow V, et al. Methylprednisolone, valacyclovir, or the combination for vestibular neuritis. N Engl J Med 2004;351: 354–361.Ⓐ

26 Ringing in Ears (Tinnitus)

David M. Barclay III

KEY POINTS

1. Subjective tinnitus is the most prevalent type and is commonly referred to as idiopathic (subjective idiopathic tinnitus).
2. Hyperacusis, the abnormally intense amplification of sound within the auditory pathways, may accompany tinnitus.
3. A complete audiologic evaluation should be performed on all patients with tinnitus.
4. The primary goal of tinnitus retraining therapy (TRT) is to induce habituation to reactions so that patients are still aware of the tinnitus but are not bothered or distressed by it.

INITIAL VISIT

Subjective

Patient Identification and Presenting Problem

John B. is a 45-year-old white man who presents with a complaint of ringing in his ears.

History of Present Illness

John states that about 3 months ago he began to hear a persistent, high-pitched ringing in both ears. The ringing has progressed into a constant, unrelenting sound that alternates between a high-pitched teakettle and the roar of a jet turbine. John has noticed that lack of sleep, stress, and caffeine make the sound louder. He has also become very sensitive to loud noises and sometimes is unable to tolerate everyday sounds, such as the car radio at a normal volume. He has not noticed any hearing loss, aural fullness, or vertigo. Falling asleep has become difficult, and his ability to concentrate during the day has suffered as

a consequence. Lately he has started to feel depressed and apathetic about the future.

Medical History

John has had no major medical illnesses or surgeries. He has no history of head trauma or recurrent ear infections. Aside from an occasional acetaminophen, he does not take any medications. He has experienced brief episodes of ringing in his ears, lasting from seconds to minutes, from the time he was a teenager. He has also experienced brief episodes of hearing his pulse in his ears.

Family History

John's father is 78, and aside from hypertension he is well. His mother is 74 and a breast cancer survivor. He has a brother and a sister, both of whom are in good health.

Social History

John has been married for 20 years and has no children. He is the headmaster of a boarding school. He eats a regular diet and enjoys bicycling and swimming. He drinks socially and does not smoke or use illegal drugs.

Review of Systems

John does not experience headaches, neck pain, shortness of breath, chest pains, palpitations, abdominal pains, or musculoskeletal problems. He has been feeling depressed for the past couple of weeks and has difficulty falling asleep.

Objective

Physical Examination

General John is a well-developed, well-nourished, alert white man in mild distress.

Vital Signs His height is 5 feet 9 inches, weight is 155 pounds, temperature is 36.9°C (98.4°F), respiratory rate is 18, blood pressure is 130/85, and pulse is 80.

Evidence levels **Ⓐ** Randomized, controlled trials (RCTs), meta-analyses, well-designed systematic reviews of RCTs. **Ⓑ** Case-control or cohort studies, nonrandomized clinical trials, systematic reviews of studies other than RCTs, cross-sectional studies, retrospective studies, certain uncontrolled studies. **Ⓒ** Consensus statements, expert guidelines, usual practice, opinion.

Head, Eyes, Ears, Nose, and Throat His head is normocephalic and atraumatic, his external ear canals and tympanic membranes are clear bilaterally, his hearing is grossly intact, and the Webber and Rinne tests are normal. His conjunctivae are pink and the pupils equal, round, and reactive to light and accommodation; extraocular movements are intact without nystagmus. His nose is clear; the maxillary and frontal sinuses are nontender. He has good dentition, and the oropharynx is clear.

Neck His neck is supple, with no lymphadenopathy, thyromegaly, or jugular venous distention.

Lungs His lungs are clear to auscultation.

Heart The heart has a normal sinus rhythm without murmurs, rubs, or gallops.

Neurologic Examination
He is alert and oriented to person, place, and time; cranial nerves II through XII are intact. Webber and Rinne tests are normal. Reflexes are 2+ throughout, motor strength is 5 out of 5 throughout, sensory examination is intact to light touch and pinprick, cerebellar function is intact, and the Romberg test is normal.

Assessment

Working Diagnosis
John's history and physical examination are most consistent with a diagnosis of subjective tinnitus.

Differential Diagnosis
Tinnitus is classified as either subjective or objective. Objective tinnitus can be heard by the examiner and is caused by an acoustic source in the body. Objective tinnitus has also been referred to as vibratory tinnitus or extrinsic tinnitus and may be heard by auscultation of the ear and surrounding vessels. It is differentiated into pulsatile and nonpulsatile tinnitus. Nonpulsatile tinnitus is further divided into mild and severe types. Mild nonpulsatile tinnitus is heard by the patient only when in a quiet environment and is usually not distressing. Severe pulsatile tinnitus is present all the time and often degrades the patient's quality of life (Heller, 2003).

Pulsatile tinnitus is classified as vascular or nonvascular. Nonvascular tinnitus is usually caused by myoclonus of the tensor tympani, stapedius muscle, or palatal musculature. Arterial causes of pulsatile tinnitus include hypertension, arteriovenous malformations, and atherosclerosis of the carotid arteries. Venous causes include benign intracranial hypertension, jugular bulb abnormalities, and hydrocephalus (Sismantis, 1998).

Subjective tinnitus is the most prevalent type and is commonly referred to as idiopathic (subjective idiopathic tinnitus). Subjective tinnitus is one of the three symptoms that constitute Ménière's disease. It has many forms, varying from a benign sound that is heard only occasionally to a constant roar that is heard 24 hours per day and is accompanied by hyperacusis and distortion of sounds. This type of tinnitus disturbs sleep and the ability to concentrate on intellectual work. It may be accompanied by phonophobia, affective disorders such as depression, and even suicide.

Hyperacusis, the abnormally intense amplification of sound within the auditory pathways, may accompany tinnitus. In this condition, the neuronal activity evoked by a given sound is significantly higher than that in a normal individual. Patients frequently experience physical discomfort in the presence of sounds that are perceived as normal to others. The secondary activation of the limbic and autonomic pathways, as well as the baseline level of activation within these systems, is normal.

Misophonia (from the Greek *miso*, "hate"), a strong aversion to sounds, can also develop. This originates from the abnormal activation of the limbic and autonomic nervous systems in the presence of a normally functioning auditory system. Misophonia is a conditioned response that depends significantly on the patient's past experiences and the context in which the sound occurs.

Conditions associated with tinnitus are listed in Table 26-1.

Plan

Diagnostic
The initial workup of tinnitus should include a self-assessment of the severity of the tinnitus, an audiologic examination, and possibly a radiographic evaluation and laboratory tests. A number of self-assessment scales have been developed to measure the intensity of the tinnitus. These scales determine the functional, physical, and psychological consequences of the tinnitus and the coping skills of the patient. One such scale, the Tinnitus Handicap Inventory, developed in 1996, is a self-report instrument that has been validated to quantify the impact

Table 26-1 Conditions Associated with Tinnitus
Ménière's disease
Presbycusis
Otitis
Otosclerosis
Ototoxicity
Vestibular schwannoma
Autoimmune hearing loss
Hormonal changes of pregnancy
Menopause

of tinnitus on daily living. It consists of 25 questions divided into three subscales: (1) functional, (2) emotional, and (3) catastrophic (Newman et al., 1996 Ⓑ). The only other scale that has been validated and shown to have good intertest reliability with the Tinnitus Handicap Inventory is the Tinnitus Questionnaire (Heller, 2003).

It is important to determine whether the tinnitus is unilateral or bilateral and hearing loss is present. The Webber and Rinne tests may be used as an initial in-office evaluation of hearing. Magnetic resonance imaging should be considered in patients with unilateral tinnitus and sensorineural hearing loss and in those with asymmetrical hearing loss suspicious for an acoustic neuroma. Patients who cannot undergo magnetic resonance imaging can have a computed tomography scan of the posterior fossa with enhancement. Computed tomography of the temporal bones should be obtained in patients suspected of hereditary hearing loss, Paget's disease, otosclerosis, and trauma (Schaber, 2003).

A complete audiologic evaluation should be performed on all patients. This testing establishes a baseline for the future and helps guide more advanced audiologic testing. Pure tone testing primarily evaluates the function of the peripheral portion of the hearing apparatus. Tympanometry may identify previously undetected middle ear effusion, stiffness of the tympanic membrane, or myoclonus of the tensor tympani, stapedius muscle, or palatal musculature. Speech reception thresholds and speech discrimination scores usually reflect pathology of the central nervous system. Other audiologic tests may include loudness matching (estimates the loudness of a pure tone necessary to extinguish the tinnitus), pitch masking (correlates the frequency of the tinnitus with a variety of stimuli), minimal masking level (determines the amount of sound necessary to mask the tinnitus), and residual inhibition (determines the tone, pitch, and intensity necessary to bring about decreased or absent tinnitus). These tests help evaluate the potential effectiveness of masking therapy (Schaber, 2003).

Laboratory testing including a complete blood count, lipid profile, chemistry panel, and thyroid function studies should be obtained in patients who may have medical abnormalities. Further testing may be indicated by the history and physical examination (Schaber, 2003).

Medications and other substances that may cause tinnitus are listed in Table 26-2.

Therapeutic

Several modalities have been used to treat tinnitus (Table 26-3) TRT is based on the neuropsychological model of tinnitus and decreased sound tolerance. It works by inducing a sustained habituation to tinnitus and/or external sounds. This habituation is

Table 26-2   Medications and Substances That May Cause Tinnitus

Analgesics
Aspirin
Nonsteroidal anti-inflammatory drugs

Antibiotics
Aminoglycosides
Chloramphenicol
Erythromycin
Tetracycline
Vancomycin

Chemotherapeutics
Bleomycin (Blenoxane)
Cisplatin
Mechlorethamine (Mustargen)
Methotrexate
Vincristine

Loop Diuretics
Furosemide
Bumetanide (Bumax)
Ethacrynic acid (Edecrine)

Others
Chloroquine (Aralen)
Heavy metals: mercury, lead
Heterocyclic antidepressants
Quinine

From Brechtelsbauer D. Adult hearing loss. Prim Care 1990;17:249–266; Schleuning AJ 2nd. Management of the patient with tinnitus. Med Clin North Am 1991;75:1225–1237; Weber P, Klein A. Hearing loss. Med Clin North Am 1999;83:125–137.

Table 26-3   Treatment Modalities Used for Tinnitus

Counseling
Medications (antidepressants, anticonvulsants, anxiolytics, local anesthetics, vasodilators)
Surgery
Masking techniques
Psychological approaches
Biofeedback
Acupuncture
Hyperbaric oxygen chamber therapy
Temporomandibular joint therapy
Tinnitus retraining therapy

From Brechtelsbauer D. Adult hearing loss. Prim Care 1990;17:249–266.

achieved through a modification of the neural connections linking the limbic and autonomic nervous systems. TRT does not "cure" tinnitus, but it can provide relief from symptoms for many patients, particularly those who suffer from hyperacusis and misophonia (Jastreboff and Jastreboff, 2003).

DISCUSSION

The overall prevalence of tinnitus in the United States is approximately 3% and varies by age with a prevalence of 1% in those younger than 45 and 9% in individuals older than 65 (Adams et al., 1999©). Approximately 80% of tinnitus cases are associated with hearing loss. When tinnitus occurs after insults to the ear, such as exposure to loud noise or ototoxic pharmacologic agents, then these factors are taken to be the cause of the tinnitus. More often, however, a cause cannot be identified, leading to the diagnosis of subjective tinnitus.

There are many theories and hypotheses regarding the mechanisms behind subjective tinnitus. The theory of discordant damage or dysfunction between the outer hair cells and the inner hair cells of the inner ear is favored by recent research. According to this theory, the perception of tinnitus is a positive phenomenon occurring within the auditory system. This explanation accounts for a number of observations about tinnitus, including the fact that 20% of patients with tinnitus have normal hearing and only 73% of deaf patients experience tinnitus (Kaltenbach et al., 2002; Jastreboff, 1990).

The phenomenon of neural plasticity and the neurophysiologic model of tinnitus have been used to explain how tinnitus affects the nonauditory areas of the brain and provide the basis for the role of TRT in treating many forms of tinnitus. Neural plasticity occurs in all parts of the central nervous system and is caused by several factors including deprivation of input, abnormal input, or injury. "Good" plasticity occurs when the functions of the injured structure are transferred to other parts of the central nervous system. "Bad" plasticity results when hyperactivity or hypersensitivity of particular neurons is transferred to other parts of the central nervous system by activating dormant synapses or forming new ones. It has been hypothesized that this rewiring is responsible not only for tinnitus but also for the symptoms associated with it, such as hyperacusis, misophonia, and affective symptoms including depression. These changes may be transient, persistent, or permanent, but most are reversible if suitable stimuli are applied (Moller, 2003).

The neurophysiologic model of tinnitus and decreased sound tolerance assumes the following four postulates: (1) in addition to the auditory system, the limbic and the autonomic systems are involved in processing tinnitus-related and sound-invoked neuronal activity, (2) the behavior-induced problems of tinnitus are largely related to sustained overactivation of the sympathetic part of the autonomic nervous system, (3) functional connections are developed between different parts of the brain in much the same way that conditioned reflexes are (Fig. 26-1), (4) it is possible to ameliorate the nega-

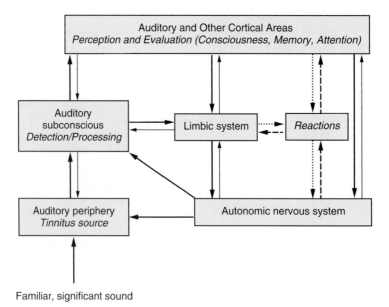

Familiar, significant sound

Figure 26-1 A block diagram of the neurophysiologic model of tinnitus and decreased sound tolerance. Note multiple functional connections between involved systems crucial in the development of conditioned reflex arcs. (Adapted from Jastreboff P, Jastreboff M. Tinnitus retraining therapy for patients with tinnitus and decreased sound tolerance. Otalaryngol Clin North Am 2003;36:321–336.)

tive impact of tinnitus and decreased sound tolerance by inducing and sustaining habituation (TRT) (Jastreboff and Jastreboff, 2003).

The plasticity of the brain must be preserved for TRT to be effective. This means that benzodiazepines, frequently prescribed to treat tinnitus, are contraindicated in patients undergoing TRT because they impair brain plasticity and reduce the ability to learn. Tinnitus masking, also a traditional form

of treatment, should be avoided because suppression of tinnitus removes the signal that needs to be habituated.

TRT invokes two types of habituation: habituation of reaction (Fig. 26-2) and habituation of perception (Fig. 26-3). The primary goal of TRT is to induce habituation to reactions and, thereby, the weakening and elimination of the connections between the auditory system and the limbic and

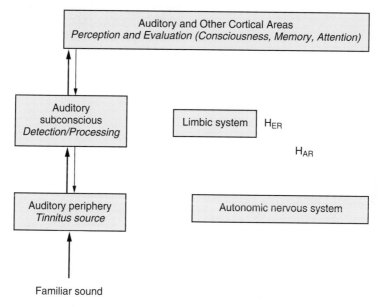

Figure 26-2 Habituation of reaction reflects lack of activation of the autonomic nervous system by the tinnitus-related neuronal activity or activity evoked by external sounds.

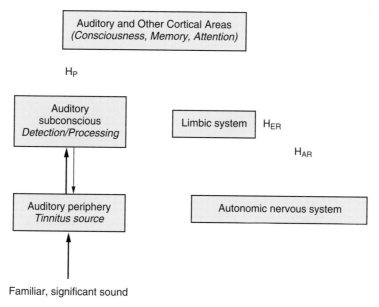

Figure 26-3 Habituation of perception reflects lack of activation of the high auditory cortical centers.

autonomic systems. When this is achieved, patients are still aware of the tinnitus but they are not bothered or distressed by it. Habituation of perception is likely to occur when habituation of reaction is sufficiently complete. The result is that patients are aware of their tinnitus a small percentage of the time.

Material Available on Student Consult
Review Questions and Answers about Tinnitus

PATIENT INFORMATION RESOURCES

American Tinnitus Association
Phone: 800-634-8978
Web: http://www.ata.org

American Academy of Audiology
Phone: 800-222-2336
Web: http://www.audiology.org

American Academy of Otolaryngology—Head and Neck Surgery
Phone: 703-836-4444
Web: http://www.ata.org

REFERENCES

Adams PF, Henderson GE, Marano MA. Current estimates from the National Health Interview Survey, 1996. National Center for Health Statistics. Vital Health Stat 1999;10:81–103.**C**

Brechtelsbauer D. Adult hearing loss. Prim Care 1990;17:249–266.

Heller A. Classification and epidemiology of tinnitus. Otolaryngol Clin North Am 2003;36:239–248.

Jastreboff PJ. Phantom auditory perception (tinnitus): Mechanisms of generation and perception. Neurosci Res 1990;8:221–254.

Jastreboff P, Jastreboff M. Tinnitus retraining therapy for patients with tinnitus and decreased sound tolerance. Otolaryngol Clin North Am 2003;36:321–336.

Kaltenbach JA, Rachel JD, Mathog TA, et al. Cisplatin-induced hyperactivity in the dorsal cochlear nucleus and its relation to outer hair cell loss: Relevance to tinnitus. J Neurophysiol 2002;88:699–714.

Moller A. Pathophysiology of tinnitus. Otolaryngol Clin North Am 2003;36:249–266.

Newman C, Jacobson G, Spitzer J. Development of the Tinnitus Handicap Inventory. Arch Otolaryngol Head Neck Surg 1996;122:143–148.**B**

Schaber M. Medical evaluation of tinnitus. Otolaryngol Clin North Am 2003;36:287–292.

Schleuning AJ 2nd. Management of the patient with tinnitus. Med Clin North Am 1991;75:1225–1237.

Sismanis A. Pulsitile tinnitus: A 15-year experience. Am J Otol 1998;19(abstract):472–477.

Weber P, Klein A. Hearing loss. Med Clin North Am 1999;83:125–137.

27

Giardiasis

John W. Tipton

INITIAL VISIT

Subjective

Patient Identification and Presenting Problem

Bob is a 29-year-old white man who presents for the first time with a complaint of diarrhea.

Present Illness

Bob states that approximately 3 weeks ago, he was awakened with the sudden onset of watery, profuse diarrhea accompanied by abdominal cramps. He initially thought this was due to something he ate or a virus and treated it by pushing fluids and avoiding solid foods. In about 3 days, he improved some but continues to have five to seven loose, semisolid stools daily. He noted the onset of fatigue after about a week. As the diarrhea continued, he noted a weight loss of 5 pounds even though he had resumed a normal diet. The diarrhea sometimes wakes him at night and seems a little worse after eating but might occur at any time. The abdominal cramping continues, and he notices a lot of stomach rumblings and flatus. Appetite is normal. There is no food intolerance, nausea, jaundice, melena, or hematochezia. He remembers a similar illness about 3 months ago that resolved after 3 to 4 weeks. This time, when his symptoms persisted, Bob sought medical care.

Medical History

Bob has had no serious medical or surgical problems. He does not take any medications and has not taken any antibiotics recently. He has no history of bowel problems other than occasional viral gastroenteritis as a child.

Family History

Bob has two younger brothers in good health. Both parents are alive and well except that his mother has essential hypertension.

Social History

Bob has been divorced for 3 years and works as a pharmacist. He has never smoked and only occasionally drinks alcohol at social gatherings. He denies illicit drug use. He is an avid camper and backpacker. His last backpacking trip was 4 months ago. He has had no recent travel out of the United States.

Review of Systems

He denies chills, fever, dysphagia, nausea, vomiting, abdominal pain other than the cramping, back pain, urinary frequency, dysuria, and depression or anxiety.

Objective

Physical Examination

Bob is a well-developed, well-nourished white man seated on the examination table in no distress. His

Evidence levels ⒶRandomized, controlled trials (RCTs), meta-analyses, well-designed systematic reviews of RCTs. ⒷCase-control or cohort studies, nonrandomized clinical trials, systematic reviews of studies other than RCTs, cross-sectional studies, retrospective studies, certain uncontrolled studies. ⒸConsensus statements, expert guidelines, usual practice, opinion.

vital signs are as follows: height, 5 feet 10 inches; weight, 165 pounds (last recorded weight, 173 pounds); blood pressure, 110/76; temperature, 98.8°F (37.1°C); pulse, 72 with regular rate and rhythm; respiratory rate, 14. There is no orthostatic change in blood pressure or pulse. Skin color is normal. Head, eyes, ears, nose, and throat are normal without any sclericterus. Neck, lungs, and heart are normal. The abdomen is flat. Bowel sounds are hyperactive. There are no masses, and the liver and spleen are normal. There is mild tenderness to deep palpation in the mid-abdomen but no guarding and no rebound tenderness. The rectal examination showed an empty rectal vault with no tenderness.

Assessment

Working Diagnosis

The working diagnosis is infectious diarrhea, probably bacterial or parasitic. The acute onset is compatible with infectious diarrhea. There is no history of bowel or other disease associated with diarrhea. Irritable bowel disease is not considered because of the nocturnal diarrhea and lack of psychological stressors.

Differential Diagnosis

The initial differential diagnosis included infectious diarrhea from bacteria, viruses, or parasites; malabsorption syndrome; inflammatory bowel disease; irritable bowel disease; and chronic diarrhea from metabolic or other disease.

1. *Infectious diarrhea* may be caused by a variety of bacteria, viruses, and parasites. The diarrhea is most commonly caused by toxic effects of exotoxins, osmotic effects, and changes in normal gut flora. Viral diarrheas are usually self-limited and short-lived. There is no history of antibiotic use that could lead to *Clostridium difficile* colitis.
2. *Malabsorption syndromes* normally cause diarrhea because of changes in the gut contents that cause increased osmotic load and water secretion and/or reduced water resorption.
3. *Inflammatory bowel diseases* such Crohn's disease and regional enteritis cause inflammatory changes in the bowel leading to a wide range of diarrhea and intestinal problems from perforation to obstruction.
4. *Irritable bowel disease* is a functional chronic disease poorly understood but generally related to stress and dietary factors that tend to cause early morning diarrhea and alternations between diarrhea and constipation.

Chronic diarrhea has a very long list of possible causes but is not likely in this patient because of the acute, recent onset. However, it is possible that his previous episode of diarrhea is related to this illness.

Plan

Diagnostic

The physician thought that infectious diarrhea was most likely considering the abrupt onset and relatively normal physical examination. The clinician initiated a series of diagnostic studies designed to confirm this suspicion.

Laboratory examination showed the following: normal complete blood count, metabolic panel, and amylase. Stool examination showed no white blood cells, blood, ova, or parasites. Stool culture was negative for pathogens. Repeat examination of the stool for ova and parasites was positive for *Giardia lamblia*.

Therapeutic

The patient was treated with metronidazole (Flagyl) 250 mg three times per day for 5 days. His symptoms of diarrhea and abdominal cramps resolved slowly over about 2 weeks.

Patient Education

Avoidance of lactose-containing foods seemed to diminish his symptoms. He was instructed on the contagious nature of his illness and proper hygienic measures to prevent future infection. The source of his infection was not clear but was surmised to be contaminated water or food. He already was aware of proper sanitizing methods for water he drinks on backpacking and camping trips.

Disposition

He regained his weight over 2 months and continued in good health over the immediate follow-up period. He was instructed to return if diarrhea became a problem again.

DISCUSSION

Giardiasis is an acute diarrhea caused by *G. lamblia* (synonyms: *Giardia intestinalis*, *Giardia duodenalis*). *G. lamblia* is a protozoal pathogen that is fairly common in all parts of the world including the United States. In the United States, it is estimated to cause approximately 2.5 million infections per year (Anonymous, 2000ⓒ). Although it is popularly thought to be primarily associated with travelers' diarrhea and drinking contaminated water from mountain streams, in reality, it is a common cause of diarrhea in all states and many venues. The parasite exists in two forms: cyst and trophozoite. The cyst is the infectious form and the trophozoite is responsible for symptoms and reproduction within the gut. The parasite stays in the trophozoite form in the small intestine and only changes back to its contagious encysted form in the large intestine. Chronic infection and shedding of the parasite is possible (Gardner, 2001 Ⓑ). The infectious cyst may survive in the environment for several weeks. It is spread by person-to-person contact and ingestion of fecally contaminated water or food. It is resistant to cold but destroyed by cooking or boiling, so contaminated food must be raw or be contaminated after cooking. It is resistant to usual levels of chlorination but can be removed from water supplies by filtration. Deep well water is usually free of the parasite, but surface water may be contaminated. It may persist in cold (Syed, 2003 Ⓑ). Domestic or wild animals, including mammals, birds, and reptiles, may be a reservoir of the infection. Person-to-person spread is seen in day care centers, nursing homes, and other sites where fecal-oral contamination is likely. Increased risk for disease is seen in infants, young children, travelers, and the immunocompromised (Leder, 2004 Ⓑ). Giardiasis is especially common in areas of the world where poor sanitation is prevalent, with infection becoming widespread or universal as early as 3 months of age in highly endemic areas. However, persons living in areas where infection is more common may build up immunity to infection and have symptom-free carrier states (Gardner, 2001 Ⓑ).

Pathology

The infection starts after oral ingestion of the infectious cyst. The incubation period ranges from 1 to 3 weeks. After ingestion of the infectious cyst, the organism changes to its trophozoite form and attaches itself to the small intestine wall. Several theories have been advanced to explain symptoms. There may be microscopic changes in the small intestine villi, and some damage may be done to the villus or its brush border leading to malabsorption, but this is not constant. There does not appear to be a significant inflammatory component. A significant number of infected persons may remain asymptomatic (Gardner, 2001 Ⓑ). The difference between symptomatic and asymptomatic states also is not apparent.

The symptoms of giardiasis are highly variable, from asymptomatic to cases of fulminate diarrhea and dehydration. The infected person may become chronically infected and remain asymptomatic and continue to shed infectious cysts. The importance to the individual of this state is unknown. Symptomatic persons tend to have an acute onset of diarrhea, which is primarily watery at first and associated with abdominal cramping and flatulence. Chronic or intermittent symptoms are highly suggestive of giardiasis (Nash, 2001 Ⓑ). Other symptoms are increased borborygmi, flatulence, and symptoms of malabsorption. Upper gastrointestinal symptoms such as nausea and vomiting may be significant. Fever and bloody diarrhea are uncommon. Chronic infections

may lead to malabsorption states, vitamin deficiencies, and failure to thrive in children, or weight loss in adults.

Differential Diagnosis

In acute diarrheas, infectious diarrhea must be considered. Bacterial causes are *Salmonella*, *Shigella*, *Yersinia*, *Campylobacter*, pathogenic *Escherichia coli*, and *C. difficile*. Viruses are common but usually self-limited over short time periods. The two common parasitic causes of diarrhea in the United States are *Giardia* and *Cryptosporidium parvum* (Verweij, 2004 Ⓑ). *Entamoeba histolytica* is common in much of the developing world but is rare in the United States. Malabsorption and inflammatory bowel disease may need to be considered. Other causes of chronic diarrhea are legion. Primary differential points for giardiasis are sudden onset, length of illness usually longer than 2 weeks, and weight loss. Chronic, intermittent diarrhea also highly favors *Giardia*. Fever and elevated white blood cell counts are not common (Nash, 2001 Ⓑ).

Laboratory Diagnosis

The parasite can be found in stool specimens. The trophozoite may be found in stools if the diarrhea is profuse, but the cyst is more commonly found. Testing for *Giardia* is historically done by searching stool samples for the parasite. This may be diagnostic for other pathogens as well. There is a high false-negative rate on examination of only one stool specimen, but the positive rate becomes high (>90%) after examining three specimens. Immunoassays and fluorescent antibodies have been used more recently. They have high sensitivity and high specificity, are inexpensive, and are relatively easy to perform (Aldeen, 1998 Ⓑ). White blood cells are usually not seen in stool samples. Blood chemistries are usually normal, except with extraintestinal complications such as hepatic or pancreatic involvement. Upper gastrointestinal series will usually be normal, except possibly for nonspecific findings such as swelling. Duodenal aspirates may show the parasite but are no longer used except in difficult to diagnose cases. Chronic cases may show signs of malabsorption of various nutrients: vitamin B_{12}, protein, and fats.

Treatment

The most commonly used treatment is metronidazole 250 mg three times daily for 5 to 7 days. In the case of relapse or incomplete remission, a repeat course of metronidazole at a higher dose can be given. Side effects are a bitter metallic taste, dyspepsia, and disulfiram-like reactions when taken with alcohol (Gardner, 2001 Ⓑ). Alternate antibiotics are available. Tinidazole (Tindamax) is highly effective as a single 2-g dose (50 mg/kg, maximum 2 g for children) and is well tolerated. It is newly available in the United States but has been widely used in other parts of the world (Anonymous, 2004 Ⓑ; Nash, 2001 Ⓑ). Nitazoxanide (Alinia) is another newly available drug that is dosed over a short interval. It appears to have higher levels of effectiveness when compared with metronidazole. The dose for adults is 500 mg twice daily for 3 days. Smaller doses are recommended for children (Ali, 2003 Ⓑ). Paromomycin (Humatin), an unabsorbed aminoglycoside, may be used when absorption is undesirable such as in early pregnancy. The usual dose is 25 to 35 mg/kg/day in three divided doses for 7 days. The use of metronidazole during pregnancy still has some controversy associated with it. Metronidazole has been shown to have teratogenic effects in rats but not in humans. Treatment during pregnancy may be postponed until after the first trimester if symptoms are mild and malabsorption is not a problem, allowing for more safety. Furazolidone (Furoxone), a nitrofuran, is available in liquid form and generally more acceptable to children but has to be dosed four times daily for 7 to 10 days. Nausea and vomiting are the most common side effects of furazolidone. Hemolysis due to glucose-6-phosphate dehydrogenase deficiency and other side effects of nitrofurans can occur. The cure rate with paromomycin and furazolidone may not be as high as with metronidazole. Quinacrine was widely used in the past but for years has been difficult to obtain in the United States. However, resistant cases may benefit from combination therapy with quinacrine and metronidazole. Albendazole (Albenza) has been used to treat giardiasis but is not approved by the U.S. Food and Drug Administration for this indication and has not been extensively tested for this diagnosis in the United States (Syed, 2003 Ⓑ). Resolution of all symptoms may be slow because the malabsorption may take several weeks to resolve. Lactose-containing foods may need to be avoided for 3 to 4 weeks as the brush border recovers.

Treatment of asymptomatic individuals is controversial and should be individualized. Certainly workers in day care or treatment centers such as nursing homes should be treated. A person who is likely to be a source of infection for people at high risk such as the immunocompromised should be seriously considered for treatment. Asymptomatic persons who are likely to be reinfected, such as those living in highly endemic areas, probably receive no benefit from treatment (Gilman, 1988 Ⓑ).

Follow-up

If symptoms resolve readily, no further follow-up is indicated. There is no need to retest for cure. Diarrhea may resolve slowly because of the persistence of malabsorption syndromes such as lactose intolerance. It may be necessary to avoid lactose-containing foods for several weeks. If symptoms persist, retesting for the causative organism may be necessary. Alternatively, empirical retreatment is an acceptable alternative. True failure of antibiotic therapy indicates the need for repeating the same antibiotic at a higher dose, switching to an alternate antibiotic, or combination antibiotic therapy. In the face of persistent symptoms, testing for concurrent disease states may be needed.

Material Available on Student Consult

Review Questions and Answers about Giardiasis

REFERENCES

Adagu IS. In vitro activity of nitazoxanide and related compounds against isolates of *Giardia intestinalis*, *Entamoeba histolytica*, and *Trichomonas vaginalis*. J Antimicrob Chemother 2002;49:103–111. Ⓑ

Aldeen WE. Comparison of nine commercially available enzyme-linked immunosorbent assays for detection of *Giardia lamblia* in fecal specimens. J Clin Microbiol 1998;36:1338–1340. Ⓑ

Ali SA. *Giardia intestinalis*. Curr Opin Infect Dis 2003;16:453–460. Ⓑ

Anonymous. Giardiasis surveillance United States. MMWR Morb Mortal Wkly Rep 2000;49. Ⓒ

Anonymous. Drugs for parasitic infections. Med Lett 2004;Aug:1–12. Ⓑ

Gardner TB. Treatment of giardiasis. Clin Microbiol Rev 2001;14:114–128. Ⓑ

Gilman RH. Rapid reinfection by *Giardia lamblia* after treatment in a hyperendemic Third World community. Lancet 1988;1:343–345. Ⓑ

Leder K. Giardiasis. Up to Date, 2004. Available at www.uptodate.com. Ⓑ

Nash TE. Treatment of *Giardia lamblia* infections. Pediatr Infect Dis J 2001;20:193–195. Ⓑ

Syed AA. *Giardia intestinalis*. Curr Opin Infect Dis 2003;16:453–460. Ⓑ

Verweij JJ. Simultaneous detection of *Entamoeba histolytica*, *Giardia lamblia*, and *Cryptosporidium parvum* in fecal samples by using multiplex real-time PCR. J Clin Microbiol 2004;42:1220–1223. Ⓑ

28

Vesicular Rash (Varicella)

David L. Gaspar

INITIAL VISIT

Subjective

Patient Identification and Presenting Problem

Linda J. is a 28-year-old patient presenting with vesicular lesions over her face and arms. Linda will soon begin to work at Hillhaven Nursing Home. As part of her pre-employment assessment, her immunizations were reviewed, and it was found she did not have a history of having had chicken pox. She had a varicella titer done that indicated she had no immunity to varicella. She received her first dose of varicella vaccine 10 days ago.

Yesterday she noted what she thought were mosquito bites on her face. By this morning, she noted more lesions on her face and arms despite staying indoors away from any apparent exposure to mosquitoes or other insects. Some of the original red lesions on her neck now have small blisters in the center of the red spots. The rash itches, and some of the scratched blisters have broken and are starting to heal by scabbing over. She took over-the-counter diphenhydramine last evening, and it helped her symptoms of itching. She feels warm and tired and has some muscle aches at the present time.

Medical and Surgical History

Linda has been very healthy in general. She had a ski injury 5 years ago and underwent a successful right anterior cruciate reconstruction. She has otherwise not been hospitalized. Her immunizations are up to date except for the need for a second dose of varicella vaccine. She takes folic acid tablets and is on a generic norethindrone and ethinyl estradiol oral contraceptive for contraception.

Family History

Her mother has had major depression but no other health issues. Her father has had prostate cancer treated with radiotherapy. She has two brothers who are alive and well.

Personal and Social History

She has been married for 2 years. She and her husband wish to start a family soon. She came in for some preconception counseling 2 months ago where she was advised to begin folate supplementation. She is a licensed practical nurse but has not worked in her field for the past 5 years.

Review of Systems

She complains of a few "canker sores" in her mouth. She has no cough or headache. Her last normal menstrual period was 2 weeks ago. A full review of systems revealed no other significant symptoms.

Objective

Physical Examination

She looks mildly ill. Her temperature is 37.0°C (98.6°F), blood pressure is 104/76, pulse is 72, and respiratory rate is 18. There are obvious vesicular lesions on her face, upper trunk, and arms. There are also small erythematous macules without vesicles and some crusted lesions on an erythematous base. Many of the lesions have a "drop of dew on a rose petal" appearance. The palms and soles of the feet are spared. There are a few shallow ulcers on the hard palate. Overall more than 50 lesions are counted. Her chest is clear, the heart examination is normal, and her abdominal examination is benign except for a few crusted lesions. There is no abdominal tenderness or organomegaly.

Assessment

Working Diagnosis

Linda appears to have varicella, or chicken pox. The clinical syndrome has appeared after her varicella immunization. It is unclear whether this is due to coincidental natural infection or occurred as a result of the vaccine.

Differential Diagnosis

The differential diagnosis of varicella can be difficult early in the illness. It may appear more localized early in the disease, and the various stages in the evolution of varicella lesions may not always be evident. Because of this, individual lesions may take on the appearance of other skin conditions including herpes simplex infection, impetigo, coxsackievirus infection, papular urticaria, insect bites, scabies, dermatitis herpetiformis, a drug rash, rickettsialpox, or contact dermatitis (Chen et al., 2002). Despite worldwide eradication, smallpox is back in the differential diagnosis of varicella in this age of fear over biologic terrorism. As the illness evolves, the distribution of lesions, the variety in their stages of development, and the rash's time course help to differentiate varicella from the other conditions.

Plan

Diagnostic

The diagnosis is clinical. In apparent naturally occurring varicella infections, no testing is necessary. In this case, Linda has developed a varicella rash after immunization. The Centers for Disease Control and Prevention (CDC) (2005 ◉) recommends strain identification testing as part of its adverse reaction surveillance. It offer's this testing free of charge. The physician phones the CDC to make arrangements for the assay. The situations in which the CDC recommends strain identification include

- Individuals who develop more than 50 lesions 7 to 42 days after vaccination
- Individuals who develop certain serious adverse experiences after vaccination including pneumonia, pneumonitis, cerebritis (encephalitis), cerebellitis (cerebellar ataxia), and aseptic meningitis
- Individuals who develop herpes zoster after vaccination
- Suspected cases of secondary transmission of the vaccine virus
- Pregnant women who inadvertently receive varicella vaccine or who have been exposed to a vaccinee and who develop a varicella rash

Therapeutic

Linda's physician prescribes acyclovir, an antiviral agent, 800 mg orally five times daily for 7 days. As an adult, Linda is at risk of having a more serious illness and is more likely to have complications if this is a coincidental natural disease. Acyclovir has been studied the most in varicella and is recommended for the following groups at high risk of developing complications from varicella (CDC, 2005 ◉):

- Healthy, nonpregnant persons 13 years and older
- Children older than 12 months with chronic cutaneous or pulmonary disorder and those receiving long-term salicylate therapy
- Consider in children receiving short, intermittent, or aerosolized courses of corticosteroids

For maximum benefit, oral acyclovir therapy should be initiated within the first 24 hours after rash onset, and Linda meets this criterion (Chen et al., 2002) There is no good evidence that treatment with antiviral agents reduces complications of varicella in healthy children between the ages of 12 months and 12 years. Treatment in this age group has been shown only to reduce the number of days of fever and the maximal number of skin lesions (Klassen et al., 2004 ◉).

Patient Education

Linda was prescribed calamine lotion to use topically for symptomatic relief. She was told she could continue to use the diphenhydramine as long as she was not going to be driving and if she did not have to be mentally alert. A second-generation nonsedating antihistamine, over-the-counter loratadine 10 mg once daily was recommended as an alternative. She is sure that her husband has had chicken pox. This makes it unlikely but not impossible for him to develop the illness again (Hall et al., 2002 ◉).

Linda was scheduled to start work in 2 days. Varicella is highly contagious, and she was told to not report to work and stay away from susceptible individuals until the scabs on her lesions had crusted over. She was advised that she should expect new crops of vesicles to appear and crust over during the next 2 to 3 days.

Should she develop new symptoms, such as a cough, become ill, or have a new fever develop, she should be seen to assess the possibility of a secondary bacterial infection or complication.

She asks whether her aunt who stopped into the house for 2 to 3 minutes to pick up a book needs to be seen or treated by her doctor. Although 90% of susceptible individuals with significant exposure will develop the disease, the aunt was not significantly exposed to Linda. "Significant exposure" is defined as 15 minutes of face-to-face contact or 60 minutes of exposure in a room (Watson et al., 2000🅑). Linda's physician might reassure Linda that her aunt probably had chicken pox as a child and is probably immune. If the aunt is concerned, she should by all means see her own family physician.

Disposition

Linda was asked to call her physician's office in 3 to 4 days to report her progress. She will need clearance to return to work and the physician asks her to return in 6 days, as most lesions will have crusted 7 days after the first appearance of the rash. Should this not be the case, she should call the office for advice, as it is important that she avoid exposing other patients in the office to varicella.

DISCUSSION

Varicella is a common disease that affects primarily children. It is caused by varicella-zoster virus, a DNA virus. Varicella-zoster virus is acquired from patients with primary varicella or herpes zoster through either direct contact with infected vesicular fluid or inhalation of aerosolized respiratory secretions. The disease has an incubation period of 11 to 22 days. In children, there may be few prodromal symptoms, whereas adults may experience myalgias, fever, and general malaise. The vesicles appear in crops over 2 to 5 days. Vesicles appear only to then ulcerate and scab over. At any one time, lesions at various stages may be seen. The lesions may commonly affect the oral mucosa, and mild liver involvement may occur. The most common complications are secondary bacterial skin infections in children and pneumonia in adults (Varicella Vaccines: WHO Position Paper, 1998 🅒). Varicella is a risk factor for invasive group A *Streptococcus* infection (CDC, 1997🅑). Other complications can affect almost any organ system and include otitis media, bacteremia, osteomyelitis, septic arthritis, encephalitis, cerebellar ataxia, Reye's syndrome, and thrombocytopenia. Following the disease, virus persists in sensory nerve ganglia where reactivation is prevented by intact cell-mediated immunity. A failure of this immunity later in life

leads to reactivation and the clinical syndrome of herpes zoster or shingles in 15% to 20% of patients (National Advisory Committee on Immunization, 2004🅒).

In adults, varicella is generally associated with a greater number of skin lesions, more systemic complaints, and a 20-fold greater risk of serious complications compared with children. Although adults make up only 1.5% of all cases of primary varicella, adults account for 17% of hospitalizations for the disease.

Of mothers who develop varicella in the immediate antepartum period (5 days before and up to 2 days after delivery), 17% to 30% of newborns will develop severe varicella with a mortality rate of 20% to 30% as a result of the intrauterine transmission of varicella-zoster virus before the transfer of protective maternal antibodies. In addition, if a mother is infected in the first two trimesters, congenital varicella syndrome (limb atrophy and scarring of the skin of the extremity) may occur in the infant. It occurs in 0.4% of births when the mother was infected in the first trimester and 2% when infected from 12 to 20 weeks' gestation (Enders et al., 1994 🅑; Harger et al., 2002 🅑).

Vaccination

The main thrust of managing this disease is immunization. At present, a live attenuated virus vaccine is available. Since the advent of varicella immunization, there has been a dramatic decrease in the incidence of the disease and the morbidity and mortality attached to the disease. Vaccination programs have reduced the number of cases by 71% to 84% and have reduced varicella-related hospitalizations and deaths (Seward et al., 2002🅑). A single dose of vaccine is recommended for children from 12 months of age to 12 years, and a two-dose regimen is recommended for individuals 13 years and older. Adults who are good candidates for immunization include health care workers, individuals such as teachers who are at higher risk of coming in contact with children with the disease, and susceptible contacts of immunocompromised individuals (Varicella Vaccines: WHO Position Paper, 1998🅒). Almost all patients with a reliable history of varicella have protective antibodies on serologic testing. Even in those without this history but who are diagnosed clinically with varicella, serology is positive in approximately 75% of patients. Because of this, even though Linda gave no history of chicken pox during her pre-employment screening visit, she underwent testing to establish susceptibility.

The following examples represent contraindications to varicella immunization (Varicella Vaccines: WHO Position Paper, 1998🅒):

- Persons who are allergic to any component of the vaccine
- Persons with cellular immunodeficiencies

- Persons taking large doses of corticosteroids (>2 mg/kg of body weight or >20 mg/day of prednisone or its equivalent)
- Persons with a moderate or severe concurrent illness
- Women who are pregnant
- Persons who have received blood products (such as whole blood or immunoglobulin) during the previous 5 months (reduces vaccine efficacy)
- Persons with a family history of congenital hereditary immunodeficiency in first-degree relatives unless they are known to be immunocompetent
- Because of the association between aspirin use and Reye's syndrome after varicella, children should avoid salicylates for 6 weeks after vaccination

Common side effects of vaccination include pain and swelling at the site of injection. In addition, 3% to 5% of vaccinees will have a rash in the area of the injection and 3% to 5% will have a generalized varicella-like rash. When occurring within 12 weeks of immunization, the majority of these rashes are found to be natural wild virus infections occurring coincidentally with the immunization (Wise et al., 2000 ⓑ). Although the risk of spread from a vaccine-induced case is very small, especially if the rash is covered, one cannot be sure that the rash is not due to natural disease. Linda was isolated from susceptibles, kept home from work, and treated with acyclovir because of this uncertainty. Special assays are needed to differentiate natural infection from vaccine-induced disease. Although the vaccine is highly effective, a breakthrough varicella rate of 3% to 4% per year is expected after vaccination. When this occurs the disease tends to be milder and more short-lived (National Advisory Committee on Immunization, 2004 ⓒ).

Postexposure Treatment

Oral acyclovir can be used in patients at high risk of developing complications, as listed previously.

Intravenous acyclovir is used in ill patients and those who are immunosuppressed.

The varicella vaccine can attenuate or prevent clinical varicella when administered as postexposure prophylaxis. The vaccine may be administered as long as 5 days after exposure but is generally ineffective when administered more than 5 days after exposure (Watson et al., 2000 ⓑ).

Varicella-zoster immune globulin (VZIG) is indicated for susceptible high-risk persons exposed to varicella. VZIG is most effective when administered within 96 hours of exposure. High-risk individuals include those with leukemia or lymphoma, congenital or acquired immunodeficiency, immunosuppressive therapy, the newborn of a mother who had the onset of varicella 5 days or less before delivery or within 48 hours after delivery, the premature infant >28 weeks' gestation whose mother lacks a history of varicella, and the premature infant <28 weeks' gestation or <1000 g (CDC, 2005 ⓒ).

VZIG has been shown to attenuate the disease in pregnant women and is used in pregnant women exposed to varicella. It should be noted the vaccine should not be used in pregnant wonen. Approximately one third of the pregnant women in a registry set up to gather data on the effect of varicella vaccine in pregnancy were given it rather than VZIG because of product confusion (Shields et al., 2001 ⓑ).

In summary, varicella is a common childhood disease that is becoming less common because of effective immunization programs. The disease is relatively mild and self-limited in children but associated with much more morbidity and mortality in adults. All children and high-risk adults without evidence of immunity should be immunized.

Material Available on Student Consult
Review Questions and Answers about Varicella

REFERENCES

Centers for Disease Control and Prevention. Outbreak of invasive group A *Streptococcus* associated with varicella in a childcare center—Boston, Massachusetts, 1997. MMWR Morb Mortal Wkly Rep 1997;46: 944–948. ⓑ

Centers for Disease Control and Prevention. Available at: www.cdc.gov/nip/vaccine/varicella/faqs-clinic-vaccine.htm#10-serious-adverse. Accessed 3/6/2005. ⓒ

Chen TM, George S, Woodruff CA, et al. Clinical manifestations of varicella-zoster virus infection. Dermatol Clin 2002;20:267–282. ⓒ

Enders G, Miller E, Cradock-Watson J, et al. Consequences of varicella and herpes zoster in pregnancy: Prospective study of 1739 cases. Lancet 1994;343:1548–1551. ⓑ

Hall S, Maupin T, Seward J, et al. Second varicella infections: Are they more common than previously thought? Pediatrics 2002;109:1068–1073. ⓑ

Harger JH, Ernest JM, Thurnau GR, et al. Frequency of congenital varicella syndrome in a prospective cohort of 347 pregnant women. Obstet Gynecol 2002;100: 260–265. ⓑ

Klassen TP, Belseck EM, Wiebe N, et al. Acyclovir for treating varicella in otherwise healthy children and adolescents (Cochrane Review). The Cochrane Library, Vol. 2. Chichester, UK, John Wiley & Sons, 2004. ⓑ

National Advisory Committee on Immunization. Update on varicella. Can Commun Dis Rep 2004;30:1–28. ⓒ

Seward JF, Watson BM, Peterson CL, et al. Varicella disease after introduction of varicella vaccine in the United States, 1995–2000. JAMA 2002;287:606–611. **B**

Shields KE, Galil K, Seward J, et al. Varicella vaccine exposure during pregnancy: Data from the first 5 years of the pregnancy registry. Obstet Gynecol 2001;98: 14–19. **B**

Watson B, Seward J, Yang A, et al. Postexposure effectiveness of varicella vaccine. Pediatrics 2000;105: 85–88. **B**

Wise RP, Salive ME, Braun MM, et al. Post-licensure safety surveillance for varicella. JAMA 2000;284: 1271–1279. **B**

Varicella vaccines: WHO position paper. Wkly Epidemiol Rec 1998;73:241–248. **C**

Chapter

29   Fever and Cough (Influenza)

Marguerite R. Duane

KEY POINTS

1. Influenza is a serious infectious disease that afflicts thousands of people each year.
2. Annual vaccination is the best way to prevent infection and minimize the effect of influenza.
3. Clinical diagnosis is difficult due to the lack of specificity and sensitivity of symptoms, but awareness of the prevalence of influenza in the community can aid in diagnosis.
4. Rapid viral tests allow early confirmation of the illness, but only viral cultures provide specific information regarding the influenza strains in circulation, which is used to formulate vaccine for the next year.
5. Antiviral agents have been shown to reduce the duration of influenza illness when given within 36 to 48 hours of symptom onset and to prevent influenza illness when used for prophylaxis.

INITIAL VISIT

Subjective

Patient Identification and Presenting Problem

Joe is a 52-year-old white man who presents with complaints of sudden onset of fever and cough last evening.

Joe reports that he had felt fine throughout the day yesterday until after dinner when he began to feel feverish. He developed a dry cough and some chest discomfort, which he attributed to the coughing spells. This morning he woke up with a severe headache and states he felt like he had "been run over by a Mack truck." He said he did not even have the energy to come to the doctor, but his wife insisted. The patient reports that his youngest daughter was ill earlier in the week with a "cold."

Medical History

Joe has a history of high blood pressure for which he takes hydrochlorothiazide 25 mg once daily. He had a hernia repair in his early 30s. Otherwise, he has had no other major illnesses, surgeries, or hospitalizations. He has never received a Pneumovax or influenza vaccine.

Family History

Joe's father is 81 years old. He has high blood pressure and chronic obstructive pulmonary disease. His mother is 78 years old and has a history of high blood pressure. Joe has two older sisters and a younger sister, one of whom has thyroid disease and another who has asthma.

Social History

Joe works full time at a print shop. He and his wife have five children, four of whom still live at home.

Evidence levels Ⓐ Randomized, controlled trials (RCTs), meta-analyses, well-designed systematic reviews of RCTs. **Ⓑ** Case-control or cohort studies, nonrandomized clinical trials, systematic reviews of studies other than RCTs, cross-sectional studies, retrospective studies, certain uncontrolled studies. **Ⓒ** Consensus statements, expert guidelines, usual practice, opinion.

Formerly, he smoked a pack of cigarettes per day for about 25 years, but he quit 3 years ago. He drinks a glass of beer or wine occasionally.

Review of Systems
In general, the patient reports feeling very fatigued and weak. He has not had much of an appetite today. He also complains of a mild sore throat but denies a runny nose or nasal congestion. In addition to the headache, Joe complains of generalized body aches. He denies chest pain, but he still has some chest discomfort. He denies shortness of breath. Further review of symptoms is negative.

Objective

Physical Examination
General Joe is a moderately ill-appearing man in no acute respiratory distress. He is 5 feet 7 inches tall and weighs 160 pounds; his temperature is 38.4°C (101.2°F), blood pressure is 140/85, respiratory rate is 22, and pulse is 96.

Head, Eyes, Ears, Nose, and Throat His head is normocephalic with no trauma. The pupils are equal, round, and reactive to light; the conjunctivae are slightly injected. There is mild erythema of the nose but no drainage; the oropharynx has slightly dry mucous membranes, mild erythema, but no exudates. The neck is supple with no lymphadenopathy.

Heart Heart rate and rhythm are regular with no murmurs.

Lungs There are decreased breath sounds at the bases, but otherwise the lungs are clear to auscultation bilaterally.

Abdomen The abdomen is soft, mildly tender, and nondistended. The skin is warm and clammy.

Assessment

Working Diagnosis
The working diagnosis is influenza given the abrupt onset and constellation of symptoms.

Differential Diagnosis
The differential diagnosis of fever and cough varies based on the patient's age and presenting symptoms. Sepsis must be considered in neonates with the sudden onset of fever and associated nonspecific symptoms. The presence of nasal discharge suggests a viral respiratory tract infection such as respiratory syncytial virus. The differential diagnosis in younger children includes bronchiolitis, bronchitis, laryngotracheitis, pneumonia, streptococcal pharyngitis,

and other upper respiratory infections. In older children and adults such as Joe, the differential diagnosis includes viral upper respiratory infections (such as parainfluenza, respiratory syncytial virus, adenovirus, and enterovirus), mononucleosis, pneumococcal pneumonia, and streptococcal pharyngitis.

Plan

Diagnostic
Joe's clinical presentation is highly consistent with influenza. Review of weekly influenza surveillance data from the Centers for Disease Control and Prevention shows more than 95% of influenza cases in the area are due to influenza A. Given the high probability that the patient has influenza as well as the prevalence of influenza in the community, further diagnostic testing is not indicated, as it would not be cost-effective (Hueston and Benich, 2004 ⑬).

Therapeutic
The patient is treated empirically with rimantadine 100 mg twice daily for 5 days.

Patient Education
The patient is informed that treatment will likely shorten the duration of his illness by about 1 day. He is educated about the highly contagious nature of the illness and is encouraged to limit contact with people who are at high risk of serious complications if they develop influenza (Table 29-1).

DISCUSSION

Influenza is a significant public health issue, with approximately 10% to 20% of the U.S. population developing the illness each year. Between 1969 and 1995, influenza accounted for an average of 114,000 hospitalizations each year, and between 1990 and 1999, it accounted for an average of 36,000 deaths per year (Prevention and Control of Influenza: Recommendations of the Advisory Committee on Immunization Practices [ACIP], 2004 ⓒ). The rate of infection is highest among children, but the rate of serious illness and death is highest among individuals older than 65 years of age and in individuals with chronic medical conditions that place them at increased risk of complications.

Influenza epidemics occur during the winter months and may be caused by the influenza A or B viruses. Influenza A is divided into subtypes based on two surface antigens, hemagglutinin and neuraminidase. Both influenza A and B viruses are further divided based on antigenic characteristics. Changes in these antigens result in new variants of the influenza virus, a process known as antigenic

Table 29-1 Individuals at Increased Risk of Complications from Influenza
Individuals 65 years and older
Residents of nursing homes and chronic care facilities
Individuals who have chronic medical conditions, such as asthma, heart disease, diabetes, renal dysfunction, or immunosuppression due to disease or medications
Individuals 6 months to 18 years of age who receive long-term aspirin therapy, as they may be at increased risk of Reye's syndrome after influenza infection
Women in their second or third trimester of pregnancy during the influenza season
Young children between 6 and 23 months of age

drift. Because infection or vaccination with one virus type may not provide protection against an antigenic variant of the same type, a major influenza epidemic may be caused by influenza virus types not included in that year's vaccine.

Prevention

Administration of the influenza vaccine is an essential component in the prevention of the disease and its complications. In the United States, an inactivated influenza vaccine and a live, attenuated influenza vaccine are available each year. The inactivated vaccine is approved for all individuals 6 months of age and older. The live, attenuated vaccine is approved only for healthy individuals between the ages of 5 and 49. The vaccine contains at least three viral strains that are expected to be present during the influenza season. The vaccine is more effective when the vaccine and epidemic strains are well matched and when persons at high risk receive the vaccine before the influenza virus has widely circulated.

The Centers for Disease Control and Prevention recommends that individuals who are at increased risk of complications from influenza receive the vaccine (see Table 29-1) (Prevention and Control of Influenza: Recommendations of the ACIP, 2004 ⓒ). Additionally, health care workers and other individuals in close contact with persons at increased risk of complications should receive the vaccine to reduce transmission rates and subsequent complications.

Diagnosis

Influenza is extremely contagious because the virus is spread from person to person via respiratory secretions. Individuals with influenza are contagious beginning approximately 1 day before the onset of symptoms until approximately 5 days into the illness. Children can spread the illness for more than 10 days after the illness begins. Symptoms typically last for 1 to 5 days, although cough and malaise may persist for more than 2 weeks (Prevention and Control of Influenza: Recommendations of the ACIP, 2004 ⓒ).

Uncomplicated influenza infection is characterized by the abrupt onset and severe nature of a constellation of symptoms. Constitutional symptoms may include fever, chills, headaches, myalgias, fatigue, weakness, malaise, and anorexia. Respiratory symptoms commonly include a dry cough and chest discomfort and may also include a stuffy nose, sneezing, and sore throat. Because the respiratory symptoms may be caused by many other respiratory pathogens, including the common cold, the diagnosis may be difficult to make.

The diagnosis of influenza is also complicated by the poor sensitivity of clinical findings and the poor specificity of clinical diagnosis. During an epidemic, studies among adults show fever and cough to be 63% to 78% sensitive for influenza. The classic triad of fever, cough, and myalgias is only 77% to 85% sensitive and 55% to 71% specific (Prevention and Control of Influenza: Recommendations of the ACIP, 2004 ⓒ). The predictive value of these symptoms depends on the level of influenza activity; therefore, awareness of influenza in the community can improve identification of the illness. The Centers for Disease Control and Prevention maintains weekly influenza surveillance data that may be obtained at its Web site (www.cdc.gov/flu).

In addition to surveillance information, laboratory testing can help in the diagnosis of influenza. As with any diagnostic test, the sensitivity and specificity may vary based on the type of test used, the type of specimen tested, and the laboratory where the test is performed. Viral culture is the most accurate method for identifying specific viral strains and subtypes. However, results are not available for 2 to 10 days, which makes it impractical to use to determine whether treatment should be initiated.

Rapid viral tests are available for use in outpatient settings, give results in less than 30 minutes, and on average cost between $12 and $24 (Montalto,

2003 **Ⓑ**). These tests vary based on the type of influenza viruses that they can detect, the types of specimens that can be used, and the complexity involved in performing the test. Some tests detect only influenza A viruses; other tests detect both influenza A and B viruses but do not distinguish between the two; finally, others detect both viruses and distinguish between influenza A and B. The tests also vary in terms of their sensitivity and specificity with sensitivities ranging from 51% to 96% and specificities ranging from 52% to 100% (Prevention and Control of Influenza: Recommendations of the ACIP, 2004 **Ⓒ**). Because the sensitivity of these tests, or their ability to rule out influenza, is lower than for viral culture, physicians may consider further testing if confirmation of a negative test is important.

Management

A rapid, accurate diagnosis is essential to initiate antiviral treatment in a timely fashion. There are four antiviral agents effective against influenza, but each is effective only when given within 36 to 48 hours after onset of symptoms. The four agents, amantadine, rimantadine, zanamivir, and oseltamivir, differ with respect to their antiviral action, age limit for use, route of administration, adverse effects, drug interactions, and cost (Table 29-2) (Montalto et al., 2000 **Ⓑ**). All four drugs are classified as pregnancy category C. In addition to these antiviral agents, patients should receive symptomatic treatment, as they would with other viral infections.

Amantadine and rimantadine are effective against influenza A. Systematic reviews show these agents reduce the duration of symptoms by approximately 1 day compared with placebo, if they are administered with 48 hours of symptom onset

(Fagan and Moeller, 2004 **Ⓐ**). When used for prophylaxis, these drugs have been shown to prevent 70% to 90% of illnesses from influenza (Couch, 2000 **Ⓑ**; Prevention and Control of Influenza: Recommendations of the ACIP, 2004 **Ⓒ**). Because these drugs are renally cleared, caution should be used when administering them in older patients and in patients with renal disease. Amantadine should also be used with caution in older patients and in patients with seizure disorders due to the central nervous system side effects (Montalto et al., 2000 **Ⓑ**).

Zanamivir and oseltamivir are neuraminidase inhibitors that are effective against influenza A and B. Both have been shown to reduce the duration of symptoms by 1 to 1.5 days as compared with placebo (Couch, 2000 **Ⓑ**; Fagan and Moeller, 2004 **Ⓐ**). Like amantadine and rimantadine, zanamivir must be given within 48 hours of symptom onset, but oseltamivir must be given within 36 hours. Although studies show both drugs are approximately 80% effective in preventing influenza illness, only oseltamivir has been approved for prophylaxis (Prevention and Control of Influenza: Recommendations of the ACIP, 2004 **Ⓒ**).Because zanamivir is administered via inhalation, caution should be used in patients with underlying airway disease due to the risk of bronchospasm and a decline in lung function.

Several important decision points occur in the evaluation and management of patients with suspected influenza. Does their clinical presentation suggest a high probability of infection with influenza? Should a rapid viral test be performed to confirm the diagnosis? If influenza infection is strongly suspected or confirmed, which medication should be prescribed? In a cost-benefit analysis of patients at high risk of influenza-related complications, rapid

Table 29-2 Comparison of Antiviral Agents Used to Treat Influenza				
Characteristics	**Amantadine (Symmetrel)**	**Rimantadine (Flumadine)**	**Zanamivir (Relenza)**	**Oseltamivir (Tamiflu)**
Antiviral action	A	A	A + B	A + B
Prophylaxis	Yes	Yes	No	Yes
Age limit for use	≥1 yr	≥18 yr for treatment ≥1 yr for prophylaxis	≥7 yr	≥18 yr
Route	Oral	Oral	Inhalation	Oral
Adverse effects	Central nervous system: insomnia, anxiety, depression; gastrointestinal effects	Gastrointestinal: dyspepsia, nausea, vomiting	Nasal/throat irritation, cough; bronchospasm in asthmatics	Nausea, vomiting
Cost for a 5-day course*	$14	$22	$57	$67

*Average wholesale cost based on *Red Book*, Montvale, NJ: Medical Economics Data, 2004.
A, influenza A; B, influenza B.

viral testing was not as cost-effective as empirical treatment alone with amantadine or rimantadine even when the probability of influenza infection was as low as 10%. Even though neuraminidase inhibitors are more expensive, rapid viral testing is not as cost-effective as empirical treatment with these agents until the prevalence of infection falls between 30% and 40% (Hueston and Benich, 2004 **B**). Therefore, from a cost-benefit perspective, rapid viral testing has a limited role in patients at high risk of complications from influenza. In deciding which medication to prescribe, consideration should be given to cost, side effect profile, patient's age, and prevalence of influenza A.

In summary, influenza is a serious infectious disease that afflicts thousands of people each year. Annual vaccination is the best way to prevent infection and minimize the effect of influenza. Clinical diagnosis is difficult due to the lack of specificity and sensitivity of symptoms, but awareness of the prevalence of influenza in the community can aid in diagnosis. Rapid viral tests allow early confirmation of the illness, but only viral cultures provide specific information regarding the influenza strains in circulation, which is used to formulate vaccine for the next year. Antiviral agents have been shown to reduce the duration of influenza illness when given within 36 to 48 hours of symptom onset and to prevent influenza illness when used for prophylaxis.

Material Available on Student Consult
Review Questions and Answers about Influenza

REFERENCES

Couch RB. Prevention and treatment of influenza. N Engl J Med 2000;343:1778–1785.**B**

Fagan HB, Moeller AH. What is the best antiviral agent for influenza infection? Am Fam Physician 2004;70: 1331–1333.**A**

Hueston WJ, Benich JJ. A cost benefit analysis of testing for influenza A in high risk adults. Ann Fam Med 2004;2:33–40.**B**

Kingston BJ, Wright CV. Influenza in the nursing home. Am Fam Physician 2002;65:75–78.**B**

Montalto NJ. An office based approach to influenza: Clinical diagnosis and laboratory testing. Am Fam Physician 2003;67:111–117.**B**

Montalto NJ, Gum KD, Ashley JV. Updated treatment for influenza A and B. Am Fam Physician 2000; 62:2467–2476.**B**

Prevention and control of influenza: Recommendations of the Advisory Committee on Immunization Practices (ACIP). MMWR Morb Mortal Wkly Rep 2004;53: 1–40.**C**

30 Sinus Congestion (Sinusitis)

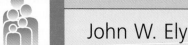

John W. Ely

INITIAL VISIT

Subjective

Patient Identification and Presenting Problem

Kathy V. is a 28-year-old kindergarten teacher who complains of sinus congestion. She was well until a week ago when she developed nasal congestion, mild sore throat, fatigue, and headache. She denied cough or fever. Initially, her nasal discharge was clear, but in the past 2 days, it has turned yellowish green. She complains of pain and fullness in both cheeks, especially when she bends forward. She tried over-the-counter decongestants, and these were somewhat helpful but did not provide complete relief. She denies pain in her maxillary teeth. She says she often gets a sinus infection in the fall and wonders whether she might be allergic to fall weeds but has never had skin testing. In the past, she has obtained relief with antibiotics for similar symptoms. She believes that she has another sinus infection and is asking for a course of antibiotics.

Medical History

Kathy had a tonsillectomy at age 5. She had two uncomplicated vaginal deliveries at age 21 and 23. She takes no other medications and has no known medication allergies.

Family History

Kathy has two sisters, who are alive and well. Her mother has hypertension and "allergies." Her father has no health problems that she is aware of.

Social History

Kathy is a nonsmoker and drinks alcohol rarely. She teaches kindergarten and is married to a restaurant manager. She has two children and lives on an acreage with her husband.

Review of Systems

Kathy denies dyspnea, chest pain, nausea, or vomiting. She has had no visual disturbance or other neurologic symptoms.

Objective

Physical Examination

General Kathy is alert but appears moderately ill and has obvious nasal congestion.

Vital Signs Her temperature is 37.6°C (99.7°F), pulse is 84, respiratory rate is 18, and blood pressure is 130/84.

Eyes, Ears, Nose, and Throat Her pupils are 3 mm, equal, and reactive to light. Her external auditory canals and tympanic membranes are normal. Her nasal mucus is clear bilaterally, turbinates are swollen bilaterally, and she cannot breathe through her left nostril at all. The nasal mucosa is pink. Maxillary sinuses are mildly tender to palpation (but probably within normal limits). There is no inflammation in her mouth and throat.

Neck Her neck is supple with no lymph node enlargement.

Lungs Her lungs are clear to percussion and auscultation.

Heart Her heart rhythm is regular with a grade II/VI systolic ejection murmur along the left sternal border.

Abdomen Her abdomen is nontender with no organomegaly or masses.

Extremities There is no edema.

Assessment

Working Diagnosis
Acute bacterial sinusitis.

Differential Diagnosis
The differential diagnosis includes other causes of nasal congestion.

The *common cold*, caused by common respiratory viruses (e.g., rhinoviruses, parainfluenza virus, influenza virus), is difficult to distinguish from bacterial sinusitis (Gwaltney et al., 1994 Ⓑ; Hickner et al., 2001Ⓑ; Williams and Simel, 1993 Ⓑ). Colds tend to produce milder symptoms and a shorter course of illness (usually less than 7 to 10 days). The mucus is likely to be clear, and fever in adults is unusual. However, there is a large overlap with the clinical findings of bacterial sinusitis, as discussed later in this chapter (Williams and Simel, 1993Ⓑ).

Allergic rhinitis is more likely to be associated with itching (itchy eyes, itchy throat, itchy nose) and with a history of atopic disease and seasonal exacerbation of symptoms. Patients often have paroxysms of sneezing and may have other evidence of atopic diseases, such as asthma or eczema. Physical findings, such as hyperlinear palms, Dennie Morgan lines (increased number of creases below the eyes), and dry skin, increase the likelihood of atopy as an explanation for nasal symptoms. However, bacterial sinusitis can be a complication of allergic rhinitis.

Vasomotor rhinitis (idiopathic rhinitis) is characterized by congestion and rhinorrhea triggered by nonspecific irritants such as odors and temperature changes. It is a chronic condition that is not associated with a purulent discharge or with systemic symptoms. It can usually be distinguished from allergic rhinitis by the absence of itching.

Rhinitis medicamentosa results from overuse of topical nasal decongestants. Patients generally admit to daily use of nose sprays and complain that they cannot function during the day or sleep at night if they stop treatment. The condition is chronic and not typically associated with other respiratory symptoms.

Plan

Diagnostic
Transillumination of the maxillary sinuses seems somewhat reduced bilaterally. However, the amount of transillumination varies depending on the exact placement of the light, and interpretation is judged unreliable. Because this is the patient's initial presentation for this illness, further diagnostic tests, such as computed tomography and sinus aspiration, are not indicated.

Therapeutic
Kathy is treated with amoxicillin 1 g three times daily for 10 days. She was advised that she could continue her over-the-counter decongestant if it seemed to help her symptoms.

Patient Education
The physician explains that Kathy probably has a viral infection, but because of her symptoms and the length of her illness, there is a moderate chance of bacterial sinusitis. Although symptomatic treatment alone is an option, the patient is convinced that she will not improve without antibiotics. She is instructed to return if she fails to improve over the next 3 to 4 days or if her symptoms worsen.

DISCUSSION

Introduction

How can bacterial sinusitis be distinguished from the common cold? This is one of the great unanswered questions in primary care and one that most family physicians grapple with every day. Sinus aspiration is onsidered the gold standard for diagnosis, but it is not a reasonable option for most patients. Sinus computed tomography scans are expensive and, even if abnormal, do not assume the diagnosis of bacterial sinusitis because viral sinusitis can cause identical findings (Gwaltney et al., 1994 Ⓑ). Therefore, bacterial sinusitis is generally diagnosed by history and physical examination findings, such as length of illness (>7 days), colored nasal discharge, maxillary pain, and so on. When the patient has all the symptoms and signs of sinusitis, the likelihood of a bacterial infection is high. When none of the signs and symptoms are present, the likelihood is low. Most patients fall between these extremes and thus have an intermediate probability of sinusitis. The question then becomes at what probability should antibiotics be prescribed. For example, if the patient has a 20% chance of bacterial sinusitis, is that high enough to justify antibiotic treatment?

In practice, the decision to treat with antibiotics depends as much on "soft" variables, such as patient wishes, physician beliefs, and community customs, as it does on the patient's clinical findings. Recent reviews and clinical guidelines have provided excellent summaries of the evidence on diagnosis and treatment of acute sinusitis (Anonymous, 1999Ⓑ; Gwaltney, 2004 Ⓒ; Hickner et al., 2001Ⓑ; Piccirillo, 2004Ⓒ). Unfortunately, the lack of reliable methods for distinguishing between common colds and bacterial sinusitis has hindered the ability of these groups to provide definitive advice. The guidelines have little to say about the real-world dilemmas faced by practicing physicians who must balance the demands of patients with concerns about the overuse of antibiotics. Physicians who are pressured by patients for antibiotics cannot say with much conviction that antibiotics are not needed because they have no practical tools for ruling out bacterial infection. Over the past 30 years, only a handful of studies have attempted to correlate clinical findings with more definitive evidence of sinusitis (Axelsson and Runze, 1976Ⓑ; Berg and Carenfelt, 1988Ⓑ; Hansen et al., 1995 Ⓑ; Lindbaek et al., 1996bⒷ; van Buchem et al., 1995 Ⓑ; van Duijn et al., 1992 Ⓑ; Williams et al., 1992Ⓑ).

Epidemiology

Only 2% of common colds are complicated by bacterial sinusitis. The maxillary sinuses are most frequently involved. The organisms most likely to cause acute sinusitis are *Streptococcus pneumoniae* and *Haemophilus influenzae* (Gwaltney, 2004 Ⓒ). In chronic sinusitis, *Staphylococcus aureus* and gram-negative rods are the predominant organisms, although anaerobes and fungi are frequently isolated also.

Risk factors for bacterial sinusitis include a preceding viral upper respiratory infection, history of nasal allergies, deviated nasal septum, nasal polyps, and swimming. Less common risk factors include cystic fibrosis, disorders of ciliary function, and immunodeficiency (e.g., human immunodeficiency virus infection).

Diagnosis

Williams et al. (1992Ⓑ) found five clinical findings that independently predicted sinusitis, when radiographic abnormalities were used as the gold standard: colored nasal discharge by history, colored nasal discharge by physical examination, maxillary tooth pain, failure to respond to decongestants, and abnormal transillumination. If all five findings were present, the patient had a high likelihood of having sinusitis, and, if none were present, the patient had a low likelihood. Most patients fell between these extremes and had intermediate probabilities. To transilluminate the maxillary sinuses, a fiberoptic light (such as an otoscope without the disposable tip) is placed on the upper cheek at the infraorbital rim. The procedure must be carried out in a completely dark room. With the patient's mouth open, the physician will observe a red glow on the hard palate if the sinus is normal. Fluid or mucosal thickening will produce various degrees of reduction in the glow. Unfortunately, the procedure is not very reliable because it depends on exact light placement, degree of dark accommodation, and intensity of the light source.

Since 1976, seven studies have attempted to correlate clinical findings with more objective evidence of sinusitis (Axelsson and Runze, 1976 Ⓑ; Berg and Carenfelt, 1988 Ⓑ; Hansen et al., 1995 Ⓑ; Lindbaek et al., 1996bⒷ; van Buchem et al., 1995 Ⓑ; van Duijn et al., 1992 Ⓑ; Williams et al., 1992Ⓑ). Based on these studies, Hickner and colleagues (2001Ⓑ) recommend withholding antibiotics for at least 7 days of typical cold symptoms because bacterial sinusitis occurs in only 20% of patients within the first 7 days. Other symptoms found to favor sinusitis include purulent nasal discharge, unilateral maxillary tooth or face pain, and worsening of symptoms after initial improvement. Current guidelines favor these findings together with the 7-day waiting period as the most clinically useful method for identifying patients who should be treated with antibiotics (Anonymous, 1999Ⓑ; Anonymous, 2001Ⓒ; Hickner et al., 2001Ⓑ).

The most accurate method for identifying bacterial sinusitis is to aspirate the involved sinus, but this procedure is too invasive for routine use. It should be reserved for research studies and in selected patients who are suspected of intracranial extension of their infection. Sinus computed tomography scanning has generally replaced plain films because of its improved accuracy and similar cost. However, imaging is not recommended for most patients because it is expensive and does not distinguish between viral and bacterial sinusitis (Gwaltney et al., 1994Ⓑ). It may be indicated for patients whose symptoms fail to respond to antibiotics or who have recurrent infections. In such patients, a normal computed tomography scan is particularly helpful in avoiding repeated courses of antibiotics. Computed tomography is also recommended in patients suspected of having intracranial or intraorbital complications, but these are rare complications.

Table 30-1 Recommendations for Managing Patients with Sinusitis and Strength of Evidence for Those Recommendations

Recommendation	Strength of Recommendation
The diagnosis of bacterial sinusitis should generally be based on clinical findings such as purulent nasal discharge, maxillary pain, and duration of illness >7 days.	B
Most patients with bacterial sinusitis should be treated with amoxicillin. In patients allergic to penicillin, doxycycline or trimethoprim/sulfamethoxazole can be used. In patients who are likely to have resistant bacteria (day care workers, patients who have recently taken antibiotics), azithromycin, levofloxacin, or high-dose amoxicillin/clavulanate should be used.	B
Radiographs should not be routinely performed to diagnose acute sinusitis. They may be indicated in patients with recurrent infection or those who fail to respond to treatment. Sinus computed tomography scanning has generally replaced plain films.	B
Decongestant/antihistamine combinations and analgesics can be offered for symptomatic treatment.	B

B, Recommendation based on inconsistent or limited-quality, patient-oriented evidence.

Treatment

The efficacy of antibiotics for acute sinusitis is controversial with some studies showing benefit and others failing to show benefit (Axelsson et al., 1970❸; Gananca and Trabulsi, 1973❸; Lindbaek et al., 1996a❸; Stalman et al., 1997❸; van Buchem et al., 1997❸). Once the decision is made to treat with antibiotics, current guidelines favor narrow-spectrum antibiotics such as amoxicillin (adult dose 1.0 g three times daily for 10 days), trimethoprim/sulfamethoxazole (one double-strength [160 mg/800 mg] tablet twice daily), or doxycycline (100 mg twice daily). Narrow-spectrum antibiotics, such as amoxicillin, are justified in patients with mild to moderate symptoms or in those who have only a moderate likelihood of bacterial infection. However, because of the increasing prevalence of resistant *S. pneumoniae* and *H. influenzae* in many communities, patients with more severe symptoms should receive broader spectrum antibiotics, such as amoxicillin/clavulanate (2000 mg/125 mg every 12 hours), cefpodoxime (200 mg every 12 hours), cefdinir (600 mg once daily), or levofloxacin (750 mg once daily). Fluoroquinolones should be avoided in patients younger than age 18 years, and doxycycline should be avoided in patients younger than age 8 years. Both should generally be avoided in pregnancy.

The duration of treatment varies. One study found that 3 days of trimethoprim/sulfamethoxazole was just as effective as 10 days' treatment (Williams et al., 1995❹). However, most physicians continue to treat for 10 days. Otolaryngologists often treat much longer (2 to 4 weeks), but they see a referral population, which includes patients who have failed shorter treatment courses. Patients who fail to respond to 10 days of a first-line antibiotic should receive a longer course of a broader spectrum antibiotic. A computed tomography scan should be obtained after one or two failed antibiotic courses (depending on severity of symptoms), and referral to an otolaryngologist should be made if the sinuses are opacified.

In patients who request antibiotics for symptoms that are most consistent with a viral infection, a compromise measure has been suggested: Couchman and colleagues (2000❸) advised patients with common respiratory symptoms to fill prescriptions for antibiotics only if their symptoms worsened or did not improve after a specified number of days (which was determined individually by the physician). In their study, only 50.2% of patients filled their prescriptions.

Symptomatic treatment with decongestant/antihistamine preparations is commonly prescribed, although evidence to support efficacy has been inconsistent. Topical decongestants can also be prescribed, but the patient should be warned not to use them for more than 4 days due to the risk of inducing rebound congestion or rhinitis medicamentosa. Patients with acute sinusitis often have severe facial pain, and analgesics should be offered in such cases.

Summary

Sinusitis should be suspected in adults who have nasal congestion lasting longer than 7 days, especially when accompanied by unilateral maxillary pain or purulent nasal discharge. In general, symptoms lasting less than 7 days can be attributed to a viral common cold unless symptoms are severe or there is a fever. Once the diagnosis is made, patients should be treated with antibiotics for 10 days. For most patients, amoxicillin 500 to 1000 mg three times daily is a reasonable choice. Alternatives include trimethoprim/sulfamethoxazole and doxycycline. For patients with severe symptoms, an antibiotic with coverage for resistant bacteria, such as amoxicillin/clavulanate, cefpodoxime, cefdinir, or levofloxacin, should be used. The main recommendations for managing patients with sinusitis are summarized in Table 30-1.

Material Available on Student Consult
Review Questions and Answers about Sinusitis

REFERENCES

Anonymous. Diagnosis and treatment of acute bacterial rhinosinusitis: Summary, evidence report/technology assessment. No. 9. Rockville, MD, Agency for Health Care Policy and Research, 1999. (AHCPR publication no. 99-E015.) Available at www.ahrq.gov/clinic/epcsums/sinussum.htm. Accessed 8/28/2004.**B**

Anonymous. Clinical practice guideline: Management of sinusitis. Pediatrics 2001;108:798–808.**C**

Axelsson A, Chidekel N, Grebelius N, Jensen C. Treatment of acute maxillary sinusitis: A comparison of four different methods. Acta Otolaryngol 1970;70:71–76.**B**

Axelsson A, Runze U. Symptoms and signs of acute maxillary sinusitis. ORL J Otorhinolaryngol Relat Spec 1976;38:298–308.**B**

Berg O, Carenfelt C. Analysis of symptoms and clinical signs in the maxillary sinus empyema. Acta Otolaryngol 1988;105:343–349.**B**

Couchman GR, Rascoe TG, Forjuoh SN. Back-up antibiotic prescriptions for common respiratory symptoms. J Fam Pract 2000;49:907–913.**B**

Gananca M, Trabulsi LR. The therapeutic effects of cyclacillin in acute sinusitis: In vitro and in vivo correlations in a placebo-controlled study. Curr Med Res Opin 1973;1:362–368.**B**

Gwaltney JM Jr. Acute Sinusitis and Rhinosinusitis, 2004. Up to Date.com. Accessed 8/21/2004.**C**

Gwaltney JM, Phillips CD, Miller RD, Riker DK. Computed tomographic study of the common cold. N Engl J Med 1994;330:25–30.**B**

Hansen JG, Schmidt H, Rosborg J, Lund E. Predicting acute maxillary sinusitis in a general practice population. BMJ 1995;311:233–236.**B**

Hickner JM, Bartlett JG, Besser RE, Gonzales R, . Hoffman JR, Sande MA. Principles of appropriate antibiotic use for acute rhinosinusitis in adults: Background. Ann Intern Med 2001;134:498–505.**B**

Lindbaek M, Hjortdahl P, Johnsen UL. Randomised, double blind, placebo controlled trial of penicillin V and amoxycillin in treatment of acute sinus infections in adults. BMJ 1996a;313:325–329.**B**

Lindbaek M, Hjortdahl P, Johnsen UL. Use of symptoms, signs, and blood tests to diagnose acute sinus infections in primary care: Comparison with computed tomography. Fam Med 1996b;28:183–188.**B**

Piccirillo JF. Acute bacterial sinusitis. N Engl J Med 2004;351:902–910.**C**

Stalman W, van Essen GA, van der Graaf Y, de Melker RA. The end of antibiotic treatment in adults with acute sinusitis-like complaints in general practice? A placebo-controlled double-blind randomized doxycycline trial. Br J Gen Pract 1997;47:794–799.**B**

van Buchem FL, Knottnerus JA, Schrijnemaekers VJ, Peeters MR. Primary-care-based randomised placebo-controlled trial of antibiotic treatment in acute maxillary sinusitis. Lancet 1997;349:683–687.**B**

van Buchem L, Peeters M, Beaumont J, Knottnerus JA. Acute maxillary sinusitis in general practice: The relation between clinical picture and objective findings. Eur J Gen Pract 1995;1:155–160.**B**

van Duijn NP, Brouwer HJ, Lamberts H. Use of symptoms and signs to diagnose maxillary sinusitis in general practice: Comparison with ultrasonography. BMJ 1992;305:684–687.**B**

Williams JW, Hollerman DR, Samsa GP, Simel DL. Randomized controlled trial of 3 vs 10 days of trimethoprim/sulfamethoxazole for acute maxillary sinusitis. JAMA 1995;273:1015–1021.**A**

Williams JW, Simel DL. Does this patient have sinusitis? Diagnosing acute sinusitis by history and physical examination. JAMA 1993;270:1242–1246.**B**

Williams JW Jr, Simel DL, Roberts L, Samsa GP. Clinical evaluation for sinusitis. Making the diagnosis by history and physical examination. Ann Intern Med 1992;117:705–710.**B**

31 Productive Cough (Acute Bronchitis)

Bruce Barrett

KEY POINTS

1. Acute bronchitis is a very common diagnosis and is usually caused by viral infection.
2. Other causes of acute cough, such as pneumonia, gastroesophageal reflux disease, and allergy, should be considered.
3. The best available evidence suggests that antibiotics may reduce symptoms and illness duration slightly. Costs and side effects make the benefit-harm trade off tenuous at best.
4. Neither age nor smoking status has been linked to antibiotic effectiveness.
5. Only doxycycline, erythromycin, and trimethoprim/sulfamethoxazole have been tested in positively reported randomized, controlled trials (RCTs); hence, these are the only antibiotics that should be considered.

6. There is very little RCT-based evidence for or against the effectiveness of antitussive treatments. However, limited use may be supported, especially when the cough is interfering with sleep.
7. Nonsteroidal anti-inflammatory drugs are effective for pain, but significant toxicity risks raise the need for caution.
8. Over-the-counter cold formulas containing decongestants and/or antihistamines are not appropriate treatments for acute bronchitis but may be helpful if nasal congestion or drainage is present.
9. Mucolytics and expectorants have not been adequately assessed for acute bronchitis, but evidence from common cold and chronic bronchitis suggests possible effectiveness.

INITIAL VISIT

Subjective

Patient Identification and Presenting Problem

Jane Doe is a 58-year-old woman who presents at your clinic with productive cough of 10 days' duration. Jane first felt ill 2 weeks ago on the first of October. She remembers feeling a scratchy throat, which progressed to sore throat, general malaise, and cough. The cough has been bothersome both during the day and at night. It has kept her awake and has awakened her out of sleep. During the past week, she has coughed up phlegm. At first, it was clear to white. Now it is green or brown. There has been no blood. She felt alternately "slightly feverish" and "chilly" during the first few days of this illness but denies high temperatures and has not felt feverish for the past several days. She denies nasal symptoms, chest pain, shortness of breath, and vomiting. She may have had some increased dyspnea on exertion, especially in the beginning of the illness. She denies sensations of maxillary pain or postnasal drip. Her sore throat has resolved. This acute illness has caused her to reduce smoking to "a few cigarettes a day." She notes that "I really should quit that stuff." She has been using an over-the-counter combination cold formula, which she believes has helped manage the cough, although it does make her "a bit groggy."

Medical History

You have known Jane since she first came to you about 4 years ago with chest pain. Previously, she had neglected her health care for many years. That original chest pain was burning in quality, bothered her most when she felt stressed, and was diagnosed empirically as reflux esophagitis when it responded to antacids. Her heartburn is now well controlled with lifestyle modifications and ranitidine (Zantac),

---

Evidence levels Ⓐ Randomized, controlled trials (RCTs), meta-analyses, well-designed systematic reviews of RCTs. Ⓑ Case-control or cohort studies, nonrandomized clinical trials, systematic reviews of studies other than RCTs, cross-sectional studies, retrospective studies, certain uncontrolled studies. Ⓒ Consensus statements, expert guidelines, usual practice, opinion.

150 mg once or twice daily. Routine health screenings revealed tobacco use (one pack per day for 30 years) and hyperlipidemia, which is now well controlled on a statin. She also takes a daily aspirin for heart attack and stroke prevention. Her blood pressure has ranged from normal to borderline. Random blood glucose screening was normal. She has had two urinary tract infections since coming to you, both of which resolved with fluids and short courses of antibiotics. With motivational counseling, she reduced her cigarette consumption to less than half a pack per day, has improved her diet, and walks a brisk mile several days per week. Mammograms, Pap smears, and a screening sigmoidoscopy have all been negative. Jane received all recommended childhood immunizations but has declined influenza vaccination. She remembers receiving antibiotics for acute coughing illnesses several years before meeting you.

Family History

Jane's father died of a heart attack at age 64. He was a smoker. Jane's mother is alive and well at 77 but was diagnosed with type 2 diabetes and hypertension in her 60s. Jane's grandparents died in their 70s and 80s of unknown causes. She has a brother and two sisters but is unaware of any major health issues.

Social History

Jane is married with three adult children. She works as an office manager. She attributes daily work stress and relationship stress as the primary obstacles to smoking cessation. Her husband nags her to quit smoking. She denies physical or sexual abuse.

Review of Systems

In addition to the acute symptoms mentioned, Jane has occasional mild heartburn, generally well controlled with antacids or ranitidine. She denies any chest pain or pressure with exercise. She also denies weight loss and feels that her general health, energy, and quality of life have improved slightly over the past 3 years. She is not aware of any significant occupational or environmental exposures but does live in a city that has occasional ozone alerts.

Objective

Physical Examination

Jane is 5 feet 10 inches and 180 pounds (body mass index = 25.8). Her blood pressure today is 128/86 mm Hg, her heart rate is 68 beats per minute, and her temperature is 37°C (98.6°F) by ear thermometer. Her respiratory rate is about 20 breaths per minute. Her mucous membranes (ocular, nasal, and oral) are moist, without any abnormal signs. Tympanic membranes are clear, with normal light reflex and no signs of middle ear fluid. Posterior pharynx is somewhat erythematous but is without exudates, swelling, or signs of postnasal drainage. There is no tenderness to maxillary percussion. There are two small, smooth, mobile, and nontender lymph nodes palpable in the anterior chain on the left side of her neck. Posterior auscultation of the lungs reveals neither rales nor rhonchi. Inspiratory effort is good, with full and symmetrical chest wall expansion. Heart sounds are normal.

Laboratory Examinations

You consider a chest radiograph, peak flow, complete blood count, C-reactive protein, and/or testing for streptococcal pharyngitis or pertussis but decide to order no tests.

Assessment

Working Diagnosis

Although you have not seen Jane before with this specific constellation of symptoms, you presumptively diagnose acute bronchitis, most likely caused by recent and perhaps ongoing upper airway viral infection with mid-airway inflammatory sequelae. Chronic exposure to tobacco smoke and possibly to other airborne pollutants is likely an underlying contributory factor.

Differential Diagnosis

The list of possible causes of acute coughing illness includes asthma, bronchiectasis, cancer, chemical bronchitis, chronic obstructive pulmonary disease, drugs (e.g., angiotensin-converting enzyme inhibitor), eosinophilic bronchitis, gastroesophageal reflux disease, interstitial lung disease, pneumonia, and sinusitis. Infectious viral respiratory pathogens include adenovirus, coronavirus, enterovirus, influenza, parainfluenza, respiratory syncytial virus, and rhinovirus. Each of these classes of virus has many subtypes; hence, there are several hundred specific viral strains that can lead to upper respiratory infection with cough. You know that influenza and respiratory syncytial virus are confined to the months November through April in your locale and thus are not in today's differential diagnosis. Last year, your state experienced an epidemic of pertussis, which was eventually controlled with an aggressive test-and-treat strategy. This year, your state public health department has reported only rare cases. Sinusitis is excluded by lack of fever, face pain, maxillary tenderness, or purulent discharge in nasal passageways or posterior pharynx. There is no history of occupational or environmental exposure. The history of esophageal reflux suggests a possible contribution, but the symptoms are much more specific for acute infectious bronchitis, presumed viral.

Plan

Diagnostic

Acute bronchitis, presumed viral, is a very common clinical diagnosis (Gonzales, 2000). There are no sensitive or specific supporting tests. The main diagnostic job of the clinician is to rule out other causes. Jane has neither paroxysmal nor whooping cough and has no known exposure risk factors. Therefore, you decide not to do the uncomfortable nasopharyngeal swab required for pertussis polymerase chain reaction testing. With normal vital signs and lung sounds and with the lack of chest pain or pressure, persistent fever, and shortness of breath, you decide the pretest probability of pneumonia is too low to order a chest radiograph. You are aware of recent research showing that C-reactive protein might be useful in the absence of a chest radiograph (Almirall et al., 2004 Ⓑ; Flanders et al., 2004 Ⓑ; Garcia et al., 2003 Ⓑ) but also know it to be too nonspecific to be helpful in this case. You do note the history of heartburn responsive to H_2 blockers and discuss the possibility that esophageal reflux disease may have contributed to Jane's symptoms. Together you decide to schedule an upper endoscopy sometime in the next month or two.

Therapeutic

After careful consideration and a detailed discussion of risks and benefits, you suggest conservative treatment: drinking lots of fluids, rest, and cough medicine. Jane will try an over-the-counter dextromethorphan-guaifenesin combination cough syrup. If that is unsuccessful, and especially if the cough keeps her awake at night, she will fill your prescription for a codeine-guaifenesin cough syrup. She will avoid cold formulas with antihistamines or decongestants, as she has neither allergic symptoms nor nasal congestion and these agents have side effect risks as well as being an expense.

Patient Education

You specifically ask Jane whether she wants or expects an antibiotic prescription. She says she would take any medicine that you think would be helpful and asks your opinion. You discuss the fact that antibiotics may be slightly better than placebo in relieving the symptom severity and duration of acute bronchitis. However, you also note the risk of side effects and touch on the societal problem of antibiotic resistance. You offer a "delayed fill" antibiotic prescription, but Jane declines. You also provide reassurance that the symptoms will go away and give her a few specific signs that would require a return visit (hemoptysis, shortness of breath or difficulty breathing, chest pain or pressure, persistent fever, cough lasting more than 6 weeks). You gently discuss the association between smoking and bronchitis and mention that more than a million Americans have kicked the habit and that you believe that she can too.

Follow-up Visit

You see Jane again for smoking cessation counseling and follow-up after an upper endoscopy performed by a gastroenterologist colleague, which showed a small hiatal hernia but no specific lesions or signs of esophageal inflammation. Although smoking cessation is initially unsuccessful, after several attempts over a few years, Jane eventually kicks the habit. In the meantime, she has two other occurrences of acute bronchitis, both of which she treats at home with fluids, rest, and over-the-counter cough suppressants.

DISCUSSION

Acute bronchitis is a very common result of upper respiratory infection. Although bacterial and chemical causes are known, the vast majority of cases of acute bronchitis stem from viral agents. There are no known effective treatments for acute bronchitis. Whether a cough is productive and the color of the phlegm are not predictive of etiologic agent (virus vs. bacteria) or response to therapy. Systematic reviews of RCTs of antibiotics suggest small but statistically significant benefits of antibiotics over placebo in terms of persistence and severity of cough (Anonymous, 1998 Ⓐ; Becker et al., 1999 Ⓐ; Bent et al., 2000 Ⓐ; Fahey et al., 1998 Ⓐ; NHS Centre for Reviews and Dissemination, 2004 Ⓐ; Orr et al., 1993 Ⓐ; Smucny et al., 2004 a Ⓐ). Combining all evaluable data, weighted mean differences suggest an approximate half day reduction in the duration of cough (Smucny et al., 2004 a Ⓐ). Of the nine published RCTs, three are "positive" in that they report statistically significant benefits of doxycycline (Verheij et al., 1994 Ⓐ) and erythromycin (Dunlay et al., 1987 Ⓐ; King et al., 1996 Ⓐ) compared with placebo. Although the other six trials testing doxycycline (Scherl et al., 1987 Ⓐ; Stott and West, 1976 Ⓐ; Williamson, 1984 Ⓐ), erythromycin (Brickfield et al., 1986 Ⓐ; Hueston, 1994 Ⓐ), and trimethoprim/sulfamethoxazole (Franks and Gleiner, 1984 Ⓐ) failed to find substantial benefit, most primary outcomes trended toward benefit, and a few secondary outcomes reached statistical significance. It should be noted that the number of unpublished RCTs is unknown. However, it is suspected that several negative trials conducted by drug companies remain unpublished. Because positive trials are more likely to be published than negative trials and because internal biases tend to favor treatment over placebo, actual benefits may be less.

There are no RCTs that specifically address the question of whether antibiotics are useful for tobacco smokers with acute bronchitis. However, Linder and Sim (2002 Ⓐ) reviewed the nine trials noted above (774 participants), looking specifically at the 276 smokers included. There were no statistically significant differences between smokers and nonsmokers. However, trends actually suggested that antibiotics were less effective for smokers than nonsmokers. This is a secondary analysis ("data dredging"); hence, conclusions are tentative but certainly do not support the widespread practice of justifying antibiotic prescriptions with smoking status.

Although it may be reasonable to prescribe antibiotics for some patients with acute bronchitis (e.g., if early pneumonia is suspected or if there is underlying chronic lung disease), most experts recommend against this practice (Anonymous, 1997Ⓐ; Gonzales et al., 2001a,bⒸ) because societal harms (antibiotic resistance) and individual adverse effects may outweigh potential benefits. Side effects of antibiotics, such as nausea, diarrhea, vaginal candidiasis, and allergic reaction, occur frequently with most antibiotics. When using antibiotics for acute bronchitis, the number needed to treat (Walter, 2001) and the number needed to harm are similar and in the range of 10 to 20 (Anonymous, 1998Ⓐ; Becker et al., 1999Ⓐ; Bent et al., 2000Ⓐ; Fahey et al., 1998Ⓐ; NHS Centre for Reviews and Dissemination, 2004Ⓐ). Nevertheless, approximately half of patients diagnosed with acute bronchitis receive a prescription for an antibiotic (Cantrell et al., 2002Ⓑ; Walter, 2001; Stone et al., 2000Ⓑ). This unfortunate situation is due both to patient demand and to physicians' beliefs and prescribing habits. Education, in the form of a pamphlet or physician advice, significantly reduces the desire for antibiotics (Macfarlane et al., 2002Ⓐ). Some evidence suggests that writing a delayed prescription may reduce antibiotic use (Arroll et al., 2004Ⓐ).

Unfortunately, there is very little reliable evidence regarding the effectiveness of cough treatments. Systematic reviews of RCTs have concluded that there is neither good evidence for nor good evidence against the effectiveness of antitussives (Anonymous, 2002a Ⓐ; Schroeder and Fahey, 2004Ⓐ; Smith and Feldman, 1993Ⓐ). However, with the definite possibility of specific effectiveness (Parvez, 1998Ⓐ) and with evidence suggesting that the placebo effect for cough treatments is substantial (Eccles, 2002; Lee et al., 1992Ⓑ), the use of over-the-counter dextromethorphan-containing formulations and/or limited use of prescription codeine or hydrocodone may be reasonable. Although benzonatate (Tessalon) has been approved as a prescription cough medicine, there is virtually no evidence for or against its effectiveness. Furthermore, the number and quality of RCTs on beta agonist (e.g., albuterol inhaler) used in the setting of acute bronchitis are limited.

Although some evidence supports use (Hueston, 1994Ⓐ), the weight of evidence currently suggests that beta agonists are not very helpful in this setting (Anonymous, 2002bⒶ; Smucny et al., 2004bⒶ).

Expectorants and mucolytics have not been adequately assessed in the setting of acute bronchitis. However, evidence from trials for common cold and in the setting of chronic lung disease suggests possible benefits and little harm (Anonymous, 2002aⒶ; Schroeder and Fahey, 2004Ⓐ; Smith and Feldman, 1993Ⓐ). Neither antihistamines nor decongestants have been shown to be helpful for bronchitis, and both carry risks. Antihistamines can cause drowsiness, which may lead to a motor vehicle accident. Decongestants are contraindicated in the settings of hypertension and heart disease. For children, there is no evidence of any benefit of any over-the-counter medicine for colds or bronchitis and reasonable evidence of potential harm (Anonymous, 2002aⒶ; Gunn et al., 2001; Schroeder and Fahey, 2004Ⓐ). Nonsteroidal anti-inflammatory drugs may help if pain is present. However, the widespread use of nonsteroidal anti-inflammatory drugs is associated with major morbidity and mortality, with more than 10,000 Americans dying each year, mostly from gastrointestinal bleeding, but also from congestive heart failure and renal failure (Fries, 1991Ⓑ; Heerdink et al., 1998Ⓑ; Page and Henry, 2000; Wolfe et al., 1999 Ⓑ). Although the effectiveness of nonsteroidal anti-inflammatory drugs appears similar, risks vary, with ibuprofen being among the safest. Acetaminophen, not a nonsteroidal anti-inflammatory drug, is even safer.

There is a broad body of robust evidence that tobacco smoking cessation can be facilitated through a variety of physician-assisted modalities (Lancaster et al., 2004Ⓐ; Park et al., 2004Ⓐ; Silagy and Stead, 2004Ⓐ; Stead et al., 2004Ⓐ). In addition to nicotine replacement, bupropion (Zyban), clonidine (Catapres), and nortriptyline (Pamelor) have all been shown to be useful in supporting smoking cessation (Gourlay et al., 2004Ⓐ; Hughes et al., 2004Ⓐ; Silagy et al., 2004Ⓐ). Although no specific evidence links acute illness with readiness to quit, it makes good sense that the occasion of an episode of acute bronchitis might provide opportunity and incentive to support active attempts at tobacco cessation or at least to "plant the seed." The fact that Jane's father smoked and died of a heart attack at age 64 might also be diplomatically used as a motivational tool.

Summary

Acute bronchitis is the most common diagnosis when a patient presents with prolonged acute cough. There are no specific methods for diagnosing bronchitis or for distinguishing bronchitis from upper respiratory infection with cough. The first job of the clinician is to rule out other causes, such as pneumonia, asthma, bacterial sinusitis, and gastroesophageal reflux disease. Once the diagnosis of acute infectious bronchitis is reached, the clinician's task turns to supporting the patient, in terms of both reassurance and selection of therapy. In most cases, antibiotics should be avoided. Until and unless better evidence emerges, the use of over-the-counter and prescription antitussives can be cautiously supported in adults. Decongestants should be avoided, especially if hypertension or heart disease is present. Beta-agonist inhalers may help those with wheezing or a history of asthma. Supportive home treatments, such as fluids, rest, and avoidance of stressors, make good sense but are largely unsupported by evidence. Unless symptoms dramatically worsen, most patients with acute bronchitis do not need a return visit.

Material Available on Student Consult

Review Questions and Answers about Acute Bronchitis

REFERENCES

Almirall J, Bolibar I, Toran P, et al. Contribution of C-reactive protein to the diagnosis and assessment of severity of community-acquired pneumonia. Chest 2004;125:1335–1342.**B**

Anonymous. Antibiotics are ineffective for acute bronchitis. ACP J Club 1997;126:39.**A**

Anonymous. Review: Antibiotics do not resolve acute cough. Evid Based Med 1998;3:183.**A**

Anonymous. Lack of evidence exists for effectiveness of over-the-counter cough preparations for children with URTI. ACP J Club 2002a;137:106.**A**

Anonymous. Beta$_2$-agonists are ineffective but increase adverse effects in acute bronchitis without underlying pulmonary disease. ACP J Club 2002b;137:72.**A**

Arroll B, Elley R, Goodyear-Smith F, Kenealy T, Kerse N. Delayed prescriptions for reducing antibiotic use in acute respiratory infections. Cochrane Database Syst Rev 2004.**A**

Becker L, Glazier R, McIsaac WJ, Smucny J. Antibiotics for acute bronchitis. The Cochrane Library. Vol. 4, 1999.**A**

Bent S, Saint S, Vittinghoff E, Grady D. Antibiotics in acute bronchitis: A meta-analysis. Am J Med 2000;107:62–67.**A**

Brickfield FX, Carter WH, Johnson RE. Erythromycin in the treatment of acute bronchitis in a community practice. J Fam Pract 1986;23:119–122.**A**

Cantrell R, Young AF, Martin BC. Antibiotic prescribing in ambulatory care settings for adults with colds, upper respiratory tract infections, and bronchitis. Clin Ther 2002;24:170–182.**B**

Dunlay J, Reinhardt R, Roi LD. A placebo-controlled, double-blind trial of erythromycin in adults with acute bronchitis. J Fam Pract 1987;25:137–141.**A**

Eccles R. The powerful placebo in cough studies? Pulm Pharmacol Ther 2002;15:303–308.

Fahey T, Stocks N, Thomas T. Quantitative systematic review of randomized controlled trials comparing antibiotic with placebo for acute cough in adults. BMJ 1998;316:906–910.**A**

Flanders SA, Stein J, Shochat G, et al. Performance of a bedside C-reactive protein test in the diagnosis of community-acquired pneumonia in adults with acute cough. Am J Med 2004;116:529–535.**B**

Franks P, Gleiner JA. The treatment of acute bronchitis with trimethoprim and sulfamethoxazole. J Fam Pract 1984;19:185–190.**A**

Fries JF. NSAID gastropathy: The second most deadly rheumatic disease? Epidemiology and risk appraisal. J Rheumatol Suppl 1991;28:6–10.**B**

Garcia VE, Martinez JA, Mensa J, et al. C-reactive protein levels in community-acquired pneumonia. Eur Respir J 2003;21:702–705.**B**

Gonzales R. Uncomplicated acute bronchitis. Ann Intern Med 2000;133:981–991.

Gonzales R, Bartlett JG, Besser RE, et al. Principles of appropriate antibiotic use for treatment of uncomplicated acute bronchitis: Background. Ann Intern Med 2001a;134:521–529.**C**

Gonzales R, Malone DC, Maselli JH, Sande MA. Excessive antibiotic use for acute respiratory infections in the United States. Clin Infect Dis 2001b;33:757–762.**B**

Gourlay SG, Stead LF, Benowitz NL. Clonidine for smoking cessation. Cochrane Database Syst Rev 2004;3.**A**

Gunn VL, Taha SH, Liebelt EL, Serwint JR. Toxicity of over-the-counter cough and cold medications. Pediatrics 2001;108:52–56.

Heerdink ER, Leufkens HG, Herings RM, Ottervanger JP, Stricker BH, Bakker A. NSAIDs associated with increased risk of congestive heart failure in elderly patients taking diuretics. Arch Intern Med 1998;158:1108–1112.**B**

Hueston WJ. Albuterol delivered by metered-dose inhaler to treat acute bronchitis. J Fam Pract 1994;39:437–440.**A**

Hughes JR, Stead LF, Lancaster T. Antidepressants for smoking cessation. Cochrane Database Syst Rev 2004.**A**

King DE, Williams WC, Bishop L, Shechter A. Effectiveness of erythromycin in the treatment of acute bronchitis. J Fam Pract 1996;42:601–605.**A**

Lancaster T, Silagy C, Fowler G. Training health professionals in smoking cessation. Cochrane Database Syst Rev 2004.**A**

Lee PCL, Jawad MS, Hull JD, West WHL, Porter K, Eccles R. The effect of placebo treatment on cough associated with common cold. Br J Clin Pharmacol 1992;51:373.**B**

Linder JA, Sim I. Antibiotic treatment of acute bronchitis in smokers: A systematic review. J Gen Intern Med 2002;17:230–234.🅐

Macfarlane J, Holmes W, Gard P, Thornhill D, Macfarlane R, Hubbard R. Reducing antibiotic use for acute bronchitis in primary care: Blinded, randomised controlled trial of patient information leaflet. BMJ 2002;324: 91–94.🅐

NHS Centre for Reviews and Dissemination. Quantitative systematic review of randomised controlled trials comparing antibiotic with placebo for acute cough in adults. Database of Abstracts of Reviews of Effectiveness 2004;3.🅐

Orr PH, Scherer K, Macdonald A, Moffatt MEK. Randomized placebo-controlled trials of antibiotics for acute bronchitis: A critical review of the literature. J Fam Pract 1993;36:507–512.🅐

Page J, Henry D. Consumption of NSAIDs and the development of congestive heart failure in elderly patients: An underrecognized public health problem. Arch Intern Med 2000;160:777–784.

Park EW, Schultz JK, Tudiver F, Campbell T, Becker L. Enhancing partner support to improve smoking cessation. Cochrane Database Syst Rev 2004;3.🅐

Parvez L. Objective evaluation of the pharmacodynamic response of 30 and 60 mg of dextromethorphan in acute cough. Eur Respir J 1998;12:413S.🅐

Scherl ER, Riegler SL, Cooper JK. Doxycycline in acutse bronchitis: A randomized double-blind trial. J Ky Med Assoc 1987;85:539–541.🅐

Schroeder K, Fahey T. Over-the-counter medications for acute cough in children and adults in ambulatory settings. Cochrane Database Syst Rev 2004;2.🅐

Silagy C, Lancaster T, Stead L, Mant D, Fowler G. Nicotine replacement therapy for smoking cessation. Cochrane Database Syst Rev 2004;3.🅐

Silagy C, Stead LF. Physician advice for smoking cessation. Cochrane Database Syst Rev 2004;3.🅐

Smith MBH, Feldman W. Over-the-counter cold medications: A critical review of clinical trials between 1950 and 1991. JAMA 1993;269:2258–2263.🅐

Smucny J, Fahey T, Becker L, Glazier R. Antibiotics for acute bronchitis. Cochrane Database Syst Rev 2004a;3.🅐

Smucny J, Flynn C, Becker L, Glazier R. Beta$_2$-agonists for acute bronchitis. Cochrane Database Syst Rev 2004b;3.🅐

Stead LF, Lancaster T, Perera R. Telephone counselling for smoking cessation. Cochrane Database Syst Rev 2004;3. 🅐

Stone S, Gonzales R, Maselli J, Lowenstein SR. Antibiotic prescribing for patients with colds, upper respiratory tract infections, and bronchitis: A national study of hospital-based emergency departments. Ann Emerg Med 2000;36:320–327.🅑

Stott NC, West RR. Randomised controlled trial of antibiotics in patients with cough and purulent sputum. BMJ 1976;2:556–559.🅐

Verheij TJ, Hermans J, Mulder JD. Effects of doxycycline in patients with acute cough and purulent sputum: A double blind placebo controlled trial. Br J Gen Pract 1994;44:400–404.🅐

Walter SD. Number needed to treat (NNT): Estimation of a measure of clinical benefit. Stat Med 2001;20: 3947–3962.

Williamson HA Jr. A randomized, controlled trial of doxycycline in the treatment of acute bronchitis. J Fam Pract 1984;19:481–486.🅐

Wolfe MM, Lichtenstein DR, Singh G. Gastrointestinal toxicity of nonsteroidal antiinflammatory drugs. N Engl J Med 1999;340:1888–1899.🅑

32

Diagnosis and Management of an Acute Exacerbation (Chronic Obstructive Pulmonary Disease)

Keith B. Holten

KEY POINTS

1. Initial evaluation of a patient with chronic obstructive pulmonary disease (COPD) presenting to the emergency department includes a chest radiograph and an arterial blood gas test.
2. Treatment for an acute exacerbation includes inhaled short-acting bronchodilators, oxygen for hypoxia, antibiotics, and corticosteroids. Mucolytics, chest physiotherapy, and methylxanthines are not effective.
3. The ongoing management of COPD can be staged, based on the forced expiratory volume in 1 second (FEV$_1$) and patient symptoms.

INITIAL VISIT

Subjective

Patient Identification and Presenting Problem

John F. is a 42-year-old white man who presents to the emergency department with shortness of breath. For 1 week, he has noticed a low-grade fever 37.9°C (100.2°F), a cough producing green sputum, and worsening dyspnea with exertion. He denies any pleuritic chest pain, nausea, diaphoresis, chills, or fatigue. There have not been any exposures to illness, including tuberculosis. He has a 2-year history of worsening dyspnea with exertion, which he attributes to being "out of condition." He notices when walking up stairs that he has to rest to "get his breath." He has smoked two packs of unfiltered cigarettes per day since he was 16 years old. He has tried to reduce the amount but has been unable to do so.

Medical History

John has been healthy and denies any treatment for medical illnesses. He has never been treated for respiratory illnesses. He has no surgical history. He is not taking medications, except for one aspirin per day because he heard it was "good for circulation." He denies any medication allergies.

Family History

His parents are living and both have type 2 diabetes. He has two siblings, both older brothers. There is no family history of chronic lung disease.

Health Habits

His cigarette smoking does increase when he is under stress. He denies alcohol or drug use. He does not exercise.

Social History

He lives with his wife, who is also a cigarette smoker. He is an insurance executive and has a sedentary job. He has not had any occupational respiratory exposures.

Review of Systems

He has morning cough and dyspnea with exertion but denies hemoptysis, weight loss, or chronic sputum production.

Objective

Physical Examination

General John is a well-nourished, alert white man in no acute distress.

Vital Signs His height is 5 feet 10 inches, weight is 210 pounds, temperature is 38.3°C (100.9°F), respiratory rate is 24, blood pressure is 136/80, and pulse is 90.

Evidence levels Ⓐ Randomized, controlled trials (RCTs), meta-analyses, well-designed systematic reviews of RCTs. Ⓑ Case-control or cohort studies, nonrandomized clinical trials, systematic reviews of studies other than RCTs, cross-sectional studies, retrospective studies, certain uncontrolled studies. Ⓒ Consensus statements, expert guidelines, usual practice, opinion.

Head, Eyes, Ears, Nose, and Throat John's head is without lesions or trauma; his pupils are equal, round, and reactive to light; and his ear canals and tympanic membranes are normal. His mouth and throat are normal.

Neck There is no cervical adenopathy and no jugular venous distention; the thyroid is nonpalpable.

Chest The anteroposterior chest wall diameter is increased; there is no chest wall tenderness.

Lungs There are decreased breath sounds diffusely, scattered ronchi that clear with coughing, and expiratory wheezes.

Heart The heart rate and rhythm are regular with no gallops, rubs, or murmurs.

Abdomen The abdomen is benign.

Lower Extremities Posterior tibial and dorsalis pedis pulses are present bilaterally and are strong. There is no edema.

Neurologic Cranial nerves II to XII are intact. There are no strength deficits.

Assessment

Working Diagnosis
COPD with acute exacerbation. An alternate term is acute bronchitis in a patient with COPD. This patient's symptoms indicate airway inflammation and infection resulting in wheezing, fever, worsening dyspnea, and purulent sputum production. The features of this illness are typical for a patient with COPD (Global Initiative for Chronic Obstructive Lung Disease [GOLD], 2001❸): onset in mid-life, significant smoking history, and dyspnea during exertion.

Differential Diagnosis (Table 32-1)
Asthma is an inflammatory airway disease with largely reversible air flow. It more commonly occurs early in life and symptoms vary from day to day. Family history is common.

Congestive heart failure is more commonly seen in the elderly and is characterized by fine basilar crackles on physical examination. A chest radiograph reveals pulmonary edema and cardiomegaly. Pulmonary function tests do not demonstrate obstruction.

Bronchiectasis is typically associated with large amounts of purulent sputum and coarse crackles on physical examination. Chest radiograph or computed

Table 32-1 Differential Diagnosis of COPD with Acute Exacerbation	
Diagnosis	**Prominent Features**
Asthma	Early life onset Positive family history Allergies Reversible obstruction
Congestive heart failure	Older adults Basilar crackles Cardiomegaly Pulmonary edema on chest radiograph
Bronchiectasis	Large volumes of purulent sputum Bacterial pathogen Bronchial dilation and thickening on chest radiograph
Pulmonary tuberculosis	All ages Infiltrate, nodular lesions on chest radiograph High local prevalence
Obliterative bronchiolitis	Younger age Nonsmokers History of rheumatoid arthritis or occupational exposure Hypodense areas on expiratory chest computed tomography
Diffuse panbronchiolitis	Males Nonsmokers Chronic sinusitis Computed tomography chest centrolobular nodular opacities and hyperinflation

Adapted from Global Initiative for Chronic Obstructive Lung Disease (GOLD), World Health Organization (WHO), National Heart, Lung, and Blood Institute (NHLBI). Global Strategy for the Diagnosis, Management, and Prevention of Chronic Obstructive Pulmonary Disease, Bethesda, MD, GOLD, WHO, NHLBI, 2001.

tomography shows bronchial wall thickening and bronchial dilation.

Pulmonary tuberculosis is seen where there is a high local prevalence or in immunocompromised patients. A chest radiograph shows an infiltrate or nodular lesion. Onset is at any age.

Obliterative bronchiolitis is usually seen in nonsmokers at a younger age. It is more common in rheumatoid arthritis or after inhaling environmental fumes.

Diffuse panbronchiolitis is mostly seen in male nonsmokers. There is a high association with chronic sinusitis. A chest radiograph shows diffuse small centrolobular densities.

Plan

Diagnostic
A chest radiograph is obtained. There is bronchial wall thickening but no evidence of an infiltrate, cardiomegaly, or pleural effusion. An arterial blood gas shows a low pH (7.32), hypercarbia ($PCO_2 = 50$), and hypoxia ($PO_2 = 72$). A complete blood count and electrolytes are normal.

Therapeutic
The patient is admitted to the hospital. Oxygen therapy at 4 L via nasal cannula is initiated, and a repeat arterial blood gas test confirms correction of the hypoxia and no change in the hypercarbia. An inhaled anticholinergic bronchodilator (ipratropium) is begun, given every 4 hours, and a corticosteroid (methylprednisolone 60 mg every 8 hours intravenously) is initiated. Antibiotics (amoxicillin 500 mg orally three times daily) are given, and because of slow progress, after 24 hours an inhaled β_2-agonist bronchodilator (albuterol) is added and given every 4 hours. A nutrition screen is negative for malnutrition. Influenza and pneumococcal vaccines are administered. After another 48 hours, the patient is discharged from the hospital; he is afebrile with a normal arterial blood gas and significant improvement in dyspnea.

Patient Education
Smoking cessation and exercise are reviewed.

Disposition
An office follow-up visit is arranged for 1 week. Completion of a 7-day course of antibiotics is recommended.

FOLLOW-UP VISIT

Subjective

John F. returns to the office for his follow-up visit 1 week later. He is free of cough and sputum produc-

tion, and his dyspnea has improved. He has not smoked since his admission to the hospital. More detailed questioning reveals no history suspicious for obstructive sleep apnea (daytime sleepiness, loud snoring, choking during sleep, or observed apnea during sleep).

Objective

His respiratory rate is 14 at rest. His lungs are clear with no crackles or wheezes. Oxygen saturation is 94% by pulse oximetry.

Assessment

COPD with an acute exacerbation is resolving. His examination is consistent with infection that cleared with treatment.

Plan

Pulmonary function studies are ordered to be done in a few weeks. Those tests show FEV_1 greater than 50% with no change after bronchodilators, consistent with mild COPD. He is counseled to avoid risk factors (smoking and airborne pollutants) and advised to get the flu vaccine yearly. He is prescribed a short-acting inhaled anticholinergic bronchodilator for use when needed. Follow-up every 3 months is scheduled.

DISCUSSION

Acute Exacerbation of Chronic Obstructive Pulmonary Disease

Evaluation of Acute Exacerbation
Physical findings are rarely diagnostic in COPD (GOLD, 2001 🄲). Findings of increased anteroposterior chest wall diameter, crackles, and wheezing support the diagnosis. Chest radiograph findings can be helpful (Snow et al., 2001 🄱), especially for patients presenting to the emergency department with acute COPD symptoms. It has been shown that 23% of patients have a change in their management based on a chest radiograph. There is not good evidence to support a chest radiograph for patients seen in the office setting. The chest radiograph can help to differentiate between pneumonia, congestive heart failure, and other differential diagnoses. Indirect findings of bullae, scarring, and bronchial wall thickening can suggest underlying COPD. Heart enlargement, fluid in the minor fissure, or pulmonary edema can support a diagnosis of congestive heart failure. Arterial blood gas analysis is helpful (Snow et al., 2001 🄰) in assessing severity of the exacerbation. The presence of hypercarbia, when associated

with hypoxia and a low pH, indicates increased risk of respiratory failure. Spirometry is not helpful to diagnose an exacerbation of COPD or to assess the severity acutely (Snow et al., 2001Ⓐ). There is little evidence that additional laboratory testing, electrocardiography, or echocardiography is useful (Snow et al., 2001Ⓒ).

Management of Acute Exacerbation

Oxygen therapy is beneficial to patients with hypoxia (Bach et al., 2001Ⓑ). Inhaled short-acting β_2-agonists and anticholinergic bronchodilators improve symptoms (Bach et al., 2001Ⓐ) in patients acutely ill with COPD. Anticholinergic bronchodilators have fewer side effects and should be used as first-line therapy. A second bronchodilator should be added if there is slow progress. Systemic corticosteroids reduce dyspnea and have been shown to reduce the relapse rate (Bach et al., 2001Ⓐ). This therapy should include 3 days of intravenous methylprednisolone, followed by oral prednisone, for a total of 2 weeks. Antibiotics are beneficial (Snow et al., 2001Ⓐ), but narrow-spectrum agents (amoxicillin, trimethoprim/sulfamethoxazole, tetracycline) should be first-line agents. No evidence is available to determine optimal length of antibiotic treatment, but generally 7 days of treatment is provided. Noninvasive positive-pressure ventilation (NPPV) decreases the risk involved in invasive mechanical ventilation (Bach et al., 2001Ⓐ). Parenteral methylxanthines and sympathomimetics are not as effective (Snow et al., 2001Ⓑ) and have potential serious cardiovascular side effects. Mucolytics and chest physiotherapy are not effective (Snow et al., 2001Ⓒ). The empirical use of diuretics has not been studied adequately (Bach et al., 2001Ⓒ).

An algorithm for the management of acute exacerbations of COPD was developed by the American College of Physicians based on the work of Snow et al. (2001Ⓒ) (Fig. 32-1). This algorithm determines the management based on the presence or absence of three criteria: increase in dyspnea, increase in sputum volume, and increase in sputum purulence. If at least one of these is present, a second level of criteria is applied: upper respiratory infection in past 5 days, fever without apparent cause, increased wheezing, increased cough, and a 20% increase of heart rate or respiratory rate over baseline. If one of these second-level criteria is present, the patient is diagnosed with a mild exacerbation. It is recommended that these patients have a chest radiograph and be treated with bronchodilators only.

Patients meeting two of the criteria (increase in dyspnea, increase in sputum volume, or increase in sputum purulence) are considered to have a moder-

ate exacerbation. The approach for these patients includes a chest radiograph, inhaled bronchodilators, systemic corticosteroids, oxygen as needed, and positive-pressure ventilation as needed.

For patients meeting three of the first-level criteria (increase in dyspnea, increase in sputum volume, and increase in sputum purulence), a severe exacerbation is diagnosed. The management includes all of the above plus antibiotics.

Long-term Management of Chronic Obstructive Pulmonary Disease

Existing medications for COPD are not shown to alter the decreasing lung function that occurs over time. A stepped approach in which treatment is increased based on severity of illness (FEV_1) can improve symptoms and the health status of sufferers (Bach et al., 2001Ⓑ; GOLD, 2001Ⓑ; Veterans Health Administration [VHA], 1999 ⒶⒷ) (Table 32-2). The most important aspect of this care is monitoring disease progression and development of complications, pharmacotherapy, exacerbation history, and comorbidities (GOLD, 2001Ⓑ). A few key areas are considered in the remainder of this section.

Smoking cessation interventions using brief strategies (ask, advise, assess, assist, and arrange) coupled with medications can be very effective (GOLD, 2001Ⓐ). Patient education and pulmonary rehabilitation, although they do not improve lung function, do improve health status by improving coping skills (GOLD, 2001Ⓑ). Inhaled corticosteroids should be prescribed only for those with proven spirometric response and FEV_1 less than 50% (GOLD, 2001Ⓑ). Systemic corticosteroids should be avoided due to an unfavorable benefit-risk ratio (GOLD, 2001Ⓐ). Long-term oxygen therapy to maintain oxygen saturation at more than 90% prolongs life (VHA, 1999Ⓐ). Influenza vaccine should be administered yearly (VHA 1999Ⓐ). Pneumococcal vaccine should be considered (VHA, 1999Ⓑ). All patients with COPD should have nutrition screening (Harmon-Weiss, 2002Ⓒ). A reasonable weight (>90% ideal) should be maintained. If food intake is inadequate, nutrition supplements should be given. Surgical management (bullectomy, lung volume reduction therapy, and lung transplantation) is still investigational and may be considered for carefully selected patients (GOLD, 2001Ⓒ).

Material Available on Student Consult

Review Questions and Answers about Chronic Obstructive Pulmonary Disease

COPD Guideline Algorithm

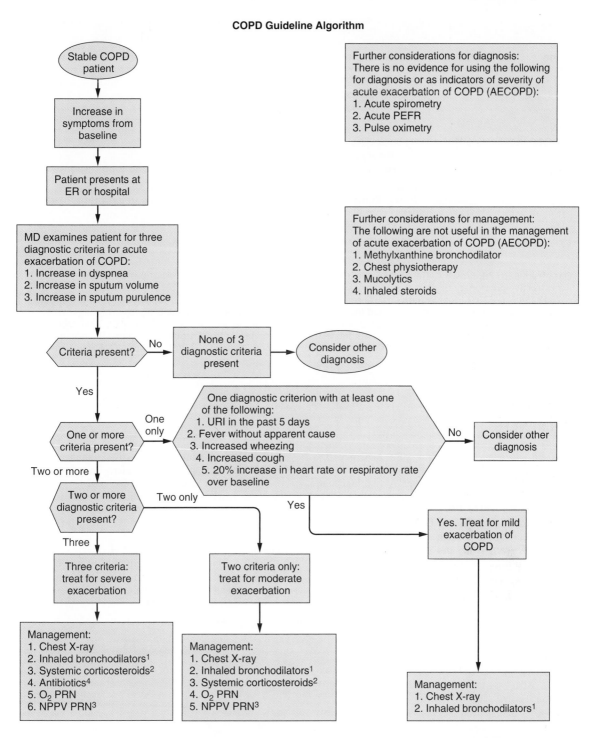

Figure 32-1 Management of acute exacerbations of chronic obstructive pulmonary disease. COPD, chronic obstructive pulmonary disease; NPPV, noninvasive positive-pressure ventilation; PEFR, peak expiratory flow rate; PRN, as needed. (Developed by American College of Physicians from Snow V, Lascher S, Mottur-Pilson C. Evidence base for management of acute exacerbations of chronic obstructive pulmonary disease. Ann Intern Med 2001;134:595–599.)

[1] Use anticholinergic bronchodilators first, once at maximum dose, then add β_2-agonist bronchodilators.

[2] Dosing regimen used in the SCOPE trial: 3 days intravenous methylprednisolone, 125 mg every 6 hours followed by oral prednisone, taper to complete the 2 week course (60 mg/day on days 4–7, 40 mg/day on days 8–11, and 20 mg/day on days 12–15).

[3] Noninvasive positive-pressure ventilation should be administered under the supervision of a trained physician.

[4] Use narrow-spectrum antibiotics; the agents favored in the trials were amoxicillin and trimethoprin-sulfamethoxazole, and tetracycline.

Table 32-2 Approach to Management of Chronic Obstructive Pulmonary Disease

Stage	FEV$_1$	Management
All	All	Avoidance of tobacco smoke, occupational dusts and chemicals, indoor and outdoor pollutants Influenza and pneumococcal vaccines
Mild	≥50%	Short-acting inhaled bronchodilator when needed
Moderate	35%–49%	Regular inhaled bronchodilator(s) Pulmonary rehabilitation Inhaled glucocorticosteroids if frequent recurrences and lung response
Severe	<35%	Regular treatment with inhaled bronchodilators Inhaled glucocorticosteroids if frequent recurrences and lung response Treat complications Pulmonary rehabilitation Long-term oxygen therapy if respiratory failure Consider surgical treatment

Data from Bach PB, Brown C, Gelfand SE, McCrory DC. Management of acute exacerbations of chronic obstructive pulmonary disease: A summary and appraisal of published evidence. Ann Intern Med 2001;134:600–620; Global Initiative for Chronic Obstructive Lung Disease (GOLD), World Health Organization (WHO), National Heart, Lung, and Blood Institute (NHLBI). Global Strategy for the Diagnosis, Management, and Prevention of Chronic Obstructive Pulmonary Disease. Bethesda, MD, GOLD, WHO, NHLBI, 2001; Veterans Health Administration. Clinical Practice Guideline for the Management of Chronic Obstructive Pulmonary Disease. Version 1.1a. Washington, DC, Department of Veterans Affairs (U.S.), Veterans Health Administration, 1999.

REFERENCES

Bach PB, Brown C, Gelfand SE, McCrory DC. Management of acute exacerbations of chronic obstructive pulmonary disease: A summary and appraisal of published evidence. Ann Intern Med 2001;134:600–620.Ⓐ Ⓑ Ⓒ

Global Initiative for Chronic Obstructive Lung Disease (GOLD), World Health Organization (WHO), National Heart, Lung, and Blood Institute (NHLBI). Global Strategy for the Diagnosis, Management, and Prevention of Chronic Obstructive Pulmonary Disease. Bethesda, MD, GOLD, WHO, NHLBI, 2001.Ⓐ Ⓑ Ⓒ

Harmon-Weiss S. Chronic Obstructive Pulmonary Disease. Nutrition Management for Older Adults. Washington, DC, Nutrition Screening Initiative, 2002.Ⓒ

Snow V, Lascher S, Mottur-Pilson C. Evidence base for management of acute exacerbations of chronic obstructive pulmonary disease. Ann Intern Med 2001;134:595–599.Ⓐ Ⓑ Ⓒ

Veterans Health Administration (VHA). Clinical Practice Guideline for the Management of Chronic Obstructive Pulmonary Disease. Version 1.1a. Washington, DC, Department of Veterans Affairs (U.S.), Veterans Health Administration, 1999.Ⓐ Ⓑ

33

Dyspnea and Confusion (Pulmonary Embolism)

Dino William Ramzi

INITIAL VISIT

Subjective

Patient Identification and Presenting Problem

Maria V. is a 72-year-old Hispanic woman who is readmitted to the hospital from a skilled nursing facility with dyspnea and confusion. Maria was well until 4 weeks earlier when she underwent a cholecystectomy for biliary colic. An incidental Dukes B carcinoma was resected by hemicolectomy. Her postoperative course was stormy, complicated by pancreatitis and a cerebrovascular accident. After a long hospitalization, she was discharged to a skilled nursing facility for rehabilitation.

Maria has been doing well since arriving at the rehabilitation wing of the skilled nursing facility. Ambulation and gait training have been difficult because of her right hemiparesis and deconditioning. Maria was started on megestrol to help her regain the weight she had lost during the hospitalization. One week later, Maria developed progressive confusion over several days. This morning, she was found to be frankly delirious and breathing rapidly.

Medical History

Maria's health problems include longstanding hypertension and congestive heart failure controlled on a loop diuretic and a β-blocker as well as bullous emphysema associated with a 30 pack-year smoking history.

Family History

Maria's father died suddenly when Maria was a child. The cause of death was never clear. One of her brothers has had problems with recurrent DVT and had a Greenfield filter placed. Maria has one daughter who is healthy. Maria suffered a series of miscarriages and never had another child.

Social History

Maria drinks socially and smoked regularly for 30 years. She quit smoking 10 years ago when her doctor told her she had emphysema. She lived with her husband until she was hospitalized this past year.

Review of Systems

Nursing home records indicate that Maria developed some lower extremity swelling over the past several days. She has been afebrile and has not been coughing.

Objective

Physical Examination

Maria is a frail elderly woman in restraints, disoriented to time, place, and person. Her vital signs are as follows: blood pressure 140/85, pulse 104, respiratory rate 24. Her oxygen saturation by pulse oximetry was

---

initially 80%, rising to 97% on an FiO$_2$ of 0.4. She is afebrile. Her head and neck examination is normal. There is no jugular venous distention. Her lung examination is normal; she has a fixed split S2. The abdomen is soft, not distended, and not tender. There is no lymphadenopathy. Her right leg shows trace edema at mid-shin, but her left leg is significantly more swollen. Her left leg measures 32 cm at a point 10 cm below the tibial tubercle as compared to 28 cm for her right leg.

Assessment

Working Diagnosis

The rapid development of dyspnea and hypoxia with asymmetrical leg swelling in a patient with multiple risk factors for the development of thromboembolic disease suggests DVT and PE.

Differential Diagnosis

The differential diagnosis of acute dyspnea includes chronic obstructive pulmonary disease exacerbation, pneumonia, pneumothorax, pulmonary edema, myocardial infarction, pericarditis, and arrhythmia, among others.

Plan

Diagnostic

A careful clinical history and examination are the first steps in the assessment of a suspected PE, with careful attention to risk factors for thromboembolism. Chest radiograph, electrocardiography, and arterial blood gas all provide important clinical information.

The use of a clinical decision rule such as the Wells rule for PE (Table 33-1) is strongly recommended. The Wells rule estimates a pretest probability of PE, which guides interpretation of further testing. Maria is clearly high risk, given her recent history of surgery and clinical findings consistent with DVT. A negative D-dimer is useful only in low-risk patients and cannot be relied on in high-risk situations.

VQ scanning has been the standard first-line investigation for many decades. The role of helical CT scanning is evolving and is commonly used as an alternative to VQ scanning. The Institute for Clinical Improvement has developed an evidence-based algorithm that uses either CT or VQ approaches to the diagnosis of PE (Fig. 33-1).

Investigations often include a Doppler ultrasound of the legs in search of a potential source of embolism. Unfortunately, PEs are frequently documented in which no evidence of an embolic source is ever found. A negative compression ultrasound is helpful in situations in which a thoracic CT is negative or a VQ scan is low or intermediate probability (see Fig. 33-1).

Table 33-1	Wells Clinical Prediction Rule for PE	
Clinical Feature		**Points**
Clinical symptoms of DVT		3
Other diagnosis less likely than PE		3
Heart rate >100 beats per minute		1.5
Immobilization or surgery within past 4 weeks		1.5
Previous DVT or PE		1.5
Hemoptysis		1
Malignancy		1
Total points		

Risk score interpretation (probability of DVT): >6 points: high risk (78.4%); 2 to 6 points: moderate risk (27.8%); <2 points: low risk (3.4%).
DVT, deep venous thrombosis; PE, pulmonary embolism.
Adapted with permission from Wells PS, Anderson DR, Rodger M, et al. Derivation of a simple clinical model to categorize patients' probability of pulmonary embolism: Increasing the model utility with the SimpliRED D-dimer. Thromb Haemost 2000;83:418.

Treatment

Immediate anticoagulation with unfractionated intravenous (IV) heparin is the treatment of choice. Maria will be switched to an oral anticoagulation regimen as soon as she is stable and will remain on warfarin for at least 6 months. The option of continuing anticoagulation beyond 6 months depends on the identification of risk factors. Maria has multiple risk factors, which may continue to influence her risk of thrombosis. One immediately remediable risk factor is megestrol, an estrogenic medication, which should be discontinued.

Patient Education

Maria should be instructed about symptoms of DVT. Any new or additional lower extremity swelling or sudden onset of chest pain and dyspnea constitutes an urgent need for consultation. Maintaining her mobility and function will be important for preventing future DVT. Additionally, she should be made aware that warfarin interacts with many medications and foods. Maria should avoid foods that contain high amounts of vitamin K, such as green leafy vegetables, cauliflower, and legumes, among others.

Disposition

Maria is returned to the nursing home once her international normalized ratio (INR) of prothrombin clotting time has reached 2.0. She is requested to

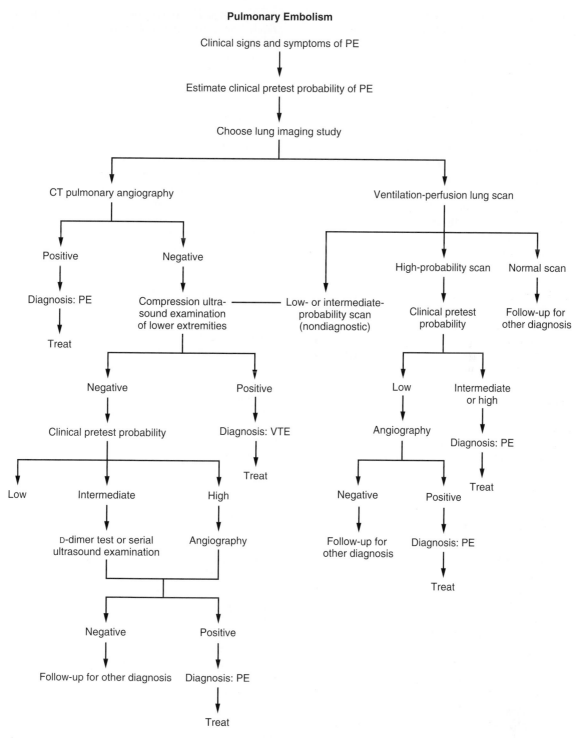

Figure 33-1 Institute for Clinical Systems Improvement evidence-based treatment algorithm for CT or VQ approaches to diagnosing pulmonary embolism (PE). (From Institute for Clinical Systems Improvement. Healthcare guidelines. Venous thromboembolism. Available at www.icsi.org/knowledge/detail.asp?catID=29&itemID=202. Accessed 10/11/2004.)

return weekly to monitor her ratio until stable and then at least monthly for periodic monitoring.

DISCUSSION

Diagnosis

PE is a potentially fatal condition that often presents suddenly, with or without evidence of prior DVT.

Patients with potential thromboembolic disease must first be evaluated for predisposing risk factors (Box 33-1). The majority of patients with PE have at least one risk factor, and 50% are hospitalized or at nursing facilities. None of the clinical findings associated with DVT or PE are specific enough to be entirely reliable. For example, a fixed split S2 may well reflect the presence of a PE, but it may also be present in pulmonary hypertension in the context of chronic obstructive pulmonary disease. Likewise, the classic electrocardiographic signs of PE such as right axis shift, P pulmonale, or right bundle branch block are present in the minority of cases. Nonspecific changes are common but do not guide the diagnosis. Chest radiograph is most commonly normal but on rare occasions demonstrates evidence of embolism or infarction. Arterial blood gas analysis is helpful in the management of hypoxemia but is not sufficiently specific to have any diagnostic use.

The use of clinical decision rules can effectively estimate the probability of PE based on a formal and standardized set of criteria. Numerous decision rules have been elaborated for use in PE. The pretest probability of PE guides the interpretation of subsequent investigations. The oldest, best validated, and most widely used clinical decision rule for pulmonary embolism is the one developed by Wells and colleagues (see Table 33-1).

Imaging technology is the backbone of investigation for PE. The definitive study to determine or refute the presence of a PE is pulmonary angiography. However, it is a dye-based and relatively invasive test that carries risk. VQ scanning has been the standard first-line investigation for many decades. The Prospective Investigation of Pulmonary Embolism Diagnosis (PIOPED) study provided landmark evidence of the usefulness of the VQ scan. The pretest probability of PE is a subjective physician determination, not a standardized set of criteria. The VQ test itself is most useful in combination with a formalized decision rule. Unfortunately, VQ scanning is difficult to interpret in the presence of other pulmonary pathology, such as chronic obstructive pulmonary disease. Results from VQ scanning frequently do not provide definitive evidence of the presence or absence of a PE.

Over the past several years, increased interest and reliance on helical CT scanning has distracted clinicians from the essential diagnosis. Helical CT scanning is technology in rapid evolution. Resolution is progressing to the point that some machines can currently discern emboli in segmental arteries but may still miss emboli in smaller, more distal vessels. In time, helical CT angiography may replace traditional angiography as the gold standard for assessing PE. However, data to validate the use of the technology in real-world clinical settings are still sparse in comparison to VQ. PIOPED II is currently

Box 33-1	Risk Factors for Thromboembolic Disease

Increasing age
Prolonged immobility
Surgery
Major trauma
Fractures
Malignancy
Pregnancy
Estrogenic medications
  Oral contraceptive pills
  Hormone therapy
  Tamoxifen (Nolvadex)
Diseases that alter blood viscosity
  Polycythemia
  Sickle cell disease
  Multiple myeloma
Inherited thrombophilia
  Lupus anticoagulant
  Antithrombin III deficiency

Fibrinogen abnormality
Plasminogen abnormality
Plasminogen activator abnormality
Protein C deficiency
Protein S deficiency
  Resistance to activated protein C
Hyperhomocystinemia
Thrombocytosis
Heparin-associated thrombocytopenia
Indwelling central catheters
Hyperlipidemias
Congestive heart failure
Obesity
Varicose veins
Venography
Chronic venous insufficiency
Venous stasis

under way and should soon provide valuable information about the true role of the current generation of CT scanners in diagnosing PE.

In recent years, refinements in D-dimer testing have spurred interest in the use of this simple blood test in the diagnosis of thromboembolic disease. For example, a D-dimer in combination with low clinical probability effectively rules out the possibility of a DVT. However, the same cannot necessarily be said for PE, in which the use of D-dimer is more limited. The D-dimer is a nonspecific marker that rises with any inflammatory condition. Thus, an elevated D-dimer has no utility when pneumonia is in the differential or in hospitalized patients in whom it is simply not sufficiently specific. The D-dimer may be useful in circumstances in which imaging has been indeterminate and there is a low clinical probability of PE. One study suggests that CT scanning in combination with D-dimer is as cost-effective as VQ scanning, in which a negative D-dimer helps reassure the clinician. It should be noted that the use of D-dimer in thromboembolic disease applies only to second-generation D-dimer tests, which are more reliable but not universally used by hospitals and laboratories.

Treatment

For patients who are hemodynamically stable, the treatment of PE is supportive and includes the administration of oxygen and IV fluids in addition to anticoagulation. Fibrinolytics, pulmonary artery catheterization, and possibly surgical embolectomy may be required in patients who are hemodynamically compromised.

Unfractionated intravenous heparin is the standard method of anticoagulation for patients with PE, although low-molecular-weight heparin is also safe and effective. Enoxaparin and tinzaparin are the only low-molecular-weight heparins currently approved for use in PE. It is not yet definitively known whether the use of low-molecular-weight heparin reduces length of hospitalization for PE.

Once the patient is fully anticoagulated with heparin, the use of warfarin follows. A nomogram for initiation of warfarin at a dose of 5 mg is presented in Table 33-2. A similar nomogram exists for the use of a 10-mg dose. Occasionally, anticoagulation does not prevent clot or embolus recurrence. In these cases, the use of an inferior vena cava filter provides some short-term benefit. Survival at 2 years does not appear to be affected by the use of an inferior vena cava filter.

Prevention

The usual duration of warfarin anticoagulation following PE is at least 6 months. Patients with PE who have ongoing risk factors need ongoing anticoagula-

Table 33-2	Initiation of Warfarin Therapy at 5 mg per Day	
Day	**INR**	**Warfarin Dose (mg/day)**
1		5
2		5
3	<1.5	10
	1.5–1.9	5
	2.0–2.9	2.5
	>3.0	0
4	<1.5	10
	1.5–1.9	7.5
	2.0–2.9	5
	>3.0	0
5	<2.0	10
	2.0–2.9	5
	>3.0	0
6	<1.5	10
	1.5–1.9	7.5
	2.0–2.9	5
	>3.0	0

INR, international normalized ratio.
Adapted with permission from Crowther MA, Harrison L, Hirsh J. Reply. Warfarin: Less may be better. Ann Intern Med 1997;127:333.

tion. Nearly 50% of episodes of DVT and PE are associated with some form of inherited or acquired thrombophilia. Patients with thrombophilias may require indefinite anticoagulation.

When there is no clinical reason for a patient to develop thromboembolic disease or when there is a strong family history, then the possibility of an inherited thrombophilia is heightened and a hematologic investigation may be considered. Multiple miscarriages may also be a clue to an underlying thrombophilia. Table 33-3 presents one author's approach to the investigation of thrombophilias in patients with PE. However, it should be noted that this approach is not validated or evidence based. It does not appear that investigation for thrombophilias reliably predicts future recurrence but may be useful in patients with a strong family history.

All patients who may be immobilized for a prolonged period of time should be considered candidates for anticoagulation in prophylactic doses. Elderly patients undergoing surgical procedures, especially orthopedic procedures, are at high risk. Young patients with major trauma or acute spinal cord injury are also at significant risk. Many critically ill and general medicine patients have risk factors associated with age and immobility, which are underrecognized.

Subcutaneously administered heparin is a simple method of prophylaxis for venous thromboembolism. Low-molecular-weight heparin is at least as effective and possibly associated with fewer

Table 33-3 Risk-Specific Investigations for Thrombophilias

Clinical Characteristics	Risk of Having a Thrombophilia	Investigations
First episode of venous thromboembolic disease with known risk factors for thromboembolism and no family history of thromboembolism*	Low	None
Age older than 50 years, idiopathic first episode of venous thromboembolic disease, and no family history of thromboembolism*	Moderate	Resistance to activated protein C with a clotting assay that dilutes patient plasma in factor V–deficient plasma or genetic test for factor V Leiden mutation Genetic test for prothrombin G20210A mutation Clotting assay for lupus anticoagulant ELISA for antiphospholipid antibodies Plasma homocysteine level
Idiopathic venous thromboembolic disease before age 50 years	High	All of the above and antithrombin assay (heparin cofactor assay)
Recurrent thrombosis		Protein C assay Protein S assay
Family history of thromboembolism*		

*Family history is defined as venous thromboembolic disease occurring in a first-degree relative before the age of 50 years.
ELISA, enzyme-linked immunosorbant assay.
Adapted with permission from Ramzi DW, Leeper KV. DVT and pulmonary embolism: Part I: Diagnosis. Am Fam Physician 2004;69:2829–2836; Ramzi DW, Leeper KV. DVT and pulmonary embolism: Part II: Treatment and prevention. Am Fam Physician 2004;69:2841–2848.

adverse events in most surgical settings. Intermittent pneumatic leg compression is useful as an adjunct or in patients who have contraindications to anticoagulation. Elastic compression stockings must be truly graded to deliver pressure of 30 to 40 mm Hg and are useful only in low-risk patients.

Material Available on Student Consult

Review Questions and Answers about Pulmonary Embolism

SUGGESTED READING

Agnelli G, Prandoni P, Becattini C, et al. Extended oral anticoagulant therapy after a first episode of pulmonary embolism. Ann Intern Med 2003;139:19–25.Ⓐ

American College of Emergency Physicians (ACEP) Clinical Policies Committee. ACEP Clinical Policies Subcommittee on Suspected Lower-Extremity Deep Venous Thrombosis. Clinical policy: Critical issues in the evaluation and management of adult patients presenting with suspected lower-extremity deep venous thrombosis. Ann Emerg Med 2003;42:124–135.Ⓑ

Bauer KA. The thrombophilias: Well-defined risk factors with uncertain therapeutic implications. Ann Intern Med 2001;135:367–373.Ⓒ

Hull RD, Raskob GE, Brant RF, et al. Low-molecular-weight heparin vs heparin in the treatment of patients with pulmonary embolism. American-Canadian Thrombosis Study Group. Arch Intern Med 2000;160:229–236.Ⓐ

Hyers TM, Agnelli G, Hull RD, et al. Antithrombotic therapy for venous thromboembolic disease. Chest 2001;119(1 Suppl):176S–193S.Ⓑ

Institute for Clinical Systems Improvement. Healthcare guidelines. Venous thromboembolism. Available at www.icsi.org/knowledge/detail.asp?catID=29&itemID=202. Accessed 12/11/2004.Ⓑ

Kovacs MJ, Rodger M, Anderson DR, et al. Comparison of 10-mg and 5-mg warfarin initiation nomograms together with low-molecular-weight heparin for outpatient treatment of acute venous thromboembolism: A randomized, double-blind, controlled trial. Ann Intern Med 2003;138:714–719.Ⓐ

Ramzi DW, Leeper KV. DVT and pulmonary embolism: Part I: Diagnosis. Am Fam Physician 2004; 69:2829–2836.B

Ramzi DW, Leeper KV. DVT and pulmonary embolism: Part II: Treatment and prevention. Am Fam Physician 2004;69:2841–2848.B

Wells PS, Anderson DR, Rodger M, et al. Derivation of a simple clinical model to categorize patients' probability of pulmonary embolism: Increasing the model utility with the SimpliRED D-dimer. Thromb Haemost 2000;83:416–420.A

Wells PS, Anderson DR, Rodger M, et al. Excluding pulmonary embolism at the bedside without diagnostic imaging: Management of patients with suspected pulmonary embolism presenting to the emergency department by using a simple clinical model and D-dimer. Ann Intern Med 2001;135:98–107.A

Chapter

34

Episodic Chest Pain (Angina Pectoris)

Ruth Falik

KEY POINTS

1. Electrocardiographic stress testing can be done in patients who are stable and able to exercise to evaluate for coronary artery disease. It is a provocative test and should be done only when trained personnel are available.
2. Exercise testing should not be done in patients with recent myocardial infarction (less than 48 to 72 hours), infective uncontrolled hypertension, severe aortic stenosis, or a history of exercise-provoked ventricular tachycardia or syncope, resting angina, decompensated heart failure, acute myocarditis or pericarditis, or significant electrolyte abnormality.
3. The presence of left bundle branch block, left ventricular hypertrophy with more than 1 mm ST depression, pre-excitation syndromes, or use of digoxin precludes accurate interpretation of electrocardiographic changes and requires an imaging stress test to evaluate for coronary artery disease.
4. In patients unable to exercise, pharmacologic agents (e.g., dipyridamole, adenosine, dobutamine) can be used to assess for evidence of provocable ischemia.

INITIAL VISIT

Subjective

Patient Identification and Presenting Problem

Richard H. is a 42-year-old white man who presents with a 2-month history of episodic chest discomfort occurring with exertion. Richard describes his discomfort as tightness in the central part of his chest that sometimes involves his left arm. These episodes resolve with rest and do not last longer than 5 minutes. He has had two episodes in the past week and is concerned. He denies cough, shortness of breath, and pain with inspiration. There is no association with eating or history of recent trauma.

Medical History

Richard has no history of diabetes or hypertension. His lipid status is unknown. He has had an appendectomy. He is on no medications.

Family History

Richard's father had a myocardial infarction at age 41 and died at age 49. His mother is alive and being treated for hypertension. His two sisters are well.

Social History

Richard is married and works in sales. He has smoked two packs of cigarettes per day since he was in his late teens. He has one or two beers per day. He denies illicit drug use. He has been trying to lose weight by walking but finds that he develops symptoms when he tries to increase his pace.

Review of Systems

The patient denies palpitations, lightheadedness, shortness of breath, and neck or back pain. His appetite is unchanged, and he denies change in bowel or bladder habits.

Objective

Physical Examination

General Richard is a well-developed overweight man in no distress.

Vital Signs He is 6 feet tall and weighs 235 pounds; his temperature is 37.1°C (98.8°F), respiratory rate is 12, blood pressure is 146/90 in the right arm and 142/88 in the left arm, and pulse is 72.

Head, Eyes, Ears, Nose, and Throat Head is without signs of trauma; eyes, ears, nose, and throat are unremarkable.

Neck The trachea is midline, neck is supple, jugular venous pulsations are of normal contour and volume, and no bruits are heard.

Chest The chest is resonant to percussion; auscultation is clear without rales, wheezes, or rubs.

Heart The rhythm is regular with normal S1 and S2, with no murmurs, rubs, or gallops heard.

Abdomen The abdomen is soft and nontender with bowel sounds in all four quadrants.

Extremities There is no cyanosis, clubbing, or edema; pulses are full and equal throughout.

Neurologic Examination A nonfocal motor and sensory examination was done, with a normal gait and intact cranial nerve assessment.

Assessment

Working Diagnosis

The working diagnosis is angina pectoris, but the differential diagnosis for chest discomfort is large; it includes conditions affecting organs of the thorax and abdomen (Table 34-1). These conditions vary from life threatening (myocardial ischemia,

Table 34-1 Differential Diagnosis of Chest Pain
Cardiac
Coronary artery disease
Aortic stenosis
Hypertrophic cardiomyopathy
Mitral valve prolapse
Pericarditis
Syndrome X
Aortic dissection
Gastrointestinal
Esophageal spasm
Esophageal reflux
Mallory-Weiss tear
Biliary disease
Peptic ulcer
Gastritis
Pancreatitis
Neurologic
Cervical disk disease
Herpes zoster
Psychiatric
Panic attacks
Pulmonary
Pulmonary embolus
Pneumothorax
Pneumonia
Pleurodynia
Pulmonary hypertension
Musculoskeletal
Costochondritis
Intercostal muscle spasm
Bicipital tendinitis

pulmonary embolism, aortic dissection, and pneumothorax) to benign (esophageal reflux or spasm, anxiety, and costochondritis). The physician needs to eliminate those conditions that place the patient in immediate jeopardy. This can be accomplished by a complete and focused history and physical examination, as well as readily available blood, electrocardiographic, and imaging tests.

Differential Diagnosis

Angina pectoris occurs when the blood supply to the myocardium is not sufficient to meet metabolic demand. The mismatch can be precipitated by an increase in demand (physical exertion, emotional stress, fever) or by a decrease in supply (obstruction to coronary flow resulting from atherosclerotic plaque, anemia, hypoxemia) or a combination of the two. The pain of angina pectoris is most frequently described as discomfort that is deep and visceral. The location is usually retrosternal and cannot be localized to a small area. It may radiate to the neck, jaw, one or both arms, and the shoulders. This reflects the common origin in the posterior horn of the spinal cord of sensory neurons to the heart, neck, shoulders, and arms. Pain is typically brought on by increased physical activity or emotional excitement, or after eating a heavy meal. Anginal pain lasts 2 to 10 minutes and is relieved with rest or sublingual nitroglycerin.

Other cardiac causes of chest pain similar to angina pectoris (a term specific to chest pain due to coronary atherosclerosis) include hypertrophic cardiomyopathy, aortic stenosis, and mitral valve prolapse; however, these cardiac lesions are associated with a systolic murmur and other characteristic findings. Syndrome X causes chest pain and electrocardiographic changes, but on angiography, patients have normal coronary arteries and an excellent prognosis.

Pericarditis causes chest pain that lasts hours to days, is positional (worse lying down, better sitting up), and has distinct electrocardiographic findings as well as a pericardial rub.

Aortic dissection, a potentially catastrophic cause of chest pain, results from a tear in the subintimal wall of the aorta or from rupture of the vasa vasorum within the aortic media. Trauma to the aorta from a motor vehicle accident or from invasive procedures, e.g., cardiac catheterization, can also cause aortic dissection. Inherited connective tissue diseases such as Marfan's and Ehlers-Danlos syndromes are associated with cystic medial degeneration and dissection of the large vessels. Acute dissection causes a sudden onset of severe chest pain, whereas angina tends to have a less abrupt onset.

Pulmonary embolism when associated with chest pain is most likely due to distention of the pulmonary artery or infarction of a segment of the lung adjacent to the pleura. The pain is typically pleuritic and often lateral. There is often tachycardia and dyspnea. When present, characteristic electrocardiographic changes (new-onset atrial fibrillation, an S wave in lead I, a Q wave in lead III, and an inverted T wave in lead III) are helpful in the diagnosis.

Pneumothorax also presents with the sudden onset of pleuritic chest pain and dyspnea and can readily be diagnosed with a chest radiograph, as can pneumonia.

Gastrointestinal conditions such as esophageal reflux, spasm, or obstruction cause chest pain that can be visceral and located in the mid-chest. These conditions can have associations with time of day, body position, or type of food ingested.

Neuromusculoskeletal conditions are the most common causes of anterior chest pain and can usually be diagnosed by the history (pain is sharp and fleeting) and the physical examination findings (reproducible pain).

Plan

Diagnostic

An electrocardiogram (ECG) is essential. The presence of electrocardiographic abnormalities consistent with acute or chronic ischemia would provide evidence that this patient is having chest pain that is due to atherosclerotic blockages of the coronary arteries, but the absence of such changes does not exclude such pathology. Richard, who does not have chest pain at this time and has a normal ECG, is a good candidate for outpatient evaluation. This should include chest radiograph, fasting lipids (to stratify risk), complete blood count, and basic metabolic profile. Only Richard's lipid profile is abnormal: Total cholesterol is 246 mg/dL, low-density lipoprotein is 149 mg/dL, and high-density lipoprotein is 32 mg/dL. A Bruce protocol electrocardiographic stress test is positive at 6 minutes (2.0 mm ST segment depression) at a heart rate of 150 beats per minute, confirming that Richard's chest discomfort is angina.

Therapeutics

Richard is started on a β-blocker, lipid-lowering drug, and aspirin without side effects. He is able to stop smoking cigarettes, although he complains of mild anxiety. He has an episode of exertional chest discomfort while on medications. The recurrence of symptoms coupled with his relative youth, his positive cardiovascular risk profile (positive family history, hyperlipidemia, and many pack-years of cigarette smoking), and strongly positive electrocardiographic stress test warrants a myocardial perfusion imaging study. It reveals a large area of anterior, septal, and apical ischemia. A cardiac catheterization is recommended. This study reveals a 90% stenosis of the proximal left anterior descending artery that is successfully stented at the time of catheterization.

Patient Education

Richard is encouraged to walk 30 minutes every day and to eat a low-fat diet.

FOLLOW-UP VISIT

Subjective

Richard is encouraged by a 15-pound weight loss over the next 3 months and notes that he is less anxious than previously, but he still misses cigarette smoking.

Objective

Richard is now able to walk 2 miles every day in 30 minutes without chest pain or shortness of breath. He has had no further episodes of chest pain since his coronary artery stent placement. His physical examination is notable for a blood pressure of 115/72 and pulse of 62. He is tolerating his medications without adverse effects.

Laboratory Tests

At 3 months on a low-fat diet and a lipid-lowering medication, Richard has a total cholesterol of 205 mg/dL, low-density lipoprotein of 112 mg/dL, and high-density lipoprotein of 38 mg/dL. Liver function testing is normal. His ECG remains entirely normal.

Plan

Richard is encouraged to continue with his dietary modifications and weight loss regimen. He will continue to take a β-blocker and aspirin. The dose of his lipid-lowering medication is increased to try to further reduce his low-density lipoprotein.

DISCUSSION

Electrocardiographic stress testing remains the most widely used test for the diagnosis of coronary artery disease (Gibbons et al., 1997 ◉). It involves the recording of a 12-lead ECG before, during, and after exercise, most commonly on a treadmill. The test consists of a standardized incremental increase in the workload while symptoms, ECG, and blood pressure are monitored. The test is stopped on complaint of chest discomfort, significant dyspnea, lightheadedness, severe fatigue, ST segment depression of more than 2 mm, a drop in systolic blood pressure of more than 10 mm Hg, or the development of ventricular tachyarrhythmia.

A test is considered positive if chest discomfort develops during testing, ST segment depression is flat and more than 1 mm below baseline (i.e., the PR segment) with a duration longer than 0.08 seconds. Upsloping or junctional ST segment changes are not considered to be diagnostic of ischemia, nor are T-wave abnormalities, conduction disturbances, or ventricular arrhythmias that occur during the test. If the target heart rate is not achieved, defined as 85% of the maximal predicted heart rate for age and gender, then an otherwise negative test is considered to be nondiagnostic. If blood pressure drops during testing, the test is considered positive because the normal response to graded exercise is a progressive increase in heart rate and blood pressure. The development of chest pain and/or severe (>2 mV) ST segment depression at a low workload (early in the test protocol) or the persistence of ST segment depression for more than 5 minutes after the termination of exercise is considered strongly positive and increases the specificity of the test for coronary artery disease.

Contraindications to exercise stress testing include rest angina within 48 to 72 hours, unstable rhythm, severe aortic stenosis, acute myocarditis, uncontrolled heart failure, and active infective endocarditis.

Major indications to perform a stress myocardial perfusion imaging study during exercise or pharmacologic stress include the following:

- Diagnosis of coronary artery disease in the patient with a positive electrocardiographic stress test without symptoms during the test or a negative electrocardiographic stress test but with symptoms suggestive of ischemia
- The presence of resting electrocardiographic abnormalities such as left bundle branch block or left ventricular hypertrophy, or use of drugs such as digoxin, all of which alter the repolarization phase of the ECG and preclude accurate interpretation of an electrocardiographic stress test
- Need to determine the functional significance of coronary artery disease

When a patient is unable to exercise due to concomitant medical conditions, e.g., peripheral vascular disease, morbid obesity, neurologic disease, poor motivation, or anti-angina medication (β-blocker or calcium channel blocker therapy), pharmacologic stress testing is done in conjunction with imaging techniques (Lee et al., 2001). Intravenous dipyridamole (Persantine) or adenosine is used in place of exercise. Dipyridamole blocks the uptake of adenosine by red blood cells and endothelium, resulting in an increase in endogenous adenosine, which in turn leads to relaxation of vascular smooth muscle and arteriolar vasodilation. The patient should be in a fasting state, having received no xanthine medications (e.g., theophylline) during the previous 36 hours and no caffeine-containing beverages in the preceding 24 hours. Dipyridamole is contraindicated in patients with reactive airways. Adenosine is a powerful vasodilator and is the mediator of dipyridamole's vasodilating action. Adenosine infusion reaches maximal effect at 2 minutes and is active for only 2 to 3 minutes postinfusion. Patient preparation and contraindications are the same as for dipyridamole.

Dobutamine is a powerful sympathomimetic drug with β_1-, β_2-, and α_1-adrenoreceptor agonist effects resulting predominantly in inotropic effects. Myocardial contractility is increased, as is systolic blood pressure. At higher doses, dobutamine causes an increase in heart rate. These effects increase myocardial oxygen requirements and in the presence of coronary artery disease may provoke ischemia. Vasodilator protocols using dipyridamole or adenosine are shorter and have a lower incidence of side effects and complications.

Two-dimensional echocardiography can assess both global and regional wall motion abnormalities of the left ventricle due to myocardial infarction or persistent ischemia. Stress (exercise or dobutamine) echocardiography may provoke akinesis or dyskinesis not present at rest. Stress echocardiography, like stress myocardial perfusion imaging, is more sensitive than exercise electrocardiography in the diagnosis of coronary artery disease (Garber and Solomon, 1999) (Table 34-2).

Coronary arteriography is indicated in patients with angina or evidence of ischemia on noninvasive testing who have evidence of ventricular dysfunction. Patients who are at high risk of sustaining coronary events based on signs of severe ischemia on noninvasive testing should also undergo coronary arteriography (Blumenthal et al., 2000). Other indications for coronary arteriography include patients with chronic stable angina pectoris who are severely symptomatic despite medical therapy and who are being considered for revascularization, i.e., percutaneous coronary intervention with stenting or coronary artery bypass grafting. Coronary arteriography is recommended for patients who present diagnostic difficulties and in whom there is a need to confirm or eliminate the diagnosis of coronary artery disease.

Coronary artery catheterization offers the option of revascularization if the vessel proves suitable, as was the case in this patient. It has the advantage of being less invasive and requiring a shorter hospitalization and hence lower cost than coronary

Table 34-2	Stress Myocardial Perfusion Imaging Versus Stress Echocardiography

Advantages of stress myocardial perfusion imaging
Greater sensitivity, especially for single-vessel coronary artery disease involving the left circumflex
Larger published database
Higher technical success rate

Advantages of stress echocardiography
Greater specificity
Provides more information of cardiac anatomy and function
Lower cost

artery bypass grafting. The disadvantages of percutaneous coronary intervention include a high incidence of incomplete revascularization, restenosis, and unknown effect on outcomes in patients with severe left ventricular dysfunction.

Material Available on Student Consult

Review Questions and Answers about Angina Pectoris

REFERENCES

Blumenthal RS, Cohn G, Schulman SP. Medical therapy versus coronary angioplasty in stable coronary artery disease: A critical review of the literature. J Am Coll Cardiol 2000;36:668–673.

Garber AM, Solomon NA. Cost-effectiveness of alternative test strategies for the diagnosis of coronary artery disease. Ann Intern Med 1999;130:719–728.

Gibbons RJ, Balady GJ, Beasley JW, et al. ACC/AHA guidelines for exercise testing: Executive summary:

A report of the American College of Cardiology/ American Heart Association Task Force on Practice Guidelines (Committee on Exercise Testing). Circulation 1997;96:345–354.ⓒ

Lee TH, Boucher CA. Noninvasive tests in patients with stable coronary artery disease. N Engl J Med 2001;344:1840–1845.

35 Palpitations (Atrial Fibrillation)

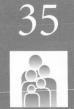

Ruth Falik

KEY POINTS

1. Rate control with chronic anticoagulation is the recommended strategy for the majority of patients with atrial fibrillation. Rhythm control is not superior.
2. Patients who are at moderate or high risk of stroke should receive long-term anticoagulation with adjusted-dose warfarin. The international normalized ratio (INR) goal is 2 to 3.
3. To achieve adequate rate control during exercise as well as at rest, use β-blockers (atenolol or metoprolol) or nondihydropyridine calcium channel blockers (diltiazem or verapamil). Digoxin is effective only for rate control at rest.
4. There is an inverse relationship between the duration of atrial fibrillation and the ability to cardiovert to sinus rhythm—the longer the duration of the dysrhythmia, the less likely cardioversion. A similar inverse relationship exists between left atrial size and successful cardioversion to sinus rhythm.

INITIAL VISIT

Subjective

Patient Identification and Presenting Problem
Howard L. is a 77-year-old man who presents with palpitations and complains of not feeling "right" for the past several days. He is unsure when this feeling began, but he states that last weekend he could not play his usual 18 holes of golf. He denies chest pain or discomfort but is aware of an irregular beating in his chest, particularly at night before falling asleep. He has no shortness of breath and continues to sleep on two firm pillows. He denies cough or fever. He has not noted heat intolerance, tremor, or weight loss.

The patient specifically denies binge drinking or stimulant drug use.

Medical History
Howard has a 35-year history of hypertension, which has been treated with hydrochlorothiazide. He has no history of rheumatic fever or recent viral illness. There are no known drug allergies.

Family History
Howard has two older sisters. Both have hypertension and one (age 66) recently had coronary artery bypass grafting for triple vessel coronary disease. His parents are dead; the causes are unknown, but they survived into their 70s.

Health Habits
Howard has never smoked cigarettes. He drinks one or two glasses of wine once or twice a week. He denies illicit drug use. Howard plays golf most weekends.

Social History
Howard lives with his wife of 49 years. He is a retired engineer. His three daughters live out of state.

Review of Systems
The patient denies a history of heart murmur, joint disease, or neurologic disorder. He denies anxiety, diarrhea, loss of consciousness, or lightheadedness.

Objective

Physical Examination
General Howard is a well-developed, well-nourished alert male sitting up on the examination table in no apparent distress.

Vital Signs He is 6 feet 3 inches tall and weighs 200 pounds. His temperature is 37°C (98.6°F), respiratory rate is 16 and unlabored, blood pressure is

---

Evidence levels Ⓐ Randomized, controlled trials (RCTs), meta-analyses, well-designed systematic reviews of RCTs. Ⓑ Case-control or cohort studies, nonrandomized clinical trials, systematic reviews of studies other than RCTs, cross-sectional studies, retrospective studies, certain uncontrolled studies. Ⓒ Consensus statements, expert guidelines, usual practice, opinion.

148/86, and pulse is irregularly irregular with a ventricular response of up to 160 beats per minute.

Head, Eyes, Ears, Nose, and Throat All are unremarkable except for male pattern baldness.

Neck The thyroid is of normal size and texture.

Cardiac There is no jugular venous distention, heart sounds are crisp and irregularly irregular, and no murmurs or gallops are heard.

Chest The chest is clear to auscultation.

Abdomen The abdomen is soft and nontender with no evidence of hepatic enlargement.

Extremities There is no edema.

Laboratory Findings
Complete blood count, partial thromboplastin time, prothrombin time, urinalysis, blood chemistry, and thyroid function studies are normal.

Chest Radiograph A normal cardiac size is seen; there is no evidence of pulmonary infiltrate.

Electrocardiogram There is atrial fibrillation with a ventricular response of 130 and nonspecific ST-T changes.

Echocardiographic and Doppler Studies There is concentric left ventricular hypertrophy with an ejection fraction of 55% and no evidence of mitral valve disease. The left atrial size is 46 mm.

Assessment

Working Diagnosis
The working diagnosis is atrial fibrillation. Atrial fibrillation is characterized by disorganized atrial electrical and mechanical activity that is manifested by the absence of P waves on the electrocardiogram and an irregularly irregular ventricular rate. It may be seen in normal individuals during acute alcoholic intoxication or it may be the presenting finding in thyrotoxicosis.

There are three major classes of atrial fibrillation: paroxysmal atrial fibrillation, in which the episodes are self-terminating, usually lasting less than 24 hours but no more than 7 days; persistent atrial fibrillation, which fails to self-terminate, lasts for more than 7 days, and requires cardioversion—if atrial fibrillation recurs postcardioversion, it is considered recurrent—and permanent atrial fibrillation which lasts longer than 1 year and cardioversion either has not been attempted or has failed.

Box 35-1	Irregularly Irregular Rhythms

Atrial fibrillation
Multifocal atrial tachycardia
Atrial flutter with variable block
Sinus rhythm with frequent ectopy

Differential Diagnosis (Box 35-1)
Frequent premature atrial depolarizations can cause an irregularly irregular rhythm, but P waves are present on the electrocardiogram. Multifocal atrial tachycardia is also an irregularly irregular rhythm with at least three different P wave morphologies and PR intervals, most typically seen in patients with chronic hypoxemic lung disease. Atrial flutter with variable atrioventricular nodal block may be perceived as having an irregular ventricular rate, but the electrocardiogram shows discrete undulations of the baseline (e.g., "sawtooth" pattern) and, most commonly, a ventricular rate of approximately 150 beats per minute as a result of a 2:1 block at the atrioventricular node. The diagnosis of atrial fibrillation can be made by correct interpretation of the electrocardiogram.

Plan

Diagnostic
The cardiac conditions most typically seen with atrial fibrillation are rheumatic mitral valve disease, coronary artery disease, atrial septal defect, congestive heart failure, pericarditis, and hypertension. These cardiac conditions can be evaluated with a thorough history, physical examination, and echocardiogram. The noncardiac associations for atrial fibrillation are hyperthyroidism, hypoxic conditions (pneumonia, pulmonary embolus), surgery (particularly cardiac, which causes pericardial inflammation), and alcohol excess. The noncardiac associations can be evaluated by simple laboratory tests and chest radiograph (spiral computed tomography scan if the clinical situation is suspicious for pulmonary embolus).

Because left ventricular function and the size of the left atrium on transthoracic echocardiography are independent predictors of thromboembolism, a strategy of performing transthoracic echocardiography on all individuals with newly diagnosed atrial fibrillation is reasonable. Left atrial size also is a predictor of the patient's ability to cardiovert to and maintain sinus rhythm; a left atrial size greater than 45 mm correlates with a poor likelihood to convert to and maintain sinus rhythm. Transesophageal echocardiography is used to identify features correlating with an increased risk of thromboembolism: the presence of left atrial thrombus, left atrial appendage size, left atrial appendage peak velocities, echocardiographic "smoke," left ventricular dysfunction, left ventricular hypertrophy, and complex aortic plaque. Transesophageal echocardiography is recommended when immediate cardioversion is considered and the duration of the arrhythmia is uncertain but likely to be longer than 48 hours, as is the case in this patient.

Therapeutic

The immediate therapeutic goals in this clinically stable patient are to provide ventricular rate control and to initiate anticoagulation. Rate control should improve hemodynamics and provide symptom relief, whereas anticoagulation diminishes the risk of thromboembolic complications. Had Howard presented with hemodynamic compromise (e.g., symptomatic low blood pressure or heart failure), immediate intervention with intravenous heparin and cardioversion, which can be pharmacologic or electrical, would have been warranted.

Because Howard has no evidence of acute decompensation and the duration of the arrhythmia is likely to be longer than 48 hours, he is started on metoprolol (50 mg orally every 12 hours) for rate control. He is instructed on the self-administration of low-molecular-weight heparin and started on oral warfarin, 5 mg per day. These agents are administered in the outpatient setting with laboratory monitoring of the prothrombin time international normalized ratio. At day 4 his international normalized ratio is 2 (goal: 2 to 3), and low-molecular-weight heparin therapy is stopped. His ventricular rate is in the 80s. He feels much better since starting the β-blocker, but he is concerned about the risk of long-term anticoagulation. After discussing the risks and benefits of attempting cardioversion versus maintaining rate control and anticoagulation, Howard chooses to attempt pharmacologic cardioversion in 3 weeks and will be electively admitted to the cardiology inpatient service at that time. He is aware that even if cardioversion is successful, he will have to remain on warfarin for an additional 4 weeks. If he cannot maintain sinus rhythm, then anticoagulation will be indefinite. He is scheduled for a recheck of his prothrombin time international normalized ratio in 1 week.

DISCUSSION

The patient's symptoms reflect decreased cardiac output due to loss of the atrial kick as well as decreased ventricular filling due to a shortened cardiac cycle. The normal echocardiogram excludes mitral valve stenosis as well as a depressed left ventricular ejection fraction. Indeed, atrial fibrillation

not associated with rheumatic heart disease or valvular abnormalities affects approximately 4% of persons older than 60 years. The prevalence of this most common arrhythmia in adults increases with age: it increases from less than 1% in persons younger than 60 years to more than 8% in those older than 80 years. The age-adjusted incidence for women is approximately half that for men.

In addition to compromised cardiac hemodynamics, the patient's cardiac arrhythmia predisposes him to thromboembolism. Compared with age-matched controls, the relative risk for stroke is increased two- to sevenfold in patients with nonrheumatic atrial fibrillation, and the absolute risk for stroke is between 1% and 5% per year, depending on associated clinical characteristics (Gage et al., 2001❸). The CHADS2 score for risk of stroke (Table 35-1) is calculated by adding 1 point each for recent congestive heart failure (i.e., active within the preceding 14 weeks or documented by echo), hypertension (systolic and/or diastolic), age (at least 75 years), and diabetes mellitus, and adding 2 points for a history of stroke or transient ischemic attack.

Because this patient is not experiencing chest pain, hypotension, or dyspnea, acute cardioversion is not indicated. The initial aim in treating this patient is to slow the ventricular rate and to start anticoagulation. This patient is without evidence of significant compromise, so this can be done in the outpatient setting with close clinical follow-up. The choice of agent for rate control is based on the Agency for Healthcare Research and Quality–funded evidence report

Table 35-1	Risk for Stroke using the CHADS2 Criteria
CHADS2 Score	**Risk Level**
0	Low
1	Low
2	Moderate
3	Moderate
4	High
5	High
6	High

The CHADS2 score is calculated by adding a point each for congestive heart failure, hypertension, age > 74, and diabetes mellitus, and adding 2 points for prior stroke or transient ischemic attack. Moderate- and high-risk patients should receive anticoagulation with warfarin.

Modified from Snow V, Weiss KB, Le Fevre M, et al. Management of newly detected atrial fibrillation: A clinical practice guideline from the American Academy of Family Physicians and the American College of Physicians. Ann Intern Med 2003;139: 1009–1017.

reviewing 48 trials assessing 17 different agents for rate control in atrial fibrillation (McNamara et al., 2003Ⓐ). Studies comparing digoxin with placebo were inconsistent, particularly during exercise. The nondihydropyridine calcium channel blockers diltiazem and verapamil were more effective than placebo or digoxin in controlling ventricular rate during exercise as well as at rest. β-Blockers atenolol and metoprolol were also found to control both resting and exertional heart rate. The Joint Panel of the American Academy of Family Physicians and the American College of Physicians recommends atenolol, metoprolol, diltiazem, and verapamil for rate control in patients with atrial fibrillation. Digoxin is effective only for rate control at rest and therefore should be used only as a second-line agent for rate control in atrial fibrillation. Digoxin may be useful in patients with concomitant heart failure.

The Joint Panel has reviewed the role of echocardiography in the acute conversion of atrial fibrillation. It based its recommendation on the Assessment of Cardioversion Using Transesophageal Echocardiography study that randomly assigned patients either to a transesophageal echocardiography–guided strategy with short-term precardioversion and 4-week postcardioversion anticoagulation or to "conventional therapy" (3 weeks of precardioversion anticoagulation and 4 weeks postcardioversion anticoagulation). The primary endpoints were stroke, transient ischemic attack, and peripheral embolism. There was no difference between patients undergoing transesophageal echocardiography and those undergoing conventional therapy. More bleeding occurred in the conventional therapy group. The transesophageal echocardiography–guided group had a shorter time to cardioversion and a higher initial success rate, but at 8 weeks, there was no difference between the groups in the number of patients still in sinus rhythm. The Joint Panel recommends that for patients who elect to undergo cardioversion, both the transesophageal echocardiography–guided approach with short-term previous anticoagulation followed by early acute cardioversion (in the absence of intracardiac thrombus) with postcardioversion anticoagulation and the delayed cardioversion with pre- and post-anticoagulation management strategies are appropriate (Klein et al., 2001Ⓐ).

The decision to pursue sinus rhythm rather than settle for rate control with long-term anticoagulation in the above case was the patient's choice. There is no evidence that rhythm control is superior to rate control with chronic anticoagulation. The Atrial Fibrillation Follow-up Investigation of Rhythm Management trial compared rhythm control and rate control (Wyse et al., 2002Ⓐ). In this multicenter, randomized controlled trial, anticoagulation was recommended in both arms. More than 4000 patients were enrolled, and the average age was 70 years. Sixty-one percent of patients were men, 89% were white, 71% had hypertension, and 38% had coronary artery disease. After patients were randomly assigned to the rhythm-control or rate-control group, physicians chose from a list of pharmacologic and nonpharmacologic therapies. Anticoagulation was continued indefinitely for the rate-control arm but could be discontinued at 4 weeks or later after conversion to sinus rhythm. The mortality rate at 5 years was essentially the same in both groups. There was no difference between the groups in terms of stroke. Analyses of other secondary endpoints, including quality of life and functional status, did not show a statistical difference between treatment groups. Of note, there were more hospitalizations in the rhythm-control group (Van Gelder et al., 2002Ⓐ).

These data were supported by a smaller study, the Rate Control versus Electrical Cardioversion for Persistent Atrial Fibrillation study. In this randomized controlled trial, 522 patients were randomly assigned to aggressive rhythm control or rate control only. Mean age was 68 years. Sixty-four percent were men, 49% had hypertension, and 27% had coronary artery disease. Endpoints including death, heart failure, thromboembolic complications, and bleeding showed no advantage to rhythm control. However, the study found rate control may be superior to rhythm control for woman and patients with hypertension. Of note, at study's end, only 39% of the rhythm control group was still in sinus rhythm.

The Joint Panel of the American Academy of Family Physicians and the American College of Physicians recommends rate control with chronic - anticoagulation for the majority of patients with atrial fibrillation. It also recommends patients with atrial fibrillation receive chronic anticoagulation with adjusted-dose warfarin, unless they are at low risk of stroke (see Table 35-1) or have a specific contraindication to the use of warfarin (e.g., thrombocytopenia, recent trauma or surgery, alcoholism).

Material Available on Student Consult

Review Questions and Answers about Atrial Fibrillation

REFERENCES

Gage BF, Waterman AD, Shannon W, Boechler M, Rich MW, Radford MJ. Validation of clinical classification schemes for predicting stroke: Results of the National Registry of Atrial Fibrillation. JAMA 2001;285: 2864–2870.[B]

Klein AL, Grimm RA, Murray RD, et al. Use of trans-esophageal echocardiography to guide cardioversion in patients with atrial fibrillation. N Engl J Med 2001; 344:1411–1420.[A]

McNamara RI, Tamariz LJ, Segal JS, Bass EB. Management of atrial fibrillation: Review of the evidence for the role of pharmacologic therapy, electrical cardioversion, and echocardiography. Ann Intern Med 2003;139: 1018–1033.[A]

Van Gelder IC, Hagens VE, Bosker HA, et al. A comparison of rate control and rhythm control in patients with recurrent persistent atrial fibrillation. N Engl J Med 2002;347:1834–1840.[A]

Wyse DG, Waldo AL, DiMarco JP, et al. A comparison of rate control and rhythm control in patients with atrial fibrillation. N Engl J Med 2002;347:1825–1833.[A]

Chapter

36

Dyspnea on Exertion (Congestive Heart Failure)

Kara L. Cadwallader

KEY POINTS

1. The incidence and prevalence of heart failure are increasing over time.
2. Heart failure has a very high associated morbidity and mortality once symptomatic.
3. Although heart failure can be difficult to diagnose, the absence of dyspnea on exertion or the presence of a normal electrocardiogram (ECG) makes it very unlikely.
4. The strongest predictors of heart failure on clinical examination are a laterally displaced point of maximal impulse and a gallop.
5. Although laboratory test results, ECG, and chest radiograph are useful, a two-dimensional echocardiogram is the gold standard of diagnosis and should be performed in all patients in whom heart failure is suspected.
6. When left ventricular (LV) dysfunction is present, an angiotensin-converting enzyme (ACE)

inhibitor and a β-blocker should be used in all patients, unless there is a contraindication. Spironolactone should be used in patients who have symptoms at rest or have had them in the past 6 months. Diuretics and digoxin should be reserved for management of symptoms.

7. Treatment of comorbid hypertension, diabetes, coronary artery disease, myocardial infarction, and tobacco and alcohol use can decrease both the risk of development as well as the progression of heart failure. Treat aggressively!

8. Close clinic and telephone follow-up, multidisciplinary team management, patient education, and patient self-monitoring of blood pressure, weight, and symptoms have been shown to be effective.

Evidence levels [A] Randomized, controlled trials (RCTs), meta-analyses, well-designed systematic reviews of RCTs. [B] Case-control or cohort studies, nonrandomized clinical trials, systematic reviews of studies other than RCTs, cross-sectional studies, retrospective studies, certain uncontrolled studies. [C] Consensus statements, expert guidelines, usual practice, opinion.

INITIAL VISIT

Subjective

Patient Identification and Presenting Problem

Mr. Clarence T. is a 64-year-old African-American man who presents to the clinic complaining of increasing dyspnea on exertion. Over the past 6 months, he has noticed generalized weakness and fatigue, intermittent nausea and anorexia, and increased swelling in his legs. Despite decreased food intake, he reports significant weight gain. He occasionally awakens in the middle of the night "gasping for air" and has had episodes of pain in his chest, mostly very early in the morning. While he used to play and run with his grandchildren, he notes that he can no longer "keep up" and has to stop frequently to "catch his breath." He believes that his fatigue is due to frequent awakenings from sleep to urinate. He has noticed some new constipation but no blood in his stools. About 6 months ago, he drove across the country to visit relatives in Mississippi and noted some leg swelling at that time. He has increased his use of ipratropium (Atrovent) and albuterol inhalers, which he was given for "smoking too much," but reports little improvement. He has been intermittently compliant with medication for hypertension.

Medical History

Mr. T. was diagnosed with hypertension at age 45. He has mild osteoarthritis in his knees and hips and was recently started on naproxen sodium (Naprosyn) for pain relief. He is overweight but is unsure whether he has been tested for diabetes. He has no history of childhood asthma or recurrent pulmonary infections. He had a cholecystectomy 1 year ago and had a prolonged recovery due to "problems with breathing."

Medications

Naprosyn, nifedipine

Family History

Mr. T.'s father died of end-stage renal disease as a complication of diabetes in his early 40s. His mother had "hardening of the arteries" and died from a heart attack in her mid-60s. He has a sister with a "clotting disorder" who is on life-long warfarin (Coumadin). He has three children who are healthy. There is no family history of thyroid disease or cancer of the colon.

Health Habits

Mr. T. began smoking at age 21 when he joined the army. He quit 2 months ago. He has a glass of bourbon each evening and sometimes drinks more on the weekends. He has never used illicit drugs. He drinks two cups of coffee in the morning. He used to walk his dog to the post office (0.5 miles) each morning but has stopped due to dyspnea.

Social History

Mr. T. is a retired auto mechanic. He is remarried to a retired nurse. He loves World War II memorabilia and hockey.

Review of Systems

Mr. T. admits to a dry cough but denies frothy sputum or hemoptysis. He has noted lightheadedness when he stands suddenly but denies syncope. He denies changes in skin or hair, diarrhea, jaundice, and abdominal pain. He denies palpitations, exertional chest pain, pleurisy, and orthopnea.

Objective

Physical Examination

Mr. T. is a well-developed man who appears slightly anxious but is speaking in full sentences and is in no acute distress. His blood pressure is 190/95, respiratory rate is 26 (without Cheyne-Stokes respiration), heart rate is 105 and regular, oxygen saturation is 91%, and temperature is 37.2°C (98.9°F). His sclerae are anicteric, and his mouth is slightly dry without lesions or evidence of bleeding. Chest examination reveals bibasilar rales, end-expiratory wheezes, and a prolonged expiratory phase. There is no dullness to percussion, egophony, or increased work of breathing. Examination of the neck reveals significant jugular venous distention, a normal carotid upstroke, and no bruits. Cardiac examination reveals a grade II/VI systolic ejection murmur that radiates into the axilla, an S3 gallop, and a laterally displaced, diffuse point of maximal impulse. Abdominal examination is positive for mild hepatomegaly and right upper quadrant tenderness but negative for a fluid wave, rebound, or guarding. His extremities have 2+ pitting edema bilaterally, but no cyanosis or clubbing in the hands or feet. His skin is not clammy or diaphoretic, and his hair appears normal in distribution. His neurologic examination is nonfocal.

Assessment

Working Diagnosis

The patient's symptoms and physical examination are most consistent with congestive heart failure (CHF). However, various pulmonary etiologies for his dyspnea are also possible.

Differential Diagnosis

A pulmonary embolism (PE) is a life-threatening potential cause of dyspnea in this patient. In the acute setting, PEs may present with chest pain (usually pleuritic), cough, hemoptysis, dyspnea, anxiety, and occasionally syncope. Physical findings may include tachycardia, fever, tachypnea, pulmonary rales, and lower extremity edema, usually unilateral.

However, chronic, recurrent PEs may present with more subtle symptoms of intermittent dyspnea, tachycardia, and pleurisy. Most emboli result from clots in the deep veins of the lower extremities. Risk factors in Mr. T. include a history of prolonged inactivity, a family history of hypercoagulability, obesity, and probable concomitant CHF.

Coronary artery disease (CAD) or an acute coronary syndrome may also present with dyspnea. Acute myocardial infarctions usually manifest with chest pain but may present painlessly with symptoms of acute heart failure. CAD may be silent or present with intermittent chest pain, usually on exertion. Any patient presenting with symptoms of CHF needs to be evaluated for CAD, as it is a common etiology of CHF. Mr. T. has multiple risk factors for CAD, including uncontrolled hypertension, obesity, family history, smoking, male gender, and African-American race.

Chronic obstructive pulmonary disease (COPD) is often difficult to distinguish from CHF. Exacerbations usually present with many similar symptoms such as anxiety, cough, dyspnea, fatigue, orthopnea, tachypnea, tachycardia, and chest pain. Hypoxia is common but may also be seen with CHF. Mr. T's major risk factor for COPD is his long history of tobacco use.

Thyroid disease may be confused with CHF or may contribute to its development. Symptoms of hyperthyroidism include anxiety, diaphoresis, tachycardia, fatigue, weight changes, and skin changes. Symptoms of hypothyroidism also include weakness, fatigue, and weight changes as well as constipation, dry skin, and edema.

Other causes of increased extracellular fluid that should be considered in a patient with dyspnea, jugular venous distention, and peripheral edema are anemia, renal failure, and liver failure.

Plan

Diagnostic

The following initial laboratory tests are performed: a complete blood count to rule out anemia and infection; electrolytes, blood urea nitrogen and serum creatinine to assess renal function and establish a baseline for potential future use of diuretic and ACE inhibitor therapies; liver function tests to assess for hepatic congestion; thyroid-stimulating hormone to rule out concomitant thyroid disease; brain natriuretic peptide (BNP) to help distinguish CHF from pulmonary disease; troponin and creatine kinase–myocardial bound (CKMB) levels drawn serially to rule out ongoing myocardial ischemia or infarction; and iron studies to rule out hemochromatosis. Other laboratory tests to consider if the history is suggestive might be an antinuclear antibody (ANA), viral serologies and antimyosin antibody (myocarditis), and laboratory tests to rule out pheochromocytosis.

A chest radiograph is obtained, which reveals cardiomegaly, cephalization of the pulmonary vessels, and bilateral pleural effusions. An ECG reveals sinus tachycardia, left atrial enlargement, LV hypertrophy (LVH), Q waves in leads II and III, and aVF consistent with an old inferior myocardial infarction. There is no evidence of current ischemia or infarction.

At this point, Mr. T. meets the Modified Framingham Clinical Criteria for diagnosis of CHF (Table 36-1). Given the suggestive clinical scenario, a Doppler echocardiogram is ordered to rule out etiologies such as valvular disease, pericarditis, and wall motion abnormalities and to assess ventricular function.

Therapeutic

The patient is admitted to the hospital and placed on oxygen and a cardiac monitor. An intravenous (IV) line is started, and IV furosemide (Lasix) is initiated with a urine output goal of more than 500 mL in 2 hours. Nitroglycerin and morphine are written to be given if there is a recurrence of chest pain. A baby aspirin is initiated, given the findings of a previous myocardial infarction on the initial ECG. The Naprosyn that Mr. T. had been taking is discontinued due to its deleterious effects on heart failure. The nifedipine is also discontinued, and a β-blocker is chosen instead for its benefits in patients with systolic heart failure as well as patients with a previous myocardial infarction. A low dose is chosen given

Table 36-1	Modified Framingham Clinical Criteria for CHF Diagnosis	
Major Criteria	**Minor Criteria**
Paroxysmal nocturnal dyspnea	Bilateral peripheral edema
Orthopnea	Nocturnal cough
Elevated jugular venous distention	Dyspnea with ordinary exertion
Pulmonary rales	Hepatomegaly
Presence of S3	Pleural effusions
Cardiomegaly on chest radiograph	Tachycardia (>120 beats/min)
Pulmonary edema on chest radiograph	Weight loss >4.5 kg over 5 days (when weight loss may be due to other conditions besides treatment of the CHF)
Weight loss (≥4.5 kg over 5 days in response to treatment of CHF)	

Diagnosis requires two major and two minor criteria; minor criteria cannot be attributable to other causes.
CHF, congestive heart failure.

Mr. T.'s probable comorbid COPD and the possibility of an exacerbation caused by the β-blocker. A low dose of an ACE inhibitor is also initiated for control of hypertension and for treatment of CHF. Mr. T. feels much better a few hours after he undergoes a brisk diuresis. His electrolytes, magnesium, blood urea nitrogen, and creatinine are carefully monitored.

Patient Education

A nutrition consult is obtained, and Mr. T. is counseled regarding a low-sodium diet and avoidance of a high intake of free water. He is also counseled regarding weight loss, exercise, and continued tobacco cessation. He is advised to avoid potentially exacerbating medications such as nonsteroidal anti-inflammatory drugs (including high-dose aspirin), corticosteroids, carbenoxolone, urinary alkalinizers, tricyclics, and calcium channel blockers (except amlodipine and felodipine). He is enrolled in a multidisciplinary outpatient disease management program that includes frequent weight, blood pressure, and medication checks.

Screening for Modifiable Risk Factors

Mr. T. is counseled about other conditions that may contribute to heart disease, and he agrees to laboratory screening for diabetes (fasting glucose) and dyslipidemia (total cholesterol, low- and high-density lipoproteins, and triglycerides).

Disposition

Serial cardiac enzymes are negative, and Mr. T.'s laboratory test results and echocardiogram confirm the diagnosis of CHF due to LV systolic dysfunction. He is also diagnosed with concomitant mitral regurgitation, dyslipidemia, and glucose intolerance. He is discharged to his home once a dry weight is achieved, his blood pressure is controlled, and he is free of dyspnea. He is sent home on Lasix, an ACE inhibitor, a β-blocker, a baby aspirin, and Tylenol for his arthritis. An outpatient cardiology referral is made for further workup of probable CAD, and he eventually undergoes cardiac catheterization. In addition, an appointment is made for pulmonary function testing to assist with the diagnosis and optimal management of his comorbid COPD.

DISCUSSION

CHF is a clinical syndrome that results when the ventricle's ability to eject and/or fill with blood is impaired. Systolic dysfunction refers to decreased ejection of blood from the ventricle or an ejection fraction of less than 40% (Chavey et al., 2001a🅐🅑). Diastolic dysfunction refers to abnormal relaxation and thus filling of the ventricle leading to increased filling pressures. The ejection fraction in pure diastolic dysfunction is greater than 50%. CHF becomes clinically apparent when the heart is no longer able to meet the metabolic needs of the body. Millions of Americans are affected by this clinical syndrome; it is a common cause of hospitalization in patients older than age 65 (Mair and Lloyd-Williams, 2002🅒). Morbidity and mortality from CHF are high, with patients at increased risk of sudden death, thromboembolism, arrhythmias, and renal insufficiency.

Many diseases place patients at an increased risk of developing CHF. The most common are CAD, hypertension, idiopathic dilated cardiomyopathy, and valvular disease. Other less common causes of cardiomyopathies that can lead to heart failure include diabetes, alcohol, hypertrophy, infiltrative processes such as sarcoidosis and amyloidosis, and infection, usually viral. Women with CHF are more likely than men to have isolated diastolic dysfunction. Common etiologies for this include hypertension with LVH, ischemia, aortic stenosis, and both restrictive and hypertrophic cardiomyopathies. There are two staging systems commonly used to grade the severity of CHF (Tables 36-2 and 36-3). These are helpful for both research and clinical purposes.

The diagnosis of CHF in its early stages can be difficult, as signs and symptoms are neither sensitive nor specific. The presence of dyspnea on exertion has almost 100% sensitivity and thus its absence virtually rules out CHF (Mair and Lloyd-Williams, 2002🅒). Weakness and fatigue due to low cardiac output are common but nonspecific. Orthopnea and paroxysmal nocturnal dyspnea are fairly specific if present but may also seen with pulmonary diseases. Gastrointestinal symptoms can confuse the clinician. Many patients with CHF have nausea due to hepatic

Table 36-2	American College of Cardiology/American Heart Association Heart Failure Staging
Stage	**Description**
A	High risk to develop heart failure; no current symptoms; no structural heart disease
B	No symptoms, but heart disease with left ventricular dysfunction is present.
C	Previous or ongoing symptoms of heart failure
D	Severe symptoms, advanced heart disease, refractory heart failure

Class	Description
1	No limitations: ordinary physical activity does not cause symptoms.
2	Mild limitations; no symptoms at rest. Ordinary physical activity causes symptoms such as dyspnea, fatigue, and angina.
3	Marked limitation; no symptoms at rest. Activities such as getting dressed cause symptoms.
4	Severe limitations; symptoms at rest; any activity worsens symptoms

Table 36-3 New York Heart Association Classification of Heart Failure

congestion and anorexia due to bowel edema and poor splanchnic circulation. Dependent edema is a common finding in CHF and many other disease states.

The physical examination can be very helpful in diagnosis. The presence of an S3 and/or S4 gallop on cardiac examination is strongly predictive of heart failure (Mair and Lloyd-Williams, 2002**©**). An abnormal apical impulse has high specificity for a decreased ejection fraction. Elevated jugular venous distention also strongly predicts heart failure and is indicative of right ventricular failure. Pulmonary findings can be misleading, as many patients with chronic heart failure will not have rales or wheezing. Similarly, dependent edema is not present until there is greater than 5 L of extracellular fluid and frequently does not correlate with the severity of symptoms.

Laboratory work similar to that done for Mr. T. is helpful to rule out many disease states that may cause heart failure. The relatively newly available BNP is one of the few laboratory tests that helps to confirm the diagnosis of CHF. Using a BNP cutoff value of 100 pg/mL gives a sensitivity of 90% and specificity of 76% for CHF. Other potential causes of increased BNP levels that must be considered include myocardial infarction, hypertension, ventricular hypertrophy, cardiomyopathies, renal failure, cirrhosis, hyperaldosteronism and Cushing's syndrome, and primary pulmonary hypertension. Thus, while an elevated BNP is helpful, it is not in itself diagnostic.

The gold standard for making the diagnosis of CHF is two-dimensional echocardiography (Mair and Lloyd-Williams, 2002**©**). All patients in whom CHF is suspected should thus have an echo. A chest radiograph is also useful. Cardiomegaly is the most common associated finding and is indicative of systolic failure. Other helpful findings of volume overload include pleural effusions, Kerley B lines, and cephalization. Radiography is also helpful to evaluate for other diagnoses such as pneumonia and COPD. Finally, the ECG is almost always abnormal if significant LV dysfunction exists. Thus, a normal ECG has a 98% negative predictive value for CHF. Common electrocardiographic findings that are helpful include dysrhythmias (atrial fibrillation, ventricular tachycardias), evidence of ischemia, left atrial enlargement, LVH, and left bundle branch block.

The acute stabilization of patients with CHF requires oxygen, cardiac monitoring, and IV access. Patients with evidence of volume overload (Mr. T.) need diuresis. If overload is mild, furosemide is used. If moderate to severe, higher dose Lasix and nitroglycerin and/or nesiritide may be required. Patients with evidence of low cardiac output (azotemia, altered mental status, cool extremities, poor response to diuretics) often require dobutamine for its inotropic effects. Dopamine and other vasopressors may be needed for severely hypotensive patients. These patients require intensive care unit monitoring, cardiology consultation, and probable placement of pulmonary artery catheters.

Once patients are stabilized, they should be started on both an ACE inhibitor and a β-blocker if there is not a contraindication (Chavey et al., 2001b**Ⓐ Ⓑ**). ACE inhibitors have been shown to decrease mortality as well as future hospitalizations and ischemic events in patients with systolic dysfunction. β-Blockers have also been shown to decrease mortality and hospitalizations. Patients often need to be maintained on diuretics to achieve a euvolemic state (Chavey et al., 2001b**Ⓐ Ⓑ**). In the setting of LV systolic dysfunction, digoxin has been shown to decrease hospitalizations but not overall mortality in CHF (Chavey et al., 2001b**Ⓐ Ⓑ**). It should be used as add-on therapy for patients already on an ACE inhibitor and diuretic. Spironolactone decreases mortality for patients with New York Heart Association class 4 CHF and requires careful monitoring of potassium and serum creatinine (Chavey et al., 2001b**Ⓐ Ⓑ**). Anticoagulation should be used only in the setting of atrial fibrillation or other indications for anticoagulation, but not for CHF alone. Calcium channel blockers are not effective and should be discontinued if not used for another indication (Chavey et al., 2001b**Ⓐ Ⓑ**; McConaghy and Smith, 2002**Ⓐ**). Nutritional supplements such as taurine, carnitine, coenzyme Q10, and antioxidants have not been shown to be effective and may be harmful. Effective nondrug interventions include exercise, a low-salt diet, multidisciplinary clinical manage-ment, and implantable defibrillators (McKelvie, 2004**Ⓐ**; McConaghy and Smith, 2002**Ⓐ**).

Prevention involves behavior modification and diagnosis and treatment of conditions that lead to heart disease. Patients should be counseled to avoid tobacco, excessive alcohol, and cocaine and to exercise regularly. Conditions such as diabetes, hypertension, dyslipidemia, thyroid disease, anemia, CAD, COPD, thiamine deficiency, and human immunodeficiency virus should be diagnosed and treated aggressively. Common medications such as nonsteroidal anti-inflammatory drugs, corticosteroids, and tricyclics may exacerbate heart failure and should be avoided.

Patients with heart failure require regular clinical follow-up and may also benefit from home nursing management and frequent telephone monitoring.

Material Available on Student Consult

Review Questions and Answers about Congestive Heart Failure

REFERENCES

Chavey WE, Blaum CS, Bleske BE, Van Harrison R, Kesterson S, Nicklas JM. Guideline for the management of heart failure caused by systolic dysfunction: Part I: Guideline development, etiology and diagnosis. Am Fam Physician 2001a;64:769–774.🅐🅑

Chavey WE, Blaum CS, Bleske BE, Van Harrison R, Kesterson S, Nicklas JM. Guideline for the management of heart failure caused by systolic dysfunction: Part II: Treatment. Am Fam Physician 2001b; 64:1045–1054.🅐🅑

McKelvie R. Heart failure. Available at www.clinical-evidence.com/ceweb/conditions/cvd/0204/0204.jsp. Accessed 10/10/2005.

Mair FS, Lloyd-Williams F. Evaluation of suspected left ventricular systolic dysfunction. J Fam Pract 2002;51:466–471.🅒

McConaghy JR, Smith SR. Outpatient treatment of heart failure. J Fam Pract 2002;51:519–525.🅐

SUGGESTED READINGS

DiDomenico RJ. Guidelines for acute decompensated heart failure treatment. Ann Pharmacother 2004;38: 649–669.

Hunt SA, Baker DW, Chin MH, et al. ACC/AHA guidelines for the evaluation and management of chronic heart failure in the adult. Bethesda, MD, American College of Cardiology Foundation, 2001.🅒

Pharmacologic Management of Heart Failure and Left Ventricular Systolic Dysfunction: Effect in Female, Black and Diabetic Patients and Cost-effectiveness. AHRQ report, publication No. 03-E044. July 2003.🅐

37 High Blood Pressure (Hypertension)

Roberto Cardarelli

INTIAL VISIT

Subjective

Patient Identification and Presenting Problem

Mr. Smith, a 62-year-old white man, presents to the office accompanied by his daughter, who is concerned about a blood pressure reading that they noticed while she was practicing using a sphygmomanometer on him for her nursing school examination. Mr. Smith states that he has not seen a physician since he was a teenager. He denies shortness of breath, chest pain at rest or with exertion, orthopnea, peripheral edema, paroxysmal nocturnal dyspnea, headaches, and urinary or visual complaints. He reports that he is physically active with construction work and has no issues with fatigue. He plans to retire in 3 years. Mr. Smith denies taking any over-the-counter or herbal medications or being exposed to any known chemicals.

Medical History

Mr. Smith has no allergies. He wears glasses only for reading. He never had a pneumococcal or influenza immunization. He reports an unremarkable childhood except for having chicken pox and believes he received all his childhood immunizations. His tetanus status is regularly monitored and updated by his employer. He has never been hospitalized and has never had surgery.

Family History

Mr. Smith is an only child and reports that his father died of a heart attack at the age of 43. His mother is still living and is in good health, except for mild glaucoma. He does not recall any other family members having medical conditions.

Social History

Mr. Smith is widowed and has one daughter, who is currently in nursing school. He has been doing construction work for 35 years and is still doing heavy manual labor. He has smoked one and a half packs of cigarettes since the age of 22 and admits to having three or four beers on weekends. He denies any illicit drug use and does not have a regular exercise regimen.

Objective

Physical Examination

Vital Signs Mr. Smith's height is 68 inches, his weight is 208 pounds, his body mass index is 31.6, and his temperature is 37°C (98.6°F). His initial blood pressure in his left arm (sitting) is 168/78 mm Hg and, repeated after 10 minutes, is 164/76 mm Hg. His initial blood pressure in his right arm (sitting) is 166/80 mm Hg and, repeated after 10 minutes, is 168/78 mm Hg. His pulse is 76 (regular) beats per minute, and his respiratory rate is 12 respirations per minute.

General Mr. Smith is a heavyset man in no acute distress who is appropriately dressed and who appears slightly older than his stated age.

Skin His skin turgor and pigmentation are normal, and no lesions are appreciated.

Head, Eyes, Ears, Nose, and Throat Mr. Smith's head is normocephalic. His eyes are anicteric. A funduscopic examination is normal. The pupils are equally reactive to light and accommodation. The nasal mucosa is normal, and the oropharynx is clear.

Neck The thyroid is not palpable and no bruits are appreciated. No jugular venous distention is noted.

Chest The lungs are clear to auscultation bilaterally.

Heart The rate and rhythm are regular with no extra heart sounds. The point of maximal impulse is auscultated slightly lateral of the mid-clavicular line. Carotid, abdominal, and femoral bruits are not appreciated. Pulses are +2 throughout.

Abdomen The abdomen is slightly obese, soft, and nontender, with normal bowel sounds. No masses are appreciated. No hepatosplenomegaly is noted.

Neurologic No focal deficits or findings are found.

Assessment

1. Elevated blood pressure without a definitive diagnosis of hypertension
2. Tobacco use

Plan

Mr. Smith is informed about his current condition and told that another elevated blood pressure reading at a separate clinic visit would give him a diagnosis of high blood pressure. Diet and exercise handouts are given to him and their contents discussed. Limiting salt intake is also discussed. He is advised to check his blood pressure daily or every other day at various times of the day for 2 weeks and to bring the readings to his next appointment.

Mr. Smith is strongly advised to quit smoking. He does not express interest in quitting, so a handout demonstrating the adverse health effects of smoking is given. He is told that help was available once he is interested in quitting.

A return appointment is scheduled for 2 weeks.

FOLLOW-UP VISIT

Mr. Smith returns with his daughter 2 weeks later. He remains asymptomatic and is irritable about the return visit since he is feeling well. He still is not interested in giving up his smoking habit. The blood pressure record shows an systolic blood pressure (SBP) range of 148 to 178 mm Hg and a diastolic blood pressure (DBP) range of 64 to 88 mm Hg. A review of symptoms remained negative, and the physical examination is unchanged. His vital signs are normal except for a blood pressure reading of 174/86 mm Hg. His diagnosis (stage 2 hypertension) and options for management are discussed, as is the need for an electrocardiogram and laboratory tests. The risks and benefits of the treatment options are further discussed, and Mr. Smith states that he is against starting a medication at this time. He agrees to regular blood pressure monitoring and to following a diet and exercise plan with the help of a nutritionist. He is reminded again about the detrimental effects of smoking to his overall health. Signs and symptoms that would require immediate attention are discussed. A follow-up visit is scheduled for 4 to 6 weeks to review the laboratory results; he is advised to make an appointment sooner if there are any significant abnormalities.

DISCUSSION

Diagnosis

The most important component of hypertension management is accurate and appropriate measurement of blood pressure. To appropriately measure the blood pressure, the patient should sit in a chair in a quiet room for 5 minutes with his feet flat on the floor, his back supported, and his arms relaxed and supported at the level of the heart (World Hypertension League, 2004). The size of the cuff bladder should be at least 80% of the size of the patient's arm. Two measurements should be made on each arm, averaged, and the readings shared with the patient. Before establishing a diagnosis of hypertension, many clinicians prefer to have at least two separate measurements at different visits and also self-monitored blood pressure readings that the patient provides. There is insufficient research to know whether self-monitored blood pressure readings predict clinical outcomes (Powers, 2003 Ⓑ). Yet they may improve patient adherence and are useful in determining response to medication. High blood pressure is established when two readings have an SBP greater than or equal to 140 mm Hg or a DBP greater than or equal to 90 mm Hg (Chobanian et al., 2003 Ⓒ).

Blood Pressure Classification

Blood pressure classification has changed based on the Seventh Report of the Joint National Committee on Prevention, Detection, Evaluation, and Treatment of High Blood Pressure (JNC-7) (Chobanian et al., 2003❻). The categories include normal (SBP ≤ 120 mm Hg and DBP ≤ 80 mm Hg), prehypertension (SBP 120–139 mm Hg or DBP 80–89 mm Hg), stage 1 hypertension (SBP 140–159 mm Hg or DBP 90–99 mm Hg), and stage 2 hypertension (SBP ≥ 160 mm Hg or DBP ≥ 100 mm Hg). It was found that patients with prehypertension were twice as likely to develop hypertension compared with those with lower blood pressures (Vasan et al., 2001❸).

Workup

Once high blood pressure has been diagnosed, the patient's lifestyle, cardiovascular risk factors, concomitant disorders, and the presence of target organ damage need to be assessed (Chobanian et al., 2003❻). In addition to hypertension, major cardiovascular risk factors include age, diabetes mellitus, decreased renal function, family history of premature heart disease (men younger than age 55 and women younger than age 65), obesity, tobacco use, and physical inactivity. Target organ damage to assess includes chest pain, history of myocardial infarction, heart failure, left ventricular hypertrophy, stroke, chronic kidney disease, peripheral arterial disease, and eye disease. In addition, causes of high blood pressure need to be evaluated, including sleep apnea, medication or illicit drug use, kidney disease, primary aldosteronism, renovascular disease, chronic steroid therapy, Cushing's syndrome, pheochromocytoma, coarctation of the aorta, and thyroid or parathyroid disease. This is accomplished by the medical history, a physical examination, and appropriate diagnostic tests. The components of the physical examination should emphasize evaluating the endocrine, cardiovascular, pulmonary, neurologic, integument, and gastrointestinal systems. The suggested laboratory and diagnostic procedures include a complete metabolic panel, fasting lipid profile, urinalysis or spot urinary albumin/creatinine ratio, hematocrit, and electrocardiogram. More extensive testing is not usually warranted unless blood pressure control is not achieved with appropriate medication (details can be found below) (Chobanian et al., 2003❻).

Treatment Goals

Cardiovascular morbidity and mortality associated with hypertension are reduced with treatment (Neal et al., 2000❹). Focus should be placed on reducing SBP, since a decrease in DBP normally follows. In addition, treating isolated SBP has been found to prevent major cardiovascular events (Ferrucci et al., 2001❹). The target blood pressure is lower than 140/90 mm Hg or lower than 130/80 mm Hg for patients with atherosclerotic disease, renal disease, and/or diabetes.

Therapy

Lifestyle modifications are a preventive and therapeutic modality in the treatment of hypertension. They should be recommended to all patients without contraindications, including those at risk of developing high blood pressure (prehypertension). A 3-month trial of lifestyle changes may be offered initially for some patients before starting a medication. Combined lifestyle changes have a cumulative effect. For example, improvements in diet and exercise decrease blood pressure better than either one alone. Weight reduction, such as using the Dietary Approaches to Stop Hypertension eating plan, can decrease blood pressure with the same magnitude of some single drug therapies (Sacks et al., 2001❹). One study found that restricted salt intake reduces blood pressure but not death or cardiovascular morbidity (Hooper et al., 2003❹).

Many clinical trials have shown how different classes of antihypertensive medications do an excellent job in reducing morbidity and mortality associated with hypertension. Table 37-1 is a simple list of the different classes of hypertensive medications. Most of the research available on antihypertensive medications has been on the thiazide-type class. The most recognized study is the Antihypertensive and Lipid Lowering Treatment to Prevent Heart Attack Trial (ALLHAT, 2002❹). Based on favorable outcomes and affordability, thiazide-type medications remain the initial medication of choice for hypertension. Another study found angiotensin-converting enzyme inhibitors have more favorable outcomes compared with diuretics (Wing et al., 2003❹). Choice of medication is also

Table 37-1	Classes of Antihypertensive Medications

Alpha agonists
  α₁
  Central α₂
Aldosterone receptor blockers
Angiotensin-converting enzyme inhibitors
Angiotensin receptor blockers
β-Blockers
Calcium channels blockers
  Dihydropyridines
  Nondihydropyridines
Combined α-blockers and β-blockers
Direct vasodilators
Diuretics
  Loop
  Potassium sparing
  Thiazide

dependent on concomitant conditions. β-Blockers are preferred for patients with a history of ischemic heart disease and stable angina, although calcium channel blockers can be used (Chobanian et al., 2003**C**). Angiotensin-converting enzyme inhibitors and β-blockers are preferred in patients with heart failure. Patients with diabetes are normally started with an angiotensin-converting enzyme inhibitor or angiotensin receptor blocker because both medications have cardiovascular benefits and slow the progression of diabetic nephropathy (Chobanian et al., 2003**C**). The JNC-7 report provides detailed information on medications that should be considered based on a patient's medical condition (Chobanian et al., 2003**C**).

As time progresses, most patients will require two or more medications. If the blood pressure at the time of diagnosis averages 20/10 mm Hg or greater above goal, the clinician should consider starting with two medications. However, it is important to consider and discuss the risks and benefits with each patient before starting two medications. Blood pressure reductions are additive when drugs are combined; however, the adverse effects may not be (Law et al., 2003**A**).

Follow-up

The management of hypertension requires regular surveillance with frequent follow-up visits. Initial monthly intervals are recommended until the blood pressure is controlled. More frequent visits should be considered in patients with poorly controlled blood pressure or other comorbid conditions. In addition, some patients become confused about the options associated with their diagnosis. Aids such as videos and pamphlets have been shown to reduce decisional conflict in patients who are newly diagnosed with hypertension (Montgomery et al., 2003 **A**). Well-controlled patients without other comorbid conditions can follow up approximately every 6 months (Birtwhistle et al., 2005 **A**). Other medical conditions

may dictate the frequency of follow-up, such as diabetes. The patient's electrolytes—especially potassium—and renal function need to be monitored on a regular basis. At each visit, lifestyle modifications, tobacco cessation, and compliance with taking medications should be encouraged. Smoking cessation in patients with coronary heart disease reduces the risk of all-cause mortality and nonfatal myocardial infarction (Critchley and Capewell, 2003**A**). Further, side effects, such as muscle cramping due to diuretics or impotence due to β-blockers, should be assessed. Aspirin therapy should be started once blood pressure is controlled, and other cardiovascular risk factors, such as weight and cholesterol levels, should be vigorously managed.

CONCLUSION

Mr. Smith eventually agrees to start a thiazide-type medication after he fails to achieve his blood pressure goal with lifestyle modifications. He continues to remain asymptomatic, and all his blood work is normal, including his cholesterol. He has cut back to a half a pack of cigarettes per day with the help of his daughter's persistence. He is encouraged to continue an exercise and diet regimen because of the beneficial health effects. After the medication is titrated over several visits, his blood pressure becomes well controlled, with an average reading of 132/82 mm Hg. After receiving the rationale for each step of his management plan, Mr. Smith has come to accept the need to manage his hypertension and to adhere to the required 6-month follow-up appointments.

Material Available on Student Consult
Review Questions and Answers about Hypertension.

REFERENCES

ALLHAT Officers and Coordinators for the ALLHAT Collaborative Research Group. Major outcomes in high-risk hypertensive patients randomized to angiotensin-converting enzyme inhibitor or calcium channel blocker vs. diuretic: The Antihypertensive and Lipid-Lowering Treatment to Prevent Heart Attack Trial (ALLHAT). JAMA 2002;288:2981–2997.**A**

Birtwhistle RV, Godwin MS, Delva MD, et al. Randomised equivalence trial comparing three month and six month follow up of patients with hypertension by family practitioners. BMJ 2005;328:204.**A**

Chobanian AV, Bakris GL, Black HR, et al. Seventh report of the Joint National Committee on the prevention,

detection, evaluation, and treatment of high blood pressure. Hypertension 2003;42:1206–1252.**C**

Critchley JA, Capewell S. Mortality risk reduction associated with smoking cessation in patients with coronary heart disease: A systematic review. JAMA 2003;290:86–97.**A**

Ferrucci L, Furberg CD, Penninx BW, et al. Treatment of isolated systolic hypertension is most effective in older patients with high-risk profile. Circulation 2001;104:1923–1926.**A**

Hooper L, Bartlett C, Davey Smith G, et al. Reduced dietary salt for prevention of cardiovascular disease. Cochrane Database Syst Rev 2003;1:CD003656.**A**

Law MR, Wald NJ, Morris JK, Jordan RE. Value of low dose combination treatment with blood pressure lowering drugs: Analysis of 354 randomized trials. BMJ 2003;326:1427–1437.Ⓐ

Montgomery AA, Fahey T, Peters TJ. A factorial randomized controlled trial of decision analysis and an information video plus leaflet for newly diagnosed hypertensive patients. Br J Gen Pract 2003;53:446–453.Ⓐ

Neal B, MacMahon S, Chapman N. Effects of ACE inhibitors, calcium antagonists, and other blood-pressure-lowering drugs: Results of prospectively designed overviews of randomized trials. Blood Pressure Lowering Treatment Trialists' Collaboration. Lancet 2000;356:1955–1964.Ⓐ

Powers DV. Review: Ambulatory blood pressure monitoring predicts clinical outcomes. Evid Based Med 2003; 8:20.Ⓑ

Sacks FM, Svetkey LP, Vollmer WM, et al. Effects of blood pressure of reduced sodium and the Dietary Approaches to Stop Hypertension (DASH) diet. DASH-Sodium Collaborative Research Group. N Engl J Med 2001;344:3–10.Ⓐ

Vasan RS, Larson MG, Leip EP, et al. Assessment of frequency of progression to hypertension in nonhypertensive participants in the Framingham Heart Study: A cohort study. Lancet 2001;358:1682–1686.Ⓑ

Wing LM, Reid CM, Ryan P, et al. A comparison of outcome with angiotensin-converting enzyme inhibitors and diuretics for hypertension in the elderly. N Engl J Med 2003;348:583–592.Ⓐ

World Hypertension League. Measuring your blood pressure. Available at www.mco.edu/org/whl/bloodpre. html. Accessed August 13, 2004.

Chapter

38

Abdominal Pain and Loose Bowel Movements (Hypercholesterolemia)

Michael Crouch

KEY POINTS

1. More than one half of U.S. adults have unhealthy levels of low-density lipoprotein (LDL) cholesterol, triglycerides, and/or high-density lipoprotein (HDL) cholesterol that place them at increased risk of coronary heart disease (CHD) and stroke—the causes of more than one half of all adult U.S. deaths. Hypercholesterolemic individuals who use tobacco, have strong family histories, or have diabetes or metabolic syndrome are at highest risk of heart attack and stroke.

2. LDL cholesterol tends to be 10 to 15 mg/dL higher when fasting than when in the postprandial state. (LDL goes up as triglycerides go down and vice versa.) This should be kept in mind when reviewing lipid results for individuals screened with nonfasting lipids for reasons of convenience and expedience.

3. With appropriate support, some patients with unhealthy baseline dietary patterns can make enough long-term modifications to their dietary intake, exercise habits, and weight status to satisfactorily improve their lipid levels and lower their CHD risk. Lifestyle change success usually requires repeated, detailed patient education, accompanied by long-term monitoring and encouragement by the primary health care provider.

4. A given amount of dietary change produces as much lipid improvement as it is ever going to provide after 4 weeks of sustained dietary change; more prolonged dietary change does not yield additional benefit unless it is accompanied by significant sustained weight loss in an overweight individual.

5. Numerous randomized controlled trials have shown statin (3-hydroxy-3-methylglutaryl

---

Evidence levels Ⓐ Randomized, controlled trials (RCTs), meta-analyses, well-designed systematic reviews of RCTs. Ⓑ Case-control or cohort studies, nonrandomized clinical trials, systematic reviews of studies other than RCTs, cross-sectional studies, retrospective studies, certain uncontrolled studies. Ⓒ Consensus statements, expert guidelines, usual practice, opinion.

KEY POINTS (Continued)

coenzyme A reductase inhibitor) therapy to be the most effective way to treat hypercholesterolemia; it lowers CHD event and stroke risk by approximately 30% to 40% in individuals with mild, moderate, or severe LDL cholesterol elevations whose estimated 10-year risk of CHD is moderately high (10% to 20%) or high (>20%).

6. Despite the overwhelming evidence of statin benefit and safety, more than one half of the persons who are considered appropriate candidates for statin therapy have never started taking a statin. The persistence rate for statin therapy in community practice in 2003

averaged approximately 60% at 1 year and less than 40% at 3 years after initiation of therapy.

7. Many patients decline or discontinue statin therapy because of procrastination, financial difficulties and priorities, exaggerated concerns about potential or perceived adverse statin side effects, minimization or denial of their CHD risk level, preference for avoiding chronic prescription medication, or the belief that statin therapy is "not natural."

8. Improving acceptance, persistence, and adherence for statin therapy often requires just as much, if not more, attitude assessment and patient education as dietary change, including provider monitoring and encouragement.

INITIAL VISIT

Subjective

Patient Identification and Presenting Problem
Gary A. is a 24-year-old white freshman medical student being seen for a preschool physical examination. Although his general health has been quite good in the past, Gary has been experiencing abdominal pain, loose bowel movements, chest discomfort, and palpitations intermittently for approximately 2 weeks.

Present Illness
Gary began experiencing cramping periumbilical pain, and loose bowel movements after a farewell weekend with college friends, just before moving to University City to begin medical school. The abdominal pain originally began while he was packing his belongings in his car. The most severe episode occurred midway through the first day of orientation week and was quite uncomfortable (8 on a scale of 10). Each episode lasts 30 to 45 minutes. The pain occurs at all different times of the day but does not awaken him from sleep. The pain is unrelated to mealtime or physical activity. Neither antacids nor bismuth subsalicylate (Pepto-Bismol) produces prompt pain relief, but a dose of bismuth subsalicylate seems to normalize his bowel movements for approximately 12 hours. His bowel movements are brown (except for being black the day after taking Pepto-Bismol), with a quite loose but not liquid consistency. The stool contains small amounts of mucus at times, without visible blood.

Gary began experiencing bilateral chest discomfort and palpitations sometime after the onset of the abdominal pain. He has had episodes lasting 5 to 10 minutes, occurring two to three times per week, and

often associated with unusually forceful and rapid heartbeat. The episodes typically occur at rest, after he has been experiencing abdominal pain for an hour or more. The symptoms are relieved by his getting up and moving around restlessly.

Medical History
Gary has had no surgery, accidents, serious injuries, or hospitalizations. He has no known medication allergies. He takes no medications on a regular basis and denies using laxatives or stool softeners.

Family History
Gary's father, a dairy farmer, died suddenly at age 48, presumably of a heart attack. His mother is in good health at age 58. His only brother has hypercholesterolemia. His only sister has had no serious health problems. His paternal grandfather died of colon cancer at age 45. His other three grandparents died of unknown causes past the age of 80. He admits to worrying quite a bit about the possibility of his having inherited a predisposition to heart disease from his father. He is also worried about getting colon cancer like his grandfather did.

Health Habits
Gary does not smoke. He drinks small amounts of alcohol on rare occasions and denies using any illicit drugs. He always wears seat belts when driving his car. For the past 5 years he has always used latex condoms when having intercourse. He exercises regularly, usually running approximately 3 to 4 miles at least three times per week. He has avoided eating red meat, pork, and whole milk dairy products for 2 years, after reading that they could increase one's risk of heart disease and cancer.

Social History

Gary is single. He has been seeing one girlfriend regularly for 2 years and is sexually active exclusively with her. They are planning to marry after his second year in medical school. He describes his relationships with his girlfriend, mother, and siblings as close and supportive. He is unsure that he will be able to compete well academically in medical school and is concerned about how he will handle the heavy academic load and mental stress that he has heard about. He made excellent grades in college while being active in intramural sports and social life.

Review of Systems

Gary has had no change in his appetite, weight, energy, or general mood. He has experienced no nausea or vomiting. He has felt somewhat jittery and restless while sitting in lectures for the past few days. He has also had uncharacteristic difficulty getting to sleep recently. He denies having thoughts of imminent life-threatening illness or death.

Objective

Physical Examination

Vital signs are all within normal limits, including blood pressure of 110/70, heart rate of 92, weight of 160 pounds, and height of 70 inches. Affect is normal except for looking mildly nervous. The physical examination is notable only for cool clammy hands, moist axillae, mild diffuse tenderness of the abdomen, and questionably diminished deep tendon reflexes. The thyroid gland and Achilles tendons are normal on inspection and palpation. Peripheral pulses are all normal.

Laboratory Tests

A multitest executive profile drawn 2 days before Gary's office visit is notable only for a total cholesterol level of 300 mg/dL (7.7 mmol/L). The panel includes normal liver and renal function test results, but does not include cholesterol subfractions or triglyceride levels.

Assessment

Working Diagnoses

Two likely diagnoses best explain the patient's symptoms and findings.

1. Adjustment disorder with anxious mood, expressed as situational anxiety, mild sleep disorder, symptoms of autonomic overactivity, and irritable bowel syndrome.
2. Familial heterozygous hypercholesterolemia (type IIa in the Frederickson classification), based on the suggestive family history and the very high total cholesterol value despite a heart healthy lifestyle.

This inherited condition is the most common cause of severe hypercholesterolemia. As is often the case, Gary's family history was a huge clue to his problem (Myers et al., 1990❸; Silberberg et al., 1998❸). Although unlikely, secondary causes of hypercholesterolemia should be kept in mind.

Differential Diagnosis

Gary's symptoms and findings suggest several other plausible possibilities.

1. Hypertriglyceridemia is a distinct possibility. Triglycerides are transported in the blood mainly in very low-density lipoprotein particles, which also contain some cholesterol. For this reason, elevated triglyceride levels raise the total cholesterol level. Triglyceride elevation of more than 150 mg/dL (1.7 mmol/L) is associated with a lesser degree of risk of heart disease than LDL cholesterol elevation.
2. Metabolic syndrome (varied combinations of central obesity, elevated triglycerides, low HDL cholesterol, insulin resistance with glucose intolerance, thrombogenic state, and proinflammatory state) is unlikely because of Greg's slenderness and high physical activity level. The prevalence of obesity and metabolic syndrome has risen alarmingly in the past several decades (to an estimated 47 million Americans in 2000), and it is a major contributor to the development of CHD and stroke (Ford and Giles, 2003❸).
3. Hypothyroidism is unlikely because of the mild tachycardia, but it is a cause of secondary hypercholesterolemia worth keeping in mind. Patients with hypothyroidism usually present with fatigue and lethargy, but some can be completely asymptomatic, especially elderly people.
4. Generalized anxiety disorder is not an appropriate diagnosis at this point because of the short duration of symptoms.
5. Somatization disorder is not an appropriate diagnosis at this point because of the relatively limited scope and duration of somatic symptoms. If this episode is not handled well, however, the patient may gradually become more preoccupied with somatic symptoms.
6. Panic disorder is unlikely because of the lack of intense acute fear of imminent personal catastrophe. If the patient were biologically predisposed to panic disorder (despite a lack of suggestive family history in this case), sustained or severely heightened concerns could eventually be expressed as panic attacks.
7. Hypochondriasis with cardiac and cancer neuroses should be kept in mind as a plausible possibility, given the patient's family history and current symptoms. If he does not already have this disorder, he may well be vulnerable to developing an exaggerated fear of heart disease as he approaches the age at

which his father died. Some degree of fear is rational, given his lipid disorder and family history.

Some other serious diagnoses are even less likely.

1. Acute pancreatitis resulting from severe hypertriglyceridemia is unlikely because of the relatively brief duration and mild severity of the pain episodes and the patient's slenderness, regular aerobic exercise, low alcohol intake, and nondiabetic status.
2. Hyperalphalipoproteinemia is unlikely, especially in a male. Patients with this condition have a very high level of HDL cholesterol (>90 mg/dL or 2.3 mmol/L and as high as 150 mg/dL or 3.9 mmol/L). High levels of HDL cholesterol are usually associated with low risk of atherosclerosis. In some cases, however, small dense HDL particles do not function normally in transporting peripheral cholesterol to the liver; such particles are proinflammatory and atherogenic, and the patient can be at risk of CHD despite having a high HDL cholesterol level.
3. Angina pectoris caused by atherosclerotic coronary artery disease is highly unlikely in such a young adult. Patients with *homozygous* familial hypercholesterolemia develop heart disease early in life, but if he had the homozygous form, he probably would have already experienced one or more atherosclerotic events (stroke or myocardial infarction).
4. Coronary vasospasm causing atypical angina is rare in this age group, especially in men.

PLAN

Diagnostic Laboratory and Special Tests

1. Fasting lipoprotein analysis (lipid profile) is the most appropriate initial test. Measurement of total cholesterol, HDL cholesterol, and triglyceride levels, and a calculated estimate of LDL cholesterol allow verification and categorization of common lipid disorders. A repeat fasting lipid profile is advisable several weeks later to examine short-term variation and establish pretreatment baseline values for LDL cholesterol level. LDL cholesterol tends to be 10 to 15 mg/dL higher when fasting than when in the postprandial state. (LDL cholesterol increases as triglycerides decrease and vice versa.) Clinicians should keep this in mind when reviewing results for individuals screened with nonfasting lipids for reasons of convenience and expedience (Weiss et al., 2003 ⓒ).
2. Thyroid-stimulating hormone level is the most cost-effective test for excluding hypothyroidism, a treatable secondary cause of high cholesterol level.
3. Electrocardiography, although very unlikely to show abnormalities, may provide useful reassurance to the patient if the reading is normal. Neither the patient nor the physician thought that electrocardiography was necessary at this point.

4. More extensive cardiovascular testing (e.g., treadmill stress test with or without contrast agent scanning, coronary artery calcium score by electron beam computed tomography) does not appear to be indicated at this time, but chest pain more typical for angina pectoris would prompt diagnostic testing.

Therapeutic Treatment Plan

1. The physician advises long-term adherence to a diet low in saturated fat and cholesterol and high in water-soluble fiber (e.g., oat bran). He asks Gary to keep a 3-day food diary, recording everything he eats and drinks for 72 hours, noting serving sizes and method of preparation. Because Gary's cholesterol is severely elevated, he is urged to follow the National Cholesterol Education Program Therapeutic Lifestyle Changes dietary guidelines (formerly known as Step 2 Diet) (National Cholesterol Education Program, 2001 ⓐ). If his cholesterol were not so high, the Heart Healthy Diet (formerly called Step 1) would be appropriate.
2. Gary is advised to continue his current aerobic exercise routine throughout medical school and residency training as much as possible. Exercise may help his anxiety and lipids.
3. Lipid-altering medication is strongly advisable if the lipid profile results show the anticipated severe LDL cholesterol elevation that is characteristic of familial heterozygous hypercholesterolemia.
4. The physician recommends the daily use of relaxation techniques to help reduce the adverse effects of stress and to help Gary deal with acute and chronic anxiety.

Patient Education

1. The physician presents and discusses both working diagnoses and answers Gary's questions.
2. The physician normalizes Gary's anxiety as an entering medical student and predicts that a good adjustment is likely. His anxiety is reframed as a useful signal of stress and as an energy-mobilizing catalyst for change.
3. The physician briefly explains and demonstrates the relaxation techniques of deep breathing, progressive muscle relaxation, and visual imagery.
4. Gary's cholesterol elevation is provisionally characterized as severe, pending confirmation of severely elevated LDL cholesterol and a normal thyroid-stimulating hormone level.
5. The strong role of cholesterol elevation as a causal risk factor for heart disease is discussed.
6. Dietary modification is emphasized as the cornerstone for hypercholesterolemia treatment. The physician gives Gary an educational pamphlet containing details of the recommended dietary changes and asks him to study it and write down any questions that he has before the next visit.

7. The physician explains that regular aerobic exercise usually improves stress coping, sometimes lowers LDL cholesterol modestly, usually increases HDL cholesterol by 5 to 15 mg/dL, and often dramatically lowers elevated triglyceride levels.
8. The physician briefly discusses the pros and cons of 3-hydroxy-3-methylglutaryl coenzyme A reductase inhibitor (statin) therapy and gives Gary a statin decision aid to study before the next visit.
9. Gary is urged to encourage his sister and fiancée to have their cholesterol checked if they have not already done so.

Disposition

Gary is asked to return to the laboratory in 4 weeks for blood tests and to the office in 5 weeks for a follow-up visit. No referral is required at this point.

FOLLOW-UP VISIT

Subjective

Gary returns for follow-up 5 weeks after his initial visit. He is feeling much better. He attributes his improvement mainly to relief from worry about his symptoms' indicating some serious underlying illness such as heart disease or cancer. His abdominal pain, chest discomfort, and palpitations have resolved. He is still having occasional loose bowel movements but is not concerned about them. Gary is anxious to discuss his lipid profile results. In the intervening month, he has discovered that a paternal aunt and a paternal uncle developed heart disease in their 50s

and 30s, respectively, and that both had high cholesterol. He has already encouraged his sister and fiancée to undergo cholesterol screening. He has increased his intake of water-soluble fiber with oatmeal for breakfasts and oat bran muffins for lunches. Gary has done some research on the Internet, and he asks about the advisability of taking fish oil capsules or red yeast rice.

Objective

The patient looks less nervous than on the first visit. His heart rate is 72 (compared with 90 on the previous visit). His 3-day food diary shows a very low intake of foods high in saturated fat and cholesterol, congruent with Therapeutic Lifestyle Change dietary guidelines.

A fasting lipoprotein analysis done the day of his first visit shows a total cholesterol of 310 mg/dL (8.0 mmol/L), HDL cholesterol of 40 mg/dL (1.0 mmol/L), triglycerides of 100 mg/dL (1.13 mmol/L), and an estimated LDL cholesterol of 250 mg/dL (6.5 mmol/L). The thyroid-stimulating hormone result is 2.0, within normal limits. A repeat lipid profile done 4 weeks after his first visit shows a total cholesterol of 302 mg/dL (7.8 mmol/L), HDL cholesterol of 44 mg/dL (1.1 mmol/L), triglycerides of 60 mg/dL (0.68 mmol/L), and an estimated LDL cholesterol of 246 mg/dL (6.4 mmol/L).

Assement

Familial heterozygous hypercholesterolemia with severely elevated total and LDL cholesterol (Fig. 38-1). He also has borderline low HDL cholesterol. The average HDL cholesterol for males is 45 mg/dL (1.15 mmol/L), and for females, the

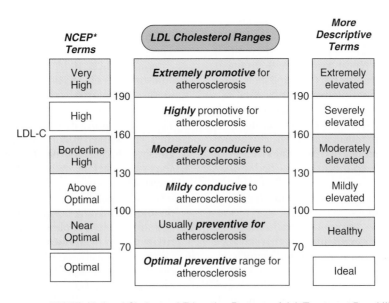

*NCEP, National Cholesterol Education Program, Adult Treatment Panel III

Figure 38-1 Prognostic range for low-density lipoprotein cholesterol (LDL-C).

average is 55 mg/dL (1.42 mmol/L). Despite his being young and having only two other risk factors (male gender and borderline low HDL cholesterol; Table 38-1), Gary's risk of atherosclerotic cardiovascular disease events over the next 10 years is high because of his particular genetic dyslipidemia (Marks et al., 2003 ◉). His LDL cholesterol level greatly exceeds the recommended cut point for considering drug therapy regardless of other risk factor status (Table 38-2).

Adjustment disorder with anxious mood of mild severity; is responding well to reassurance and education about stress-coping strategies.

Plan

Diagnostic Laboratory and Special Tests

1. A repeat lipid profile should be obtained to monitor treatment response approximately 4 to 6 weeks after each change in the regimen is made. Once a regimen has achieved satisfactory results, a lipid profile should be repeated every 6 to 12 months to monitor the ongoing response.

2. Numerous more sophisticated tests are becoming available for measuring other independent risk factors for CHD. Although none are indicated for this very high risk patient, they can be helpful to refine 10-year CHD risk estimates for selected patients with marginal low-intermediate or intermediate-high risk levels based on the major risk factors. Abnormal values for any of them indicate increased risk of CHD events.

   a. C-reactive protein is a moderate, independent CHD predictor when it persists in the moderately elevated range (3 to 10 mg/L). Higher values (>10 mg/L) are occasionally seen in asymptomatic persons and in chronic illness, but severe C-reactive protein elevation usually indicates the presence of an acute or subacute infection or inflammatory condition (Pearson, 2004).

   b. Lp(a) lipoprotein is a relatively uncommon independent predictor of CHD.

   c. Homocysteine is a relatively uncommon CHD risk predictor; high levels predict risk.

   d. Apolipoprotein B is the main protein in LDL; high levels predict risk.

   e. Apolipoprotein A is the main protein in HDL; low levels predict risk.

Table 38-1 Other Risk Factors for Coronary Heart Disease

Factors cited by National Cholesterol Education Program (NCEP) Adult Treatment Panel (ATP) III
Male gender
Cigarette smoking
Diabetes mellitus
Hypertension
Low high-density lipoprotein cholesterol
Obesity
Personal history of atherosclerotic disease
Family history of lipid disorder
Family history of atherosclerotic disease
   (especially men age <55 and women <65)

Other Coronary Heart Disease Risk Factors (not cited by NCEP ATP III)
C-reactive protein elevation
Homocysteine elevation
Lip (a) elevation
Apolipoprotein B elevation
Low apolipoprotein A-I level
Postmenopausal status for females
Lipoprotein-associated phospholipase-2 elevation
   (PLAC test)
Small dense low-density and high-density
   lipoprotein particles
Proinflammatory high-density lipoprotein
Coronary-prone (type A) behavior or personality
Old age (risk increases with increasing age)

Table 38-2 LDL Cholesterol Cut Points Recommended for Considering Drug Therapy by the National Cholesterol Education Program Adult Treatment Panel III

Risk *Category*	10-Year Estimated *Risk for CHD*	LDL Level (mg/dL [mMol/L]) for *Considering Drug Therapy*
CHD or CHD risk equivalent (diabetes, stroke)	>20%	≥100 mg/dL (2.6 mMol/L) (70–100 mg/dL or 1.8–2.6 mMol/L: drug optional)
2+ risk factors	10–20%	≥130 mg/dL (3.35 mMol/L)
	<10%	>160 mg/dL (4.2 mMol/L)
0–1 risk factor (not diabetes)	Usually <10%	>190 mg/dL (4.9 mMol/L) (160–189 mg/dL or 4.2–4.9 mMol/L:drug optional)

CHD, Coronary heart disease; LDL, low-density lipoprotein.

f. LDL and HDL particle size and number predict CHD. Small dense particles are atherogenic.

g. Lipoprotein-associated phospholipase A2, measured by the phospholipase-associated complex (PLAC) test, predicts CHD events when elevated.

h. Proinflammatory HDL is an abnormal HDL type that is atherogenic, not protective.

i. Interleukin-6 is another indicator of inflammation that correlates with C-reactive protein.

j. Serum amyloid A (SAA) predicts CHD risk when elevated.

k. Two identified serum adhesion molecules predict CHD risk-soluble intercellular adhesion molecule and soluble vascular cell adhesion molecule.

Therapeutic Treatment Plan

The physician again advises close adherence to a lifelong Therapeutic Lifestyle Change dietary pattern by restricting foods high in saturated fat and cholesterol. Whole milk dairy products and fatty cuts of beef and pork are the main sources of saturated fat for the average person. The physician recommends using nonhydrogenated corn, safflower, soybean, olive, or flaxseed oil in cooking and avoiding oils high in saturated fat (coconut and palm) and trans fat (most commercial fried foods). The goal is to restrict saturated fat to less than 7% of daily caloric intake, with total fat providing a maximum of 25% to 35% of caloric intake, and less than 200 mg/day of dietary cholesterol, less than 2400 mg/day of sodium, and just enough calories to maintain a healthy weight. Carbohydrates are to provide 50% to 60% of total calories, mainly in the form of slowly digested starches (whole wheat bread, brown rice), with minimal intake of sugars and white starches. The recommended goal for fiber intake is 20 to 30 g/day (preferably mostly viscous soluble fiber from such foods as oat bran, whole grain bread and cereal, brown rice, apples, pears, prunes, beans, peas, Brussels sprouts, broccoli, and cauliflower). Protein intake is best limited to 15% of total calories; long-term high-protein intake may harm the kidneys.

Additional dietary recommendations are made to maximize LDL cholesterol lowering (Hu and Willett, 2002Ⓐ; Jenkins et al., 2003Ⓑ):

1. Cold water fish: two servings per week (salmon, mackerel, sardine, herring, bluefish) (AHA, 2002Ⓐ). Gary is cautioned to limit swordfish to once per month because of its high mercury content.

2. Nuts with healthy fat ratios (almonds, peanuts, pecans, walnuts): one 2-oz serving per day.

3. Soy products (tofu, soy burgers/dogs/milk): two servings per day in lieu of animal protein.

4. Plant sterol/stanol product as margarine/butter substitute: two to three servings per day; brands include Benecol, Take Control, and Smart Balance Omega Plus.

5. Omega-3 fatty acids supplementation (fish oil rich in eicosapentaenoic acid and docosahexaenoic acid): two to three capsules per day if not eating fish regularly (reduces triglycerides but can increase LDL cholesterol). Gary is cautioned that intake of more than 3 g/day may increase stroke risk.

Other dietary supplements were *not* recommended because they have been less studied.

1. Linolenic acid supplementation is converted to eicosapentaenoic acid in the body.

2. Garlic has produced mixed results in clinical trials. It sometimes lowers LDL cholesterol 10% to 15%.

3. Fenugreek, 50 to 100 g/day, can lower LDL 20% to 35%. Its safety is not established.

4. Gugulipids, 25 mg, three times per day, can reduce LDL by 15% to 35%. Its safety is not established.

5. Red yeast rice contains nine natural statin compounds. It lowers LDL 15% to 30%, but its safety is not established. Red yeast rice products containing statins were removed from the U.S. market in 2000.

6. Flavonoids contain antioxidants from green and black teas, grape juice, and wine. Lipid effects and safety are not established.

Gary is encouraged to bring his fiancée along to the next visit for a more detailed discussion of food selection and preparation. A referral to a dietitian is offered for more detailed dietary education.

Lipid altering medication is strongly recommended to lower LDL cholesterol at least to below 100 mg/dL (2.6 mmol/L) and ideally below 70 mg/dL (1.8 mmol/L), in accordance with National Cholesterol Education Program Adult Treatment Panel guideline recommendations (Table 38-3) (Grundy et al., 2004Ⓐ) and American Heart Association Evidence-Based Guidelines for Cardiovascular Disease Prevention (Table 38-4) (Mosca et al., 2004Ⓐ). Gary is advised to keep his LDL cholesterol lowered lifelong. Pros and cons of lipid drugs in general and specific drugs are discussed. Because his LDL cholesterol is so high and his family history so concerning, immediate drug therapy is recommended.

The statin (3-hydroxy-3-methylglutaryl coenzyme A reductase inhibitor) atorvastatin is recommended as the medication most likely to produce good results with monotherapy because of its superior efficacy (40% to 50% reduction of LDL cholesterol compared with 25% to 35% with most other "statins") and excellent results in multiple clinical trials (Colhoun et al., 2004Ⓑ; Koren et al., 2004Ⓑ). Gary has checked with his health insurance plan and found that atorvastatin is one of the preferred medications on the second lowest tier of his plan's formulary and that he

Table 38-3	LDL Cholesterol Treatment Goals Recommended by the National Cholesterol Education Program Adult Treatment Panel III		
	Treatment Goal for LDL Cholesterol, mg/dL (mmol/L)		
Known CAD or diabetes	<100 (<2.6)	Optional goal is <70 (<1.8)	
No known CAD 10-year risk >20%	<100 (<2.6)	Optional goal is <70 (<2.6)	
10-year risk 10–20%	<130 (<3.35)	Unlikely to occur	
10-year risk <10%	≥2 risk factors: <160 (<4.2)	<2 risk factors: <190 (<4.9) Optional goal is <160 (<4.2)	

CAD, Coronary artery disease; LDL, low-density lipoprotein.

can get a month's supply for a $20 copayment (compared to the $95 retail cost [Table 38-5]). A newer statin, rosuvastatin, is mentioned as an option to consider if atorvastatin results are not satisfactory. At the time of this visit, rosuvastatin's superior efficacy (50% to 60% reduction of LDL chole1sterol) is offset by its short time on the market and controversy about its safety (Jones et al., 2003 **B**).

Niacin is presented as an inexpensive ($10 to $20 per month) over-the-counter choice for adjunctive treatment. Sustained release niacin (Slo-Niacin) gives good results at 1 to 2 g/day. The usual side effects of flushing and itching can be minimized by taking one aspirin one to three times daily, but many patients do not tolerate niacin well. Liver toxicity should be watched for, especially during the first few months, by monitoring the liver enzyme alanine aminotransferase periodically. Patients with diabetes mellitus or prediabetes or who are at increased risk of diabetes should be periodically screened for glucose intolerance (fasting or random glucose).

Ezetemibe was presented as a useful adjunctive drug to add to a statin instead of increasing statin dose, if the usual therapeutic dose does not produce satisfactory results (Table 38-6) (Gagne et al., 2002 **B**).

Cholestyramine and colestipol are presented as costly adjunctive treatment options for use at a low to medium dose to avoid the constipation caused by a high dose.

Relaxation techniques are discussed. The physician explains deep breathing, progressive muscle relaxation, and visual imagery in more detail, encourages Gary to try them, and lends Gary an audiotape with relaxation instructions.

Patient Education

The physician discusses the general pros and cons of the over-the-counter and prescription medications for lowering LDL cholesterol. He also elicits Gary's preferences and priorities related to taking prescription drugs. (Gary states a preference for not taking long-term prescription drugs but a willingness to waive that preference in this instance in favor of reducing his risk of heart attack and stroke.) The physician discusses statins' generally excellent safety record (Ballantyne, 2003 **B**). Three potential side effects are discussed: (1) mild elevation of the liver enzyme alanine aminotransferase, which occurs in approximately 10% of patients and is virtually always benign; (2) muscle discomfort or weakness (occurs in approximately 10% of patients); and (3) the only serious potential side effect, rhabdomyolysis (rare, occurring in approximately one in 10,000 to 100,000 patients) (Graham et al., 2004 **B**). The physician answers Gary's questions and then strongly recommends statin therapy. Gary agrees to start on statin therapy right away. He says that he had minimal reservations about potential side effects compared with potential benefits. The physician emphasizes the noncurative nature of statin therapy and the need to continue taking a statin long-term to minimize CHD risk (unless a better treatment comes along).

The physician discusses the genetic inheritance pattern of familial hypercholesterolemia and the reproductive implications of the patient's marrying someone who also has familial hypercholesterolemia. He suggests that Greg watch for new developments from human genome research that might pertain to his cholesterol problem.

The dietary information is discussed and Greg's nutrition questions are answered. The physician stresses the importance of maintaining a healthy diet long term to help the medication do a good job.

Disposition

The patient is asked to return to the laboratory in 6 weeks for a fasting lipid profile and alanine aminotransferase and to schedule an office visit for 7 weeks to discuss his response to treatment.

DISCUSSION

Gary's symptoms are quite common expressions of anxiety related to difficulty coping with stress at home, school, or work. Most patients in this situation respond well to simple reassurance, normalization, and empathic support, coupled with developing an effective repertoire of strategies for preventing and coping with stress and anxiety. Gary's anxiety appears to stem partly from irrational fear about acute heart disease and a more rational fear of eventually having heart disease. Discussing and treating his major risk factor for

Table 38-4 American Heart Association Evidence-based Guidelines for Cardiovascular Disease Prevention (2002)

Measure	Description	Class of Evidence	Level of Evidence	Generalizability to Women
Lifestyle Interventions				
Cigarette smoking	Consistently encourage women not to smoke and to avoid environmental tobacco	I	B	1
Physical activity	Consistently encourage women to accumulate a minimum of 30 min of moderate-intensity physical activity (e.g., brisk walking) on most, and preferably all, days of the week	I	B	1
Heart healthy diet	Consistently encourage an overall healthy eating pattern that includes intake of a variety of fruits, vegetables, grains, low-fat or nonfat dairy products, fish, legumes, and sources of protein low in saturated fat (e.g., poultry, lean meats, plant sources) Limit saturated fat intake to <10% of calories, limit cholesterol intake to <300 mg/d, and limit intake of trans fatty acids	I	B	1
Weight maintenance/ reduction	Consistently encourage weight maintenance/reduction through an appropriate balance of physical activity, caloric intake, and formal behavioral programs when indicated to maintain/achieve a body mass index between 18.5 and 24.9 kg/m^2 and a waist circumference <35 in.	I	B	1
Psychosocial factors	Women with cardiovascular disease (CVD) should be evaluated for depression and referred/treated when indicated	IIa	B	2
Omega-3 fatty acids	As an adjunct to diet, omega-3 fatty acid supplementation may be considered in high-risk* women	IIb	B	2
Folic acid	As an adjunct to diet, folic acid supplementation may be considered in high-risk* women (except after revascularization procedure) if a higher than normal level of homocysteine has been detected	IIb	B	2
Cardiac rehabilitation	Women with a recent acute coronary syndrome or coronary intervention, new-onset or chronic angina should participate in a comprehensive	I	B	2

Table 38-4 American Heart Association Evidence-based Guidelines for Cardiovascular Disease Prevention (2002) (Continued)

Measure	Description	Class of Evidence	Level of Evidence	Generalizability to Women
	risk-reduction regimen, such as cardiac rehabilitation or a physician-guided, home- or community-based program			
Major Risk Factor Interventions				
Blood pressure: lifestyle	Encourage an optimal blood pressure of <120/80 mm Hg through lifestyle approaches	I	B	1
Blood pressure: drugs	Pharmacotherapy is indicated when blood pressure is ≥140/90 mm Hg or an even lower blood pressure in the setting of blood pressure–related target-organ damage or diabetes. Thiazide diuretics should be part of the drug regimen for most patients unless contraindicated	I	A	1
Lipids, lipoproteins	Optimal levels of lipids and lipoproteins in women are low-density lipoprotein cholesterol (LDL-C) <100 mg/dL, high-density lipoprotein cholesterol (HDL-C) > 50 mg/dL, triglycerides <150 mg/dL, and non–HDL-C (total cholesterol minus HDL cholesterol) <130 mg/dL and should be encouraged through lifestyle approaches	I	B	1
Lipids: diet therapy	In high-risk* women or when LDL-C is elevated, saturated fat intake should be reduced to <7% of calories and cholesterol to <200 mg/days, and trans fatty acid intake should be reduced	I	B	1
Lipids: pharmacotherapy, high risk*	Initiate LDL-C–lowering therapy (preferably a statin) simultaneously with lifestyle therapy in high-risk women with LDL-C ≥100 mg/dL	I	A	1
	Initiate statin therapy in high-risk women with an LDL-C <100 mg/dL unless contraindicated	I	B	1
	Initiate niacin[†] or fibrate therapy when HDL-C is low or non–HDL-C elevated in high-risk women	I	B	1
Lipids: pharmacotherapy, intermediate risk[‡]	Initiate LDL-C–lowering therapy (preferably a statin) if LDL-C level is ≥130 mg/dL on lifestyle therapy or	I	A	1

Continued

Table 38-4 American Heart Association Evidence-based Guidelines for Cardiovascular Disease Prevention (2002) (Continued)

Measure	Description	Class of Evidence	Level of Evidence	Generalizability to Women
	Initiate LDL-C–lowering therapy with niacin[†] or fibrate therapy when HDL-C is low or non–HDL-C elevated after LDL-C goal is reached	I	B	1
Lipids: pharmacotherapy, lower risk[§]	Consider LDL-C–lowering therapy in low-risk women with 0 or 1 risk factor when LDL-C level is >190 mg/dL or if multiple risk factors are present when LDL-C is >160 mg/dL or	IIa	B	1
	Consider niacin[†] or fibrate therapy when HDL-C is low or non-HDL-C elevated after LDL-C goal is reached	IIa	B	1
Diabetes	Lifestyle and pharmacotherapy should be used to achieve near-normal glycosylated hemoglobin (HbA1C) (<7%) in women with diabetes	I	B	1
Preventive Drug Interventions				
Aspirin, high risk[*]	Aspirin therapy (75–162 mg) or clopidogrel if patient is intolerant to aspirin, should be used in high-risk women unless contraindicated	I	A	1
Aspirin, intermediate risk[‡]	Consider aspirin therapy (75–162 mg) in intermediate-risk women as long as blood pressure is controlled and benefit is likely to outweigh risk of gastrointestinal side effects	IIa	B	2
β-Blockers	Should be used indefinitely in all women who have had a myocardial infarction or who have chronic ischemic syndromes unless contraindicated	I	A	1
Angiotensin-converting enzyme (ACE) inhibitors	Should be used (unless contraindicated) in high-risk[*] women	I	A	1
Angiotensin-receptor blockers	Should be used in high-risk[*] women with clinical evidence of heart failure or an ejection fraction <40% who are intolerant to ACE inhibitors	I	B	1
Atrial Fibrillation/Stroke Prevention				
Warfarin	Among women with chronic or paroxysmal atrial fibrillation, warfarin should be used to maintain the international normalized ratio at 2.0–3.0	I	A	1

Table 38-4 American Heart Association Evidence-based Guidelines for Cardiovascular Disease Prevention (2002) (Continued)

Measure	Description	Class of Evidence	Level of Evidence	Generaliz-ability to Women
Aspirin	unless they are considered to be at low risk of stroke (<1%/yr) or high risk of bleeding			
	325 mg should be used in women with chronic or paroxysmal atrial fibrillation with a contraindication to warfarin or at low risk of stroke (<1%/yr).	I	A	1
Class III Interventions				
Hormone therapy	Combined estrogen plus progestin hormone therapy should not be initiated to prevent CVD in postmenopausal women	III	A	—
	Combined estrogen plus progestin hormone therapy should not be continued to prevent CVD in postmeno-pausal women	III	C	—
	Other forms of menopausal hormone therapy (e.g., unopposed estrogen) should not be initiated or continued to prevent CVD in postmeno-pausal women pending the results of ongoing trials	III	C	—
Antioxidant supplements	Antioxidant vitamin supplements should not be used to prevent CVD pending the results of ongoing trials	III	A	1
Aspirin, lower risk§	Routine use of aspirin in lower risk women is not recom-mended pending the results of ongoing trials	III	B	2

*High risk is defined as coronary heart disease (CHD) or risk equivalent or a 10-year absolute CHD risk >20%.
†Dietary supplement niacin must not be used as a substitute for prescription niacin, and over-the-counter niacin should only be used if approved and monitored by a physician.
‡Intermediate risk is defined as a 10-year absolute CHD risk of 10% to 20%.
§Lower risk is defined as a 10-year absolute CHD risk <10%.
Strength of Recommendations: classification—class I, intervention is useful and effective; class IIa, weight of evidence/opinion is in favor of usefulness/efficacy; class IIb, usefulness/efficacy is less well established by evidence/opinion; class III; intervention is not useful/effective and may be harmful; level of evidence— A, sufficient evidence from multiple randomized trials; B, limited evidence from single randomized trial or other nonrandomized studies; C, based on expert opinion, case studies, or standard of care; Generalizability Index—1, very likely that results generalize to women; 2, somewhat likely that results generalize to women; 3, unlikely that results generalize to women; 0, unable to project whether results generalize to women.

heart disease could greatly reduce his anxiety, if the treatment is successful and well tolerated. If treatment does not go well, however, his anxiety could escalate.

More than one half of U.S. adults have unhealthy levels of LDL cholesterol, triglycerides, and/or HDL cholesterol that place them at increased risk of CHD and stroke, the causes of more than one half of all adult U.S. deaths. Hypercholesterolemic individuals who use tobacco, have strong family histories, or have diabetes or metabolic syndrome are at highest risk of heart attack and stroke.

Gary's lipid disorder, familial heterozygous (Type IIa) hypercholesterolemia, is generally asymptomatic until atherosclerotic lesions progress to a

Table 38-5 Retail Cost of Therapeutic Equivalent Doses of HMG-CoA Reductase Inhibitors (Statins) as Monotherapy or Combination Therapy

Medication	Trade Name	Dose	Monthly Retail Cost
OTC Niacin	**Slo-Niacin**	**1000–2000 mg**	**$10–20**
Lovastatin	Generic	10 mg	$20
Lovastatin	Generic	20 mg	$26
Lovastatin	Generic	40 mg	$32
Fluvastatin	Lescol	20 mg	$64
Fluvastatin	Lescol	40 mg	$64
Simvastatin	Zocor	10 mg	$79
Pravastin	Pravachol	20 mg	$101
Lovastatin + OTC niacin	**Generic + Slo-Niacin**	**20 mg, 500 mg**	**$36**
Lovastatin-niacin	Advicor	20–500 mg	$75
Lovastatin	Altoprev	40 mg ER	$75
Fluvastatin	Lescol	80 mg XL	$77
Atorvastatin	Lipitor	10 mg	$78
Rosuvastatin	Crestor	5 mg	$94
Pravastatin	Pravachol	40 mg	$103
Simvastin	Zocor	20 mg	$125
Lovastatin + OTC niacin	**Generic + Slo-Niacin**	**40 mg + 1000 mg**	**$42**
Lovastatin	Altoprev	60 mg ER	$78
Rosuvastatin	Crestor	10 mg	$94
Lovastatin-niacin	Advicor	20–1000	$95
Atorvastatin	Lipitor	20 mg	$108
Simvastatin	Zocor	40 mg	$125
Pravastatin	Pravachol	80 mg	$138
Lovastatin + OTC niacin	**Generic + Slo-Niacin**	**40 mg + 2000 mg**	**$52**
Simvastatin-ezetemibe	Vytorin*	10–10 mg	$90*
Rosuvastatin	Crestor	20 mg	$94
Simvastatin-ezetemibe	Vytorin*	20–10 mg	$106*
Atorvastatin	Lipitor	40 mg	$108
Simvastatin	Zocor	80 mg	$125
Fluvastatin + ezetemibe	Lescol + Zetia	80 mg XL, 10 mg	$156
Rosuvastatin	**Crestor**	**40 mg**	**$94**
Rosuvastatin + OTC niacin	Crestor + Slo-Niacin	5 mg, 1000 mg	$104
Atorvastatin	Lipitor	80 mg	$108
Simvastatin-ezetemibe	Vytorin*	40–10 mg	$113*
Simvastatin-ezetemibe	Vytorin*	80–10 mg	$113*
Atorvastatin + ezetemibe	Lipitor + Zetia	10 mg, 10 mg	$157
Rosuvastatin + ezetemibe	Crestor + Zetia	5 mg, 10 mg	$173
Rosuvastatin + OTC niacin	**Crestor + Slo-Niacin**	**10 or 20 mg, 2000 mg**	**$114**
Atorvastatin + OTC niacin	Lipitor + Slo-Niacin	20 or 40 mg, 2000 mg	$128
Rosuvastatin + ezetemibe	Crestor + Zetia	10 mg, 10 mg	$173
Rosuvastatin + ezetemibe	Crestor + Zetia	20 mg, 10 mg	$173
Atorvastatin + ezetemibe	Lipitor + Zetia	20 mg, 10 mg	$187
Atorvastatin + ezetemibe	Lipitor + Zetia	40 mg, 10 mg	$187
Rosuvastatin + OTC niacin	**Crestor + Slo-Niacin**	**40 mg, 2000 mg**	**$114**
Atorvastatin + OTC niacin	Lipitor + Slo-Niacin	80 mg, 200 mg	$128
Rosuvastatin + ezetemibe	Crestor + Zetia	40 mg, 10 mg	$173
Atorvastatin + ezetemibe	Lipitor + Zetia	80 mg, 10 mg	$187

*Based on retail price quotes from community pharmacies, December 20, 2004, survey, Houston, TX, for whole tablets of 3-hydroxy-3-methylglutaryl coenzyme A (HMG-CoA) reductase inhibitors (statins), except for Vytorin prices, which, because Vytorin was not on local pharmacy Web sites, are from a Canadian Internet pharmacy www.abconlinepharmacy.com&/ns/customer/home.php?cat=27&page=4.

ER, extended release; OTC, over-the-counter.

Table 38-6 Cost-effective Medication Regimens for Treating Elevated LDL Cholesterol

	LDL-C Treatment Goal	
Baseline LDL-C (mg/dL)	**<130 mg/dL**	**<100 mg/dL**
100–159	Lovastatin, generic, one 10- or 20-mg tab, qd, $20–26/mo or fluvastatin (Lescol), one half 40-mg tab, qd, $32/mo or simvastatin (Zocor), one half 10-mg or one half 20-mg tab, qd, $40-65 mo or lovastatin-niacin (Advicor), one 20-500-mg tab, qd, $75/mo	Lovastatin, generic, one 20-mg, plus OTC niacin (Slo-Niacin), one 500 mg, qd, $36/mo or simvastatin (Zocor), one half 40-mg tab, qd, $65/mo or lovastatin (Altoprev), one 40-mg ER tab, qd, $75/mo or lovastatin-niacin (Advicor), one 20–500-mg tab, qd, $75/mo or fluvastatin (Lescol XL), one 80-mg ER tab, qd, $77/mo or atorvastatin (Lipitor), one 10-mg tab, qd, $78/mo or rosuvastatin (Crestor), one 5-mg tab, qd, $94/mo
160–189	Lovastatin, generic, one 20-mg, qd, plus OTC niacin (Slo-Niacin), one 500-mg, qd, $36/mo or simvastatin (Zocor), one half 40-mg tab, qd, $65/mo or lovastatin (Altoprev), one 40-mg ER tab, qd, $75/mo or lovastatin-niacin (Advicor), one 20–500-mg tab, qd, $75/mo or fluvastatin (Lescol XL), one 80-mg ER tab, qd, $77/mo or atorvastatin (Lipitor), one 10-mg tab, qd, $78/mo or rosuvastatin (Crestor), one 5-mg tab, qd, $94/mo	Lovastatin (generic), one 40-mg, plus OTC niacin (Slo Niacin), one to two 500-mg, bid, $42-52/mo or simvastatin (Zocor), one half to one 80 mg tab, qd, $65–125/mo or lovastatin (Altoprev), one 60-mg ER tab, qd, $78/mo or rosuvastatin (Crestor), one 10-mg tab, qd, $94/mo or lovastatin-niacin (Advicor), one 20–1000-mg tab, qd, $95/mo or atorvastatin (Lipitor), one 20-mg tab, qd, $108/mo
≥190	Lovastatin (generic), one 40-mg plus OTC niacin (Slo-Niacin), one or two 500-mg, qd, $42-52/mo or simvastatin (Zocor), one half to one 80-mg tab, qd, $65-130/mo or lovastatin (Altoprev), one 60-mg ER tab, qd, $78/mo or rosuvastatin (Crestor), one 10-mg tab, qd, $94/mo or lovastatin-niacin (Advicor), one 20–1000-mg tab, qd, $95/mo or atorvastatin, one 20-mg tab Lipitor, $108/mo	Rosuvastatin (Crestor), one 20- or 40-mg tab, qd, $94/mo or atorvastatin (Lipitor), one 40- or 80-mg tab, qd, $108/mo or rosuvastatin (Crestor), one 20- or 40-mg tab, qd, plus OTC niacin (Slo Niacin), four 500-mg, qd, $114/mo or simvastatin (Zocor), one 80-mg tab, qd, $125/mo or atorvastatin (Lipitor), one 40- or 80-mg tab, qd, plus OTC niacin (Slo Niacin), two 500-mg, bid, $128/mo or simvastatin (Zocor), one half 40- or 80-mg tab, qd, plus ezetemibe (Zetia), one 10-mg tab, qd, $144/mo or atorvastatin (Lipitor), one 10-mg tab, qd, plus ezetemibe (Zetia), one 10-mg tab, qd, $157/mo or rosuvastatin (Crestor), one 5-mg tab, qd, plus ezetemibe (Zetia), one 10-mg tab, qd, $173/mo

ER, extended release; LDL-C, low-density lipoprotein cholesterol; OTC, over-the-counter.

critical extent or until a plaque ruptures and triggers formation of a coronary thrombus. This usually occurs after the age of 30. For persons with this disorder, the average age of developing clinical heart disease is 42 for men and 52 for women. Although the likelihood of Gary's having symptomatic coronary artery disease now is quite low, he most likely already has some degree of coronary atherosclerosis. His concern about developing early heart disease in his 30s or 40s is well founded. The severity of cholesterol elevation might be exacerbated by the stress of beginning medical school and ambivalence about his ability to succeed academically and cope well with the demands of his chosen profession. It would be important to clarify that his long-term LDL cholesterol range is the important determinant of prognosis, not any particular LDL cholesterol level.

Familial heterozygous (Type IIa) hypercholesterolemia is not uncommon, with a prevalence of approximately one in 400 in the general population. Mild and moderate degrees of hypercholesterolemia are extremely common. More than 50% of American adults have levels of LDL cholesterol high enough to promote coronary atherosclerosis, especially in the presence of other identified risk factors. More than one half of patients who experience myocardial infarctions have total cholesterol values between 200 and 239 mg/dL (5.2 to 6.1 mmol/L) and LDL cholesterol levels below the National Cholesterol Education Program cut point for defining high LDL cholesterol (160 mg/dL [4.1 mmol/L]). Individuals with diabetes, hypertension, or tobacco abuse (cigarette smokers and users of oral tobacco) are at especially high risk if their LDL cholesterol levels are even mildly elevated (100 to 159 mg/dL or 2.6 mmol/L) and/or their HDL cholesterol levels are below average. After menopause, women's risk of CHD rapidly catches up to men's.

When starting a program of dietary change to lower LDL cholesterol, it can be very helpful to ask patients to bring in their spouse, children, and other key family members for a family conference to discuss the rationale and details of a heart healthy diet. Teaching patients and spouses how to interpret the information on food labels is an important component of patient education. Figuring out ways to deal with ethnic food preferences and customs is an important need for some families.

Patients who have an average American intake of saturated fat and cholesterol usually respond to persistent dietary modification by lowering their total and LDL cholesterol levels by approximately 10% to 30% of the baseline value. Patients who already have a low intake of saturated fat do not respond well to dietary modification because they have so little room for change. Cholesterol lowering medication usually lowers the LDL cholesterol an additional 25% to 60% below the level achieved by dietary modification, depending on the medication and dose.

Multiple large randomized clinical trials have established that lowering elevated LDL cholesterol with statin medication is the most cost-effective way to substantially lower the risk of CHD events (myocardial infarction and CHD death) in both men and women and in the elderly (who are at higher risk of a CHD event) (National Cholesterol Education Program, 2001Ⓐ). While patients with severe LDL elevation (>190 mg/dL) and/or low HDL cholesterol (<40 mg/dL) are most likely to benefit from treatment, statins have also shown primary prevention benefit in individuals with moderate LDL cholesterol elevation (130 to 189 mg/dL) and secondary prevention benefit in high-risk individuals with LDL cholesterol levels above 100 mg/dL. For elderly patients, the estimated potential benefit of treatment (enhanced quality of life for more of the remaining life span) must be weighed for each individual against the expense and possible adverse effects of medications being considered.

The National Cholesterol Education Program Adult Treatment Panel guidelines for lifestyle change and drug therapy (see Fig. 38-1) (Grundy et al., 2004 Ⓐ) and the American Heart Association Guidelines for Primary Prevention of Cardiovascular Disease and Stroke (see Table 38-4) (Mosca et al., 2004Ⓐ) are based on the evidence from these studies. Many patients prefer to delay starting lipid-lowering medication until persistently elevated values on several lipid profiles convince them that they cannot obtain satisfactory results with dietary change, regular exercise, and sustained weight loss. Despite the overwhelming evidence of statin benefit and safety, more than one half of the persons who are considered appropriate candidates for statin therapy have never started taking a statin. Worse, the persistence rate for statin therapy in community practice in 2003 averaged approximately 60% at 1 year and less than 40% at 3 years after initiation of therapy (Ellis et al., 2004Ⓐ). The main patient obstacles to statin acceptance and persistence are (1) misunderstanding or denying the seriousness of their risk of CHD, (2) failing to appreciate the noncurative nature of statin therapy, (3) being distrustful of statins because of their "not being natural," (4) worrying inordinately about potential or perceived adverse side effects of statins, (5) wishing to avoid acknowledging and accepting their physical frailty and mortality, and (6) the added short-term health care costs entailed with statin therapy (LaRosa and LaRosa, 2000Ⓒ; Morris and Schulz, 2003 Ⓒ). The impact of cost on compliance can be minimized by careful selection of statin and by having patients split pills into halves to save money (see Table 38-6) (Crouch, 2001Ⓐ). The risk of serious adverse side effects from statin therapy can be minimized by instructing patients about medications to avoid while on a statin (Table 38-7) and by monitoring patients' other medications closely and avoiding or using great caution when prescribing medications that tend to raise statin blood levels when taken concomitantly.

Table 38-7 Drugs and Other Substances That Interact with Statins*

Grapefruit juice
Niacin, also called nicotinic acid (Slo-Niacin, Niacor, Niaspan, Nico-400, Niadelay, Endur-Acin)
Gemfibrozil (Lopid)
Femfibrate (Tricor)
Itraconazole (Sporonox)
Amlodopine (Norvasc)
Diltiazem (Cardizem, Cartia, Dilacor, Diltia, Tiazac)
Verapamil (Calan, Covera, Isoptin, Verelan)
Amiodarone (Cordarone)
Cimetidine (Tagamet)
Erythromycin (EES, E-Mycin, Eryc, PCE, Ery-Tab)
Clarithromycin (Biaxin)
Clindamycin (Cleocin)
Cyclosporine
Indinavir (Crixivan)
Nelfinavir (Viracept)
Ritonavir (Norvir)
Saquinavir (Invirase)
Tacrolimus (Prograf)

*Some statins (atorvastatin, simvastatin, and lovastatin, but not pravastatin, rosuvastatin, or fluvastatin) interact with other drugs metabolized by the cytochrome P-450 3A4 liver enzyme system.

Studies continue to show that physicians have not done well managing dyslipidemia in accordance with treatment guidelines (Eaton and Stamp, 2002 ◎; McBride et al., 1998◎). The main physician obstacles to prescribing statin therapy are (1) unfamiliarity with the details of lipid guidelines, (2) complexity of the recommendations for lipid assessment and treatment, (3) skepticism about guideline validity and insufficient familiarity with the outcomes of statin clinical trials, (4) logistical difficulties with applying the guidelines in a busy primary care practice, (5) time pressure, and (6) inadequate reimbursement for time spent doing patient education (Powell-Cope et al., 2004◎).

Guidelines are also available for diagnosing and managing hypercholesterolemia in children. Dietary prevention should ideally begin relatively early in life in all individuals at increased risk of CHD to mini-mize or postpone the development of atherosclerosis in adulthood (AHA, 1997). Although many clinicians are reluctant to use lipid-altering drugs in children, medication should be considered if a child has severely elevated LDL cholesterol that does not respond well to dietary modification.

Triglyceride elevation increases the risk of heart disease in female patients, especially those with diabetes. Patients with mild triglyceride elevations often benefit from restriction of carbohydrates and alcohol, weight loss, exercise, and improved control of diabetes. Severe or persistent hypertriglyceridemia should be treated with niacin, fenofibrate, or gemfibrozil, and/or a statin. The goal of treatment is to reduce the triglyceride level to below 150.

Low HDL cholesterol is a powerful independent risk factor, even if LDL cholesterol is only mildly elevated (100 to 159 mg/dL). Although National Cholesterol Education Program guidelines have not yet recommended medical management for low HDL cholesterol per se, the results of the Helsinki study suggest that treating low HDL cholesterol is at least as beneficial as lowering elevated LDL cholesterol. Hygienic approaches, including regular aerobic exercise, weight loss, and smoking cessation, tend to raise HDL cholesterol by 5 to 15 mg/dL, as does treatment with niacin, gemfibrozil, or fenofibrate. Statins sometimes elevate HDL cholesterol slightly.

The Prevention Challenge

The prognosis for patients with lipid problems can be greatly improved by lasting lifestyle changes, long-term lipid-lowering medication, and diligent follow-up care. Creative solutions are needed to improve the level of acceptance and trust in the efficacy and safety of statin therapy among both patients and physicians, so that more of the statins' preventive potential can be realized.

Material Available on Student Consult

Review Questions and Answers about Hypercholesterolemia

RESOURCES

American Heart Association. Available at www.americanheart.org
National Cholesterol Education Program. Available at www.nhlbi.nih.gov/about/ncep/index.htm
Therapeutic Lifestyle Change diet. Available at www.nlhbi.nih.gov/cgi-bin/chd/step2intro.cgi
10-Year CHD Risk Estimate Calculator. Available at www.nhlbi.nih.gov/atpiii/calculator.asp?usertype=prof
10-Year CHD Risk Estimate Calculator (downloadable Excel 95 and 2000 spreadsheet versions for Palm or MAC OS version). Available at http://hp2010.nhlbihin.net/atpiii/riskcalc.htm
Third Report of Expert Panel on Detection, Evaluation, and Treatment of High Blood Cholesterol in Adults (Adult Treatment Panel III) Executive Summary. Available at www.nhlbi.nih.gov/guidelines/cholesterol/atp_iii.htm
Implications of Recent Clinical Trials for the National Cholesterol Education Program Adult Treatment Panel III Guidelines. Circulation 2004 July 13;110:227–239.

Available at www.nhlbi.nih.gov/guidelines/cholesterol/atp3upd04.htm

HeartAge (online alternative way of expressing CHD risk). Available at www.heartage.com.

NCEP ATP III: X. Adherence. Available at www.nhlbi.nih.gov/guidelines/cholesterol/chap_9.pdf

All resources accessed November 29, 2005

REFERENCES

AHA Compliance Action Program. Available at www.americanheart.org/CAP/patient/con_quiz.html, www.americanheart.org/CAP/pro/prof_pledge.html, www.americanheart.org/CAP/pro/prof_quiz.html

American Heart Association (AHA). Nutrition and Children. A Statement for Healthcare Professionals from the Nutrition Committee, 1997.

AHA Scientific Statement: Fish consumption, fish oil, omega-3 fatty acids and cardiovascular disease, #71-0241. Circulation 2002;106:2747–2757.Ⓐ

Ballantyne CM. Current and future aims of lipid-lowering therapy: Changing paradigms and lessons from the Heart Protection Study on standards of efficacy and safety. Am J Cardiol 2003;92:3K–9K.Ⓑ

Colhoun HM, Betteridge DJ, Durrington PN, et al. Primary prevention of cardiovascular disease with atorvastatin in type 2 diabetes in the Collaborative Atorvastatin Diabetes Study (CARDS): Multicentre randomized placebo-controlled trial. Lancet 2004; 364:685–696.Ⓑ

Crouch MA. Effective use of statins to prevent coronary heart disease. Am Fam Physician 2001;63:309–320, 323–324.Ⓒ

Eaton CB, Stamp MJ. National Cholesterol Education Program (NCEP): The Adult Treatment Panel III Guidelines. Practice patterns related to the Adult Treatment Panel III guidelines in primary care. Am J Cardiol 2002;90:687.Ⓒ

Ellis JJ, Erickson SR, Stevenson JG, et al. Suboptimal statin adherence and discontinuation in primary and secondary prevention populations. J Gen Intern Med 2004;19:638–645.Ⓐ

Ford ES, Giles WH. A comparison of the prevalence of the metabolic syndrome using two proposed definitions. Diabetes Care 2003;26:575–581.Ⓒ

Gagne C, Bays HE, Weiss SR, et al. Efficacy and safety of ezetimibe added to ongoing statin therapy for treatment of patients with primary hypercholesterolemia. Am J Cardiol 2002;90:1084–1091.Ⓑ

Graham DJ, Staffa JA, Shatin D, et al. Incidence of hospitalized rhabdomyolysis in patients treated with lipid-lowering drugs. JAMA 2004;292:2585–2590.Ⓒ

Grundy SM, Cleeman JI, Merz NB, et al. Implications of recent clinical trials for the National Cholesterol Education Program Adult Treatment Panel III Guidelines. Circulation 2004;110:227–239.Ⓐ

Hu FB, Willett WC. Optimal Diets for prevention of coronary heart disease. JAMA 2002;288:2569–2578.Ⓐ

Jenkins DJA, Kendall CWC, Marchie A, et al. Effects of a dietary portfolio of cholesterol-lowering foods vs lovastatin on serum lipids and C-reactive protein. JAMA 2003;290:502–510.Ⓑ

Jones PH, Davidson MH, Stein EA, et al. Comparison of the efficacy and safety of rosuvastatin versus atorvastatin, simvastatin, and pravastatin across doses (STELLAR Trial). Am J Cardiol 2003;92:152–160.Ⓑ

Koren MJ, Hunninghake DB. Clinical outcomes in managed-care patients with coronary heart disease treated aggressively in lipid-lowering disease management clinics. The ALLIANCE Study. J Am Coll Cardiol 2004; 44:1772–1779.Ⓑ

LaRosa JH, LaRosa JC. Enhancing drug compliance in cholesterol-lowering treatment. Arch Fam Med 2000; 9:1169–1175.Ⓒ

Marks D, Thorogood M, Neil HA, Humphries SE. A review on the diagnosis, natural history, and treatment of familial hypercholesterolaemia. Atherosclerosis 2003; 168:1–14.Ⓒ

McBride P, Schrott HG, Plane MB, Underbakke G, Brown RL. Primary care practice adherence to national cholesterol education program guidelines for patients with coronary heart disease. Arch Intern Med 1998; 158:1238–1244.Ⓒ

Morris LS, Schulz RM. Medication compliance: The patient's perspective. Clin Ther 1993;15:593–606.Ⓒ

Mosca L, Appel LJ, Benjamin EJ, et al. Evidence-based guidelines for cardiovascular disease prevention in women. Circulation 2004;109:672–693.Ⓐ

Myers RH, Kiely DK, Cupples LA, Kannel WB. Parental history is an independent risk factor for coronary artery disease: The Framingham Study. Am Heart J 1990;120:963–969.Ⓑ

National Cholesterol Education Program, Adult Treatment Panel III. Summary of the third report of the National Cholesterol Education Program (NCEP) Expert Panel on Detection, Evaluation, and Treatment of High Blood Cholesterol in Adults (Adult Treatment Panel III). JAMA 2001;285:2486–2497.Ⓐ

Pearson TA, Mensah GA, Hong Y, Smith SC. CDC/AHA workshop on markers of inflammation and cardiovascular disease: Application to clinical and public health practice: Overview. Circulation 2004;110:e543–e544.

Powell-Cope GM, Luther S, Neugaard B, Nelson VJ. Provider-perceived barriers and facilitators for ischaemic heart disease (IHD) guideline adherence. J Eval Clin Pract 2004;10:227–239.Ⓒ

Silberberg JS, Wlodarczyk J, Fryer J, Robertson R, Hensley MJ. Risk associated with various definitions of family history of coronary heart disease. The Newcastle Family History Study II. Am J Epidemiol 1998;147: 1133–1139.Ⓑ

Weiss R, Harder M, Rowe J. The relationship between non-fasting and fasting lipid measurements in patients with or without type 2 diabetes mellitus receiving treatment with 3-hydroxy-3-methylglutaryl-coenzyme A reductase inhibitors. Clin Ther 2003;25:1490–1497.Ⓒ

39

Bilateral Leg Pain (Peripheral Arterial Disease)

Kalyanakrishnan Ramakrishnan

KEY POINTS

1. Clinical presentation of peripheral arterial disease (PAD) ranges from asymptomatic stenosis to intermittent claudication (IC) and critical limb ischemia (CLI).
2. Many patients with PAD are asymptomatic (less than 50% of patients with an abnormal ankle/brachial index [ABI] have claudication). Individuals with even asymptomatic PAD have a reduced functional capacity, a lower quality of life, a sixfold increase in cardiovascular morbidity and mortality, carotid artery stenosis, and cognitive dysfunction.
3. Smoking, diabetes mellitus, and hypertension have the greatest association with and an additive effect on the risk of PAD.
4. The ABI (normal ≥ 1) is a simple, painless, highly reproducible test performed to document PAD, and values less than 0.9 correlate well with 50% or greater stenosis of one or more major lower limb arteries.
5. Treatment aims to relieve lower extremity symptoms, increase functional walking capacity and quality of life, prevent progression of disease and ulcer formation, and preserve the limb. Lifestyle changes and medications result in improvement in most patients.
6. Revascularization (endovascular or surgical) is reserved for short-distance IC, rest pain (CLI), nonhealing ulcers, or threatened limb loss.

INITIAL VISIT

Subjective

Patient Identification and Presenting Problem
John B. is a 60-year-old man who presents with a history of bilateral leg pain described as a cramping discomfort in both calves and right thigh after walking two blocks. The pain is relieved after a minute or two of rest. Other symptoms include charley horses, occasional tingling and numbness in his right foot, and fatigue in the legs on walking around the house or on standing for 15 minutes. He has no nocturnal pain or rest pain. He denies any change in color of the legs or any sores, chest pain, shortness of breath, dizziness, numbness in his upper limbs, or transient loss of vision. He also denies any abdominal discomfort after meals, anorexia, weight loss, or erectile dysfunction.

Medical History
Medical history is significant for hypertension, non–insulin-dependent diabetes mellitus, and hypercholesterolemia. His comorbid illnesses are well controlled on metoprolol (Lopressor) 50 mg twice daily, lisinopril (Zestril) 20 mg daily, atorvastatin (Lipitor) 20 mg daily, and metformin (Glucophage) 1000 mg twice daily. Three years ago, he was admitted with an episode of congestive heart failure, thought to be ischemic in origin. Since then, however, his cardiorespiratory status had been stable. He had also undergone a cholecystectomy and an appendectomy in the early 1980s.

Social History
He has a 40-pack-year smoking history. He denies any alcohol or drug use. He professes to "eat whatever he wants." He enjoyed walking 2 miles every day until his leg cramps prevented this continued activity.

Family History
Both his parents had died of myocardial infarction.

Objective

Physical Examination
On physical examination, his pulse is 70 beats per minute and regular, blood pressure is 140/90, and weight is 220 pounds. There are no carotid bruits

---

Evidence levels Ⓐ Randomized, controlled trials (RCTs), meta-analyses, well-designed systematic reviews of RCTs. Ⓑ Case-control or cohort studies, nonrandomized clinical trials, systematic reviews of studies other than RCTs, cross-sectional studies, retrospective studies, certain uncontrolled studies. Ⓒ Consensus statements, expert guidelines, usual practice, opinion.

or jugular venous distention. Cardiorespiratory examination shows no evidence of congestive heart failure. Abdominal examination is negative for organomegaly, palpable aortic aneurysm, and renal bruits. On examination of his lower extremities, the right femoral pulse is weak with a bruit. No distal pulses are palpable on the right. The left femoral pulse is normal; popliteal and pedal pulses are absent on the left. Power, sensations, and reflexes are normal in both lower limbs. No areas of skin breakdown are noticed.

Assessment

Working Diagnosis
Intermittent claudication due to right common iliac artery stenosis and bilateral superficial femoral artery occlusion.

Differential Diagnosis (Table 39-1)
1. *Intermittent claudication.* This is defined as reproducible lower limb discomfort during exercise, relieved within minutes by rest or reduction in walking pace. It is the most common symptom of mild to moderate atherosclerotic PAD and affects 3% to 5% of adults (five million people) in the United States. Claudication most frequently localizes to the calf muscles due to their relatively greater metabolic demand, and the superficial femoral arteries are a common site of atherosclerosis. Buttock or thigh claudication may result from atherosclerotic narrowing of the aortoiliac segment. Patients may quantify their exercise capacity in walking distance or time to the onset of claudication (claudication distance) (Brook et al., 2002Ⓑ).
2. *Lumbosacral radiculopathy due to degenerative joint disease, spinal stenosis, and herniated intervertebral disks* cause pain in the buttock, hip, thigh, calf, and/or foot with walking, often after very short distances, or even with standing (neurogenic pseudoclaudication). Fatigue, numbness, or paresthesias in the legs and feet may also be present. The pain is made worse on lying prone or extension of the spine and is relieved by sitting or bending forward. Sensorimotor deficits may be

noticed in the lower limbs. In cauda equina syndrome (central disk herniation), saddle anesthesia and bladder or bowel incontinence may be present.
3. *Osteoarthritis of the hips and knees* causes discomfort in the area of the buttock, groin, thigh, or knee, typically worse with movement and alleviated by rest. Severe osteoarthritis may present with rest pain or nocturnal pain. Morning stiffness lasting less than 30 minutes is common. Knee instability or buckling while descending stairs or stepping off curbs may be noticed. The pain is usually localized to the affected joint and may be elicited by palpation and range-of-motion maneuvers. Crepitation or effusion may be present in the knee.
4. *Skeletal muscle disorders such as myositis* can cause exertional leg pain. Muscle tenderness, abnormal neuromuscular examination findings, elevated skeletal muscle enzymes, and a normal pulse examination should distinguish myositis from PAD.
5. *Chronic venous insufficiency* due to deep vein thrombosis may cause exertional leg pain (venous claudication) due to the rapid increase in venous pressure and congestion due to exercise-induced hyperemia and outflow obstruction. This is seen most commonly following iliofemoral venous thrombosis without adequate collateralization. Patients often experience aching sensations at rest and bursting cramps on ambulation. They may also have peripheral edema, venous stasis pigmentation, varicosities, ulcers, or lipodermatosclerosis (induration and scarring of the lower leg leading to a champagne-bottle deformity). The discomfort is relieved by frequent leg elevation, avoiding prolonged standing or sitting, and wearing graduated compression stockings.
6. *Chronic compartment syndrome* seen in young well-conditioned athletes may present as agonizing pain, tense swelling, paresthesias, or weakness of the calf or feet brought on by exercise or passive stretching of the muscles post-exercise and relieved by rest and elevation. Muscle swelling and increased osmotic pressure in an unyielding compartment result in decreased blood flow and acute myoneural ischemia. Foot drop may be

Table 39-1 Differential Diagnosis of Claudication

Vascular	Musculoskeletal	Neurologic
Atherosclerosis	Herniated disk	Lumbosacral radiculopathy
Thrombosis	Spinal canal stenosis	
Embolism	Osteoarthritis of hips or knees	Myositis
Thromboangiitis obliterans	Baker's cysts	Compartment syndrome
Arterial entrapment	Ligament/tendon injury	
Venous insufficiency		

From Lesho EP, Manngold J, Gey DC. Management of peripheral arterial disease. Am Fam Physician 2004;69:525–532.

present. The anterior compartment of the leg is most commonly involved (45%), followed closely by the deep posterior compartment (40%).

7. *Popliteal artery entrapment* is a rare cause of exercise-induced leg pain in young men. An abnormal relationship between the popliteal artery and the surrounding myofascial structures in the popliteal fossa results in entrapment and arterial insufficiency in the affected limb, causing leg symptoms with exertion.

8. *Buerger's disease* (thromboangiitis obliterans) occurs predominantly in young men of age 20 to 40 who smoke. It involves small- and medium-sized arteries and superficial veins of the extremities in a segmental pattern. Patients notice coldness, numbness, tingling, or burning of the involved extremity. Intermittent claudication of the foot or leg, rest pain, ulceration, or gangrene may occur.

Plan

Diagnostic Testing

John B. had normal blood counts and liver and kidney function tests. His total cholesterol was reported as 240 mg/dL, and low-density lipoprotein level was 148 mg/dL. Segmental pressure measurements showed a sharp drop in the right thigh and both legs and feet. The ABI measured 0.65 in the right thigh, 0.95 in the left thigh, and 0.5 in both legs and feet. An arteriogram showed some insignificant plaques in the aorta and both common iliac arteries, a 3-cm occlusion of the right external iliac artery, bilateral superficial femoral artery occlusions, normal popliteals, and three-vessel runoff in both legs.

Treatment

John B. was started on aspirin 81 mg/day and cilostazol (Pletal) 100 mg twice daily. He was advised to enter a smoking cessation program and to exercise on a treadmill 30 minutes daily at least three times per week or until claudication limited his exercise. He was also counseled about "eating right." Tight control of his sugars was recommended, and the doses of both the blood pressure and cholesterol medications were adjusted to aim for a target blood pressure of 130/80 and a low-density lipoprotein level lower than 100 mg/dL (Regensteiner and Hiatt, 2002Ⓑ).

FOLLOW-UP VISIT

When seen 6 weeks later, John B. was still smoking a pack daily. His claudication distance was decreasing, although he had not experienced any rest pain. Angioplasty was therefore advised, and he underwent an uneventful angioplasty and stenting of the right external iliac artery. Three months later, he underwent a femoropopliteal bypass on the left due

to worsening rest pain in his left lower limb. Unfortunately, the graft clotted, and he subsequently required a left above-knee amputation for spreading gangrene. He still continues to smoke, takes his medications indifferently, is not motivated to use his prosthesis, and is wheelchair bound.

DISCUSSION

PAD results from chronic narrowing of the distal abdominal aorta or iliac or lower extremity arteries. Most lesions in the lower limbs develop in the posterior aspects of the proximal portions of the major arteries, bifurcation sites, or specific areas of high atherogenesis (distal superficial femoral artery at the Hunter's canal) (Levy, 2002Ⓑ). An area of stenosis becomes hemodynamically significant at rest when the arterial diameter is reduced by greater than 80%. The clinical presentation of PAD ranges from asymptomatic stenosis to IC and CLI. Eight to 12 million people in the United States have PAD; its prevalence increases with age and affects 12% to 17% of those older than age 50 and almost 20% of people older than age 70. Many patients with PAD are asymptomatic. Less than half of patients with an abnormal ABI have IC.

Individuals with PAD have a reduced functional capacity, lower quality of life, an extremely high risk (sixfold) of cardiovascular morbidity and mortality, carotid artery stenosis, and cognitive dysfunction (Criqui et al., 1992Ⓐ).

Risk factors for PAD include smoking, diabetes mellitus, and hypertension (Table 39-2). Others include advancing age, family history, hyperlipidemia, renal dysfunction, previous myocardial infarction, heart failure or stroke, elevated homocysteine and C-reactive protein levels, and previous

Table 39-2 Risk Factors for Peripheral Arterial Disease
Smoking
Diabetes mellitus
Hypertension (systolic blood pressure)
Previous myocardial infarction, stroke, heart failure
Chronic renal insufficiency
Positive family history
Chronic infections
Age (~75 yr)
Fibrinogen level
African-American race
Hyperhomocysteinemia

From Regensteiner JG, Hiatt WR. Treatment of peripheral arterial disease. Clin Cornerstone 2002;4:26–40.

infections (pneumonia, chronic bronchitis, peptic ulcer, and periodontal infections). PAD has a higher prevalence in African Americans. The distribution of PAD is similar for men and women, although its frequency is much higher in women with diabetes mellitus. Smoking, diabetes mellitus, and hypertension have an additive effect on the risk of PAD.

Most patients with PAD are asymptomatic. Apart from IC (described previously), patients may present with persistent rest pain, nonhealing ulcers, or gangrene. Leriche syndrome refers to bilateral lower limb claudication and impotence due to aortoiliac occlusion. On examination, trophic changes (dry skin, thickened nails, and loss of hair and subcutaneous fat), ulcers, or gangrene may be noticed in the lower limbs. Ischemic ulcers are usually located on the plantar surface of the foot, over the first and fifth metatarsal heads. Peripheral pulses may be reduced or absent; bruits may be present over stenotic vessels (carotid, femoral, iliac).

The ABI (normal ≥ 1) is a simple, painless, highly reproducible test performed with a handheld, continuous-wave Doppler probe that compares the blood pressure obtained in the dorsalis pedis or posterior tibial artery (whichever is higher) with the higher of the two brachial artery pressures (Fig. 39-1). Resting ABI values less than 0.9 correlate well with 50% or greater stenosis of one or more major lower limb arteries. An ABI of 0.71 to 0.9 indicates mild PAD, 0.41 to 0.70, moderate PAD, and ABI less than 0.40 indicates severe PAD (Belch et al., 2003 Ⓑ). The ABI may be high if the vessels are calcified and incompressible (as in diabetes mellitus and renal failure) and does not define the site of the lesion or differentiate between stenosis and total occlusion. The ABI may be repeated after exercise (treadmill or

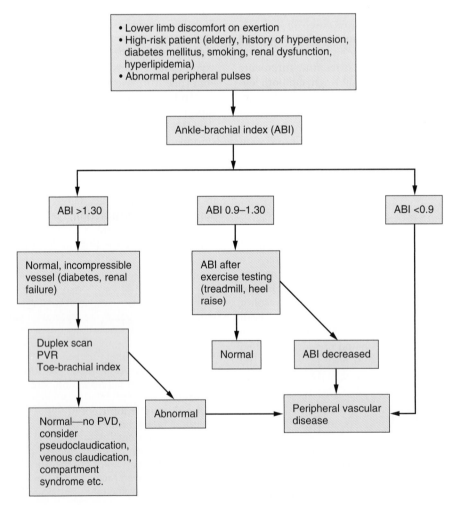

Figure 39-1 Evaluation of peripheral arterial disease. PVD, peripheral vascular disease; PVR, peripheral vascular resistance. (From Hiatt WR. Medical treatment for peripheral arterial disease and intermittent claudication. N Engl J Med 2001;344:1608–1621.)

heel raise) in symptomatic patients with a normal ABI at rest (Pellerito, 2001 Ⓑ).

Measurement of segmental lower limb pressures helps to localize the site of the PAD. A decrease in pressure between two consecutive levels (thigh, leg, or foot) of greater than 30 mm Hg suggests proximal arterial occlusive disease (Jaff, 2002 Ⓑ). Ultrasound duplex scanning detects arterial wall thickness, degree of stenosis, and changes in flow velocity and has higher sensitivity in detecting lesions in the more proximal arteries (iliac and superficial femoral). Peak systolic velocity determination and Doppler waveform analyses also help localize and quantify PAD. Significant PAD shows elevated peak systolic velocity, marked spectral broadening, and loss of diastolic reversal (Pellerito, 2001 Ⓑ). Transcutaneous measurement of oxygen tension denotes adequacy of tissue perfusion. Values greater than 40 mm Hg predict healing of foot ulcers or primary forefoot amputations; values less than 10 mm Hg are associated with failure to heal. Angiography is useful in defining the anatomy of the aorta, iliac arteries and their branches, and the peripheral arteries. Magnetic resonance angiography is a cost-effective, noninvasive alternative, as accurate and reliable as conventional angiography in imaging inflow vessels and grading stenosis severity. Using gadolinium minimizes contrast nephrotoxicity and enhances the accuracy of imaging.

The goals of treatment include relief of lower extremity symptoms, increasing functional walking capacity and quality of life, preventing the progression of disease and ulcer formation, and preservation of the limb (Brook et al., 2002 Ⓑ). Smoking cessation slows the progression of IC to CLI, reduces the need for revascularization, and improves graft patency (Hiatt, 2001 Ⓑ). Diabetics should maintain glycohemoglobin levels below 7% (Table 39-3). Blood pressure should be maintained at 130/80 to minimize cardiovascular morbidity and mortality. Low-density lipoprotein cholesterol levels should be reduced to lower than 100 mg/dL. Exercise programs improve oxygen consumption, skeletal muscle metabolism, and endothelial vasodilator function and reduce blood viscosity and ischemia (Regensteiner and Hiatt, 2002 Ⓑ). Sessions should last longer than 30 minutes and be carried out at least three times every week. Ideally the patient should walk until near-maximal pain is reached in each session, and the program should last at least 6 months. Aspirin, in doses between 81 and 325 mg/day, or clopidogrel 75 mg/day should be commenced (Fig. 39-2). Cilostazol, a phosphodiesterase 3 inhibitor, at 100 mg twice daily relieves IC, improves walking time and distance, and enhances of quality of life. Common side effects include headache, loose stools, and dizziness. It should not be administered to patients with heart failure of any severity or when the ejection fraction is less than 40%. Ticlopidine, another antiplatelet agent, is associated with serious hematologic side effects that preclude its use. Pentoxifylline (Trental), at a dose of 400 mg three times daily with meals, or naftidrofuryl (a serotonin antagonist) 100 to 200 mg three times daily are other options. Adequate pain control in CLI often requires narcotics. Feet are evaluated periodically to minimize trauma, and ulcers should be kept clean, infections

Table 39-3 Nonoperative Management Strategies for Peripheral Arterial Disease

Risk Factor	Goal	Treatment
Smoking	Cessation	Counseling; nicotine patch, gum, spray; bupropion
Hypertension	SBP ≤ 130/80	ACE inhibitors, β-blocker (if CAD, no rest pain or CLI)
Diabetes mellitus	Glycohemoglobin < 7.0%	Oral hypoglycemics, insulin, exercise, diet
Hyperlipidemia	LDL < 100 mg/dL	Statins ± niacin or fibric acid derivatives
Platelet aggregation	Antiplatelet therapy	Aspirin 81–325 mg/day Cilostazol 100 mg twice daily Clopidogrel 75 mg/day Pentoxyfilline 400 mg three times daily Naftidrofuryl 100–200 mg three times daily
Lack of exercise	Exercise therapy	30-min sessions at least three times per week until near-maximal pain is reached for 6 mo

ACE, angiotensin-converting enzyme; CAD, coronary artery disease; CLI, critical limb ischemia; LDL, low-density lipoprotein; SBP, systolic blood pressure.
From Regensteiner JG, Hiatt WR. Treatment of peripheral arterial disease. Clin Correstone 2002;4:26–40.

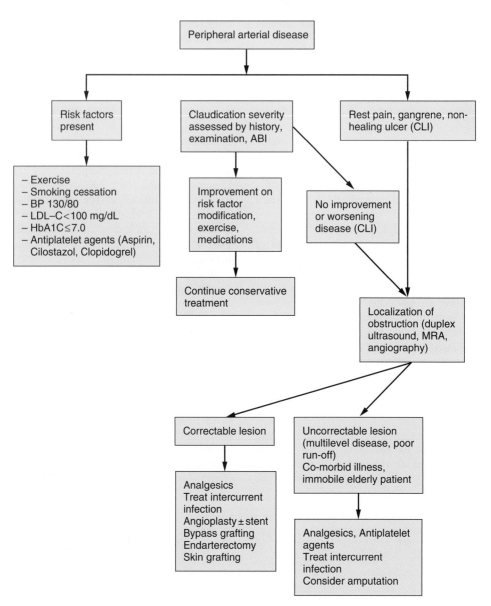

Figure 39-2 Treatment of peripheral arterial disease. ABI, ankle/brachial index; BP, blood pressure; CLI, critical limb ischemia; HbA1C, hemoglobin A$_{1c}$; LDL-C, low-density lipoprotein cholesterol; MRA, magnetic resonance angiography. (From Hiatt WR. Medical treatment for peripheral arterial disease and intermittent claudication. N Engl J Med 2001;344:1608–1621.)

treated, and ongoing pressure minimized (Rajagopalan and Grossman, 2002 Ⓑ).

Revascularization (endovascular or surgical) is reserved for short-distance IC, rest pain (CLI), non-healing ulcers, or threatened limb loss (Brook et al., 2002Ⓑ). Patients who exercise regularly derive the most benefit. Angioplasty with or without stenting for lower extremity ischemia is appropriate for short common iliac or femoropopliteal artery stenoses or occlusions. Surgical endarterectomy or bypass (aortoiliac, femoro-popliteal) is indicated in the presence of long-segment stenosis or occlusion, associated aneurysmal dilatation of the vessel, or lesions causing distal embolization and

benefits most patients (85%) with threatened limb loss (see Fig. 39-2). Continuing antiplatelet agents or oral anticoagulants postoperatively maximizes the patency of the reconstructed vessel or the bypass. The absence of patent distal vessels with a low ABI (<0.3) in the setting of CLI makes amputation inevitable (Rajagopalan and Grossman, 2002 Ⓑ).

Material Available on Student Consult

Review Questions and Answers about Peripheral Arterial Disease

REFERENCES

Belch JJF, Topol EJ, Agnelli G, et al. Critical issues in peripheral arterial disease detection and management: A call to action. Arch Intern Med 2003;163:884–892.**Ⓑ**

Brook RD, Weder AB, Grossman PM, Rajagopalan S. Management of intermittent claudication. Cardiol Clin 2002;20:521–534.**Ⓑ**

Criqui MH, Langer RD, Fronek A, et al. Mortality over a period of 10 years in patients with peripheral arterial disease. N Engl J Med 1992;326:381–386.**Ⓐ**

Hiatt WR. Medical treatment for peripheral arterial disease and intermittent claudication. N Engl J Med 2001;344:1608–1621.**Ⓑ**

Jaff MR. Lower extremity arterial disease: Diagnostic aspects. Cardiol Clin 2002;20:491–500.**Ⓑ**

Lesho EP, Manngold J, Gey DC. Management of peripheral arterial disease. Am Fam Physician 2004;69:525–532.**Ⓑ**

Levy PJ. Epidemiology and pathophysiology of peripheral arterial disease. Clin Cornerstone 2002;4:1–15.**Ⓑ**

Pellerito JS. Current approach to peripheral arterial sonography. Radiol Clin North Am 2001;39:553–567.**Ⓑ**

Rajagopalan S, Grossman PM. Management of chronic critical limb ischemia. Cardiol Clin 2002;20:535–545.**Ⓑ**

Regensteiner JG, Hiatt WR. Treatment of peripheral arterial disease. Clin Cornerstone 2002;4:26–40.**Ⓑ**

Chapter

40

Leg Pain and Swelling (Venous Thrombosis)

Jennifer DeVoe

KEY POINTS

1. Patients with deep vein thrombosis (DVT) (and/or pulmonary embolism [PE]) should be treated urgently with low-molecular-weight (LMW) heparin, unfractionated intravenous heparin, or adjusted-dose subcutaneous heparin.

2. Continue treatment with chosen heparin product for at least 5 days. Check a platelet count between day 3 and day 5 of therapy to monitor for heparin-induced thrombocytopenia. If the patient remains on heparin, check another platelet count between days 7 and 10, and another at day 14. Stop the heparin product if the patient experiences a precipitate or sustained decrease in the platelet count, or if the platelet count is less than 100,000/μL.

3. Overlap oral anticoagulation with the chosen heparin product for at least 4 to 5 days. Warfarin can usually be initiated simultaneously with the heparin. The heparin product can be discontinued on day 5 or 6 after at least two consecutive days of a therapeutic International Normalized Ratio (INR). (In a few cases, such as massive PE or severe iliofemoral thrombosis, continue heparin therapy for approximately 10 days.)

4. While the patient is taking warfarin, the INR target range should be 2.0 to 3.0. In some cases in which warfarin is contraindicated or not tolerated, LMW heparin or adjusted-dose unfractionated heparin can be continued.

5. The use of thrombolytic agents requires further investigation.

6. Consider inferior vena caval filter placement in some individuals who are unable to take long-term anticoagulant therapy or in patients with recurrent thromboembolism despite adequate anticoagulation.

7. If a first thromboembolic event is due to a reversible or time-limited factor, continue anticoagulation therapy for at least 3 months. Until recently, a first idiopathic event was usually treated for 3 to 6 months. Several trials now

Continued

Evidence levels Ⓐ Randomized, controlled trials (RCTs), meta-analyses, well-designed systematic reviews of RCTs. **Ⓑ** Case-control or cohort studies, nonrandomized clinical trials, systematic reviews of studies other than RCTs, cross-sectional studies, retrospective studies, certain uncontrolled studies. **Ⓒ** Consensus statements, expert guidelines, usual practice, opinion.

KEY POINTS (Continued)

suggest that prolonged anticoagulation is beneficial in patients with a first idiopathic thromboembolic event (Kearon et al., 2003 Ⓐ; Ridker et al., 2003 Ⓐ; Schulman et al., 2003 Ⓐ). No clear guidance has yet emerged as to the optimal length of time for anticoagulation, but suggested length has been extended to 6 to 12 months in most recent writings. However, treatment decisions must still take into account the unique factors present in each individual case.

8. Prolonged anticoagulation, for at least 12 months, also appears to be beneficial in second cases (Ridker et al., 2003 Ⓐ). Indefinite anticoagulation is recommended for patients with three or more episodes or earlier in some patients with confirmed thrombophilias who have had massive or unusual clots.

9. Use caution in treating cancer patients with anticoagulant therapy, which is associated with both benefit and a high rate of complications.

10. In patients who will be at risk for developing a clot (e.g., surgery, prolonged immobilization), remember to consider primary prophylaxis with either anticoagulant medications or physical methods (e.g., intermittent pneumatic compression) that are effective for preventing DVT.

INITIAL VISIT

Subjective

Patient Identification and Presenting Problem
Mrs. Val B. is a 70-year-old woman who is seen in the clinic with left leg pain and swelling.

Present Illness
Val reports that she started noticing swelling in her left leg 2 nights ago. She initially thought it was due to standing on her feet for several hours while volunteering at the fair. Despite elevating her feet and staying off her leg yesterday, she noticed that the swelling persisted and that her leg was more painful. It is now warmer than her right leg and seems to be showing some discoloration. She has not taken any recent airplane flights or experienced a long period of immobilization. She has never used hormone replacement therapy. She denies acute shortness of breath or hemoptysis; however, she has had dyspnea on exertion over the past 4 months, especially while going up one flight of stairs. She also reports a chronic cough productive of clear sputum. She has a 100-pack-year smoking history and is currently trying to quit.

Medical History
Her history is significant for coronary artery disease, and she is status post myocardial infarction and stent placement in the left anterior descending artery in 1999. She has occasional angina and palpitations with exertion, relieved with nitroglycerin. She also has chronic obstructive pulmonary disease, managed with daily inhalers, occasional nebulizer treatments, and steroid bursts; however, she does not require supplemental oxygen. Her gastroesophageal reflux disease responds well to a proton-pump inhibitor. She also has osteoporosis and hypercholesteremia. She denies any history of blood clots or stroke.

Surgical History
Mrs. B. had a total abdominal hysterectomy at age 58 years.

Medications
She is using ipratropium + albuterol (Combivent) metered-dose inhaler, fluticasone + salmeterol (Advair Diskus), albuterol (Ventolin) nebulizer as needed, isosorbide mononitrate (Imdur), aspirin, atorvastatin (Lipitor), lisinopril (Zestril), alendronate (Fosamax), and esomeprazole (Nexium).

Habits
She has smoked two packs of cigarettes per day for the past 50 years.

Family History
Val's father had coronary artery disease and died of a myocardial infarction at age 72 years, and her two younger brothers have coronary artery disease. Her mother died of colon cancer at age 65 years. Her daughter and son currently have no health problems. No family history is known of blood clots or stroke.

Social History
Mrs. B. was born and raised in Washington State and is a retired dairy farmer. She recently moved into town to be closer to her daughter. Her husband is currently dying of lung cancer.

Review of Systems
Mrs. B. has had occasional nausea, vomiting, and diarrhea over the past 7 months since her husband's cancer diagnosis. She reports a 5-pound weight loss over that same time period. The patient also

reports frequent postnasal drip and sinus congestion. She denies fevers, chills, headaches, bladder changes, arthralgias, or myalgias.

Objective

Physical Examination

General Mrs. B. is a well-nourished, well-developed woman sitting comfortably in the chair, breathing comfortably, and in no acute distress, speaking in full sentences. She has notable kyphosis.

Vital Signs

Blood pressure, 110/70
Heart rate, 90
Respirations, 16
Height, 61 inches
Weight, 99 pounds
O_2 saturation, 96% on room air

Head, Eyes, Ears, Nose, and Throat Pupils are equal, round, and reactive to light and accommodation. Extraocular movements are intact. Sclerae are noninjected and anicteric. Tympanic membranes are clear bilaterally. Nares and oropharynx are mildly erythematous with no exudate.

Lungs Good breath sounds are present bilaterally. She has a prolonged expiratory phase and an occasional wheeze.

Cardiovascular Regular rate and rhythm are noted without audible murmur.

Abdomen Bowel sounds are normoactive. The abdomen is soft and nondistended, with no ascites or hepatosplenomegaly.

Genitourinary No pelvic masses are palpated.

Rectal No rectal masses are palpated; stool is light brown and guaiac negative.

Extremities No clubbing or cyanosis is seen. Ipsilateral calf swelling is noted (left calf circumference measures 4 cm larger than the right calf), with mild erythema and warmth. A 3+ pitting edema is found up to the left tibial tuberosity, with no edema in the right leg. Tenderness appears on deep palpation of the left calf muscles, with no palpable cord. Equivocal Homan's sign is noted. The legs are warm and well perfused, with symmetrical 2+ distal arterial pulses. No skin vesicles or open sores are seen.

Initial Laboratory and Radiology Examination

Mrs. B.'s initial laboratory evaluation includes a normal complete blood count, normal serum chemistries including liver- and renal-function tests,

and a normal urinalysis. Her coagulation studies (including prothrombin time, activated partial thromboplastin time, and D-dimer) are all normal, except an elevated D-dimer of 1500 ng/mL by enzyme-linked immunosorbent assay. Chest radiograph shows no elevation of the hemidiaphragm, infiltrate, or effusion; lung parenchyma is consistent with severe emphysema.

Recent Studies

Pulmonary-function tests 6 months ago: FEV_1 of 1.01, 52% of predicted value; FVC, 2.32, 93% of predicted value, with a ratio of 4.3. After bronchodilators, FEV_1 increased to 1.13, 58% predicted value, and FVC, to 2.58, or 103% of predicted value. Mammogram 6 months ago: negative. Colonoscopy 2 years ago: negative.

Assessment

Working Diagnosis

Ipsilateral lower extremity edema, possibly due to deep vein thrombosis (DVT).

Differential Diagnosis

A wide differential diagnosis exists for lower extremity edema associated with warmth, redness, and pain (Landaw, 2004 Ⓐ). Table 40-1 outlines some of the most common causes.

Plan

When evaluating a patient with possible DVT, a pretest probability scoring system can be a helpful guide in the diagnostic process. A score devised by Wells and colleagues is commonly used (Wells et al., 1997 Ⓑ; Wells et al., 2003 Ⓐ). Table 40-2 summarizes the features of this pretest probability score and how it applies to Mrs. B.

Diagnostic

In this case, Mrs. B. has a pretest probability score of 4, indicating a high clinical probability of DVT, so Doppler compression ultrasonography of the lower extremities is immediately performed. Her ultrasound reveals a large DVT in the left lower extremity. Although she does not have acute respiratory symptoms, she does have concerning dyspnea on exertion and a positive D-dimer. It is important to rule out a pulmonary embolism. A helical computed tomography (CT) scan is negative for pulmonary embolism or evidence of malignancy but confirms significant emphysema. Because she is older than 50 years with an idiopathic first episode of venous thrombosis and no family history, she is considered to be "weakly thrombophilic" and will be advised to undergo a limited screening for inherited hypercoagulable conditions including activated protein C resistance, prothrombin mutation, antiphospholipid antibodies, and plasma homocysteine. If a DVT had developed

Table 40-1 Differential Diagnosis for Unilateral Lower Extremity Edema

1. *Popliteal (Baker's) cyst.* A popliteal cyst usually causes calf symptoms when it is leaking or has ruptured. Leg swelling can occur when the popliteal vein is compressed and may ultimately result in a DVT.
2. *Knee injury.* Pain, inflammation, and swelling of the calf can accompany knee joint pathology.
3. *Drug-induced edema.* Some drugs, such as calcium channel blockers, cause leg swelling. Although the edema is usually bilateral, it can be asymmetric, especially when there is underlying venous pathology.
4. *Calf muscle pull or tear.* Calf muscle injuries are frequently sustained during unusual physical activity. Ecchymosis may be present as a sign of bleeding within muscle compartments of the affected leg.
5. *Superficial thrombophlebitis.* It is common to find a palpable, tender cord in superficial vein phlebitis.
6. *Venous valvular insufficiency.* Chronic venous insufficiency can cause unilateral leg edema, especially when there is a past history of DVT in the affected extremity.
7. *Lymphedema.* Lymphedema also causes chronic edema of the extremities and can be unilateral in some cases.
8. *Cellulitis.* Cellulitis is commonly associated with edema, warmth, pain, and discoloration.

From Landaw SA. Approach to the diagnosis and therapy of suspected deep vein thrombosis: UpToDate. Available at www.uptodate.com, last revised May 14, 2004. Accessed October 5, 2004.

before age 50 years, if she had a recurrent DVT or a family history of thromboembolic disease or both, additional tests would be recommended to check for deficiencies of antithrombin, protein C, and protein S (Bauer, 2001❸). Although her cancer screening tests have recently been negative and her chest CT scan did not show evidence of malignancy, any DVT recurrence will warrant a further malignancy workup.

Therapeutic

Mrs. B. is started on low-molecular-weight heparin subcutaneous injections (1 mg/kg twice daily) and warfarin (Coumadin) oral therapy (5 mg daily, orally). Her heparin will be discontinued after approximately 5 days, when her International Normalized Ratio (INR) of prothrombin clotting time exceeds 2.0.

Patient Education

Mrs. B. is instructed about the three primary goals of treatment for DVTs: (1) to stop clot propagation in the leg, (2) to stop embolic disease to the lungs, and

Table 40-2 Wells Revised Model for Determining Pretest Probability of Deep Vein Thrombosis (DVT)		
Clinical Feature	**Score***	**Does Mrs. B. Have This Clinical Feature?**
Active cancer (treatment within past 6 months or current palliative treatment)	1	No
Paralysis, paresis, or recent plaster immobilization of the lower extremity	1	No
Recently bedridden for more than 3 days or major surgery within the past 12 weeks	1	No
Localized tenderness along the distribution of the deep venous system	1	Yes
Entire leg swollen	1	Yes
Calf swollen to more than 3 cm larger than the asymptomatic side (measured 10 cm below tibial tuberosity)	1	Yes
Pitting edema confined to the symptomatic leg	1	Yes
Collateral superficial veins (nonvaricose)	1	No
Previously documented deep-vein thrombosis	1	No
Alternative diagnosis at least as likely as deep-vein thrombosis	−2	No
Mrs. B.'s Score*	4	

*A score greater than or equal to 2 indicates a high probability of DVT; a score less than 2 indicates that DVT is unlikely.
Data from Wells PS, Anderson DR, Rodger M, et al. Evaluation of D-dimer in the diagnosis of suspected deep vein thrombosis. N Engl J Med 2003;349:1227–1235.

(3) to prevent DVT recurrence. Mrs. B. is told that a recent evidence-based guideline recommends that she remain on anticoagulation therapy for 6 to 12 months (Hyers et al., 2001 ❹). She is counseled regarding smoking cessation.

Disposition

Mrs. B. will make regular visits to the anticoagulation clinic for warfarin dosing to keep her INR between 2.0 and 3.0. A visiting nurse will administer her low-molecular-weight heparin twice-daily injections for at least 5 days. She will have a follow-up physician visit in 2 to 3 days. She is instructed to return immediately if signs or symptoms of pulmonary embolism develop, such as acute shortness of breath, tachypnea, tachycardia, distended neck veins, or hemoptysis.

DISCUSSION

DVT falls within the spectrum of venous thromboembolic disease, which includes both DVT and pulmonary embolism (PE). In people younger than 60 years, the annual incidence of venous thromboembolism is 117 cases per 100,000 persons. By age 85 years, the incidence may be as high as 900 cases per 100,000 (Ramzi and Leeper, 2004a Ⓐ). Improved diagnostic strategies and treatment guidelines have contributed to a significant decrease in mortality from venous thromboembolic disease in the past 10 to 20 years (Ramzi and Leeper, 2004b Ⓐ). When faced with a patient who has a suspected DVT or PE or both, clinicians must consider the best approaches to diagnosis, evaluation, and treatment.

Diagnosis

In diagnosing DVT, a careful history and physical examination must first be performed. Several common risk factors should be addressed when taking a history, including recent surgery or immobilization, previous history of DVT, malignancy, stroke, estrogen therapy, lower extremity trauma, pregnancy or postpartum state, and obesity. Classic symptoms of DVT include swelling, pain, and discoloration in the involved extremity. Physical examination may reveal a palpable cord (reflecting a thrombosed vein), ipsilateral edema, erythema, warmth, superficial venous dilation, or a combination of these (Ramzi and Leeper, 2004a Ⓐ). Examination maneuvers, such as Homan's sign, can be done but are not highly sensitive or specific. Because of the inaccuracies of physical examination, at least one imaging study is generally indicated to confirm or exclude the diagnosis (Hirsh and Lee, 2002).

Contrast venography is the "gold standard" for the diagnosis of DVT (Hull et al., 1981 Ⓑ). However, venography is usually not the initial diagnostic study performed because of patient discomfort and difficulty in obtaining an adequate study. In one study comparing venography with noninvasive studies, venography could not be performed in 20% of cases because of contraindications or technical factors (Heijboer et al., 1992 Ⓑ). Although several combinations of noninvasive studies are acceptable, Doppler ultrasonography is usually the first-line noninvasive diagnostic procedure for patients with suspected DVT. Compression ultrasonography has a positive

predictive value of 94% (95% confidence interval, 87% to 98%) (Cogo et al., 1998 Ⓑ). If an initial ultrasound study is negative and the clinical suspicion of DVT is high, a repeat study should be obtained 5 to 7 days later. If results from the second study are equivocal, venography can be used.

Several algorithms have been developed to diagnose DVT accurately by using a clinical pretest probability and noninvasive imaging. Recently, algorithms have been revised to include D-dimer laboratory analysis, when available and reliable. D-Dimer is a degradation product of cross-linked fibrin that is detectable at levels greater than 500 ng/mL of fibrinogen equivalent units in nearly all patients with venous thromboembolism. A positive D-dimer cannot establish the diagnosis of venous thromboembolism because it is nonspecific and commonly elevated in many patients hospitalized for other conditions. The highly sensitive D-dimer test is useful to rule-out DVT because of its high negative predictive value in cases in which DVT is unlikely. A recent systematic review assessed the sensitivity, specificity, likelihood ratios, and variability among D-dimer assays (Stein et al., 2004Ⓐ). Enzyme-linked immunosorbent assays (ELISA) and quantitative rapid ELISA are the most clinically useful because they have the highest sensitivities (0.96 for both) and negative likelihood ratios (0.12 and 0.09, respectively) for excluding DVT. A negative quantitative rapid ELISA result is as diagnostically useful as a negative duplex ultrasound for excluding DVT, especially in patients with a low pretest probability. In contrast, whole-blood agglutination and quantitative and semi-quantitative latex agglutination assays had lower sensitivities.

Two additional noninvasive studies have shown promise: magnetic resonance venography and lower extremity CT scans; however, these diagnostic studies are still under active investigation. Figure 40-1 outlines a summary of one common diagnostic algorithm.

Evaluation

Once a diagnosis of DVT is made and treatment is initiated, the second step is to conduct an evaluation of possible causes. The thrombophilic state that leads to a DVT can be inherited or acquired. In some acquired cases, the etiology can be easily identified, such as immobilization after surgery or long airplane trips. Other acquired causes, such as malignancy and the inherited conditions usually require further investigation. An extensive evaluation for malignancy should be undertaken if a patient has a recurrent thrombosis or has abnormal clinical findings. In selected subsets of patients in whom no obvious acquired cause is evident, a screen for hereditary thrombophilias should be performed. The likelihood

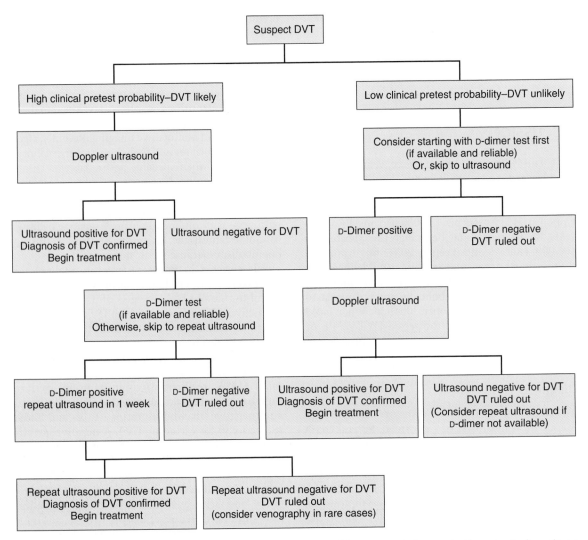

Figure 40-1 New suggested diagnostic algorithm for patients with suspected deep vein thrombosis, by using a D-dimer laboratory test. DVT, deep vein thrombosis.

of identifying a coagulation abnormality in appropriate screening has been estimated to be as high as 30% to 40% (Bauer and Lip, 2004Ⓐ).

No consensus exists on thrombophilia screening guidelines; however, most recommendations are based on the prevalence of inherited causes of hypercoagulability and the patient's history. If an acquired cause is identified, it is usually not necessary to screen unless the thrombosis occurs in association with oral contraceptive use or pregnancy; in unusual vascular beds such as portal, hepatic, mesenteric, or cerebral or in patients with a history of warfarin-induced skin necrosis (Bauer and Lip, 2004Ⓐ). A "strongly" thrombophilic patient has a first idiopathic venous thrombosis before age 50 years, a history of recurrent thromboses, or at least one first-degree relative with

thromboembolism before age 50 years. A "weakly" thrombophilic patient has no family history and a first thrombophilic event after age 50 years. In both strong and weak patients, screening tests should be done for activated protein C resistance, prothrombin mutation, antiphospholipid antibodies, and plasma homocysteine. Additional tests for deficiencies of antithrombin, protein C, and protein S are recommended only for individuals who fall into the strongly thrombophilic category (Bauer, 2001 Ⓑ).

Once screening tests have been chosen, it is important to be aware of timing considerations. Acute thrombosis, comorbid illness, and anticoagulant therapy can affect the results; therefore confirmative testing should be done at least 2 weeks after completion of anticoagulant therapy.

Treatment

Most treatment protocols follow evidence-based recommendations that were put forth at the Sixth American College of Chest Physicians Consensus Conference on Antithrombotic Therapy and published in January 2001 (Lip and Hull, 2004 ◎). Since the publication of these recommendations, guidelines for the patient with a first idiopathic venous thromboembolic event have been revised (Hirsh et al., 2003).

Material Available on Student Consult

Review Questions and Answers about Venous Thrombosis

REFERENCES

Bauer KA, Lip GYH. Evaluation of the patient with established venous thrombosis. Available at www.uptodate.com, last revised May 14, 2004. Accessed October 5, 2004.◎

Bauer KA. The thrombophilias: Well-defined risk factors with uncertain therapeutic implications. Ann Intern Med 2001;135:367–373.◎

Cogo A, Lensing AW, Koopman MM, et al. Compression ultrasonography for diagnostic management of patients with clinically suspected deep venous thrombosis: Prospective cohort study. BMJ 1998;316:17–20.◎

Heijboer H, Cogo A, Buller HR, Prandoni P, ten Cate JW. Detection of deep vein thrombosis with impedance plethysmography and real-time compression ultrasonography in hospitalized patients. Arch Intern Med 1992;152:1901–1903.◎

Hirsh J, Fuster V, Ansell J, Halperin JL. American Heart Association/American College of Cardiology Foundation guide to warfarin therapy. J Am Coll Cardiol 2003;41:1633–1652.

Hirsh J, Lee AY. How we diagnose and treat deep vein thrombosis. Blood 2002;99:3102–3110.

Hull RD, Hirsh J, Sackett DL, et al. Clinical validity of a negative venogram in patients with clinically suspected venous thrombosis. Circulation 1981;64:622–625.◎

Hyers TM, Agnelli G, Hull RD, et al. Antithrombotic therapy for venous thromboembolic disease. Chest 2001;119:176S–193S.◎

Kearon C, Ginsberg JS, Kovacs MJ, et al. Comparison of low-intensity warfarin therapy with conventional-intensity warfarin therapy for long-term prevention of recurrent venous thromboembolism. N Engl J Med 2003;349:631–639.◎

Landaw SA. Approach to the diagnosis and therapy of suspected deep vein thrombosis: UpToDate. Available at www.uptodate.com, last revised May 14, 2004. Accessed October 5, 2004.◎

Lip GYH, Hull RD. Treatment of deep vein thrombosis: UpToDate. Available at www.uptodate.com, last revised May 13, 2004. Accessed October 5, 2004.◎

Ramzi DW, Leeper KV. DVT and pulmonary embolism: Part I: Diagnosis. Am Fam Physician 2004a;69:2829–2836.◎

Ramzi DW, Leeper KV. DVT and pulmonary embolism: Part II: Treatment and prevention. Am Fam Physician 2004b;69:2841–2848.◎

Ridker PM, Goldhaber SZ, Danielson E, et al. Long-term, low-intensity warfarin therapy for the prevention of recurrent venous thromboembolism. N Engl J Med 2003;348:1425–1434.◎

Schulman S, Wahlander K, Lundstrom T, Clason SB, Eriksson H. Secondary prevention of venous thromboembolism with the oral direct thrombin inhibitor ximelagatran. N Engl J Med 2003;349:1713–1721.◎

Stein PD, Hull RD, Patel KC, et al. D-Dimer for the exclusion of acute venous thrombosis and pulmonary embolism: A systematic review. Ann Intern Med 2004;140:589–602.◎

Wells PS, Anderson DR, Bormanis J, et al. Value of assessment of pretest probability of deep-vein thrombosis in clinical management. Lancet 1997;350:1795–1798.◎

Wells PS, Anderson DR, Rodger M, et al. Evaluation of D-dimer in the diagnosis of suspected deep vein thrombosis. N Engl J Med 2003;349:1227–1235.◎

41 Tiredness (Anemia)

Paul Paulman

KEY POINTS

1. Anemia should be considered not a primary diagnosis, but a marker for other disease processes.
2. The most common symptoms of anemia are dyspnea with exertion, weakness, headache, lethargy, and palpitation.
3. Most causes of anemia can be determined in a primary care office through history, physical examination, and judicious use of standard laboratory tests.

INITIAL VISIT

Subjective

Patient Identification and Presenting Problem

Sandy is a 64-year-old white American woman who appears for an office visit with the complaint of "just feeling tired."

Present Illness

Sandy has been fatigued for more than 12 months with gradual worsening. Her husband states that she "looks pale." She has had no depressive symptoms and no symptoms to suggest a sleep disorder. She has had no wheezing or chest pain but does become dyspneic after climbing two flights of stairs. No changes have occurred in her diet; she eats a "standard American diet." She has no history of thyroid disease and no nausea, vomiting, or diarrhea. She has had no blood loss and no fevers, chills, or joint pain.

Medical History

Operations Abdominal hysterectomy 4 years ago for postmenopausal bleeding, no endometrial hyperplasia or malignancies were found.

Allergies No medication or seasonal allergies are present.

Illnesses Hyperlipidemia, postmenopausal bleeding, mild arthritis in both knees.

Hospitalizations She had two normal vaginal deliveries and a hysterectomy.

Medications She is taking atorvastatin (Lipitor), 10 mg/day, glucocosamine and chondroitin sulfate, aspirin (81 mg/day), and over-the-counter vitamins with iron.

Family and Social History

Sandy is a vice president in charge of operations at a local telemarketing firm. She is married, with two children and two grandchildren. She does not smoke or use illicit drugs and drinks less than one alcoholic beverage per day on average. She exercises 30 minutes aerobically per day. Sandy's parents were first-generation immigrants from Sweden. The family history is positive for thyroid disease (mother) and colon cancer (father). No family history is known of anemia, depression, sleep disorders, collagen vascular disease, breast cancer, or arthritis.

Review of Systems

Sandy denies any blood loss, pain, nausea, vomiting, fever, chills, or diarrhea. She has not had any heat or cold intolerance. She has had no cough or headache and has not been exposed to tuberculosis or other infectious diseases. No one else at her workplace has

Evidence levels Ⓐ Randomized, controlled trials (RCTs), meta-analyses, well-designed systematic reviews of RCTs. Ⓑ Case-control or cohort studies, nonrandomized clinical trials, systematic reviews of studies other than RCTs, cross-sectional studies, retrospective studies, certain uncontrolled studies. Ⓒ Consensus statements, expert guidelines, usual practice, opinion.

experienced similar symptoms. She has not used new herbal or over-the-counter preparations. She has had no changes in her sleep patterns and has not experienced any emotional trauma or family discord. She denies loss of appetite or feelings of sadness.

Objective

Physical Examination
Vital Signs
Height, 66 inches
Weight, 148 pounds
Blood pressure, 126/62 mm Hg
Pulse, 102 and regular
Temperature, 98.2°F (36.8°C) (oral)
Respirations, 16 per minute, unlabored

General Alert, very pleasant and cooperative, well oriented.

Integument Marked pallor, no rashes.

Lymph No adenopathy.

Head, Eyes, Ears, Nose, and Throat Palpebral conjunctivae are pale; otherwise no abnormalities.

Neck Trachea midline, thyroid not palpable, carotids full.

Lungs Clear.

Heart Tachycardia; regular and rhythmic with no murmurs or rubs.

Breasts No masses, tenderness, or nipple discharge.

Neurologic Mild decrease in vibratory sense in both lower extremities.

Abdomen Soft, normoactive bowel sounds, with no masses, tenderness, or organomegaly.

Pelvic Normal external genitalia, vagina normal, cervix and uterus surgically absent, adnexa not palpable, no masses. Stool test negative for blood.

Extremities Loss of color in palmar creases with no clubbing, cyanosis, or edema.

Laboratory Tests
Office laboratory hemoglobin level is 5.4 g/dL. A stat complete blood count (CBC) run at the hospital shows a hemoglobin of 5.3 g/dL with macrocyctic indices, a white blood cell (WBC) level of 7200/μL, and adequate platelets. A thyroid-stimulating hormone, complete metabolic profile including electrolytes, B_{12} level, red blood cell (RBC) and serum folate levels, and intrinsic factor antibody assay are pending.

Assessment

Working Diagnosis
Macrocytic anemia. Given Sandy's age, symptom complex, including the gradual onset of symptoms, the hemoglobin level, and her ethnic background, pernicious anemia (B_{12} deficiency) must be considered.

Differential Diagnosis
1. *Alcoholism.* Alcohol has direct toxic effects on bone marrow and can decrease red cell folic acid, leading to a macrocytic anemia. Sandy has no history of excessive or problematic alcohol intake.
2. *Medications.* Several medications, most notably anticonvulsants, antineoplastics, oral contraceptives, and sulfa-derived medications, can cause macrocytic anemia. None of Sandy's medications have been closely associated with macrocytic anemia.
3. *Thyroid disorders.* Hypothyroidism causes a decrease in red cell production and can affect release of erythropoietin from the kidneys. Sandy has no symptoms to suggest a thyroid disorder.
4. *Liver disease.* Hepatic dysfunction also can affect erythropoietin release, as well as disrupting iron metabolism. Sandy has no symptoms of liver disease.
5. *Bone marrow disorders.* Primary bone marrow disorders, including marrow replacement and malignancies, can cause a macrocytic anemia. The presence of a normal WBC and platelet count makes a bone marrow disorder unlikely.
6. *Folic acid deficiency.* Because of the relatively low level of folic acid reserves in the human body (4 to 5 months' supply), folic acid deficiency is a common cause of macrocytic anemia. Folic acid deficiency can occur because of increased requirement (pregnancy, malignancy, hemodialysis, or decreased absorption or intake of folic acid [e.g., malabsorptive syndromes, alcoholism, or eating disorder]). Sandy has no symptoms suggestive of conditions causing folic acid deficiency.

Plan and Treatment

Sandy is hospitalized for monitored transfusion of 2 units of packed red blood cells after blood has been drawn for diagnostic studies.

Patient Education

Causes of macrocytic anemia and risks and benefits of transfusion were discussed with Sandy.

Disposition

Sandy was discharged to home the following morning with a hemoglobin of 8.8 g/dL and was asked to return to the office in 3 days for laboratory results and further treatment. She is instructed in home fecal occult blood testing and given three test cards.

FOLLOW-UP VISIT

Subjective

Sandy returns to the office in 3 days and reports that she feels much better. Her exercise tolerance has improved. She experienced no problems with the transfusion.

Objective

Sandy's tachycardia (heart rate, 72 beats/min) and her pallor have improved. No other major changes in her physical examination were found. Her hemoglobin is 8.6 g/dL; her thyroid stimulating hormone (TSH) is 2.1 in mIU/L (normal range, 0.4 to 5.0 mIU/L); her metabolic profile is normal, serum folic acid level is 10 μg/L (normal range, 5.0 to 25 μg/L), red blood cell folic acid level is 310 μg/L (normal range, 166 to 690 μg/L), B_{12} level is 35 mg/L (normal range, 200 to 800 mg/L), intrinsic factor antibody assay is positive (normal value, negative). All three fecal occult blood tests are negative.

Assessment

Sandy has pernicious anemia (vitamin B_{12} deficiency).

Plan

After discussing treatment options, Sandy chose weekly intramuscular injections of 1000 μg of vitamin B_{12} for 4 weeks, followed by 1000 μg of vitamin B_{12} orally every day. She will return to the office in 2 weeks for hemoglobin and vitamin B_{12} levels.

DISCUSSION

Anemia is a common problem seen in primary care practices, and the most common cause of anemia is iron deficiency. Anemia is an absolute or relative reduction of hemoglobin or red blood cells (RBCs). Normal hemoglobin values are listed by age and gender in Table 41-1. Anemias are classified by RBC size

Table 41-1 Normal Hemoglobin Values

Age	Male	Female
Newborn	15.0–21 g/dL	15.0–21.0 g/dL
3 months	9.5–12.5 g/dL	9.5–12.5 g/dL
1 year to		
puberty	11.0–13.5 g/dL	11.0–13.5 g/dL
Adults	13.5–17.5 mg/dL	11.5–15.5 g/dL

(microcytic, normocytic, or macrocytic) and can be caused by decreased RBC production, increased RBC destruction, an increase in plasma volume (Table 41-2), or a combination of causes. Anemia should not be considered a primary diagnosis, but rather a sign of nutritional deficiency (e.g., iron, folate, B_{12}) or other pathologic processes (e.g., microcytic anemia is often seen in elderly patients with colon cancer). The signs and symptoms seen in anemia are caused by decreased delivery of oxygen to peripheral tissues, or by the deficiency of the nutrient causing the anemia.

Signs and Symptoms of Anemia

Mild anemia may cause few or no symptoms. The most common symptoms of anemia are dyspnea with exertion, weakness, headache, lethargy, and palpitations. Older patients may experience angina pectoris, heart failure, claudication, confusion, or retinal hemorrhage. Physical signs include pallor of the skin or mucous membranes, tachycardia, systolic heart

Table 41-2 Common Causes of Anemia

Decreased RBC Production	Increased RBC Destruction	Increased Plasma Volume
Iron deficiency (microcytic)	Hemolytic anemias (normocytic)	Pregnancy (normocytic)
Sideroblastic (microcytic)		
Thalassemias (microcytic)		
Lead poisoning (microcytic)		
Anemia of chronic disorders (normocytic or microcytic)		
Vitamin B_{12} or folate deficiency (macrocytic)		
Bone marrow failure (normocytic)		

murmur, jaundice, or loss of color of the palmar flexion creases (if the hemoglobin level is 7 g/dL or less). The severity of signs and symptoms of anemia depends on the degree and rapidity of onset of the anemia and the age and the general medical condition of the patient. Sandy exhibited weakness, dyspnea on exertion, skin pallor, loss of color of palmar creases, and tachycardia as manifestation of her anemia. Her neurologic findings in her lower extremities are likely due to her B_{12} deficiency.

Causes of Anemia

Anemia Due to Decreased Production of RBCs

Sideroblastic Anemia Sideroblastic anemia is characterized by hypochromic RBCs, increased marrow iron, and ringed sideroblasts in the bone marrow. Ringed sideroblasts are abnormal erythroblasts with iron granules surrounding the nucleus. Sideroblastic anemia can be hereditary, caused by a defect in heme synthesis, or acquired from bone marrow dysfunction or replacement. Some patients with hereditary sideroblastic anemia respond to pyridoxine therapy. Folic acid therapy also is recommended. In acquired sideroblastic anemia, treatment is aimed at correcting the cause of the bone marrow failure. For some patients, the only treatment is repeated blood transfusions, sometimes resulting in iron overload requiring chelation therapy. Erythropoietin has been used in some cases of sideroblastic anemia.

Thalassemia The thalassemias (alpha and beta) are a group of genetic disorders characterized by a reduced rate of production of α- or β-globin chains. The severity of the disease is dependent on the number of genes affected. Thalassemia is seen most commonly in patients from the "thalassemia belt" (southern Europe, northern Africa, the Middle East, Indian subcontinent, and Southeast Asia, including Indonesia). Patients with thalassemia are first seen with microcytic hypochromic RBCs with or without anemia, depending on the severity of the genetic defect. Hemoglobin electrophoresis is usually required to make the diagnosis. Treatment depends on the severity of the illness and is aimed at maintaining the hemoglobin at 10 g/dL or more. Treatment modalities include regular blood transfusions (with iron chelation if iron overload occurs), folic acid supplementation, splenectomy if hemolysis is a problem, and bone marrow transplantation in very severe cases (Schrier, 1994 Ⓐ).

Lead Poisoning Lead causes a microcytic hypochromic anemia by inhibiting heme and globin synthesis. Children are at highest risk for lead poisoning from various sources including ingestion of lead-containing paint chips. Signs and symptoms of lead

poisoning include pallor, abdominal pains, irritability followed by lethargy, anorexia, ataxia, slurred speech, and convulsions. Laboratory findings include basophilic stippling of RBCs, elevated lead level, and elevated free erythrocyte protoporphyrin level. The treatment of lead poisoning consists of removing the source of exposure and removal of lead through chelation when clinically indicated. Because lead poisoning is very widespread, screening is recommended for any child at risk for lead exposure and for any child who demonstrates cognitive, language, or learning deficits.

Anemia of Chronic Disorders A number of chronic infections, connective tissue diseases, renal failure, and malignancies can cause a microcytic hypochromic anemia by blocking erythropoietin response, decreasing RBC life span, and decreasing iron release from macrophages. The characteristics of anemia of chronic disorders include mild anemia (hemoglobin level rarely less than 9.0 g/dL), decreased serum iron and total iron-binding capacity levels, and normal or increased ferritin level. Treatment of the anemia usually depends on treatment of the underlying cause. Erythropoietin has been successfully used in some cases of anemia of chronic disorders (Krantz, 1994 Ⓐ).

B_{12} and Folate Deficiency Deficiencies of both vitamin B_{12} and folate can cause a macrocytic anemia. The most common cause of B_{12} deficiency is malabsorption (including that due to pernicious anemia). The most common causes of folate deficiency include dietary deficiency, malabsorption, excessive folate demand, and drugs (including alcohol and chemotherapeutic agents). The diagnosis can be made through blood levels of vitamin B_{12} or folate or both, and replacement therapy can be instituted. Vitamin B_{12} is usually replaced by the parenteral route (500 to 1000 µg/month), because malabsorption is the leading cause of vitamin B_{12} deficiency. Oral B_{12}, given at dose of 1000 µg/day, has been successfully used to treat pernicious anemia (Oh and Brown, 2003 Ⓐ). Folate can usually be replaced via the oral route (5 mg/day). Signs and symptoms include mild jaundice, glossitis, angular stomatitis, and peripheral sensory neuropathy. Folate deficiency does not cause neurologic symptoms. Laboratory findings include macrocytic RBCs, hypersegmented neutrophils, and elevated bilirubin level.

The intrinsic factor antibody assay is often positive in pernicious anemia; this assay has decreased the need to perform the Schilling test to diagnose pernicious anemia (Davenport, 1996 Ⓐ). In patients with vitamin B_{12} deficiency, both vitamin B_{12} and serum folate levels can be low. A low RBC folate level is a more precise indicator (less than 150 µg/dL) of chronic folate deficiency than is a serum folate level (Schrier, 2005).

Bone Marrow Failure Replacement or an intrinsic defect of bone marrow usually is the cause of normocytic anemia. Treatment is aimed at correcting the cause of the marrow replacement or defect, if possible, or maintaining an acceptable hemoglobin level via transfusion.

Anemia Due to Increased RBC Destruction

A number of intrinsic and acquired illnesses including splenomegaly, hemoglobinopathies (e.g., sickle cell disease), infections, drug effects, collagen vascular diseases, and tumors can cause an increase in RBC destruction. Laboratory findings include an elevated reticulocyte count, abnormal RBC morphology, increased unconjugated bilirubin level, decreased haptoglobin level, and increased plasma hemoglobin level. Treatment is aimed at correcting the cause of hemolysis or at maintaining an acceptable hemoglobin level through transfusion.

Anemia Due to Increased Plasma Volume

A relative anemia due to hemodilution from increased plasma volume can be seen in various conditions including pregnancy. This disease responds to treatment of the underlying condition.

Initial Evaluation of Anemia in the Office

A cause for most cases of anemia can be determined by a thorough history and physical examination and judicious use of the clinical laboratory. Patients with anemia from suspected underproduction of RBCs should be screened for gastrointestinal blood loss; iron studies are indicated if RBC indices are microcytic. Vitamin B_{12} and folate levels should be obtained in patients with macrocytic RBC indices, with or without anemia. Bone marrow examination may be helpful in some patients with anemia from RBC underproduction, especially those for whom standard treatment protocols fail. If hemolysis is suspected, a reticulocyte count, haptoglobin level, and examination of the peripheral blood smear for abnormal cell forms are reasonable screening tests. Lead screening is recommended for children with microcytic anemia. Other tests are indicated based on the history and results of screening laboratory evaluations. Further testing may be indicated to evaluate uncommon causes of anemia.

Material Available on Student Consult

Review Questions and Answers about Anemia

REFERENCES

Davenport, J. Macrocytic anemia. Am Fam Physician 1996;53:155–162.◐

Krantz SB. Pathogenesis and treatment of the anemia of chronic diseases. Am J Med Sci 1994; 307:353–359.◐

Oh RC, Brown DL. Vitamin B_{12} deficiency. Am Fam Physician 2003;67:979–986.◐

Schrier SL. Thalassemia: Pathophysiology of red cell changes. Annu Rev Med 1994;45:211–218.◐

Schrier SL. Diagnosis and treatment of vitamin B_{12} and folic acid deficiency. Available at www.uptodate.com/physicians/hematology_toclist.asp, Accessed 9/14/2005.

SUGGESTED READINGS

Brill JR, Baumgardner DJ. Normocytic anemia. Am Fam Physician 2000;62:2255–2264.

Centers for Disease Control and Prevention. Recommendation to prevent and control iron deficiency in the United States. Min Recomm Rep 1998;47:1–29.

Hoffman R, Benz E, Shattell S, eds. Hematology: Basic Principles and Practice. New York: Churchill-Livingstone, 2000.

42

Right Upper Quadrant Abdominal Pain (Cholelithiasis)

Joel J. Heidelbaugh

KEY POINTS

1. Gallstones are extremely common in our society, with a 35% lifetime prevalence for women, compared with a 20% lifetime prevalence for men.
2. Cholesterol stones are the most common form of gallstones in the Western world.
3. Observational studies on the natural history of asymptomatic gallstones report a complication rate of 1% to 2% per year.
4. Because the incidence of the development of biliary complications as the presenting complaint of gallstone disease is rare (0 to 5.5%), the recommendation is for expectant management of asymptomatic gallstones.
5. Transabdominal ultrasonography is the gold standard for diagnosing gallstones in most patients.
6. Laparoscopic cholecystectomy is the gold standard for the treatment of acute cholelithiasis.
7. Laparoscopic cholecystectomy and endoscopic stone extraction via either pre- or postoperative endoscopic retrograde cholangiopancreatography together make up the gold standard for treatment of choledocholithiasis.

INITIAL VISIT

Subjective

Patient Identification and Presenting Problem

Sherrie M. is a 29-year-old African-American with the complaint of right upper quadrant (RUQ) abdominal pain that occasionally radiates to her right shoulder, as well as episodic nausea. She has been evaluated in the office of her family physician and by other providers over the past few months for similar complaints, which were thought to be "the stomach flu," "reflux disease," and "all in my head," according to the patient.

Present Illness

Sherrie states that this episode of RUQ abdominal pain began to develop 2 days ago after she consumed beef tacos, nachos, hot salsa, and a caffeinated beverage. She has experienced similar pain numerous times in the past, and it has always resolved on its own over several days to weeks, or with antacids. At a previous visit, she was advised to try Prilosec (omeprazole) on demand for symptomatic relief and has seen only a slight improvement of her symptoms after this treatment. In this instance, the RUQ abdominal pain gradually progressed to 10/10, is radiating to her right shoulder, and she has become nauseated with several episodes of nonbloody, nonbilious emesis yesterday. Sherrie is uncertain whether she has been febrile at home. She complains that her pain becomes more severe when she takes a deep breath.

Medical History

Sherrie has a medical history significant for a mixed anxiety/depression disorder since her teenage years and post-traumatic stress disorder (PTSD) resulting from a domestic assault by her boyfriend, the father of her two children, several months ago. She is currently under the care of both a psychiatrist and a psychologist. Sherrie has had two normal spontaneous vaginal deliveries at term without any complications, and no surgical history other than vaginal laceration repairs subsequent to her deliveries. Currently, she takes Ortho-Novum 7/7/7 daily for contraception, as well as clonazepam (Klonopin), 0.5 mg twice daily; bupropion (Wellbutrin), 100 mg twice daily; and paroxetine (Paxil), 40 mg daily for her psychiatric disorders.

Evidence levels Ⓐ Randomized, controlled trials (RCTs), meta-analyses, well-designed systematic reviews of RCTs. Ⓑ Case-control or cohort studies, nonrandomized clinical trials, systematic reviews of studies other than RCTs, cross-sectional studies, retrospective studies, certain uncontrolled studies. Ⓒ Consensus statements, expert guidelines, usual practice, opinion.

Family History
Sherrie is unaware of her father's medical history, as he has only rarely been involved in her life. Her mother has hypertension, has poorly controlled type 2 non–insulin-requiring diabetes mellitus, and is morbidly obese. Sherrie has two younger sisters who are alive and well without any significant medical problems.

Social History
Sherrie has 2 boys, ages 4 years and 19 months. She works part-time as a cashier at a fast-food restaurant. She has smoked approximately 1/2 pack of cigarettes per day since she was age 15 years, denies any current alcohol or illicit drug use, but has consumed alcohol on occasion in the past. Her boyfriend, the father of her two children, is now in jail on account of spousal abuse.

Review of Systems
Sherrie admits sporadic nausea and nonbloody, nonbilious emesis, but denies diarrhea or constipation; bloody, dark, or tarry stools; abdominal trauma; headache; chest pain; palpitations; syncope; cough; or any genitourinary symptoms. Her last normal menstrual period was 1 week ago. She admits occasional anorexia secondary to epigastric and RUQ pain after eating hot, spicy, and fatty foods, and does not think that she has lost any weight recently. Sherrie denies any other constitutional symptoms or other recent illness. She denies taking any nonsteroidal anti-inflammatory drugs or aspirin in the recent past.

Objective

Physical Examination
General Sherrie is an obese woman sitting on the examination table in mild distress.

Vital Signs
Height, 5 feet 3 inches tall
Weight, 254 pounds
Body mass index, 45
Temperature, 37.6°C (99.6°F)
Blood pressure, 139/87
Pulse, 88 and regular
Respiratory rate, 18

Head, Eyes, Ears, Nose, and Throat Head is normocephalic, atraumatic; pupils are equally round and reactive to light; extraocular movements are full; sclerae are anicteric; external auditory canals and tympanic membranes are clear bilaterally; oropharynx is without significant lesions; dentition is good.

Neck Supple, with full range of motion and no cervical lymphadenopathy, jugular venous distention, thyromegaly, or carotid bruits.

Lungs Clear to auscultation bilaterally without wheezes, rales, or rhonchi.

Heart Regular rate and rhythm, S_1, S_2, no murmurs, rubs, or gallops.

Abdomen Obese, soft, with marked tenderness during deep inspiration along the ninth right costal margin in the midclavicular line (a positive Murphy's sign). The liver percusses to approximately 10 cm below the last rib in the midclavicular line. Although the abdominal examination is difficult because of the patient's body habitus, the abdomen was felt to be nondistended, with positive bowel sounds, no hepatosplenomegaly, bruits, masses, ascites, or fluid wave. Abdominal and inguinal hernias appeared to be absent. Pelvic examination was deferred.

Extremities Warm and well perfused, without cyanosis, clubbing, or edema.

Neuromuscular Cranial nerves II to XII are grossly intact, with no focal deficits on strength and sensory testing.

Rectal Guaiac negative, no masses, fissures, fistulae, or hemorrhoids.

Skin No significant lesions.

Laboratory Studies
A complete blood count revealed 12,200/mm³ white blood cells, with a differential of 67% neutrophils, 24% leukocytes, and 9% monocytes. Serum amylase is 42 IU/L; lipase is 17 IU/dL; alkaline phosphatase is 93 IU/L; alanine aminotransferase (ALT) is 39 IU/L; aspartate aminotransferase (AST) is 26 IU/L; and total bilirubin is 0.5 mg/dL. Serum chemistries were otherwise normal. A urinalysis and a urine pregnancy test were normal.

Radiographic Studies
An abdominal ultrasound revealed multiple hyperechoic, mobile gallstones and a moderate amount of gallbladder sludge. A positive sonographic Murphy's sign was noted. The common bile duct (CBD) measured 0.5 mm in diameter (within normal limits), with no evidence of gallbladder wall thickening or pericholecystic fluid. The remainder of the ultrasound evaluation was within normal limits. A cholescintigraphy (HIDA) scan was negative for CBD obstruction.

Assessment

Working Diagnosis
The working diagnosis for Sherrie is acute calculous cholecystitis.

Differential Diagnosis (Box 42-1)

1. *Dyspepsia.* This term is used to describe a constellation of symptoms including heartburn, regurgitation, reflux, and epigastric abdominal pain. Patients may describe this term as "gas," "bloating," "frequent belching," and "stomach pain." Dyspepsia can be associated with numerous gastrointestinal (GI) disorders, including gastric or duodenal ulcers or both, gastroesophageal reflux disease, upper GI malignancies, pancreatitis, hiatal hernia, cholelithiasis, choledocholithiasis, as well as psychiatric disorders including anxiety and depression, medication side effects, acute myocardial infarction, and angina.

2. *Choledocholithiasis.* CBD stones are found in up to 10% of patients with symptomatic cholelithiasis, yet routine ultrasonography may miss up to one third of stones present in the CBD as a result of overlying loops of bowel (Avunduk, 2002Ⓑ). CBD stones can be either primary (those that develop in the duct itself) or secondary (those that originate in the gallbladder and migrate). Approximately 95% of patients with cholesterol gallstones also have stones in the CBD (Avunduk, 2002Ⓑ). If these stones are discovered after a cholecystectomy, they may have been overlooked (retained) or may have formed after the surgery (recurrent). Bile stasis associated with partial obstruction or marked dilation of the duct may promote choledocholithiasis. Patients with choledocholithiasis often appear similar to patients with cholelithiasis, but they may also have concomitant obstructive jaundice, cholangitis, pancreatitis, hemobilia, or a combination of these.

3. *Perforated peptic ulcer.* A perforated gastric or duodenal ulcer often is first seen with epigastric or upper quadrant abdominal pain or both with radiation to the back or upper extremities, nausea, and vomiting. Most patients with this syndrome will have a gradually worsening case of epigastric abdominal pain that may become unrelenting, leading to generalized peritonitis, abdominal rigidity, the disappearance of bowel sounds, and the increased probability of cardiovascular collapse and sepsis. If the suspicion for a perforated ulcer is high, then plain film radiographs should be obtained to evaluate for the presence of free air under the diaphragm. Prompt surgical evaluation should be obtained, and the patient should be hemodynamically stabilized.

4. *Acute appendicitis.* The diagnosis of appendicitis is usually made on a clinical basis, considering the combination of the patient's presenting physical signs and symptoms. Often this includes a sudden onset of epigastric or periumbilical pain that will eventually migrate to the right lower quadrant (RLQ). The characteristic findings in a patient with acute appendicitis include a low-grade fever, leukocytosis, and tenderness over McBurney's point (the junction of the middle and outer thirds of the line from the umbilicus to the anterior superior iliac spine). Rovsing's sign (pain sensed in the RLQ after deep palpation in the left lower quadrant), the psoas sign (worsening of pain with extension of the ipsilateral hip joint, which stretches the iliopsoas muscle), the obturator sign (pain produced by internal rotation of the ipsilateral flexed thigh), or

---

Box 42-1	Differential Diagnosis of Cholelithiasis

Gastrointestinal

Acute acalculous cholecystitis
Appendicitis
Choledocholithiasis
Dyspepsia
Gastroesophageal reflux disease (GERD)
Gastrointestinal malignancy
Hiatal hernia
Hepatitis (acute)
Intestinal ischemia
Intestinal obstruction/ileus
Peptic ulcer disease
Perforated peptic ulcer
Pancreatitis

Cardiovascular

Acute myocardial infarction
Angina (unstable)
Ruptured aortic aneurysm

Psychiatric

Anxiety
Major depressive disorder
Panic disorder
Post-traumatic stress disorder

Pulmonary

Pleurisy
Pneumonia
Pneumothorax

Renal

Pyelonephritis
Renal colic

Other

Abdominal muscle strain
Abdominal trauma

a combination of these may suggest irritation or rupture of the appendix and peritonitis. Atypical presentations of appendicitis are exceedingly common, especially in obese patients, as not all appendicitis appears with RLQ pain. Plain radiographs, abdominal/pelvic ultrasonography, computerized tomography (CT), or a combination of these may be useful in locating an appendicolith, abscess, regional inflammation, or signs of perforation.

5. *Pancreatitis.* This condition, in both its acute and chronic forms, usually is first seen with epigastric or upper quadrant abdominal pain or both that may radiate to the midthoracic area of the back, chest, flanks, and lower abdomen, and is associated with nausea, vomiting, anorexia, and abdominal distention secondary to ileus. Leukocytosis and elevations in serum amylase, lipase, glucose, and lactate dehydrogenase are common, depending on the time of the clinical presentation.

6. *Intestinal obstruction/gallstone ileus.* Mechanical obstruction may occur in the setting of a large gallstone that has traveled into the small bowel (usually the ileum) by way of a cholecystenteric fistula. The *Mirrizzi syndrome* occurs when a gallstone becomes impacted in the cystic duct and may obstruct the common hepatic duct either from direct obstruction or from inflammatory changes around the duct itself (Avunduk, 2002Ⓑ). A high level of suspicion should prompt the clinician to evaluate the patient

for these conditions and make an expedient referral for radiographic and surgical evaluations.

7. *Acute acalculous cholecystitis.* A severe form of gallbladder inflammation, this condition occurs in the absence of gallstones. Most patients who experience this condition are elderly or debilitated as a result of comorbid disease or trauma, in the intensive care unit, in the postoperative period, receiving total parenteral nutrition or a combination of these. With this condition, a high incidence is seen of gallbladder necrosis, gangrene, perforation of the gallbladder, sepsis, and potentially death (Avunduk, 2002Ⓑ).

8. *Anxiety/depression/post-traumatic stress disorder.* Many patients with any or a combination of these disorders have a variety of vague systemic complaints, with one of the more common complaints being episodic "stomach pain." This complaint is frequently associated with nausea, vomiting, anorexia, and dyspepsia, and it may wax and wane with the patient's psychological symptoms.

Plan

Diagnostic

Risk factors for cholelithiasis are presented in Box 42-2. When a physician encounters a patient with abdominal pain, the first step in diagnostic planning is to determine the severity of the pain and the

Box 42-2	Risk Factors for the Development of Cholelithiasis
Age: incidence increases with age in both women and men	*Ileal disease, bypass, or resection:* Crohn's disease or surgical resection of distal small bowel leads to the impairment of bile acid reabsorption
Cystic fibrosis with pancreatic insufficiency: largely due to malabsorption of bile salts	
Diabetes mellitus: due to increased biliary cholesterol secretion and obesity, if applicable	*Medications:* ceftriaxone, clofibrate, estrogens, octreotide, progestogens
Diet: high in calories, refined carbohydrates, polyunsaturated fats, and cholesterol	*Obesity:* bile in people who are obese is more lithogenic
Dyslipidemia: decreased low-density lipoproteins with increased hepatic uptake, increased serum triglycerides, decreased serum high-density lipoproteins	*Pregnancy:* the increase of estrogens and progesterone leads to impaired gallbladder emptying
	Rapid weight loss: cholesterol is mobilized from peripheral adipose tissue and is secreted into bile, leading to cholesterol supersaturation
Family history: prevalence varies in different populations (i.e., >75% of Pima Indian women have gallstones by age 30 yr)	*Spinal cord injury:* depending on level of injury (i.e., thoracic), may lead to gallbladder stasis
Gender: 2 to 3 times higher risk in women	*Total parenteral nutrition:* promotes gallbladder sludge and stasis
Genetic predisposition: greater in Native American Pima Indians, Chileans, Scandinavians, those with apolipoprotein E_4/E_4 alleles	*Truncal vagotomy:* may decrease gallbladder motility

Adapted from Avunduk C. Gallstones. In Avunduk C (ed): Manual of Gastroenterology, Diagnosis and Therapy, 3rd ed. Philadelphia, Lippincott Williams & Wilkins, 2002, pp 340–350.

potential for complications from underlying pathology. The physician must then determine whether the patient warrants an emergency workup with laboratory tests, radiographic imaging, expectant management, or a prompt surgical evaluation (Table 42-1).

Serum bilirubin, alkaline phosphatase, amylase, alanine aminotransferase, and aspartate aminotransferase may be elevated in patients with acute cholecystitis, and the patient may exhibit a leukocytosis with a left shift with or without the presence of ascending cholangitis. The evaluation of gallstones via abdominal ultrasonography is currently the best screening modality, with sensitivity and specificity above 90% (Horton and Bilhartz, 2002 Ⓐ). A CT scan of the upper abdomen is more sensitive than conventional plain film radiography, yet it may miss a significant amount of cholesterol gallstones and biliary sludge readily seen on ultrasonography. Biliary scintigraphy (HIDA scan) uses technetium-99m–labeled derivatives of excreted bile acids to determine CBD obstruction. This test is generally reserved for those patients for whom a definitive diagnosis cannot be reached after routine abdominal ultrasonography. False-positive scans may occur in patients with chronic cholecystitis, and false-negative scans may occur in cases of acute acalculous cholecystitis (Horton and Bilhartz, 2002Ⓑ).

Endoscopic retrograde cholangiopancreatography (ERCP) with sphincterotomy is useful in identifying and treating CBD stones but is invasive, expensive, and often fraught with complications, including iatrogenic pancreatitis. Endoscopic ultrasonography is a noninvasive method for evaluating CBD stones that is becoming more widely used and has excellent sensitivity and specificity in detecting these stones. Magnetic resonance cholangiopancreatography is another noninvasive modality for identifying gallstones and CBD stones, but it often has a lower sensitivity and specificity as compared with ultrasound and is more costly (Horton and Bilhartz, 2002Ⓐ).

Therapeutic

Both surgical and nonsurgical approaches exist for the patient with symptomatic cholelithiasis. The laparoscopic cholecystectomy is the recommended treatment of choice for long-term management of symptomatic biliary colic. When it is suspected that the operation may be complicated, or if the patient is morbidly obese, the open form of the procedure is often preferred, yet the complication rate is higher. Nonsurgical treatments include pain relief with narcotic analgesics, excluding morphine and its derivatives (which may precipitate spasm of the sphincter of Oddi and worsen symptoms), extracorporeal shockwave lithotripsy, and gallstone dissolution via oral bile acid therapy and contact solvents such as methyl-tert-butyl ether (Ransohoff and Gracie, 1993Ⓑ).

Disposition

The plan for Sherrie was to undergo a surgical evaluation for a laparoscopic cholecystectomy. Within 1 week after her surgery, she is to return to our office for postsurgical evaluation.

Patient Education

Sherrie was educated on the importance of proper dietary modifications, including the minimization of saturated fats and foods high in cholesterol. Our office provided a referral to a dietitian to assist Sherrie in making the proper modifications in her diet. In addition, she was instructed on an exercise program to follow after she is fully recovered from her surgery in an attempt to reach an ideal weight. Smoking cessation and the avoidance of alcohol were also strongly encouraged.

Table 42-1	Comparison of Diagnostic Methods for Cholelithiasis and Choledocholithiasis	
Modality	**Sensitivity (%)**	**Specificity (%)**
Abdominal radiographs[*†]	<50	<50
Abdominal CT[*†]	60–70	60–70
Ultrasonography[*]	90–95	98
Ultrasonography[†]	25–58	68–91
HIDA scan[†]	85–90	80–90
MRCP[†]	70–100	80–100
EUS[†]	94–100	>90

[*]Cholelithiasis.

[†]Choledocholithiasis.

CT, computed tomography; HIDA scan, biliary scintigraphy using dimethylphenylcarbamyl methyliminodiacetic acid (HIDA); MRCP, magnetic resonance cholangiopancreatography; EUS, endoscopic ultrasonography.

Adapted from Avunduk C. Gallstones. In Avunduk C (ed): Manual of Gastroenterology, Diagnosis and Therapy, 3rd ed. Philadelphia, Lippincott Williams & Wilkins, 2002, pp 340–350.

FOLLOW-UP VISIT

Sherrie underwent an uncomplicated laparoscopic cholecystectomy 1 week before her follow-up visit. She admits complete symptom relief, except for one episode of postprandial nausea in the postoperative period. She plans to meet with a dietitian and to commence an exercise program to foster weight loss.

DISCUSSION

Gallstones are extremely common among both young and older patients, in both male and female patients, and affect approximately 20% of all Americans. Population-based studies indicate that the prevalence for women between the ages of 20 and 55 years ranges from 5% to 20% and increases to 25% to 30% after the age of 50 years. It has been estimated that by the age of 75 years, gallstones will develop in up to 35% of women and 20% of men, either symptomatically or asymptomatically (Attili et al., 1995 ⓒ). The prevalence of gallstones for men is approximately one-third to one-half that for women in any given age group.

Gallstones are formed from the precipitation of the insoluble bile constituents cholesterol, polymerized bilirubin, bile pigments, calcium salts, and proteins. They are classified into cholesterol, black pigment, and brown pigment stones. Cholesterol stones are the most commonly occurring gallstones in the Western world; black pigment stones generally occur in patients with chronic hemolytic disorders, and brown pigment stones, which are more common in Asia, are associated with impaction of the biliary tract (Avunduk, 2002 ⓒ) (Figs. 42-1 to 42-5).

Results from observational studies on the natural history of asymptomatic gallstones suggest that serious complications develop in 1% to 2% of cases per year and that this rate decreases over time (Kragg et al., 1995 ⓑ). The Rome Group for the Epidemiology and Prevention of Cholelithiasis (GREPCO) study found that the overall cumulative probability of developing biliary colic over time was 11.9% at 2 years, 16.5% at 4 years, and 25.8% at 10 years, with a cumulative probability of 3% of developing complications at 10 years (GREPCO, 1984 ⓑ). The incidence of the development of biliary complications as the presenting complaint of gallstone disease is rare, ranging from none to 5.5% (GREPCO, 1984 ⓑ). Based on these data, evidence from well-designed cohort and case-controlled studies is summarized by GREPCO to weigh in favor of expectant treatment of asymptomatic gallstones.

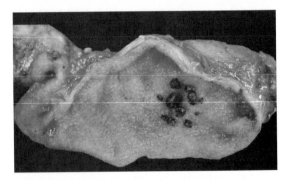

Figure 42-2 Gallbladder with black-pigment gallstones. (Courtesy of Dr. Henry D. Appelman, Professor of Pathology, University of Michigan Medical School, Ann Arbor, Michigan.)

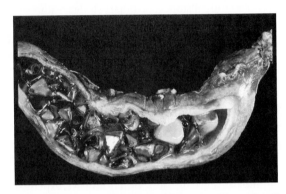

Figure 42-3 Gallbladder with multiple cholesterol gallstones. (Courtesy of Dr. Henry D. Appelman, Professor of Pathology, University of Michigan Medical School, Ann Arbor, Michigan.)

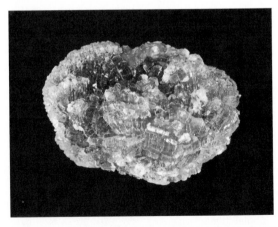

Figure 42-4 Gallbladder with multiple cholesterol gallstones. (Courtesy of Dr. Henry D. Appelman, Professor of Pathology, University of Michigan Medical School, Ann Arbor, Michigan.)

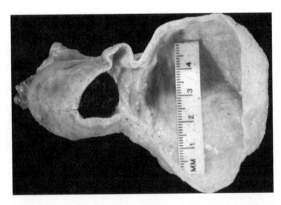

Figure 42-1 Gallbladder hydrops with black-pigment gallstone obstructing the cystic duct. (Courtesy of Dr. Henry D. Appelman, Professor of Pathology, University of Michigan Medical School, Ann Arbor, Michigan.)

In the approach to the patient with symptomatic gallstones, the clinician must entertain and effectively rule out other potential causes of RUQ localized abdominal pain, distinguishing biliary from nonbiliary

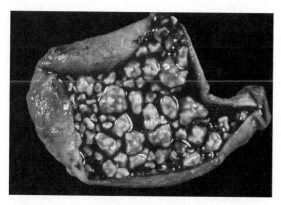

Figure 42-5 Cholesterol gallstone (Courtesy of Dr. Henry D. Appelman, Professor of Pathology, University of Michigan Medical School, Ann Arbor, Michigan.)

etiologies as the primary source of pain and disease. For example, it is often a challenge to differentiate between dyspepsia and biliary colic. Population-based studies have failed to show any significant difference in the prevalence of patients with dyspepsia with and without gallstones (Abraham et al., 2001Ⓑ). One meta-analysis found that heartburn, flatulence, regurgitation, and fatty food intolerance were not associated with gallstones, but that epigastric pain, nausea, and vomiting were associated with a higher odds ratio of having gallstones (Kragg et al., 1995Ⓐ).

Patients suspected to have biliary disease should undergo a targeted workup, and those with nonbiliary symptoms should not be treated for gallstones. Cohort studies have suggested that patients with both biliary and nonbiliary symptoms should be given realistic expectations for the management of their complaints, specifically regarding the level of anticipated symptomatic improvement, and continued follow-up with their primary care provider should be strongly encouraged (Abraham et al., 2001Ⓑ).

Numerous randomized controlled trials have confirmed the adoption of laparoscopic cholecystectomy as the gold standard for the treatment of gallstone disease over the open procedure. The most serious complication of this procedure is CBD injury, occurring in approximately 0.1% to 0.2% of cases, and it is directly related to the surgeon's skill and experience, anatomic variation, and local inflammatory conditions. The main advantages of this procedure include the avoidance of a large abdominal incision through the skin and muscles of the RUQ, and a decrease in hospital stay, convalescence, and postoperative pain (Abraham et al., 2001Ⓑ; Ransohoff and Gracie, 1993Ⓑ).

Randomized trials have examined the treatment options for choledocholithiasis and have shown that the treatment of choice is laparoscopic cholecystectomy and pre- or postoperative endoscopic stone extraction via ERCP. Open cholecystectomy and CBD exploration, usually via an intraoperative cholangiogram, are reserved for patients with contraindications to the laparoscopic procedure, or who require abdominal exploration. In approximately 2% of patients, a residual CBD stone is demonstrated on postoperative cholangiograms. In these rare cases, the stones may be extracted by ERCP with sphincterotomy or dissolved via MBTE infusion (Abraham et al., 2001Ⓑ; Ransohoff and Gracie, 1993Ⓑ).

Material Available on Student Consult

Review Questions and Answers about Cholelithiasis

REFERENCES

Abraham NS, Romagnuolo J, Barkun A. Gallstone disease. In Irvine EJ, Hunt RH (eds): Evidence-Based Gastroenterology. Hamilton, Canada, Decker, 2001, pp 360–376. ⒶⒷⒸ

Attili AF, DeSantis A, Capri R, et al. The natural history of gallstones: The GREPCO experience. Hepatology 1995;21:656–659. ⒶⒷⒸ

Avunduk C. Gallstones. In Avunduk C (ed): Manual of Gastroenterology, Diagnosis and Therapy, 3rd ed. Philadelphia, Lippincott Williams & Wilkins, 2002, pp 340–350. ⒷⒸ

Horton JD, Bilhartz LE. Gallstone disease and its complications. In Feldman M, Friedman L, Sleisenger M (eds): Sleisenger and Fordtran's Gastrointestinal and Liver Disease: Pathophysiology/Diagnosis/Management, 7th ed. Philadelphia, Elsevier, 2002, pp 1065–1086. ⒶⒷⒸ

Kragg N, Thijs C, Knipschild P. Dyspepsia: How noisy are gallstones? A meta-analysis of biliary pain, dyspeptic symptoms, and food intolerance. Scand J Gastroenterol 1995;30:411–421. Ⓐ

Ransohoff DF, Gracie WF. Treatment of gallstones. Ann Intern Med 1993;119:606–619. ⒶⒷⒸ

Rome Group for the Epidemiology and Prevention of Cholelithiasis (GREPCO). Prevalence of gallstone disease in an adult female population. Am J Epidemiol 1984;119:796–805. ⒷⒸ

43

Cramping Abdominal Pain (Irritable Bowel Syndrome)

Scott E. Moser

INITIAL VISIT

Subjective

Patient Identification and Presenting Problem

Susan M. is a 41-year-old woman who complains of intermittent abdominal cramps that have been worsening over the past several months.

Present Illness

Susan describes her pain as "crampy" and occasionally like a "sharp knife." It is so severe that it doubles her over. It most often strikes in the right upper quadrant but also can be in other parts of the abdomen; no radiation to the back occurs. The pain usually occurs a few minutes to a few hours after meals and is worse if she eats "too much," although no specific relation to fatty or spicy foods is noted. Antacids have had no effect. Susan gets the most relief from a bowel movement but often has to try several times before she senses she has fully evacuated her stool. Her bowels have never moved very regularly. Sometimes she has two or three bowel movements per day, and other times she goes 2 to 3 days between bowel movements. During flare-ups of the pain, she often has multiple, thin, small-volume "diarrhea" stools accompanied by mucus but no blood. She is nauseated with the abdominal cramps but has not vomited. She cannot remember the cramps ever waking her at night but notes that they often come at the most inopportune times at her job, such as before and during important presentations. She has not noticed any relation to her menstrual cycle, which has a regular 28- to 30-day pattern. She wears loose-fitting dresses to work because slacks feel tight, especially when the abdominal pain starts.

Medical History

Susan is G2P1AB1, with one vaginal delivery and one early miscarriage. She has had no other surgery, medications, or allergies.

Family History

Susan's 63-year-old father is 4 years status post partial colectomy for colon cancer and doing well without evidence of recurrence. Her mother and siblings have no serious illnesses. Susan has been divorced for 5 years and has a 16-year-old daughter who lives with her and who has no medical problems.

Social History

Susan is a loan officer at a bank, a job she enjoys but finds very stressful. She does not smoke. She has a glass of wine several times per year on special occasions. She denies sexual intercourse since her divorce, noting that she endured years of verbal abuse and occasional physical abuse before leaving her ex-husband.

Review of Systems

Susan has obtained Pap tests every 2 to 3 years with no abnormal findings. She is actively trying to lose weight through a nonspecific low-calorie diet. She feels fatigued and is tired of dealing with her pain but denies feeling depressed. Her knees ache when she tries to exercise, but she denies other joint or muscle pain. She denies any urinary symptoms.

Objective

Physical Examination

Susan is a somewhat anxious, moderately overweight woman with normal vital signs. Her general physical examination, including pelvic, is normal except for the abdomen. The abdomen appears distended, and borborygmus is noted without aid of a stethoscope. She is moderately tender to palpation in all quadrants with some voluntary guarding but no rebound. She has no masses or hepatosplenomegaly.

Laboratory Tests

Complete blood count, serum electrolytes, and liver function tests are normal. A gallbladder ultrasound is normal.

Assessment

Working Diagnosis

Irritable bowel syndrome (IBS), mixed constipation and diarrhea type.

Differential Diagnosis

1. *Cholelithiasis.* The pain of IBS can be in any part of the abdomen, and it is often global, but it is most frequently in the lower abdomen. The right upper quadrant location of some of Susan's pain, along with her age and weight, are suggestive enough of gallbladder disease to warrant a nonurgent ultrasound at presentation.
2. *Isolated constipation.* If the "diarrhea" represents small-volume discharge leaking around an obstipating stool, she may have isolated constipation. The distinction is clinically important in that isolated constipation should have a more aggressive "clean-out phase" than IBS with constipation symptoms.
3. *Lactose intolerance.* The prevalence of lactose intolerance is 7% to 20% in adults of northern European extraction and much higher among other ethnic groups. The symptoms of cramping, flatulence, bloating, and diarrhea are very similar to those of IBS. Milk products are common enough in processed foods that patients may not make the association with their symptoms for themselves. A lactose tolerance test or lactose breath hydrogen test can make the diagnosis in cases in which the dietary history is suggestive.
4. *Colon cancer.* A change in bowel pattern can be a sign of colon cancer, although abdominal pain is rare. Minimal evaluation should include a rectal examination and appropriate screening based on age and family history.
5. *Thyroid disease.* In cases with a marked predominance of either diarrhea or constipation, a thyroid-stimulating hormone level can make the diagnosis.
6. *Celiac disease.* Gluten-sensitive enteropathy may have an incidence as high as about 1 in 200 patients of northern European extraction. This autoimmune disease is characterized by variable levels of diarrhea and malabsorption that improve after complete discontinuation of dietary gluten. Screening for this condition with specific autoantibody studies should be considered in patients with diarrhea-predominant symptoms.
7. *Infectious bowel disease.* Parasitic infestations are characterized by diarrhea-predominant symptoms without nighttime relief, usually accompanied by weight loss, and may have other features of inflammation such as hematochezia or fever.
8. *Inflammatory bowel disease.* Ulcerative colitis and Crohn's disease would have features similar to those described for infectious bowel disease and may exhibit the systemic findings associated with these conditions.
9. *Somatization.* Psychosocial factors frequently play an important role in IBS and could be the primary issue in treatment. More than half of women with chronic abdominal or pelvic pain have a significant history of physical or sexual abuse.
10. *Medications.* Susan's history does not suggest a medication as the etiology of her symptoms, but it is important to remember that many commonly prescribed drugs cause IBS-like symptoms. Examples include diarrhea from selective serotonin reuptake inhibitors (SSRIs), gastrointestinal distress from tetracycline and erythromycin, and constipation from calcium channel blockers.
11. *Dietary indiscretion.* Irregular eating patterns can cause or exacerbate IBS symptoms. The Institute of Medicine report on dietary recommendations published in 2002 encouraged men to consume 38 g of total dietary fiber per day and women to

consume 25 g. Median intake in the United States at the time of the report was 12 to 18 g/day, with many people taking in less than 10 g/day.

Plan

Diagnostic

Even though Susan has classic IBS symptoms, she is older than 40 years with a family history of colon cancer, so she is scheduled for colonoscopy. She is given a pain diary to elicit relations with foods, stressors, or other activities that may not be apparent to her now. Because she has no weight loss and her diarrhea seems to be of small volume, no further tests are ordered.

Therapeutic

Susan is offered psychotherapy regarding her history of abuse, but she declines. She is started on psyllium, 1 Tbsp per day, and given a prescription for hyoscyamine, 0.125-mg tablets, one by mouth every 4 hours as needed for cramps.

Patient Education

Susan is instructed regarding the current recommendations for dietary fiber intake and given a patient guide listing fiber contents of common foods. She is given reassurance about the likelihood that her symptoms represent a medically benign although often uncomfortable problem. She is instructed about the importance of colon cancer screening, given her family history.

FOLLOW-UP VISIT

Susan's colonoscopy was normal. She made a discovery as she reviewed the dietary fiber list: her diet was extremely low in fiber. She ate lots of tossed salads, thinking they were high in "roughage." She learned that lettuce and other salad ingredients are poor sources of fiber compared with legumes, whole grains, and many other fruits and vegetables. She noted some improvement in bowel regularity and cramps with the medications, but her symptoms are still interfering with her job. She indicates a readiness to talk with a counselor regarding her job stress and history of abuse.

DISCUSSION

IBS is the most commonly diagnosed gastrointestinal condition and the second highest cause of work absenteeism (behind the common cold). Its prevalence in North America is 10% to 15% of the population, with a female predominance of 2:1. IBS accounts for as many as 25% to 50% of referrals to gastroenterologists. Onset is usually before age 35

years and often dates back to childhood. It is characterized by periodic exacerbations of chronic abdominal pain accompanied by altered bowel habits and bloating in the absence of an organic cause. Considerable overlap of IBS is found with fibromyalgia, interstitial cystitis, and chronic fatigue syndrome, suggesting a possible unifying explanation of muscle hypersensitivity. Recent evidence suggests that small-intestinal bacterial overgrowth might serve as an explanation that meets this unifying principle (Lin, 2004). Psychiatric comorbidity is very common, with 94% of IBS patients exhibiting depression, anxiety, a somatoform disorder, or a combination of these.

Because no specific biologic marker is known for IBS, several authors have attempted to standardize the criteria to make the diagnosis clinically (Table 43-1). The predictive value of Manning's criteria depends on the number of criteria met and the patient's age and gender (Table 43-2). In the absence of alarm features, a presumptive diagnosis of IBS can be made on the basis of these clinical criteria, avoiding extensive diagnostic testing. Alarm features include (1) age older than 50 years, (2) persistent diarrhea, (3) significant weight loss, (4) fever, (5) blood in stools, (6) anemia, (7) abnormal physical findings or blood studies, (8) family history of irritable bowel disorders or cancer, and (9) failure to respond to initial IBS treatment. Screening for these alarm features can be accomplished with the history and physical examination followed by a complete blood count, routine blood chemistries, and stool Hemoccult. Patients with chronic diarrhea should be considered for additional evaluation as outlined earlier for celiac disease, thyroid disease, lactose intolerance, and parasitic infection. Patients with persistent constipation should undergo screening for hypothyroidism and further evaluation if initial treatment of constipation fails. Screening for colon cancer is as per guidelines for the general population. A history of physical or sexual abuse is common in patients with IBS, and exploration of this possibility should be a routine part of the evaluation.

Treatment goals include (1) establishment of an effective therapeutic relationship, (2) patient understanding of and reassurance regarding IBS, (3) control of predominant symptoms, and (4) identification and reduction of precipitating or exacerbating factors with the overall goal of return to a comfortable daily routine. Anticholinergics (dicyclomine, hyoscyamine, and others) can control spasmodic pain and are available in both immediate-release formulations for acute pain relief and long-acting preparations for prolonged or recurrent pain relief. Tricyclic antidepressants also are useful for chronic control of frequent or severe pain, probably because of their anticholinergic and antidepressant activity.

Table 43-1 Symptom-based Criteria for Irritable Bowel Syndrome

Symptom-based Criteria	Symptoms	Sensitivity (%)	Specificity (%)	Positive Predictive Value (%)
Manning	Abdominal pain Pain relief with bowel movement More frequent stools with pain Looser stools with pain Mucus in stools Feeling of incomplete evacuation	42–90	70–100	74

Rome I	>3 mo of continuous or recurrent abdominal pain relieved with defecation or associated with change in stool consistency
	Plus: >2 of the following on 25% of days
	  Altered stool frequency
	  Altered stool form
	  Altered stool passage
	  Passage of mucus
	  Bloating or abdominal distention
		65–84	100	69–100

Rome II	Abdominal discomfort or pain for ≥12 wk (not necessarily consecutive) in the preceeding 12 mo and having two of the three following features:
	  Relieved with defecation
	  Onset associated with a change in frequency of stool
	  Onset associated with a change in form (appearance) of stool
	Supportive symptoms:
	  Fewer than three bowel movements per wk
	  More than three bowel movements per day
	  Hard or lumpy stools
		49–65*	100*	69–100*

*Found to have sensitivity and specificity similar to Rome I.
From Holten KB. Irritable bowel syndrome: Minimize testing, let symptoms guide treatment. J Family Pract 2003;52:942–950.

Additional treatment of IBS is based on whether the predominant symptom is constipation, diarrhea, or alternating constipation and diarrhea. Dietary-fiber supplements (bran, psyllium, methylcellulose, polycarbophil) to increase total daily fiber intake above 25 g/day are mainstays of IBS therapy. Dietary fiber helps with constipation, but evidence that it reduces pain is mixed. Cathartics are useful for acute constipation but should be used with caution in IBS patients because they can precipitate diarrhea. Tegaserod, a $5HT_4$-receptor agonist, is the only agent approved specifically for treating constipation-predominant IBS (Holten, 2003). The approval is for use in women only; severe diarrhea and ischemic colitis are serious potential side effects.

Table 43-2	Predicted Percentage Probability of Irritable Bowel Syndrome as a Function of Age, Gender, and Number of Manning Criteria Present		
	Predicted Probability of IBS vs. Those Without		
Number of Manning Criteria (1–6)	**At age 20 yr**	**At age 40 yr**	**At age 60 yr**
Men			
Any 2	51	38	26
Any 4	72	61	48
All 6	87	80	70
Women			
Any 2	64	51	38
Any 4	82	73	61
All 6	92	87	80

From Talley NJ, Phillips SF, Melton LJ, Mulvihill C, Wiltgen C, Zinsmetster AR. Diagnosing value of Manning Criteria in irritable bowel syndrome. Gut 1990;31:77–81.

For diarrhea-predominant IBS, alosetron, a $5HT_4$-receptor antagonist, has been demonstrated to be effective in women (Holten, 2003). Its use is restricted because of potential severe constipation and ischemic colitis. Loperamide is effective for control of diarrhea but is no more effective than placebo at relieving global symptoms of IBS.

Other medications, including the SSRIs, peppermint oil, lactobacillus, pancreatic enzymes, and ginger, are commonly used for IBS but have minimal evidence to support their effectiveness. Narcotics should be used with extreme caution if at all because of precipitation of constipation and potential habituation.

Psychological approaches seem of greatest benefit in patients who relate exacerbations of their IBS to specific stressors, demonstrate associated anxiety or depression, have relatively short duration of symptoms, or have intermittent symptoms rather than chronic pain (American Gastroenterological Association, 2002ⓒ).

IBS is usually considered a problem that can be very distressing but is medically benign. However, recent evidence suggests that IBS is an independent risk factor for ischemic colitis. Excluding patients taking alosetron or tegaserod, patients with IBS were more than 3 times as likely to develop ischemic colitis as the general population in two large studies (Cash, 2004).

Material Available on Student Consult

Review Questions and Answers about Irritable Bowel Syndrome

REFERENCES

American Gastroenterologic Association. Medical position statement: Irritable bowel syndrome. Gastroenterology 2002;123:2105–2107.ⓒ

Cash BR, Chey WD. A clinical and safety update on serotonergic agents for the treatment of irritable bowel syndrome and chronic constipation. Express Report, a supplement to Family Practice Recertification, September 2004.

Holten KB. Irritable bowel syndrome: Minimize testing, let symptoms guide treatment. J Family Pract 2003; 52:942–950.

Lin HC. Small intestinal bacterial overgrowth: A framework for understanding irritable bowel syndrome. JAMA 2004;292:852–859.

Talley NJ, Phillips SF, Melton LJ, Mulvihill C, Wiltgen C, Zinsmeister AR. Diagnosing value of the Manning criteria in irritable bowel syndrome. Gut 1990;31:77–81.Ⓑ

44

Heartburn (Gastroesophageal Reflux Disease)

Brian S. Bacak

KEY POINTS

1. Heartburn is the most common symptom of gastroesophageal reflux disease (GERD).
2. Heartburn and acid regurgitation symptoms (belching, exacerbation by spicy and fatty foods, sour taste) are highly specific but poorly sensitive for the diagnosis of GERD.
3. GERD can be diagnosed based on history; for uncomplicated GERD, diagnostic imaging is not necessary.
4. Dyspepsia refers to episodic midepigastric pain that can be accompanied by esophageal reflux symptoms, nausea, and bloating.
5. The differential diagnosis for dyspepsia includes GERD.
6. Peptic ulcer disease, biliary tract disorders, medication side effects, underlying malignancies, pancreatic disease, and cardiac ischemia can present with symptoms similar to those of GERD.
7. The presence of dysphagia, unexplained weight loss, early satiety, gastrointestinal bleeding, anemia, vomiting, odynophagia, or onset of GERD symptoms after the age of 50 years suggests complicated GERD or an underlying pathology that needs further investigation.
8. For uncomplicated GERD, initial medical therapy with either a proton-pump inhibitor or an H2RA is preferred over endoscopy.
9. Patients with documented esophagitis on endoscopy should be continued on maintenance medical therapy after resolution of their symptoms.
10. Lifestyle modifications are an important component of GERD management.
11. Complications from GERD include Barrett's esophagus, esophageal strictures, bleeding, and adenocarcinoma.
12. No role for *Helicobacter pylori* testing exists in the management of GERD.

INITIAL VISIT

Subjective

Patient Identification and Presenting Problem

Bob R. is a 38-year-old white man who complains of heartburn and is seeking relief. Bob complains of heartburn and belching. The pain is burning, episodic, and occurs at night and in the early morning. The pain has been present for the past 4 to 6 months. It occurs after he eats spicy food. He complains of an acidic taste associated with the belching. He initially had some relief with over-the-counter antacid medications, but now the burning sensation occurs more frequently.

Medical History

Bob has hypertension. He takes hydrochlorothiazide, 25 mg by mouth once a day. He is not diabetic. He has had no surgeries.

Family History

Bob has one sister, who is 40 years old and in good health. No family history of heart disease or colorectal disease, peptic ulcer disease, or other gastrointestinal disorders is known.

Social History

Bob works as a dispatcher for a trucking company. He is married, with two children in junior high. Bob is an ex-smoker. He stopped smoking 4 months ago, and as part of his management strategy, he has been

---

Evidence levels ⒶRandomized, controlled trials (RCTs), meta-analyses, well-designed systematic reviews of RCTs. Ⓑ Case-control or cohort studies, nonrandomized clinical trials, systematic reviews of studies other than RCTs, cross-sectional studies, retrospective studies, certain uncontrolled studies. Ⓒ Consensus statements, expert guidelines, usual practice, opinion.

sucking on peppermint candies. He drinks four beers a week and denies illicit substance use. He is on an exercise program that involves walking through the hills near his house for 1 hour, 3 nights a week.

Review of Systems
Bob feels at his baseline. He denies any recent increases in stress and says that he does not feel depressed. He denies nausea, difficulty swallowing, or changes in his appetite or bowel habits. The pain is not colicky, is nonradiating, and is unchanged by exertion. He denies shortness of breath, diarrhea, vomiting, and diaphoresis.

Objective

Physical Examination
General Bob is an overweight man in no acute distress.

Vital Signs
Height, 5 feet 9 inches
Weight, 200 pounds
Body mass index, 29.5
Blood pressure, 132/82
Pulse, 76
Respiratory rate, 14
Temperature, 37.1°C (98.8°F)
No orthostatic change is found in blood pressure or pulse.

Head, Eyes, Ears, Nose, and Throat Anicteric sclerae, no conjunctival pallor; oropharynx shows no tonsillar erythema or oral lesions; dentition notable for moderate erosions with loss of enamel and exposed dentin.

Cardiovascular Heart sounds have a regular rate and rhythm, with no murmur, gallop, or rub; no carotid, abdominal, or femoral bruits.

Lungs Clear to auscultation with good air movement.

Abdomen With minimal midepigastric tenderness to palpation; no hepatomegaly or splenomegaly; no Murphy's sign, ascites, or overlying skin changes.

Rectal Normal tone, no masses; stool testing negative for occult blood.

Skin No jaundice.

Assessment

Working Diagnosis
Bob's sensation of midsternal burning in his chest is referred to as *heartburn*. His complaints of frequent belching, an acidic taste, and symptom exacerbation with spicy foods suggest acid regurgitation. Together, these symptoms suggest a working diagnosis of *gastroesophageal reflux disease* (GERD) and are highly suggestive of and specific for GERD (Klauser, 1990Ⓑ).

Differential Diagnosis
The differential diagnosis for Bob's symptoms falls within the larger category of dyspepsia. Episodic, epigastric pain accompanied by heartburn, regurgitation, and other symptoms is known as dyspepsia and can be caused by several different pathologic processes. After investigation, a majority of patients will not have a specific pathologic process identified and will be diagnosed with nonulcer or "functional" dyspepsia (Bazaldua, 1999 Ⓒ). The remaining causes include GERD and other structural conditions.

Peptic ulcer disease occurs in up to 25% of persons with dyspepsia. A prior diagnosis of a peptic ulcer greatly increases the likelihood of a recurrence. Other risk factors for peptic ulcer disease include a family history of ulcers, current cigarette smoking, and a history of nonsteroidal anti-inflammatory drug (NSAID) use. Orthostatic symptoms, anemia, and the presence of blood in the stool suggest a peptic ulcer with accompanying blood loss.

An *underlying malignancy* such as gastric cancer, esophageal cancer, or pancreatic or abdominal cancer rarely is first seen as dyspepsia without accompanying "warning symptoms" (Box 44-1). Underlying malignancies are more common in the elderly and typically have a shorter presenting history (Bazaldua, 1999 Ⓒ).

Biliary tract disease can cause dyspepsia. Gallstones produce pain located in the right upper quadrant that is episodic, severe, and temporally related to

Box 44-1	Warning Signs and Symptoms of Dyspepsia and GERD That Suggest Complicated Disease or More Serious Underlying Process

Dysphagia
Unexplained weight loss
History of gastrointestinal bleeding
Early satiety
Iron-deficiency anemia
Vomiting
Odynophagia (sharp substernal pain on swallowing)
Initial onset of heartburn-like symptoms after age 50 years
History of immunocompromised state
Anorexia

the ingestion of a high-fat meal. Biliary disease is frequently accompanied by acholic stools, dark-colored urine, and jaundice and is associated with a positive Murphy's sign on physical examination.

Medication-induced dyspepsia can be associated with multiple agents. Dyspepsia is classically associated with the use of NSAID agents, which can cause mucosal injury to the esophagus and stomach lining. Dyspepsia also has been attributed to alendronate, oral iron, and macrolide antibiotics such as erythromycin. Certain herbal medications also cause dyspepsia (Bazaldua, 1999 Ⓒ).

Ischemic heart disease can appear as dyspepsia. Most typically, patients characterize the pain of heart disease as radiating substernal chest pressure, rather than the burning, nonradiating pain of esophageal reflux disease. Ischemic symptoms should be considered more likely in anyone with a history of multiple cardiac risk factors (Bazaldua, 1999 Ⓒ). Diagnostic testing and risk stratification can aid in distinguishing between cardiac and noncardiac causes of dyspepsia.

Plan

Diagnostic

Bob's symptom history is highly suggestive of and specific for GERD. His physical examination findings of dental erosions and dentin exposure support prolonged oral exposure to acidic stomach acids (Bazaldua, 1999 Ⓒ). Bob denies any of the warning signs and symptoms that might suggest a more serious underlying process.

Given Bob's symptom complex, no further testing is necessary to assign the working diagnosis of GERD (Heidelbaugh, 2003 Ⓑ).

Therapeutic

Bob is started on a histamine H_2-receptor antagonist (H2RA), ranitidine (Zantac), 150 mg by mouth on a twice-daily basis.

Patient Education

Bob is given information on lifestyle modification that he should attempt to follow, along with his medication (Box 44-2). He is counseled specifically on his diet, and he is given a patient handout with instructions for elevating the head of his bed by 4 to 6 inches by using blocks placed under the bed supports. His use of peppermint candies may be exacerbating his symptoms; he is instructed to switch to a nonmint candy such as root beer or lemon drops.

Disposition

Bob is instructed to make a follow-up appointment in 2 months and to call if any new symptoms or problems arise.

Box 44-2 | **Lifestyle Modifications That *ASSIST ME* in the Management of GERD**

Avoid medications that can make reflux worse
Slim down (modest weight reduction)
Smaller meal portions
Ingest less alcohol
Sit up after eating (avoid recumbency for 2–4 hr after eating)
Tobacco cessation

Meals: acidic and spicy foods such as caffeine, chocolate, alcohol, mints, garlic, and tomato-based items should be avoided
Elevate the head of the bed 6 to 8 inches

FOLLOW-UP VISIT

Subjective

After 7 weeks, Bob telephones for an appointment because of continued heartburn. On evaluation, Bob states that the ranitidine has helped, but that he still has midsternal burning and belching in the morning. He is abstinent from smoking and has improved his diet. However, he has not attempted to raise the head of his bed, and he admits to eating snacks occasionally within 1 hour before his usual bedtime.

Objective

Bob's blood pressure is 128/82 mm Hg, his pulse is 80, and he has normal respirations. He is afebrile. His weight is 197 pounds. Abdominal examination reveals no epigastric tenderness to palpation and no masses. His conjunctivae and skin show no pallor, icterus, or jaundice.

Assessment

Bob has GERD with poor initial response to a trial of an H2RA. He has been partially compliant with the recommended lifestyle modifications. He has no new complaints and has no apparent warning signs or symptoms of more serious underlying disease.

Plan

Diagnostic

No current indications exist for imaging, endoscopy, or 24-hour pH monitoring.

Therapeutic

Bob is asked to discontinue the ranitidine and to begin an 8-week trial of a proton-pump inhibitor

(PPI). Bob will begin rabeprazole (Aciphex), 20 mg by mouth, 30 to 60 minutes before his first meal of the day, as part of an 8-week trial. He will continue with the lifestyle modifications previously suggested.

Disposition

Bob is asked to schedule an appointment at the conclusion of his 8-week PPI trial. At that time, further treatment will be dictated by his response to the PPI.

DISCUSSION

Epidemiology

GERD is a very common entity in family medicine, and it is the most common upper gastrointestinal disorder in the Western world. Among the adult population of the United States, 20% experience heartburn and symptoms of GERD at least once per week, with almost half experiencing symptoms on a monthly basis. Patients with GERD consistently report low quality-of-life scores (Heidelbaugh and Nostrant, 2004🅑).

Pathophysiology

The development of GERD has been associated with the presence of hiatal hernias, abnormal lower-esophageal sphincter pressures, delayed gastric emptying, and gastric acid–secretion abnormalities. As the medical understanding of GERD has evolved, theories behind the pathophysiology have changed. Currently, up to 80% of episodes of GERD are thought to be associated with transient lower-esophageal sphincter relaxation (TLESR) episodes (Modlin, 2004🅑). Hiatal hernias are associated with TLESR episodes, as is gastric distention. Sphincter relaxations allow the reflux of acidic stomach contents into the esophagus. The presence of acid in contact with the esophageal mucosa causes irritation and inflammation. Damage to this stratified squamous epithelium can be accelerated by prolonged acid-contact time resulting from sphincteric relaxation, delayed gastric emptying with subsequent reflux, or ineffectual esophageal motility. A direct correlation exists between the exposure of the esophagus to acid and the severity of GERD. Heartburn and regurgitation symptoms are highly specific for the presence of GERD. However, GERD with esophageal mucosal injury can often be documented in persons without the presence of symptoms, and poor correlation is found between the presence or absence of a hiatal hernia and GERD (Modlin, 2004🅑).

Diagnosis

In the absence of warning signs or alarm symptoms (see Box 44-1), the diagnosis of GERD can be made clinically without additional testing. In the presence of warning signs, upper endoscopy is recommended. It allows direct visualization of the esophageal mucosa (Eisen, 2001🅒). If extraesophageal manifestations of GERD, such as cough, asthma, laryngitis, and hoarseness, are suspected, ambulatory 24-hour pH monitoring can be helpful to confirm GERD. Ambulatory monitoring also can be helpful in patients who fail to respond to initial treatment with a PPI. A negative pH study does not preclude the diagnosis of GERD. Barium contrast radiology can be useful if other causes of dyspepsia are sought, such as peptic ulcers, malignancy, or esophageal strictures, but it has no role in the initial evaluation of uncomplicated GERD (Eisen, 2001🅒). Esophageal motility testing also has no role in the diagnosis of GERD, unless achalasia or dysmotility disorders are suspected. It is useful in the preoperative evaluation for antireflux surgery (Eisen, 2001🅒).

Historically the diagnosis of GERD was thought to require the presence of documented mucosal abnormalities on endoscopy. Often, endoscopy in symptomatic individuals fails to show visible mucosal damage. This subset of GERD is known as nonerosive reflux disease (NERD). It is managed similarly to traditional GERD. Patients with NERD may show abnormal pH testing, or they may show normal pH monitoring along with normal endoscopy. This variant is referred to as *functional heartburn* (Modlin, 2004 🅑).

Therapy

Bob's initial treatment plan parallels the most commonly advocated approach for GERD. Several studies have shown that antacid therapy is more effective than placebo in the relief of GERD symptoms. Treatment with oral sucralfate (Carafate) has not been shown to be more beneficial than that with placebo (Heidelbaugh, 2004🅑).

Lifestyle modifications are an important part of therapy (see Box 44-2). Weight loss is often advocated, although the reduction of symptoms shown in clinical trials with weight loss has not been associated with a corresponding decrease in pH testing. Certain foods, such as chocolate, coffee, peppermint, and alcohol, are thought to transiently decrease lower esophageal sphincter pressure and should be reduced or eliminated from the diet (Eisen, 2001🅐).

Initial treatment with an H2RA or a PPI is indicated. As in Bob's case, treatment with an H2RA can be initiated as part of step-up therapy. Currently four H2RA medications are available (Box 44-3). They are considered equally efficacious. To initiate therapy, the chosen H2RA is begun at the standard prescription dosage for an 8-week trial. H2RA medications have been shown to be more effective

Box 44-3	Histamine H$_2$-Receptor Antagonists (H2RAs)
Cimetidine (Tagamet) Famotidine (Pepcid) Nizatidine (Axid) Ranitidine (Zantac)	

Box 44-4	Proton Pump Inhibitors (PPIs)
Lansoprazole (Prevacid) Omeprazole (Prilosec) Pantoprazole (Protonix) Rabeprazole (Aciphex) Esomeprazole (Nexium)	

than placebo in the control of symptoms for GERD and in esophageal healing times for documented esophagitis. Tachyphylaxis with the H2RAs during prolonged use can occur (Eisen, 2001Ⓐ). As in Bob's treatment plan, failure to improve after a trial of a H2RA then prompts a change to a once-daily dosage of a PPI.

Step-down therapy for GERD involves initial treatment with a PPI medication (Box 44-4). The PPI of choice is started at the standard daily dose and prescribed for an 8-week trial. In comparisons with placebos, PPI medications are shown to be markedly more effective in symptom relief and healing of esophagitis. They also have proved to be superior to treatment with antacids and H2RA medications. All PPIs have been considered equally efficacious, although the newest PPI, esomeprazole, has shown faster healing rates of documented esophagitis when compared to other PPIs. Its benefit in symptom reduction in GERD is less clear. Long-term therapy with a PPI does not appear to increase the incidence of malignancies or interfere with vitamin absorption. Step-down therapy may be more cost effective than step-up therapy, but studies have yielded conflicting results. At the end of the 8-week trial, the PPI can then be dosed on an as-needed basis, or the patient can be changed to a daily or as-needed H2RA. Patients who have documented esophagitis on endoscopy should be monitored for healing and should remain on maintenance therapy to prevent recurrence (Eisen, 2001Ⓐ).

Refractory GERD exists when symptoms are not controlled by initial medical management or when symptom relapse occurs after initial control. Endoscopy should be performed in these patients to evaluate for esophagitis. Monitoring with pH testing will typically show evidence of acid reflux. These patients are offered additional options to include medical management or laparoscopic fundoplication. Antireflux surgery can be offered to those patients who have normal gastric emptying, normal esophageal manometry, and have had a partial response to acid-suppression therapy. It also may be useful in those patients with a coexistent hiatal hernia. When compared with PPI therapy, antireflux surgery performed by experienced surgeons has long-term success rates that equal or exceed medical therapy. In other settings,

the outcome of surgery is inferior to medical management. Endoscopic treatments that seek to increase lower-esophageal sphincter tone should be considered experimental and not pursued as treatment options (Modlin, 2004Ⓒ).

Complications

Complications associated with GERD include esophageal strictures, bleeding, Barrett's esophagus, and adenocarcinoma. Barrett's esophagus is caused by prolonged exposure to gastric acid and is characterized by a transformation of the normal squamous epithelium to metaplastic columnar epithelium. This markedly increases the risk of esophageal adenocarcinoma over the general population. For this reason, screening endoscopy is recommended every 5 to 10 years for persons with long-term GERD symptoms (Eisen, 2001Ⓒ).

Other

There is no role for *Helicobacter pylori* testing in patients with GERD unless a coexisting peptic ulcer is present. *Helicobacter pylori* infection is implicated in the development of peptic ulcers and is a primary risk factor for gastric cancer. Its role in GERD, however, is less clear. Some studies have shown an association between therapy for *H. pylori* and an increased occurrence of refractory GERD (Cremonini, 2003 Ⓐ).

Summary

GERD is a common problem in the general population. Uncomplicated GERD can be managed medically, by using either PPI or H2RA agents in an initial trial. After initial treatment, patients should be maintained on the lowest dose of the chosen agent to prevent relapse. The presence of alarm symptoms or refractory GERD dictates further investigation to include endoscopy or pH monitoring.

Material Available on Student Consult

Review Questions and Answers for Gastroesophageal Reflux Disease

REFERENCES

Bazaldua OV, Schneider FV. Evaluation and management of dyspepsia. Am Fam Physician 1999;60:1773–1787.**C**

Cremonini F. Meta-analysis: The relationship between *Helicobacter pylori* infection and gastro-oesophageal reflux disease. Aliment Pharmacol Ther 2003;18:279–289.**A**

Eisen GM. An evidence-based approach to gastro-esophageal reflux disease: Evidence-based. Gastro-enterology 2001;2:160–168.**C**

Heidelbaugh JJ, Nostrant TT, Kim C, et al. Management of gastroesophageal reflux disease. Am Fam Physician 2003;68:1311–1321.**B**

Heidelbaugh JJ, Nostrant TT. Medical and surgical management of gastroesophageal reflux disease. Clin Fam Pract 2004;6:547–568.**B**

Klauser AG, Schindlbeck NE, Muller-Lissner SA, et al. Symptoms in gastro-oesophageal reflux disease. Lancet 1990;335:205–208.**B**

Modlin IM, Moss SF, Kidd M, et al. Gastroesophageal reflux disease: Then and now. J Clin Gastroenterol 2004;38:390–402.**B**

C h a p t e r

45 Pancreatitis (Acute Pancreatitis)

Leslie Brott

KEY POINTS

1. The diagnosis of pancreatitis is based on clinical presentation, supported by elevated levels of lipase and/or amylase and, in some cases, radiographic evaluation of the pancreas.
2. The severity of pancreatitis can be assessed early using staging systems such as APACHE (Acute Physiology, Age and Chronic Health Evaluation) II and multiple organ system failure scales. Patients with severe pancreatitis should be monitored in the intensive care unit. Those with mild pancreatitis can usually be managed in the general medical ward.
3. The mainstays of treatment include fluid resuscitation and pain management.
4. The most common causes of acute pancreatitis are gallbladder disease and ethanol ingestion.
5. Early complications of acute pancreatitis include pancreatic necrosis and secondary infection. Late complications include pancreatic pseudo-cyst and abscess.

INITIAL VISIT

Subjective

Patient Identification and Presenting Problem

Mike V. is a 55-year-old man who presents with a 24-hour history of abdominal pain. Mike is an otherwise healthy man who developed epigastric pain yesterday. The constant, dull pain radiates into his back and worsens with deep breathing. He feels more comfortable sitting up, as lying flat accentuates the pain. He has nausea but denies vomiting and is, in fact, able to eat small amounts. His last normal bowel movement was yesterday, before the onset of his pain. He took ibuprofen once yesterday for his pain, but it provided no relief. He has had no fever or chills. There has been neither heartburn nor urinary complaints. He drinks three or more alcohol drinks daily and has for many years. He has never had abdominal surgery.

Medical History

Mike has no known chronic medical problems. He has had two orthopedic surgeries. He is on no chronic medications and has no drug allergies.

Family History
There is no family history of pancreatitis. The patient believes that his mother has had gallbladder problems.

Social History
Mike has a female significant other. He works in computer operations for an insurance company in town. He does not smoke and denies current or past use of illicit drugs.

Review of Systems
The patient denies dizziness, cough, shortness of breath, chest pain, and palpitations. He has not experienced easy bleeding or bruising or bloody stools. He has never had seizures or signs of delirium tremens when abstaining from alcohol.

Objective

Physical Examination
General Mike is a well-developed man sitting hunched over on the examination table. He is alert and conversant but in moderate distress. He weighs 196 pounds (stable over the past 2 years) and is 6 feet tall.

Vital Signs His blood pressure is 112/78, heart rate is 82, and temperature is 37.1°C (98.7°F).

Head, Eyes, Ears, Nose, and Throat His pupils are equal, round, and reactive to light. Tympanic membranes are normal. The oropharynx is without erythema or exudates. There is good dentition.

Neck The neck is supple with no lymphadenopathy.

Heart The rate and rhythm are regular with no murmurs.

Lungs The lungs are clear bilaterally, but breathing is shallow.

Back The back is straight. There is a well-healed vertical lumbar incision. Bilateral costovertebral angle tenderness is found.

Abdomen There are hypoactive bowel sounds. The abdomen is distended and diffusely tender but more exquisitely in the epigastrium. There is no hepatosplenomegaly or masses and no rebound or involuntary guarding.

Genitourinary He has normal male genitalia with no hernia.

Rectal There is normal tone; stool is brown and guaiac negative. The prostate is of normal size.

Extremities There is no clubbing, cyanosis, or edema.

Laboratory Data
The patient's complete blood count is remarkable for an elevated white count of 17,300 with 92% neutrophils and 1% bands. Hemoglobin, hematocrit, and platelets are normal. The complete metabolic panel is within normal limits including serum transaminases. His amylase is 2182 U/L (normal 25 to 125 U/L), and lipase is 7200 U/L (normal 10 to 140 U/L).

Radiographic Studies
Plain films of the abdomen show a nonspecific abdominal gas pattern. There are no abnormal air-fluid levels, calcifications, or distended bowels. The chest radiograph is normal as well.

Assessment

Working Diagnosis
Acute pancreatitis, most likely due to gallstones or alcohol.

Differential Diagnosis
Other causes of acute upper abdominal pain include the following:

1. *Peptic ulcer disease with perforation* presents with an abrupt onset of epigastric pain versus pancreatitis in which the pain may be more gradual, reaching peak severity in 10 to 20 minutes. The patient with a perforated ulcer will experience initial nausea and vomiting, but this will resolve quickly. Movement does not relieve the pain, whereas in pancreatitis, the fetal or sitting positions seem to lessen the intensity of the pain.
2. *Biliary colic* and *acute cholecystitis* cause a very similar epigastric pain as pancreatitis, but it is of shorter duration, lasting hours rather than days. The pain will wax and wane as opposed to the constant, unremitting pain of pancreatitis.
3. *Mesenteric ischemia* and *infarction* occur more often in elderly patients who have a history of cardiovascular disease. These patients' sudden onset of abdominal pain is accompanied by nausea, vomiting, and bloody diarrhea.
4. *Intestinal obstruction* presents as cyclic pain with associated vomiting. There is abdominal distention with hyperactive, high-pitched bowel sounds.
5. An *inferior myocardial infarction* can present with epigastric pain. However, the pain usually radiates into the chest, jaw, and left upper extremity. Patients classically have diaphoresis, nausea, and shortness of breath, and cardiac risk factors can often be identified (family history, tobacco use, hyperlipidemia, hypertension). Electrocardiographic and cardiac enzyme elevations differentiate it from pancreatitis.

6. A patient with a *dissecting aortic aneurysm* suffers the abrupt onset of severe, tearing chest and/or abdominal pain. His or her vital signs are often remarkable for hypotension. Chest radiographs may show a widened mediastinum, cardiomegaly from heart failure, or pericardial effusion or possibly a left pleural effusion.

7. *Ruptured ectopic pregnancy* is included in the differential, although obviously is not a consideration in our patient. As many as one half of women with a ruptured ectopic pregnancy will present with diffuse abdominal pain. They will often have other signs of early pregnancy as well, including breast tenderness and nausea. Approximately 75% will have vaginal bleeding. A positive pregnancy test will often differentiate these patients from those with acute pancreatitis.

Plan

Diagnostic

Based on history, physical examination and laboratory studies (particularly the high levels of amylase and lipase), Mike is diagnosed with acute pancreatitis. Identifying the cause of his pancreatitis is important in preventing recurrent episodes. The two most common causes of pancreatitis are gallstones, which cause more than half the cases, and alcohol, constituting approximately 30% of the cases. Laboratory studies and ultrasound scans are commonly used to differentiate the two. In gallstone pancreatitis, the serum alanine aminotransferase and aspartate aminotransferase are generally elevated. In alcoholic pancreatitis, it is thought that a serum lipase/amylase ratio of greater than 2.0 occurs, although this is not particularly specific. A transabdominal ultrasound scan was performed in our patient immediately after diagnosis. No gallstones or common duct stones were identified nor was there evidence of biliary tract obstruction. With the negative results of the ultrasound scan, the high serum lipase/amylase ratio, and a history of significant alcohol use, our patient is diagnosed with alcoholic pancreatitis.

Therapeutic

Mike is admitted as an inpatient to our community hospital. He is started on intravenous fluids and is kept NPO. His pain is initially treated with meperidine, but due to inadequate pain relief, he is placed on a patient-controlled anesthetic device with hydromorphone. His pain gradually resolves over the next 4 or 5 days. He suffers no systemic complications of pancreatitis and is hemodynamically stable throughout his hospitalization. He is monitored closely for evidence of alcohol withdrawal using the Clinical Institute Withdrawal Assessment for Alcohol scale. Once his pain has resolved, oral feeding is started. This is tolerated well, and Mike is discharged home.

Patient Education

Mike is taught that alcohol use is the most likely cause of his pancreatitis. He is advised to abstain from further alcohol use, as it may cause recurrent episodes of pancreatitis. He is offered information on alcohol rehabilitation. In the weeks following discharge, he is to monitor for a return of epigastric pain, which may indicate a late complication of acute pancreatitis such as formation of a pseudocyst.

Disposition

The patient is to follow up at the clinic in 1 week following discharge, sooner if pain, fever, nausea, or vomiting develops.

DISCUSSION

Acute pancreatitis can cause significant morbidity and mortality. Its incidence is increasing worldwide for unclear reasons. It is important for family physicians to identify pancreatitis early and treat it appropriately to avoid serious sequelae. It is estimated that 40% of all cases of pancreatitis are missed, only to be found at autopsy.

Acute pancreatitis can be divided into mild and severe disease. Mild pancreatitis accounts for 80% of all cases and is defined as interstitial edema of the pancreas with minimal distal organ involvement. Severe pancreatitis is distinguished by pancreatic necrosis with possible infection and multiorgan failure. The inappropriate activation of trypsin, a pancreatic enzyme, is the pathophysiologic basis for acute pancreatitis. When the resultant inflammation is localized to the pancreas, mild disease results. If the inflammation extends into the space surrounding the pancreas, a systemic inflammatory response ensues, resulting in severe disease.

Clinical Presentation

The patient with acute pancreatitis presents with the acute onset of severe upper abdominal pain, which is characterized as boring and steady. Approximately half the patients will experience radiation of the pain in a bandlike pattern to the back. Ninety percent experience nausea and vomiting. On examination, the patient with mild pancreatitis will have abdominal tenderness but rarely guarding; bowel sounds will be diminished. Those with severe pancreatitis will appear toxic and will exhibit abdominal guarding and distention. They are more likely to have tachycardia, hypotension, and fever.

There are two examination findings that are described classically as indicative of pancreatitis:

Cullen's sign (ecchymosis of the periumbilical area) and Grey Turner's sign (ecchymosis of the flank). These signs are quite rare (less than 1% of all cases) and are not specific for pancreatitis.

Laboratory Studies

Several laboratory studies are helpful in diagnosing pancreatitis and identifying the etiology, but none are diagnostic in isolation. An elevated white blood cell count and elevated serum glucose level are common. Liver enzymes may be elevated, especially in gallstone pancreatitis.

Serum amylase and lipase are key laboratory indices in the evaluation of pancreatitis. Amylase is produced by both the pancreas and salivary glands. Although there are assays that differentiate the two, a total serum amylase can be obtained quickly and cheaply and is helpful in the diagnosis of pancreatitis. After the onset of pancreatic inflammation, the amylase rises within 6 to 12 hours and will remain elevated for 3 to 5 days in mild cases. However, serum amylase is not completely sensitive nor specific. There are many nonpancreatic causes of an elevated amylase. Therefore, it is used as one element in the diagnosis of pancreatitis.

Another element is the lipase level. Lipase is produced almost entirely by the pancreas. Its sensitivity and specificity, however, are similar to amylase. Like amylase, it rises early in the course of pancreatitis but stays elevated as long as 14 days. Opinions differ on the value of either the lipase or amylase level. Some experts argue that taken together, they differentiate pancreatitis from other acute abdominal processes, particularly if their values are three times normal.

There are additional laboratory markers that are in development as markers for pancreatitis. C-reactive protein is readily available and is valuable in determining prognosis, if not diagnosis. Serum levels of trypsin and elastase also have value in detecting pancreatitis but are not readily available to most hospitals and clinics.

Radiographic Studies

Radiographic studies are used in the workup of pancreatitis to determine both its etiology and prognosis. Plain films of the abdomen are often normal, thus excluding other causes of intra-abdominal pain. A transabdominal ultrasound scan is useful early in the diagnosis of pancreatitis to identify gallstones, biliary duct dilation, common duct stones, and ascites. It should be performed within 24 hours of presentation. One pitfall of ultrasonography, however, is that the pancreas is often not well visualized because as much as 35% of the time, it is obscured by bowel gas. Nevertheless, it is useful in differentiating gallstone from alcoholic pancreatitis.

A more valuable imaging test for the diagnosis and staging of pancreatitis is contrast-enhanced computed tomography (CT). CT gauges the severity of the pancreatitis as well as excludes other intra-abdominal pathology and should be used in patients whose diagnosis is in question, who present with severe symptoms, or who have evidence of infection (fever, persistent leukocytosis). CT is helpful in staging the severity of pancreatitis and, in fact, forms the basis of one of the staging systems (see later).

Prognosis

Identifying the patient with acute pancreatitis is much easier than predicting the prognosis of the disease. Much work has been done over the years to develop systems to stage acute pancreatitis to predict severity and mortality. Approximately 20% of patients with pancreatitis are graded as severe, and the mortality rate can be as high as 10%. Staging systems attempt to identify early those patients who are most likely to develop severe pancreatitis.

One of the first staging systems reported was that of Ranson. Eleven criteria are used to predict the severity of disease (Box 45-1). The criteria are divided into signs at admission and at 48 hours. Traditionally, if fewer than three signs are noted, mortality is less than 1%. Mortality rises to 100% if more than six signs are found. Unfortunately, the system is neither very sensitive (57% to 85%) nor specific (68% to 85%), and it takes 48 hours to complete staging. It is valuable, however, in excluding severe disease, as its negative predictive value is approximately 90%.

Two newer staging systems, the APACHE II and multiple organ system failure scale, are improvements over Ranson's criteria. Unlike Ranson's, they can be used at admission and then on a daily basis to assess progression of disease. APACHE II uses

---

Box 45-1	**Ranson's Criteria**

At initial presentation:
- Older than 55 years
- White blood cell count >16,000/mm^3
- Low-density lipoprotein >350 IU/L
- Aspartate aminotransferase >250 IU/L
- Glucose >200 mg/dL

At 48 hours:
- Decrease of hematocrit >10%
- Increase in blood, urea, nitrogen >5 mg/dL
- Serum calcium <8 mg/dL
- Arterial Po$_2$ <60 mm Hg
- Base deficit >4 mEq/L
- Fluid sequestration >600 mL

age, presence of chronic disease and 12 physiologic parameters including vital signs (i.e., temperature, heart rate, respiratory rate) and laboratory values (i.e., serum sodium, creatinine, hematocrit, arterial pH) to determine a severity score. The multiple organ system failure system assesses the cardiovascular, pulmonary, renal, neurologic, hepatic, and gastrointestinal systems separately to stage pancreatitis. Any significant abnormality in a system qualifies as a point, and severity is based on total points obtained on a daily basis.

CT is the basis of yet another system of staging pancreatitis. Using a 5-point severity scale based on the pancreas' appearance on CT, along with the percentage of pancreatic necrosis, the Computed Tomography Severity Index predicts morbidity and mortality. This scale reflects the importance of CT in the management of pancreatitis.

Management

Management of pancreatitis is dependent on the severity of disease. Almost all patients need to be admitted to the hospital. Those with severe disease or poor prognostic indicators should be monitored in the intensive care unit. All patients need fluid resuscitation and bowel rest. Cardiac, renal, and pulmonary status should be monitored closely. Pain control is best with meperidine or hydromorphone. An antiemetic is also usually necessary. There is no evidence that proton pump inhibitors, H_2 blockers, or antibiotics are routinely necessary. Nasogastric tubes are needed only if an ileus is present and decompression is needed, but they are not routinely used.

Patients with mild cases can be expected to improve in 3 to 7 days. Once their pain has diminished, oral feedings may begin with small amounts of noncaloric liquid. Their diet is advanced as tolerated.

Complications

The complications of pancreatitis usually occur within 2 weeks of the onset of symptoms. Seventy percent to 80% of all deaths from acute pancreatitis are attributed to secondary infection of the pancreas. Necrosis of the pancreas can lead to multiorgan failure including acute renal failure, hypovolemia and circulatory shock, sepsis, and acute respiratory distress syndrome.

Beyond the acute period, late-presenting complications of pancreatitis include pancreatic pseudocysts and abscesses. Patients will often present weeks after their initial episode with new complaints of abdominal pain. Abdominal CT will identify these findings.

Causes

The majority of cases of acute pancreatitis are due to two main causes: gallbladder disease, accounting for more than 50% of all cases, and alcohol use, implicated in approximately 30% of all cases. Other less common causes include hereditary pancreatitis, hypertriglyceridemia (>1000 mg/dL), hypercalcemia/hyperparathyroidism, infection (viral or bacterial), medications, iatrogenic (e.g., endoscopic retrograde cholangiopancreatography), α_1-antitrypsin deficiency, anatomic abnormalities, pregnancy, and trauma, among others.

Material Available on Student Consult
Review Questions and Answers about Acute Pancreatitis

SUGGESTED READINGS

Balthazar E. Staging of acute pancreatitis. Radiol Clin North Am 2002;40:1199–1209.

Munoz A, Katerndahl D. Diagnosis and management of acute pancreatitis. Am Fam Physician 2000;62:164–174.

Orbuch M. Optimizing outcomes in acute pancreatitis. Clin Fam Pract 2004;6:607.

Feldman M, Friedman L, Sleisenger M, eds. Sleisenger and Fordtran's Gastrointestinal and Liver Disease, 7th ed. Philadelphia, Elsevier, 2002, pp 913–941.

46

Swollen Foreskin (Diabetes Mellitus Type 2)

Cheng-Chieh Chuang

KEY POINTS

1. Diabetes mellitus type 2 usually does not produce symptoms for years before the diagnosis is made. Screening all people 45 years and older, and those younger than 45 with risk factors, is recommended.
2. Screening can be done using the fasting glucose or 2-hour postprandial blood glucose level tested using 75 g of anhydrous glucose.
3. The management of diabetes mellitus type 2 has three major components: nutrition, physical activity, and medication. The goals are to lower the blood glucose level and decrease hemoglobin A1C to less than 7%.
4. Medical nutrition therapy is a concept that incorporates nutrition and physical activity. It includes carbohydrate counting, calorie restriction, weight reduction, and exercise. Medical nutrition therapy may decrease the hemoglobin A1C by 1% to 2%.
5. There are two main defects in glucose metabolism in diabetes, insulin resistance and insulin deficiency. A high fasting glucose level reflects

insulin resistance, and postprandial hyperglycemia reflects the insulin deficiency.
6. Secretagogues (sulfonylureas, meglitanide, d-phenylalanine derivative) work primarily to enhance the body's production of insulin in response to glucose intake.
7. Insulin sensitizers (biguanide, thiazolidinediones) treat insulin resistance.
8. Insulin is the most potent of all medications. The goal of using insulin is to duplicate the natural physiologic insulin and glucose level, in which basal insulin supplies half of the body's needs and insulin secreted in response to meals supplies the rest.
9. Individuals with type 2 diabetes tend to have lipid disorders and hypertension.
10. Diabetes is considered a coronary heart disease risk equivalent. Aspirin should be considered for all individuals with diabetes mellitus type 2.
11. Potential microvascular complications from diabetes mellitus type 2 include nephropathy, retinopathy, and neuropathy.

INITIAL VISIT

Subjective

Patient Identification and Presenting Problem

David M. is a 37-year-old white man of Portuguese descent who says with some embarrassment that he is here for a second opinion. He saw a urologist 1 week ago because of difficulty retracting his foreskin for the past 3 to 4 weeks. The urologist suggested circumcision. Not satisfied with this proposal, Mr. M. decided to see a primary care physician.

History of Present Illness

Mr. M. was in his usual state of health until 3 to 4 weeks ago, when he began experiencing increasing discomfort and then pain while retracting his foreskin to urinate or have sex. He reports no dysuria, no urethral discharge, no history of sexually transmitted disease, no increase in urinary frequency, and no changes in foreskin color. This is the first time in his life he has had a problem with his foreskin.

Medical History

Mr. M. states that he has been in excellent health.

Evidence levels Ⓐ Randomized, controlled trials (RCTs), meta-analyses, well-designed systematic reviews of RCTs. Ⓑ Case-control or cohort studies, nonrandomized clinical trials, systematic reviews of studies other than RCTs, crosssectional studies, retrospective studies, certain uncontrolled studies. Ⓒ Consensus statements, expert guidelines, usual practice, opinion.

Family History

Mr. M.'s parents have diabetes mellitus type 2 and hypertension. His father had a heart attack at age 53. His mother also takes thyroid medication. He has no siblings.

Social History

Mr. M. has been married for the past 15 years and works as a truck driver. He reports a monogamous sexual relationship with his wife since marriage. He has never had sex with another woman or man. He has two healthy teenage children. He does not smoke, but drinks one glass of red wine with his dinner. He denies any illicit drug use. He feels that loading and unloading cargos for his truck is enough exercise for him. On average, he watches 4 hours of television a day. He notes that in his early 20s he used to lift weights and play soccer, but after marriage he stopped these activities.

Review of Systems

The review of systems is negative other than for the complaints already noted. Specifically, Mr. M. reports no fatigue, no malaise, no polydypsia, no polyuria, no nocturia, no recurrent infection, no visual changes, no dental problems, no numbness or paresthesia anywhere, and no abnormal nodes, especially in his groin.

Objective

Mr. M. is obese and pleasant. His blood pressure is 150/90, pulse is 80 and regular, weight is 258 pounds, height is 5 feet 8 inches, and body mass index (BMI) is 39.3. Genital examination reveals an edematous foreskin, which on slight retraction discloses a white, cheesy discharge. No inguinal lymphadenopathy is palpable bilaterally. The rest of the genital examination is negative. Normal saline and KOH slide of the discharge shows elongated pseudohyphae and budding spores. An office fingerstick blood test shows a glucose concentration of 250 mg/dL. Urinalysis of a clean catch urine specimen shows a high glucose concentration but is otherwise negative, including for ketones. The specimen is sent for culture, gonorrheal, and chlamydial studies. Mr. M. declines HIV and syphilis testing, saying that he has no risk factor for them. He is asked to return for fasting blood tests for glucose, hemoglobin A1C, a lipid panel (total cholesterol, high-density lipoprotein [HDL] level, low-density lipoprotein [LDL] level, and triglycerides), a complete blood cell count, determination of electrolyte, blood urea nitrogen, creatinine, and thyroid-stimulating hormone levels, and liver function tests. A spot urine is also ordered to check for microalbuminuria. He is instructed not to drink alcoholic beverages for 3 days before the blood tests.

Assessment

Working Diagnosis

The working diagnosis is *Candida* balanitis, most likely associated with hyperglycemia of diabetes mellitus.

Differential Diagnosis

Nonketotic hyperglycemia can be due to diabetes mellitus type 2. It can also be caused by acute pain from trauma, myocardial ischemia or infarction, other critical illnesses, steroid use or Cushing's disease, hypothyroidism, and hemochromatosis.

Plan

Mr. M. chooses to take one dose of oral fluconazole, 150 mg, for the balanitis. The high glucose level comes as a shock to Mr. M. He maintains that it is impossible for him to have diabetes as his parents do, because he feels great except for the foreskin problem. He is to return in 1 week after the test results are ready.

FIRST FOLLOW-UP VISIT

Subjective

At his 1-week visit Mr. M. is happy that the candidiasis has cleared. He is somewhat distraught, however, because he used his parents' glucometer a day before returning to the office and found his fasting glucose concentration to be 165 mg/dL. He is very anxious about the full blood test results.

Objective

His blood pressure is 145/95 and his pulse is 85. The results of the blood tests are within normal range except for a fasting glucose concentration of 154 mg/dL, a hemoglobin A1C value of 11.4%, a total cholesterol concentration of 250 mg/dL, an HDL concentration of of 44 mg/dL, an LDL concentration of 169 mg/dL, and a triglyceride concentration of 256 mg/dL. A spot urine test shows no microalbuminuria. He has no thyromegaly. Results of the cardiac examination, external genitals examination, bilateral foot examination, and neurologic examination, including the monofilament test, are all normal. The electrocardiogram is also normal.

Assessment

The physician's assessment is diabetes mellitus type 2, presumptive hypertension, and dyslipidemia.

Plan

A long discussion with Mr. M. about lifestyle modification (medical nutrition therapy), including increasing physical activities and sensible nutrition, ensues. Mr. M. insists that he does not want any medication at present and that he will try lifestyle modification first. Because he enjoys watching television, which helps relax him after a full day's work, the physician suggests he obtain a stationary bicycle to use while watching television. A few other exercises that can be done in front of the television are also explored. He is referred for a dilated diabetic eye examination. He is also referred to a nutritionist for detailed meal and food planning needed for medical nutrition therapy, and to a diabetic nurse for further education on diabetes and the use of a glucometer. The physician suggests that his wife also attend the meeting with the nutritionist because she cooks for the family. Because Mr. M. takes a glass of wine with his evening meal, he is instructed to be on the watch for hypoglycemia and always to drink with food. The possible effect of alcohol on his blood pressure is discussed. He is to return in 2 weeks and bring with him daily fasting glucose readings.

SUBSEQUENT FOLLOW-UP VISITS

At his return visit in 2 weeks' time, Mr. M.'s fasting glucose readings show a gradual decrease during that period, with last 2 days' readings in the 110s. In addition to working out on the stationary bicycle, Mr. M. has joined one of his old buddies in weight training.

Three months after his initial visit Mr. M. has lost 18 pounds, and his hemoglobin A1C value has come down to 6.5%. His home blood pressure readings range from 110-140/70-85. His lipid profile has also improved to within normal limits, although his blood pressure is still in the high normal range. Mr. M is still not interested in any medication.

At his 6-month visit Mr. M. has lost an additional 15 pounds, for a total of 33 pounds since his first visit. His blood pressure numbers at home range from 110–130/70–85. His hemoglobin A1C value is 6.1%.

Mr. M. continues to do well until 3 years after diagnosis, when his hemoglobin A_{1c} value hovers in the low 7s with medical nutrition therapy alone. Medication therapy with metformin is started. His blood pressure also has increased slightly to 110–140/70–90, and an ACE inhibitor is started. His lipid panel is still within normal limits.

DISCUSSION

Up to half of patients with diabetes mellitus type 2 are diagnosed after complications develop. Unlike most of these individuals, who present with cardiovascular complications, Mr. M. presented with candidiasis. It is possible that the candidiasis contributed further to the hyperglycemia, which would explain the initial hemoglobin A1c value of 11.4%.

Symptoms

Classic symptoms of diabetes mellitus type 2 include fatigue, polydypsia, polyuria, unexplained weight loss, and blurred vision. Because the majority of those with undiagnosed diabetes mellitus type 2 are without symptoms, screening individuals at high risk is recommended.

Screening

In contrast to the current recommendation by the U.S. Preventive Services Task Force, which recommends screening only those who have hypertension or hyperlipidemia, the American Diabetes Association and the U.S. Department of Health and Human Services recommend screening all people 45 years and older, and those younger than 45 with the following risk factors: obesity, a family history of diabetes, member of a high-risk ethnic group (African American, Latino, Native American), polycystic ovary disease, hypertension, or dyslipidemia. Other risk factors include acanthosis nigricans, associated with insulin resistance, components of metabolic syndrome (central obesity, hypertension, dyslipidemia), and preexisting cardiovascular disease (American Diabetes Association Expert Committee, 2004 ⟲).

Screening can be done using fasting glucose or 2-hour postprandial blood glucose using 75 g of anhydrous glucose. The latter test may be abnormal before the first one, but the convenience of the fasting glucose test makes it the more practical method. With either method, a second, confirmatory test is needed before the diagnosis can be made.

Management

Once diabetes mellitus type 2 has been diagnosed, management has three major components: nutrition, physical activity, and medical management. The goals are to lower the glucose concentration and to decrease the hemoglobin A1C value to less than 7%, thereby minimizing or preventing the microvascular and macrovascular complications of diabetes. Each percentage point reduction in A1C corresponds to a 30 mg/dL reduction in fasting glucose levels (Table 46-1).

Patient education and an emphasis on the patient's own involvement in disease management are crucial. In addition, the patient may need support to deal with the anger and frustration of living with a chronic condition. The primary care physician's main functions are to facilitate these efforts and to coordinate care among a formal or informal team consisting of a dietician, an ophthalmologist or optometrist, and other specialists, such as an exercise physiologist, podiatrist, nephrologist, cardiologist, and psychologist or psychiatrist, depending on the severity of the illness and the associated

Table 46-1	Hemoglobin A1C Level and Corresponding Average Glucose Value
Hemoglobin A1C* (%)	**Average Blood Glucose Level (mg/dL)**
4	60
5	90
6	120
7	150
8	180
9	210
10	240
11	270
12	300
13	330

*Glycosylated hemoglobin, also known as %A1C, is a measure of average blood glucose level over the preceding 8 to 12 weeks.

complications. Negotiating with patients changes in lifestyle, diet, exercise, and tobacco cessation is important and necessary. Resources available to help patient and physician are listed in Box 46-1.

Table 46-2 lists items important in the management of diabetes mellitus type 2.

Medical Nutrition Therapy

Medical nutrition therapy is a concept that incorporates nutrition and physical activity. It includes carbohydrate counting, calorie restriction, weight reduction, and exercise (Franz, 2004Ⓐ ⒷⒸ). The recommended macronutrient intake central to medical nutrition therapy is listed in Table 46-3.

Medical nutrition therapy may decrease the hemoglobin A1C value by 1% to 2%. It improves insulin resistance and may control the hypertension and dyslipidemia associated with diabetes mellitus type 2. It is reasonable to attempt a trial of medical nutrition therapy without medication in patients with hemoglobin values at or below 8.5%, and in individuals who, like Mr. M., insist on no medication initially and who are not at immediate risk of severe hyperglycemia.

Box 46-1	**Patient Education Resources**

American Diabetes Association
800-232-6733
www.diabetes.org

National Diabetes Information Clearinghouse
301-654-3327
www.niddk.nihgov/health/diabetes/ndic.htm

National Diabetes Education Program
www.ndep.nih.gov

Carbohydrate Counting Carbohydrate counting involves counting carbohydrate intake, focusing more on the total amount of carbohydrate than on the type of food. The convention now is that one carbohydrate choice is equal to 15 g of carbohydrates (Table 46-4). Individuals plan their total daily personal carbohydrate needs with the help of a dietician. The goal is to have an even intake throughout the day of carbohydrates coming from starchy foods, meat and meat substitutes, and fats. Although the emphasis in carbohydrate counting is on total carbohydrate intake, discrimination among food sources is ultimately necessary, as calories from other nutrients such as fats will affect calorie restriction and weight reduction.

Fat Reduction Reduction of fat intake is part of calorie restriction. Distinguishing among different types of fats is also important. Saturated fat increases LDL concentrations and total cholesterol levels. Polyunsaturated fats that contain omega-3 fatty acids decrease LDL levels, increase HDL levels, and decrease triglyceride levels. Monounsaturated fats such as canola and olive oils decrease LDL concentrations and protect HDL cholesterol. Trans fats (partially hydrogenated vegetable oils), used in most restaurants and confectioneries, increase LDL concentrations and lower HDL concentrations, and now are recognized as detrimental to health.

Physical Activities

Exercise, or adequate physical activy, is not only important for glucose control; it also confers many other health benefits, such as increasing HDL, weight reduction, and enhancing the sense of well-being. Exercise at least once every 2 to 3 days is needed for these benefits to appear. Cumulative exercise, such as three 10-minute sessions, may be as beneficial as one 30-minute session.

Weight Reduction Insulin resistance typically starts at a BMI of 27. The ideal goal for weight reduction is a BMI of less than 25. However, it may not be possible to achieve this ideal, for a variety of reasons. If the patient agrees that weight loss is a goal, a gradual loss of about 10% of current weight, or 20 pounds, at the rate of 1/2 to 1 pound a week, may be reasonable.

Medical Management

Medical management for diabetes mellitus type 2 not only aims to contain hyperglycemia, it also involves preventing and controlling comorbid conditions (hypertension, dyslipidemia) and diabetic complications (neuropathy, retinopathy, nephropathy, and cardiovascular disease).

Containing Hyperglycemia There are two main defects in glucose metabolism in diabetes, insulin resistance and insulin deficiency. A high fasting glucose concentration reflects insulin resistance, and postprandial hyperglycemia reflects insulin deficiency. The U.K.

Table 46-2 Taking Care of Patients with Diabetes Mellitus Type 2

	Interval	Goal
Physical and Emotional Assessment		
Blood pressure	Every visit	Target goal < 130/80
Weight	Every visit	BMI < 27, or 10% less than the original weight
Foot examination		
Visual inspection	Every visit	
Pedal pulses, neurologic examination	Yearly	
Dilated eye examination	Upon diagnosis and every year	
Screening for depression	At least yearly	
Dental examination	At least twice yearly	
Prophylaxis	2–4 x per year	
Laboratory Studies		
Hemoglobin A1C	Every 3 months 1–2 x per year if stable	<7%
Microalbuminuria (albumin/ creatinine ratio)	At diagnosis Every year till proteinuria is documented	
Blood lipid	At diagnosis and yearly	Triglyceride < 200 mg/dL HDL > 45 (men), >55 (women) LDL < 100 mg/dL
Self-Management Training		
Assess knowledge of diabetes, medications, self-monitoring, complications, and problem-solving skills	Initially and yearly	
Self-glucose monitoring	As needed	
Medical nutrition therapy	Ongoing	
Physical activity	Ongoing	
Weight management	Ongoing	
Interventions		
Medication	As needed	A1C < 7%
Aspirin therapy	Unless contraindicated	81 mg/day to 325 mg/day
Smoking cessation	Encourage at every visit	
Immunization	Influenza yearly Pneumococcal at diagnosis if not done already	

Prospective Diabetes Study (1995 Ⓐ) suggested that at the time of diagnosis, individuals with type 2 diabetes have about half of their beta-cell function remaining, as the real onset of the diabetes occurred around 10 to 11 years earlier. Six years after diagnosis, beta-cell function decreases further to about a quarter of its original function. Therefore, after some time with medical nutrition therapy, it is often necessary to start medication to achieve good glycemic control.

Oral Glucose-Lowering Agents There are several classes of oral glucose-lowering agents (Lebovitz, 2001 Ⓐ Ⓑ). Some are secretagogues (sulfonylureas,

meglitanide, *d*-phenylalanine derivative) that function primarily to enhance the body's production of insulin in response to glucose intake. These drugs may induce hypoglycemia. Others are insulin sensitizers (biguanide, thiazolidinediones) that treat insulin resistance and in general do not induce hypoglycemia. There is also a third class of agents, a-glucosidase inhibitors, which delay carbohydrate absorption.

The major action, efficacy, indication, and side effects of each class of oral agent are listed in Table 46-5. Metformin, a secretagogue, or a thiazodinedione is often used for initial monotherapy for diabetes mellitus type 2.

Table 46-3 Macronutrient Composition Recommended for Medical Nutrition Therapy

Nutrient	Recommended Intake
Carbohydrate	50–60% of total calories
Protein	Ca. 15% of total calories
Total fat	25–35% of total calories
Saturated fat	<7% of total calories
Polyunsaturated fat	Up to 10% of total calories
Monounsaturated fat	Up to 20% of total calories
Trans fatty acids	Minimum
Cholesterol	<200 mg/day
Fiber	20–30 g/day

About half of individuals with diabetes mellitus type 2 need another agent added after 3 years of monotherapy. Two-drug therapy should also be considered for patients whose A1C value is above 8% after medical nutrition therapy. The addition of a second agent may decrease A1C by 1% to 2%. There is no evidence that any one combination is better than another. The addition of a third agent may further decrease A1C by about 1% to 1.5%. Insulin may be considered for A1C values above 8% on two agents.

Sulfonylurea Sulfonylurea stimulates beta cells to secrete more insulin in response to elevated glucose levels. It is used in patients with a BMI less than 27, an A1C value less than 9%, and/or a postprandial glucose level of 200 to 300 mg/dL. Second-generation sulfonylureas are better tolerated and are preferred. About 85% of the clinical effectiveness of glyburide and glipizide is achieved with half the recommended maximal dose. Once daily preparations appears to be clinically

superior and cause less hypoglycemia. An individual's response to the medication may take place within days.

The most important side effect is hypoglycemia. Other side effects include weight gain and gastrointestinal symptoms. Sulfonylureas need to be used with caution in the presence of renal disease.

Other Secretagogues Meglitinide and nateglinide are rapid-acting secretagogues with a short duration of action. Either is taken with meals. They do not have a renal contraindication.

Biguanides Biguanides targets fasting glucose. They reduce hepatic glucose production and improve insulin action to increase glucose uptake at the muscle level.

Metformin is the only biguanide used in the United States. It may reduce A1C values by up to 2.2%. It also reduce weight and reduce cholesterol and triglyceride concentrations. It is the only oral agent shown thus far to reduce cardiovascular complications.

Meformin is indicated for a BMI greater than 27, an A1C value less than 9%, and a blood glucose concentration of 160 to 250 mg/dL. Care should be taken in patients with renal disease and liver disease, excessive alcohol intake, metabolic acidosis, and active cardiac or pulmonary disease. Meformin should be stopped before contrast dye use or surgery. The most common side effects are gastrointestinal distress and a metallic taste.

Thiazolidinediones Rosiglitazone and pioglitazone are the thiazolidinediones used in the United States. They enhance insulin-sensitizing effect on muscles, adipose tissue, and liver cells. They may also increase HDL concentrations, decrease blood pressure, decrease inflammation (CRP), and effect better fat distribution. Hemoglobin A1C may be reduced by up to 2.6% with a thiazolidinedione.

Table 46-4 Food Servings Equivalent to 15 g of Carbohydrate

1 small apple (4 oz)	1 cup milk
¼ large bagel (1oz)	½ cup orange juice
1 small banana (4 oz)	⅓ cup cooked pasta
1 biscuit	1 medium peach (4 oz)
1 slice of bread	½ cup peas
2-inch-square unfrosted cake	½ cup pinto beans or kidney beans
¾ cup ready-to-eat cereal	3 cups popped popcorn
½ cup cooked cereal	½ cup mashed potato
2 small cookies (2/3 oz)	15–20 potato chips (3/4 oz)
½ cup corn	¾ oz pretzels
6 saltine crackers	⅓ cup rice
½ cup canned fruit	1 tablespoon sugar
½ hamburger bun	½ cup sweet potato
½ cup light ice cream	2 taco shells (6-inch size)
1 tablespoon jam	1 tortilla (6-inch size)

Table 46-5 The Effect of Various Treatments on the Reduction of Hemoglobin A1C Values

Treatment	Medical Nutrition Therapy	Sulfonylurea	Biguanide	Thiazolidinedione Inhibitor	α-Glucosidase	Insulin
Reduction in hemoglobin A1C	1%–2%	Up to 2.3%	Up to 2.2%	Up to 2.6%	0.5%–1%	Unlimited
Action		Secretagogue	Insulin sensitizer	Insulin sensitizer		
Monotherapy indication	A1C < 8.5%	BMI < 27, A1C < 9%	BMI = 27, A1C < 9%	BMI > 27, A1C < 9%	A1C < 8%	
Major side effect		Hypoglycemia	Metabolic acidosis, gastrointestinal symptoms	Weight gain, edema	Gastrointestinal symptoms	Hypoglycemia, weight gain
Caution		Hypoglycemia, renal disease	Stop before contrast dye use; renal or hepatic disease, cardiac or pulmonary disease	Congestive heart failure; monitor liver function	Renal or hepatic disease	

In general, thiazolidinedione is indicated for insulin resistance, a BMI greater than 27, an A1C value less than 9%, a glucose concentration of 160 to 250 mg/dL, and metabolic syndrome. Liver function should be monitored regularly, and thiazolidinedione should be discontinued if the alanine transaminase level is more than 2.5 times normal. It also should not be used in individuals with New York Heart Association functional status class II to IV.

The side effects of thiazolidinediones include volume expansion leading to weight gain, edema, and a mild reduction in hemoglobin values.

a-Glucosidase Inhibitors This class includes acarbose (Precose) and miglitol (Glyset). They target postprandial glucose by delaying the absorption of disaccharides and complex carbohydrates, and to a lesser degree lactose. If acarbose or miglitol is used in combination with sulfonylureas or insulin, then hypoglycemia can be managed with glucose or milk.

a-Glucosidase inhibitors are less potent than sulfonylureas or biguanides, with the usual A1C reduction of 0.5% to 1%. They are indicated for insulin resistance or deficiency, an A1C value less than 8%, and a postprandial glucose concentration of 180 to 225 mg/dL. They need to be used with caution in patients with liver or renal disease. The most common side effects are diarrhea and flatulence.

Insulin Insulin has the greatest blood sugar lowering potency of all medications. The goal of using insulin is to duplicate the natural physiologic insulin and glucose level, in which basal insulin supplies half of the body's needs while insulin secreted in response to meals fills the rest. The insulin regimen should start simple and advance as needed (Mayfield et al., 2004Ⓒ).

Insulin is usually divided into two major types. Background insulin includes NPH, lente, ultralente, and glargine. Glargine is preferred as it provides the most consistent results. It can be given at bedtime or in the morning to accommodate the patient's lifestyle. Bolus insulin includes regular, Aspart, and Lispro. Aspart or Lispro is preferred as they provide more flexibility.

There are several ways in which insulin may contribute to the management of diabetes mellitus type 2. It can be used briefly for 2 to 3 months upon diagnosis to stabilize the hyperglycemia before transitioning to an oral agent. Patients taking several combination oral agents may want to switch to a combination of an oral agent and long-acting glargine, or just combinations of short-acting and long-acting insulins in place of oral agents.

Common side effects of insulin are hypoglycemia, local skin reactions, weight gain, systemic allergic reactions, and lipodystrophy.

New Agents Injectable glucose lowering agents from two new classes were approved by the U.S. Food and Drug Administration (FDA) in 2005 for treatment of type 2 diabetes. Exenatide (Byetta) is an incretin mimetic that stimulates insulin secretion, slows gastric emptying, and reduces hunger. Pramlintide (Symlin) is a synthetic amylin, which along with insulin, is secreted by the pancreas to reduce postprandial glucose.

Inhaled insulin may also receive FDA approval soon. It was approved in the European Union in 2005.

Another class of glucose lowering agent, glitazars, is under investigation. It improves blood glucose like the thiazolidinediones and improves lipids like a fibrate. The first glitazar is muraglitazar, which is pending FDA approval but has raised some safety concerns regarding the cardiovascular system.

Complications and Comorbid Conditions

Macrovascular Complications, Dyslipidemia, and Hypertension

Individuals with diabetes mellitus type 2 tend to have lipid disorders and hypertension (National Cholesterol Education Program Expert Panel, 2001Ⓐ Ⓑ; Stratton et al., 2000Ⓐ). The lipid disorders include hypertriglyceridemia, low HDL concentration, and an increase in atherogenic small, dense LDL particles. The management goals are to achieve HDL concentrations above 40 mg/dL, triglyceride levels below 150 mg/dL, and LDL concentrations below 100 mg/dL (<70 for individuals with high cardiac risks). There are several classes of medication for these goals. Statins lower LDL concentrations. Fibrate increases HDL concentrations and lowers triglyceride levels. Combinations of these two alone or with niacin, nicotinic acid, thiazolidinedione, and ezetimebe are also used.

The aim of blood pressure control is to achieve a systolic blood pressure of less than 130 mm Hg and a diastolic blood pressure of less than 80 mm Hg, according to the American Diabetes Association (2003Ⓒ) and the National Kidney Foundation (2004Ⓒ), or a diastolic blood pressure of less than 85, according to the Joint National Committee VII (2003Ⓒ). ACE inhibitors or thiazide diuretics are usually the first choice for those with no nephropathy. For individuals with nephropathy, ACE inhibitors are preferred if tolerated. Angiotensin-receptor blockers are used if ACE inhibitors are not tolerated.

According to the National Cholesterol Education Program Expert Panel on Detection, Evaluation and Treatment of High Blood Cholesterol in Adults (2001Ⓐ Ⓑ) (Adult Treatment Panel III), diabetes is considered a coronary heart disease risk equivalent.

Aspirin should be considered for all individuals with diabetes mellitus type 2.

Preventing Microvascular Complications

Potential microvascular complications from diabetes mellitus type 2 include nephropathy, retinopathy, and neuropathy. An annual microalbuminuria screen with spot urine (albumin/creatinine ratio) is used for monitoring early signs of nephropathy. An ACE inhibitor is often used for prevention and treatment for nephropathy. An annual dilated eye examination screens for and prevents diabetic retinopathy. Screening for peripheral neuropathy entails a comprehensive foot examination, including inspection of skin and nails, palpation for pedal pulses, and checking for reflexes, light touch sensation, and vibration.

Preventing and Forestalling the Development of Diabetes Mellitus

Lifestyle changes such as sensible nutrition and physical activity as discussed in medical nutrition therapy can prevent and forestall diabetes. Identifying and educating individuals at risk are important. Metformin, thaizoidinediones, and antihypertensives such as ACE inhibitors and ARBs may prevent the complex interaction among diabetes, hyperlipidemia, and hypertension.

Material Available on Student Consult

Review Questions and Answers about Diabetes Mellitus Type 2

REFERENCES

American Diebetes Association. Clinical practice recommendations 2003. Diabetes Care 2003;26(Suppl 1): S1–S156.Ⓐ Ⓑ Ⓒ

American Diabetes Association Expert Committee. Diagnosis and classification of diabetes mellitus. Diabetes Care 2004;27(Suppl 1):S5–S10.Ⓒ

Franz MJ, Bantle JP, et al. Nutrition principles and recommendations in diabetes. Diabetes Care 2004;27(Suppl 1): S36–S46.Ⓐ Ⓑ Ⓒ

Joint National Committee on Prevention, Detection, Evaluation, and Treatment of High Blood Pressure. The seventh report. JAMA 2003;289:2560–2571.Ⓒ

Lebovitz HE. Oral therapies for diabetic hyperglycemia. Endocrinol Metab Clin North Am 2001;30:909-933.Ⓐ Ⓑ

Mayfield JA, White RD, et al: Insulin therapy for type 2 diabetes: Rescue, augmentation, and replacement of beta-cell function. Am Fam Physician 2004;70:489–500.Ⓒ

National Cholesterol Education Program Expert Panel on Detection, Evaluation and Treatment of High Blood Cholesterol in Adults (Adult Treatment Panel III):

Executive summary of the third report of the National Cholesterol Education Program (NCEP) Expert Panel on Detection, Evaluation and Treatment of High Blood Cholesterol in Adults (Adult Treatment Panel III). JAMA 2001;285:2486-2497.Ⓐ Ⓑ

National Kidney Foundation. Kidney Disease Outcome Quality Initiative (K/DOQI). K/DOQI clinical practice guidelines on hypertension and antihypertensive agents in chronic kidney disease. 2004. Available at www.kidney.org/professionals/kdoqi/guidelines_bp/index.htm. Accessed 1/6/2006.

Stratton IM, Adler AI, et al. Association of glycemia with macrovascular and microvascular complications of type 2 diabetes (UKPDS 35): Prospective observational study. BMJ 2000;321:405–412.Ⓐ

U.K. Prospective Diabetes Study 16. Overview of 6 years' therapy of type 2 diabetes: A progressive disease. U.K. Prospective Diabetes Study Group. Diabetes 1995;44:1249–1258 [erratum in Diabetes 1996; 45:1655].Ⓐ

SUGGESTED READINGS

Diabetes Coalition of California, California Diabetes Prevention and Control Program. Basic Guidelines for Diabetic Care. Sacramento, California Diabetes Prevention and Control Program, Department of Health Services, 2003.Ⓐ Ⓑ Ⓒ

Thiedke CC. From page to practice: Improving care of type 2 diabetes. American Academy of Family Physicians Monograph, April, 2004.

47

Obesity and Elevated Blood Pressure (Metabolic Syndrome)

Anna Mies Richie

KEY POINTS

1. The combination of visceral adiposity, poor nutrition, inactivity, and a genetic predisposition leads to insulin resistance.
2. Type 2 diabetes is a two-hit disorder: insulin resistance and beta cell toxicity.
3. Waist circumference is measured at the iliac crest, with the patient gently exhaling.
4. In certain populations, waist circumference may be a more sensitive measure of relative disease risk than body mass index (BMI).
5. Successful management of the patient with metabolic syndrome should focus on weight reduction and modification of the patient's lifestyle.

INITIAL VISIT

Subjective

Patient Identification and Presenting Problem

Suzanne S. is a 36-year-old white woman who presents to the clinic for her annual physical and Pap examination. She has no concerns or problems to discuss. Her last Pap was 1 year before.

Medical History

Suzanne has no major medical illnesses. A tubal ligation is her only surgery. She has had two normal spontaneous vaginal deliveries 4 and 7 years ago. During the last pregnancy, Suzanne had gestational diabetes that was controlled with diet. On her 6 week postpartum visit, her blood sugar was normal.

Family History

Both parents are living. Her mother is obese, has type 2 non–insulin-dependent diabetes, hypertension, and high cholesterol. Her father has hypertension. She has two younger sisters, both alive and well. There is no family history of breast or colon cancer. Her two children are healthy.

Health Habits

Suzanne denies using tobacco products, alcohol, or illicit drugs. She has had no exercise routine for more than 5 years.

Social History

Suzanne lives with her husband and two children. She enjoys singing in the church choir and reading.

Review of Systems

A 12-point review of systems is negative except for an 8-pound weight gain in the past year. The patient admits to only 1 day per week or less of physical activity. The patient also states she has been eating more fast food for lunch and eating out more for dinner due to time constraints and increased stress from a new job. Nighttime snacking is common. Fruits and vegetables are consumed only once or twice daily.

Objective

Physical Examination

Suzanne is a pleasant woman who appears her stated age. Her blood pressure is 138/88 (recheck 136/88), pulse is 78 and regular, weight is 190 pounds, and height is 5 feet 5 inches. BMI is 32, and waist circumference is 37 inches. The physical examination is normal except for abdominal obesity. A Pap smear is done.

Evidence levels **A** Randomized, controlled trials (RCTs), meta-analyses, well-designed systematic reviews of RCTs. **B** Case-control or cohort studies, nonrandomized clinical trials, systematic reviews of studies other than RCTs, cross-sectional studies, retrospective studies, certain uncontrolled studies. **C** Consensus statements, expert guidelines, usual practice, opinion.

Assessment

Working Diagnosis
Obesity, elevated blood pressure, hypothyroidism, metabolic syndrome.

Plan

Diagnostic
Fasting plasma cholesterol, high-density lipoprotein (HDL), low-density lipoprotein (LDL), triglycerides, fasting glucose, liver, kidney, and thyroid function studies (aspartate aminotransferase, alanine aminotransferase, creatinine, blood urea nitrogen, and thyroid-stimulating hormone) were performed.

Patient Education
The 8-pound weight gain since last year and the 28-pound weight gain since her first child 7 years ago were discussed. A physical activity prescription, including 30 minutes of activity at least 3 days per week, was given; both cardiovascular and resistance training were recommended. Increasing fruits and vegetables and decreasing portion sizes were recommended.

FOLLOW-UP VISIT

Subjective

Suzanne returned in 2 weeks to follow up on her laboratory test results. She reports that she has started improving her diet and has walked several times since the last patient encounter, although finding time to work out routinely is still difficult.

Objective

Her blood pressure is 138/86, pulse is 70 and regular, and weight is 188 pounds. BMI and waist circumference have not changed (32 and 37, respectively).

Laboratory Tests
The results of the lipid panel were triglycerides, 180 mg/dL; HDL cholesterol, 40 mg/dL; LDL cholesterol, 130 mg/dL; fasting glucose, 116 mg/dL; thyroid-stimulating hormone 1.2 µIU/mL (normal). Liver function studies and creatinine were also normal.

Assessment

Metabolic syndrome is most likely due to visceral obesity, inactivity, excess caloric consumption, and age.

Plan

A strict weight loss program was recommended concentrating on the triad of nutrition, physical activity, and behavioral modification. The risks of developing hypertension, diabetes mellitus, heart disease, and stroke were discussed. A follow-up visit in 1 month was recommended for a blood pressure and weight check. Periodic cholesterol and glucose assessment will be made; further action will depend on the amount of weight loss.

DISCUSSION

Metabolic syndrome is the product of primary insulin resistance of tissues and secondary defects of free fatty acid (FFA), carbohydrate, and lipoprotein metabolism. The constellation of increased abdominal obesity, elevated triglycerides, hyperglycemia, and elevated blood pressure is related to the underlying insulin resistance. This ultimately predisposes to the development of diabetes mellitus type 2, dyslipidemia, hypertension, and cardiovascular disease (CVD). Metabolic syndrome provides a common clustering of these diseases (Fig. 47-1).

The relationship between these findings has been described throughout the 20th century (Table 47-1). In 2001, the National Cholesterol Education Program Adult Treatment Panel (ATP) III published guidelines defining metabolic syndrome (Table 47-2). Although the new guidelines are specific, the disease itself should be understood as a progression of vague and complex interactions between the elevated FFAs and target organs.

Assessing U.S. Census 2000 data, approximately 47 million adults in the United States manifest metabolic syndrome. The prevalence of metabolic syndrome is also high among obese children and adolescents. Factors associated with increased expression of metabolic syndrome include excess caloric and carbohydrate consumption, visceral obesity, physical inactivity, advancing age, family history, and medications (some atypical antipsychotics).

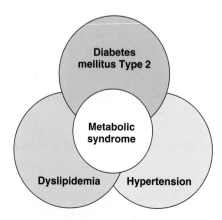

Figure 47-1 The clustering of metabolic syndrome.

Table 47-1	Recognition of Insulin Resistance throughout the Past Century	
1923	Kylin	Described clustering of hypertension, hyperglycemia, and gout
1936	Himsworth	Recognized class of diabetes related to a lack of an "insulin-sensitizing" factor
1947	Vague	Recognized the high risk of "android" (upper body) obesity compared with "gynoid" (gluteofemoral) obesity
1988	Reaven	Syndrome X (hyperinsulinemia, high blood pressure, elevated triglycerides, low HDL)
1989	Kaplan	The Deadly Quartet—Recognized the relationship of syndrome X with upper body obesity
1999	World Health Organization	Hypertension, dyslipidemia, obesity, elevated fasting insulin, microalbuminuria
2001	NCEP ATP III	Waist circumference, HDL, triglycerides, blood pressure, fasting glucose (see Table 47-2)

HDL, high-density lipoprotein; NCEP ATP III, National Cholesterol Education Program Adult Treatment Panel III.

Table 47-2	NCEP ATP III Diagnostic Factors for Metabolic Syndrome in Adults
Risk Factor	**Defining Level**
Abdominal obesity (waist circumference)	
Men	>102 cm (>40 inches)
Women	>88 cm (>35 inches)
Triglycerides	≥150 mg/dL (1.69 mmol/L)
HDL cholesterol	
Men	<40 mg/dL (1.04 mmol/L)
Women	<50 mg/dL (1.29 mmol/L)
Blood pressure	≥130/85 mm Hg
Fasting glucose	≥110 mg/dL (6.1 mmol/L)

Diagnosis is established when three or more risk factors are present.
HDL, high-density lipoprotein; NCEP ATP III, National Cholesterol Education Program Adult Treatment Panel III.
From Executive Summary of the Third Report of the National Cholesterol Education Program (NCEP) Expert Panel on Detection, Evaluation, and Treatment of High Blood Cholesterol in Adults (Adult Treatment Panel III). JAMA 2001;285: 2486–2497.

In the United States, Mexican Americans have the highest age-adjusted prevalence of metabolic syndrome (31.9%). The prevalence in whites is the same in both men and women (24%). However, African-American women and Mexican-American women have a much higher prevalence than men of the same ethnic background.

Visceral Adiposity and Free Fatty Acids

Visceral adipose tissue may be categorized as an endocrine organ because of its regulation and production of hormones. It appears that visceral adipose tissue differs significantly from other adipose tissue because of the larger cell size, greater insulin resistance, increased adrenergic receptors, impaired insulin-mediated antilipolysis, and increased catecholamine-mediated lipolysis. These differences increase the FFAs in circulation.

The increase in FFAs contributes to insulin resistance and vice versa. FFAs impair the insulin mediated glucose transport at muscle tissue and also cause beta-cell lipotoxicity in the pancreas resulting ultimately in hyperglycemia. As the peripheral tissues become more resistant to insulin, glucose disposal declines and the FFA level continues to increase. As the FFA level and insulin resistance increase, hepatic glucose and lipoprotein production increase, contributing to the hyperglycemia and dyslipidemia (Fig. 47-2).

One study of women of similar body fat used magnetic resonance imaging to characterize them by percentage of visceral adiposity. Women with larger amounts of visceral adipose tissue had higher levels of fasting insulin and triglycerides and lower levels of HDL cholesterol.

Pathophysiology of Insulin Resistance

Under normal conditions, plasma insulin regulates the release of FFAs from adipocytes, glucose disposal in skeletal muscle, and glucose and lipid metabolism in the liver. A variety of theories are thought to underlie the defects in insulin-stimulated glucose transport in the peripheral tissue and liver (Box 47-1).

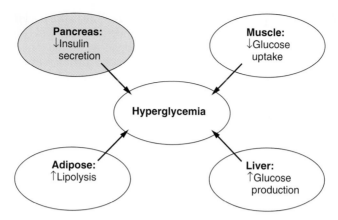

Figure 47-2 The progression from visceral adiposity to metabolic syndrome.

In the earliest phases, most of the insulin resistance appears to be concentrated in the peripheral tissue (adipose and skeletal muscle), the site responsible for approximately 70% to 90% of glucose disposal following a carbohydrate load. Loss of insulin sensitivity in the liver is believed to be a later stage of insulin resistance. The liver is an important site for glucose clearance, storage, gluconeogenesis, insulin clearance, and lipid metabolism.

Diabetes Mellitus

The combination of visceral adiposity, poor nutrition, inactivity, and a genetic predisposition leads to insulin resistance and the clinical diagnosis of diabetes mellitus type 2. The progression of abnormal glucose begins with postprandial hyperglycemia from peripheral tissue resistance and develops to fasting hyperglycemia. Fasting hyperglycemia is more closely associated with hepatic resistance.

In an effort to improve the peripheral and hepatic resistance, release of insulin from the pancreas progressively increases. As long as the beta-cell function is adequate, the patient will be normoglycemic from compensatory hyperinsulinemia. Once the beta-cell function is inadequate, there is a relative insulin deficiency resulting in diabetes mellitus (fasting glucose >126 mg/dL) (Fig. 47-3).

Box 47-1	Possible Theories and Mechanisms for Insulin Resistance

1. The hormone resistin, secreted from adipocytes, has been shown to impair glucose tolerance.
2. The "thrifty genotype" hypothesis proposes that evolving from a harsh environment and unstable food supply causes efficient fat storage, leading to weight gain, thus predisposing a person to metabolic syndrome.
3. Defects in the genes that code for: glycogen synthase, hexokinase, the insulin receptor substrate (IRS) isomer, glucose transporter 4 (GLUT 4), tumor necrosis factor α, and/or peroxisome proliferators activated receptor (the target of the diabetic drug class thiazolidinediones).
4. There may be a link between insulin resistance and leptin resistance, a protein encoded by the obese gene in adipocytes that is thought to signal a decrease in ingestive behavior.
5. Chronic elevations of free fatty acids have been shown to inhibit the phosphatidyl-

inositol 3 kinase (PI3K) activity, leading to decreased glucose transport into muscle.
6. Chronic hyperglycemia causing interference or toxicity to the insulin-stimulated glucose transport.
7. Tumor necrosis factor (TNF) may be overexpressed in the muscle and adipose tissue and is negatively correlated with insulin stimulated glucose metabolism.
8. Alterations in the hypothalamic–pituitary-adrenal axis, possibly in diurnal cortisol kinetics in response to stress.
9. Receptor knockout models suggest the liver may have a greater role in whole-body insulin sensitivity.
10. Defects in the β_3-adrenergic receptor have been associated with increased lipolysis in visceral fat tissue and features of metabolic syndrome.
11. Low birth weight predisposes to increased risk of diabetes.

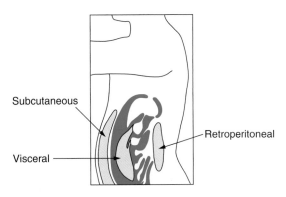

Figure 47-3 Etiology of type 2 diabetes mellitus: insulin resistance and diminished insulin secretion.

Therefore, type 2 diabetes is a two-hit disorder: insulin resistance and beta-cell toxicity. Because insulin resistance is related to three areas (adipose, skeletal, and hepatic tissue) and beta-cell toxicity occurs in the pancreas, the development of hyperglycemia has been referred to as the "dyshormonious quartet" (Fig. 47-4).

Dyslipidemia

Elevated serum triglycerides, decreased HDL cholesterol, normal to minimally increased LDL cholesterol, and small LDL particles define atherogenic dyslipidemia, a characteristic feature associated with metabolic syndrome. This lipid profile is related to the overproduction, impaired clearance, and abnormal regulation of the lipoprotein particle and composition (variation in the amount of cholesterol carried per particle).

Triglyceride and very low density lipoprotein particle production increases in response to increased FFA delivery to hepatic tissue. Normally, very low density lipoprotein particles are cleared by lipoprotein lipase. Increased levels of FFAs, apolipoprotein C-III, and decreased physical activity impair lipoprotein lipase and result in insulin resistance. The makeup of the LDL and HDL particles may also become triglyceride enriched and cholesterol depleted, making them less stable in the presence of insulin resistance.

Hypertension

Because resistance to insulin-mediated glucose disposal and compensatory hyperinsulinemia are common in patients with hypertension, the possibility has been raised that insulin resistance causes hypertension. There may be a relationship between eating, especially carbohydrate and fat consumption, and increased sympathetic activity. Obesity-related hypertension may also be a byproduct of mechanisms to restore energy balance and stabilize body weight.

Waist Circumference

Measurement of the waist circumference with a tape measure can be used to assess visceral adiposity (Fig. 47-5) and risk of CVD. The measurement should be at the iliac crest, not at the belt line, with the patient gently exhaling. Men are more apt to develop the classic "apple" shape, whereas women tend to have lower body obesity or the "pear" shape. This body fat distribution may be influenced by androgens, corticosteroids, and growth hormones. Women with polycystic ovarian syndrome are also more likely to develop the characteristic visceral obesity.

In certain populations, such as Asian Americans and older women of normal weight, waist circumference may be a more sensitive measure of relative disease risk than BMI. For patients with a BMI between 25 and 34.9 kg/m^2, a high waist circumference increases the risk of type 2 diabetes mellitus, dyslipidemia, hypertension, and CVD. However, with a BMI greater than 35 kg/m^2, waist circumference may not be as significant to the risk of morbidity and mortality (Table 47-3).

The National Institutes of Health (NIH) developed evidence-based waist circumference cutoff points that assist with identifying those at increased health risk. Those with high waist circumference values are

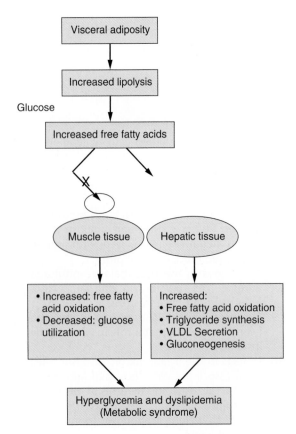

Figure 47-4 The dyshormonious quartet. VLDL, very low density protein.

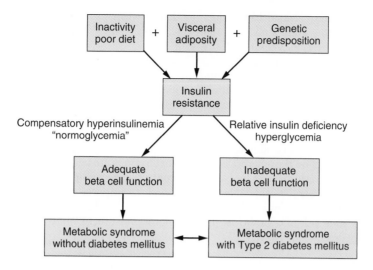

Figure 47-5 Location of visceral adipose tissue.

more likely to have hypertension, diabetes, dyslipidemia, and metabolic syndrome compared with those with normal waist circumference values. Many associations remained significant after adjusting for confounding variables (age, race, poverty, physical activity, smoking, and alcohol intake) in normal weight, overweight, and obese women and overweight men. In this study, the adverse effects of a high waist circumference were more apparent in women than men.

Cardiovascular Disease

Individuals with metabolic syndrome are at increased risk of CVD and overall mortality. In the Kuoppio Ischemic Heart Disease Risk Factor Study, a prospective cohort of 1209 Finnish men of age 42 to 60 years without known CVD, cancer, or diabetes were followed for an average of 11.4 years to determine CVD, coronary heart disease (CHD) death, and all-cause mortality among those with and without defined metabolic syndrome. After adjustment for conventional cardiovascular risk factors, CHD death was 2.9- to 4.2-fold higher for subjects with ATP III defined metabolic syndrome. Data from the Framingham Heart Study reported that the presence of metabolic syndrome alone predicts approximately 25% of all new-onset CVD. The 4S (Scandinavian Simvastatin Survival Study) and the Air Force/Texas Coronary Atherosclerosis Prevention Study (AFCAPS/TexCAPS) both showed that patients with metabolic syndrome showed an increased risk of major coronary events.

Table 47-3 Classification of Overweight and Obesity by BMI, Waist Circumference, and Associated Disease Risk

| | | Disease Risk (Relative to Normal Weight and Waist Circumference) | |
| | | Men: ≤40 inches (102 cm) Women: ≤35 inches (88 cm) | Men: >40 inches (102 cm) Women: >35 inches (88 cm) |
Classification	BMI (kg/m²)		
Underweight	<18.5	—	—
Normal	18.5–24.9	—	Increased
Overweight	25.0–29.9	Increased	High
Obesity	30.0–34.9	High	Very high
Morbid obesity	35.0–39.9	Very high	Very high
Supermorbid obesity	≥40	Extremely high	Extremely high

BMI, body mass index.

Adapted from National Heart, Lung, and Blood Institute. Clinical Guidelines on the Identification, Evaluation, and Treatment of Overweight and Obesity in Adults. Available at www.nhlbi.nih.gov/guidelines/obesity/ob_home.htm. Accessed 1/24/2006.

Besides dyslipidemia and elevated blood pressure, there may be many other factors involved that independently increase the risk of CVD. For example, increased levels of asymmetric dimethylarginine are associated with endothelial dysfunction and increased risk of CVD. There is a significant relationship between insulin resistance and plasma concentration of dimethylarginine.

It is believed that long before diabetes becomes manifest, the clustering of metabolic abnormalities seems to exert an additive effect on the atherosclerotic process. The relationship between diabetes and CVD is so profound that approximately 75% of people with diabetes will die of CVD complications. Also, those with diabetes have the same risk of a cardiovascular event as do people with already established CHD.

Management of Metabolic Syndrome

Successful management of the patient with metabolic syndrome should focus on weight reduction and modification of the patient's lifestyle (diet, physical activity). Behavior modification techniques may include self-monitoring, stimulus control, cognitive restructuring, stress management, and social support.

From the Nurses Health Study, almost 90,000 women were followed to examine the association of lifestyle and CHD. Adherence to lifestyle guidelines involving diet, exercise, and abstinence from smoking was associated with a very low risk of CHD, more than 80% lower than that in the rest of the population.

Physical activity is an important predictor of weight maintenance. Several studies suggest that physically activity, even in obese patients, may substantially reduce the risk of cardiovascular events and all-cause mortality.

Exercise has been shown to improve lipoprotein production and concentration. Using conventional lipid analysis, exercise may not show a significant change in the lipid profile. However, using nuclear magnetic resonance spectroscopy, exercise can be shown to positively affect the concentration and size of LDL, HDL, and very low density lipoprotein, making these particles more stable and less atherogenic.

Exercise can also increase insulin sensitivity in muscle cells by increasing the mitochondrial oxidation.

Pharmacotherapy

Beyond lifestyle changes, aggressive pharmacologic treatment is frequently necessary. Because of the high risk of CVD, all patients with metabolic syndrome, unless there is a contraindication, should be prescribed aspirin for antiplatelet therapy. Frequently, medications are needed for hyperlipidemia, glycemic control, hypertension, and weight loss.

It is important to remember that, although a number of medications may lower blood sugar, lower blood pressure, or improve lipids, the overall goal is to decrease mortality. For example, if the medication has been shown to increase HDL but has not been shown to decrease mortality, then treatment with this medication would be treating a disease, not the patient. For example, estrogen therapy has been shown to favor lipid profiles; however, the current evidence suggests estrogen therapy may lead to an increase in cardiovascular events. Generally, patient-oriented medical practice is the goal over disease-oriented medicine. This may require some difficult decision making and analysis of the evidence.

Conclusion

CHD remains the leading cause of death among men and women in the United States. Much effort has focused on the pharmacologic management of hypertension, hyperlipidemia, CHD, and congestive heart disease. These treatments are of proven benefit but costly and are secondary and tertiary prevention. Addressing a healthy BMI early in a disease process by promoting healthy lifestyle practices is important in stopping the disease process of metabolic syndrome that ultimately will lead to the diseases associated with CVD.

Material Available on Student Consult

Review Questions and Answers about Metabolic Syndrome

SUGGESTED READINGS

Depres JP, Lemieux I, Prud'homme D. Treatment of obesity: Need to focus on high risk abdominally obese patients. BMJ 2001;322:716–720.

Ford ES, Giles WH, Dietz WH. Prevalence of the metabolic syndrome among US adults: Findings from the Third National Health and Nutrition Examination Survey. JAMA 2002;287:356–359.

Ginsberg HN. New perspectives on atherogenesis: Role of abnormal triglyceride-rich lipoprotein metabolism. Circulation 2002;106:2137–2142.

Isomaa B, Almgren P, Tuomi T, et al. Cardiovascular morbidity and mortality associated with the metabolic syndrome. Diabetes Care 2001;24:683–689. ⑧

Janssen I. Body mass index, waist circumference, and health risk. Arch Intern Med 2002;162:2074–2079. ⑧

Lakka H, Laaksonen DE, Lakka TA, et al. The metabolic syndrome and total and cardiovascular disease mortality in middle aged men. JAMA 2002;288: 2709–2716. ⑧

Report of the Expert Committee on the Diagnosis and Classification of Diabetes Mellitus. Diabetes Care 2003;26(Suppl 1):S5–S20.❸

The Sixth Report of the Joint National Committee on Prevention, Detection, Evaluation, and Treatment of High Blood Pressure. NIH/NHLBL (NIH publication no. 98-4080). Washington, DC, Government Printing Office, 1997.❸

Third Report of the National Cholesterol Education Program Panel. Executive Summary (NIH publication no. 01-3670). Washington, DC, Government Printing Office, 2001.❸

Tuomilehto J, Lindstrom J, Eriksson JG, et al. Prevention of type 2 diabetes mellitus by changes in lifestyle among subjects with impaired glucose tolerance. N Engl J Med 2001;344:1343–1350.❹

Weiss, R, Dziura J, Burgert T, et al. Obesity and the metabolic syndrome in children and adolescents. N Engl J Med 2004;350:2362–2374.❸

Chapter

48 Abdominal Obesity (Metabolic Syndrome)

Darwin Deen

KEY POINTS

1. Metabolic syndrome (MES) is associated with insulin resistance and predicts risk of diabetes mellitus and myocardial infarction.
2. MES is associated with an atherogenic dyslipidemia and a prothrombotic state.
3. Polycystic ovary syndrome and nonalcoholic steatohepatitis are also associated with insulin resistance.
4. Exercise and a weight reduction diet reduce insulin resistance.
5. Assessment of and attention to stage of behavior change will help physicians be more effective at stimulating behavior change in their patients.

INITIAL VISIT

Subjective

Patient Identification and Presenting Problem

Eric V. is a 37-year-old man who presents at his wife's urging for a physical examination. Eric denies any current complaints but reports that during a

health screening at his job a few months ago, he was told that his blood pressure was elevated. The reading was 138/90. At the time, he was advised to see his personal physician to have his blood pressure rechecked, but he was feeling fine and forgot about it. Eric reports a 10- to 15-pound weight gain over the past 2 years—since he got married and his wife had their daughter. On further questioning, he admits that his pants waist size has increased from 36 to 40 inches and that his wife has commented on his "beer belly." He also feels that his physical activity level has declined since the birth of his 8-month-old daughter.

Medical History

Eric denies any significant medical history. He had asthma as a child but has had no problems related to his breathing since he was about 14 years old. He has occasional eczema for which he uses hydrocortisone cream as needed. He reports some seasonal allergy symptoms.

Family History

Eric is an only child. His father died suddenly at the age of 62 (he thinks he was told his father had a heart attack). His mother is 77 and has had diabetes for approximately 15 years ago.

Evidence levels ❹ Randomized, controlled trials (RCTs), meta-analyses, well-designed systematic reviews of RCTs. ❸ Case-control or cohort studies, nonrandomized clinical trials, systematic reviews of studies other than RCTs, cross-sectional studies, retrospective studies, certain uncontrolled studies. ❸ Consensus statements, expert guidelines, usual practice, opinion.

Social and Occupational History

Eric is married and has one child. He works as a police officer. He smoked as a teen but stopped more than 10 years ago. He drinks one to two beers nightly (12-oz. cans) and more on social occasions when he and his wife get together with coworkers. He has never used recreational drugs.

Review of Systems

Eric denies headache, blurry vision, chest pain, or shortness of breath. He has no polyuria or polydipsia.

Objective

Physical Examination

Eric is a well-developed overweight but not obese-appearing young man with a mildly protruding abdomen. He sits on the examination table in no apparent distress. He is 70 inches tall and weighs 216 pounds. His blood pressure is 135/88, and his resting pulse is 80. There is no significant difference in his blood pressure when he is standing or lying down or between his right and left arms. On inspection of his skin, some hyperpigmentation around his neck and under his axillae consistent with acanthosis nigricans is noted (Figs. 48-1 and 48-2). His head, ears, eyes, nose, and throat examination is entirely within normal limits. His neck is supple with no palpable thyroid gland. His heart sounds are normal, and his PMI is not displaced. His lungs are clear bilaterally, and his abdominal examination reveals no masses or palpable organomegaly. When he is both sitting and standing, his subcutaneous abdominal fat flows over his belt in front and on both sides. His extremities and peripheral pulses are unremarkable. There is no palpable adenopathy. His neurologic examination is normal. His waist circumference measures 41 inches. His body mass index is calculated at 31.

Assessment

Working Diagnosis

Based on his blood pressure and waist circumference, you suspect that Eric has metabolic syndrome (MES) (Table 48-1). You discuss with him the possibility that his weight and specifically his abdominal obesity are putting him at risk of future diabetes and heart disease and ask him to return in 1 week for fasting blood sugar and lipid profile measurements.

Differential Diagnosis for Acanthosis Nigricans

1. *Pseudoacanthosis nigricans.* Same clinical appearance as acanthosis nigricans but no underlying

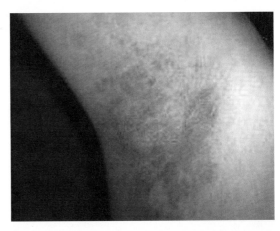

Figure 48-1 Brown, velvety plaques in the axilla of a patient with acanthosis nigricans. (From Levine NL, Baron JB. Acanthosis nigricans. E-medicine, July 2002. Available at www.emedicine.com/derm/topic1.htm.)

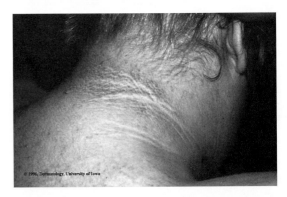

Figure 48-2 Syndromes associated with acanthosis nigricans. (From Department of Dermatology, University of Iowa College of Medicine. Available at www.tray.dermatology.uiowa.edu/AcanNigr01.htm.)

insulin resistance. Dominant mode of inheritance (also called hereditary benign acanthosis nigricans).
2. *Malignant acanthosis nigricans.* Lesions are occasionally associated with an underlying malignancy.
3. *Drug-induced acanthosis nigricans.* Drugs that produce or aggravate insulin resistance have been associated with acanthosis nigricans, for example, niacin, oral contraceptive, methyltestosterone, atypical antipsychotics.
4. *Acanthosis nigricans associated with insulin resistance type A.* A rare inherited form of severe insulin resistance associated with hyperandrogenism in females. Cause unknown. Diabetes invariably develops.
5. *Acanthosis nigricans associated with insulin resistance type B.* A rare inherited form of severe insulin resistance abnormality characterized by insulin antireceptor autoantibodies.

Table 48-1 Adult Treatment Panel III Criteria for Metabolic Syndrome

Component	Criteria (Any Three)
Abdominal/central obesity	Waist circumference: >102 cm (40 inches) in men, >88 cm (35 inches) in women
Hypertriglyceridemia	≥150 mg/dL
Low HDL cholesterol	<40 mg/dL (<1.036 mmol/L) for men, <50 mg/dL (<1.295 mmol/L) for women
High blood pressure	≥130/85 mm Hg or documented use of antihypertensive therapy
High fasting glucose	≥110 mg/dL (≥6.1 mmol/L)

HDL, high-density lipoprotein.
Adapted from National Cholesterol Education Panel. Adult treatment panel III report. Available at www.nhlbi.gov/guidelines/cholesterol/index.htm. Accessed 8/28/2002.

Eric is not certain how to respond to the information that you have given him but promises to return for the requested blood work and to read the information in the educational handout that you have provided (www.aafp.org/afp/20040615/2887ph.html).

FOLLOW-UP VISITS

Two weeks later he returns for the results of his laboratory work:

Laboratory Test	Result (mg/dL)
Fasting glucose	100
Total cholesterol	237
Triglycerides	467
High-density lipoprotein	31
Alanine aminotransferase, aspartate aminotransferase, total and direct bilirubin	Within normal limits
Complete blood count	Within normal limits

Low-density lipoprotein is not calculated because his triglyceride level is too high. His non–high-density cholesterol level is calculated at 206.

Although MES is a reflection of insulin resistance, which can be measured using a ratio of fasting insulin to glucose, you have decided not to draw a fasting insulin level because, according to the National Cholesterol Education Program's Adult Treatment Panel III, the methodology for this test is poorly standardized. In addition, it adds little to making the diagnosis of MES.

You go over the results of these laboratory tests with Eric, who is upset at how high his triglycerides are and does not understand how his blood work can be so abnormal when he feels fine. You explain to him that this is a risk assessment and indicates a metabolic abnormality that will take years to have an effect on how he feels and that the good news is that because he is aware of the problem, he has an opportunity to do something about it before it causes any permanent damage.

You take a 24-hour recall of activity and diet from him and learn the following information. Breakfast is usually a cup of coffee and a bagel with cream cheese or butter or a croissant with jelly. He frequently has a snack consisting of a muffin or donut and another cup of coffee before lunch. He uses whole milk and sugar in his coffee. Lunch is two slices of pepperoni pizza or fast food and a large soda. He eats dinner at home with his wife, who often makes fried chicken or steak or occasionally fish. He likes rice or potatoes as a side dish and usually has a vegetable or salad. He is sedentary on most days of the week but plays softball with his coworkers on weekends in the spring and summer. Although he enjoys this leisure time activity, he admits that he is not in the kind of shape that he used to be in and that it takes him a few weeks each spring to get back to being able to run the bases without getting seriously short of breath. You ask him "stages of change" questions (Box 48-1) to assess his readiness to make lifestyle changes. He seems more ready to change his exercise habits than his diet.

DISCUSSION

Metabolic Syndrome

MES has been called by a variety of names, including syndrome X and insulin resistance syndrome. This cluster of risk factors is responsible for much of the excess cardiovascular disease morbidity among overweight and obese patients and those with type 2 diabetes mellitus (DM) (Vega, 2001 **B**). The National Cholesterol Education Program's Adult Treatment Panel III report (2002 **C**) identified MES as an independent risk factor for cardiovascular disease and considers it an indication for intensive lifestyle modification; this conclusion is based on numerous nonintervention trials.

Although definitions have varied, the major characteristics of MES include insulin resistance, abdominal obesity, elevated blood pressure, and lipid abnormalities including elevated triglycerides

Box 48-1	Assessing Readiness to Change

Stage of change can be determined using the following series of questions:

1. Have you *ever* changed or tried to change the way you eat to lose weight or improve your health?
   If "no," skip to question 4.
   If "yes," proceed to question 2.
2. Are you currently following a dietary plan to lose weight or for other health related reasons?
   If "no," skip to question 4.
   If "yes," proceed to question 3.
3. How long have you been following this plan?
   If less than a month, the patient is in **action** stage.
   If longer than 6 months, the patient is in **maintenance** stage.
4. During the past month, have you thought about dietary changes you could make to lose weight or improve your health?
   If "yes," the patient is in **contemplation** stage. If the plan is specific and will be implemented within a month, then the patient is in **preparation** stage.
   If no, the patient is in **precontemplation** stage.

and low high-density lipoprotein levels (Deen, 2004❸). MES is also associated with a proinflammatory/prothrombotic state that may include coagulation abnormalities, elevated uric acid levels, microalbuminuria, and a shift toward small dense low-density lipoprotein particles. The proinflammatory state characterized by elevated levels of C-reactive protein has been recognized as a stronger predictor of sudden cardiac death than elevated lipid levels (Albert et al., 2002❸). The coagulation abnormalities include endothelial dysfunction, hyperfibrinogenemia, increased platelet aggregation, and increased levels of plasminogen activator inhibitor 1. Insulin resistance has been implicated in the polycystic ovarian syndrome and nonalcoholic steatohepatitis. Using the definition of the Adult Treatment Panel III of MES, a review of data from the Third National Health and Nutrition Examination Survey estimated that 22% of U.S. adults (24% after age adjustment) have MES.

At this time no randomized controlled trials aimed specifically at treating MES have been published. Therefore, current treatment for MES consists of aggressive management of the individual components of the syndrome. Anything that reduces insulin

resistance has the potential to successfully address MES. Expending more calories through exercise and consuming fewer calories by eating less are the most obvious and most successful interventions. The type of exercise or the specific type of diet is of secondary importance. Starting slowly and gradually increasing exercise duration and intensity are associated with greater long-term compliance with an exercise regimen. Any diet that leads patients to consume fewer calories will be effective, but saturated fat intake and simple carbohydrate intake deserve specific attention. Although pharmacotherapy needs to be considered for some components, all patients diagnosed with MES should be encouraged to attempt to change their diet and exercise habits as primary therapy. There is no question that weight loss improves most (if not all) aspects of MES as well as reduces obesity-related morbidity and mortality (Williamson et al., 1999❸). Unfortunately, most patients find weight loss very difficult to achieve. The good news is that dietary changes and increased exercise levels can be effective therapy, even in the absence of weight loss.

Behavior Change

The transtheoretical model of behavior change is well suited to assessing a patient's motivation and readiness to make lifestyle changes to reduce obesity, diabetes, and cardiovascular-related risks. According to the transtheoretical model, the stages that individuals go through are precontemplation (not considering making a change in the target behavior), contemplation (considering the pros and cons of making a behavior change), preparation (planning steps to make a change), action (actually changing the targeted behavior), maintenance (making the changed behavior habitual), and relapse (when a formerly altered behavior pattern returns). Appropriate provider responses to a patient depend on the stage that the patient is in (Table 48-2).

PLAN

Eric is started on an angiotensin-converting enzyme inhibitor medication that will lower his blood pressure while not interfering with other aspects of his lifestyle (he sits for many hours in a patrol car daily and is concerned about the impact of a diuretic). You counsel him about diet and exercise and discuss glucose-sensitizing medication. You assure him that exercise and dieting for weight loss is more effective than medication (Diabetes Prevention Program Research Group, 2002❹). You review his goals with him, and he seems to understand that there is no "quick fix" to this problem and that improvement is up to him. You reassure him that while it will not be

Table 48-2   Stage-Specific Interventions

Client Stage	Clinician's Motivational Tasks
Precontemplation	Raise doubt: increase the client's perception of the risks and problems of current behavior
Contemplation	Tip the balance: discuss reasons to change, risks of not changing; strengthen the client's self-efficacy for change
Determination (preparation)	Help determine the best course of action
Action	Help patient take steps toward change, build multiple small steps
Maintenance	Help patient to identify and use strategies to prevent relapse
Relapse	Help patient renew the process, avoid being judgmental

easy, he does not have to be "perfect," that you are confident that he can succeed, and that you will be there to help him in any way that you can. He makes an appointment for his wife and himself to see a dietitian in their community for dietary advice, and he promises to begin your exercise prescription by walking daily for 25 to 30 minutes.

NEXT FOLLOW-UP VISIT

Eric returns in 1 month. He is disappointed because he has not lost any weight, but he reports that he and his wife have tried a number of the suggestions made by the dietitian and that most of them have been quite positive. He has started walking more, and although he usually walks only 3 to 4 days a week, he feels bet-ter the day after he walks (better sleep, more energy), and he is motivated to try to find the time to walk on the other days. His wife and daughter usually walk with him, so they spend family time together. He has switched his milk to 2% and will try changing to 1% in a few more weeks. He is avoiding his second breakfast in the morning and has started bringing a piece of fruit with him for a snack. If he is really hungry, he has an energy bar or a handful of nuts. He no longer has pizza or fast food for lunch, opting instead for a brown bag lunch of a turkey sandwich with light mayonnaise, lettuce, and tomato, as well as yogurt and a few baby carrots. His wife has stopped frying foods in oil for dinner, and they are eating broiled or sautéed chicken breast or fish one to two nights per week. You congratulate him on the many positive changes that he has made and assure him that if he keeps up like this, he will begin to see changes in his weight and waist circumference. You also challenge him to try to reduce his beer consumption to three to four cans per week rather than the same quantity per day. He denies any problems with his antihypertension medication, and his blood pressure is 135/85.

Eric returns in 2 months. He and his wife have continued seeing the dietitian, and he reports that he enjoys a number of new recipes using whole grains that his wife has found. He has continued his walking regimen and has increased his pace when his wife and daughter are not along. He drinks beer only on Friday and Saturday nights, and he has noticed that his pants are looser. He weighs 210 pounds, and his waist circumference is 39 inches. You ask him about his plans for the future, and he says that he wants to start running as soon as he feels up to it and that he would like to get off the medication for his blood pressure if he can. You assure him that his goal is achievable.

Material Available on Student Consult

Review Questions and Answers about Metabolic Syndrome

REFERENCES

Albert CM, Ma J, Rifai N, Stampfer MJ, Ridker PM. Prospective study of C-reactive protein, homocysteine, and plasma lipid levels as predictors of sudden cardiac death. Circulation 2002;105:2595–2599.**B**

Deen D. Metabolic syndrome: A time for action. Am Fam Physician 2004;69:2875–2882.**B**

Diabetes Prevention Program Research Group. Reduction in the incidence of type 2 diabetes with lifestyle intervention or metformin. N Engl J Med 2002;346: 393–403.**A**

Levine NL, Baron JB. Acanthosis nigricans. E-medicine, July 2002. Available at www.emedicine.com/derm/topic1.htm. Accessed 1/8/2006.

Vega GL. Obesity, metabolic syndrome, and cardiovascular disease. Am Heart J 2001;142:1108–1116.**B**

National Cholesterol Education Project. Adult treatment panel III report. Available at www.nhlbi.nih.gov/guidelines/cholesterol/index.htm. Accessed 8/28/2002.**C**

Williamson DF, Pamuk E, Thun M, Flanders D, Byers T, Heath C. Prospective study of intentional weight loss and mortality in overweight white men aged 40–64 years. Am J Epidemiol 1999;149:491–503.**B**

Chapter

49

Irregular Menstruation and Fatigue (Cushing's Syndrome)

David M. Barclay III

KEY POINTS

1. Most women who present with Cushing's syndrome also have clinical features of polycystic ovary syndrome, suggesting that Cushing's syndrome should be ruled out in these patients.
2. Cushing's syndrome may be diagnosed using 24-hour urinary free cortisol (UFC) in combination with an overnight 1 mg dexamethasone suppression test (DST).
3. Hypertension, abdominal obesity, glucose intolerance, and psychological disturbances are common presenting symptoms of Cushing's syndrome.
4. Metabolic syndrome shares many features in common with Cushing's syndrome.
5. Primary care providers should treat the secondary conditions associated with hypercortisolism while a definitive treatment is pursued.

INITIAL VISIT

Subjective

Patient Identification and Presenting Problem

Katie B. is a 29-year-old white woman who presents as a new patient complaining of irregular menses.

History of Present Illness

Katie had her first period at the age of 14, and until about a year ago, they came regularly every 28 days, lasted 4 to 5 days, and had an "average" flow. She is a gravida 0, para 0. Katie is sexually active with her husband only. He had a vasectomy so she is sure she is not pregnant. During the past year, her periods have become less frequent, occurring every 6 to 8 weeks, and her last period was 3 months ago. In addi-

tion, she feels tired all the time and finds it difficult to go about her usual daily routine. Activities that used to excite her, such as her passion for kickboxing, no longer interest her, and even if she had the energy to box, excessive bruising has prevented her from participating in the sport. She believes that her lack of activity is responsible for the 15-pound weight gain she has experienced over the past year.

Medical History

Other than one or two urinary tract infections as a teenager, Katie's health has been excellent until recently. Two months ago she went to the emergency department with unbearable lower abdominal pain and was diagnosed with a kidney stone. She was given antibiotics and pain medication and the stone passed on its own 3 days later.

Family History

Katie's mother is 68 years old and has arthritis. Her father is 74 years old. He has hypertension and diabetes. She has two sisters and one brother, who are in good health as far as she knows.

Social History

Katie has been married for 5 years and has no children. She works as a guidance counselor at the local high school. She eats a regular diet and until recently enjoyed running, swimming, and kickboxing. She drinks socially and does not smoke or use illegal drugs.

Review of Systems

Katie has gained 15 pounds in the past year with no noticeable change in eating habits. Constipation has also become a problem. She feels slow and lethargic on most days, and she describes her mood as "blue." She does not consider herself depressed but admits that many activities that used to be enjoyable are no longer interesting. She has no trouble falling asleep, but getting up in the morning is very difficult. She has noticed that she bruises easily and often notices

Evidence levels (A) Randomized, controlled trials (RCTs), meta-analyses, well-designed systematic reviews of RCTs. (B) Case-control or cohort studies, nonrandomized clinical trials, systematic reviews of studies other than RCTs, cross-sectional studies, retrospective studies, certain uncontrolled studies. (C) Consensus statements, expert guidelines, usual practice, opinion.

new bruises during her morning shower. She has had no headaches, shortness of breath, chest pains, abdominal pains, or muscle aches.

Objective

Physical Examination

General Katie appears anxious and alert. Her arms and legs appear thin while her trunk appears mildly obese.

Vital Signs Her height is 5 feet 4 inches, weight is 138 pounds, temperature is 37.2°C (98.9°F), respiratory rate is 18, blood pressure is 150/97 mm Hg, and pulse is 84.

Head, Eyes, Ears, Nose, and Throat Katie's face appears rounded (moon face); external ear canals and tympanic membranes are clear bilaterally; hearing is grossly intact; conjunctivae are pink; pupils are equal, round, and reactive to light and accommodation; extraocular movements are intact without nystagmus; nose is clear; maxillary and frontal sinuses are nontender; mouth has good dentition; and the oropharynx is clear.

Neck A prominent hump (buffalo hump) is present on her posterior neck; there is no lymphadenopathy, thyromegaly, or jugular venous distention.

Lungs The lungs are clear to auscultation.

Heart There is normal sinus rhythm without murmurs, rubs, or gallops.

Neurologic Katie is alert and oriented to person, place, and time; cranial nerves II through XII are intact; reflexes are 2+ throughout; motor strength is 5/5 throughout; however, the proximal musculature of all extremities appears atrophied relative to the distal musculature. The sensory examination is intact to light touch and pinprick; cerebellar function is intact.

Skin Sun-exposed areas are darkly tanned. There are purple striae on the medial and proximal thighs and lower abdomen.

Assessment

Working Diagnosis

The presence of mild hypertension, moon face, a buffalo hump on the posterior neck, proximal muscle wasting, striae, oligomenorrhea, neuropsychiatric problems, and a history of nephrolithiasis are all findings that warrant an evaluation for the presence of hypercortisolism or overt Cushing's syndrome. Most women who present with Cushing's syndrome also have clinical features of polycystic ovary syndrome, suggesting that Cushing's syndrome should be ruled

Table 49-1 Features of Cushing's Syndrome and Metabolic Syndrome X

Cushing's Syndrome	Metabolic Syndrome X
Hypertension	Hypertension
Diabetes/insulin resistance	Diabetes/insulin resistance
Dyslipidemia	Dyslipidemia
Osteoporosis	PCOS/hyperandrogenism
PCOS/hyperandrogenism	Oligomenorrhea/hypogonadism
Oligomenorrhea/hypogonadism	Abdominal obesity
Myopathy/cutaneous wasting	Nodular adrenal disease
Abdominal obesity	
Kidney stones	
Neuropsychiatric problems	
Nodular adrenal disease	

PCOS, polycystic ovary syndrome.

out in these patients. In addition, several characteristics of the metabolic syndrome are shared with Cushing's syndrome (Table 49-1), presumably because of the hyperactivity of the hypothalamic-pituitary-adrenal axis found in both. The differential diagnosis of Cushing's syndrome is found in Box 49-1.

Box 49-1 Differential Diagnosis of Cushing's Syndrome

Metabolic syndrome X
Obesity
Chronic alcoholism
Depression
Iatrogenic Cushing's syndrome
Subclinical hypercortisolism
Acute illness

Plan

Diagnostic

The first step in Katie's workup is to establish a diagnosis of Cushing's syndrome. Several diagnostic tests have been used over the years, and no single test has proven fully capable of distinguishing all cases of Cushing's syndrome from normal and obese individuals.

The 24-hour urinary free cortisol (UFC) gives an integrated index of the amount of free (unbound) cortisol in the blood during this period and is considered by most experts to be the most useful initial test at this time. Urinary cortisol levels, unlike plasma cortisol levels that measure total cortisol, both unbound and bound, are not influenced by factors that affect corticosteroid-binding globulin. Because some individuals have intermittent hypercortisolism, if the initial test is normal and there is a high index of suspicion, as many as three 24-hour urine collections should be performed. Urinary creatinine should also be measured to verify the adequacy of the urine collection. If the glomerular filtration rate is less than 30 mL/min, the UFC level may be falsely decreased. In children, the UFC level should be corrected by dividing the body surface area by 1.72 m^2.

The most widely available measurement of UFC is by immunoassays (e.g., radioimmunoassay, immunometric assays). These assays may be influenced by various metabolites of cortisol and some synthetic glucocorticoids. The reference range for UFC depends on the type of assay used. The introduction of high-performance liquid chromatography allows the separation of various urinary glucocorticoids and metabolites; however, some substances such as carbamazepine and digoxin can coelute with cortisol and cause false elevations of the UFC. Although this technology is more sensitive and specific, it is more expensive and is not widely available. The recent addition of mass spectrometry combined with high-performance liquid chromatography may overcome these problems in the future. UFC levels in excess of four times normal are considered diagnostic for Cushing's syndrome. Milder elevations may be seen in conditions such as depression, chronic anxiety, and alcoholism and in normal pregnant women. UFC may not identify early or subclinical cases of Cushing's syndrome and is often used in conjunction with other tests.

A low-dose dexamethasone suppression test (DST) has been used to evaluate patients with suspected Cushing's syndrome for more than four decades. The overnight low-dose DST consists of a 1-mg oral dose of dexamethasone taken between 11 PM and 12 AM, followed by a fasting plasma cortisol measurement between 8:00 and 9:00 AM the following morning. The old cutoff value for this test of 5 μg/dL has recently been reduced to 1.8 μg/dL, greatly enhancing the sensitivity of this test for mild hypercortisolism. The specificity of the 1.8 μg/dL cutoff is limited due to the misclassification of patients with increased corticosteroid-binding globulin, acute and chronic illness, pseudo-Cushing's syndrome (e.g., alcoholism), and the otherwise healthy individual who fails to suppress cortisol to this level. Another increasingly recognized problem is the suppression of steroids by dexamethasone in patients with proven Cushing's syndrome. Some experts believe that the low sensitivity and specificity of this test do not justify its continued use.

The classic 2-day DST is another way to perform this test (dexamethasone 0.5 mg is given every 6 hours for 48 hours with measurement of urine steroids). This test has been shown to have a sensitivity of 79%, a specificity of 74%, and a diagnostic accuracy of 71% in patients with mild Cushing's syndrome. Factors that can cause an apparent lack of suppression for any DST include decreased intestinal absorption of dexamethasone, drugs that enhance hepatic metabolism of dexamethasone (carbamazepine, phenytoin, barbiturates, rifampin, meprobamate, aminoglutethimide, methaqualone), elevated concentrations of corticosteroid-binding globulin (exogenous estrogen therapy, pregnancy), and pseudo-Cushing's conditions. Any cortisol assay used for this test must have a sensitivity of at least 1 μg/dL.

Late-night salivary cortisol testing appears to be a promising first-line screening test for Cushing's syndrome in the future. Cortisol concentrations in saliva are independent of salivary flow rate and are highly correlated with free plasma cortisol. Late-night (11 PM) salivary cortisol is a simple way to screen for Cushing's syndrome and has been found to have a high diagnostic sensitivity and specificity. Larger studies of this technique and more widely available commercial assays may make it an alternative first-line screening test in the future.

Katie undergoes a 24-hour UFC, and the result is positive with a level of 150 μg/dL. An overnight 1-mg DST is also abnormal at 7.2 μg/dL.

FOLLOW-UP VISIT

Subjective

Katie returns for her follow-up visit 2 weeks later. She reports no change in her symptoms, and having done an Internet search on Cushing's syndrome, she is not surprised to learn that her tests were diagnostic for the condition.

Objective

Her blood pressure is 160/97 mm Hg, and her pulse is 86. The rest of her examination is unchanged.

Assessment

Cushing's syndrome is established.

Plan

The next step in Katie's workup is to establish the cause of her disease. Figure 49-1 outlines a straightforward approach to the differential diagnosis of Cushing's syndrome.

An endocrinologist experienced in the diagnosis and management of Cushing's syndrome should be

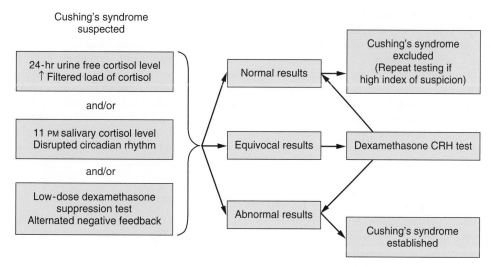

Figure 49-1 Differential diagnosis of Cushing's syndrome. (Reproduced with permission from Ruff HR, Findling FW. A physiologic approach to diagnosis of Cushing's syndrome. Ann Inter Med 2003;138:980–991.)

consulted to manage her disease at this point. In the meantime, she should be placed on antihypertensive medication to control her blood pressure and have an evaluation for insulin resistance/diabetes with an oral glucose tolerance test while a definitive cure for her disease is pursued.

DISCUSSION

The mortality rate for patients with Cushing's syndrome is four times higher than that of age- and gender-matched controls, largely due to the complications caused by glucocorticoid excess. The primary goal of management is therefore to properly identify the condition and eliminate the hypercortisolism.

Obesity

Excess glucocorticoids bring about a redistribution of body fat from peripheral to more central parts of the body, primarily the abdominal region. Abdominal obesity (visceral obesity) is now recognized as an independent risk factor for increased mortality and is one of the four key components of the metabolic syndrome (abdominal obesity, hypertension, insulin resistance/diabetes, hyperlipidemia).

Hypertension

Hypertension is present in 70% to 80% of patients with Cushing's syndrome and may be the presenting sign. Although patients with Cushing's syndrome usually have mild hypertension, it may be severe and accompanied by organ damage, particularly cardiac hypertrophy. It is thought that the concentric remodeling of the left ventricle seen in some patients may be due to prolonged exposure to excess circulating cortisol. Hypertension is treated using conventional medications (thiazides, calcium channel blockers, and angiotensin-converting enzyme inhibitors). In most patients, successful treatment of Cushing's syndrome eliminates hypertension, but in some it persists, likely secondary to microvascular remodeling and/or underlying essential hypertension.

Impaired Glucose Tolerance/Diabetes

It is estimated that approximately 20% to 50% of patients with Cushing's syndrome have overt diabetes, and 30% to 60% have some degree of glucose intolerance. These estimates may actually be low, as the oral glucose tolerance test is not often performed in patients with Cushing's syndrome.

Hyperlipidemia

The insulin resistance induced by hypercortisolism also contributes to the development of lipid abnormalities. Very-low-density lipoproteins and low-density lipoproteins are elevated, leading to an elevation of total triglycerides and cholesterol, whereas high-density lipoproteins are not affected.

Gonadal Axis

Females with Cushing's syndrome may display several of the characteristics of polycystic ovary disease, including oligomenorrhea or amenorrhea and the effects of hyperandrogenism (acne, hirsutism, metabolic syndrome). Hyperprolactinemia may also be present. Males usually develop features of hypogonadotropic hypogonadism. Restoration of the gonadal axis in men and premenopausal women is variable, and thus patients should be evaluated 3 months after successful cure. If gonadal function has not returned, steroid replacement may be considered.

Thyroid Axis

Thyroid function is suppressed by hypercortisolism through inhibition of thyrotropin-releasing hormone and thyroid-stimulating hormone and decreased conversion of thyroxine to triiodothyronine. After surgical cure of Cushing's syndrome, hypothyroidism may persist for at least 3 months. Patients with persistently subnormal free thyroxine levels should receive replacement therapy titrated according to the free thyroxine, not the thyroid-stimulating hormone. Occasionally, curing Cushing's syndrome may unmask a preexisting primary autoimmune thyroid disease presenting as either hypothyroidism or hyperthyroidism.

Psychological Disturbances and Cognitive Disturbances

Fifty percent to 80% of patients with Cushing's syndrome meet *Diagnostic and Statistical Manual of Mental Disorders IV* criteria for major depression. Other symptoms including mania, anxiety, and suicidal ideations may also be present. Patients with hypercortisolism also have impaired cognitive function, often specific to the medial temporal lobe declarative memory system, associated with reversible apparent loss of brain volume. One year after surgical cure, the loss of brain volume and mood disorders usually improve, but there is no change in cognitive function. Many patients, however, have residual symptoms and may need continued psychological and pharmacologic support.

Coagulopathy

Hypercortisolism stimulates the synthesis of several clotting factors by the liver, creating a hypercoagulable state and predisposing patients to thromboembolic events.

Osteoporosis

Glucocorticoids inhibit bone mineralization at many levels, from decreased calcium absorption to altered metabolism at the level of the osteoblasts and osteoclasts. This places patients with Cushing's syndrome at increased risk of fracture and the complications thereof, including back pain from vertebral fractures, kyphosis, height loss, and nonvertebral fractures. Deficits in bone mineralization are partially reversible to varying degrees in any given patient with the reversal of hypercortisolism. Some patients may require pharmacologic intervention to improve bone density both before and after cure of the disease.

Nephrolithiasis

Patients with Cushing's syndrome have an increased prevalence of nephrolithiasis compared with the general population. The reason for this is not completely clear but it probably is because of the synergistic effect of various hypercortisolism-dependent hemodynamic and metabolic abnormalities, particularly excessive uric acid excretion and systemic arterial hypertension.

Somatotropic Axis

Hypercortisolism reduces the secretion of growth hormone and the response of growth hormone to various stimuli. This may lead to growth retardation in children due to inhibition of the epiphyseal cartilage. Children's growth curve should be monitored after reversal of hypercortisolism, and children should be treated with growth hormone in selected cases.

Hyperpigmentation

Hyperpigmentation is seen in Cushing's syndrome that is secondary to adrenocorticotropic hormone–producing pituitary tumors. Adrenocorticotropic hormone is a precursor of melanocyte-stimulating-hormone and, as such, stimulates the production of melanin by melanocytes. Increased skin pigmentation, especially in the creases, pressure areas, new scars, and nipples, is common. Patients may present simply with a complaint of "getting darker."

Material Available on Student Consult

Review Questions and Answers about Cushing's Syndrome

SUGGESTED READINGS

Arnaldi G, Angeli A, Atkinson AB, et al. Diagnosis and complications of Cushing's syndrome: A consensus statement. J Clin Endocrinol Metab 2003;88:5593–5602.🅒

Findling JW, Raff H. Diagnosis and differential diagnosis of Cushing's syndrome. Endocrinol Metab Clin North Am 2001;30:729–747.

Findling J, Raff H, Aron D. The low-dose dexamethasone suppression test: A reevaluation in patients with

Cushing's syndrome. J Clin Endocrinol Metab 2004; 89:122–126.🅑

Papanicolaou D, Mullen N, Kyrou I, Nieman L. Nighttime salivary cortisol: A useful test for the diagnosis of Cushing's syndrome. J Clin Endocrinol Metab 2002; 87:4515–4521.🅑

Chapter

50

Fatigue (Hypothyroidism)

Sarah Ellen Lesko

KEY POINTS

1. Think of hypothyroidism when encountering unexplained constitutional symptoms or hyperlipidemia, especially in an older woman.
2. Do not screen everyone for thyroid disease; keep your eye out for future recommendations.
3. Be patient when treating hypothyroidism; do not expect rapid correction of thyroid-stimulating hormone (TSH) level.
4. Approach subclinical hypothyroidism with a watchful waiting approach; for a detailed risk/benefit discussion with your educated patients, discuss the evidence found at www.ahrq.gov/clinic/3rduspstf/thyroid/thyrrs.htm.

INITIAL VISIT

Subjective

Patient Identification and Presenting Problem

Christine G. is a 53-year-old white woman who presents to her regular clinic complaining of fatigue.

Present Illness

Christine describes a slowly increasing sensation of tiredness that has progressed over at least 2 months. She finds it difficult to get up to go to work and has little energy once there. Her sleep has been normal. She has noticed a weight gain of about 5 pounds, although she denies any change in eating habits. Her bowel movements are less frequent and harder than usual. She has decreased the distance of her daily walks due to new leg cramps, and she feels like she needs to "bundle up" more. Her menstrual periods, previously light and somewhat irregular, have become heavier and longer. Her mood is "okay," although she is more worried than usual. She has normal enjoyment of her favorite activities. She has tried taking ginkgo supplements for the past month but has had no relief.

Medical History

Christine has been coming to the clinic regularly for 15 years. She had mildly elevated cholesterol 3 years ago (total cholesterol 221, high-density lipoprotein 55, low-density lipoprotein 148, triglycerides 90), which she attempted to manage with diet. Her last mammogram 9 months ago was normal; her last Pap smear 2½ years ago was normal with the exception of yeast. She had three negative fecal occult blood tests 9 months ago as well but has

---

Evidence levels 🅐 Randomized, controlled trials (RCTs), meta-analyses, well-designed systematic reviews of RCTs. 🅑 Case-control or cohort studies, nonrandomized clinical trials, systematic reviews of studies other than RCTs, cross-sectional studies, retrospective studies, certain uncontrolled studies. 🅒 Consensus statements, expert guidelines, usual practice, opinion.

not yet had a flexible sigmoidoscopy. Surgical history is notable only for a tonsillectomy/adenoidectomy at age 3.

Family History
Mrs. G.'s father died at age 78 in a motor vehicle accident; her mother, who has mild to moderate Alzheimer's dementia, lives in an assisted-living facility. Mrs. G.'s two older sisters are well; they experienced menopause at ages 58 and 56. A brother died in infancy due to a congenital heart defect. Mrs. G.'s two children are well.

Social History
Mrs. G. is an elected state official with a demanding work and social schedule. She is married and has two children in college. She is a nonsmoker and drinks one to two glasses of wine daily.

Review of Systems
Mrs. G. denies shortness of breath, chest pain, dizziness, visual changes, voice changes, galactorrhea, recent viral infection, fever, radiation exposure, snoring, headaches, nausea, and vomiting.

Objective

Physical Examination
General Christine is a well-groomed woman who looks her stated age. Blood pressure is 120/90 mm Hg, pulse is 60 and regular, weight is 160 pounds (previous weight 9 months ago was 152 pounds), and height is 5 feet 4 inches.

Head, Eyes, Ears, Nose, and Throat Her pupils are equally round and reactive to light; extraocular movements are intact; and conjunctivae are pink.

Neck Her neck is supple, with no lymphadenopathy; her thyroid is smooth and mobile without nodularity.

Heart Her heart rate is 60, with a regular rhythm, no murmurs, rubs, or gallops.

Lungs The lungs are clear to auscultation.

Extremities There are no cords, clubbing, or edema.

Skin There are no rashes; her hands feel slightly rough.

Neurologic Cranial nerves II through XII are grossly intact; patellar and ankle reflexes are present with a slightly prolonged relaxation phase; gait is normal.

Laboratory Studies
A laboratory test is sent after the visit.

Assessment

Working Diagnosis
Fatigue, possibly secondary to hypothyroidism. Fatigue is a common presenting complaint (accounting for 10% to 20% of primary care visits), as it is a common final pathway of a host of problems. It can be very difficult to identify the cause of fatigue. Medical causes may account for only 10% of fatigue complaints. History can help sort out the broad differential diagnosis (Table 50-1). Fatigue that lasts more than 6 months or varies in severity is more likely to be functional. Fatigue that is worse in the morning is often psychiatric. The history should focus on evaluating the timing, severity, and symptoms associated with fatigue as well as a detailed sleep and drug history.

Table 50-1	Differential Diagnosis of Fatigue as Presenting Complaint in the Primary Care Office
Psychological	Depression, anxiety, eating disorder, substance abuse, somatization, seasonal affective disorder
Pharmacologic	Check side effect profiles; many antihypertensives and sleeping aids
Endocrine	Hypothyroidism, diabetes, hypoadrenal states
Reproductive	Pregnancy
Neoplastic	All types
Hematologic	Anemia
Infection	Chronic infection, Lyme disease
Cardiopulmonary	Heart failure, mitral regurgitation or stenosis, chronic lung disease
Connective tissue disease	Polymyalgia rheumatica, rheumatoid arthritis, sarcoidosis
Disturbed sleep	Sleep apnea
Renal	Renal insufficiency or failure
Gastrointestinal	Liver disease
Neurologic	Multiple sclerosis

Table 50-2 Symptoms and Signs of Hypothyroidism Present at Time of Diagnosis

Coarse skin/dry skin/coarse hair	Possible statistical significance*
Bradycardia	Possible statistical significance*
Abnormal or delayed relaxation of ankle reflexes	Possible statistical significance*
Hoarse voice/deep voice	Possible statistical significance*
Cold sensitivity	
Fatigue	
Puffy eyes	Possible statistical significance*
Weight gain	
Irregular menses/heavy menses	
Muscle cramps/weak muscles	Possible statistical significance*
Slow thinking/poor memory/math difficulty	
Decreased hearing	
Diastolic hypertension	
Pretibial edema	
Carpal tunnel syndrome	
Depression/dementia	
Constipation	

*In one or more studies, shown to be present more frequently in patients with hypothyroidism than in a control population.

Hypothyroidism can be similarly elusive to pinpoint. Presenting symptoms for hypothyroidism may include a large variety of complaints (Table 50-2), only a few of which have been found to be possibly statistically significant for biochemical hypothyroidism. Physical examination also has a poor diagnostic accuracy for hypothyroidism. No single sign effectively rules hypothyroidism in or out, although a combination of coarse skin, bradycardia, and delayed ankle reflex may increase the likelihood of biochemical hypothyroidism. However, due to the poor prognosis of untreated disease, clinicians need to test at-risk patients. If it is not caught and treated, hypothyroidism can progress to myxedema with lethargy, generalized edema, severe obstructive sleep apnea, and, ultimately, coma. Side effects of untreated hypothyroidism include all the previously mentioned symptoms as well as hypercholesterolemia (increased low-density lipoprotein and decreased high-density lipoprotein due to decreased catabolism of very low density lipoprotein and intermediate density lipoprotein), normocytic anemia, and pernicious anemia.

Causes of hypothyroidism can be separated into primary hypothyroidism (impaired thyroid function), which accounts for 95% of patients with hypothyroidism (Table 50-3), and secondary hypothyroidism (impaired hypothalamic-pituitary function). Secondary hypothyroidism is the result of

Table 50-3 Causes of Primary Hypothyroidism

Type of Hypothyroidism	Expected Prognosis/Course
Hashimoto's thyroiditis: immune mediated; antimicrosomal antibodies are a marker	Transient hyperthyroidism followed by hypothyroidism; majority of cases are mild and do not require thyroid hormone replacement
Postpartum thyroiditis; variant of Hashimoto's	Usually resolves over 2–3 mo
Radiation-induced hypothyroidism	Usually requires hormone replacement
Subacute thyroiditis: follows viral upper respiratory infection	Resolves over weeks to months
Subtotal thyroidectomy	Transient hypothyroidism; becomes permanent in half of cases
Drugs: lithium (5% clinically hypothyroid), propylthiouracil, methimazole	Medication dependent
Iodide excess: impairs thyroxine synthesis/release	Correct excess
Iodide deficiency: inhibits thyroxine synthesis	Correct deficiency
Infiltrative disease: hemochromatosis, amyloidosis, scleroderma	Address underlying disease

injury to the thyrotropic cells, most often by pituitary adenoma. In cases of secondary hypothyroidism, the TSH will be low.

Key points of Mrs. G.'s history include weight gain, inability to tolerate cold, menorrhagia, constipation, and muscle cramps. Key components of her physical examination are borderline bradycardia, documented weight gain, delayed relaxation phase of reflexes, and rough skin on her hands. A past significant laboratory test is her abnormal lipid profile. Given this combination of symptoms and physical findings, a measurement of TSH is warranted. The clinician could consider checking a hematocrit as well.

Plan

Diagnostic

TSH alone is the recommended screening tool to detect hypothyroidism. It has a sensitivity of 89% to 95% and a specificity of 90% to 96%. TSH and thyroid hormone (thyroxine) concentrations are related by inverse log. Therefore, a 50% decrease in free thyroxine concentration causes a 90-fold increase in TSH concentration. For this reason, TSH is the much more sensitive detector of primary hypothyroidism. Mrs. G.'s TSH result returns at 22.4 mIU/L (normal for this laboratory, 0.50 to 5.10 mIU/L). A free thyroxine measurement, added on by automatic clinical laboratory algorithm when TSH is high, is low-normal at 0.85 ng/dL. Mrs. G. has overt hypothyroidism and needs thyroid hormone replacement.

Therapeutic

Mrs. G. is prescribed a starting dose of 50 μg levothyroxine (Synthroid) per day (usual starting dose 25 to 50 μg in elderly patients or those with comorbidities, 100 μg in young patients). This dose may be increased by 25 to 50 μg every 4 to 8 weeks to a typical dose of 1.7 μg/kg body weight/day. (In this patient, 100 to 125 μg/day).

Patient Education

Mrs. G. is educated on the expected course of treatment (likely permanent) and symptom resolution (should improve within 3 to 4 weeks and resolve within 3 months). She is warned about the potential unmasking of silent coronary artery disease as well as other possible side effects of the medication. The etiology of her hypothyroidism is likely Hashimoto's thyroiditis; it is not necessary to definitively test for the causative factor, as it will not affect treatment decisions.

FOLLOW-UP VISIT

Subjective

Mrs. G. returns for re-evaluation 5 weeks after her original visit. She reports that she is feeling better although not yet back to baseline. Her bowel habits have returned to normal and her fatigue level has improved significantly. She had mild insomnia the first week that she took the levothyroxine. She had one menstrual period that was still heavier than usual. She has experienced no chest pain or palpitations.

Objective

Her pulse is 75 and regular, blood pressure is 125/80, and weight is 156 pounds. Her gait and reflexes are normal.

Laboratory Testing

Repeat TSH is 10.2 mIU/L; free thyroxine is 1.29 ng/dL.

Assessment

Mrs. G. has had a good initial response to treatment with thyroid replacement hormone. Her subjective complaints have improved, her weight is down, her reflexes are normal, and her pulse has returned to normal.

Plan

The advisability of maintaining the current dose of levothyroxine and rechecking the TSH in 6 weeks—due to the common lag of TSH returning to normal—is discussed with Mrs. G. The option of increasing the dose by 25 μg/day is also discussed, with the risk of overtreatment and future need to decrease her levothyroxine dose. The patient prefers to increase her dose and is scheduled for repeat TSH, fasting cholesterol, and follow-up visit in 6 weeks.

DISCUSSION

Hypothyroidism, although not difficult to diagnose once the laboratory test is ordered, presents many dilemmas in clinical practice. The prevalence of hypothyroidism in the general population increases with age and disproportionately affects women. Prevalence in women 60 and older approaches 5%. The core clinical question often becomes: Whom to test? Referencing the nonspecific symptom information given above, the physician is clearly asked to invoke the art of medicine. The U.S. Preventive Services Task Force states, "Clinicians should remain alert for subtle or nonspecific symptoms of thyroid dysfunction when examining such patients, and maintain a low threshold for diagnostic evaluation of thyroid function."

Table 50-4   Recommendations Regarding Thyroid Screening

U.S. Preventive Services Task Force	Insufficient evidence to recommend for or against routine screening in adults (yield of screening may be greater in postpartum women, patients with trisomy 21, and the elderly)
American Academy of Family Physicians	Recommends against routine screening in asymptomatic patients younger than 60
Canadian Task Force on the Periodic Health Examination	No screening; have a high index of suspicion for nonspecific symptoms in perimenopausal and postmenopausal women
American College of Physicians	Screen women older than 50 with one or more symptoms that could be caused by thyroid disease
American College of Obstetricians and Gynecologists	Apply knowledge of the symptoms for postpartum thyroid dysfunction; test as indicated
American Association of Clinical Endocrinologists	Screen all women of childbearing age before pregnancy or during the first trimester
American Thyroid Association	Measure thyroid function in all adults beginning at age 35 and every 5 years thereafter

Screening

By definition, screening tests are performed on asymptomatic populations. Because the symptoms of hypothyroidism can be vague or multifactorial, several groups have studied the utility of generalized screening for thyroid dysfunction. Principles of a good screening test include good detection rate (sensitivity) of the screening test (with an acceptable false-positive rate) as well as evidence that treatment improves clinically important outcomes. TSH testing can detect asymptomatic thyroid disease; however, the U.S. Preventive Services Task Force recently concluded that there is insufficient evidence to establish the benefits versus harms of treatment for screening-detected hypothyroidism. Current recommendations for population-based screening for thyroid disease are listed in Table 50-4.

Subclinical Hypothyroidism

Invariably, even when applying the best clinical algorithms, the clinician will have to analyze indeterminate results. This occurs in thyroid function testing when the TSH result returns in the mildly elevated range (generally 5 to 10 mIU/L) with a normal free thyroxine and with no clearly attributable symptoms of hypothyroidism. This is termed subclinical hypothyroidism and has a prevalence of 7% in women (approaching 20% in women older than age 60) and 2.5% in men. Of patients with an abnormally high TSH, approximately 75% will have values lower than 10 mIU/L. The clinical course of subclin-

ical hypothyroidism shows that approximately 20% of these patients will develop clinically symptomatic hypothyroidism within 5 years. Patients with high titers of antithyroid antibodies are at greatest risk (implicating Hashimoto's thyroiditis). However, there is no evidence to recommend treatment of subclinical hypothyroidism to prevent overt hypothyroidism. "The USPSTF estimates that in a reference population of 1,000 women screened, 3 cases of overt hypothyroidism would be prevented in 5 years, but 40 people would have taken medication for 5 years without a clear benefit." Subclinical hypothyroidism does not appear to be associated with an abnormal lipid panel when adjusted for confounding factors. Treatment of patients with subclinical hypothyroidism with thyroid hormone replacement, hypothesized to improve lipid profiles, myocardial function, adverse cardiac endpoints, and neuropsychiatric function, has not proved to be clinically beneficial. In addition, there are potential harms of overtreatment, including osteoporosis, palpitations, and worsening coronary artery disease. Therefore, although each case should be approached on an individual basis, subclinical hypothyroidism should in general be followed by laboratory testing but not treated with thyroid replacement hormone.

Material Available on Student Consult

Review Questions and Answers about Hypothyroidism

SUGGESTED READINGS

Agency for Healthcare Research and Quality: Screening Thyroid Disease: Recommendation Statement, January, 2004. Available at www.ahrq.gov/clinic/3rduspstf/thyroid/thyrrs.htm. Accessed 9/1/2004.Ⓐ

Canaris Gay J, Steiner JF, Ridgway EC. Do traditional symptoms of hypothyroidism correlate with biochemical disease? J Gen Intern Med 1997;12: 544–550.Ⓑ

Hueston WJ, Pearson WS. Subclinical hypothyroidism and the risk of hypercholesterolemia. Ann Fam Med 2004;2:351–355.Ⓑ

Indra R, Patil SS, Joshi R, Pai M, Kalantri SP. Accuracy of physical examination in the diagnosis of hypothy- roidism: A cross-sectional, double-blind study. J Postgrad Med 2004;50:7–10.Ⓑ

Sharpe M, Wilks D. Fatigue: Clinical review. BMJ 2002;325:480–483.

Surks MI, Ortiz E, Daniels GH, et al. Subclinical thy- roid disease: Scientific review and guidelines for diagnosis and management. JAMA 2004;291: 228–238.Ⓐ

U.S. Preventive Services Task Force. Screening for thyroid disease. In Guide to Clinical Preventive Services, 2nd ed. Baltimore, Williams & Wilkins, 1996, p 209.Ⓐ

Chapter

51 Unexplained Weight Loss (Hyperthyroidism)

Barbara A. Majeroni

KEY POINTS

1. Hyperthyroidism should be considered in the differential of unexplained weight loss. Check a thyroid-stimulating hormone (TSH) level.
2. The most common cause of hyperthyroidism is Graves' disease.
3. A very low or undetectable TSH is the hallmark of thyrotoxicosis.
4. In the pregnant patient, iodine 131 is con- traindicated. Propylthiouracil is generally the preferred treatment. In severe cases, subtotal thyroidectomy can be performed in the second trimester.
5. Because lean body mass declines with age, weight loss in the elderly may be of greater clinical significance.
6. A single measurement of low serum TSH in indi- viduals age 60 years or older has been associated with increased mortality, particularly due to circu- latory and cardiovascular disease.
7. A study of cancer incidence in patients treated with iodine 131 found significant decreases in the incidence of cancers of the pancreas, bronchus, trachea, bladder, and lymphatic and hematopoietic systems. Although a threefold increase in the risk of thyroid cancer was found, the absolute risk remained small.
8. TSH should be measured in elderly patients with systolic hypertension, a widened pulse pressure, recent-onset angina, atrial fibrillation, or an exacer- bation of underlying ischemic heart disease.

Evidence levels Ⓐ Randomized, controlled trials (RCTs), meta-analyses, well-designed systematic reviews of RCTs. Ⓑ Case-control or cohort studies, nonrandomized clinical trials, systematic reviews of studies other than RCTs, cross-sectional studies, retrospective studies, certain uncontrolled studies. Ⓒ Consensus statements, expert guidelines, usual practice, opinion.

INITIAL VISIT

Subjective

Patient Identification and Presenting Problem

Mrs. P. is a 53-year-old married white woman who was in her usual state of good health until about 6 months ago. At that time, she noticed that she was losing weight. She began to pay more attention to her eating habits and believes she has a good appetite and eats a well-rounded diet, but she has continued to lose weight. By her scale at home, she has lost 30 pounds over the past 6 months. She initially attributed the problem to nervousness and stress at work, where she is in a supervisory position at a nursing home, but the problem has continued despite her efforts to delegate more at work. Now she is experiencing excessive fatigue and difficulty sleeping, as well as continued weight loss. Her sister was recently diagnosed with breast cancer, and she worries that this might be the problem, although she has not noted any changes on her monthly breast self-examination.

Medical History

Mrs. P. has been in good health. She had a tubal ligation at age 32 years and cholecystectomy at age 48 years. Her two pregnancies resulted in normal spontaneous vaginal deliveries. She stopped menstruating 2 years ago. No history of diabetes, heart disease, hypertension, cancer, gastrointestinal (GI), or psychiatric illness is known. She has no known allergies. Her only medication is an over-the-counter multiple vitamin and mineral supplement, which she started about 4 months ago. Her last Pap test was 5 years ago. She has never had a mammogram.

Family History

Mrs. P.'s father died at age 76 years of prostate cancer. Her mother is living and well at age 74 years. One older sister had surgery for breast cancer. Another sister and brother are well. No family history of heart disease, respiratory disease, renal, hematologic, GI, or endocrine disease is known. Her children and grandchildren have no medical problems.

Social History

Mrs. P. lives with her husband, who works as a computer consultant. One daughter lives upstairs. The other is married and lives with her husband and two children about an hour away. Mrs. P. has never smoked and denies any past or present use of alcohol or illicit drugs. She enjoys her work as a nursing supervisor and is able to take some time off occasionally to travel with her husband to various cities in the United States. She has always been physically active, biking or swimming several times a week. Her husband is her only sexual partner, and she feels sure that he does not see anyone else.

Review of Systems

She has no headaches, visual disturbances, hearing problems, or dizziness. She denies chest pain, but admits to occasional palpitations, not necessarily associated with activity. No shortness of breath, cough, or sputum; no abdominal pain, diarrhea, or constipation; and no blood in stools is reported. She has soft bowel movements 2 or 3 times a day. She has had no vaginal bleeding or discharge. She notes some vaginal dryness and complains of excessive sweating, which she attributes to hot flashes. No rashes or skin changes, and no jaundice or pruritis is found. She denies feeling hopeless or suicidal, but states she has felt very tense and anxious lately. She has had no hallucinations or delusions.

Objective

Physical Examination

Mrs. P. is well groomed, pleasant, and cooperative. She appears tense and worried. Her height is 68 inches; weight, 120 pounds. Weight at last visit, 1 year ago, was 158 pounds. Blood pressure is 128/80; pulse, 100; respirations, 16; oral temperature, 37.6°C (99.7°F). Hair is normal. Head is normocephalic. Her eyes are normal in configuration. Sclerae are clear, extraocular movements are intact. Pupils are equally round and reactive to light and accommodation; fundi show no hemorrhages or vascular changes. Tympanic membranes are clear. Pharynx is clear. Teeth are in good condition. No lymphadenopathy is appreciated; thyroid is diffusely enlarged, with no nodules or tenderness. Heart is regular with normal S_1 and S_2 and no murmur. Lungs are clear to examination. Breasts are symmetrical, with no masses, skin changes, or nipple discharge, and with no axillary adenopathy. Her abdomen is soft and nontender with no organomegaly. Bowel sounds are active in all quadrants. On pelvic examination, the vaginal mucosa is atrophic; no skin lesions are present. The cervix has no lesions or discharge. Pap smear is taken from the cervix. No masses or tenderness of the uterus or adnexae are found. Rectal examination: normal tone, no lesions, heme-negative, soft brown stool. Extremities: No edema, clubbing, or cyanosis. Hands are warm and moist. Distal pulses are normal. Neurologic examination reveals no focal abnormalities except for a symmetrical fine tremor of the hands. Deep tendon reflexes are brisk and symmetrical. Cranial nerves II through XII are intact. Gait and station are normal. No deficits are observed in strength or sensation. Memory, thought processes, and speech patterns are normal.

Assessment

Unexplained weight loss results from either decreased intake (or absorption) or increased output (or metabolism) of caloric energy. A loss of more than 5% of total body weight within a 6- to 12-month period suggests underlying pathology, especially when progressive. Low body weight and weight loss are powerful indicators of morbidity and mortality (Bouras et al., 2001).

Differential Diagnosis (Box 51-1)

1. *Decreased intake.* Common causes of weight loss that result from social isolation, problems with finances, problems with dentition, inability to shop, or loneliness are unlikely in this woman, who has a job and family support. She is taking no drugs that would be likely to cause nausea or anorexia, and no suspicion of alcoholism exists.

2. *Psychiatric disorders.* Because of her age and the history of good appetite, the diagnosis of anorexia nervosa is unlikely. Loss of appetite due to mood disorders occurs in depression and in bipolar disorder. Psychotic patients may stop eating because of delusions, such as fear of being poisoned. This patient has been worried and is concerned about her sister, but she denies feeling sad or hopeless and continues to take pleasure in activities such as traveling with her husband. She does not fulfill criteria for a diagnosis of depression.

3. *Cancer.* Malignancies account for about one third of all patients with unintentional weight loss, which may be the presenting complaint. In a woman of this age, common cancers would include lung, breast, and GI cancers. Because the patient never smoked, lung cancer is less likely, although not impossible. The absence of cough or sputum production is reassuring. A first-degree relative with breast cancer increases her risk for this. A mammogram is indicated despite a normal examination. A single heme-negative stool does not rule out colon cancer, and if no other cause is found for the weight loss, further GI workup with an upper GI endoscopy and colonoscopy would be considered.

4. *Gastrointestinal disorders.* GI disorders are the most common nonmalignant organic causes identified in patients with unintentional weight loss. Upper tract disorders such as reflux, gastritis, and peptic ulcer disease may result in reduced intake. Decreased absorption of calories can occur with chronic pancreatitis, short-bowel syndrome, sprue, inflammatory bowel disease, or parasitic infection. Mrs. P. has no symptoms to suggest an intestinal disorder. If no cause for her weight loss is found in her initial evaluation, further GI evaluation will be considered.

Box 51-1	**Differential Diagnosis of Involuntary Weight Loss**

Reduced Intake

Social isolation
Financial limitations
Problems with dentition
Inability to obtain food, mobility, transportation restrictions
Alcohol or drug abuse
Drugs that alter appetite, cause nausea, or affect taste

Psychiatric Disorders

Anorexia nervosa
Depression, anxiety, bereavement
Dementia
Psychosis

Cancer

Gastrointestinal tact is most common site for occult tumors
Hepatobiliary
Hematologic
Lung
Breast
Genitourinary
Ovarian
Prostate

Infection

Tuberculosis
Fungal disease
Amebic abscess
Subacute bacterial endocarditis
Human immunodeficiency virus

Endocrine/Metabolic Diseases

Diabetes mellitus
Hyperthyroidism
Apathetic hypothyroidism

Gastrointestinal Disorders

Peptic ulcer disease
Gastroesophageal reflux
Pancreatitis
Sprue
Short bowel syndrome
Inflammatory bowel disease

Chronic Illnesses

Congestive heart failure
Renal or hepatic disease
Connective tissue disease
Pulmonary disease

Idiopathic (25%)

5. *Infection.* Chronic infectious processes such as subacute bacterial endocarditis, tuberculosis, or acquired immunodeficiency syndrome (AIDS) can result in weight loss. This patient has no lifestyle risk factors for AIDS. Because she works in a health care facility, she has an annual purified protein derivative (PPD) skin test, and all have been negative. No physical signs of infection are noted.

6. *Endocrine diseases.* Diabetes mellitus causes weight loss, initially due to osmotic diuresis, and in insulin-dependent forms, due to caloric wastage. Weight loss in diabetes is frequently associated with increased food intake. Increased metabolism resulting in weight loss can be caused by hyperthyroidism. Signs and symptoms are variable and may be subtle. This patient's symptoms of nervousness, weight loss, palpitations, increased sweating, and fatigue could be secondary to hyperthyroidism, even in the absence of exophthalmos and heat intolerance. Although it is more commonly associated with weight gain, patients with hypothyroidism sometimes initially have apathy and weight loss. This is more common in patients older than 65 years.

7. *Chronic disease.* In addition to cancer, other chronic disease can result in increased metabolic demands and decreased caloric intake, resulting in weight loss. Some examples are congestive heart failure, renal failure, cirrhosis, and chronic obstructive pulmonary disease. In some neurologic diseases, functional limitations reduce caloric intake. This patient's physical examination does not point to any of these.

8. *Idiopathic.* In approximately 25% of patients evaluated for weight loss, the problem remains unexplained despite extensive evaluation and prolonged follow-up.

Plan

Because the cause of Mrs. P.'s weight loss has not been clearly defined by the history and physical, further evaluation is indicated (Box 51-2). Laboratory values ordered included a complete blood count (CBC), glucose, electrolytes, blood urea nitrogen (BUN), creatinine, amylase, liver enzymes, albumin, free thyroxine (T_4), and thyroid-stimulating hormone (TSH). A mammogram was scheduled. Further testing will be determined based on these results.

FOLLOW-UP

Laboratory Tests

A normal CBC made infection unlikely. A fasting glucose of 100 ruled out diabetes. Normal electrolytes, BUN, and creatinine suggested normal renal function. Amylase and liver enzymes were also within normal range. Albumin was 2.5 g/100 mL (0.385 mmol/L),

Box 51-2	Evaluation for Unexplained Weight Loss

Complete history and physical
Labs: Complete blood count, electrolytes, blood urea nitrogen, creatinine, glucose, free thyroxine, thyroid-stimulating hormone, liver function tests, amylase, urinalysis
Stool hemoccult ×3.
Further studies based on symptoms: chest radiograph, upper gastrointestinal studies, barium enema, or colonoscopy
If these do not reveal a cause, and social factors have been corrected, close follow-up is recommended rather than extensive undirected testing.

suggesting chronic malnutrition. T_4 was elevated at 19.5 µg/100 mL (251.5 nmol/L), and TSH was 0.03 mU/L. Mammogram and Pap test were normal.

Diagnosis

The combination of low TSH with an elevated T_4 is diagnostic of *hyperthyroidism*. This is consistent with the patient's symptoms of weight loss with nervousness, palpitations, fatigue, and sweating, and the physical findings of enlarged thyroid and a higher-than-expected heart rate. A radioactive iodine-uptake scan was ordered.

DISCUSSION

Most common in white women, hyperthyroidism affects up to 2% of women and 0.2% of men. Prevalence increases with age and is highest in patients older than 80 years. In this age group, the female predominance becomes less marked (1:2 compared with 1:8 in younger groups) (Flynn et al., 2004❷). Although signs and symptoms are variable, the most common signs of thyrotoxicosis include resting tachycardia, atrial fibrillation in the elderly, thyroid gland enlargement, tremor, exophthalmos, lid lag, warm moist skin, and muscle weakness. More than 50% of patients exhibit some of the common symptoms, which include nervousness, increased sweating, heat intolerance, palpitations, dyspnea, fatigue, weight loss, diarrhea, polyuria, oligomenorrhea, loss of libido, and eye complaints.

Sinus tachycardia is the most common rhythm disturbance in patients with hyperthyroidism (Klein and Ojamaa, 2001❸). Atrial fibrillation occurs in 5% to 15% of patients with hyperthyroidism and may be the presenting problem. The risk of atrial fibrillation or atrial flutter is higher in men than in women and increases with age (Frost et al., 2004❸). Treatment of the hyperthyroidism alone reverts atrial fibrillation to sinus rhythm in fewer than half of the cases. Hyperthyroidism is associated with a risk of worsening of existing heart disease but can also, by itself, cause cardiac disease. Excess thyroid hormone causes palpitations with some degree of exercise intolerance and a widened pulse pressure. In patients with hyperthyroidism, cardiac output is increased because of a decrease in systemic vascular resistance, an increase in resting heart rate, increased left ventricular contractility, and increased blood volume. In older patients with heart disease, the increased workload that results from hyperthyroidism may further impair cardiac function.

More than 50% of thyrotoxic men report sexual dysfunction associated with decreased libido, which is improved after 6 months of treatment for hyperthyroidism. Thirty percent of hyperthyroid patients in this study had lower-than-normal semen volumes and sperm densities than did controls. Sperm motility also was significantly lower. After treatment, sperm density and motility improved (Krassas et al., 2002❸).

Testing

Measurement of serum thyrotropin (TSH) by using at least a second-generation assay (detection limit, approximately 0.05 mIU/L) is the most sensitive test for screening for hyperthyroidism, a normal result virtually excluding hyperthyroidism, except in the rare instance in which it is due to thyrotropin hypersecretion (Woeber, 2000). An undetectable value is the hallmark of hyperthyroidism. Confirmation is by measuring the free thyroxine (T_4). If the free T_4 is normal and suspicion is high for thyrotoxicosis, a serum free triiodothyronine (T_3) should also be measured to rule out T_3 thyrotoxicosis.

Misleading laboratory results may occur. Drugs such as glucocorticoids, levodopa, and dopamine can cause a low TSH in patients who are euthyroid. Estrogen in pregnancy, hormone replacement therapy, or oral contraceptives may cause an increased T_4, but free T_4 will be normal, and the patient is euthyroid. Causes of thyrotoxicosis are summarized in Box 51-3.

The usual pattern in hyperthyroidism is a high free T_4 with a low TSH. A thyroid scan with radioactive iodine (RAIU) can help differentiate the causes of hyperthyroidism. Factitious or iatrogenic hyperthyroidism can be differentiated by the RAIU, which is suppressed to less than 5% in the presence of excess exogenous thyroid hormone. In endogenous disease, the RAIU is elevated. In toxic adenoma or toxic multinodular goiter, the radioisotope is concentrated in one or more areas, whereas in Graves' disease, diffuse uptake may occur throughout the gland. In thyroiditis, the

Box 51-3	Causes of Thyrotoxicosis

Graves' disease (most common)
Iatrogenic (overtreated hypothyroidism)
Thyroiditis
    Hashimoto's (autoimmune) thyroiditis,
        subacute thyroiditis, silent thyroiditis,
        postpartum thyroiditis
Toxic multinodular goiter
Toxic adenoma
Factitious hyperthyroidism (patient taking
    excess thyroid hormone)
Excess exogenous iodine
Rare causes
    TSH-secreting pituitary adenoma
    Trophoblastic tumor
    Struma ovarii
    Thyroid cancer
    Activating mutation of the TSH receptor
    Thyroid hormone–resistance syndrome

TSH, thyroid-stimulating hormone.

RAIU may be reduced when T_4 is high and increased when T_4 is low, in a patchy nonhomogeneous pattern. The RAIU also is reduced, at times to zero, in patients with hyperthyroidism due to excess iodine (Jod-Basedow disease). These patients have goiter, but no image on thyroid scan. Trophoblastic tumors are rare, but they can cause a low TSH because of tumor secretion of excess β-human chorionic gonadotropin, which interacts with TSH receptors in the thyroid. Another rare cause of hyperthyroidism is struma ovarii, in which thyroid nests in the ovary become hyperplastic and produce thyroxine. If no other cause for the hyperthyroidism is found, focusing the gamma camera on the ovaries at the thyroid scan will reveal increased radioactive iodine uptake in this condition.

Results

Mrs. P.'s thyroid scan showed diffuse increased uptake, suggestive of Graves' disease. Although the classic triad of Graves' disease includes hyperthyroidism with diffuse thyroid enlargement, ophthalmopathy, and dermopathy, the three major manifestations need not appear together, and some patients exhibit only one of the three.

Treatment

Hospitalization is required only in the case of serious arrhythmias, congestive heart failure, or impending thyroid storm. Mrs. P. can be treated as an outpatient.

Symptoms of nervousness and palpitations may be controlled with a β-blocker while awaiting definitive treatment. In acute thyroiditis, symptomatic treatment may be used alone in anticipation of spontaneous remission. Graves' disease may be treated with propylthiouracil, methimazole, or carbimazole (not available in the United States) in the hope of remission or to achieve a euthyroid state before ablative treatment with radioactive iodine (Pearce and Braverman, 2004). In the case of Mrs. P., the history suggested a long duration of hyperthyroidism. Definitive treatment with iodine 131 was administered. The patient was informed before the treatment that in as many as 40% to 70% of patients treated with this modality, hypothyroidism will develop within 10 years, requiring life-long hormone replacement therapy.

Follow-up

After her treatment with radioactive iodine, Mrs. P. will be monitored by her family doctor, who will watch carefully for signs of hypothyroidism and monitor her T_4 and TSH to determine whether she has obtained a euthyroid state. The β-blocker will be tapered as symptoms permit. Health-maintenance issues that will continue to be addressed include the advisability of annual mammograms, regular Pap tests, and consideration of calcium supplementation.

Material Available on Student Consult

Review Questions and Answers about Hyperthyroidism

REFERENCES

Bouras EP, Lang SM, Scalapio JS. Rational approach to patients with unintentional weight loss. Mayo Clinic Proc 2001;76:923–929.

Flynn RWV, MacDonald TM, Morris AD, et al. The thyroid epidemiology, audit, and research study: Thyroid dysfunction in the general population. J Clin Endocrinol Metab 2004;89:3879–3884. Ⓑ

Frost L, Vestergaard P, Mosekilde L. Hyperthyroidism and the risk of atrial fibrillation or flutter: A population based study. Arch Intern Med 2004;164:1675–1678. Ⓑ

Klein I, Ojamaa K. Mechanisms of disease: Thyroid hormones and the cardiovascular system. N Engl J Med 2001;344:501–509. Ⓑ

Krassas GE, Pontikides N, Deligianni V, Miras K. A prospective, controlled study of the impact of hyperthyroidism on reproductive function in males. J Clin Endocrinol Metab 2002;87:3667–3671. Ⓑ

Pearce EN, Braverman LE. Hyperthyroidism: Advantages and disadvantages of medical therapy. Surg Clin North Am 2004;84:833–847.

Woeber KA. Update on the management of hyperthyroidism and hypothyroidism. Arch Intern Med 2000; 1060:1067–1071.

52

Dysuria and Urinary Frequency (Urinary Tract Infection)

Kurt Kurowski

INITIAL VISIT

Subjective

Patient Identification and Presenting Problem

Amber L. is a 30-year-old white woman who complains of frequency and burning on urination.

Present Illness

The patient states that she began to notice dysuria and frequency of urination yesterday but without urgency or hematuria. She has no vaginal discharge or dyspareunia. She also denies noticing any fever or back pain. She has had two episodes of similar symptoms in the past 6 months. She was told on these previous episodes that she had a bladder infection and was given 3-day courses of antibiotics with resolution of her symptoms. Her last episode was 1 month ago. Before the past 6 months, she had only two urinary tract infections (UTIs), and neither of these was during childhood. She has not had any recent instrumentation of her urinary tract and has not been hospitalized.

Her last menstrual period was 1 week ago. She has no history of vaginal spermicide use or immunocompromise.

Medical History

She had an appendectomy at age 15 years. The only medication she takes is Ortho Evra patch for birth control.

Family History

No history of urinary tract abnormalities is known in her parents or her two siblings. Her maternal grandmother has diabetes mellitus.

Social History

She was married for 2 years and has no children. She has been divorced for the past 3 years and is currently living with her boyfriend of 8 months. She is a receptionist in a primary care medical office. She tries to avoid eating meat, as she is opposed to the killing of animals, but she does consume milk and cheese. She does not smoke but has two to three glasses of wine each week.

Review of Systems

The patient denies any nausea, vomiting, fever, or chills.

Objective

Physical Examination

General The patient appears in no distress, but she did have to make a quick trip to the bathroom to urinate just before you came into the room.

Vital Signs

Temperature, 37.3°C (99.2°F)
Blood pressure, 128/80
Pulse, 86 and regular
Respiratory rate, 16
Height, 5 feet 6 inches
Weight, 120 pounds

Head, Eyes, Ears, Nose, and Throat Pharynx reveals a moist mucosa.

Abdomen Her abdomen has active bowel sounds and is scaphoid, with suprapubic tenderness to deep palpation but no guarding or rebound. No palpable masses in the abdomen or palpable kidneys are found.

Back No dimpling or skin defects overlie the spine, and no costovertebral angle tenderness is seen.

Pelvic On pelvic examination, no external vaginal lesions are found. A scant amount of yellowish white discharge is present in the vagina. The cervix appears smooth, with no cervical motion tenderness. The fundus is smooth and nontender, and no adnexal masses are appreciated.

Neurologic Motor strength and sensation to pain and touch are normal in both legs.

Assessment

Working Diagnosis

The working diagnosis is recurrent cystitis. Recurrent cystitis is defined as three or more UTIs in the course of 1 year (or two episodes in 6 months). Although she has had multiple recent infections, she has an uncomplicated infection. Complicated infections are more likely to be caused by resistant organisms and occur when the urinary tract is abnormal or when the infection occurs in an environment where resistant organisms are more likely to be present, such as hospitals, nursing homes, Foley catheters, etc. (Tables 52-1 and 52-2).

Differential Diagnosis

1. *Pyelonephritis.* The hallmarks of pyelonephritis are high fever, chills, back or flank pain, and nausea and vomiting. Of these, the single best predictor of pyelonephritis is a temperature greater than 38.9°C (102°F). However, the presence or absence of these clinical indicators is not always reliable, and the mislabeling of cystitis as pyelonephritis and vice versa occurs in about 30% of patients. Pregnant women

Table 52-1	Bacterial Prevalence in Uncomplicated Urinary Tract Infection	
Bacteria	**Prevalence (%)**
Escherichia coli	≥80
Staphylococcus saprophyticus	10–15 (20% in college-aged population)
Proteus species	3
Klebsiella species	3
Enterobacter species	1.5
Citrobacter species	0.8
Enterococcus species	0.5

Table 52-2	Bacterial Prevalence in Complicated Urinary Tract Infection	
Bacteria	**Prevalence (%)**
Escherichia coli	30
Proteus species	13
Enterobacter species	3
Staphylococcus epidermidis	12
Staphylococcus aureus	4
Enterococcus species	16
Pseudomonas species	5
Others (Serratia, Streptococci, Actineobacter, and Citrobacter species)	17

and those with diabetes mellitus or tract abnormalities have an increased risk of pyelonephritis with UTIs, even if the hallmark symptoms are not present.

2. *Interstitial cystitis.* This patient is in the age range and of the gender in which interstitial cystitis predominates. Previous UTIs also are considered to be a risk factor for interstitial cystitis. However, the asymptomatic periods in her recent history strongly speak against this diagnosis. Patients with interstitial cystitis typically have severe combinations of dysuria, frequency, and suprapubic pain, which vary from day to day but are usually disabling in severity.

3. *Relapsing cystitis.* Reinfections are much more common than relapsing infections, even when symptoms recur shortly after previous episodes. A relapsing infection is caused by the same organism because it was not eradicated with the first treatment and typically occurs within 2 weeks of treatment. In contrast to reinfection, an abnormality in the urinary tract is common when a UTI relapses.

4. *Bladder cancer.* Risk factors for bladder carcinoma are cigarette smoking and exposure to industrial dyes or solvents. Bladder cancer is more common in men. Most patients have at least intermittent hematuria, either gross or microscopic, but some have pyuria, and occasional patients are initially seen with urinary frequency and urgency. Urine cytology has been useful in the diagnosis of higher-stage and more undifferentiated tumors, in which sensitivity approaches 90%, but ultimate diagnosis and staging of bladder carcinoma is by cystoscopy and transurethral resection.

5. *Vaginitis.* Bacterial vaginitis is most commonly caused by altered vaginal flora but also can be caused by the direct introduction of organisms. Candida and Trichomonas vaginitis are more inflammatory than bacterial vaginosis and therefore more likely to produce dysuria. Among noninfectious etiologies, atrophic vaginitis in postmenopausal women and chemical vaginitis from vaginal products and scented toilet paper must be considered.

6. *Viral cystitis.* Adenovirus type II is a recognized cause, most typically producing a spontaneously resolving hemorrhagic cystitis in children.

7. *Chemical cystitis.* Cyclophosphamide is the most common cause. Initial symptoms are similar to those of bacterial cystitis, but microscopic and gross hematuria can develop, particularly with prolonged courses and higher doses.

8. *Radiation cystitis.* This should be suspected as the cause in any patient with a previous history of radiation to nearby structures (prostate, uterus) who has cystitis symptoms but no evidence of infection on culture.

9. *Urethral diverticulum.* During physical examination, milking of the urethra will reveal a palpable mass, and pus will be seen at the urethral meatus.

Plan

Diagnostic

Because Ms. L. has symptoms suggestive of an uncomplicated cystitis, a urinalysis (dipstick would be adequate) is the only test indicated. Despite a history suggestive of recurrent infections, no history suggests a complicated infection or pyelonephritis, both of which would warrant urine cultures with sensitivity. A complete blood count (CBC) with differential and blood cultures (blood cultures are positive in about 20% of cases of pyelonephritis) would be appropriate only if the patient appeared septic. Urine Gram stains are appropriate to guide initial antibiotic choices in patients with urosepsis but are not necessary for uncomplicated cystitis.

Therapeutic

The patient is given nitrofurantoin sustained release, 100 mg twice daily for 3 days, for the acute infection and then 50 mg after intercourse for prophylaxis.

Patient Education

The patient is instructed to urinate after intercourse and to avoid vaginal spermicides. She is to stop the nitrofurantoin and contact the office if any fever, cough, or skin reactions develop. The beneficial role of daily cranberry juice also is discussed.

Disposition

The patient is sent home. She is instructed to make an appointment in 6 months, at which time a trial off the prophylactic antibiotic is planned, even if it has suppressed repeated infections. She will return sooner if UTI symptoms appear despite receiving prophylaxis.

DISCUSSION

Two basic goals exist in the approach to a patient with dysuria. The first goal is to determine whether the cause is a UTI or one of the other causes listed in the differential diagnosis section. The second goal, if the diagnosis is UTI, is differentiation between upper or lower tract infection and complicated or uncomplicated infection.

Cystitis is an extremely common infection in women, with 40% of women experiencing at least one episode in their lifetimes. It is rare in men unless at least partial obstruction or some other anatomic abnormality occurs in their urinary tract. Male infants who have not been circumcised also have an 8 times higher relative risk. In some men, the infection is acquired through intercourse. If present, the triad of symptoms of dysuria, frequency, and urgency is particularly predictive of cystitis. The dysuria of cystitis is sensed as more internal than is that of vaginitis. Associated hematuria is common. Many UTIs are associated with intercourse, with symptoms developing approximately 24 hours later. Vaginal spermicides kill protective lactobacilli but are not bactericidal against *Escherichia coli* and thus are risk factors. In smaller children or infants who cannot describe dysuria, the presence of an otherwise unexplained fever is the most typical presentation. Visible discomfort with urination, falling off height curves with chronic infection, and nausea, vomiting, or diarrhea can suggest UTI in these age groups.

Infectious vaginitis is associated with a vaginal discharge, and the dysuria is described as more external. Risk factors such as recent antibiotic use, sexual activity, and diabetes mellitus should be elicited. Dyspareunia is frequently present with vaginitis. Atrophic vaginitis is a consideration in any postmenopausal woman complaining of dysuria. Previous vaginal dryness and dyspareunia are typically present, and frequently systemic features such as hot flashes are found.

Urethritis is the most common cause of dysuria in young adult men, but it is usually asymptomatic in women. Men often notice a urethral discharge and can have urethral pruritus.

Painless hematuria (gross or microscopic), especially in patients with risk factors, suggests bladder carcinoma. However, bladder carcinoma is not an initial concern if symptoms of infection are found with the hematuria.

Interstitial cystitis should be suspected with chronic symptoms. Often severe, they can include any combination of dysuria, urgency, frequency, and suprapubic pain that cannot be otherwise explained by infection or the other presented differential diagnoses for dysuria.

Pyelonephritis is suggested when back/flank pain, nausea and vomiting, or high fever is reported. Although low-grade temperature elevations can be seen with cystitis, a fever of greater than 38.9°C (102°F) has been shown to be the best indicator. Pyelonephritis also is more likely (even if these other features are not present) if the patient has had previous episodes of pyelonephritis, has an abnormal urinary tract, is pregnant, or has delayed (for longer than 1 week) getting treatment for the cystitis. In about 20% of pyelonephritis cases, no cystitis symptoms are present.

Even with use of these criteria, however, about one third of cystitis cases and one third of pyelonephritis cases are misclassified. Because of this, any woman who notices a quick return of symptoms, even though these symptoms initially improved on a 3- or even 7-day antibiotic course, should be assumed to have pyelonephritis and given a 14-day course of antibiotics after urine culture.

The physical examination needed in assessing a patient with possible UTI is focused, but important. Vital signs, especially temperature and blood pressure, should be obtained. Cystitis patients are typically afebrile, but some have a low-grade temperature elevation (less than 38.9°C [102°F]). Patients with interstitial cystitis, chemical or radiation cystitis, or viral cystitis or urethritis are afebrile. Costovertebral angle tenderness should be evaluated for evidence of pyelonephritis. About 20% of patients with UTIs will have suprapubic tenderness. In UTIs, this tenderness is mild to moderate and not associated with guarding or rebound. The remainder of the abdomen should be palpated for evidence of hydronephrosis or other tract abnormalities (e.g., polycystic kidneys).

Pelvic examination can be omitted if symptoms of UTI are obvious and supported by urinalysis results. Lower back inspection for dimples or hairy patches and motor and sensory examinations of the lower extremities are appropriate for recurrent infections in which spina bifida or neurogenic bladder may be predisposing to infection. Prostate examination is indicated in men with suspected UTI, as prostatitis can occur with dysuria, and prostatic urethral obstruction from benign prostatic hypertrophy or localized adenocarcinoma of the prostate is a major predisposing factor to UTI development.

A dipstick urinalysis is an inexpensive and useful test in assessing for possible UTIs. In nonpregnant adults, the sensitivity of urine leukocyte esterase is greater than 90% for a UTI. Urinary nitrite is only about 30% sensitive (although this improves to 60% if the first void of the morning is used) but is a highly specific test for UTI. White blood cell casts on a microscopic urinalysis are highly specific for pyelonephritis, but sensitivity is poor. The presence of bacteriuria on Gram stain is very specific for UTI but is not sensitive (especially for infections with colony counts of less than 10^5). Gram-positive cocci on Gram stain can give presumptive clues as to enterococci to guide empirical antibiotic therapy in urosepsis. Urine culture is not necessary in uncomplicated cystitis in nonpregnant adult women. Urine culture should be obtained if pyelonephritis is suspected or if the UTI is complicated. Urine cultures are indicated in children, even

in uncomplicated cystitis, as the sensitivity (about 88%) and specificity of a positive leukocyte esterase are slightly poorer than those in adults (American Academy of Pediatrics, 1999 Ⓐ). Blood cultures are positive in about 20% of pyelonephritis cases. They should be obtained in suspected urosepsis and can be obtained in any patient hospitalized for pyelonephritis. Although a CBC is appropriate for patients in urosepsis, elevated white blood cell counts and sedimentation rates are not adequately specific to be useful in the differentiation of pyelonephritis from cystitis. Imaging studies are not needed in the vast majority of cases. Indications for urgent imaging are symptoms that suggest ureteral obstruction in association with the UTI. Other situations in which imaging is appropriate are to assess for perinephric abscess in patients who remain febrile after 3 days of treatment with an appropriate antibiotic, and to rule out vesico-ureteral reflux in children (especially preschoolers) in whom voiding cystourethrograms (VCUGs) are indicated (Hoberman et al., 2003Ⓑ). See Box 52-1 for VCUG indications.

Treatment choices for uncomplicated cystitis in nonpregnant women include 3-day courses of trimethoprim-sulfa-DS, twice daily, or nitrofurantoin, 100 mg four times daily, or an oral first-generation cephalosporin or amoxicillin with clavulanate (500/125 mg twice daily). Oral fluoroquinolones should be reserved for high local trimethoprim-sulfa resistance (greater than 20%) (Gupta et al., 1999 Ⓑ). Fosfomycin in a single 3-g dose is another option but is less effective than the 3-day courses. Children, men, and pregnant women should receive 7-day antibiotic courses, and sensitivity should be confirmed with culture (Keren and Chan, 2002 Ⓐ). Fluoroquinolones and tetracyclines are contraindicated in children and during pregnancy. Trimethoprim-sulfa has particular safety concerns in pregnancy. Pyelonephritis is treated with the same antibiotics (except for fosfomycin) for 14-day courses, but if a fluoroquinolone is chosen, this can be reduced to 7 days (Talan et al., 2000 Ⓐ).

Box 52-1	Indications for Voiding Cystourethrograms in Urinary Tract Infections

Children
    Any UTI in boy
    One UTI in girl younger than 5 years or two
      or more infections in girl younger than 5 yr
Adults or children
    Symptom of flank pain that occurs only with
      micturition
    Otherwise unexplained renal scarring or
      poor renal growth

Table 52-3	Antibiotic Choices for Complicated Urinary Tract Infection
Antibiotic	**Comments**
Ampicillin and gentamicin	Ampicillin, 1g IV q6h; gentamicin, 1 mg/kg IV q8h
Piperacillin and tazobactam (Zosyn)	3.375 g IV q6h or 4.5 g IV q8h
Ticarcillin and clavulanate (Timentin)	3.1 g IV q6h
Meropenem (Merrem IV)	1 g IV q8h
Fluoroquinolone	Ciprofloxin (Cipro), 400 mg IV or PO twice daily, or gatifloxacin (Tequin), 400 mg q day, or levofloxacin (Levaquin), 500 mg q day, or ofloxacin (Floxin), 400 mg PO twice daily

Table 52-4	Prophylactic Antibiotics for Recurrent Urinary Tract Infection
Antibiotic	**Dose**
Daily Administration	
Trimethoprim-sulfa (Bactrim)	1 single-strength (400 mg/80 mg) tab each day
Nitrofurantoin (Furadantin)	50–100 mg qhs
Postcoital Administration	
Trimethoprim-sulfa	One double-strength (800 mg/160 mg) tab after coitus
Nitrofurantoin	One 100-mg tablet after coitus

Complicated infections require 2 weeks of therapy. See Table 52-3 for options. Perinephric abscesses require surgical or percutaneous drainage as well as antibiotics. Treatment for recurrent UTIs should first try to correct factors that may be adversely affecting vaginal flora. Alternative contraceptive methods should be used if the patient is using a spermicide. Postmenopausal women increase their vaginal lactobacilli and decrease their frequency of UTIs with vaginal estrogens (Raz and Stamm, 1993[A]); however, this decrease does not occur with oral estrogens (Brown et al., 2001[A]). Cranberry products have been shown to reduce the incidence of UTIs in women (Jepson et al., 2004[A]). If such factors are not present or if recurrences continue, daily or intermittent antibiotics, as in Table 52-4, can be used. The need for continued prophylaxis should be assessed at 6 to 12 months, as spontaneous resolution is common.

Material Available on Student Consult

Review Questions and Answers about Urinary Tract Infection

REFERENCES

American Academy of Pediatrics: Committee on Quality Improvement and Subcommittee on Urinary Tract Infection Practice Parameter. The diagnosis, treatment, and evaluation of the initial urinary tract infection in febrile infants and young children. Pediatrics 1999;103:843–852.[A]

Brown JS, Vittinghoff E, Kanaya AM, et al., for the Heart and Estrogen/Progestin Replacement Study Group. Urinary tract infections in postmenopausal women: Effect of hormone therapy and risk factors. Obstet Gynecol 2001;98:1045–1052.[A]

Gupta K, Scholes D, Stamm WE. Increasing prevalence of antimicrobial resistance among uropathogens causing acute uncomplicated cystitis in women. JAMA 1999;281:736–738.[B]

Hoberman A, Charron M, Hickey RW, Baskin M, Kearney DH, Wald ER. Imaging studies after a first febrile urinary tract infection in young children. N Engl J Med 2003;348:195–202.[B]

Jepson RG, Mihaljevic L, Craig J. Cranberries for preventing urinary tract infections. Cochrane Database Syst Rev 2004;CD001321.[A]

Keren R, Chan E. A meta-analysis of randomized, controlled trials comparing short- and long-course antibiotic therapy for urinary tract infections in children. Pediatrics 2002;109:e70.[A]

Raz R, Stamm WE. A controlled study of intravaginal estriol in postmenopausal women with recurrent urinary tract infections. N Engl J Med 1993;329:753–756.[A]

Talan DA, Stamm WE, Hooton TM, et al. Comparison of ciprofloxacin (7 days) and trimethoprim-sulfamethoxazole (14 days) for acute uncomplicated pyelonephritis in women: A randomized trial. JAMA 2000;283:1583–1590.[A]

53 Bedwetting (Childhood Nocturnal Enuresis)

Jennifer DeVoe

KEY POINTS

1. Reassurance that enuresis will spontaneously resolve is usually the best approach in children younger than 7 years.
2. Once the child is old enough to be partially responsible for treatment, motivation and simple behavior therapies are usually the first line of treatment (including reinforcement for dry nights, bladder-training exercises, fluid management, or a combination of these therapies).
3. Enuresis alarms or pharmacologic therapy or both should be considered in children who have failed to improve after 3 to 6 months of behavioral interventions. In systematic reviews, enuresis alarms are superior to pharmacologic therapy because their effects are sustained after

discontinuation and because they are associated with fewer adverse effects.
4. Desmopressin acetate (DDAVP) is an effective short-term alternative to the enuresis alarm in patients who are unresponsive to the alarm. It also may be used as an adjunct to the alarm and as a short-term solution for camp attendance or sleepovers.
5. Tricyclic antidepressants (TCAs) are an effective short-term therapy for nocturnal enuresis. However, TCAs have a high relapse rate and potentially severe adverse effects.
6. A primary care provider can effectively manage nocturnal enuresis. On occasion, children with refractory nocturnal enuresis may benefit from referral to a pediatric urologist.

INITIAL VISIT

Subjective

Patient Identification and Presenting Problem

Bob L. is a 9-year-old boy who reports nighttime enuresis. He is accompanied by his father, who reports that Bob has been wetting his bed since he was an infant. Bob is currently wetting nearly every night and has never had a period of dryness. He denies daytime wetting. He has not complained of polydypsia, polyuria, dysuria, hematuria, or urinary urgency. His parents have tried limiting his evening fluid intake and waking him at night to urinate. Despite these measures, he is still wetting the bed on most nights.

Medical History

Bob has no history of bladder infections or diabetes mellitus. He has had no hospitalizations and takes no medications.

Family History

Bob is the youngest of four children. He has two sisters and one brother. His father reports that all three of his siblings had problems with nocturnal enuresis but with only occasional frequency. Bob's father also wet the bed regularly until age 8.

Social History

Bob's parents are getting divorced, and Bob recently started seeing a counselor.

Review of Systems

Bob denies insomnia, abdominal pains, headaches, constipation, diarrhea, or encopresis.

Objective

Physical Examination

General Bob is a well-nourished 9-year-old boy who appears to be healthy.

Evidence levels Ⓐ Randomized, controlled trials (RCTs), meta-analyses, well-designed systematic reviews of RCTs. Ⓑ Case-control or cohort studies, nonrandomized clinical trials, systematic reviews of studies other than RCTs, cross-sectional studies, retrospective studies, certain uncontrolled studies. Ⓒ Consensus statements, expert guidelines, usual practice, opinion.

Vital Signs
Blood pressure, 106/70
Heart rate, 84
Respirations, 16
Height, 52.5 inches
Weight, 95.1 pounds

Head, Eyes, Ears, Nose, and Throat Tympanic membranes are clear. Pupils are equal, round, and reactive to light. Mucous membranes are moist with no erythema in the pharynx.

Neck No lymphadenopathy or thyromegaly.

Cardiovascular Heart sounds are regular with no murmurs; 2+ distal pulses.

Lungs Clear to auscultation bilaterally.

Abdomen Soft and nontender with no masses.

Genitourinary He has a circumcised penis; both testes are descended. No evidence of wetness is seen in undergarments; Tanner stage II; no hernias.

Back No clefts or tufts of hair, no scoliosis.

Extremities Warm and well perfused with no edema.

Musculoskeletal Gait and physical mobility are within normal range.

Neurologic Normal strength, sensation, and deep tendon reflexes throughout.

Skin Mild facial acne.

Laboratory Examination
Urinalysis is negative for blood, glucose, ketones, leukocyte esterase, and nitrites. Basic metabolic panel is normal.

Assessment

Working Diagnosis
Bob is diagnosed with *primary monosymptomatic nocturnal enuresis*. Urinary incontinence at night is a common problem in children. Fifteen percent of 5-year-old children remain incompletely continent of urine. Most of these children have isolated nocturnal enuresis (monosymptomatic nocturnal enuresis). Monosymptomatic nocturnal enuresis is usually divided into primary and secondary forms.

- *Primary enuresis.* Children who have never achieved a satisfactory period of nighttime dryness have primary enuresis. An estimated 80% of children with monosymptomatic nocturnal enuresis have this form (Gonzalez, 2004Ⓐ).
- *Secondary enuresis.* Approximately 20% of children with monosymptomatic nocturnal enuresis have had a period of dryness, usually for at least 6 months, before the onset of wetting begins; these children have secondary enuresis. Secondary enuresis is often associated with an unusually stressful event (e.g., parental divorce, birth of a sibling, death of a family member) at a time of vulnerability in a child's life (Gonzalez, 2004Ⓐ). However, the exact cause of secondary enuresis remains unknown.

A small percentage of children who have nighttime wetting also have significant daytime problems. The daytime symptoms usually include urgency, frequency, and occasionally daytime incontinence (diurnal enuresis). Urologic and neurologic disorders (e.g., detrusor instability, recurrent urinary tract infection, spinal dysraphism) are more common among children with diurnal symptoms than in those with isolated nocturnal enuresis. In addition, some children also have troublesome encopresis (incontinence of stool). Patients who have nocturnal enuresis with daytime symptoms are described as having complex or complicated enuresis (also called dysfunctional voiding), whereas those who have associated bowel symptoms are often described as having dysfunctional elimination syndrome (Feng and Churchill, 2001Ⓑ).

Epidemiology
The prevalence of monosymptomatic nocturnal enuresis slowly declines with age, as outlined in Table 53-1 (Gonzales, 2003Ⓑ; Howe and Walker, 1992Ⓐ). The disorder is twice as common among boys as among girls and resolves spontaneously in most children (Forsythe and Redmond, 1974Ⓑ; Klackenberg, 1981Ⓑ). The longer the enuresis persists, the lower the probability that it will resolve spontaneously (Bakker et al., 2002Ⓑ; Forsythe and Redmond, 1974Ⓑ; Klackenberg, 1981Ⓑ).

Table 53-1 Prevalence of Nocturnal Enuresis in Children, by Age

Child's Age (yr)	Prevalence of Nocturnal Enuresis among All Children (%)
5	16
6	13
7	10
8	7
10	5
12 to 14	2–3
≥15	1–2

Differential Diagnosis and Possible Causes for Nocturnal Enuresis

When presented with a child who is bedwetting, the clinician should consider diagnoses other than enuresis. In some cases, further evaluation and treatment are required to determine the exact diagnosis. See Box 53-1 for a list of alternative diagnoses (Gonzalez, 2003 Ⓐ).

Nocturnal childhood enuresis may be caused by several different factors. In any given child, several of these factors may occur simultaneously. Maturational delay, genetics, small bladder capacity, decreased nocturnal secretion of antidiuretic hormone, detrusor instability, sleep disorders, and psychological problems have been considered as major contributors to nocturnal enuresis (Gonzales, 2003 Ⓐ). No consensus exists about the exact combination of causes or the validity of an exact relation between each cause and childhood nocturnal enuresis.

Plan and Discussion

Diagnostic

Because Bob does not have daytime symptoms of urinary incontinence, no urologic imaging studies (renal sonogram or voiding cystourethrogram) are indicated at this time. His neurologic examination is normal, so neuroimaging (usually magnetic resonance imaging of the spine) also is not recommended.

Patient Education

Bob is given information about how to manage his fluid intake. Normal bladder capacity (in ounces) can be estimated by adding 2 to a child's age in years, up to age 10. Thus Bob is given a visual demonstration of 11 ounces of liquid. His father asks about the times when Bob is most likely to wet the bed, and he is told that enuretic episodes occur at random throughout the night and can occur in all stages of sleep. In most cases, enuresis occurs during non–rapid eye movement (REM) sleep (mainly in the early part of the sleep cycle), but some children wet during phases of early awakening.

Therapeutic

After a discussion of various approaches to treatment, the patient and his father agree first to try some nonpharmacologic interventions. Bob and his father make a plan for a stepwise approach to these therapies, described in succeeding sections and outlined in Figure 53-1.

1. *Motivational therapy.* Bob agrees to keep a record of progress, and his father will give him awards for periods of dryness, with larger awards for longer dry periods. Motivational therapy is a good first-line therapy for primary nocturnal enuresis, particularly in younger children (Cendron, 1999 Ⓐ). In a Cochrane systematic review, children using reward systems (e.g., star charts) had significantly fewer wet nights, higher cure rates, and lower relapse rates compared with those of controls (Glazener and Evans, 2004 Ⓐ).

2. *Bladder-retention training.* Bob will try holding his urine for successively longer intervals ("as long as possible") after first sensing the urge to void. His father will record his volume of voided urine once per week to evaluate success. The target volume is 11 ounces, based on the calculated bladder capacity for Bob's age. In Cochrane systematic reviews of simple behavioral and physical interventions for nocturnal enuresis in children, not enough evidence was available to evaluate bladder retention used either in isolation or in addition to other interventions (Glazener and Evans, 2004 Ⓐ). Nonetheless, a trial of this simple behavioral method is recommended before use of alarms and pharmacologic agents, which may be more demanding and have adverse effects (Jalkut et al., 2001 Ⓑ; Koff, 1983 Ⓑ).

3. *Fluid management.* A review of Bob's previous diary showed that he was drinking a disproportionate amount of fluid in the evening hours, so he will try to drink 40% of his total daily fluid in the morning (7 AM to 12 PM), 40% in the afternoon (12 PM to 5 PM), and only 20% in the evening (after 5 PM). In addition, he agrees to drink only non-caffeinated beverages in the evening (Jalkut et al., 2001 Ⓑ). This fluid-management program permits Bob to drink as much as he wants throughout the day. Encouraging fluid intake in the morning and afternoon reduces the need for significant intake later in the day. It also increases daytime urinary flow and may assist in bladder training to increase functional bladder capacity (Jalkut et al., 2001 Ⓑ).

Box 53-1	Differential Diagnosis for Childhood Nocturnal Enuresis

Unrecognized underlying medical disorders (e.g., sickle cell disease, seizures, hyperthyroidism)
Encopresis or constipation
Dysfunctional voiding (usually associated with daytime symptoms)
Urinary tract infection
Chronic renal failure
Spinal dysraphism
Upper airway obstruction
Pinworms
Chronic renal failure
Diabetes mellitus
Diabetes insipidus
Psychogenic polydipsia

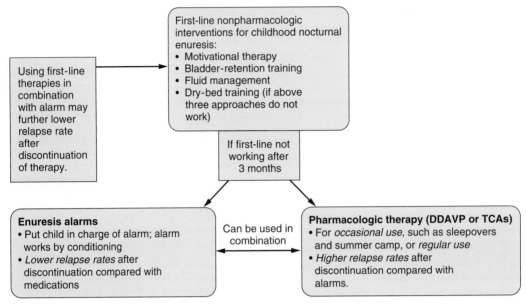

Figure 53-1 Stepwise approach to the management of childhood nocturnal enuresis. DDAVP, desmopressin acetate; TCAs, tricyclic antidepressants.

4. *Dry-bed training.* If motivational therapy, bladder training, and fluid management do not work for Bob, his family will try intensive dry-bed training and may consider purchasing an alarm. During the first night, Bob will be awakened frequently and taken to the toilet. Even if an accident occurs before the time of awakening, Bob must still practice getting up and going to the toilet. On subsequent nights, Bob will be awakened once, at progressively earlier times, and taken to the toilet.

5. *Enuresis alarms.* Because an alarm costs between $40 and $90, Bob and his father will not immediately buy one. They are aware, however, that conditioning therapy with an enuresis alarm is the most effective means of controlling nocturnal enuresis (Glazener et al., 2004Ⓐ; Moffatt et al., 1993Ⓐ). The alarm works through conditioning: the patient learns to wake or inhibit bladder contraction in response to the neurologic conditions present before wetting.

Disposition

Bob and his father understand that nonpharmacologic therapies should be tried for approximately 3 to 6 months. They will return for a follow-up visit after 3 months.

FOLLOW-UP VISIT

Subjective

Bob and his father return 3 months later. His father reports that Bob continues to wet his bed nearly every night, despite trying a combination of the first three approaches (motivational therapy, bladder-retention training, and fluid management). They have started dry-bed training; however, Bob's continued enuretic episodes are starting to cause major embarrassment, and Bob has become more withdrawn. He refused to go to summer camp and had a miserable summer. He continues to deny polydypsia, polyuria, dysuria, hematuria, or urinary urgency. They have not yet tried an enuresis alarm, but they request a trial of medications for the bedwetting.

Objective

Physical Examination

General Bob, a well-nourished, healthy-appearing 9-year-old boy, is more withdrawn, avoids eye contact, and offers minimal verbal responses to examiner questions. He is responsive and interactive with his father.

Vital Signs
Blood pressure, 110/72
Heart rate, 80
Respirations, 16
Height, 53.0 inches
Weight, 97.1 pounds

The remainder of the physical and laboratory examinations is unchanged from the previous visit.

Assessment

The assessment is primary monosymptomatic nocturnal enuresis unresponsive to nonpharmacologic therapies. Bob and his father consider the continued enuresis to be a "big problem" and are eager to try other interventions (see Fig. 53-1 for a stepwise approach to the management of nocturnal enuresis in children).

Plan

Therapeutic Interventions

Bob and his father agree to buy an enuresis alarm for nightly use. Bob will be in charge of the alarm. Each night before he goes to sleep, he will test the alarm; with the sound (or vibration) in mind, he will imagine in detail, for 1 to 2 minutes, the sequence of events that should occur when the alarm sounds (or vibrates) during sleep. In one Cochrane systematic review, approximately two thirds of children using alarms became dry for 14 consecutive nights (compared with children with no alarm, relative risk (RR) for failure, 0.36; 95% confidence interval, 0.31 to 0.43) (Glazener et al., 2003a ⓐ). Forty-five percent of children who continued to use the alarm remained dry after treatment, compared with only 1% in the no-treatment group (Glazener et al., 2003a ⓐ). Bob also requests a medication to help him stay dry during sleepovers and summer camp. This pharmacologic intervention is sought because Bob is getting older and experiencing social pressures and self-esteem problems linked to the enuresis. He is counseled about desmopressin acetate (DDAVP), with a starting dose of 0.2 mg per night, increasing to 0.6 mg over a 2-week trial period. He is warned about relapse if the medication is stopped and is strongly encouraged first to try consistent alarm therapy, which has been shown to be the most effective long-term treatment.

Patient Education Regarding Alarms and Medications to Treat Childhood Nocturnal Enuresis

Bob and his father are educated about the pitfalls in treatment of childhood enuresis and the latest evidence. Most of the efforts surrounding childhood enuresis have focused on finding a treatment with long-term benefits. Two medications have been promising in the short term: tricyclic antidepressants and DDAVP. Tricyclic antidepressants (TCAs) have been used to treat enuresis since 1960. TCAs decrease the amount of time spent in REM sleep, stimulate vasopressin secretion, and relax the detrusor muscle. DDAVP, in tablet and intranasal forms, was approved as a treatment option for nocturnal enuresis in 1990. Twenty-five percent of patients achieve total dryness by using DDAVP, whereas another 50% show a significant decrease in nighttime wetting (Moffatt et al., 1993 ⓐ). However, discontinuation of medications is associated with high rates of relapse (60% to 70%) (Wille, 1986 ⓐ). Cochrane systematic reviews comparing DDAVP with TCAs or alarms in the treatment of nocturnal enuresis showed the following:

- Compared with placebo, DDAVP (20-μg nasal spray) reduced bedwetting by 1.34 nights per week (95% confidence interval, 1.11 to 1.57) (Glazener and Evans, 2002 ⓐ).
- Compared with placebo, children treated with DDAVP (20-μg nasal spray) were more likely to be dry for 14 nights (RR, 1.19; 95% confidence interval, 1.10 to 1.27) (Glazener and Evans, 2002 ⓐ).
- DDAVP and TCA appear to be equally effective (Glazener and Evans, 2002 ⓐ).
- Although alarms appear to be less immediately effective than DDAVP, alarms are more effective in preventing relapse. Alarms also are more effective than TCAs during and after treatment. Relapse can occur after the alarm unit is discontinued. However, the relapse rate after discontinuation of therapy is much lower with alarms than with DDAVP (RR, 0.11; 95% confidence interval, 0.02 to 0.78) or TCAs (Glazener et al., 2003b ⓐ; Glazener et al., 2004 ⓐ).
- The combination of alarm therapy with a complex behavioral intervention, such as dry-bed training or full-spectrum home training, may further decrease the relapse rate (Glazener et al., 2004 ⓐ).

Many other drugs, including phenmetrazine, oxybutinin, indomethacin, amphetamine sulfate, ephedrine, atropine, furosemide, and diclofenac have been tried. A systematic review of randomized trials of drugs other than TCAs and DDAVP in the treatment of nocturnal enuresis found that although indomethacin and diclofenac were better than placebo, none of the drugs was better than DDAVP (Glazener et al., 2003c ⓐ).

Summary

Childhood nocturnal enuresis is common and has a high spontaneous resolution rate. Evidence supports a genetic link between parents who had childhood enuresis and their children. Most treatment should be delayed until the child is at least age 7. Simple behavioral methods are usually tried first, but more active intervention should be recommended as the child gets older, because social pressures increase, and self-esteem is affected. In Cochrane systematic literature reviews, arousal alarm systems are the most effective long-term therapy. Fluid management and bladder training may be helpful supplemental approaches. Pharmacologic agents can be effective in the short term, especially for children who want to participate in age-specific social activities, such as camping or sleepovers with friends. Refer to the Key Points in the treatment of childhood nocturnal enuresis.

Material Available on Student Consult

Review Questions and Answers about Childhood Nocturnal Enuresis

REFERENCES

Bakker E, van Sprundel M, van der Auwera JC, van Gool JD. Voiding habits and wetting in a population of 4,332 Belgian schoolchildren aged between 10 and 14 years. Scand J Urol Nephrol 2002;36:354–362. **B**

Cendron M. Primary nocturnal enuresis: Current. Am Fam Physician 1999;59:1205–1214, 1219–1220. **A**

Feng WC, Churchill BM. Dysfunctional elimination syndrome in children without obvious spinal cord diseases. Pediatr Clin North Am 2001;48:1489–1504. **B**

Forsythe WI, Redmond A. Enuresis and spontaneous cure rate: Study of 1129 enuretics. Arch Dis Child 1974;49:259–263. **B**

Glazener C, Evans J. Desmopressin for nocturnal enuresis in children. Cochrane Database Syst Rev 2002;CD002112. **A**

Glazener C, Evans J. Simple behavioural and physical interventions for nocturnal enuresis in children. Cochrane Database Syst Rev 2004;CD003637. **A**

Glazener C, Evans J, Peto R. Alarm interventions for nocturnal enuresis in children. Cochrane Database Syst Rev 2003a;CD002911. **A**

Glazener C, Evans J, Peto R. Tricyclic and related drugs for nocturnal enuresis in children. Cochrane Database Syst Rev 2003b;CD002117. **A**

Glazener C, Evans J, Peto R. Drugs for nocturnal enuresis in children (other than desmopressin and tricyclics). Cochrane Database Syst Rev 2003c;CD002238. **A**

Glazener C, Evans J, Peto R. Complex behavioural and educational interventions for nocturnal enuresis in children. Cochrane Database Syst Rev 2004;CD004668. **A**

Gonzales ET. Approach to the child with nocturnal enuresis. Available at www.uptodate.com, last revised September 2, 2003. Accessed 9/29/2004. **A**

Gonzales ET. Management of nocturnal enuresis in children. Available at www.uptodate.com, last revised March 4, 2004. Accessed 9/29/2004. **A**

Howe AC, Walker CE. Behavioral management of toilet training, enuresis, and encopresis. Pediatr Clin North Am 1992;39:413–432. **B**

Jalkut MW, Lerman SE, Churchill BM. Enuresis. Pediatr Clin North Am 2001;48:1461–1488. **B**

Klackenberg G. Nocturnal enuresis in a longitudinal perspective: A primary problem of maturity and/or a secondary environmental reaction? Acta Paediatr Scand 1981;70:453–457. **B**

Koff SA. Estimating bladder capacity in children. Urology 1983;21:248. **B**

Moffatt ME, Harlos S, Kirshen AJ, Burd L. Desmopressin acetate and nocturnal enuresis: How much do we know? Pediatrics 1993;92:420–425. **A**

Wille S. Comparison of desmopressin and enuresis alarm for nocturnal enuresis. Arch Dis Child 1986;61:30–33. **A**

54 Nausea, Vomiting, and Lethargy (Acute Renal Failure)

Kurt A. Lindberg

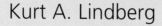

KEY POINTS

1. Acute renal failure (ARF) is caused by prerenal, intrarenal, and postrenal etiologies.
2. Differentiating between prerenal and intrarenal pathology can usually be done by relying on a careful history supplemented by evaluating serum and urine laboratory values.
3. Postrenal causes of renal failure are readily ruled out by using a Foley catheter and renal ultrasound.
4. Prerenal ARF is caused by decreased perfusion of the glomerulus.
5. The most common cause of intrarenal failure is acute tubular necrosis (ATN).
6. Prerenal ARF and ischemic ATN represent two ends of a continuum. The more severe the decrease of glomerular perfusion, the more prolonged the recovery will be.
7. Treatment of renal failure focuses on reversing the underlying cause and managing fluid and electrolyte abnormalities.

INITIAL VISIT

Subjective

Patient Identification and Presenting Problem

Mary D. is a 58-year-old woman complaining of nausea, vomiting, and lethargy. She was in her usual state of health until about 2 weeks ago, when she slipped on some ice and twisted her left knee. She went to the emergency room, where she had normal radiographs and was determined to have a strained knee. She was given ibuprofen, 800 mg, to use for the discomfort and discharged home. Approximately 2 days later, she began having gradually worsening nausea. This was not associated with fever, diarrhea,

or abdominal pain. The symptoms worsened over the subsequent week to the point at which she is unable to hold down any fluids, is lightheaded and weak, and is beginning to slur words and wax and wane in her cognition.

Medical History

The patient has adult-onset diabetes, which is usually controlled well with oral medication. Her husband reports that her sugars have been running in the 100s through the past 2 days. She has hypertension that has been well controlled and chronic renal insufficiency with a baseline creatinine of 1.8 mg/dL.

Medications

She takes glipizide (Glucotrol), 10 mg twice a day; pravastatin (Pravachol), 20 mg daily; lisinopril (Zestril), 40 mg daily; hydrochlorothiazide, 25 mg daily; and now ibuprofen, 800 mg 3 times a day as needed. She has no known medical allergies.

Family History

Mary's father died at age 70 of complications of diabetes, and her mother died at age 74 of a stroke and congestive heart failure (CHF). She has one sister, who has diabetes and early heart disease. Her three adult children are healthy.

Social History

Mary was divorced and has recently remarried. She has been a one-pack-a-day smoker for more than 40 years. She does not drink alcohol or use drugs. She has had no exposure to anyone with a similar illness.

Review of Systems

As stated, she has had no fever or upper respiratory symptoms. She reports no shortness of breath, cough, or sputum production. She has had no chest pain or palpitations. She has had two loose stools in the past several days but no signs of melena or blood. Her urine has been normal in color and has been

---

Evidence levels ⒶRandomized, controlled trials (RCTs), meta-analyses, well-designed systematic reviews of RCTs. Ⓑ Case-control or cohort studies, nonrandomized clinical trials, systematic reviews of studies other than RCTs, cross-sectional studies, retrospective studies, certain uncontrolled studies. Ⓒ Consensus statements, expert guidelines, usual practice, opinion.

slightly decreased from her usual output. She has had no dysuria or urinary frequency, no peripheral swelling or skin changes, and no changes in her joints or muscles. According to her husband, she has been intermittently uncoordinated during the past several days, having difficulty walking, speaking, and remembering where she is or what is happening around her. At other times, she seems quite clear. She has had no localized numbness or weakness.

Objective

Physical Examination

Mary is a middle-aged obese woman who is lethargic with no signs of acute distress. She is 5 feet 8 inches tall and weighs 225 pounds (down about 10 pounds from her last visit a month ago). Her temperature is 36.6°C (97.8°F); respiratory rate, 14; pulse, 115; and blood pressure, 98/50 while reclined. She is unable to co-operate with a standing blood pressure. Her head examination is normal, with somewhat dry mucous membranes and no oral lesions. Her neck is supple with no jugular venous distention, lymphadenopathy, or thyromegaly. Lungs are clear to auscultation bilaterally. Her heart is tachycardic but regular with no murmur. Abdomen is diffusely tender, worse in the epigastrium, with normal bowel sounds. She has no abdominal mass or organomegaly. Peripheral examination reveals no edema and no rashes. She has no joint pain or swelling. Neurologically she has difficulty maintaining eye contact, is somewhat confused, but is able to answer simple questions appropriately. She is unable to stand or ambulate and has been brought to the examination room in a wheelchair. Cranial nerves are intact, and symmetrical strength and sensation are noted in her periphery.

Laboratory Tests

Blood chemistries obtained this morning show the following values.

Sodium: 133 mmol/L (normal [nl], 136 to 144)
Potassium: 5.5 mmol/L (nl, 3.6 to 5.1)
Chloride: 104 mmol/L (nl, 101 to 111)
Carbon dioxide: 17 mmol/L (nl, 22 to 32)
Blood urea nitrogen (BUN): 88 mg/dL (nl, 7 to 19)
Creatinine (Cr): 3.5 mg/dL (nl, 0.4 to 1.0)
BUN/Cr ratio: 25.1

A complete blood count is within normal limits. A urinalysis shows urine concentration of 1.020 with no sediment, a few ketones, and no other abnormalities. Urine electrolytes are pending.

Assessment

Working Diagnosis

Acute renal failure, predominantly prerenal but may have components of intrinsic renal disease.

Differential Diagnosis

1. *Dehydration due to emesis.* Mary may have gastroenteritis, acute cholecystitis, or another primary cause of nausea and vomiting, causing hypovolemia. This state of decreased intravascular volume may have decreased perfusion of the kidneys, leading to accumulation of waste products (e.g., BUN and Cr).

2. *Ibuprofen effect.* The recent addition of ibuprofen, a nonsteroidal anti-inflammatory drug (NSAID), seemed to coincide with the patient's onset of symptoms. NSAIDs can cause gastrointestinal side effects, which can result in nausea and hypovolemia such as that described earlier. NSAIDs can have a direct effect on decreasing glomerular filtration rate (prerenal). NSAIDs also can cause allergic interstitial nephritis (intrarenal) (Albright, 2001**Ⓑ**).

3. *Other medication effect.* The patient is taking an angiotensin-converting enzyme inhibitor (ACE-I) medication, lisinopril, which has been known to reduce glomerular filtration rate (GFR) and cause renal failure. Similarly, hydrochlorothiazide may have caused dehydration, leading to decreased renal perfusion. However, these two medications have been present over a long period and are less likely to be at fault for her current presentation.

4. *New intrinsic renal disease.* Although statistically less common, intrinsic renal disease is still a consideration. With this degree of prerenal azotemia, a component of acute tubular necrosis (ATN) may be present. It is the most common intrarenal cause of acute renal failure (ARF) (Brady et al., 2004**Ⓐ**).

5. *Postrenal obstruction.* The etiologies that result in postrenal obstruction (Box 54-1) are usually simply diagnosed and remedied and should always be a consideration. The relatively normal urine production in this patient's history makes this an unlikely possibility.

Plan

Therapeutic

Mary is admitted to the hospital for control of her vomiting, evaluation of the etiology of the renal failure, and hydration. Her examination is most suggestive of hypovolemia at this time, and correcting this condition may result in resolution of her renal failure and symptoms. Care should be taken, however, to avoid overcorrection of her dehydrated state. If her kidneys are sufficiently damaged, they may be unable to manage a significant fluid bolus, and *hyper*volemia may ensue. Judicious use of normal saline or lactated Ringer's solution is appropriate.

Any medications that result in decreased renal perfusion should be discontinued until the etiology of her condition can be better ascertained and her condition improved. Because hydrochlorothiazide, lisinopril, and

Box 54-1	Etiologies of Acute Renal Failure

Prerenal

Loss of intravascular volume
- Fluid loss (vomiting, diarrhea, overdiuresis, skin losses)
- Hemorrhage
- Third spacing (congestive heart failure, pancreatitis, hypoalbuminemia)
- Ineffective cardiac output (congestive heart failure)

Hypotension
- Antihypertensive medications or anesthesia
- Sepsis
- Cardiogenic shock

Loss of glomerular pressure
- NSAID medications
- ACE inhibitors
- Renal vasoconstriction (e.g., with use of norepinephrine, ergotamine, hypercalcemia)

Intrarenal

Diseases of large vessels
- Thrombosis of renal arteries or veins
- Atheroembolism or thromboembolism
- Arterial dissection

Diseases of glomerulus/small blood vessels
- Acute or rapidly progressive glomerulonephritis

Vasculitis
Scleroderma
Hemolytic-uremic syndrome, TTP, or DIC
Toxemia of pregnancy

Diseases of renal tubules
- Acute tubular necrosis (ATN)
  - Ischemic (usually the result of the conditions listed in PRERENAL)
  - Toxic (e.g., caused by antibiotics, IV contrast, myoglobin, or hemoglobin deposition)
- Obstruction of tubules (e.g., uric acid, calcium oxalate, light chains)

Diseases of interstitium
- Infection (bacterial pyelonephritis, fungal, or viral)
- Allergic interstitial nephritis
- Infiltration (e.g., lymphoma, leukemia, sarcoidosis, allograft rejection)

Postrenal

Ureteral (tumors, calculi, clot, sloughed papillae, retroperitoneal fibrosis)
Bladder (prostate enlargement/cancer, bladder tumor, neurogenic, clotted blood)
Urethral (stricture, tumor, malfunctioning catheter)

ACE, acute tubular necrosis; DIC, disseminated intravascular coagulation; NSAID, nonsteroidal anti-inflammatory drug; TTP, thrombotic thrombocytopenic purpura.

ibuprofen are all problematic, they should be stopped. If the patient's blood pressure or pain becomes uncontrolled, other medications that do not affect the kidney's performance should be used instead.

The placement of a Foley catheter is useful to rule out some causes of postrenal obstruction and to monitor closely the patient's fluid status and renal function.

Mary does not have a significant electrolyte problem at this time. Close observation of her electrolytes will be necessary as fluid resuscitation, pH, and renal function evolve.

Diagnostic

This patient has already had some of the basic investigations that must take place when one suspects renal failure. These are a urinalysis, complete blood count, serum electrolytes, BUN, and Cr. Urine electrolytes will provide more insight into whether she has predominantly a prerenal or intrarenal pathology. Mary's decreased serum carbon dioxide suggests some acute acidosis. Obtaining an arterial blood gas would be more definitive in assessing her acid/base condition, if it is thought to be appropriate. A renal

ultrasound should be ordered to assess the presence of postrenal obstruction and to assess the general appearance of her kidneys. Shrunken, hardened kidneys would suggest a chronic loss of renal function, whereas enlarged or inflamed kidneys would suggest an acute etiology. It is rare that any more invasive testing would be required, such as a renal biopsy.

DISCUSSION

ARF is defined as a significant decline in GFR over a course of hours to weeks, which results in the accumulation of nitrogenous waste products (e.g., BUN and Cr). No absolute criteria exist for what constitutes "a significant decline" in the GFR, nor does the increase of BUN and serum Cr levels always indicate the severity of this decline. Some commonly used objective standards are an increase in serum Cr of 0.5 mg/dL, an increase of 50% over the baseline Cr level, or a decline in the Cr clearance of at least 25% (Albright, 2001❺). In patients for whom no baseline laboratory values are available, ARF is difficult to differentiate from chronic renal failure. ARF is most common in the inpatient setting, where the majority of the research on this topic has been performed. It has been estimated that in hospitalized patients, the mortality of ARF is 20% to 70%, depending on the specific population tested and the criteria for ARF used (Singri et al., 2003❸). It also has been estimated that up to 30% of patients with ARF will require some form of long-term dialysis (Albright, 2001❸).

ARF is rarely diagnosed without the assistance of laboratory testing of BUN and Cr. This is primarily because the symptoms of ARF are nonspecific. An absence or significant reduction of urine output (less than 400 mL/day) may herald the condition. However, approximately half of ARF presentations involve normal or even increased urine flow. Patients with ARF will frequently have symptoms of fatigue, nausea, pruritus, shortness of breath, edema, flank pain, confusion, and so forth. The clinical examination may reveal signs of hypovolemia or hypervolemia, hypertension or hypotension, mental status changes, a distended bladder, or skin changes due to an underlying systemic cause (e.g., vasculitis, lupus, or scleroderma). A routine urinalysis may appear normal or may be filled with sediment. Because of this wide variety of presenting signs and symptoms, the condition of ARF becomes evident only on review of screening blood work (Singri et al., 2003 ❸).

Once the condition of ARF is recognized, a determination of its most likely etiology will help to guide therapy. The causes of ARF are best considered by the site of pathology in relation to the nephron (Fig. 54-1). *Prerenal* causes of ARF are those affecting the amount or pressure of blood flow across the glomerulus. *Intrarenal* etiologies are those that affect the function of the nephron itself (e.g., the small blood vessels, glomerulus, tubules, or interstitium). *Postrenal* causes are primarily obstruction of the urine flow away from the nephron. The most frequent etiologies of ARF based on this classification are presented in Box 54-1.

Although a thorough history and physical are usually adequate to determine the likely cause of ARF, some laboratory testing may be useful to help delineate prerenal versus intrarenal causes (Table 54-1). Some of the most common causes of postrenal obstruction may be diagnosed (and corrected) by the placement of a Foley catheter into the bladder. This procedure is an excellent first step in the evaluation and treatment of ARF. Most other causes of postrenal obstruction may be assessed by using a renal ultrasound (Albright, 2001❸).

Prerenal causes of ARF predominate in the outpatient setting, accounting for approximately 70% of cases (Singri et al., 2003 ❸). Frequently, such a patient has a condition of quantitative loss of intravascular volume (e.g., hemorrhage or dehydration) or loss of "effective" circulation to the kidneys (e.g., CHF). This depleted state results in a direct decrease of GFR with resultant increases in waste products. This condition is often referred to as *prerenal azotemia*. In these situations, reinstituting adequate vascular perfusion will result in an immediate return to normal GFR and a gradual return to baseline BUN and Cr. Adequate vascular perfusion is accomplished by the addition of fluids in the case of hypovolemia, but it may require diuresis in the case of volume overload (e.g., CHF).

Lack of flow across the glomerulus also may occur when the kidney's own methods to preserve GFR are inhibited. For example, NSAID medications inhibit the production of prostaglandins, which are responsible for maintaining dilation of the afferent (incoming) arteriole in the glomerular complex (refer to Fig. 54-1). When this happens, the amount of pressure producing a flow of filtrate across the glomerulus is diminished (i.e., decreased GFR). Conversely, ACE inhibitors block angiotensin II (a vasoconstrictor) at the efferent arteriole. This too results in decreased pressure and flow across the glomerulus (Albright, 2001❸).

When the blood flow into the kidneys is reduced for a long enough period or to a large enough degree, damage to the cells that line the tubules will occur. These cells have a high metabolic activity rate, which makes them prone to anoxic stress. Damage of the tubules due to ischemia, or similar damage due to nephrotoxins, is referred to as ATN. This intrarenal pathology is the most common cause of ARF in the inpatient setting and is a significantly more severe problem than is prerenal azotemia. In ATN, the damaged cells must regenerate before normal function of the kidneys may return. This may take days to weeks to occur, even if normal perfusion of the kidneys has returned. No treatment is available to speed this process (Brady et al., 2004❹).

The transition from mildly decreased blood flow causing prerenal azotemia to severely limited flow resulting in ATN represents a continuum. The worse the ischemic insult, the worse the tubular damage, and the longer the recovery. Some tubules may be so severely damaged that the patient's kidneys may never fully recover function.

Damage to other parts of the nephron also will result in ARF with intrarenal indices. Malfunction of the glomerulus is often caused by inflammation, which appears with abnormal urine sediment or signs of a systemic disease. Such urine abnormalities may include severe proteinuria (nephrotic category) or hemoglobinuria (erythrocytes and red cell casts; nephritic category). Systemic diseases that may occur with glomerulonephritis are lupus, hepatitis, vasculitis, and pulmonary renal syndromes. If glomerulonephritis is suspected, specialized renal biopsies and serologic assays (antinuclear antibody, anti-double stranded [ds] DNA, etc.) will usually identify

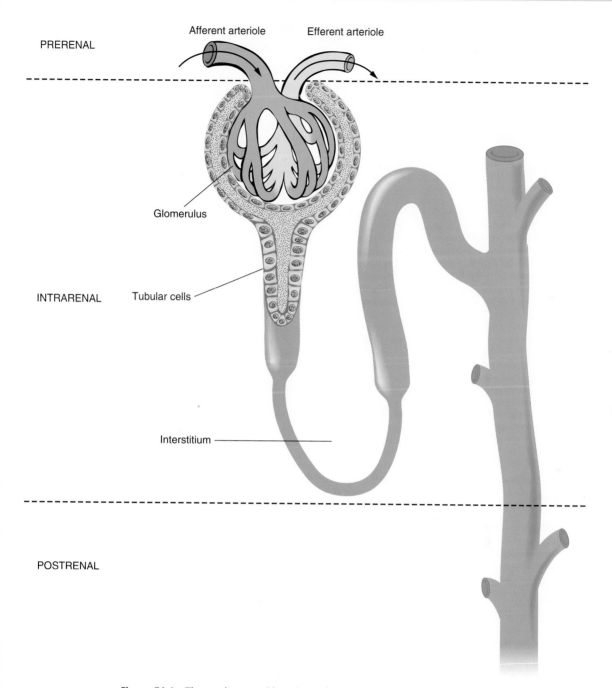

PRERENAL

Afferent arteriole

Efferent arteriole

Glomerulus

INTRARENAL

Tubular cells

Interstitium

POSTRENAL

Figure 54-1 The nephron and locations of pathology in acute renal failure.

the underlying cause. These causes are important in that they are frequently reversible with immunosuppressive therapy (Albright, 2001 Ⓑ).

Damage to the interstitium of the nephron resulting in ARF may be caused by infection (pyelonephritis) or inflammation due to an allergic response from medications. The hallmark of allergic interstitial nephritis is the presence of eosinophils in the blood or urine and a rash. Frequently, one or more of these signs may be absent. Thus the practitioner should

have a high index of suspicion in considering this as a possibility.

Sometimes the exact etiology of a patient's ARF is not initially apparent. Regardless of the ability to identify or reverse the etiology of renal pathology, the most important therapy to provide for a patient with ARF is the maintenance of fluid balance, acid/base balance, and serum electrolytes. As has already been discussed, a patient who has hypovolemia should receive intravenous fluids (i.e., normal

Table 54-1 Laboratory Values Differentiating Prerenal versus Intrarenal Causes of Acute Renal Failure

	Prerenal	Intrarenal
Serum BUN/ creatinine ratio	>20	10–20
Urine specific gravity	>1.020	~1.010
Urine osmolality (mOsm/kg)	>350	~300
Urinary Na concentration (mEq/L)	<10	>20
*FeNa (%)	<1	>1
Urine sediment	Hyaline casts	Granular casts, red cells or casts, white cells or casts, eosinophils, etc.

*The "fractional excretion of sodium" (FeNa) is one of the most sensitive tests to differentiate these two conditions.

FeNa = ([urine sodium] × [plasma creatinine])/([urine creatinine] × [plasma sodium]) × 100

BUN, blood urea nitrogen.

Box 54-2 **Indications for Hemodialysis**

Severe derangements in electrolyte concentration (potassium or sodium)
Volume overload unable to be corrected by diuretics
Severe acid base imbalance
Florid symptoms of uremia (pericarditis, encephalopathy, bleeding, nausea)
Very elevated blood urea nitrogen (approx. BUN, >100)

Bun, blood urea nitrogen.

saline or lactated Ringer's solution) to maximize perfusion of the kidneys. Diuretics should be used in increasing doses to treat a patient with significant hypervolemia. Failure of these medications to stabilize patients with signs of fluid overload is an indication for hemodialysis (Box 54-2). In patients who appear to be euvolemic, the use of diuretics or "renal dose" dopamine to increase urine production is not recommended because neither has been shown to make a difference in clinical outcomes (Brady et al., 2004Ⓐ).

Hyperkalemia is another common problem in patients with ARF. If the level of potassium is very high and resulting in significant electrocardiographic changes, the patient should be treated with calcium gluconate or calcium chloride to stabilize cardiac function. Temporary shifts of potassium out of the serum and into cells can be accomplished with intravenous insulin, which requires concomitant dextrose administration. Total body potassium may be reduced with the use of furosemide (Lasix) if sufficient urine is being produced. Sodium polystyrene sulfonate (Kayexalate) can be used to bind potassium enterically. This may be given orally or as an enema. Recent studies have suggested, however, that colonic necrosis may occur in patients who are severely ill if they are treated with this medication (Albright, 2001Ⓑ). Thus it should be used with some amount of caution. As listed in Box 54-2, uncontrolled hyperkalemia is an indication for dialysis.

Material Available on Student Consult

Review Questions and Answers about Acute Renal Failure

REFERENCES

Albright RC Jr. Acute renal failure: A practical update. Mayo Clin Proc 2001;76:67–74.Ⓑ
Brady HR, Clarkson MR, Lieberthal W. Acute renal failure. In Brenner BM, Rector FC (eds): Brenner and Rector's The Kidney, 7th ed. Philadelphia, Saunders, 2004, pp 1215–1292.Ⓐ
Singri N, Ahya S, Levin ML. Acute renal failure. JAMA 2003;289:747–751.Ⓑ

55

Multiple Allergies (Allergic Rhinitis Asthma)

Greg L. Ledgerwood

KEY POINTS

1. Remember to include the diagnosis of asthma in a differential when it presents in an atypical fashion, such as a postinfectious cough.
2. Gastroesophageal reflux disease is a frequent companion in asthmatics.
3. Classify asthma in the correct severity category.
4. Use inhaled corticosteroid (ICS) therapy in all patients, including women who are pregnant.
5. Obta in consultation for any patient with asthma that becomes difficult to control or who becomes pregnant.
6. Remember that ICSs are the preferred first-line therapy for children of all ages.
7. Perform pulmonary-function tests.
8. Review patient medications, albuterol use, and proper metered-dose inhaler use, and re-evaluate the patient's current asthma-severity classification with each visit.

INITIAL VISIT

Subjective

Patient Identification and Presenting Problem

Emily C. is a 26-year-old married woman with a history of allergic rhinitis and asthma for her "entire" life. She also complains of dry, itchy skin. She has one child and is contemplating another pregnancy. Since a sinus infection 3 weeks ago, she awakens nightly with shortness of breath and coughing. Using her inhaler allows her to return to sleep.

Present Illness

Emily has had respiratory problems "as long as [she] can remember." She was told by her mother that at age 2, she was admitted to a hospital because of her asthma and required a nebulizer at least daily until around age 11, when she says her breathing problems "just got better." As a child, she thinks she tried "every medication under the sun" to treat her asthma. She carried a hand-held inhaler from that time on and continues to do so today. She uses this medicine at least daily, more so since the weather has turned cold. She was seen by an allergist at age 17 and was skin tested. She states that she was positive to "everything," particularly molds and dust mites. She received allergy shots for $2\frac{1}{2}$ years and thought that they helped her eye and nasal allergies. She stopped immunotherapy when she went to college because it was "too much of a hassle."

She uses over-the-counter allergy medications during the spring and fall but states that certain ones make her very sleepy. She was given a prescription allergy medication in the past, but her insurance would not cover it; it was very expensive. She remembers getting a chest radiograph when she started college but does not believe she has ever had a "breathing" test.

Her first child, a boy, seems to "catch" every infection in the community, even though she breast-fed until he was 12 months old; he also wheezes when ill. Emily is concerned that any future children might have the same problem. She worries about this and the fact that her health seems to be getting worse. Before her first pregnancy, Emily worked as a news producer for the local television station. She now only does volunteer work at her son's preschool. She believes that she had fewer problems when she was working. Her husband has had "mild hay fever" since his teenage years. Tobacco smoke really bothers her, as do some other odors such as certain perfumes and cleaning solutions.

They have recently moved into a newer home. The previous owners had dogs and cats that stayed indoors during the winter months. Although she believes the home is basically clean, when the forced-air furnace is running, she notices worsening

---

Evidence levels Ⓐ Randomized, controlled trials (RCTs), meta-analyses, well-designed systematic reviews of RCTs. Ⓑ Case-control or cohort studies, nonrandomized clinical trials, systematic reviews of studies other than RCTs, cross-sectional studies, retrospective studies, certain uncontrolled studies. Ⓒ Consensus statements, expert guidelines, usual practice, opinion.

"allergy" problems and also thinks she uses her inhaler more. Neither Emily nor her husband was raised with pets in the home, but they have been entertaining the idea of getting a cat for their young son. She wonders if this will be a problem.

Emily does not use any medications other than her albuterol inhaler on a regular basis. She was given an inhaled steroid before her first pregnancy, but she stopped using this when she became pregnant because she had heard about steroids and their "bad" effects. She occasionally takes aspirin for headaches but prefers acetaminophen (Tylenol). She denies any drug allergies, although she will not take penicillin because her mother was "allergic" to it, and she believes she might be as well.

She thinks she had fewer problems during her pregnancy. Over the past several months, she has experienced more allergy and asthma problems. She does not believe that they are well controlled. Contemplating another pregnancy, she is worried about how her asthma and any medications she might need will affect it. She also is afraid that her children will become asthmatic.

Medical History
Emily had her tonsils removed at age 6 because of snoring and difficulty swallowing. Her ear infections, which had been frequent, seemed to become less of a problem after this. She thinks she had a "pneumonia shot" in the past; however, she thinks it did not work because she had pneumonia while she was in college. Other than her respiratory problems, she is in good health. She has used "birth control pills" in the past. She denies experiencing any drug allergies.

Family History
Emily has two brothers, one with "mild" asthma. Both parents are alive without significant health problems except that her mother also has asthma and, unfortunately, smokes. Emily's mother does require oxygen at bedtime. Her paternal grandmother had diabetes before she died.

Health Habits
Neither she nor her husband smokes. She has an occasional alcoholic beverage, mostly wine with a meal. She did not consume any alcohol when pregnant. She stays very active and exercises at least 3 times per week, either jogging or cycling. She always uses her albuterol inhaler before running or bicycling. If she forgets, she "runs out of air" very quickly. She enjoys gardening and sewing.

Social History
Emily has been happily married for the past 5 years. Before her first pregnancy, she worked with the local television station in news production. After her first child, she became a stay-at-home mom, recently vol-

unteering at her son's preschool. She denies any significant stress in her life, except that she is becoming more discouraged about her health. She wonders whether she will have to quit exercising because of her asthma.

Review of Systems
Emily has not experienced a change in appetite or weight. Energy levels and sleep patterns have become a problem recently. She denies headaches or visual changes. She has had problems with "heartburn" since her teenage years. The rest of her review of systems is noncontributory except for a problem with dry, itchy skin on her face, arms, and behind her knees.

Objective

Physical Examination
Emily is a pleasant, well-developed white woman who is alert, cooperative, and gives a good and very complete medical history.

Vital Signs
Blood pressure, 112/60, left arm, sitting
Pulse, 68 and regular
Respiration rate, 15, with a prolonged expiratory phase

Head, Eyes, Ears, Nose, and Throat Nose shows boggy inferior turbinates with clear rhinorrhea bilaterally. Tympanic membranes show peripheral scarring without acute changes. Scleral membranes demonstrate mild injection.

Chest Chest wall looks normal, and the chest is currently clear to percussion and auscultation.

Heart Cardiac sounds are normal.

Abdomen Abdomen is currently unremarkable.

Skin Skin is dry, with mild excoriations at the popliteal areas bilaterally.

Laboratory Tests
A complete blood count (CBC) shows a white count of 6300 with 9% eosinophils and 3% basophils. Nasal cytology shows only neutrophils. Induced sputum cytology demonstrates mild to moderate eosinophils. Pulmonary-function tests done without a bronchodilator reveal a decrease of her forced expiratory volume (FEV_1) to 75% of predicted, a normal forced vital capacity (FVC), and a reduced forced expiratory flow (FEF) of 25/75, only 60% of predicted.

Assessment

Working Diagnosis
1. *Allergic rhinosinusitis.* This is supported by history and physical findings.

2. *Asthma of moderate severity.* This probably has a significant allergic component.
3. *Atopic dermatitis*
4. *Gastroesophageal reflux disease*

Differential Diagnosis

1. Respiratory distress associated with gastroesophageal reflux and frequent aspiration
2. "Cardiac" asthma
3. Congenital bronchiectasis
4. Pulmonary embolism, chronic and recurrent
5. Psychosocial adjustment disorder
6. Contact dermatitis
7. Vasomotor rhinitis

Plan

Therapeutic/Patient Education

1. Discuss asthma and allergic rhinitis and factors that cause and influence these diseases.
2. Explain severity levels of asthma and how these determine the appropriate medication use.
3. Prescribe a low-dose inhaled steroid with a long-acting β-agonist.
4. Continue short-acting β-agonist; ask patient to track frequency of use.
5. Consider using an intranasal steroid for upper airway allergic disease.
6. Discuss dust and dander control in the home and the possibility that animal exposure in the home might contribute to increased difficulty now and in the future.
7. Review correct use of metered-dose inhalers with a spacer; discuss and demonstrate use of a peak flow meter, how to record the personal best, and how these values relate to the action plan that also has been developed.
8. Prescribe low-potency steroid ointment for atopic dermatitis.
9. Update influenza vaccination if needed, and suggest pneumococcal vaccine booster every 7 to 10 years.
10. Follow-up visit recommended in 4 to 6 weeks.

FIRST FOLLOW-UP VISIT

Subjective

Emily returns after making the medication changes recommended. She also spent time cleaning her home, paying particular attention to the heating and cooling system and her bedroom and that of her child. After several days, her awakening at night stopped, and her need for rescue albuterol almost disappeared. She believes this is the best she has felt in a very long time. She wonders if she will have to use these medications for the "rest of my life."

Objective

Physical Examination

The data reveal a normal examination. Repeated spirometry shows her FEV_1 to be 94% of predicted, and her FEF of 25/75 is 90% of predicted. This is approximately 3 hours after her prescribed inhaled steroid/long-acting β-agonist use.

Assessment

The patient has become stable.

Plan

1. Discuss the importance of continued regular use of medication, even with pregnancy.
2. Review proper use of inhalers.
3. Update influenza vaccination if indicated.
4. Review peak expiratory flow values, and reinforce the importance of instituting the action plan when needed. See physician if action plan is instituted.
5. Suggest follow-up visit to discuss potential medication reduction in 4 to 6 months.
6. Continue to track frequency of albuterol use.
7. See sooner if conception occurs to discuss therapy and for an obstetrics/gynecology consult.

DISCUSSION

Asthma is a reversible obstructive airway disorder of the tracheobronchial tree characterized by paroxysmal episodes of respiratory distress, often interspersed with periods of apparent well-being (Ledgerwood, 2002 ◉). Physiologic changes include smooth muscle spasm, mucus plugging, edema, inflammation of the bronchial wall, and potential thickening of the basement membrane or smooth muscle or both, so-called remodeling. The history often provides the diagnosis. Asthma should be considered in any person with unexplained episodes of dyspnea, cough, recurrent "colds," or bronchitis. Specific diagnostic studies are occasionally helpful. Often a chest radiograph is normal, except in acute episodes, in which hyperinflation is seen. Serum immunoglobulin E (IgE) levels and CBCs also can be normal, except in allergic patients, in whom IgE levels can be elevated and WBC differentials show elevated eosinophils and perhaps basophils. Baseline pulmonary-function tests (PFTs) are mandated. These can be normal as well, but serve as a baseline for future events. Differences between obstructive/restrictive diseases, however, can be determined. Methacholine challenge should be used only by providers experienced with this procedure.

In the past several years, much has been learned about the relation of environment and genetics and how these two elements interact in any given asthmatic patient (Taussig et al., 2003 Ⓐ). Information from the National Heart, Lung, and Blood Institute (NHLBI), under the guidance of the National Institutes of Health and the National Asthma Education and Prevention Program (NAEPP), used both evidence-based information and scientific data (ranked according to level of scientific validity) to change previous recommendations pertaining to therapy for both acute and chronic asthma. These were published in the autumn of 2002 (NAEPP Expert Panel Report, 2002 Ⓒ). These principles have been used to stratify asthma severity in both children and adults, based not only on objective data (PFTs) but also on symptoms: albuterol use, nocturnal awakenings, and so forth (Tables 55-1 and 55-2). From these recommendations, different therapeutic interventions have evolved. These are significantly different from previous treatment modalities, particularly in the case of children. Long-term management of asthma dictates that the correct level of severity be recognized: mild intermittent, mild persistent, moderate persistent, and severe persistent. Goals of asthma therapy now include minimal or no chronic symptoms day or night; minimal or no exacerbations; no limitations on activities (no school/work missed); minimal use of short-acting β-agonists (fewer than once per day, fewer than one canister per month); minimal or no adverse effects from medications (Table 55-3) (NAEPP Expert Panel Report, 2002 Ⓒ).

The Tucson Children's Respiratory Study (Taussig et al., 2003 Ⓐ) has helped define not only those children at risk for asthma but also those who potentially are subject to permanent decline in lung function without proper intervention (see Table 55-1). Inhaled corticosteroid (ICS) therapy has been shown to be the only medication to prevent relapse and improve quality of life (NAEEP Expert Panel Report, 2002 Ⓒ). With data showing no adverse effects on the hypothalamic-pituitary-adrenal axis, growth, bone mineral density, or subcapsular cataracts, ICSs are now considered the first line of therapy in the treatment of asthma for children younger than 5 years (Childhood Asthma Management Program Research Group, 2000 Ⓐ; NAEPP Expert Panel Report, 2002 Ⓒ). Inhaled sodium cromolyn also can be used but is not the preferred drug. Leukotriene inhibitors also are indicated in the treatment of asthma, but data supporting these as first-line therapy are not as plentiful. Because low-dose ICS therapy is still preferred in all patients, especially children, the issue of how to deal with the loss of asthma control also has been updated. Excellent evidenced-based data demonstrate that adding a long-acting β-agonist to low-dose ICS therapy allows control to be achieved without increasing the risk of side effects sometimes seen in high-dose ICS therapy (Nelson et al., 2000 Ⓐ). With the newer ICS products, the difference between high- and low-dose ICSs should be reviewed (Table 55-4). The "step-up/step-down" approach is still recommended, with a re-evaluation every 1 to 6 months, depending on control. A parent (especially the mother) who has asthma presents the greatest risk of asthma developing in any offspring. Other issues that may contribute to the potential future diagnosis of asthma include male gender, parental smoking, atopic dermatitis, allergic rhinitis, wheezing apart from colds, sensitization to *Alternaria* sp., obesity in prepubertal girls, and frequent lower respiratory tract infections before age 3 (Fig. 55-1). Of the early childhood infections, only *respiratory syncytial virus* has been associated with the development of asthma. Recent data suggest that *rhinovirus* sp. might also be involved in both children and adults (Jacoby, 2002 Ⓑ).

The NAEPP expert panel states that the use of antibiotics during acute flares is *not* associated with outcome improvement unless substantial evidence of bacterial involvement exists. It is therefore recommended that these agents not be used routinely. Action plans continue to be valuable, but primarily in patient education, and the 1997 NHLBI recommendations remain unchanged (Gibson and Powell, 2004 Ⓐ).

Adult asthma therapy parallels that of children (see Table 55-2). The only really significant difference is being able to obtain more objective information, specifically PFTs. It is recommended that PFTs be done with an initial evaluation and at any time medication changes occur or control is of concern (both before and after use of small-volume nebulization of albuterol). It is impractical to do PFTs on children, with perhaps the exception of peak flow readings. Even then, children younger than 5 present a challenge. It is important to observe the correct use of metered-dose inhalers, whether they are aerosol driven or the dry-powder type. Use of spacer devices is recommended on all propellant units. In several years, chlorofluorocarbon propellant devices will be unavailable.

The NAEPP database has been developed in such a way that updated recommendations will be made by using computer data banking. These excellent scientific databases will allow a more rapid response to evolving studies dealing with asthma. Issues that must be addressed concerning control include the following.

1. How does β_2-receptor genetics influence therapy?
2. What objective laboratory information can be used in a practical fashion? (Nitrous oxide–exhalation concentration measurement is expensive.)
3. Will sputum eosinophils and CD8 lymphocytes identification be anything but a research tool (both cell types are associated with control when decreased or absent) (Childhood Asthma Management Program Research Group, 2000 Ⓐ)?
4. What is the role of viral infections as they pertain to initiation/exacerbation of asthma (Nelson et al., 2000 Ⓐ)?

Text continued on page 444

Table 55-1 Stepwise Approach for Managing Infants and Young Children (5 Years of Age and Younger) with Acute or Chronic Asthma

Classify Severity: Clinical Features before Treatment or Adequate Control		Medications Required to Maintain Long-Term Control
	Symptoms/Day Symptoms/Night	Daily Medications

Step 4: Severe persistent	Continual
	Frequent
		• Preferred treatments:
		  – High-dose inhaled corticosteroids
		   and
		  – Long-acting inhaled beta$_2$-agonists
		   and, if needed,
		  – Corticosteroid tablets or syrup long term (2 mg/kg/day, generally do not exceed 60 mg per day). (Make repeat attempts to reduce systemic corticosteroids and maintain control with high-dose inhaled corticosteroids.)

Step 3: Moderate persistent	Daily
	>1 night/week
		• Preferred treatments:
		  – Low-dose inhaled corticosteroids and long-acting inhaled beta$_2$-agonists
		   or
		  – Medium-dose inhaled corticosteroids
		• Alternative treatment:
		  – Low-dose inhaled corticosteroids and either leukotriene receptor antagonist or theophylline
		
		If needed (particularly in patients with recurring severe exacerbations):
		• Preferred treatment:
		  – Medium-dose inhaled corticosteroids and long-acting beta$_2$-agonists
		• Alternative treatment:
		  – Medium-dose inhaled corticosteroids and either leukotriene receptor antagonist or theophylline

Step 2: Mild persistent	>2/week but <1 x/day
	>2 nights/month
		• Preferred treatment:
		  – Low-dose inhaled corticosteroid (with nebulizer or MDI with holding chamber with or without face mask or DPI)
		• Alternative treatment (listed alphabetically):
		  – Cromolyn (nebulizer is preferred or MDI with holding chamber) *or* leukotriene receptor antagonist

Step 1: Mild intermittent	≤2 days/week ≤2 nights/month	• No daily medication needed.

Quick Relief: All patients		• Bronchodilator as needed for symptoms. Intensity of treatment will depend upon severity of exacerbation.
		  – Preferred treatment: Short-acting inhaled beta$_2$-agonists by nebulizer or face mask and space/holding chamber
		  – Alternative treatment: Oral beta$_2$-agonist
		• With viral respiratory infection
		  – Bronchodilator q 4–6 hours up to 24 hours (longer with physician consult); in general, repeat no more than once every 6 weeks
		  – Consider systemic corticosteroid if exacerbation is severe or patient has history of previous severe exacerbations
		• Use of short-acting beta$_2$-agonists >2 times a week in intermittent asthma (daily, or increasing use in persistent asthma) may indicate the need to initiate (increase) long-term control therapy

Continued

Table 55-1 Stepwise Approach for Managing Infants and Young Children (5 Years of Age and Younger) with Acute or Chronic Asthma (Continued)

Step down
Review treatment every 1 to 6 months; a gradual stepwise reduction in treatment may be possible.

Step up
If control is not maintained, consider step up. First, review patient medication technique, adherence, and environmental control.

Goals of Therapy: Asthma Control
- Minimal or no chronic symptoms day or night
- Minimal or no exacerbations
- No limitations on activities; no school/parent's work missed
- Minimal use of short-acting inhaled beta$_2$-agonist (< 1x per day, <1 canister/month)
- Minimal or no adverse effects from medications

Notes
The stepwise approach is intended to assist, not replace, the clinical decisionmaking required to meet individual patient needs.
Classify severity: assign patient to most severe step in which any feature occurs.
There are very few studies on asthma therapy for infants.
Gain control as quickly as possible (a course of short systemic corticosteroids may be required); then step down to the least medication necessary to maintain control.
Provide parent education on asthma management and controlling environmental factors that make asthma worse (e.g., allergies and irritants).
Consultation with an asthma specialist is recommended for patients with moderate or severe persistent asthma. Consider consultation for patients with mild persistent asthma.
DPI, dry powder inhaler; MDI, metered-dose inhaler.
Adapted from National Asthma Education and Prevention Program Expert Panel Report. Guidelines for the Diagnosis and Management of Asthma: Update on Selected Topics. Bethesda, MD, National Institutes of Health. NIH Publication No. 02-5075, 2002.

Table 55-2 Stepwise Approach for Managing Asthma in Adults and Children Older Than 5 Years of Age: Treatment

Classify Severity: Clinical Features before Treatment or Adequate Control			Medications Required to Maintain Long-Term Control
	Symptoms/Day Symptoms/Night	PEF or FEV$_1$ PEF Variability	Daily Medications
Step 4: Severe persistent	Continual Frequent	≤60% >30%	• Preferred treatment: – High-dose inhaled corticosteroids *and* – Long-acting inhaled beta$_2$-agonists *and*, if needed, – Corticosteroid tablets or syrup long term (2 mg/kg/day, generally do not exceed 60 mg per day). (Make repeat attempts to reduce systemic corticosteroids and maintain control with high-dose inhaled corticosteroids.)
Step 3: Moderate Persistent	Daily >1 night/week	>60% – < 80% >30%	• Preferred treatment: – Low-to-medium dose inhaled corticosteroids and long-acting inhaled beta$_2$-agonists • Alternative treatment (listed alphabetically): – Increase inhaled corticosteroids within medium-dose range *or* – Low-to-medium dose inhaled corticosteroids and either leukotriene modifier or theophylline

Table 55-2 Stepwise Approach for Managing Asthma in Adults and Children Older Than 5 Years of Age: Treatment (Continued)

			If needed (particularly in patients with recurring severe exacerbations):
			▪ Preferred treatment:
			  – Increase inhaled corticosteroids within medium-dose range and add long-acting inhaled beta$_2$-agonists
			▪ Alternative treatment:
			  – Increase inhaled corticosteroids within medium-dose range and add either leukotriene modifier or theophylline

Step 2: Mild persistent	>2/week but < 1x/day >2 nights/month	≥80% 20%–30%	▪ Preferred treatment: – Low-dose inhaled corticosteroids ▪ Alternative treatment (listed alphabetically): cromolyn, leukotriene modifier, nedocromil, *or* sustained release theophylline to serum concentration of 5–15 mcg/mL
Step 1: Mild intermittent	≤2 days/week ≤2 nights/month	≥80% < 20%	▪ No daily medication needed ▪ Severe exacerbations may occur, separated by long periods of normal lung function and no symptoms. A course of systemic corticosteroids is recommended.
Quick Relief: All patients	▪ Short-acting bronchodilator: 2–4 puffs short-acting inhaled beta$_2$-agonists as needed for symptoms. ▪ Intensity of treatment will depend on severity of exacerbation; up to 3 treatments at 20-minute intervals or a single nebulizer treatment as needed. Course of systemic corticosteroids may be needed. ▪ Use of short-acting beta$_2$-agonists >2 times a week in intermittent asthma (daily, or increasing use in persistent asthma) may indicate the need to initiate (increase) long-term control therapy.		

Step down
Review treatment every 1 to 6 months; a gradual stepwise reduction in treatment may be possible.

Step up
If control is not maintained, consider step up. First, review patient medication technique, adherence, and environmental control.

Goals of Therapy: Asthma Control
▪ Minimal or no chronic symptoms day or night
▪ Minimal or no exacerbations
▪ No limitations on activities; no school/work missed
▪ Maintain (near) normal pulmonary function
▪ Minimal use of short-acting inhaled beta$_2$-agonist (< 1x per day, < 1 canister/month)
▪ Minimal or no adverse effects from medications

Notes
The stepwise approach is meant to assist, not replace, the clinical decisionmaking required to meet individual patient needs.

Classify severity: assign patient to most severe step in which any feature occurs (PEF is % of personal best; FEV$_1$ is % predicted).

Gain control as quickly as possible (consider a short course of systemic corticosteroids); then step down to the least medication necessary to maintain control.

Provide education on self-management and controlling environmental factors that make asthma worse (e.g., allergens and irritants).

Refer to an asthma specialist if there are difficulties controlling asthma or if step 4 care is required. Referral may be considered if step 3 care is required.

FEV$_1$, forced expiratory volume; PEF, peak expiratory flow.

Adapted from National Asthma Education and Prevention Program Expert Panel Report. Guidelines for the Diagnosis and Management of Asthma: Update on Selected Topics. Bethesda, MD, National Institutes of Health. NIH Publication No. 02-5075, 2002.

Table 55-3 Usual Dosages for Long-Term-Control Medications

Medication	Dosage Form	Adult Dose	Child Dose
Inhaled Corticosteroids *(See Table 55-4)*			
Systemic Corticosteroids		*(Applies to all three corticosteroids)*	
Methylprednisolone	2, 4, 8, 16, 32 mg tablets	• 7.5–60 mg daily in a single dose in AM or qod as needed for control	• 0.25–2 mg/kg daily in single dose in AM or qod as needed for control
Prednisolone	5 mg tablets, 5 mg/5 cc, 15 mg/5 cc	• Short-course "burst" to achieve control: 40–60 mg per day as single or two divided doses for 3–10 days	• Short-course "burst": 1–2 mg/kg/day, maximum 60 mg/day for 3–10 days
Prednisone	1, 2.5, 5, 10, 20, 50 mg tablets; 5 mg/cc, 5 mg/5 cc		
Long-Acting Inhaled Beta$_2$-Agonists *(Should not be used for symptom relief or for exacerbations. Use with inhaled corticosteroids.)*			
Salmeterol	MDI 21 mcg/puff DPI 50 mcg/blister	2 puffs q 12 hours 1 blister q 12 hours	1–2 puffs q 12 hours 1 blister q 12 hours
Formoterol	DPI 12 mcg/single-use capsule	1 capsule q 12 hours	1 capsule q 12 hours
Combined Medication			
Fluticasone/ Salmeterol	DPI 100, 250, or 500 mcg/50 mcg	1 inhalation bid; dose depends on severity of asthma	1 inhalation bid; dose depends on severity of asthma
Cromolyn and Nedocromil			
Cromolyn	MDI 1 mg/puff Nebulizer 20 mg/ampule	2–4 puffs tid–qid 1 ampule tid–qid	1–2 puffs tid–qid 1 ampule tid–qid
Nedocromil	MDI 1.75 mg/puff	2–4 puffs bid–qid	1–2 puffs bid–qid
Leukotriene Modifiers			
Montelukast	4 or 5 mg chewable tablet, 10 mg tablet	10 mg qhs	4 mg qhs (2–5 yrs) 5 mg qhs (6–14 yrs) 10 mg qhs (> 14 yrs)
Zafirlukast	10 or 20 mg tablet	40 mg daily (20 mg tablet bid)	20 mg daily (7–11 yrs) (10 mg tablet bid)
Zileuton	300 or 600 mg tablet	2,400 mg daily (give tablets qid)	
Methylxanthines *(Serum monitoring is important [serum concentration of 5–15 mcg/mL at steady state]).*			
Theophylline	Liquids, sustained-release tablets, and capsules	Starting dose 10 mg/kg/ day up to 300 mg max; usual max 800 mg/day	Starting dose 10 mg/kg/ day; usual max: • <1 year of age: 0.2 (age in weeks) + 5 = mg/kg/day • ≥1 year of age: 16 mg/kg/day

DPI, dry powder inhaler; MDI, metered-dose inhaler.
Adapted from National Asthma Education and Prevention Program Expert Panel Report. Guidelines for the Diagnosis and Management of Asthma: Update on Selected Topics. Bethesda, MD, National Institutes of Health. NIH Publication No. 02-5075, 2002.

Table 55-4 Estimated Comparative Daily Dosages for Inhaled Corticosteroids

Drug	Low Daily Dose		Medium Daily Dose		High Daily Dose	
	Adult	Child*	Adult	Child*	Adult	Child*
Beclomethasone CFC: 42 or 84 mcg/puff	168–504 mcg	84–336 mcg	504–840 mcg	336–672 mcg	>840 mcg	>672 mcg
Beclomethasone HFA: 40 or 80 mcg/puff	80–240 mcg	80–160 mcg	240–480 mcg	160–320 mcg	>480 mcg	>320 mcg
Budesonide DPI: 200 mcg/inhalation	200–600 mcg	200–400 mcg	600–1,200 mcg	400–800 mcg	>1,200 mcg	>800 mcg
Inhalation suspension for nebulization (child dose)		0.5 mg		1.0 mg		2.0 mg
Flunisolide: 250 mcg/puff	500–1,000 mcg	500–750 mcg	1,000–2,000 mcg	1,000–1,250 mcg	>2,000 mcg	>1,250 mcg
Fluticasone MDI: 44, 110, or 220 mcg/puff	88–264 mcg	88–176 mcg	264–660 mcg	176–440 mcg	>660 mcg	>440 mcg
DPI: 50, 100, or 250 mcg/inhalation	100–300 mcg	100–200 mcg	300–600 mcg	200–400 mcg	>600 mcg	>400 mcg
Triamcinolone acetonide: 100 mcg/puff	400–1,000 mcg	400–800 mcg	1,000–2,000 mcg	800–1,200 mcg	>2,000 mcg	>1,200 mcg

*Children ≤12 years of age

CFC, chlorofluorocarbons; DPI, dry powder inhaler; HFA, hydrofluoroalkane.

Adapted from National Asthma Education and Prevention Program Expert Panel Report. Guidelines for the Diagnosis and Management of Asthma: Update on Selected Topics. Bethesda, MD, National Institutes of Health. NIH Publication No. 02-5075, 2002.

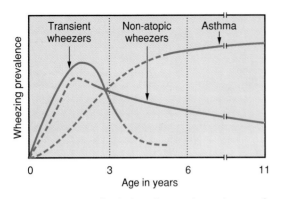

Figure 55-1 Hypothetical peak prevalence by age for the three different wheezing phenotypes. The prevalence for each age interval should be the area under the curve. This does not imply that the groups are exclusive. (Modified from Figure 2 in Stein RT, Holberg CJ, Morgan WJ, et al. Peak flow variability, methacholine responsiveness and atopy as markers for detecting different wheezing phenotypes in childhood. Thorax 1997;52: 946–952.)

5. Can immunoregulation be manipulated to change the lymphocytic immune response from a TH_2 (allergic) to a TH_1 (nonallergic) response?

The advances in detecting and treating asthma in the past several years are dramatic. Omalizumab, a murine-derived anti-IgE antibody, has shown excellent promise in treating the most severe forms of allergic asthma (Spector, 2004Ⓐ). The goals of the NAEPP expert panel seem likely to be achieved with aggressive applications of knowledge already obtained. We hope that future discoveries relating to genetics and environment will lead to complete understanding of factors that currently are obstacles to asthma control.

Material Available on Student Consult

Review Questions and Answers about Allergic Rhinitis Asthma

REFERENCES

Childhood Asthma Management Program Research Group. Long-term effects of budesonide or nedocromil in children with asthma. N Engl J Med 2000;343:1054–1063.Ⓐ

Gibson PG, Powell H. Written action plans for asthma: An evidence-based review of the components. Thorax 2004;59:87–88.Ⓐ

Jacoby DB. Virus-induced asthma attacks. JAMA 2002;287: 755–761.Ⓑ

Ledgerwood GL. Allergy. In Rakel RE (ed): Textbook of Family Practice, 6th ed. Philadelphia, WB Saunders, 2002, pp 473–493.Ⓒ

NAEPP Expert Panel Report. Guidelines for the Diagnosis and Management of Asthma: Update on Selected Topics. Bethesda, MD, National Institutes of Health. NIH Publication No. 02-5075, 2002.Ⓒ

Nelson HS, Busse WW, Kerwin E, et al. Fluticasone propionate/salmeterol combination provides more effective asthma control than low-dose inhaled corticosteroid plus montelukast. J Allergy Clin Immunol 2000; 106:1088–1095.Ⓐ

Spector S. Omalizumab: Efficacy in allergic disease. Panminerva Med 2004;46:141–148.Ⓐ

Stein RT, Holberg CJ, Morgan WJ, et al. Peak flow variability, methacholine responsiveness and atopy as markers for detecting different wheezing phenotypes in childhood. Thorax 1997;52:946–952.

Taussig LM, Wright AL, Holberg CJ, Halonen M, Morgan WJ, Martinez FD. Tucson Children's Respiratory Study: 1980 to present. J Allergy Clin Immunol 2003; 111:661–676.Ⓐ

56

Widespread Pruritic Rash (Adverse Drug Reaction)

Rahul Gupta

KEY POINTS

1. Types of Adverse Drug Reaction (ADR)
   A. Type A: Nonimmunologic (75% to 80%)—Predictable
      i. Side effects
      ii. Toxicity
      iii. Drug-drug interactions
      iv. Overdoses
   B. Type B: Immunologic or nonimmunologic (20% to 25%)—Unpredictable
      i. Immune mediated
         a. Type I to IV hypersensitivity reaction
         b. Morbilliform rash
         c. Stevens-Johnson syndrome (SJS), toxic epidermal necrolysis (TEN)
         d. Drug-induced lupus
         e. Anticonvulsant hypersensitivity syndrome
      ii. Nonimmune mediated
         a. Idiosyncratic reactions: Hemolytic anemia in patients with glucose-6-phosphate dehydrogenase deficiency treated with primaquine
         b. Drug intolerance

   c. Anaphylactoid reactions after contrast media
2. Diagnostic Tests for ADRs
   A. Comprehensive history and physical examination
   B. Discontinuation of drug and reassessment
   C. Complete blood count, chemistry
   D. Drug levels (if indicated)
   E. Drug-specific skin tests (if indicated)
3. Treatment of ADRs
   A. Discontinue the offending drug
   B. Administer epinephrine for anaphylaxis
   C. Administer antihistamines and/or corticosteroids, supportive care
   D. Treat SJS/TEN as burn injury
   E. Note that corticosteroids are controversial in SJS, contraindicated in TEN
   F. Avoid using chemically similar compounds
   G. Desensitization if the drug must be used again (only for type 1 reaction)
   H. Provide patient education
   I. Keep risk factors for ADR in mind

INITIAL VISIT

Subjective

Patient Identification and Presenting Problem

Kathy W. is a 47-year-old white woman and homemaker who complains of a skin lesion. Kathy was doing well until 4 weeks ago, when she noticed a rash over her chest and face. The rash began as being diffusely red, raised, and pruritic. She applied hydrocortisone cream to the lesion for several days. Instead of resolving, the rash spread to her trunk, back, and face and across both arms. Furthermore, Kathy states that the rash now involves her whole body, including her palms and the soles of her feet. Her scalp is pruritic as well.

Medical History

Kathy has had hypertension for the past 20 years. She was diagnosed with elevated cholesterol and osteoarthritis 4 years ago. Recently her physician notified her that she has developed stage I chronic kidney disease from long-standing hypertension. About 4 weeks ago her physician discontinued

---

Evidence levels Ⓐ Randomized, controlled trials (RCTs), meta-analyses, well-designed systematic reviews of RCTs. Ⓑ Case-control or cohort studies, nonrandomized clinical trials, systematic reviews of studies other than RCTs, cross-sectional studies, retrospective studies, certain uncontrolled studies. Ⓒ Consensus statements, expert guidelines, usual practice, opinion.

celecoxib (Celebrex) and started her on sulindac (Clinoril). She observed that the rash and pruritus started at that time, but she has not discontinued any of her medications.

Family History
Kathy's father was an electrician and died from his first heart attack at age 51. Her mother is 70 years old and has coronary artery disease, osteoarthritis, and hypertension.

Social History
The patient does not smoke or drink alcohol. She denies any illicit drug use. She has been happily married for the past 20 years. Kathy and her husband both walk 2 miles each day and follow a heart-healthy diet. She does not remember any such skin problem in the past. She enjoys outdoor activities such as gardening and fishing.

Medications
Kathy takes metoprolol (Lopressor), aspirin, and sulindac (Clinoril). She also uses acetaminophen (Tylenol) occasionally.

Review of Systems
Kathy can recall no recent changes in the use of skin or hair products. She has not changed her detergent. Because of the rash she has stopped wearing jewelry and wears only cotton clothing. She reports no changes in weight or sleep patterns. She denies any fever, shortness of breath, cough, palpitations, chest pain, or anxiety.

Objective

Physical Examination
General Kathy is a healthy-appearing, well-developed white woman. She is observed to be somewhat uncomfortable due to intense pruritus. She is nicely dressed and has tanned skin. She is wearing no makeup.

Vital Signs Kathy is afebrile. Vital signs are within normal limits.

Skin Her skin displays facial erythema with macules and papules along with some exfoliation. There are no erosions of the mucous membranes. Symmetrically arranged, intensely pruritic papules with confluent erythema are noted diffusely throughout the trunk, back, and on all four extremities. There are several crops, ranging from fresh lesions to old healing ones (Fig. 56-1). Purulent discharge and weeping are also observed from some lesions on the lower extremities. Minimal bilateral axillary lymphadenopathy is also noted.

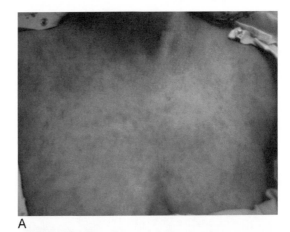

A

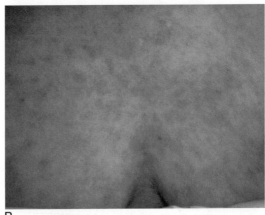

B

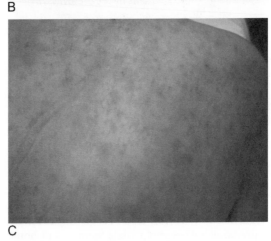

C

Figure 56-1 Symmetrical, intensely pruritic papules throughout the trunk with confluent erythema in several craps (**A** and **B**). Some weeping is also noted. **C**, Similar lesions cover the upper back.

Chest Breath sounds are normal. Both heart sounds are normal, without murmurs or clicks.

Abdomen Scaphoid and soft without tenderness. Bowel sounds are normal.

Laboratory Tests

None were done at this visit. The patient had her cholesterol level and chemistry profile done a week before her visit. Her cholesterol level was 225 mg/dL. Her aspartate transaminase and alanine transaminase levels were twice the normal range.

Assessment

Differential Diagnosis

The cause of this generalized pruritic, erythematous and papular-type rash with what seems to be a secondary bacterial infection can be established by Kathy's history. She notes that it all really began when she started taking sulindac approximately 4 weeks ago. Such a pattern is consistent with drug eruption associated with nonsteroidal anti-inflammatory drugs (NSAIDs), which has progressed because the patient did not discontinue the offending agent. The patient's condition could be confused with atopic dermatitis, psoriasis, and contact dermatitis.

1. *Drug eruption with secondary bacterial infection.* NSAIDs such as sulindac may cause cutaneous drug eruption, which may be associated with or followed by secondary bacterial infection. One percent to 5% of people using NSAIDs may develop a drug eruption. The common serious and distinctive drug reaction patterns of the skin are described in the Discussion section.
2. *Atopic dermatitis.* This is a chronic inflammatory dermatosis that is considered familial, and patients commonly exhibit additional symptoms of atopic disorders such as allergic rhinitis or asthma. Altogether the atopic disorders affect 8% to 25% of the total population worldwide. Therefore, the diagnosis is based on a personal and family history of atopy, pruritus, and physical eczema. This disorder commences at age 5 to 7 years. Examination reveals recurrent excoriated, scaling papules and plaques with erythema, and intense pruritus located commonly at flexural areas such as the antecubital and popliteal fossa. Secondary bacterial infection can occur. The approach to treatment includes skin hydration, topical corticosteroids, and the elimination of precipitating irritants. Current evidence suggests that immunomodulators that work by blocking T-cell activation such as tacrolimus 0.1% ointment or pimecrolimus 1% cream when applied twice daily may be advantageous compared to corticosteroids because they do not induce systemic immunosuppression or cutaneous atrophy.
3. *Psoriasis.* This condition affects 1% to 2% of the U.S. population. It is a chronic inflammatory disorder characterized by symmetric, erythematous, sharply demarcated papules and rounded plaques with silvery scales. Commonly affected areas include elbows, knees, scalp, and hands. Patients often complain of pruritus. Several variants of classic psoriasis are described including guttate, pustular, and erythrodermic types. Joint and nail involvement, such as pitting of nails, can be seen in 25% to 50% of patients with psoriasis. Although the cause of psoriasis remains unknown, some drugs such as lithium, β-blockers, and NSAIDs have been known to induce or aggravate the condition. Psoriasis may develop in an area of previous trauma, a process known as the Koebner phenomenon. Treatment of psoriasis involves topical therapies such as corticosteroids, calcipotriene (vitamin D_3 analog), anthralin, tazarotene (retinoid), coal tar preparations, and keratolytics. Natural sunlight, phototherapy, and systemic treatments such as sulfasalazine, methotrexate, cyclosporine, and oral retinoids have been demonstrated efficacious. The application of biologic therapies currently in use for other diseases such as rheumatoid arthritis and Crohn's disease is currently being evaluated.
4. *Contact dermatitis.* This is an inflammatory response of the skin to an allergen or irritant. It accounts for 4% to 7% of dermatology referrals. In the United States, 90% of worker's compensation claims in dermatology are for contact dermatitis. Allergic contact dermatitis results from direct skin contact with a substance that the body recognizes as foreign. This is a delayed type of hypersensitivity reaction in contrast to irritant contact dermatitis, which is a nonimmunologic-type reaction resulting from direct insult to the tissues. As an example, poison ivy exposure leads to allergic contact dermatitis. Both types of contact dermatitis are localized to the area of contact with the offending agent. Treatment requires avoidance of the inciting agent. Symptomatic treatments range from topical corticosteroids, calamine lotion, and cold compresses to systemic corticosteroids, depending on the severity of the reaction and the site on the body.

Plan

Diagnostic

No testing is required at this time.

Therapeutic

1. Discontinue the offending agent (sulindac).
2. Start hydroxyzine HCl (Atarax) 25 mg four times daily by mouth. Hydroxyzine antagonizes H1 receptors in the periphery and reduces the histamine activity.
3. Start topical corticosteroids such as triamcinolone acetonide (Aristocort), which decrease inflammation by suppressing migration of poly-

morphonuclear leukocytes and reversing capillary permeability.
4. Administer cephalexin (Keflex) 500 mg twice daily for 1 week.
5. Provide patient education and prevention. Have patient avoid NSAIDs. Provide a list to the patient and advise him or her to use hypoallergenic soap and detergents.

FOLLOW-UP VISIT

Subjective

Kathy returned 1 month later and was ecstatic about the improvement in her rash and pruritus. She has not used any NSAIDs but continues her other medications. She states that because the diet and exercise trial recommended previously has not helped with her cholesterol levels, she would like to initiate therapy. Also, a repeat chemistry done 2 days ago, including liver function tests, is normal.

Objective

Kathy's skin examination reveals mostly healing and dry skin lesions. There is minimal scaling and erythema. No significant desquamation is noted. The rest of the examination is normal.

Plan

The patient is started on atorvastatin 10 mg daily. She is advised to follow up in 3 months for repeat liver function tests.

DISCUSSION

About 10% to 20% of hospitalized patients and 2% to 5% of outpatients develop adverse effects while taking medications. Epidemiologic studies indicate that a small group of frequently used drugs accounts for the majority of ADRs, and therefore familiarity with some of these drugs as well as the type of adverse reactions is imperative in clinical practice (Table 56-1 and Box 56-1).

Definition and Classification

The term adverse drug reaction incorporates all the adverse events related to drug administration. The World Health Organization defines an ADR as any noxious, unintended, and undesired effect of a drug that occurs at doses used for prevention, diagnosis, or treatment. Drug hypersensitivity is defined as an immune-mediated response to a drug formulation in a sensitized patient. Drug allergy is a response medi-

Table 56-1 Adverse Drug Reactions to Commonly Used Drugs

Drug	Adverse Reaction or Effect
β-Lactam antibiotics	Hypersensitivity reactions such as urticaria, anaphylaxis, serum sickness, neutropenia, interstitial nephritis, pseudomembranous colitis
Sulfonamides	Skin rash including exfoliation, nausea, diarrhea, neutropenia, thrombocytopenia, and renal failure
Nonsteroidal anti-inflammatory drugs	Skin rash, nausea, diarrhea, epigastric discomfort, gastritis, hepatitis, headache, neutropenia, and thrombocytopenia
Aspirin	Urticaria, angioedema, nausea, gastritis, tinnitus, prolonged bleeding time, and dizziness
Acetaminophen	Hepatic necrosis and neutropenia
Warfarin	Fatal or nonfatal hemorrhage from any tissue or organ, skin necrosis, nausea, and hepatitis
Digoxin	Anorexia, nausea, vomiting, diarrhea, visual disturbance, cardiac arrhythmias, headache, and dizziness
Loop diuretics	Hypovolemia, hypokalemia, hyperuricemia, hyponatremia, hyperglycemia, and ototoxicity
Prednisone	Fluid retention, hypertension, proximal muscle weakness, peptic ulcer, pancreatitis, osteoporosis, skin atrophy, adrenal suppression, hyperglycemia, hyperlipidemia, psychosis, cataracts, glaucoma, and hirsutism
β-Blockers	Fatigue, bradycardia, bronchospasm, depression, and impotence

Box 56-1	Drugs That Rarely Cause Rashes

Acetaminophen
Antihistamines: diphenhydramine
Atropine
Benzodiazepines
Digoxin
Insulin
Prednisone
Propanolol
Theophylline
Thyroid hormones
Spironolactone

ated by drug-specific immunoglobulin E (IgE) antibodies.

ADRs are broadly divided into two categories. Type A reactions are common, nonimmunologic, and predictable and may include toxicity, overdoses, side effects, and drug interactions. Approximately 75% to 80% of ADRs fall into this category. Type B reactions account for the remaining 20% to 25% of ADRs. These are unpredictable, often are not manifest until after a drug is marketed, and may be immune mediated. Examples in this category include drug intolerance, idiosyncratic reactions, and allergic or hypersensitivity (immunologic) reactions. Immune-mediated reactions account for 5% to 10% of all drug reactions and constitute true drug hypersensitivity, including IgE-mediated drug allergies.

The Gell and Coombs classification system separates drug hypersensitivity reactions into four types depending on the mechanism, time of onset, and clinical manifestations (Table 56-2). However, some allergic reactions may not be associated with a single mechanism alone. Examples include fixed drug eruption, maculopapular rash, erythema multiforme, exfoliative dermatitis, vasculitis, and specific drug hypersensitivity syndromes.

Although it is not possible to determine which individual will develop a drug reaction, some risk factors have been identified that appear to contribute to such reactions (Box 56-2). These risk factors have been divided into those related to the patient and those related to the drug. Patient-related factors that may increase the likelihood of a drug hypersensitivity reaction include older age, family history of drug allergy, personal history of drug reaction to a chemically related compound, concurrent illness, female gender, slow acetylator type, and history of atopy. Although atopy has no effect on induction of a drug-specific IgE response, it is associated with increased risk of serious reactions once an IgE response has been generated. A large molecular weight and multivalency are the most important drug-related factors to influence the development of a drug hypersensitivity reaction. Smaller molecular weight compounds may also become immunogenic by their ability to covalently link to carrier proteins such as albumin.

Diagnosis

Most allergic reactions have dermatologic manifestations with or without other immunologic features. Maculopapular or morbilliform eruption is the most common dermatologic drug-induced reaction. The actual pathogenesis is unclear, although a T cell–mediated process is likely, as there is a 2-day to 2-week delay in onset. The erythematous, maculopapular rash commences over the trunk and soon spreads to the extremities. It is usually symmetrical, confluent, and spares the palms and soles. Urticaria is usually an IgE-mediated (type I) reaction, occurring minutes to hours after drug exposure and may

Table 56-2 Gell and Coombs Classification of Drug Hypersensitivity Reactions

Reaction Type	Mechanism	Clinical Characteristics	Time of Onset
Type I	Drug–IgE complex mediated	Urticaria, angioedema, bronchospasm, hypotension, nausea, vomiting, diarrhea	Minutes to hours after drug exposure
Type II	Direct cytotoxic: drug-specific IgG or IgM antibodies mediated	Hemolytic anemia, neutropenia, thrombocytopenia	Variable
Type III	Drug–antibody immune complex deposition on tissues	Serum sickness, fever, rash, arthralgias, urticaria, vasculitis, lymphadenopathy	1–3 wk after drug exposure
Type IV	Delayed, T-cell mediated	Allergic contact dermatitis	24–72 hr after topical drug exposure

Ig, immunoglobulin.

Box 56-2	**Risk Factors for Development of Drug Reactions**

Patient-Related Factors

Older age
Female
Personal history of atopy
Personal or family history of previous drug allergy
Use of β-blockers
Concurrent illness (liver disease, renal disease, human immunodeficiency virus, Epstein-Barr infection, cytomegalovirus infection, systemic lupus erythematosus
Slow acetylator phenotype

Drug-Related Factors

Large molecular weight and multivalent compound
Topical, intravenous, or intramuscular route
Frequent, short courses of therapy

also be observed in immune complex disease (type III). Allergic contact dermatitis is an example of delayed hypersensitivity (type IV). It presents as a papulovesicular eruption caused by a medication applied topically to the skin. TEN, SJS, and erythema multiforme describe severe erythematous, polymorphic eruptions associated with urticaria, vesicles, and epidermal detachment. Mucous membranes are commonly involved. In TEN, full-thickness epidermal necrosis involves more than 30% of the body surface area. Drugs such as penicillins and sulfonamides cause approximately 65% of TEN cases, and the mortality rate is 40%. SJS presents as widespread erythematous or purpuric macules and targetoid lesions. The same drugs may be involved as well as infections such as mycoplasma and viruses such as herpes. As the rate of epidermal detachment in SJS is much less compared with TEN, the mortality rate is also much lower, approximately 5%. Drug rash with eosinophilia and systemic symptoms syndrome is a discrete drug reaction distinguished by a morbilliform rash, fever, lymphadenopathy, eosinophilia,

and atypical lymphocytes. The rash may change to an exfoliative type. Varying organ system involvement may include liver, kidney, intestinal tract, lungs, and bone marrow.

No further diagnostic workup is usually required for an ADR because the condition is primarily a clinical diagnosis. A skin or patch test is a useful diagnostic procedure to confirm suspected type I hypersensitivity reaction. A positive test in the presence of antigen-specific IgE is supportive of the diagnosis. A skin biopsy may help establish a diagnosis by showing both superficial and deep perivascular inflammatory cell infiltrates. Eosinophils may be present as well. Laboratory evaluation may reveal eosinophilia, atypical lymphocytes, neutropenia, nephritis, vasculitis, hemolytic anemia, and hepatitis.

Management

The first step in management is obtaining a good history because this will usually suggest the culprit drug. A physical examination should be able to further confirm the type of rash and to rule out features of anaphylaxis such as hypotension, upper airway edema, and acute urticaria. Other serious drug reactions can be suggested by the presence of fever, lymphadenopathy, arthralgias, and bronchospasm.

Treatment requires discontinuing the offending agent. If the patient is on multiple drugs, reduce the number to as few as possible and re-evaluate. Further therapy for drug hypersensitivity is mostly supportive and symptomatic. Topical corticosteroids and oral antihistamines may help. Systemic corticosteroids may help speed recovery in severe cases. TEN and SJS frequently require hospitalization and intensive therapy. Use of corticosteroids in SJS is controversial because it has been found to be helpful in some studies but has been shown to delay healing in others. Corticosteroids are contraindicated in TEN, which should be treated similar to a burn injury.

Material Available on Student Consult
Review Questions and Answers about Adverse Drug Reaction

SUGGESTED READINGS

Demoly P. Classification and epidemiology of hypersensitivity drug reactions. Immunol Allergy Clin North Am 2004;24:345–356.[B]

Gruchalla RS. Drug allergy. J Allergy Clin Immunol 2003;111(2 Suppl):S548–S559.[B]

Habif TP. Clinical Dermatology, 4th ed. St. Louis, Mosby, 2004.[C]

Joint Task Force on Practice Parameters, the American Academy of Allergy, Asthma and Immunology, and the Joint Council of Allergy, Asthma and Immunology. Executive summary of disease management of drug hypersensitivity: A practice parameter. Ann Allergy Asthma Immunol 1999;83:665–700.[C]

Schmader KE, Hanlon JT, Pieper CF, et al. Effects of geriatric evaluation and management on adverse drug reactions and suboptimal prescribing in the frail elderly. Am J Med 2004;116:394–401.Ⓐ

Volcheck GW. Clinical evaluation and management of drug hypersensitivity. Immunol and Allergy Clin North Am 2004;24:357–371.Ⓐ

Chapter

57 Acne (Acne Vulgaris)

Scott Kinkade

KEY POINTS

1. Acne is common and distressing to patients but can almost always be well controlled.
2. The pathogenesis of acne starts with androgenic stimulation of the pilosebaceous unit causing increased sebum and hyperkeratinization that leads to follicular plugging and a comedone. *Propionibacterium acnes* then proliferates within the comedone and releases inflammatory mediators and chemoattractants.
3. Topical retinoids are an excellent cornerstone for all facets of acne therapy.
4. Patients should be reassessed after a minimum of 6 to 8 weeks to give the medications adequate time to work.
5. Patient education should be targeted toward dispelling acne myths, instructions on how to use the medications, expected side effects, and expected efficacy.

INITIAL VISIT

Subjective

Patient Identification and Presenting Problem

Sara is an 18-year-old young woman home from college on Christmas break. You have seen her a few times in the past for minor illnesses and injuries. Today she is seeing you for "worsening acne." Sara states that she has had "mild acne" for several years. When it has become noticeable, usually around the time of her menses, she has applied an over-the-counter benzoyl peroxide 5% cream. She says that this first semester of college has been stressful and has caused her acne to worsen significantly. She attributes the condition to increased stress from tests, too much greasy food in the dormitory cafeteria, not washing her face often enough, and not getting enough sleep. She has been using the benzoyl peroxide product daily for several months but does not feel that it is controlling the acne.

Medical History

Sara has had no surgeries, hospitalizations, or significant medical illnesses. Her immunizations are up to date.

Family History

Family history is noncontributory. Specifically, no one has had severe, scarring acne.

Health Habits

Sara does not take any medicines. She does not smoke or use alcohol. She exercises a few times per week.

Social History

Sara is a freshman in college. She is making good grades and has a strong peer network.

Review of Systems

Sara reports no excessive fatigue except when she stays up late studying. Her mood is good, and she does not feel depressed. Her menstrual cycles have been regular. She denies any polydipsia, polyuria, or polyphagia.

Objective

Physical Examination

Vital Signs Sara's vital signs are normal. Her weight is 128 pounds, and her height is 67 inches.

General She is an alert white female who appears comfortable.

Skin The hair pattern is normal with no signs of virilization. She has 30 to 40 scattered inflamed papules and pustules and a few noninflamed comedones (all <4 mm) on the chin, cheeks, and forehead. There are three to four excoriated lesions on the upper back and none on the chest. There are no nodules or cysts, and there is no evidence of scarring or changes in the pigmentation.

Assessment

Working Diagnosis

Acne vulgaris.

Differential Diagnosis

Rosacea usually begins after age 30. It can appear very similar to acne vulgaris. Patients typically have facial flushing and can have telangiectasias. These features help distinguish it from acne.

Folliculitis is distinguished by small perifollicular pustules that more commonly affect the trunk and extremities in addition to the chest, back, and face. One variant, gram-negative folliculitis, occurs in patients on long-term antibiotics. The pustules are usually concentrated around the nares and central face.

Steroid acne, mechanical acne, pomade acne, and *acne cosmetica* are variants of acne that are distinguished mainly by the history.

Steroid acne occurs after systemic or prolonged topical corticosteroid therapy. There are numerous small papules and pustules on the face in the case of topical steroids or on the trunk and upper arms in the case of systemic steroids.

Mechanical acne is due to trauma and occlusion from things such as a phone receiver, bra straps, or a chin strap on a helmet.

Pomade acne results from hair oils and usually occurs along the hairline. It is more common in black males and females.

Acne cosmetica is due to greasy, occlusive cosmetics and moisturizers. It is most common in females.

Plan

Therapeutic

Given that Sara has tried benzoyl peroxide 5% cream, it would be reasonable to step up the therapy targeting various components of the pathogenesis of acne.

Her benzoyl peroxide is mainly an antibiotic, although it has some comedolytic activity. Adding another or different antibiotic and a more powerful comedolytic would be helpful. Sara is given a prescription for tretinoin (Retin-A) 0.025% cream and tetracycline 500 mg to be taken twice daily on an empty stomach. She is given extensive counseling on the pathogenesis and treatment options for acne as well as expectations of therapy.

Patient Education

Patients can have significant emotional distress from their acne and, at times, are pessimistic about the ability to treat it, given past failures. Patients should understand that although acne is a chronic disease, it can almost always be well controlled. Many of the medications have side effects and must be used as directed. If the side effects can be anticipated, compliance increases. Finally, therapies should be given sufficient time to work before re-evaluation. When starting a new therapy, the minimum time needed before assessing efficacy is 6 to 8 weeks.

Sara can be told that stress (such as around the time of examinations) can exacerbate acne. Many women also experience premenstrual flares of their acne. Research on various diets has not shown a link between consumption of greasy foods or chocolate and acne. Tetracycline must be taken on an empty stomach to be effective. It can cause some gastrointestinal upset and photosensitivity and can stain the teeth of children younger than age 12. It cannot be given to pregnant women. Retin-A can cause irritation, transient worsening of acne, and photosensitivity. It should be applied at night, with a pea-sized dose spread evenly over the face. If it is too irritating, a smaller dose can be used, or it can be used every other night. Because many patients get frustrated with tretinoin when their face gets irritated or when their acne worsens, it is not uncommon for patients to stop using it after a week. Encouragement and patient education are essential components of patient therapy and can help patients overcome side effects of medications.

DISCUSSION

Acne affects almost 80% of adolescents and young adults. It can be well controlled in almost all cases. Because some adolescents may feel ashamed about their acne or may feel resigned to the fact that it is incurable, the doctor may need to encourage patients to try acne medications. An excellent approach is during well-child, sports, or school physical exami-

Table 57-1 Treatment Based on Pathophysiologic Target

Medication	Decrease Androgen-Mediated Sebum Production	Decrease Hyperkeratinization and Follicular Plugging (Comedone Formation)	Decrease *Propionibacterium acnes* Bacteria	Decrease Inflammation
Topical Therapies				
Topical retinoids	—	++	—	(+)
Benzoyl peroxide	—	+	++	—
Topical erythromycin or clindamycin	—	(+)	++	+
Azelaic acid	—	+	+	+
Salicylic acid	—	+	—	—
Systemic Therapies				
Oral antibiotics	—	–	++	(+)
Oral contraceptives	+	(+)	—	—
Oral corticosteroids	+	—	—	+
Isotretinoin	++	+	+	++

++, Strong activity, +, moderate activity, (+), weak activity.

nations. The provider can note the presence of acne, ask the patient whether he or she would like to try to control it, and then have the patient come in for an appointment dedicated to formulation and discussion of an acne treatment plan.

The precursor lesion of acne is the microcomedone, which forms in the pilosebaceous unit. Androgens stimulate the sebaceous gland and cause increased sebum production. In acne, the keratinocytes within the follicle hyperproliferate and clump together, plugging the follicle. The resulting microcomedone matures into either an open comedone (blackhead) or closed comedone (whitehead). With the retained sebum and relatively anaerobic environment, the bacteria *Propionibacterium acnes* flourish. The sebum and the *P. acnes* generate inflammatory mediators and cause an inflammatory lesion to develop.

Therapy is guided by the severity of the acne and by targeting different components of the pathogenesis of acne lesions (Tables 57-1 and 57-2). Mild acne can be comedonal, inflammatory, or mixed. In mild acne there are no cysts or scarring and usually fewer than 20 lesions. Moderate acne is easily visible, usually with more than 20 lesions or covering about half of the face, with no scarring or cysts. Severe acne involves more than half of the face, has a cystic component, or causes scarring.

For purely comedonal acne or mild cases, a topical retinoid is the preferred therapy. Alternatives or additional therapy include topical antibiotics such as benzoyl peroxide, clindamycin, erythromycin, azelaic acid, or a benzoyl peroxide/topical antibiotic combination.

Careful instruction in the use of topical retinoids is required to increase patient compliance and achieve

Table 57-2 Treatment Based on Severity

Acne Classification	Initial Treatments	If Inadequate Response
Mild comedonal	Topical retinoid	Add topical antibiotic or BPO
Mild inflammatory	Topical antibiotic (BPO, clindamycin, erythromycin, azelaic acid, and BPO/Abx) or topical retinoid	Add topical retinoid or topical antibiotic
Moderate inflammatory	Topical retinoid ± oral antibiotic or BPO or topical BPO/Abx	Oral antibiotic; oral contraceptive for females; increase strength of retinoid or change type; consider referral to dermatologist
Severe	Oral antibiotic and topical retinoid ± oral contraceptive for females ± BPO/Abx	Refer to dermatologist; isotretinoin

BPO, benzoyl peroxide; BPO/Abx, topical product containing benzoyl peroxide and either erythromycin or clindamcyin.

the best outcome. For patients who are sensitive to topical retinoids, there are several strategies that can be tried, based on the following. First, the creams are less drying and irritating than gels or solution. Second, the lowest possible formulation can be used. Third, tretinoin is available in alternate vehicles, a microsphere (Retin-A Micro) and a polyolprepolymer (Avita), which are less irritating. Fourth, adapalene (Differin) is usually less irritating than tretinoin or tazarotene. Finally, these can be used sparingly or every other day until tolerated or applied and washed off after a short time.

Benzoyl peroxide is inactivated by topical retinoids, so they should not be used together. Typically, the topical retinoid is used at night and the benzoyl peroxide is used in the morning. Benzoyl peroxide is unique in that it does not induce resistance in *P. acnes*, unlike the other oral and topical antibiotics. Side effects of benzoyl peroxide include facial irritation and bleaching of clothes, towels, and bed linens.

Topical antibiotics include erythromycin and clindamycin (Cleocin T). They are available as solutions, lotions, ointments, and gels. In addition, they are available as combination products with either benzoyl peroxide or tretinoin. Combination products can increase patient compliance, decrease bacterial resistance, and enhance penetration. Side effects of topical antibiotics are predominantly due to local irritation. There have been a few reports of systemic side effects from topical antibiotics.

Azelaic acid (Azelex) is not as potent an antibiotic as benzoyl peroxide, erythromycin, or clindamycin, but it does not induce resistance in *P. acnes*. It also has mild comedolytic, anti-inflammatory, and hypopigmenting properties. The ability to decrease some postinflammatory hyperpigmentation from acne lesions is unique to azelaic acid. Salicylic acid is available over the counter in various acne washes and creams. It is a mild keratolytic. Side effects to azelaic acid and salicylic acid are primarily due to local irritation.

Moderate acne and severe acne require systemic therapy. Topical preparations can still be used, but an oral antibiotic, oral contraceptive, or isotretinoin is required. Oral tetracyclines (tetracycline, doxycycline, and minocycline) are first-line therapies. Erythromycin leads to higher rates of resistant *P. acnes* and trimethoprim-sulfamethoxazole (Bactrim), while effective, has a higher rate of severe side effects. Oral antibiotics are used at full strength for 6 to 8 weeks or until there is an improvement in the acne. They can then be decreased to maintenance doses but should not be used longer than needed due to bacterial resistance. A typical course of antibiotics is 6 to 9 months. Tetracycline is the least expensive but must be taken 1 to 2 hours before meals, which decreases patient compliance. A usual starting dose is 500 mg twice daily. It is contraindicated in children younger than age 12 and in pregnancy and can cause photosensitivity and gastrointestinal upset. Doxycycline is usually started at a dose of 100 mg twice

daily and can be taken with foods. It can cause photosensitivity but less than with tetracycline. It should not be used in children or in pregnancy. Minocycline (Minocin) is the most expensive but also probably the most effective because it is very lipophilic and concentrates in the sebaceous glands. The usual starting dose is 50 to 100 mg twice daily, and it can be taken with food. There are fewer gastrointestinal problems and less phototoxicity than with the other tetracycline derivatives. Minocycline has some severe but rare side effects, including central nervous system disturbances (headache, vertigo, and pseudotumor cerebri), blue-gray discoloration of the skin and oral mucosa, autoimmune hepatitis, and drug-induced lupus.

Combination oral contraceptives are an option for females, particularly when contraception is desired. They suppress ovarian and peripheral androgen metabolism and increase sex hormone–binding globulin, resulting in a net reduction in free testosterone. Several oral contraceptives, including those containing the progestins norethindrone, desogestrel, norgestimate, and drospirenone, have been studied and found to be effective.

Products containing the progestins norgestrel, levonorgestrel, and norethindrone are not as efficacious because of their androgenic effects.

Isotretinoin (Accutane) is a powerful and effective medicine for controlling acne and may cause remission. It is indicated for severe nodular acne unresponsive to conventional therapy. It should also be considered for scarring acne and other moderate to severe acne cases that do not respond well to conventional treatments. Because of severe side effects, including teratogenicity and possible increases in depression and suicide, it should be prescribed only by physicians experienced with the use of the drug. In addition, the manufacturer requires prescribers to be enrolled in a special program that outlines specific protocols for use. Common but less severe side effects include dry skin and mucous membranes, hyperlipidemia, myalgias, arthralgias, and headaches.

Patients should be reassessed after at least 6 to 8 weeks of therapy and encouraged to continue therapy, even if their acne seems to transiently worsen at the beginning. Maintenance of acne therapy is best managed with a topical retinoid or benzoyl peroxide. Continuous, long-term use of topical or oral antibiotics leads to resistance and treatment failures. In the case of worsening acne while on an antibiotic, one should consider gram-negative folliculitis, or, more commonly, antibiotic resistance.

Material Available on Student Consult

Review Questions and Answers about Acne Vulgaris

SUGGESTED READINGS

Feldman S, Careccia RE, Barham KL. Diagnosis and treatment of acne. Am Fam Physician 2004;69: 2123–2130.**C**

Gollnick H, Cunliffe W, Berson D, et al. Management of acne: A report from a Global Alliance to Improve Outcomes in Acne. J Am Acad Dermatol 2003;49: S1–S37.**C**

Haider A, Shaw JC. Treatment of acne vulgaris. JAMA 2004;92:726–735.**A**

Katsambas A, Papakonstantinou A. Acne: Systemic treatment. Clin Dermatol 2004;22:412–418.**C**

Katsambas AD, Stefanaki C, Cunliffe WJ. Guidelines for treating acne. Clin Dermatol 2004;22:439–444.**C**

Krautheim A, Gollnick HP. Acne: Topical treatment. Clin Dermatol 2004;22:398–407.**C**

Rigopoulos D, Ioannides D, Kalogeromitros D, Katsambas AD. Comparison of topical retinoids in the treatment of acne. Clin Dermatol 2004;22:408–411.**C**

Smolinski KN, Yan AC. Acne update: 2004. Curr Opin Pediatr 2004;16:385–391.**C**

Thiboutot D. Acne: Hormonal concepts and therapy. Clin Dermatol 2004;22:419–428.**C**

Chapter

58

Genital Warts (Condyloma Acuminata)

Richard P. Usatine and Heidi Chumley

KEY POINTS

1. Condyloma acuminata (genital warts) are caused by human papillomavirus (HPV) and are sexually transmitted.
2. The differential diagnosis for condyloma acuminata includes condyloma lata, molluscum contagiosum, and pearly penile papules.
3. Any person with genital warts should be tested for sexually transmitted diseases including syphilis and human immunodeficiency virus (HIV). Women with genital warts should have Pap smear screening.
4. Genital warts may be treated by the application of topical medications such as imiquimod or podofilox or by the destruction of wart tissue with cryotherapy, electrotherapy, or surgery.

5. When choosing which treatments to prescribe, the physician should consider the size, keratinization, location and number of genital warts, patient preferences, treatment costs, convenience, and adverse effects.
6. Treatment of genital warts improves symptoms from the warts and induces wart-free periods but does not necessarily prevent transmission of HPV to a partner.
7. While condom use may not prevent transfer of the HPV, it does prevent the occurrence of genital warts in partners of persons with HPV and does reduce the transmission of other sexually transmitted diseases (STDs).

Evidence levels **A** Randomized, controlled trials (RCTs), meta-analyses, well-designed systematic reviews of RCTs. **B** Case-control or cohort studies, nonrandomized clinical trials, systematic reviews of studies other than RCTs, cross-sectional studies, retrospective studies, certain uncontrolled studies. **C** Consensus statements, expert guidelines, usual practice, opinion.

INITIAL VISIT

Subjective

Patient Identification and Presenting Problem

Fred B. is a 32-year-old white man who presents for the first time concerned that he may have warts on his penis (Figs. 58-1 and 58-2). He believes that the warts started about 4 months ago. He has been married for 2 years. He denies having sexual relationships outside of his marriage and believes his wife is also not having sex with anyone else. Fred admits to having other sexual partners before meeting his wife but does not understand how he could have contracted this now.

Medical History

Fred denies any history of STDs and had a negative HIV test before he got married. The patient has no other symptoms and no chronic illnesses.

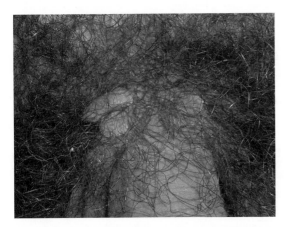

Figure 58-1 Condyloma acuminata at the base of the penis.

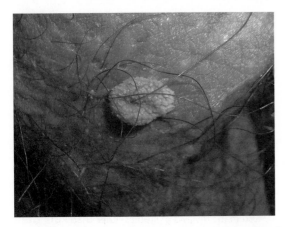

Figure 58-2 Close-up of a genital wart on the shaft of the penis.

Family History

Both parents are alive and well. A full family history is not essential for this particular case.

Health Habits

Fred generally lives a healthy lifestyle and denies drug and tobacco use. He likes to have wine with dinner when he goes out but does this less than twice a week.

Social History

Fred is married and has no children.

Review of Systems

He denies fevers, urethral discharge, and burning on urination.

Objective

Physical Examination

The patient has no fever or lymphadenopathy. A genital examination (see Fig. 58-1) reveals skin-colored verrucous lesions at the base of the penis. A close-up photograph of one of the lesions on the shaft of the penis clearly shows the cauliflower look of condyloma acuminata (see Fig. 58-2).

Assessment

Working Diagnosis

These large verrucous lesions are most likely condyloma acuminata. These are caused by the HPV and are sexually transmitted. It is possible to contract HPV and not develop warts until much later.

Differential Diagnosis

Other causes of genital lesions that may be confused with condyloma acuminata include:

1. *Condyloma lata.* Lata means flat, and this type of flat wart occurs in secondary syphilis. Condyloma lata are teeming with spirochetes, and a dark-field microscopy can be used to visualize the *Treponema pallidum*. These lesions are much less common than condyloma acuminata and can be distinguished with a markedly positive Venereal Disease Research Laboratories (VDRL) test or rapid plasmin reagin test.
2. *Molluscum contagiosum.* The papules of molluscum contagiosum are smooth and pearly with central umbilication. They look stuck on the surface and range from 1 to 5 mm. The papules can be found anywhere on the body except for the scalp and can vary from a few isolated papules to many widespread lesions. Molluscum contagiosum is caused by three different DNA poxviruses

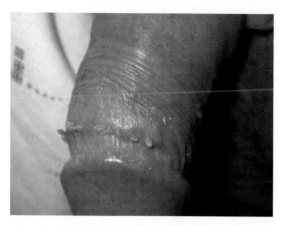

Figure 58-3 Pearly penile papules on the corona of the glans and genital warts on the shaft.

and is spread through person-to-person contact, autoinoculation, or contact with fomites. In adults, these lesions may be sexually transmitted and found in the genital area.

3. *Pearly penile papules.* Figure 58-3 shows a patient with pearly penile papules on the corona of the glans and genital warts on the shaft of the penis. The pearly penile papules are a variation of the normal male anatomy. The main reason to recognize these papules is to reassure worried men that they are normal and to avoid removing them with unnecessary invasive treatments (Usatine, 2004).

Plan

Diagnostic

Since Fred likely has one type of STD, he should be tested for syphilis and HIV regardless of other risk factors (Centers for Disease Control and Prevention, 2002◕). In this case, testing for syphilis with either a rapid plasmin reagin or VDRL test will be helpful to rule out condyloma lata. These specific condyloma lesions do not resemble molluscum contagiosum and do not need to be biopsied to establish the diagnosis.

There are no data to support the use of type-specific HPV nucleic acid tests in the routine diagnosis or management of visible genital warts (Centers for Disease Control and Prevention, 2002◕).

Therapeutic

The primary goal of treating visible genital warts is the removal of symptomatic warts (Centers for Disease Control and Prevention, 2002◕). Treatment can induce wart-free periods. Available therapies for genital warts may reduce, but probably will not eradicate, infectivity (Centers for Disease Control and Prevention, 2002◕). There is no evidence that suggests that one single treatment is ideal for all patients or all warts. The natural history of genital warts is benign, and the types of HPV that cause external genital warts (HPV 6 and 11) are not associated with cancer.

The Centers for Disease Control and Prevention 2002 treatment guidelines for STDs recommend the following options:

Patient-Applied Treatments (See Table 58-1 for Cost Data)
Podofilox 0.5% solution or gel (Condylox). Patients should apply podofilox solution with a cotton swab or podofilox gel with a finger to visible genital warts twice daily for 3 days, followed by 4 days of no therapy. This cycle may be repeated, as necessary, for up to four cycles. The health care provider should apply the initial treatment to demonstrate the application technique and identify the warts to be treated.

Imiquimod 5% cream (Aldara). Patients should apply imiquimod cream once daily at bedtime, three times weekly for up to 16 weeks. The treatment area should be washed with soap and water 6 to 10 hours after the application.

Provider-Administered Treatments
Cryotherapy. Cryotherapy is applied with liquid nitrogen, a chemical refrigerant, or a cryoprobe using CO_2 or nitrous oxide gas (Usatine, 1998). Providers

Table 58-1	Self-Administered Medications for Human Papillomavirus	
Medication	**Method**	**Cost**
Podofilox 0.5% solution or gel (podophyllotoxin)	Apply twice daily for 3 days, then off 4 days. May repeat cycle total of 4 times.	Generic topical solution, 3 mL, $90.85 Condylox gel, 3.5 g (1 tube), $164 Condylox solution, 3.5 mL, $121
Imiquimod 5% cream	Apply once daily 3 times/wk. Wash off after 6–10 hr. May use up to 16 wk.	12 packets for $159 (for 4 wk of therapy if one packet is used per application; using a packet for more than 1 day is possible)

Prices from ePocrates. Available at www.epocrates.com. Accessed 10/30/2005.

should freeze each lesion for about 5 to 15 seconds with 2-mm margins, as HPV is present in normal-appearing tissue surrounding each lesion (Usatine, 1998). Freeze time is the amount of time that the lesion remains frozen and not the amount of time the cryogen is applied. These times will vary depending on the cryogen, the delivery method, the size of the lesion, and the patient's tolerance. The coldest cryogen is liquid nitrogen; it is delivered most efficiently with a cryogun. Other cryogens include nitrous oxide and chemical refrigerants. Fewer complications will occur with shorter freeze times, and the freeze times can always be increased at the next visit if needed. No current evidence indicates that double freeze/thaw cycles are superior to a single freeze and thaw. Providers can repeat applications every 1 to 2 weeks. Cryosurgery is ideal for isolated lesions on the penile shaft or on the vulva (Usatine, 1998). Figure 58-4 shows the genital wart in Figure 58-2 undergoing treatment with liquid nitrogen in a cryogun.

For patients with multiple lesions that make up a considerable extent of the surface area of the penis or the vulva, patient-administered topically applied medications are better tolerated than cryotherapy.

Podophyllin resin 10% to 25% (Podifin) in a compound tincture of benzoin. A small amount should be applied to each wart and allowed to air dry. The treatment can be repeated weekly, if necessary. To avoid the possibility of complications associated with systemic absorption and toxicity, some specialists recommend that application be limited to <0.5 mL of podophyllin or an area smaller than 10 cm² of warts per session. Some specialists suggest that the preparation should be thoroughly washed 1 to 4 hours after application to reduce local irritation. Avoid using podophyllin during pregnancy.

Trichloroacetic acid (TCA) (Tri-chlor). A small amount should be applied only to the warts and allowed to dry, at which time a white "frosting" develops. This treatment can be repeated weekly, if necessary. Figure 58-5 shows the white frosting that is visible on penile warts right after treatment with topical TCA.

Surgical removal. Surgical removal is achieved by tangential scissor excision (snip excision), curettage, or electrosurgery. These methods usually require local anesthetic unless the lesion is tiny or on a tiny base. When using electrosurgery, the physician should use a smoke evacuator and surgical mask to avoid inhaling smoke with viral particles.

When choosing the type of therapy for each patient, it is helpful to note that the soft nonkeratinized warts respond well to the various forms of podophyllin and trichloroacetic acid, while the more keratinized lesions respond better to physical ablative methods such as cryotherapy, excision, and electrocautery. Imiquimod appears to work well for both types of lesions but is more effective for the nonkeratinized warts. The softer nonkeratinized warts are often found on the softer mucosa around the anus, under the foreskin, and around the female introitus. The firmer, more keratinized warts are often found on more keratinized skin such as on the shaft of the penis.

Patient Education

Patient education should include information about transmission and outcomes.

- Advise patients that genital warts are transmitted sexually and encourage testing for other STDs, including cervical cytology screening in women.
- Reassure women that the risk of cervical cancer is low even with genital warts and that yearly Pap smears can detect early changes that can be treated before cancer develops.

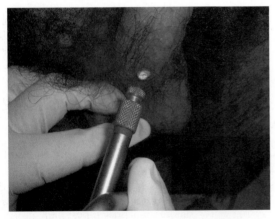

Figure 58-4 Genital wart undergoing treatment with liquid nitrogen in a cryogun.

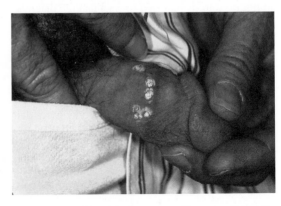

Figure 58-5 White frosting on penile warts right after treatment with topical trichloroacetic acid.

- Encourage patients to use condoms, particularly if the patient is not in a monogamous relationship. Condoms may reduce the risk of a partner developing warts but probably do not reduce transmission of HPV.
- Clarify that HPV has a long latency period and that the development of genital warts in only one partner does not indicate sexual contact outside that relationship.
- Encourage current partners and recent partners to be assessed for genital warts and advised about STDs and their prevention.
- Reassure patients that these warts typically resolve, although it may take up to 6 months, and recurrences may occur (von Krogh et al., 2001❸).

Disposition

The treatment options were discussed with the patient. A process of shared decision making was used to come up with the treatment plan. The patient decided to have cryotherapy performed in the office and was given a prescription for imiquimod cream to be used on any remaining warts. The patient tolerated the cryotherapy with an acceptable level of temporary discomfort. His HIV and rapid plasmin reagin tests were negative. While still using the imiquimod cream, he returned with his wife to discuss the implications of his infection for her. Her physical examination and Pap smear were normal. After long discussions and much reassurance, they both understood that he was probably infected before their marriage.

DISCUSSION

HPV causes many types of warts in humans, including common warts (verruca vulgaris), flat warts (verruca plana), plantars warts, and genital warts (condyloma acuminata). The common and flat warts found on hands, feet, and other locations can be a cosmetic and functional nuisance. These warts are most often treated with cryotherapy and topical acids. Genital warts can be physically and psychologically distressing; however, the most deadly consequence of HPV infection is cervical cancer. The detection and treatment of cervical dysplasia and cancer involve using the Pap smear, the colposcope, and treatment with surgical means when indicated.

HPV can be divided into high-risk (oncogenic) and low-risk (noncogenic) types. High-risk HPV (such as HPV 16 and 18) may actually lead to cancers of the cervix, vulva, vagina, anus, or penis. Low-risk HPV (such as HPV 6 and 11) can cause genital warts and may cause abnormal Pap results without causing cancer.

The most important predictors of any HPV infection are lifetime number of sexual partners, young age,

and, for men, being uncircumcised (Svare et al., 2002❸). The most important risk factor for oncogenic HPV types is lifetime number of partners. Risk factors for the noncogenic HPV types include number of partners in the past year and ever having genital warts (Svare et al., 2002❸). Fortunately, a vaccine that targets oncogenic HPV subtypes 16 and 18 has shown promise in decreasing infection and cervical dysplasia in women and is in late clinical trials (Harper et al., 2004❹).

Genital HPV infection or genital warts are not nationally reportable diseases. Therefore, comprehensive surveillance data are not available for HPV infections. If age-specific incidence estimates for cervical HPV infection among women reflect the HPV incidence rates among men, then approximately 6.2 million new HPV infections occurred in the year 2000 among Americans age 15 to 44; of these infections, 74% (4.6 million) occurred among 15- to 24-year-old persons (Myers, 2000; Weinstock et al., 2004).

There is no single first-line treatment option for genital warts, in part because each therapy has less than optimal cure and recurrence rates. The treatment guidelines from the Centers for Disease Control and Prevention are based on a limited number of clinical trials. One double-blind, randomized, multicenter, vehicle-controlled study demonstrated that 0.5% podofilox gel was significantly better than vehicle gel for successfully eliminating and reducing the number and size of anogenital warts. In the intent-to-treat population, 37% treated with podofilox gel had complete clearing of the treated areas compared with 2% who had clearing of warts with the vehicle gel after 4 weeks (Tyring et al., 1998❹) ($P < 0.001$, number needed to treat = 3).

Imiquimod has been shown to be effective in many studies, including three randomized controlled trials in which clearance rates were 37% to 52% after 8 to 16 weeks of treatment (Maw, 2004). One study found that clearance rates were twofold higher in women than in men (72% and 33%, respectively) (Sauder et al., 2003❹). This is probably because genital warts in females are less keratinized than the most commonly found warts on the penile shaft in males. Similarly, clearance rates with imiquimod seem to be higher in uncircumcised men (62%) than in circumcised men (33%), probably due to the degree of keratinization (Maw, 2004). However, uncircumcised men are at higher risk of acquiring genital warts and other STDs independent of other sexual risk factors (Svare et al., 2002❸).

Recurrence rates for sole therapy with imiquimod (9% to 19%) are substantially lower than for most other genital wart treatments including podophyllin (Maw, 2004). Imiquimod may even be effective in reducing wart recurrence rates when used as an adjunct to surgical treatment (Maw, 2004).

Figure 58-6 shows condyloma acuminata around the anus of a 2-year-old girl. The mother had common

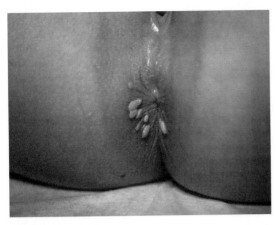

Figure 58-6 Condyloma acuminata around the anus of a 2-year-old girl.

In summary, genital warts bring up complicated social and personal issues that need to be addressed with the patients and their partners. Medical or surgical treatment should be determined using informed consent and shared decision making. When choosing which treatments to prescribe for patients, the clinician should consider the size, keratinization, location and number of genital warts, patient preferences, treatment costs, convenience, and adverse effects. Most treatments take months to work. If one treatment does not work, other options should be considered.

Material Available on Student Consult

Review Questions and Answers about Condyloma Acuminata

warts (verruca vulgaris) on her fingers and believed that these warts were the result of her diapering her child. Genital warts in children should prompt investigation for child abuse, as was done in this case.

REFERENCES

Centers for Disease Control and Prevention. 2002 Sexually transmitted diseases treatment guidelines. MMWR Recomm Rep 2002;51:1–80.**ⓒ**

Harper DM, Franco EL, Wheeler C, et al. Efficacy of a bivalent L1 virus-like particle vaccine in prevention of infection with human papillomavirus types 16 and 18 in young women: A randomised controlled trial. Lancet 2004;364:1757–1795.**ⓐ**

Maw R. Critical appraisal of commonly used treatment for genital warts. Int J STD AIDS 2004;15:357–364.

Myers ER. Mathematical model for the natural history of human papillomavirus infection and cervical carcinogenesis. Am J Epidemiol 2000;151:1158–1171.

Sauder DN, Skinner RB, Fox TL, Owens ML. Topical imiquimod 5% cream as an effective treatment for external genital and perianal warts in different patient populations. Sex Transm Dis 2003;30:124–128.**ⓐ**

Svare EI, Kjaer SK, Worm AM, Osterlind A, Meijer CJ, van den Brule AJ. Risk factors for genital HPV DNA in men resemble those found in women: A study of male attendees at a Danish STD clinic. Sex Transm Infect 2002;78:215–218.**ⓑ**

Tyring S, Edwards L, Cherry LK, et al. Safety and efficacy of 0.5% podofilox gel in the treatment of anogenital warts. Arch Dermatol 1998;134:33–38.**ⓐ**

Usatine RP. Pearly penile lesions. J Fam Pract 2004;53:885–888.

Usatine R. Cryosurgery. In Usatine R, Moy R, Tobinick E, Siegel D, (eds): Skin Surgery: A Practical Guide. St. Louis, Mosby-Year Book, 1998, pp 137–164.

von Krogh G, Lacey CJ, Gross G, Barrasso R, Schneider A. European Course on HPV Associated Pathology (ECHPV), European Branch of the International Union against Sexually Transmitted Infection and the European Office of the World Health Organization. European guideline for the management of anogenital warts. Int J STD AIDS 2001;12(Suppl 3):40–47.**ⓒ**

Weinstock H, Berman S, Cates W. Sexually transmitted diseases among American youth: Incidence and prevalence estimates, 2000. Perspect Sex Reprod Health 2004;36:6–10.

59 Pigmented Thumbnail (Nail Lentigo)

Robert S. Fawcett

KEY POINTS

1. Longitudinal melanocytic bands are almost ubiquitous in dark-skinned adults, which makes the diagnosis of malignant melanoma of the nail problematic in those individuals.
2. Risk factors making biopsy of a new band necessary include the usual ABCDE criteria for melanoma as well as Hutchinson's sign (skin involvement at the proximal or distal nail fold); family history of dysplastic nevi or melanoma; single nail involvement, particularly of the thumb or index finger; sudden change in appearance; association with trauma; nail dysplasia; or onset after age 60.
3. Biopsy of possible melanoma is done by removing the nail and excising the skin involved with the pigmentation, being sure to include the most proximal area, and warning the patient in advance of the likelihood of resultant nail dysplasia.

INITIAL VISIT

Subjective

Patient Identification and Presenting Problem
Jadyra G. is a 65-year-old Hispanic woman who presents to the office complaining of an expanding streak on her right thumb. The streak itself has been present for about 10 years but has recently gotten broader. Jadyra also notes that the notching of the distal nail plate is new.

Medical History
The patient has hypertension that is well controlled with hydrochlorothiazide and an angiotensin-converting enzyme inhibitor. She is moderately overweight but not diabetic. There is no history of cancer, heart disease, or skin problems.

Family History
The patient's mother died of a stroke at age 72. Her father died in an accident at age 35. The woman has three brothers and two sisters with whom she has little contact, but she is not aware that any have chronic medical problems. She knows of no cancers in the family, although one sister had a breast biopsy for what turned out to be benign disease. Several children and grandchildren are alive and well.

Social History
The patient does not drink or smoke. She lives with her husband and stays active caring for a number of grandchildren.

Review of Systems
There is nothing of significance to the case. The patient complains of some aches in her knees and back for which she takes occasional acetaminophen and ibuprofen with some relief. She takes milk of magnesia for occasional constipation. She denies taking other over-the-counter medications or herbal supplements.

Objective

Physical Examination
Jadyra G. is a healthy-appearing, moderately obese Hispanic woman in no distress. Her blood pressure is 140/75, pulse is 76 and regular, temperature is 36.9°C (98.4°F), and respiratory rate is 16. The examination is unremarkable aside from the right thumb. There she has pigmentation on the radial two thirds of the thumbnail, with a 4-mm darkly banded area to the radial side (Figs. 59-1 and 59-2). The pigmentation extends onto the proximal nail fold and eponychium (Hutchinson's sign) and into the distal nail fold beneath the free edge of the nail. Nail dystrophy is manifest by slight thickening over the most darkly pigmented area and by notching at the free edge of the nail plate. No inflammation is seen, and scraping the surface of the nail plate with a no. 15 blade does not affect the coloration of the nail. No other nails show pigmented bands.

Assessment

Working Diagnosis
Rule out subungual melanoma.

Differential Diagnosis
1. *Melanoma* is relatively rare in darkly pigmented individuals, but approximately half of the melanomas that do occur are in the nail bed, and

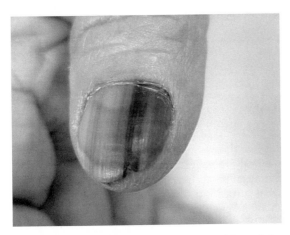

Figure 59-1 Dysplasia of the nail (see notching of the distal plate), broadness of the pigmented band (>3 mm), and Hutchinson's sign (extension of pigment onto proximal nail fold) make malignancy more likely. (Reproduced with permission from Fawcett RS, Linford S, Stulberg DL. Nail abnormalities: Clues to systemic disease. Am Fam Physician 2004;69:1422. Copyright © 2004 American Academy of Family Physicians. All Rights Reserved.)

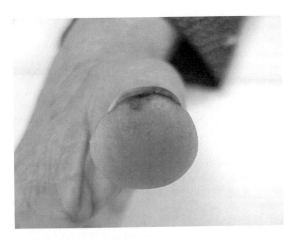

Figure 59-2 Extension of the pigmented area to the distal nail fold makes malignancy more likely. (Reproduced with permission from Fawcett RS, Linford S, Stulberg DL. Nail abnormalities: Clues to systemic disease. Am Fam Physician 2004;69:1422. Copyright © 2004 American Academy of Family Physicians. All Rights Reserved.)

most of those are on the index finger or thumb. Melanoma of the nail is usually seen in older individuals in the sixth or seventh decade of life. Nail dystrophy and single nail involvement as well as Hutchinson's sign and the recent change in the lesion all make this the diagnosis to consider most strongly and, because of the consequences of missing it, to rule out.

2. *Longitudinal melanonychia* is almost universally seen in older darkly pigmented individuals. It is totally benign and usually affects several fingers or toes.

3. *Acanthosis nigricans* can cause some variable brown discoloration of the nail plate, but this patient does not have the velvety, thickened, darkly pigmented skin in the axilla or neck that suggests that condition.

4. *Adrenal insufficiency* can cause longitudinal brown lines. This patient feels well, however, and her blood pressure is slightly elevated. She does not have any overall increase in pigmentation.

5. *Drugs.* Adriamycin, bleomycin, hydroxyurea, and minocycline can all cause brown discoloration, although all nails would likely be affected.

6. *Lentigo.* Brown pigmentation from lentigo simplex can affect the nail, just as it can other sun-exposed areas. Lentigo maligna and lentigo maligna melanoma are also possible, however, and need to be ruled out through biopsy.

7. *Nevus.* Nevi can occur on the nail bed, as they can anywhere else, and may give a streaked appearance as the nail grows distally. It would be unusual, however, for nevi to appear de novo in this age group without a potential for malignancy. Biopsy would be warranted here as well.

Plan

After visual inspection with both the naked eye and 10× magnification, noting the extension of the lesion onto not only the proximal but also the distal nail fold, the patient is referred to a dermatologist for biopsy. The dermatologist removes the nail and biopsies the nail bed. Because the patient is otherwise healthy, no additional workup is thought to be immediately indicated.

Disposition

The biopsy is returned with a diagnosis of lentigo. The patient is reassured regarding the benignity of this diagnosis but educated regarding the necessity of self-evaluation for any changes in the lesion. Arrangements are made to see the patient back in the family doctor's office in 6 months.

At the return visit, the nail has completely regrown, although with a prominent longitudinal depression in the area of the previous procedure. Pigmentary streaking remains, although it is considerably narrower and lighter than at the previous visit. Continued surveillance and 6-month follow-up are recommended

DISCUSSION

Nails are laid down by the nail matrix at the proximal end of the nail bed. As the nail plate is formed, it moves distally, and the more distal cells of the nail matrix lay down additional layers to the undersurface of the plate. If the cells of the nail matrix are more pigmented than surrounding cells, the keratin that they lay down on the underside of the nail plate might well retain some of that pigment, giving rise to a longitudinal striation in the nail. In fact, such lines are quite common among more highly pigmented individuals. One may observe them in 77% of African Americans older than the age of 20. They usually involve multiple nails, although the color variations may be subtle.

The chief problem with such stripes is in distinguishing them from malignant melanoma, which can also give rise to pigmented longitudinal bands. There are a number of factors that may increase the likelihood of malignancy in a patient with these bands. They are outlined in Box 59-1.

Nevi and lentigo can cause similar changes. The latter is thought to represent actinic change, often stemming from significant sun exposure in childhood. Again, the problem is in distinguishing benign from malignant lesions, which can arise from either lesion.

The evaluating physician should think of the usual ABCDE risk factors for melanoma in these situations as well (as adapted from the article by Levit et al. in the Suggested Reading list). *Asymmetry* is applicable in that a single nail being affected increases risk. *Border* irregularities and *color* variegation could apply to blurring and indistinct margins of the streak. *Diameter* could apply to width of the band greater than 3 to 4 mm or a widening band, and *enlargement* might be viewed as extending onto the skin at the distal nail fold or the proximal nail bed and eponychium (Hutchinson's sign).

If melanoma is suspected, biopsy should be performed. Simple punch biopsy including the nail plate can be done if the band is 3 mm or narrower, with good cosmetic result. If a wider band is present, the nail plate should be removed, and an elliptical or punch biopsy can then be performed over the area of pigmentation. Such a biopsy is likely to result in permanent dysplasia of the nail plate when it regrows, so one should consider referring the patient for the procedure. The physician performing the biopsy must also exercise caution so as

---

Box 59-1	**Risk Factors for Melanoma in a Nail with Longitudinal Pigmented Striation**

1. Sudden change in appearance of band (wider, darker, blurred border)
2. Single nail involvement (especially thumb, index finger, or great toe)
3. Pigmentation of skin of nail fold or proximal nail bed (Hutchinson's sign)
4. New pigmentation in older individual (60s and 70s)
5. Association with history of digital trauma
6. Family history of melanoma or dysplastic nevi
7. Abnormal nail structure (destruction or disruption of nail plate)

Adapted from Fawcett RS, Linford S, Stulberg DL. Nail abnormalities: Clees to systemic disease. Am Fam Physician 2004;69:1417–1424.

---

not to disrupt the extensor tendon. Procedures involving the proximal nail bed should be oriented with the long axis across the finger; those involving the lateral or distal region should be longitudinal.

Other causes for longitudinal stria should also be ruled out. Temporary staining can occur with tobacco and podophyllin. Shelling walnuts can also result in dark brown stains over the nails. Staining may be differentiated from pigmentation by simply scraping the nail. More generalized brown nail discoloration may be seen with long-term hydroxyurea administration and with hyperthyroidism.

Material Available on Student Consult

Review Questions and Answers about Nail Lentigo

SUGGESTED READINGS

Fawcett RS, Linford S, Stulberg DL. Nail abnormalities: Clues to systemic disease. Am Fam Physician 2004;69: 1417–1424.

Habif TP. Nail diseases. In Clinical Dermatology: A Color Guide to Diagnosis and Therapy. Philadelphia, Mosby, 2004, pp 864–868.

Levit EK, Kagan MH, Scher RK, Grossman M, Altman E. The ABC rule for clinical detection of sub-ungual melanoma. J Am Acad Dermatol 2000:42:269–274.

Mayeaux EJ. Nail disorders. Primary Care 2000;27: 333–350.

60

Rash and Fever (Rocky Mountain Spotted Fever)

Walter D. Leventhal

KEY POINTS

1. A high degree of suspicion in any patient who develops an unusual flu-like illness with minimal respiratory symptoms during the spring and summer months.
2. A history of tick bite or environmental exposure to ticks.
3. A willingness to begin doxycycline, especially in the absence of confirmatory laboratory evidence.
4. A maculopapular rash on the forearms and/or ankle areas in a patient with fever and severe headache during the summer months.

INITIAL VISIT

Subjective

Patient Identification and Presenting Problem

Kathy T. is a 33-year-old white woman from Chicago who presents to her family physician in May with a 1- to 2-day history of flu-like illness: headache, myalgia, nausea, and a temperature that has ranged between 37.8°C and 38.3°C (100°F and 101°F). About 10 days earlier, she and her husband had gone to their mountain cabin in North Carolina to clear out the underbrush. While there she found a tick on her abdomen one evening, and she removed it. Kathy is examined briefly, and antipyretics and antiemetics are prescribed. Over the next several days, her condition changes, with development of swollen cervical glands and continued nausea and vomiting.

SECOND VISIT

Kathy returns to her physician 3 days later. Examination fails to show any signs of pulmonary, cardio-vascular, or abdominal infection, and there is no hepatosplenomegaly. A diagnosis of a viral syndrome is made. A complete blood count shows a hemoglobin of 11.3 g/dL and a white blood cell count of 9500/mm^3: 65% polymorphonuclear leukocytes, 30% lymphocytes, and 5% monocytes. Platelets are noted to be 90,000/mm^3. The patient mentions the tick bite again, but only supportive therapy is prescribed.

Within 36 hours, Kathy's condition has worsened and her musculoskeletal pain has increased. The fever has persisted, and she has developed a reddish purple macular rash on her forearms and legs. Overnight, Kathy's level of consciousness has diminished to the point that she does not respond to verbal stimuli. The rash has developed into purpura, some parts of which are palpable, spreading centrally to involve her thighs and trunk.

Kathy is immediately admitted to an intensive care unit with a presumptive diagnosis of sepsis of uncertain cause. Her platelet count now is 9000/mm^3, and her white blood cell count has risen to 26,500/mm^3. Cultures are drawn, and intravenous chloramphenicol and gentamicin are administered. She has begun to have seizures and has developed renal and hepatic failure. The patient became hypotensive, and all resuscitative efforts failed. She died within 24 hours after admission.

An autopsy has determined her death to be due to disseminated intravascular coagulation, probably caused by rickettsial disease or meningococcemia. Cultures for meningococcus are negative and complement fixation titers and indirect fluorescent antibodies are negative for *Rickettsia* infection, but the diagnosis is later confirmed as *Rickettsia* by immunofluorescent staining of skin biopsies.

DIFFERENTIAL DIAGNOSIS

The combination of fever and rash presents the practitioner with a difficult and common problem. Although many conditions may present initially with

---

fever and rash, one can subdivide these by considering their potential severity, for example, life threatening or minor.

Life-threatening conditions associated with fever and rash include:

1. *Rocky Mountain spotted fever.* See diagnosis of Kathy's case in Discussion section.
2. *Meningococcemia.* Meningococcemia tends to occur in late winter and early spring and often in crowded conditions, e.g., barracks or schools. The patient may present with petechiae initially on the trunk and extremities, but in fulminating cases, petechiae can spread visibly over several hours. Shock and disseminated intravascular coagulation are associated clinical manifestations. Diagnosis is confirmed by Gram stain of skin lesions, blood cultures, and spinal fluid examination. A chronic form of meningococcemia associated with rash has also been described.
3. *Disseminated gonococcemia.* There is a much higher incidence in women. The rash consists of pustules on an erythematous base, usually over the extremities. It is often associated with migratory polyarthralgia, arthritis, and pelvic inflammatory disease. Diagnosis can be confirmed by a Gram stain of the lesions as well as culture and sensitivity of the blood, joint fluid, or cervical secretions.
4. *Toxic shock syndrome.* Toxic shock syndrome occurs predominantly in women, with the rash preceded by a flu-like illness and diarrhea associated with mucus. The rash is macular, giving a sunburned appearance. It occurs over the whole body but is seen mainly on the hands and feet. The clinical presentation is that of multisystem involvement. The diagnosis is confirmed by history, physical examination, and isolation of a toxin-producing strain of *Staphylococcus aureus.*
5. *Bacterial endocarditis.* Bacterial endocarditis is often associated with a history of valvular heart disease, prosthetic valves, and recent dental or surgical procedures. The rash is petechial and associated with Osler's nodes and Janeway's lesions. The rash is found in the palate and upper chest and may be present on the palms, fingers, soles, and toes. A heart murmur, splenomegaly, hematuria, and metastatic abscesses may be present. Diagnosis is by echocardiography and serial blood cultures.
6. *Lyme disease.* Lyme disease is caused by exposure to ticks in endemic areas—the Northeast, Midwest, or West—in the summer. The rash classically manifests as erythema migrans, often on the thigh, groin, or axillae. Clinically, the patient presents with a flu-like syndrome, later developing central nervous system, cardiac, or joint involvement. The diagnosis is confirmed by history and serology.

The preceding differential diagnosis does not include many other minor conditions associated with fever and rash often found in children—that is, the viral exanthems associated with measles, chicken pox, roseola, rubella, and fifth disease (erythema infectiosum). One should also consider in this category the rashes associated with drug reactions, which also may be associated with fever (Table 60-1).

DISCUSSION

This case illustrates many of the characteristics of Rocky Mountain spotted fever. Unfortunately, it also demonstrates the rapid course of the infection from the time of first exposure to the tick to prodrome and ultimately to fulminating multi-organ failure and shock when not recognized and treated (American Academy of Pediatrics, 2003 ◐).

The patient lived in Chicago but had vacationed in North Carolina, and this particular area typifies the most common area of cases reported, that is, the south Atlantic, southeastern, and south central states. The name Rocky Mountain spotted fever is misleading because even though the condition has been reported in every state, after the Carolinas and Tennessee, Oklahoma is the state with the most other cases reported (Gubler et al., 1994 ◐). A clue to the etiology is that the majority of these cases appear between April and late September (that is, the spring and summer), which is when ticks are most prevalent. This is also the time when people are active outdoors and therefore more prone to exposure. The main vector for this condition is the American dog tick, which transmits the offending organism, *Rickettsia rickettsii.*

After the tick has bitten its human host, organisms are usually disseminated through the bloodstream during the first 6 to 12 hours, when the tick is still attached to the host. Attachment by the tick to the host is usually painless, and the tick is often discovered only accidentally at the end of the day when the patient undresses.

This patient also showed the initial symptoms of a flu-like illness, fever, headache, myalgia, and sometimes vomiting within 4 to 20 days after being bitten.

Usually the rash occurs on the fourth to the sixth day after the patient first complains of the systemic symptom; it begins on the wrist and ankles. It can then involve the palms and soles and later becomes more generalized. Initially, the rash is erythematous and macular but can become petechial if untreated (Habif, 2004 ◐). The rash is difficult to see in African Americans. It is also important to note that the rash does not develop in approximately 15% of cases. The infection is then referred to as Rocky Mountain spot-*less* fever. The spotless type of rash appears to be more common in adults.

Table 60-1 Some Major Diseases Associated with Fever and Rash

Disease	Morphology of Rash	Distribution of Rash	Diagnostic Method	Treatment
Ecthyma gangrenosum and *Pseudomonas* septicemia	Erythematous to purpuric macules, hemorrhagic vesicles, bullae, nodules, painless ulcers with central necrotic, black eschar	Especially in axillae and anogenital regions	Blood culture; biopsy with tissue culture	Admit to hospital; aminoglycoside plus an antipseudomonal penicillin or antipseudomonal cephalosporin (e.g., ceftazidime or cefepime)
Meningococcemia and purpura fulminans	Petechiae, macules, papules, purpura (may become ecchymotic)	Generalized; especially on lower extremities; neck and face usually spared	Blood culture	Admit to hospital; penicillin G or third-generation cephalosporin (e.g., ceftriaxone)
Vibrio vulnificus infection	Large, hemorrhagic bullae are characteristic; also cellulitis, lymphangitis	Especially on lower extremities	Blood and wound cultures	Admit to hospital; doxycycline plus ceftazidime; débridement often necessary
Staphylococcal toxic shock syndrome	Scarlatiniform rash (diffuse erythema), strawberry tongue; desquamation late in course	Generalized	Clinical assessment of diagnostic criteria	Admit to hospital; appropriate antibiotic (e.g., nafcillin); supportive care
Staphylococcal scalded skin syndrome	Diffuse, ill-defined erythema with fine sandpaper appearance; peeling of skin; Nikolsky's sign present	Generalized; especially in perineal and periumbilical regions (in neonates) and extremities (in older children)	Blood cultures	Admit to hospital; antistaphylococcal antibiotics (e.g., nafcillin)
Streptococcal toxic shock syndrome	Localized area of cellulitis or necrotizing fasciitis; sometimes generalized erythema as well	Localized or generalized	Clinical assessment; blood cultures; culture of local primary lesion if present; CT scan to evaluate for necrotizing fasciitis	Admit to hospital; penicillin G plus clindamycin
Disseminated candidiasis	Erythematous papules and nodules	Trunk and extremities	Blood and tissue cultures	Admit to hospital; amphotericin B or fluconazole
Stevens-Johnson syndrome	Macules, plaques, target lesions (both typical and atypical), vesicles, bullae, erosions and blisters of mucous membranes	Generalized	Fulfillment of clinical and histopathologic criteria	Admit to hospital; supportive care; discontinuation of unnecessary drugs; antibiotic therapy for *Mycoplasma pneumoniae* if indicated
Toxic epidermal necrolysis	Macules, target lesions, large bullae, severe mucosal erosions	Generalized; especially on trunk and proximal extremities	Fulfillment of clinical and histopathologic criteria	Same as for Stevens-Johnson syndrome

Table 60-1 Some Major Diseases Associated with Fever and Rash (Continued)

Disease	Morphology of Rash	Distribution of Rash	Diagnostic Method	Treatment
Infective endocarditis	Petechiae, purpura, Osler's nodes, Janeway's lesions, splinter hemorrhages	Petechiae and purpura on heels, shoulders, legs, oral mucosa, conjunctivae; Osler's nodes on digits (especially pulps of fingers and toes); Janeway's lesions on palms and soles; splinter hemorrhages on nail plates	Blood cultures; echocardiography; clinical presentation	Admit to hospital; appropriate antibiotic therapy
Scarlet fever (usually *Streptococcus pyogenes* [group A streptococcus])	Diffuse erythema with punctate elevations ("sand paper skin"); linear striations (Pastia's lines) of confluent petechiae (which can be demonstrated on arms by applying a tourniquet)	Generalized, with sparing of area around mouth ("circumoral pallor")	Clinical assessment; throat culture; blood cultures	Penicillin
North American blastomycosis	Inflammatory papules and nodules with crusts; hyperkeratotic plaques with central ulceration	Face and extremities	Blood culture; biopsy with tissue culture	Itraconazole or amphotericin B
Histoplasmosis	Ulcers, papules, plaques, purpura, abscesses, nodules, mucosal ulcerations	Generalized	Blood cultures; biopsy and tissue cultures	Itraconazole or amphotericin B
Coccidioidomycosis	Papules, nodules, plaques, ulcers, papulopustules	Head	Blood cultures; biopsy and tissue cultures	Fluconazole or amphotericin B
Cryptococcosis	Papules, plaques, nodules, palpable purpura, cellulitis, pyoderma gangrenosum–like ulcers	Head and neck	Blood and tissue cultures	Amphotericin B
Rocky Mountain spotted fever	Macules, papules; later becomes petechial	Wrists and ankles initially, then palms and soles; finally, centripetal spread to face, trunk, and more proximal aspects of extremities	Fourfold increase in antibody titers between acute and convalescent phases	Doxycycline
Primary HIV infection	Macules, papules, mucocutaneous ulcers, palatal papules	Face, trunk	HIV-1 RNA testing and HIV antibody testing (ELISA)	See Chapter 17

Continued

Table 60-1   Some Major Diseases Associated with Fever and Rash (Continued)

Disease	Morphology of Rash	Distribution of Rash	Diagnostic Method	Treatment
Leptospirosis	Macules, papules, urticaria (wheals), purpura	Trunk	Four-fold increase in antibody titers between acute and convalescent phases	Doxycycline or penicillin G
Disseminated gonococcal infection	Macules, papules, vesicles, and petechiae initially, which may evolve into hemorrhagic vesicopustules	Distal extremities, typically near an involved joint	Blood cultures; biopsy with tissue cultures; cultures of urethra, cervix, rectum, and pharynx	Ceftriaxone
Lyme disease	Macules, papules, erythema chronica migrans	Trunk, lower extremities; classically a single lesion but multiple lesions can be present	Serologic tests 4–6 wk after onset	Doxycycline
Typhoid fever (*Salmonella typhi*)	Slightly raised pink macules that blanch on pressure (rose spots)	Trunk, anteriorly and posteriorly (typically in crops of about 10–20 lesions)	Blood cultures; urine and stool cultures; smear and culture of rose spots	Ciprofloxacin, trimethoprim-sulfamethoxazole, or third-generation cephalosporin (ceftriaxone or cefotaxime)
Mycoplasma pneumoniae infection	Maculopapular or morbilliform rash most common; a variety of rashes can be seen, including urticaria, erythema multiforme (including Stevens-Johnson syndrome), erythema nodosum, and papulovesicular lesions	Variable	Fourfold increase in antibody titers between acute and convalescent phases, or demonstration of high IgM antibody titer	Doxycycline or a macrolide antibiotic (erythromycin, azithromycin, or clarithromycin)
Rat-bite fever caused by *Spirillum minus*	Maculopapular, later becoming petechial	Begins on abdomen; progresses to extremities; may involve palms and soles	Inoculation of blood or wound aspirate into mice or guinea pigs; darkfield examination of bite, rash, or aspirate from lymph node; RPR (VDRL) often false positive (50%)	Penicillin G
Rat-bite fever caused by *Streptobacillus moniliformis*	Maculopapular or petechial	Most extensive on extremities; typically around joints; may become generalized	Blood, wound, or joint fluid cultures; serologic tests may be helpful (fourfold increase in antibody titers between acute and convalescent phases)	Penicillin G

Table 60-1 Some Major Diseases Associated with Fever and Rash (Continued)

Disease	Morphology of Rash	Distribution of Rash	Diagnostic Method	Treatment
Epidemic typhus	Macules, papules, petechiae	Axillary folds, trunk, extremities (characteristically the face, palms, and soles are spared)	Fourfold increase in antibody titers between acute and convalescent phases	Doxycycline
Murine typhus	Macules, papules, morbilliform rash	Begins on inner surfaces of arms and axillae; quickly becomes generalized, involving especially the trunk (limited involvement of face, palms, and soles)	Fourfold increase in antibody titers between acute and convalescent phases	Doxycycline
Acute rheumatic fever	Macules, erythema marginatum, subcutaneous nodules	Erythema marginatum on trunk, extremities; subcutaneous nodules on extensor surfaces near joints	Fulfillment of Jones' criteria	Benzathine penicillin G
Secondary syphilis	Macules, papules, mucous patches, condylomata lata; rash is sometimes pustular	Usually generalized, with involvement of palms and soles; sometimes confined to palms and soles or to face	RPR (VDRL) is nearly always positive in secondary syphilis (in contrast to other stages of syphilis); confirmed by FTA-ABS (or MHA-TP) assays; dark-field microscopy	Benzathine penicillin G
Herpes zoster (shingles and disseminated herpes zoster)	Grouped vesicles on an erythematous base; hemorrhagic bullae; in disseminated form, large ulcers and plaques	Shingles has dermatomal distribution; disseminated herpes zoster is generalized	Tzanck smear or direct fluorescent antibody test	Acyclovir
Babesiosis	Petechiae, purpura, ecchymoses	Generalized	Giemsa-stained blood smear or indirect immunofluorescence	Clindamycin and quinine
Ehrlichiosis	Usually, macules and papules; may be petechial; diffuse erythema sometimes seen	Trunk	Fourfold increase in antibody titers between acute and convalescent phases; indirect immunofluorescence	Doxycycline

Continued

Table 60-1 Some Major Diseases Associated with Fever and Rash (Continued)

Disease	Morphology of Rash	Distribution of Rash	Diagnostic Method	Treatment
Kawasaki disease	Erythema (most often, raised, deep red, plaquelike eruption; sometimes morbilliform); swelling of hands and feet; involvement of mucous membranes (dry, fissured lips, strawberry tongue; oropharyngeal erythema; conjunctival suffusion; later, desquamation)	Generalized, especially on trunk and extremities; accentuation in perineal area	Clinical criteria with exclusion of other etiologies	Aspirin; IV immune globulin

CT, computed tomography; ELISA, enzyme-linked immunosorbent assay; FTA-ABS, fluorescent treponemal antibody, absorbed; HIV, human immunodeficiency virus; IgM, Immunoglobulin M; IV, intravenous; MHA-TP, microhemagglutination–*Treponema pallidum*; RPR, rapid plasma reagin; VDRL, Venereal Disease Research Laboratory.
From Longshore S, Camisa C. Fever with rash and other skin lesions. In Bryan CS (ed): Infectious Diseases in Primary Care. Philadelphia, WB Saunders, 2002, pp 181–184.

The fact that systemic symptoms frequently develop before the rash appears is important in considering preventive and early treatment modalities. Rocky Mountain spotted fever should be suspected in any patient who presents with a flu-like illness with headache and who has been in the endemic areas, especially during the summer. The physician should be particularly suspicious when the patient reports removing a tick. Unfortunately, in the case presented, despite the fact that the history of the tick bite was given repeatedly, it was ignored, with deadly consequences. The overall mortality for an untreated individual may be as high as 30% (Braunwald et al., 2002; Habif, 2004). The mortality is usually higher for individuals who are 40 years or older and for African Americans. Most of the delays in initiating appropriate treatment result from failure to recognize the significance of the history of a tick bite in an endemic area.

The diagnosis must rely on a high degree of suspicion and on familiarity with the clinical presentation and the epidemiologic criteria for the area. This case also illustrates the importance of a physician's asking about and paying attention to a patient's history of travel and insect bites, especially when a patient presents with a flu-like illness in the summer. When this patient presented to her physician with a flu-like illness, thrombocytopenia was noted, but no intervention was initiated.

Laboratory diagnosis is usually confirmed serologically with fourfold increases or decreases in antibody titer between acute and convalescent sera by indirect immunofluorescence, complement fixation, indirect hemagglutination, or latex agglutination (Centers for Disease Control and Prevention, 2004).

In practical terms, the decision to treat the patient suspected of having Rocky Mountain spotted fever should not await the result of a laboratory test. Only on the very rarest of occasions is culture from blood or tissue obtained. Complement fixation and microagglutination tests are specific for the disease but lack sensitivity, especially when the patient has received antibiotic treatment. In the case described, confirmation of the diagnosis was obtained by immunofluorescent staining of the skin biopsy specimen.

Treatment in the early phases of the suspected illness is very effective. Drugs of choice are tetracycline and doxycycline. Doxycycline is given in the following recommended doses: 100 mg twice daily for adults and children weighing more than 100 pounds (45 kg) and 2.2 mg/kg twice daily for children weighing less than 100 pounds. Duration is 7 to 10 days, and in the severely compromised, the dose may be given parenterally. Tetracycline would still be a reasonable alternative. Chloramphenicol is no longer considered appropriate (American Academy of Pediatrics, 2003; Centers for Disease Control and Prevention, 2004).

Given the widespread range of illnesses that can result from tickborne diseases, including Lyme disease, relapsing fever, ehrlichiosis, tularemia, tick fever, and babesiosis, this case also provides an opportunity to consider the control of all tickborne infections.

Physicians and local communities should be aware of the prevalence of tickborne infections in their areas. The onset of spring each year should provide a reminder to everyone to promulgate precautions through the summer. Some specific suggestions include the following (Gubler et al., 1994©):

1. Widespread education, especially in endemic areas by all the media from early spring through summer.
2. The avoidance of known tick-infested areas.
3. Use of protective clothing to cover the arms, legs, and other exposed areas.
4. Permethrin spray to decrease tick attachment may be employed, and tick repellents containing diethyltoluamide may also be used to limit exposure to ticks. Great care especially with children should be employed in using diethyltoluamide-containing repellents.
5. Regular body checks for tick attachment by people who have been possibly exposed in endemic areas should be performed. Adults should inspect themselves and their children's bodies regularly for potential tick exposure. The more frequently this is done, the better. It is generally thought that the longer the tick remains attached, the higher the inoculum will be.
6. Tick removal should also be taught with an emphasis on removing all the mouth parts with curved forceps or tweezers and avoidance of squeezing tick body parts. A simple plastic tool called Ticked Off is now available. It consists of a small plastic spoon-shaped instrument with a V shaped notch cut into the distal part of the spoon. If the mouth parts are placed in the notch, the tick and all its body parts may be removed with careful pressure and traction (Gubler et al., 1994©).

This case of Rocky Mountain spotted fever embodies many of the basic principles of modern family medicine, namely the prevention of a serious illness, the ability to make an early and accurate diagnosis and provide effective treatment, and the opportunity to educate our patients and communities.

Material Available on Student Consult

Review Questions and Answers about Rocky Mountain Spotted Fever

REFERENCES

American Academy of Pediatrics. 2003 Redbook: Report of the Committee on Infectious Diseases, 26th ed. Elk Grove, IL, American Academy of Pediatrics, 2003, pp 532–534.©

Braunwald E, Fauci A, Kasper D, Hauser S, Longo D, Jameson JL. Harrison's Principles of Internal Medicine. Companion Handbook, 15th ed. New York, McGraw-Hill, 2002, pp 465–474.©

Gubler D, Koster F, Legters L, et al. A field guide to animal-borne infections. Patient Care 1994;28:23–44.©

Habif T. Clinical Dermatology, 4th ed. St. Louis: Mosby-Year Book, 2004.©

Longshore S, Camisa C. Fever with rash and other skin lesions: Infectious Diseases in Primary Care. In Bryan CS (ed): Philadelphia, WB Saunders, 2002, pp 181–184.©

Centers for Disease Control and Prevention. Fatal cases of Rocky Mountain spotted fever in family clusters—Three states, 2003. MMWR Morb Mortal Wkly Rep 2004;53:407–410. Reprinted in JAMA 2004;292:31–33.©

61 Red Area on Left Temple (Basal Cell Carcinoma)

Mark Andrews

INITIAL VISIT

Subjective

Patient Identification and Presenting Problem

Jane S. is a 76-year-old white woman who presents with a complaint of a puffy red area on her left temple, noted for the past several months, that seems to be slowly growing (Fig. 61-1).

Present Illness

Mrs. S. states that the lesion arose gradually as a small red spot and later became a little larger and elevated. She denies similar rashes, trauma to the area, or previous insect bites. No associated pruritus, pain,

crusting, or drainage is noted. There is no immediate family history of similar skin problems.

Medical History

Mrs. S. has a history of hypertension, for which she is taking lisinopril. She is also taking ibuprofen to manage the symptoms of degenerative joint disease in her knees. She has no history of significant dermatologic problems or recurrent skin infections. She has not taken antibiotics recently. She states she has not been using new cosmetics or soaps. There is no history of major previous surgery.

Family History

Mrs. S. has one sister who has multiple health problems but no history of chronic skin problems. Her parents died a number of years ago and their health problems are not well known.

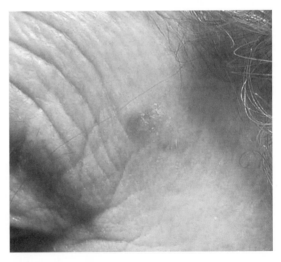

Figure 61-1 The timed spot freeze technique demonstrated on a superficial nodular basal cell carcinoma on the left temple. The lesion is approximately 10 mm.

Evidence levels Ⓐ Randomized, controlled trials (RCTs), meta-analyses, well-designed systematic reviews of RCTs. **Ⓑ** Case-control or cohort studies, nonrandomized clinical trials, systematic reviews of studies other than RCTs, cross-sectional studies, retrospective studies, certain uncontrolled studies. **Ⓒ** Consensus statements, expert guidelines, usual practice, opinion.

Social History

Mrs. S. is widowed and has been retired from the accounting field for more than 15 years. She has no smoking history and denies alcohol use. There is no history of illicit drug use.

Review of Systems

The patient denies fever, chills, pruritus, cough or cold symptoms, or rash in other body areas. She has had no sore throat or localized facial pain.

Objective

Physical Examination

Mrs. S. is a well-developed, well-nourished, alert woman. She is not in distress. Her height is 5 feet 1 inch, and her weight is 145 pounds. Her temperature is 37°C (98.6°F), respiratory rate is 16, blood pressure is 148/84, and pulse is 80. A focused skin examination reveals an approximately round, 1-cm, slightly raised red nodule on the left temple. There is no similar skin lesion identified elsewhere. The area in question is well demarcated and without ulceration, crusting, or bleeding. On examination with a hand lens, the tissue is opalescent, with increased vascularity and some vessel tortuosity. The area is nontender, but the raised tissue is firm and palpable.

Assessment

Working Diagnosis

The working diagnosis, based on clinical appearance and the patient's history, is an early primary nodular basal cell carcinoma. Other possibilities in the differential diagnosis, although much less likely, include a squamous cell carcinoma or—least possible—an inflamed seborrheic keratosis.

Seborrheic keratoses tend to have a rougher, gritty surface without inflammation and a more stuck-on appearance with darker pigmentation. On close observation, small, clear pseudocysts can often be seen in the body of the lesion.

Squamous cell cancer, on the other hand, is often more distorted on the surface and has a greater tendency to ulcerate and crust and invade tissue, except for the in situ form (Bowen's disease), which is indolent and flat and often appears like a chronic fungal or eczematous red patch, occasionally with some crusting.

Plan

Diagnostic

The current working diagnostic possibilities are discussed with Mrs. S. She agrees to undergo a shave biopsy under local lidocaine anesthesia, with the biopsy performed using a sterilized razor blade and postprocedural hemostasis achieved with aluminum chloride

Table 61-1 Efficacy of Cryosurgery

Lesion	Cure Rate (%)
Viral warts (hands)	75
Dermatofibroma	90
Actinic keratosis	99
Bowen's disease	>95
Basal cell carcinoma	>95
Squamous cell carcinoma	>95

Modified from Dawber R. Cryosurgery. In Lask G, Moy R (eds): Principles and Techniques of Cutaneous Surgery. New York, McGraw-Hill, 1996.

solution (Drysol). A Polysporin dressing is applied after the procedure. The various options for management of the presumed basal skin cancer are discussed.

Patient Education

Mrs. S. is informed of the various treatment options and allowed to select among the reasonable alternatives. Primary excision might be considered first, but this would require excising an elliptical area approximately 1.5 to 2 cm by 5 to 6 cm, which is a considerable size excision on the temple region for a neoplasm of fairly low aggressiveness. There is also the option of performing electrodesiccation and curettage under local anesthesia, and finally the option of cryosurgery, which offers some compelling advantages, including lack of prep time and expensive supplies, no need for injection anesthesia, and minimal postprocedural infection risk, wound care, or need for suture removal. Cure rates are about 97% in experienced hands compared with 98% for primary excision and 99% for Mohs' technique (which is not strictly indicated for small primary basal cell lesions that are well demarcated and not in areas that are difficult to treat; it is more aggressive and costly than needed) (Graham, 1994❸, 2001❸; Kuflik and Gage, 1991❸) (Table 61-1).

FOLLOW-UP VISIT

Subjective

Mrs. S. returns for definitive treatment and is considering cryosurgical intervention if needed. The shave biopsy site has healed well, without evidence of secondary bacterial infection or significant irritation.

Objective

Physical Examination

Her vital signs are stable and the biopsy site is healing nicely. The minimal crusting is removed easily, and no ulceration or bleeding is noted.

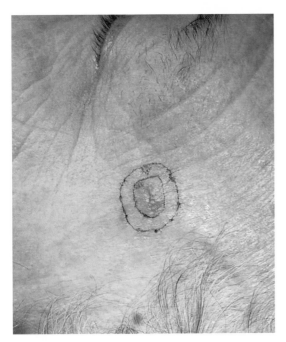

Figure 61-2 The lesion with an appropriate margin of normal skin outlined, about 5 additional millimeters.

Laboratory Tests

Her biopsy result reveals histologic changes consistent with a nodular basal cell carcinoma, with the tumor extending to the bottom of the shave specimen.

Assessment

Mrs. S. has a small, localized, superficial but nodular-type basal cell carcinoma of the left temple area.

Plan

Therapeutic

The cryosurgery option for management is again discussed with the patient, and informed consent is

obtained. The perimeter of the basal cell cancer is outlined with a surgical marking pen, and then 5 mm further out a perimeter is also marked for delineating the outer border of the eventual freeze halo (Fig. 61-2). The liquid nitrogen spray is then begun using a timed spot freeze technique with the gun 1 cm away from the center of the lesion. The spray is continuously administered until the freeze zone extends to the outer marked margin of the halo zone, and then the spray is pulsed to maintain the freeze area for 30 seconds (Fig. 61-3). The freezing is then stopped and the area is allowed to completely thaw over 3 to 4 minutes. The process is repeated once for a total of two complete freeze-thaw cycles (Graham, 2001❻; Kuflik and Gage, 1991❺). The treatment at this point is complete. Follow-up care instructions are given to the patient (Box 61-1). Cosmesis with cryosurgery is quite satisfactory compared with the cosmetic effect remaining after other treatment modalities (Fig. 61-4). Common side effects are hypopigmentation (more of a concern in darker pigmented individuals), hair loss, and slightly

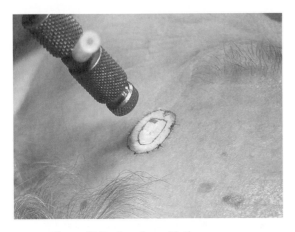

Figure 61-3 Freezing with the cryogun.

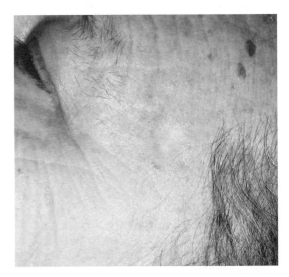

Figure 61-4 Follow-up image of treatment site healing at 5 months.

Table 61-2   Contraindications to Cryosurgery

Absolute Contraindications
Proven sensitivity or adverse reaction to cryosurgery
Melanoma
Areas of compromised circulation
Sclerosing basal cell or recurrent basal cell/squamous cell carcinoma, particularly in high-risk areas
   (temples, nasolabial groove)
Patient nonacceptance of potential pigment changes
Lesions in which tissue pathology is required (In these situations biopsy specimens should be obtained
   before cryosurgery treatment is undertaken)

Relative Contraindications
Cold intolerance
Raynaud's disease
Multiple myeloma
Cryoglobulinemia
Collagen and autoimmune diseases
Cold urticaria
Concurrent treatment with immunosuppressive drugs
Pyoderma gangrenosum

Modified from Andrews M. Cryosurgery for common skin conditions. Am Fam Physician 2004;69:2365–2372.

slower initial healing due to the local inflammation resulting from the freezing process (Heidenheim and Jemec, 1991). Scarring is a rare complication of cryosurgery unless continuous freezing at one location is maintained for more then 30 seconds after an adequate freeze ball has formed around the target area; longer freezing can result in disruption of the collagen matrix of the skin and possible scarring (Andrews, 2004 ⓒ). Table 61-2 lists contraindications to cryosurgery and Table 61-3 lists common side effects.

DISCUSSION

Although family physicians are not routinely trained in the cryotherapy management of skin cancers, the principles and techniques involved are not complex or difficult to master. Workshops are offered at a number of national meetings that will assist clinicians in developing the basic skills needed to begin selectively treating more superficial cutaneous malignancies as their experience develops.

Achieving an adequate, usually 3- to 5-mm, halo of frozen tissue around a lesion and utilizing a repeat freeze-thaw cycle for deeper tumors should yield a cure rate of 97% to 99% in appropriately selected tumors (Graham, 2001 ⓒ; Graham and Clark, 1990 ⓒ). The surgeon's preoccupation with always obtaining clear tissue margins with malignant lesions has pervaded training programs but is not borne out as definitely superior in light of the similar low recurrence rates achieved with cryosurgical techniques. This may be partially attributable to patient selection, but it could also reflect the immunologic activation that occurs with inflammation arising from the freezing itself.

Cryosurgery has proved competitive with other techniques in the management of skin cancers such as basal cell and squamous cell carcinomas. It is also commonly used in the treatment of premalignant lesions and in situ malignancies such as actinic

Table 61-3   Complications and Side Effects of Cryosurgery

Acute
Pain
Edema
Blister formation
Bleeding (at the freeze site)
Syncope (rare—vasovagal)
Headache (after treatment of facial lesions)

Delayed
Infection (rare)
Bleeding
Excess granulation tissue (rare)

Protracted—Temporary
Hyperpigmentation
Milia
Hypertrophic scars
Altered sensation

Protracted—Permanent
Hypopigmentation
Hair and hair follicle loss
Atrophy (rare)

Modified from Andrews M. Cryosurgery for common skin conditions. Am Fam Physician 2004;69: 2365–2372.

keratosis, lentigo maligna, Bowen's disease, keratoacanthoma, and actinic cheilitis (Andrews, 2004©; Graham, 1994©).

Tumor Selection

Well-defined or well-demarcated basal cell or squamous cell carcinomas less than 1 to 2 cm in size and 3 mm in depth respond most favorably to cryosurgical intervention (Graham, 2001©). Superficial spreading and smaller noduloulcerative basal cell cancer subtypes are some of the most readily amenable to treatment with this modality. Squamous cell carcinoma in situ (Bowen's disease) and squamous cell carcinoma arising in hypertrophic actinic keratosis, which are less aggressive variants of this type of skin cancer, are particularly ideal for cryosurgery (Cooper, 2001©; Dawber et al., 1997). Tumors of the ear or nose overlying cartilage or bone respond well, with excellent healing. Sclerosing or morpheaform basal cell carcinomas, because of their ill-defined margins, should probably not be treated with cryosurgery. Neither should larger lesions of the scalp and nasolabial folds. Many clinicians avoid cryosurgical treatment of tumors in the lower extremities, particularly in the elderly, because of issues of delayed healing and higher rates of wound infections (Dawber et al., 1997).

Material Available on Student Consult

Review Questions and Answers about Basal Cell Carcinoma

REFERENCES

Andrews M. Cryosurgery for common skin conditions. Am Fam Physician 2004;69:2365–2372.©

Cooper C. Cryotherapy in general practice. Practitioner 2001;245:954–956.©

Dawber R, Cryosurgery. In Lask G, Moy R (eds): Principles and Techniques of Cutaneous Surgery. New York, McGraw-Hill, 1996.

Dawber R, Colver G, Jackson A. Equipment and techniques. In Cutaneous Cryosurgery: Principles and Clinical Practice. London, Martin Dunitz, 1997, pp 28–36.

Graham G. Cryosurgery for benign, premalignant, and malignant Lesions. In Wheeland R (ed): Cutaneous Surgery. Philadelphia, WB Saunders, 1994.©

Graham G. Cryosurgery in the management of cutaneous malignancies. Clin Dermatol 2001;19:321–327.©

Graham G, Clark L. Statistical analysis in cryosurgery of skin cancer. Clin Dermatol 1990;8:101–107.©

Heidenheim M, Jemec GBE. Side effects of cryosurgery. J Am Acad Dermatol 1991;4:653.

Kuflik EG, Gage AA. The five-year cure rate achieved by cryosurgery for skin cancer. J Am Acad Dermatol 1991; 24:1002–1004.®

SUGGESTED READINGS

Dawber RPR. Cryosurgery: Complications and contraindications. Clin Dermatol 1991;8:96–100.©

Kuflik EG. Cryosurgery updated. J Am Acad Dermatol 1994;31:25–44.®

Luba M, Scott B, Andrew M, Stulberg D. Common benign skin tumors. Am Fam Physician 2003;67:729–738.

Usatine R, Moy R. Cryosurgical technique. In Skin Surgery: A Practical Guide. St. Louis, Mosby, 1998, pp 137–164.©

Zacarian SA. Cryogenics, the cryolesion and the pathogenesis of cryonecrosis. In Zacarian SA (ed): Cryosurgery for Skin Cancer and Cutaneous Disorders. St. Louis, Mosby, 1985, pp 1–30.®

62

Thorn in Bottom of Foot (Plantar Wart)

Daniel L. Stulberg

INITIAL VISIT

Subjective

Patient Identification and Presenting Problem

Wendy R. is a 32-year-old woman who presents with the chief concern of a thorn in the bottom of her foot.

Present Illness

Wendy reports that approximately 4 weeks ago she had been pruning Pyracantha bushes in her yard. The following day she went outside barefooted and stepped on a thorn from the trimmed branches. With some difficulty, she used a razor blade, needle, and tweezers to remove what she thought was the whole thorn from the bottom of her right foot. Two weeks later, after the initial inflammation and pain had subsided, she noticed that the area of the wound had thickened skin and was not returning to a normal appearance. She again attempted home surgery to remove the remaining portion of the thorn but was unable to identify or extract any more material. She now presents to the office to have the area evaluated and the thorn removed.

Medical History

Wendy reports that she is in good health. She had her appendix removed at age 12 and had a tubal ligation after the birth of her fourth child. She reports that she had routine childhood illnesses but no hospitalizations other than for childbirth.

Family History

Wendy's parents are both alive and in good health. Her maternal grandfather had a long history of type 2 diabetes and died of a myocardial infarction at the age of 72. Her paternal grandmother is a survivor of postmenopausal breast cancer.

Health Habits

Wendy is a nonsmoker and drinks no alcohol. She walks regularly for exercise but notes that this has become difficult due to the pain in her foot.

Medications

Wendy takes multivitamins.

Social History

Wendy is married and a full-time homemaker with four school-age children. She is very active in her community.

Review of Systems

Wendy reports that she has not purchased any new shoes in the past 6 months, and her shoes are in good condition. She denies arthritis, arthralgias, or history of foot fractures. She gets dry skin in the winter, which responds to moisturizers. The only other skin concern she has had was warts when she was in grade school.

Evidence levels Ⓐ Randomized, controlled trials (RCTs), meta-analyses, well-designed systematic reviews of RCTs. Ⓑ Case-control or cohort studies, nonrandomized clinical trials, systematic reviews of studies other than RCTs, cross-sectional studies, retrospective studies, certain uncontrolled studies. Ⓒ Consensus statements, expert guidelines, usual practice, opinion.

Objective

Physical Examination

Wendy's vital signs are all within normal limits. She is alert and appropriately and neatly dressed. Examination of her skin reveals several benign-appearing moles on the trunk. Both of her heels have some thickening overlying the Achilles tendons. The plantar surface of her right foot is notable for a raised 7-mm lesion just lateral to the fifth metatarsal head. There is slight irregularity and peeling of the epidermis at that site with diminished normal skin lines. It is firm to the touch, with no erythema, warmth, fluctuance, or drainage. Direct pressure causes moderate discomfort. There are no other skin lesions of note.

Laboratory Tests

No radiographic or laboratory testing is done at the time of visit. A no. 15 blade scalpel is used to shave down the thickened lesion, revealing multiple pinpoint bleeding spots.

Assessment

Working Diagnosis

Plantar wart, based on the location, symptoms, and clinical appearance. There is no evidence of bacterial infection or remaining foreign body to justify a wound exploration.

Differential Diagnosis

1. *Foreign body reaction due to retained thorn.* The history pointed the patient in this direction, but clinical examination failed to support this diagnosis. The inflammatory nature of wood leads to erythema, fluctuance, and even purulent drainage subacutely when it is retained as a foreign body.
2. *Granuloma or cyst due to a foreign body.* This would be a similar possibility but would more likely present later and with deeper findings.
3. *Callus.* In response to excessive pressure, recurrent friction, or poorly fitting shoes, the normal response is to develop a very thickened epidermis in the affected area. Factors incongruous with this diagnosis are the diminished normal skin lines and the pinpoint bleeding spots revealed on paring the lesion.
4. *Corn.* As the result of an underlying bony prominence, there can be excessive callous response and even erosions. This patient has no significant bony abnormalities.
5. *Skin cancer.* Squamous cell cancers can sometimes develop in warts or appear verrucous. This lesion was not present long enough to suggest malignancy; however, if it does not respond to therapy as anticipated, then a biopsy would be prudent.

Plan

Diagnostic

The physical examination and the paring down of the lesion as noted above make the diagnosis. No viral cultures, biopsy, or other laboratory testing is indicated.

Therapeutic

Multiple treatment modalities are available for the destruction of warts. Treatment decisions are based on patient age, location, extent, pain tolerance, risk of scarring, inconvenience, and patient's desires. Cryotherapy can lead to blistering, which could increase the patient's discomfort when walking. After a thorough discussion of the options, Wendy chose over-the-counter topical salicylic acid applied at bedtime after soaking the lesion for 10 minutes. The soaking facilitates penetration of the salicylic acid. Peeling away the dead skin can also aid in the local tissue destruction.

Patient Education

Warts are the outward sign of a viral infection by the human papillomavirus (HPV). The virus can be passed from person to person via direct contact or from contact with a contaminated surface. After infection, the virus lives inside the body and can cause characteristic thickening of the skin, resulting in a wart.

Over-the-counter salicylic acid liquids or patches are reasonably effective for destroying the wart but will not take away the viral infection. Therefore, warts can recur later in life in the same or different areas. Over-the-counter topical treatment usually takes weeks to months to work.

Warts will often go away without treatment, explaining why so many odd "folk remedies" are reported to work.

The body's immune system plays a major role in whether people have warts. That is why people with human immunodeficiency virus or those taking immunosuppressant drugs often develop warts and have a hard time getting rid of them.

Physicians can use many different procedures to destroy warts but there is always the chance of recurrence.

Disposition

Wendy was advised to follow up at the clinic if the wart did not clear up in 2 to 3 months with daily application of salicylic acid or if she desired more aggressive treatment.

FOLLOW-UP VISIT

Subjective

Wendy is seen 2 months after her initial visit. She reports using the salicylic acid daily for 1 month with mild improvement but no resolution of her wart. She then became discouraged and stopped treatment. She states that the wart is back to its previous size and is causing increasing pain with walking.

Objective

Examination of Wendy's foot again shows a thickened, firm epidermal lesion without any evidence of bacterial infection. She has no other significant skin lesions and no indications of other systemic illnesses.

Assessment

Plantar wart with no significant improvement.

Plan

Diagnostic

Since her examination and history indicate no risk factors or indications of an immune system problem, no laboratory testing is indicated.

Therapeutic

Multiple treatment options are discussed with Wendy, including cryotherapy, curettage with electrodesiccation, injection with bleomycin, application of duct tape, laser destruction, or local injection with *Candida albicans* antigen. Wendy chooses to have her wart injected with *Candida albicans* antigen, which is based on the theory that it will induce an immune system reaction locally to the antigen. The warty tissue gets caught up in the associated immune response and is gradually destroyed.

Patient Education

Treating warts can be a very frustrating and time-consuming process. Multiple treatments may be tried before the wart resolves either from the treatment or spontaneously. Many warts will disappear on their own within 1 to 2 years.

Disposition

Wendy is advised to follow up in 2 to 3 months if the wart persists, sooner if there are any signs of infection, increased pain, or other complaints.

DISCUSSION

Wendy's diagnosis of plantar wart is common in family medicine. Prevalence studies have yielded conflicting results, but most data suggest that at any given time approximately 5% of the population has warts, with estimates of occurrence in the school-age population reaching as high as 24% (Allen, 2000Ⓑ). The incidence of true infectivity with HPV is proba-

bly higher, as cells can be infected asymptomatically and the latency period between infection and the display of disease can be as long as 6 months. In general, warts are rarely present in infancy, have a peak incidence in the teen years, and then become less common with age.

Warts are benign neoplasms of the epidermis caused by the HPV. The virus is a double-stranded DNA virus that infects the keratinocytes, causing hyperproliferation and mass effect. The mass is confined to the epidermis, although it may appear to invade the dermis because of downward displacement (Habif, 2004Ⓒ). The category of warts is often further subdivided into common warts, filiform warts, flat warts, and plantar warts. More than 80 types of HPV have been characterized (Gibbs, 2004Ⓑ). Most often, HPV types 1 and 2 are responsible for common and plantar warts. HPV types 2, 4, and 27 have also been implicated in common warts (Gibbs, 2004Ⓑ).

Common Warts (Verruca Vulgaris)

Common warts typically present as flesh-colored papules, starting out as small, pin-sized papules representing discrete hyperkeratosis. They gradually evolve over a period of weeks to months to rough gray, brown, or black dome-shaped, solitary nodules or clusters, often with black dots on their surface (Fig. 62-1). These black dots are thrombosed capillaries. Warts also obscure normal skin lines, which is an important diagnostic feature (Habif, 2001Ⓒ) (Fig. 62-2).

Treatment

Two thirds of common warts resolve spontaneously within a 2-year period. Nongenital warts in the immunocompetent person are usually harmless and medically require no treatment unless associated with pain or disfigurement, which is rare. Still, patients often seek treatment because of the social

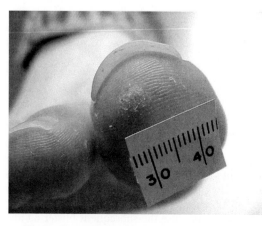

Figure 62-1 Wart with thrombosed capillaries.

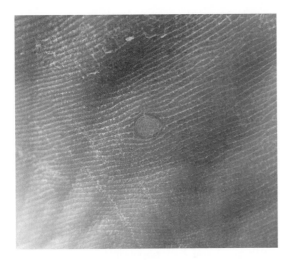

Figure 62-2 Wart displacing normal skin lines.

stigma associated with warts and find themselves having to choose from a wide selection of over-the-counter or physician-recommended treatment options (Gibbs, 2004**B**).

First-line treatments for the common wart include topical salicylic acid and cryotherapy with liquid nitrogen. Wendy opted for topical salicylic acid as her first treatment choice. Therapy with topical solutions containing salicylic acid is clearly superior to treatment with placebo (Gibbs, 2004**B**). Typically, a 17% over-the-counter solution is applied daily until the wart disappears. This requires not only diligence but patience, as it can take weeks to months, even with consistent application. Efficacy is enhanced by paring the superficial layers of the wart with a scalpel, pumice stone, or sandpaper (emery board) as well as occlusion by a nonpermeable membrane. The 40% films or plaster (Duofilm, Mediplast) are cut to the exact size of the wart and then left in place for 48 to 72 hours. They are applied weekly until the wart disappears. Efficacy is again improved by paring the wart before treatment and between applications of the topical patches. The films can be used on common warts and are particularly effective on solitary plantar warts (Barone, 2000**C**).

Cryotherapy with liquid nitrogen is also a common treatment method. Liquid nitrogen can be applied to the surface of a wart through direct application with a cotton-tipped swab or through a spray nozzle mechanism. The goal is a 10- to 15-second freeze with a "freeze halo" extending beyond the margin of the wart by 2 mm. It is less desirable for treatment of periungual warts because postprocedure swelling under the nail can be quite painful. It also must be used with caution in the treatment of plantar warts because the subsequent blistering and swelling can make ambulation extremely painful.

A clinical trial comparing the local application of duct tape with cryotherapy in the treatment of common warts suggested that occlusion with duct tape for 6 of 7 days for as long as 8 weeks was as effective or more effective in the short-term cure of the common wart (Focht, 2002**B**).

Other treatments for common warts that are possibly effective include the daily application of mild corticosteroid cream under an occlusive dressing, electrosurgery after local anesthesia, and, in adults, oral vitamin A 50,000 U/day for no longer than 3 months (contraindicated in pregnancy) (Sauer, 1996**C**).

Flat Warts (Verruca Plana)

These typically present as pink, light brown, or yellow papules that are relatively flat in appearance and typically do not exceed 3 to 4 mm in diameter. They sometimes occur in clusters of 20 to 30 or more and most often are found on the dorsum of the hand, the forehead, and the beard area.

Treatment

Groups of flat warts can sometimes be successfully treated with tretinoin cream 0.025% to 0.1%. This is the preferred method when treating facial warts because of its low risk of scarring. Isolated lesions can be treated by cryotherapy.

Plantar Warts (Verruca Plantaris)

Plantar warts occur on the soles of the foot along pressure points such as the heel or the metatarsal heads (Fig. 62-3). Paring back the epidermal hypertrophy of a plantar wart produces a surface studded with black dots (thrombosed capillaries) that bleed with deeper debridement (Fig. 62-4), whereas paring a simple callus or corn often produces a pale, translucent central core.

Treatment

Treatment of plantar warts is not necessary unless the warts are painful and result in disability. Wendy initially underwent treatment with salicylic acid. Additional treatment options could include cryotherapy or blunt dissection, which is often used by podiatrists. However, when choosing a treatment option for plantar warts, physicians should seek therapies that limit any scarring or inflammation to reduce subsequent disability.

Wendy next chose local injection with *Candida albicans* antigen into the base of her wart (Fig. 62-5). It is theorized that local injection of 1:1000 *Candida albicans* antigen (the author uses Candin for dermal skin testing, 0.1 mL mixed with 0.9 mL of 1:1,000,000 lidocaine, injecting 0.5 mL per wart up to two warts per session and then repeatedly stabs the wart with the injecting needle) stimulates a local immune response resulting in resolution of warts. An unpublished double-blind, placebo-controlled trial in 1999 suggested a

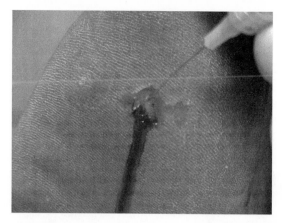

Figure 62-5 Injection of plantar wart with *Candida albicans* antigen mixed with lidocaine.

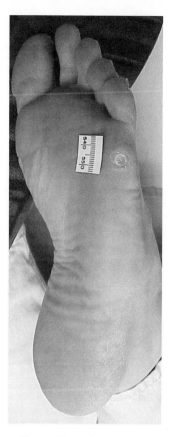

Figure 62-3 Plantar wart.

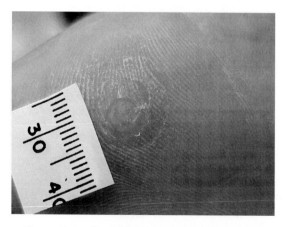

Figure 62-4 Thrombosed capillaries after paring.

superior response to antigen when compared with placebo. Possible complications include potential risk of stimulating an immunologic response to normal gastrointestinal tract floral organisms and the potential risk of triggering a *Candida* hypersensitivity syndrome (Allen, 2000Ⓑ).

Other less common or more invasive treatment options are sometimes used by other specialties.

Treatment of warts is varied and requires much patience as well as persistence. Topical, surgical, and oral therapies have all been used with varying degrees of success. The right treatment plan for any one patient depends on the partnership between physician and patient in reaching a common goal. In the vast majority of cases, warts will resolve spontaneously over the course of months to years, but achieving earlier resolution can be even more satisfying for the patient as well as his or her physician.

Material Available on Student Consult

Review Questions and Answers about Plantar Warts

REFERENCES

Allen AL. What's new in human papillomavirus infection. Curr Opin Pediatr 2000;12:365–369.Ⓑ

Barone EJ. Skin Disorders: The Academy Collection Quick Reference Guides for Family Physicians. New York, Lippincott Williams & Wilkins, 2000.Ⓒ

Focht DR. The efficacy of duct tape vs cryotherapy in the treatment of verruca vulgaris (the common wart). Arch Pediatr Adolesc Med 2002;156:971–974.Ⓑ

Gibbs S. Local treatment for cutaneous warts (review). Cochrane Database Syst Rev 2004;3.Ⓑ

Habif TP. Skin Disease: Diagnosis and Treatment. St. Louis: Mosby, 2001.Ⓒ

Habif TP. Clinical Dermatology: A Color Guide to Diagnosis and Therapy, 4th ed. St. Louis, Mosby, 2004.Ⓒ

Sauer GC. Manual of Skin Diseases, 7th ed. New York, Lippincott–Raven, 1996.Ⓒ

Stulberg DL, Hutchinson AG. Molluscum contagiosum and warts. Am Fam Physician 2003;67:1233–1240.Ⓒ

Verbov J. How to manage warts. Arch Dis Child 1999; 80:97–99.Ⓒ

Chapter

63 Changing Nevus (Melanoma)

Cheng-Chieh Chuang

KEY POINTS

1. Early detection of curable primary melanoma can be lifesaving for patients, and as a result, gratifying to physicians.

2. Personal risk factors for melanoma include light complexion, inability to tan, blond or red hair, blue eyes, presence of many pigmented lesions, and immunocompromised status. The presence of many clinically atypical moles, a prior history of melanoma, or a family history of melanoma confers the greatest risk.

3. Familial atypical mole syndrome is an autosomal dominant syndrome characterized by multiple nevi and atypical nevi, with significant risk for development of melanoma.

4. Increased exposure to ultraviolet radiation (UVA and UVB) is a major environmental contributor to the risk of developing melanoma.

5. About half of melanomas develop de novo, the others from an existing lesion. Although nevi can be precursors to melanomas, they more often indicate an increased risk; the greater the number of nevi, the greater the risk for melanoma.

6. Early signs of melanoma include asymmetry, border irregularity, color variation, diameter enlargement (greater than 6 mm), and elevation. These elements are usually referred to as the "ABCDE" rule of melanoma. Recent change in a mole in these areas should prompt attention. Bleeding is a late sign of melanoma and usually portends a poor prognosis.

7. There are several benign lesions that may resemble melanoma. Among these are nevi, seborrheic keratoses, angiomas, and dermatofibromas. All suspicious lesions should be excised with narrow margins.

8. Melanoma is generally classified, on the basis of the tumor's microscopic anatomy, as superficial spreading melanoma, nodular melanoma, lentigo maligna melanoma, and acral-lentiginous melanoma. There are two types of local growth in a melanoma: radial and vertical.

9. Breslow's depth of invasion number is the thickness in millimeters from the top of the granular cell layer or base of superficial ulceration to the deepest part of the tumor, and is the most important prognostic variable.

10. The presence of histologic ulceration places the tumor in a later stage.

INITIAL VISIT

Subjective

History of Present Illness

Ms. M. is a 40-year-old sales representative whose sister, while applying sunscreen for her on the beach, noticed a mole that had changed in color.

Ms. M. and her sister have spent summers by the ocean every year since childhood. They use a lot of sunscreen with an SPF of 30 because their skin burns very easily. Ms. M. has always had moles, especially on her back, since her teenage years. Other than this finding, the review of systems is negative.

Family History

Both parents had skin cancer, although the types are unknown.

Medical History

The patient's medical history is negative.

Objective

Physical Examination

The patient has blond hair and blue eyes. She has multiple lentigines on sun-exposed areas. There are many nevi ranging from 2 to 7 mm on her body, mostly on her upper trunk. There are at least 40 nevi on her back alone, 4 of which appear atypical, including the lesion in question. The mole in question is on the right upper back near the axilla. It is asymmetric in shape, slightly raised, about 7 mm in diameter, with an irregular border and variation of dark pigmentation within. There is neither ulceration nor bleeding. No axillary lymphadenopathy is found.

Assessment

The diagnostic assessment is atypical nevus or melanoma with recent changes.

This patient possibly has familial atypical nevi syndrome. She has many nevi, several of which are atypical. Her family history of skin cancer (though type unknown) and increasing numbers of nevi since adolescence also point to this possibility.

Plan

The mole is excised with a narrow margin and sent for pathologic examination.

FOLLOW-UP VISIT

The pathology report suggests superficial spreading melanoma with Breslow's thickness of 0.6 mm without ulceration. The margin is reported to be free of tumor cells.

A second excision with the margin of 1 cm is performed, with the pathologist reporting margins free of tumor cells.

The patient's answers to a review of systems focusing on symptoms in Table 63-1 are negative. A full physical exam does not suggest any signs of metastasis (Johnson et al., 2000 ©).

With the information that Ms. M.'s mother also has a history of melanoma, it was possible to make a clinical diagnosis of familial atypical nevi syndrome for Ms. M.

Ms. M. is instructed on self-examination of her skin using the ABCDE rule (Table 63-2). She is advised that she should never sunbathe and never do outdoor work without appropriate clothing and

---

Table 63-1 Review of Systems for Visceral Melanoma Metastases

Constitutional	Hepatic	Paralysis	Skin
Weight loss	Abdominal pain	Local weakness	Color change
Fatigue	Jaundice		Easy bruising
Malaise		**Musculoskeletal**	New pigmented
Fever	**Neurologic**	Bone pain	skin lesion(s)
Decreased appetite	Headache		Nonhealing/bleeding
Weakness	Focal CNS symptoms	**Gastrointestinal**	skin lesion(s)
	Balance problems	Cramping	
Respiratory	Memory disturbance	Anorexia	**Lymphatics**
Cough	Visual disturbances	Abdominal pain	Lumps
Chest pain	Blackouts	Vomiting	"Swollen glands"
Hemoptysis	Depression	Bleeding	
Dyspnea	Seizures	Constipation	
Pneumonia	Numbness	Nausea	
Pleurisy	Mood swings		

CNS, central nervous system.
Adapted from Johnson TM, Chang A, Redman B, et al. Management of melanoma with a multidisciplinary melanoma clinic model. J Am Acad Dermatol 2000;42:820–826.

Table 63-2	ABCDE Rule of Melanoma Screening

Asymmetry in shape
Border irregularity
Color haphazardly displayed
Diameter enlargement in recent time (>6 mm)
Elevation of the lesion

Any of these may be a sign of melanoma. Often it is not possible to distinguish between an atypical nevus and a melanoma until after biopsy.

Table 63-3	Risk Factors for Developing Cutaneous Melanoma	

Risk Factor	Risk Ratio
Personal history of atypical moles, family history of melanoma, and more than 75 to 100 moles	35
Previous nonmelanoma skin cancer	17
Congenital nevus >20 cm	5–15
History of melanoma	9–10
Family history of melanoma in first-degree relatives	8
Immunosuppression	6–8
2–9 atypical nevi without family history	4.9–7.3
51–100 nevi	3–5
26–50 nevi	1.8–4.4
Chronic tanning with UVA, treatment with PUVA	5.4
Up to three repeated blistering sunburns	1.7–3.8
Freckling	3
Fair skin, inability to tan	2.6
One atypical nevus	2.3
Red or blond hair	2.2

PUVA, oral methoxalen and UVA.
Adapted from Robinson JK. Early detection and treatment of melanoma. Dermatol Nurs 2000; 12:397–402, 441–442.

sunscreen with an SPF of greater than 30. Photographs of her skin are taken for future comparison. She is to be followed every 3 months for 3 years. Thereafter she is to be seen every 6 months.

Ms. M.'s family is advised of their increased risk of melanoma, need for everyday sun protection, the ABCDE rule of screening (see Table 63-2), and regular screening exams with a physician. Specifically, those family members found to have atypical nevi are to be checked every 6 months and those without atypical nevi every year.

DISCUSSION

Melanoma is a malignant proliferation of melanocytes that has the potential to metastasize to any organ. Melanomas may originate in skin, eyes, ears, gastrointestinal tract, leptomeninges, and oral and genital mucous membranes. This chapter focuses on cutaneous melanoma. Table 63-3 lists risk factors for developing cutaneous melanomas.

In the United States melanoma ranks fifth in incidence of all cancers among men and seventh among women. It is the most common cancer in women 20 to 29 years of age, and it occurs 20 times more commonly in whites than in African Americans.

Individuals at a high risk for melanoma should be counseled in the primary care setting with respect to preventive measures, self-examination, and regular medical surveillance. Because the prognosis of melanoma is related to the depth of the lesion, and examination of the skin is easily performed, early detection of curable primary melanoma can be lifesaving for patients, and as a result, gratifying to physicians.

Risk Factors

Personal risk factors for melanoma include light complexion, inability to tan, blond or red hair, blue eyes, presence of numerous nevi, and immunocompromised status (Rhodes et al., 1987[A][B]). The presence of many clinically atypical moles, a prior history of melanoma, or a family history of melanoma confers the greatest risk.

Increased exposure to ultraviolet radiation (UVA and UVB) is a major environmental contributor to the development of melanoma. Intermittent sun exposure and severe sunburns, especially during childhood, are considered more dangerous than chronic exposure. Certain sunscreens block UVB, the cause of sunburn, but are not as effective against UVA, which has also been shown to promote melanoma. Sunscreens such as zinc oxide, titanium dioxide, benzophenones, oxybenzones, sulisobenzone, and avobenzone (Parsol 1789), block both UVA and UVB, and are thus more effective at preventing the development of melanoma.

Some studies suggest that PUVA (oral methoxalen and UVA) treatment for various skin conditions including psoriasis confers risk for the development of melanoma. Tanning beds emit UVA, and therefore their use can be a risk factor.

Origin

Roughly half of melanomas develop de novo, the others from existing lesions such as benign nevi, atypical nevi, or congenital nevi. Although nevi can be precursors to melanomas, they more often are markers for an increased risk. The greater the number of nevi present, the greater the risk for melanoma.

Identification

Early signs of melanoma include asymmetry, border irregularity, color variation, diameter enlargement, and elevation. These elements are usually referred to as the ABCDE rule of melanoma (see Table 63-2). Recent change in a mole in these areas should prompt attention. Bleeding is a late sign of melanoma and usually portends a poor prognosis.

Examination can be done by simple visual observation, magnification with a 10× ocular hand lens, or with a dermatoscope.

Benign Lesions That Resemble Melanomas

There are several benign lesions that may resemble melanoma: nevi, seborrheic keratoses, angiomas, and dermatofibromas. A biopsy should be performed on all suspicious lesions.

Nevi

Nevi are classified as acquired (benign), congenital, and atypical. Table 63-4 lists the differences between benign and atypical nevi.

Acquired Nevi Acquired nevi, also known as benign nevi, usually appear after 6 months of age (Color Plates 63-1 to 63-8). Most are less than 5 mm in diameter. They may be junctional, compound, or dermal nevi.

A junctional nevus is located at the dermoepidermal junction and tends to be flat. When some nevus cells of a junctional nevus migrate to the dermis, the nevus becomes a compound nevus. Dermal nevi are the result of complete migration of nevus cells into the dermis and tend to be elevated.

Shave excision, or simple excision with suture closure, can be done for nevi that do not appear suspicious. Small dark spots within nevi may be melanoma. Biopsy with excision should be performed on all suspicious-appearing nevi.

Congenital Nevi Congenital nevi are present at birth (Color Plates 63-9 to 63-11). The malignant potential of congenital nevi may be dependent on the depth of penetration of the nevus cells into the dermis and subcutaneous tissues. Cells of larger nevi tend to penetrate deeper and are thus more prone to become malignant.

Atypical Nevi Atypical nevi are also known as dysplastic nevi, or atypical moles (Naeyaert and Brochez, 2003**🅐 🅑**) (Color Plates 63-12 to 63-17). They may be familial or sporadic. Atypical nevi are

Table 63-4 Differences between Atypical Nevi and Common Nevi

Characteristics	Atypical Nevi	Common Nevi
Distribution	Back most common Extremities Sun-protected areas Female breasts, scalp, buttocks, groin	Sun-exposed areas Most above the waist
Age at onset	Appear as normal nevi at age 2–6 years	Absent at birth, appear at age 2–6 years
	New nevi appear throughout life	Grow in uniform manner throughout life Several may appear at puberty
Size	Usually >5 mm	Usually <6 mm
Shape	Irregular	Round and symmetric
Color	Variable within a single lesion	Uniform within a single lesion

usually larger than 5 mm, irregularly pigmented and/or irregularly shaped, and tend to appear in puberty or later rather than in childhood. In contrast to common nevi (acquired or congenital), atypical nevi continue to develop after the fourth decade. They may appear on the scalp, buttocks, and breasts, in addition to sun-exposed areas.

Atypical nevi are a risk factor for melanoma and can be precursor lesions to melanomas. At present there are no data available on the effect of prophylactic removal on decreasing risk for melanoma.

Familial atypical mole/nevi syndrome is an autosomal dominant syndrome characterized by multiple nevi and atypical nevi, with significant risk for development of melanoma.

Table 63-4 lists general differences between common nevi and atypical nevi.

Other Melanocytic Lesions Halo nevus is a compound or dermal nevus with a white border. The average age of onset is 15 years. Lymphocytic involvement is associated with the depigmentation and development of the halo. A symmetric halo surrounding a typical nevus rarely requires removal except for cosmetic reasons (Color Plate 63-18).

Spitz nevus is most common in children. Though known as benign juvenile melanoma, it should be removed for microscopic examination, because the clinical and histologic appearances are similar to melanoma (Color Plate 63-19).

Labial melanotic macules are brown macules on the lower lip most commonly found in women. Similar lesions can occur in the vulvar region and glans penis, and are more common in dark-skinned persons. They are benign if not atypical in appearance. Cryotherapy or laser surgery may be performed for cosmetic reasons.

Seborrheic Keratoses

Seborrheic keratosis is the most common of the benign epithelial tumors (Color Plates 63-20 and 63-21). It tends to appear after the age of 30 and is hereditary. Lesions start as macules and become more pigmented, taking on a "stuck-on" appearance in the form of a plaque. Later on the surface becomes "warty." Horn cysts on the surface are plugged follicles and are virtually pathognomonic of the lesion. Treatment for non-suspicious lesions is with electrocautery or cryotherapy.

Angiomas

Cherry angiomas usually appear in the third decade of life and increase in number (Color Plates 63-22 and 63-23). They are made up of many moderately dilated capillaries. Apart from cosmetic concerns, they are of no clinical consequence. Sometimes they can mimic melanoma in appearance. Treatment is by electrocoagulation or laser coagulation for small lesions, excision for large ones.

Dermatofibromas

Dermatofibromas are common button-like dermal nodules of variable colors appearing mostly on the extremities (Color Plates 63-24 to 63-27). Pigmented versions may be confused with melanoma. Lateral compression with two fingers produces a retraction or "dimple" (retraction or dimple sign). Treatment can be either by cryotherapy or excision.

Freckles

Freckles are also known as ephelides. They are associated with sun exposure and fade without it. They also decrease with age. The tendency to have freckles is an autosomal dominant trait. Treatment and prevention are with sunscreen.

Lentigines

Lentigines, also known as liver spots, range from 2 to 20 mm in diameter (Color Plate 63-28). They occur in sun-exposed areas and increase with age. Lentigines are the predominant component of photoaging in people of Chinese and Japanese descents. Cryotherapy, topical retinoids, tazarotine cream, and/or hydroquinone can be used for treatment.

Classification of Melanomas

Based on the microscopic anatomy of the tumor, melanoma is generally classified as superficial spreading melanoma, nodular melanoma, lentigo maligna melanoma, and acral-lentiginous melanoma. There are two types of local growth in a melanoma: radial and vertical. Radial growth confines the neoplastic melanocytes in the basal layer of the epidermis, and the tumor for the most part spreads horizontally along the plane of the skin. The lesion usually presents as a macule or a patch. The melanocytes in the vertical growth phase invade deeper than the basal layer of the epidermis into the dermis and/or the subcutaneous layer, and the lesion more often presents as a papule or a nodule than as a macule. Vertical growth in general confers much greater risk for metastasis. Table 63-5 lists the distinguishing characteristics of the different melanomas.

Superficial Spreading Melanoma

Superficial spreading melanoma constitutes 70% of melanomas (Color Plate 63-29). Although it can occur anywhere, the most common site is on the

Table 63-5 Types of Melanomas				
	Superficial Spreading	**Nodular**	**Lentigo Maligna Melanoma**	**Acral-Lentiginous**
Percentage of all melanomas	70%	15% to 20%	4% to 15%	30% to 75% in nonwhites 2% to 8% in whites
Location	Trunk in both sexes, legs in women	Trunk and legs	Head, neck, and trunk (sun-exposed areas)	Palms, soles, under nail plates

upper back of both sexes and the legs of women. It is characterized by irregular radial growth and usually is larger than 6 mm in diameter. It often begins as a flat or elevated brown lesion and evolves into black, blue, red, or white colors.

Nodular Melanoma

Nodular melanoma occurs most often in the fifth and sixth decades of life (Color Plate 63-30). The frequency of nodular melanomas is 15% to 20%, and men have twice the risk of women for developing this type of melanoma. It is dome-shaped and grows rapidly in weeks or months. The nodular appearance derives from its rapid vertical growth.

Lentigo Maligna Melanoma

Lentigo maligna melanoma occurs most often in the sixth and seventh decades of life and makes up 4% to 15% of melanomas (Color Plate 63-31). It occurs on exposed areas, especially the face.

A precursor for this melanoma, melanotic freckle of Hutchinson (also known as lentigo maligna), is confined to radial growth, may last for years, and may never evolve into the vertical growth phase to become lentigo maligna melanoma.

Acral-Lentiginous Melanoma

Acral-lentiginous melanoma occurs on the palms, soles, terminal phalanges, and mucous membranes (Color Plates 63-32 to 63-35). It accounts for 30% to 75% of melanomas in African Americans, Asians, and Hispanics. In whites, 2% to 8% of melanomas are of this type. The foot is the most common site for nonwhites. Periungual spread of pigmentation from melanoma to the proximal and lateral nail fold is called Hutchinson's sign.

Management

Initial Biopsy

All suspicious lesions should be excised with narrow margins (1–3 mm of normal skin). A wider margin may impede later identification of sentinel node(s).

When the suspicion is low, when the lesion is too large, or when it is impractical to perform excision, a punch biopsy through the thickest and darkest part of the lesion is done. Repeat biopsy is needed if the specimen is inadequate for accurate histologic staging. Incisional biopsy does not affect survival (Bong et al., 2002🅑).

Shave biopsy often does not permit Breslow's depth of invasion measurement and, therefore, is usually not recommended.

Prognostic Factors

Breslow's depth of invasion number is the thickness in millimeters from the top of the granular cell layer or base of superficial ulceration to the deepest part of the tumor. Because tumor thickness is the most important prognostic factor, this number is essential for the evaluation and management of melanoma (Negin et al., 2003🅐 🅑)

The presence of histologic ulceration is the second most important prognostic factor. It places the tumor in a later stage.

Clark levels, which indicate the anatomic depth of tumor invasion, do not seem to provide as good a correlation with prognosis as Breslow's thickness, though they may help differentiate between 1a and 1b in staging (Kim et al., 2002).

Excision after Biopsy

The entire lesion of the melanoma must be excised and confirmed by histologic verification. The margin of resection is based on the depth of the tumor (Breslow's number), as listed in Table 63-6. The margins for excision for lesions on the face and digits may have to be compromised.

Metastatic Staging

Melanoma tends to metastasize to the lungs, liver, and brain.

Sentinel lymph node micrometastasis is considered by some to be an important factor for recurrence and a powerful predictor of survival (Brady and Coit, 1997🅐). The sentinel lymph node is the first node in the lymphatic chain that drains the lesion. Biopsy is considered for melanomas with Breslow's thickness between 1 and 4 mm (Balch et al., 1996🅐). Radiographic mapping (lymphoscintigraphy) is used preoperatively to identify the sentinel lymph node. Sentinel lymph node biopsy is not indicated if there is clinically evident notal metastasis. In this case, nodal dissection is indicated.

Table 63-7 lists the tumor-node-metastasis (TNM) staging system for cutaneous melanoma as classified by the American Joint Committee on Cancer (Balch et al., 2001🅐 🅑). Survival rates for melanoma TNM and staging categories are listed in Table 63-8.

In the TNM system, the T category reflects the Breslow's thickness, not the Clark level. The N category reflects the number of metastatic lymph nodes discovered either microscopically by sentinel node biopsy or macroscopically by physical examination.

Table 63-6	Surgical Margins for Cutaneous Melanoma
Tumor Thickness	**Excision Margins**
In situ	0.5 cm
<2 mm	1 cm
≥2 mm	2 cm

From Sober AJ, Chuang Y, Duric M, Guidelines of care for primary cutaneous melanoma. J Am Acad Dermatol 2001;45:579–586.

Table 63-7 Melanoma Tumor-Node-Metastasis Classification		
T Classification	**Thickness (Breslow)**	**Ulceration Status**
T1	≤1.0 mm	a: Without ulceration and level II/III
		b: With ulceration or level IV/V
T2	1.01–2.0 mm	a: Without ulceration
		b: With ulceration
T3	2.01–4.0 mm	a: Without ulceration
		b: With ulceration
T4	>4.0 mm	a: Without ulceration
		b: With ulceration
N Classification	**No. of Metastatic Nodes**	**Nodal Metastatic Mass**
N1	One node	a: Micrometastasis*
		b: Macrometastasis†
N2	Two to three nodes	a: Micrometastasis*
		b: Macrometastasis†
		c: In-transit metastasis(es)/ satellite(s) without metastatic node(s)
N3	Four or more metastatic nodes, or matted nodes, or in-transit metastasis(es)/satellite(s) with metastatic node(s)	
M Classification	**Site**	**Serum Lactate Dehydrogenase**
M1a	Distant skin, subcutaneous, or nodal metastases	Normal
M1b	Lung metastases	Normal
M1c	All other visceral metastases	Normal
	Any distant metastasis	Elevated

*Micrometastases are diagnosed after sentinel or elective lymphadenectomy.
†Macrometastases are defined as clinically detectable nodal metastases confirmed by therapeutic lymphadenectomy or when nodal metastasis shows gross extracapsular extension.
From Balch CM, Buzaid AC, Soong SJ. Final version of the American Joint Committee on Cancer staging system for cutaneous melanoma. J Clin Oncol 2001;19:3635–3648. © 2001 American Society for Clinical Oncology.

The M category represents distant metastasis and the presence of elevated serum lactate dehydrogenase. Ulceration in general places the melanoma in a higher stage.

Melanoma in situ is also known as stage 0 melanoma and is a very early stage in the disease in which the tumor is confined strictly in the epidermis in the radial growth phase. It is considered to have very low potential for disease recurrence or spread to lymph nodes.

Initial Diagnostic Workup and Follow-up
Table 63-9 provides guidelines for initial workup and follow-up visits.

For lesions less than 4 mm in thickness with negative nodal involvement, chest radiography and blood work for initial staging or routine follow-up have limited value for asymptomatic patients but may alleviate the patient's anxiety. In general, the Breslow's thickness number and the presence of nodal involvement, guided by a review of systems and a complete physical examination with attention to the skin, lymph nodes, liver, and spleen, direct the need for laboratory tests and imaging studies.

Individuals with a history of melanoma should be able to perform a self-examination of skin and lymph nodes. Photographing the skin may be useful. At least an annual exam with the physician is needed, and the follow-up interval depends on Breslow's thickness.

Medical Treatment
Besides surgery, chemotherapy is usually not effective for melanoma. Interferon alfa-2b (IntronA) was approved adjuvent treatment to surgery in patients with high risk of systemic recurrence. Several vaccine and biologic modifiers are under investigation for their use in the treatment of metastatic melanoma.

Table 63-8 Survival Rates for Melanoma Tumor-Node-Metastasis and Staging Categories

Pathologic Stage	TNM	Thickness (mm)	Ulceration	No. + Nodes	Nodal Size	Distant Metastasis	No. of Patients	Survival ± Standard Error				
								1-Year	2-Year	5-Year	10-Year	
IA	T1a	1	No	0	—	—	4,510	99.7 ± 0.1	99.0 ± 0.2	95.3 ± 0.4	87.9 ± 1.0
IB	T1b	1	Yes or level IV, V	0	—	—	1,380	99.8 ± 0.1	98.7 ± 0.3	90.9 ± 1.0	83.1 ± 1.5
IIA	T2a	1.01–2.0	No	0	—	—	3,285	99.5 ± 0.1	97.3 ± 0.3	89.0 ± 0.7	79.2 ± 1.1
	T2b	1.01–2.0	Yes	0	—	—	958	98.2 ± 0.5	92.9 ± 0.9	77.4 ± 1.7	64.4 ± 2.2
IIB	T3a	2.01–4.0	No	0	—	—	1,717	98.7 ± 0.3	94.3 ± 0.6	78.7 ± 1.2	63.8 ± 1.7
	T3b	2.01–4.0	Yes	0	—	—	1,523	95.1 ± 0.6	84.8 ± 1.0	63.0 ± 1.5	50.8 ± 1.7
IIC	T4a	>4.0	No	0	—	—	563	94.8 ± 1.0	88.6 ± 1.5	67.4 ± 2.4	53.9 ± 3.3
	T4b	>4.0	Yes	0	—	—	978	89.9 ± 1.0	70.7 ± 1.6	45.1 ± 1.9	32.3 ± 2.1
IIIA	N1a	Any	No	One	Micro	—	252	95.9 ± 1.3	88.0 ± 2.3	69.5 ± 3.7	63.0 ± 4.4
	N2a	Any	No	Two to three	Micro	—	130	93.0 ± 2.4	82.7 ± 3.8	63.3 ± 5.6	56.9 ± 6.8
IIIB	N1a	Any	Yes	One	Micro	—	217	93.3 ± 1.8	75.0 ± 3.2	52.8 ± 4.1	37.8 ± 4.8
	N2a	Any	Yes	Two to three	Micro	—	111	92.0 ± 2.7	81.0 ± 4.1	49.6 ± 5.7	35.9 ± 7.2
	N1b	Any	No	One	Macro	—	122	88.5 ± 2.9	78.5 ± 3.7	59.0 ± 4.8	47.7 ± 5.8
	N2b	Any	No	Two to three	Macro	—	93	76.8 ± 4.4	65.6 ± 5.0	46.3 ± 5.5	39.2 ± 5.8
IIIC	N1b	Any	Yes	One	Macro	—	98	77.9 ± 4.3	54.2 ± 5.2	29.0 ± 5.1	24.4 ± 5.3
	N2b	Any	Yes	Two to three	Macro	—	109	74.3 ± 4.3	44.1 ± 4.9	24.0 ± 4.4	15.0 ± 3.9
	N3	Any	Any	Four	Micro/macro	—	396	71.0 ± 2.4	49.8 ± 2.7	26.7 ± 2.5	18.4 ± 2.5
IV	M1a	Any	Any	Any	Any	Skin, SQ	179	59.3 ± 3.7	36.7 ± 3.6	18.8 ± 3.0	15.7 ± 2.9
	M1b	Any	Any	Any	Any	Lung	186	57.0 ± 3.7	23.1 ± 3.2	6.7 ± 2.0	2.5 ± 1.5
	M1c	Any	Any	Any	Any	Other visceral	793	40.6 ± 1.8	23.6 ± 1.5	9.5 ± 1.1	6.0 ± 0.9
Total							17,600				

SQ, squamous cell carcinoma.

From Balch CM, Buzaid AC, Soong SJ. Final version of the American Joint Committee on Cancer staging system for cutaneous melanoma. J Clin Oncol 2001;19:3635–3648. © 2001 American Society for Clinical Oncology.

Table 63-9 Follow-up Guidelines for Cutaneous Melanoma

Breslow Depth (mm)	History and Physical Exam	Radiography/Laboratory
Stage IA	Every 6 months for 2 years Every 12 months thereafter	No
Stage I/II	Every 4–6 months for 3 years Every 12 months thereafter	Initial: CXR, optional CBC, LFTs Follow-up: yearly CXR, optional CBC, LDH
Stage III/IV	Every 3–4 months for 3 years Every 12 months thereafter	Initial: CXR, CT scans; CBC, LFTs Follow-up: every 6–12 months CXR and LFTs

CBC, complete blood count; CXR, chest radiogram; LDH, lactate dehydrogenase; LFTs, liver function tests (lactate dehydrogenase [LDH], aspartate aminotransferase [AST], alanine aminotransferase [ALT], and alkaline phosphatase).
Adapted from Robinson JK. Early detection and treatment of melanoma. Dermatol Nurs 2000;12:397–402, 441–442.

Prevention

Prevention of melanoma may include avoiding excessive exposure to sun and using sunblocks effective against UVA as well as UVB. Frequent regular screening of individuals at high risk to detect early curable lesions is essential.

Material Available on Student Consult

Review Questions and Answers about Melanoma

REFERENCES

Balch CM, Buzaid AC, Soong SJ, et al. Final version of the American Joint Committee on Cancer staging system for cutaneous melanoma. J Clin Oncol 2001;19:3635–3648.🅐🅑

Balch CM, Soong SJ, Bartolucci AA, et al. Efficacy of an elective regional lymph node dissection of 1 to 4 mm thick melanomas for patients 60 years of age and younger. Ann Surg 1996;224:255–263.🅐

Bong JL, Herd RM, Hunter JA, et al. Incisional biopsy and melanoma prognosis. J Am Acad Dermatol 2002; 46:690–694.🅑

Brady MS, Coit DG. Sentinel lymph node evaluation on melanoma. Arch Dermatol 1997;133:1014–1020.🅐

Habif TP. Clinical Dermatology: A Color Guide to Diagnosis and Therapy. St. Louis, Mosby, 2004, pp 773–813.🅒

Johnson TM, Chang A, Redman B, et al. Management of melanoma with a multidisciplinary melanoma clinic model. J Am Acad Dermatol 2000;42:820–826.🅒

Kim CJ, Reintgen DS, Balch CM. The new melanoma staging system. Cancer Control 2002;9:9–15.

Naeyaert JM, Brochez L. Clinical practice. Dysplastic nevi. N Engl J Med 2003;349:2233–2240.🅐🅑

Negin BP, Riedel E, Oliveira SA, et al. Symptoms and signs of primary melanoma: Important indicators of Breslow depth. Cancer 2003;98:344–348.🅐🅑

Rhodes AR, Weinstock MA, Fitzpatrick TB, et al. Risk factors for cutaneous melanoma. JAMA 1987;258: 3146–3154.🅐🅑

Robinson JK. Early detection and treatment of melanoma. Dermatol Nurs 2000;397–402,441–442.🅐🅑

Sober AJ, Chuang TY, Duric M, et al. Guidelines of care for primary cutaneous melanoma. J Am Acad Dermatol 2001;45:579–586.🅐 🅑🅒

SUGGESTED READINGS

Stulberg DL, Clark N, Tovey D. Common hyperpigmentation disorders in adults: Part I and Part II. Am Fam Physician 2003;68:1955–1968.🅒

Tsao H, Atkins MB, Sober AJ. Management of cutaneous melanoma. N Engl J Med 2004;351:998–1012.🅐🅑

Color Plates

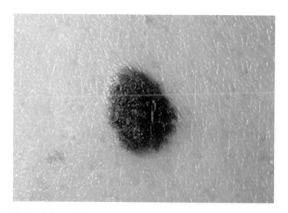

Color Plate 63-1 Junction nevus. The lesion is slightly raised, dark, and uniform.

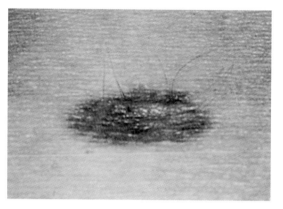

Color Plate 63-2 Compound nevus. The surface is covered with uniform brown-black dots.

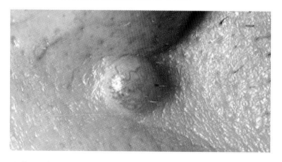

Color Plate 63-3 Dermal nevus. Flesh-colored with surface vessels; resembles basal cell carcinoma.

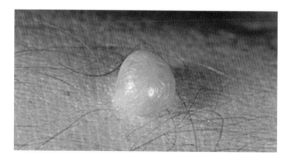

Color Plate 63-4 Dermal nevus. Dome shaped.

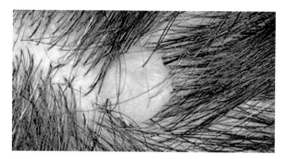

Color Plate 63-5 Dermal nevus. Flesh colored and dome shaped.

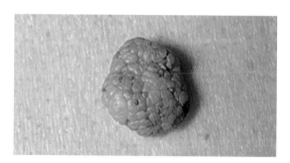

Color Plate 63-6 Dermal nevus. Warty (verrucous) surface.

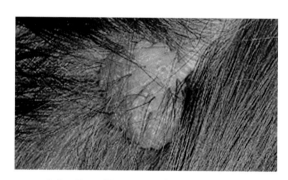

Color Plate 63-7 Dermal nevus. Polypoid.

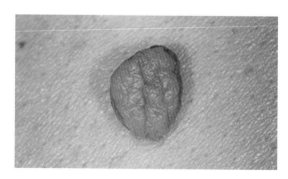

Color Plate 63-8 Dermal nevus. Pedunculated with a soft, flabby, wrinkled surface.

Color Plates 63-1 through 63-35 from Habif TP: Clinical Dermatology: A Color Guide to Diagnosis and Therapy, 4th ed. Philadelphia, Mosby, 2004, with permission.

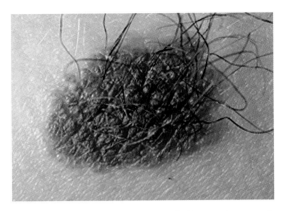

Color Plate 63-9 A small congenital nevus has a uniform cobblestone surface and is covered with hair.

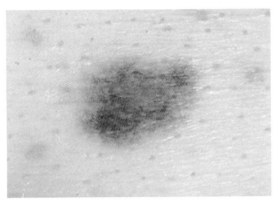

Color Plate 63-12 Atypical mole. Macular, variable pigmentation, ill-defined borders.

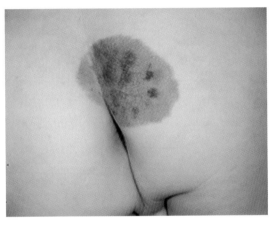

Color Plate 63-10 Medium-sized congenital nevus. Pigmentation is variable and nonuniform, but a biopsy showed all such areas were benign.

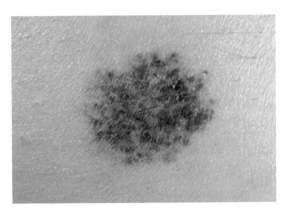

Color Plate 63-13 Atypical mole. Macular, complex pigmentation, notched border.

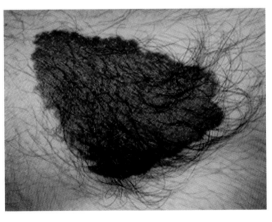

Color Plate 63-11 Medium-sized congenital nevus. The border is irregular and appears notched, but that characteristic is maintained in a uniform manner around the entire border.

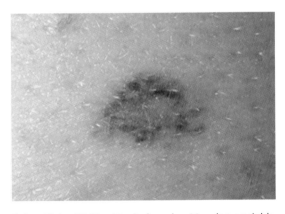

Color Plate 63-14 Atypical mole. Macular, variable pigmentation, fades at border.

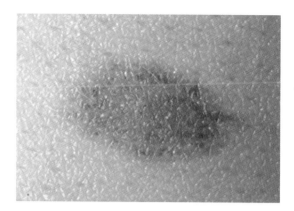

Color Plate 63-15   Atypical mole. Papular, large lesion.

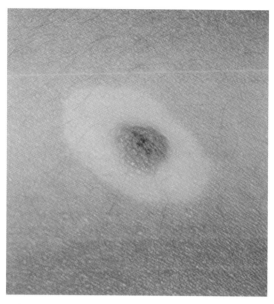

Color Plate 63-18   Halo nevus. A sharply defined, white halo surrounds this compound nevus.

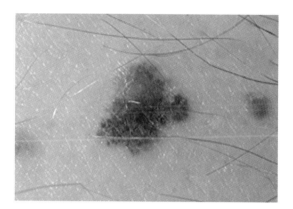

Color Plate 63-16   Atypical mole. Macular, papular, variable pigmentation, irregular border.

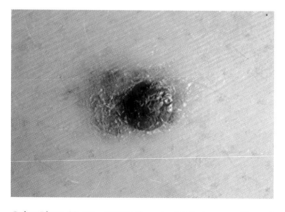

Color Plate 63-17   Atypical mole. "Fried egg pattern," raised with dark center, macular periphery, pigmentation fades at border.

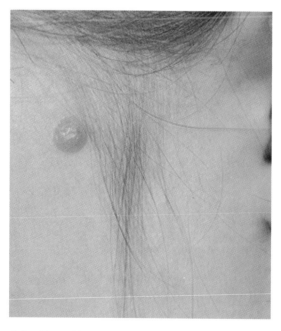

Color Plate 63-19   Benign juvenile melanoma (Spitz nevus). A reddish, dome-shaped nodule that generally appears in children.

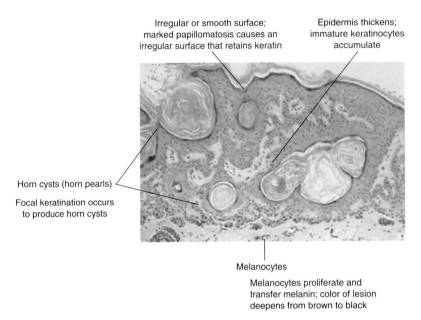

Irregular or smooth surface; marked papillomatosis causes an irregular surface that retains keratin

Epidermis thickens; immature keratinocytes accumulate

Horn cysts (horn pearls)

Focal keratination occurs to produce horn cysts

Melanocytes

Melanocytes proliferate and transfer melanin; color of lesion deepens from brown to black

Color Plate 63-20   Seborrheic keratosis. Cross-section shows embedded horn cysts.

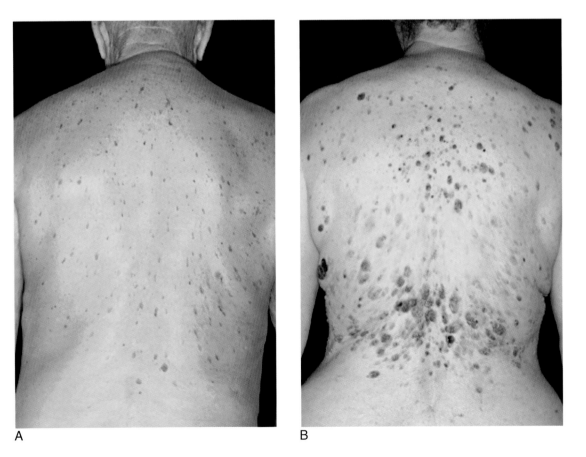

A

B

Color Plate 63-21   Seborrheic keratosis. Lesions are very common on the back; an individual may have numerous lesions on the sun-exposed back and none on the buttocks.

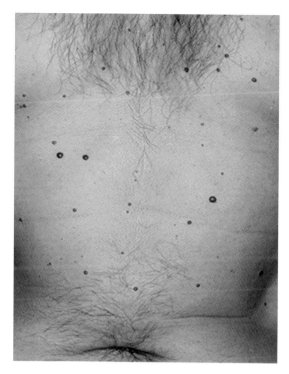

Color Plate 63-22 Cherry angioma. Multiple small, red papules commonly occur on the trunk.

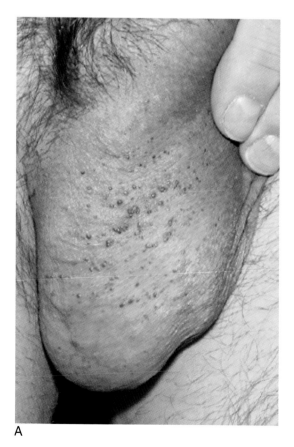

A

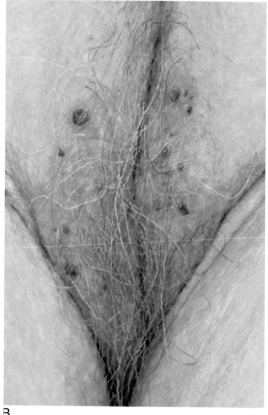

B

Color Plate 63-23 Angiokeratomas (Fordyce). Multiple red-to-purple papules consisting of multiple small blood vessels.

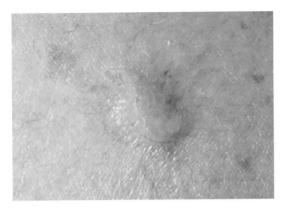

Color Plate 63-24 Dermatofibroma. Early lesions have a well-defined border with an irregular red surface. Brown pigmentation may occur at the periphery after months or years. Pigmentation may extend onto the lesion but almost never reaches the center. Patients often suspect melanoma at this stage.

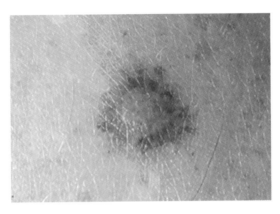

Color Plate 63-25 Dermatofibroma. A typical lesion on the lower leg that is slightly elevated, round, and hyperpigmented, with a scaling surface.

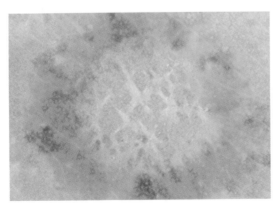

Color Plate 63-26 Dermatofibroma. Dermoscopy reveals a white lacy center surrounded by a uniform network.

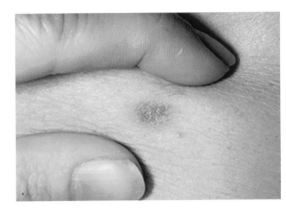

Color Plate 63-27 Retraction sign. Dermatofibromas retract beneath the skin during attempts to compress and elevate them.

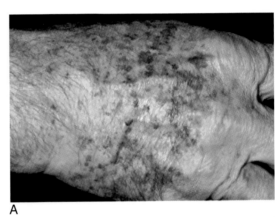

A

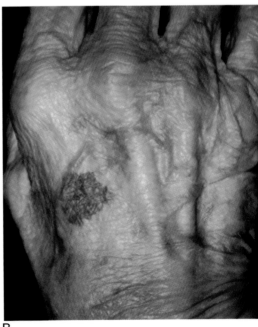

B

Color Plate 63-28 Lentigo (liver spots). Brown macules that appear in chronically sun-exposed areas.

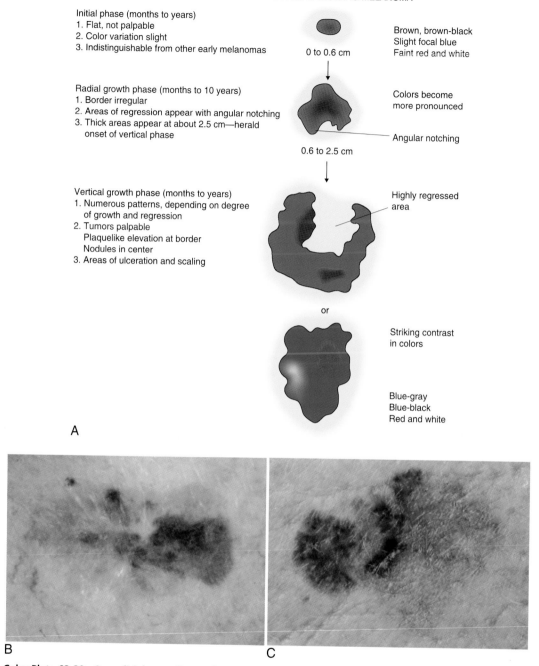

SUPERFICIAL SPREADING MELANOMA

Initial phase (months to years)
1. Flat, not palpable
2. Color variation slight
3. Indistinguishable from other early melanomas

Brown, brown-black
Slight focal blue
Faint red and white

0 to 0.6 cm

Radial growth phase (months to 10 years)
1. Border irregular
2. Areas of regression appear with angular notching
3. Thick areas appear at about 2.5 cm—herald onset of vertical phase

Colors become more pronounced

Angular notching

0.6 to 2.5 cm

Vertical growth phase (months to years)
1. Numerous patterns, depending on degree of growth and regression
2. Tumors palpable
   Plaquelike elevation at border
   Nodules in center
3. Areas of ulceration and scaling

Highly regressed area

or

Striking contrast in colors

Blue-gray
Blue-black
Red and white

A

B

C

Color Plate 63-29 Superficial spreading melanomas in all stages of development. The small early lesions have irregular borders, irregular pigmentation, and small white areas indicating regression. The largest tumors show an accentuation of all of these features.

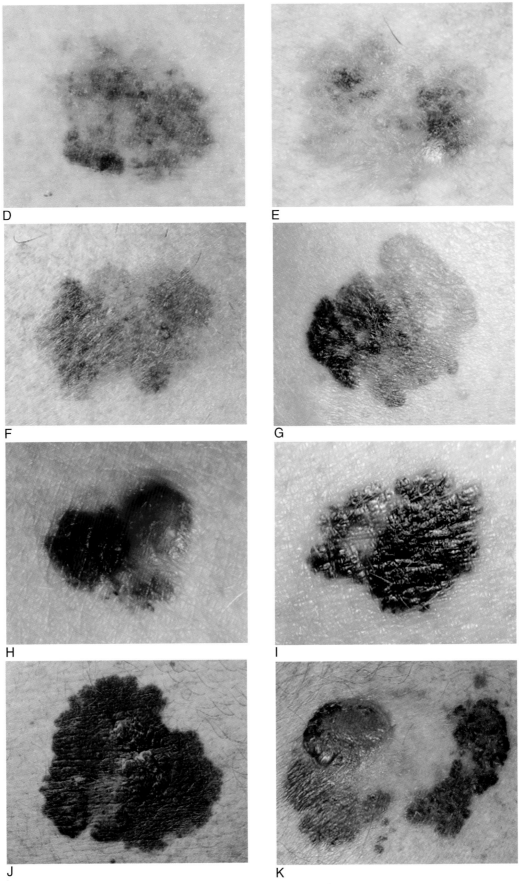

D

E

F

G

H

I

J

K

Color Plate 63-29 Continued

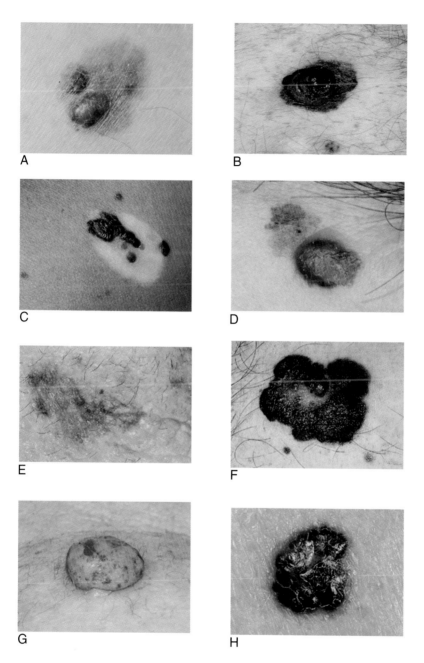

Color Plate 63-30 Nodular melanoma.

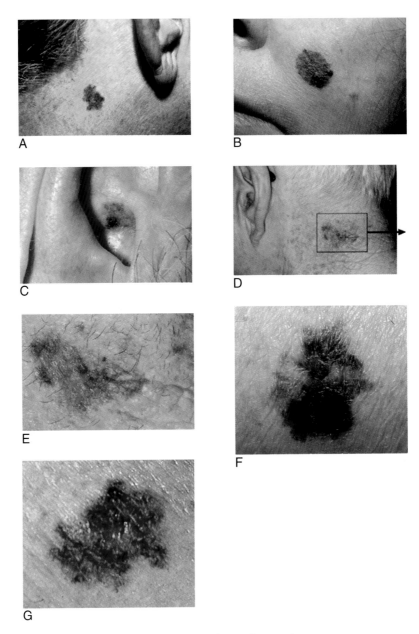

Color Plate 63-31 Lentigo maligna melanoma.

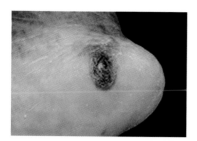

Color Plate 63-32 Acral lentiginous melanoma. A large, dark, flat lesion.

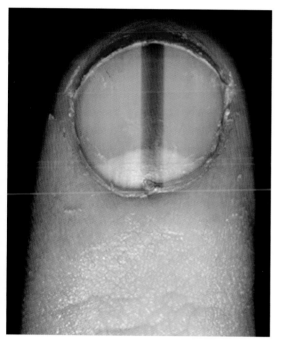

Color Plate 63-33 Acral lentiginous melanoma. The sudden appearance of a pigmented band at the proximal nail fold is suggestive of melanoma.

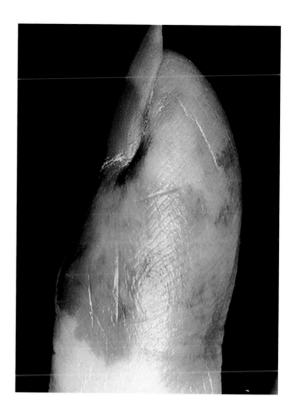

Color Plate 63-34 Acral lentiginous melanoma. Periungual spread of pigmentation from a melanoma to the proximal and lateral nail folds is called Hutchinson's sign.

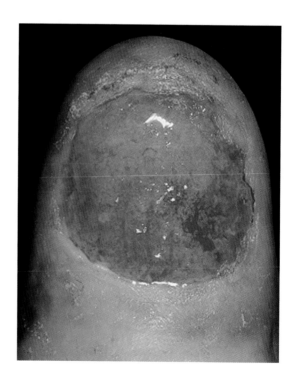

Color Plate 63-35 Acral lentiginous melanoma. Melanoma involving the entire nail bed.

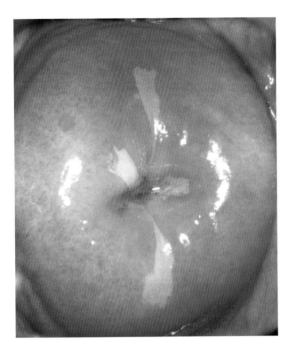

Color Plate 86-1 Colposcopic findings for patient, Aletha. Acetic acid has been applied, demonstrating acetowhite epithelium in a geographic pattern. (From Apgar BS, Brotzman G, Spitzer M, eds. Colposcopy: Principles and Practice. Philadelphia, WB Saunders, 2002.)

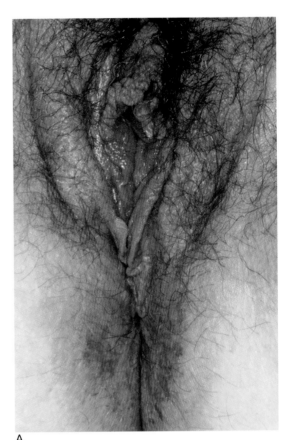

A

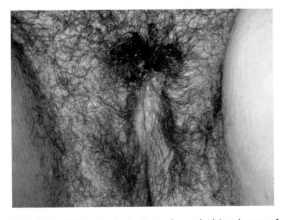

Color Plate 86-2 Psoriasis. Note the red, thin plaque of erythema in a horseshoe pattern around the labia majora and mons pubis. No scaling is visible. (From Apgar BS, Brotzman G, Spitzer M, eds. Colposcopy: Principles and Practice. Philadelphia, WB Saunders, 2002.)

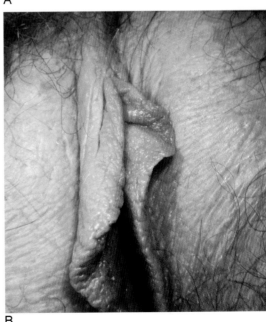

B

Color Plate 86-3 A, Lichen simplex chronicus. Note marked lichenification, erythema, and swelling of labia majora with excoriations, erosions, and perianal crusting. B, Lichen simplex chronicus. Lichenification of medial aspects of the labia majora is evident. (From Apgar BS, Brotzman G, Spitzer M, eds. Colposcopy Principles and Practice. Philadelphia, WB Saunders, 2002.)

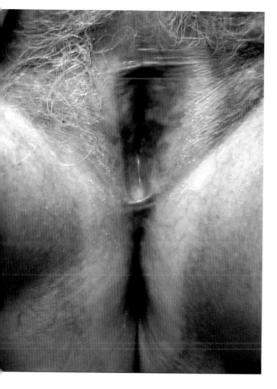

Color Plate 86-4 Lichen sclerosus. This is the classic "figure-eight" pattern with abnormal skin changes surrounding the vaginal opening (upper part of the "8") and similar skin changes surrounding the anal opening (lower part of the "8"). The skin is pale and thin, with a shiny lichenified (cellophane-like) appearance. Agglutination of the labia minora to labia majora and clitoral folds to each other results in a loss of labia minora and most of the clitoris. (Courtesy of Jon C. Calvert, MD.)

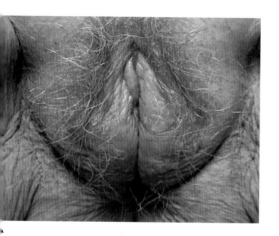

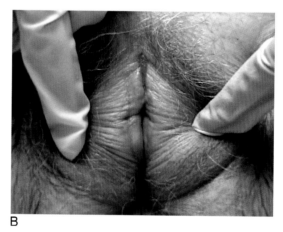

B

lor Plate 86-5 Lichen sclerosus. **A,** Thinning of the vulvar epithelium is noted with a pale shiny appearance to the in. **B,** With retraction of labia the demarcation between the normal-appearing, pink labial skin and the thin, cello-ane-like skin representing lichen sclerosus is evident. Agglutination between the right labia minor and the labia ajora is also noted. (Courtesy of Jon C. Calvert, MD.)

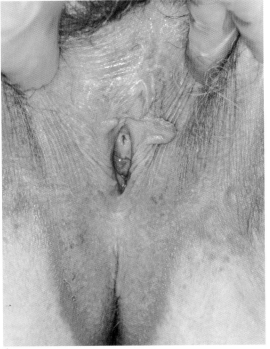

A

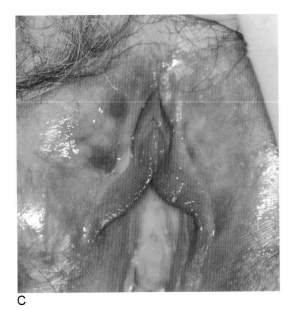

B

C

Color Plate 86-6 **A,** Lichen planus. Note diffuse, whitish pink involvement of the whole vulvar, perineal, perianal are with extension into the labiocrural area and small erosions secondary to scratching. There is scarring with loss of mo of the clitoris and right labium minus in a patient with severe pruritus and secondary candidiasis. **B,** Whitish, scarre vulva with complete loss of the clitoris and labia minora and partial vaginal stenosis. **C,** Periclitoral erosions with su rounding whitish, scarred areas with no loss of architecture. (From Apgar BS, Brotzman G, Spitzer M, eds. Colposcop Principles and Practice. Philadelphia, WB Saunders, 2002.)

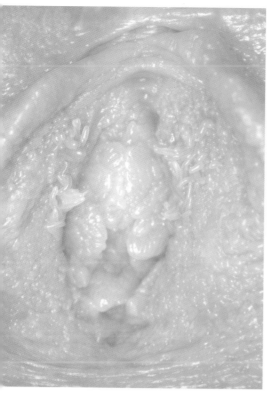

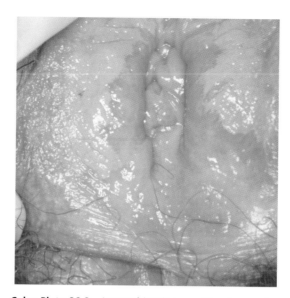

Color Plate 86-8 Acetowhitening resulting from suba-cute or chronicinflammation. (From Apgar BS, Brotzman G, Spitzer M, eds. Colposcopy: Principles and Practice. Philadelphia, WB Saunders, 2002.)

olor Plate 86-7 Squamous vestibular micropapillo-atosis. (From Apgar BS, Brotzman G, Spitzer M, eds. olposcopy: Principles and Practice. Philadelphia, WB aunders, 2002.)

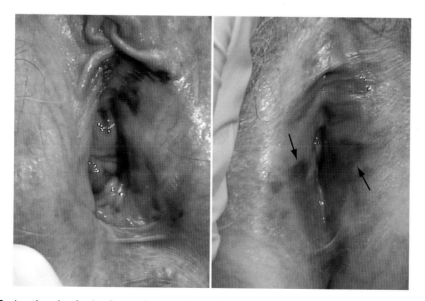

lor Plate 86-9 Lentigo simplex is a hyperpigmented macular lesion most commonly seen on the vulvar skin of older omen. Lesions are frequently multiple and flat, with irregular borders. They may vary in size from 1 to 2 mm to more an 1 cm (*arrows*). Biopsy may be used to exclude atypical nevi and melanoma. (Courlesy of Jon C. Calvert, MD.)

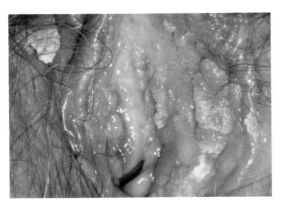

Color Plate 86-10 Multiple condyloma of the introitus, raised, "cauliflower-like," varying in color from white (leukoplakia) to pearly-pink-white. (Courtesy of V. Cecil Wright, MD.)

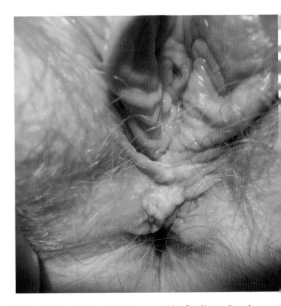

Color Plate 86-12 This is a subtle finding. On the perineum between the fourchette and the anal opening, in the midline there is an area of thickening fine nodularity with central leukoplakia. The skin surrounding the raised lesion is slightly reddened. Palpation of this lesion reveals it to be about 1–1.5 cm in diameter, firm, and extending just beneath the epithelium. Biopsy revealed VIN III (carcinoma in situ of the perineum). (Courtesy of Jon C. Calvert, MD.)

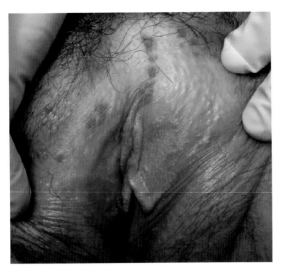

Color Plate 86-11 The vulva is dotted with pigmented raised lesions varying in diameter from 1 mm to 6 mm. These lesions extend from the hair line of the mons superiorly laterally and inferiorly to the perineum. There are lesions on the clitoral hood, on the skin of the fourchette, and on the perineal body down to just superior to the perineal body. Biopsy of these lesions revealed VIN III (carcinoma in situ of the vulva). (Courtesy of Jon C. Calvert, MD.)

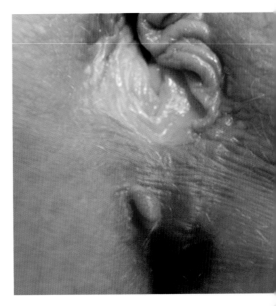

Color Plate 86-13 Patient presented concerned a "skin tag" near the opening of the vagina. Palpation of the "skin tag" found it to be firm, with thickening of the skin at the base of the tag extending out from the point of attachment. Biopsy revealed VIN III (carcinoma in situ of the vulva) with microscopic invasion at the margins of the biopsy. (Courtesy of Jon C. Calvert, MD.)

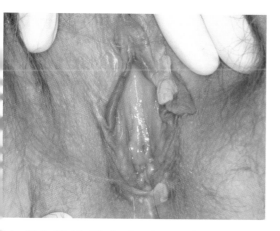

Color Plate 86-14 Viral vulvar intraepithelial neoplasia grade 3 involving the clitoral prepuce, labia minora, and introitus. Human papillomavirus studies were positive. (From Apgar BS, Brotzman G, Spitzer M, eds. Colposcopy: Principles and Practice. Philadelphia, WB Saunders, 2002.)

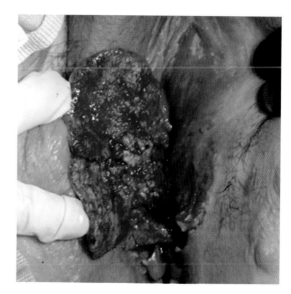

Color Plate 86-15 Large eroding squamous cell carcinoma of the vulva in a 23-year-old drug addict whose presenting symptom was foul-smelling discharge. The cancer had eroded into the perineum and capsule of the anal sphincter. (Courtesy of Jon C. Calvert, MD.)

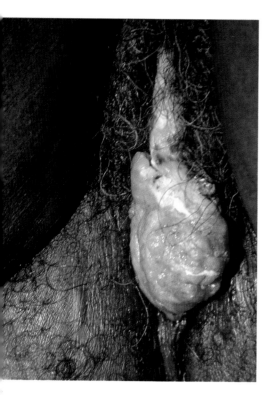

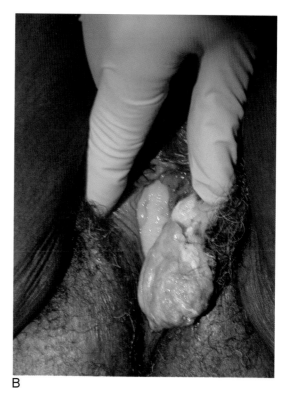

B

Color Plate 86-16 **A,** Exophitic squamous cell caracinoma of the vulva displaying the three skin color changes most commonly associated with advanced vulvar dysplasia or cancer (red, black, and white). **B,** The pedunculated exophytic cancer is attached to the left labia minora. Palpation reveals it to have an irregular surface and to be rubber hard in consistency. The surface also has areas of erosion/infection, where the tumor has been "rubbed raw." (Courtesy of Jon Calvert, MD.)

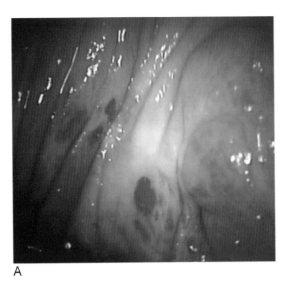

A

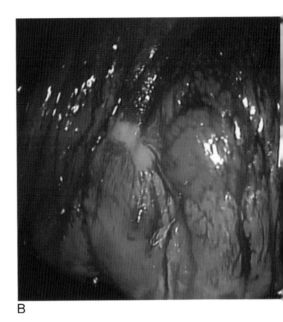

B

Color Plate 86-17 **A,** In the center of the picture of the apex of this posthysterectomy vagina there is a small area o thickened white skin (postapplication of 3% acetic acid), just above the red area of erosion at 6 o'clock. **B,** Followin the application of Lugol's, the normal vaginal epithelium has taken up the dye. In the center of the picture there is linear area that has not taken up the dye. It is smooth and appears slightly raised with well-defined margins. Biops revealed VAIN III (carcinoma in situ of the vagina). (Courtesy of Jon C. Calvert, MD.)

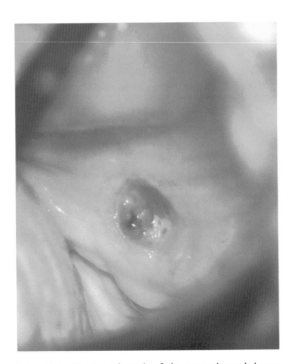

Color Plate 86-18 Adenosis of the posterior cul-de-sac. (From Apgar BS, Brotzman G, Spitzer M, eds. Colposcopy: Principles and Practice. Philadelphia, WB Saunders, 2002.)

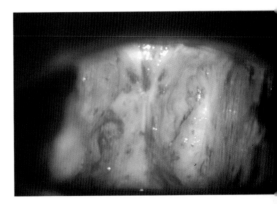

Color Plate 86-19 Vaginal atrophy: Loss of normal pir color, loss of circular rugation and vaginal dryness a characteristic of vaginal atrophy. If atrophy is marke petechial lesion of varying sizes can be noted and m be exacerbated by trauma such as speculum placemen (Courtesy of V. Cecil Wright, MD.)

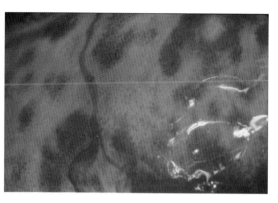

Color Plate 86-20 Vagina, near vaginal cuff, demonstrating "strawberry" pattern of ulceration of epithelium associated with vaginal infections such as trichomoniasis. (Courtesy of V. Cecil Wright, MD.)

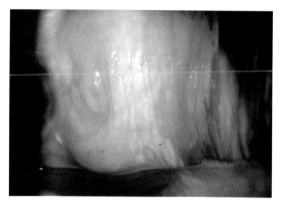

Color Plate 86-22 Deep white thickened vaginal epithelium after application of acetic acid. Biopsy revealed vaginal intraepithelial neoplasia grade 3, VAIN III. (Courtesy of V. Cecil Wright, MD.)

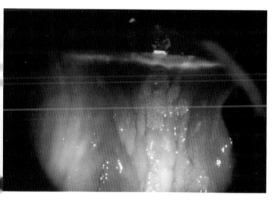

Color Plate 86-21 Vaginal condyloma. After application of acetic acid multiple white, flat condyloma are noted to be present on the vaginal wall. (Courtesy of V. Cecil Wright, MD.)

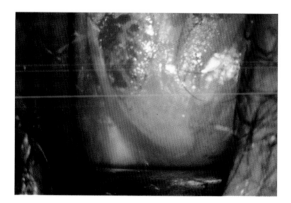

Color Plate 86-23 Two different, adjacent vaginal wall lesions. The first is acetowhite in appearance and the second is raised and deep red. Biopsy of the first revealed vaginal intraepithelial neoplasia grade 3, VAIN III, and biopsy of the second revealed adenocarcinoma. (Courtesy of V. Cecil Wright, MD.)

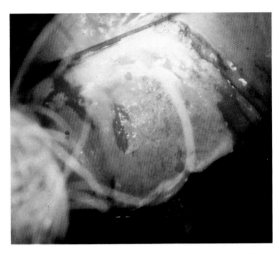

Color Plate 86-24 Vaginal cuff of a woman who had a hysterectomy for carcinoma in situ of the cervix. The majority of the lesion is acetowhite. Biopsy of the areas that bled easily revealed squamous cell carcinoma of the vagina. (Reproduced with the permission of V. Cecil Wright, MD.)

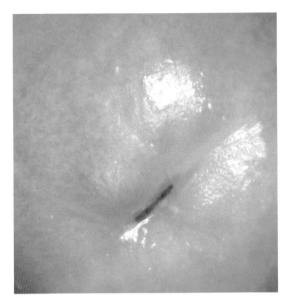

Color Plate 86-25 Ectocervix (exocervix), the portion of the cervix covered by stratified squamous epithelium. (From Apgar BS, Brotzman G, Spitzer M, eds. Colposcopy: Principles and Practice. Philadelphia, WB Saunders, 2002.)

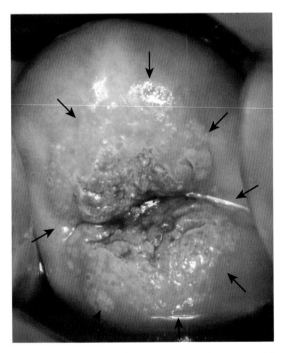

Color Plate 86-26 Transformation zone: the geographic area of transformation or metaplasia between the original (old) squamocolumnar junction and the new squamocolumnar junction. Nabothian cysts, mature squamous epithelium, squamous metaplasia, mature columnar epithelium, and gland crypts may be present. Practically speaking, once the transformation is complete, no remnants of the metaplastic process remain (such as gland openings and nabothian cysts), and the original squamocolumnar junction may be unidentifiable. (From Apgar BS, Brotzman G, Spitzer M, eds. Colposcopy: Principles and Practice. Philadelphia, WB Saunders, 2002.)

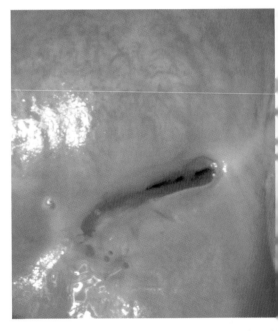

Color Plate 86-27 This cervix, portio, and external os do not demonstrate ectropion. Though the cervical opening is small, the demarcation between the squamous epithelium of the portio and the columnar epithelium of the cervical canal can be identified. This demarcation is termed the new squamocolumnar junction. (From Apgar BS, Brotzman G, Spitzer M [eds]. Colposcopy: Principles and Practice. Philadelphia, WB Saunders, 2002.)

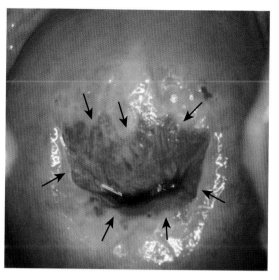

Color Plate 86-28 The "new" squamocolumnar junction. The current junction where the squamous and columnar cells meet on the surface of the cervix at the time the patient is being evaluated, it demarcates the junction of the endocervical glandular epithelium and the squamous epithelium after squamous metaplasia is completed. (From Apgar BS, Brotzman G, Spitzer M, eds. Colposcopy: Principles and Practice. Philadelphia, WB Saunders, 2002.)

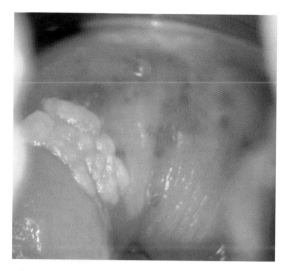

Color Plate 86-30 Leukoplakia: an elevated white plaque seen before the application of 3% to 5% acetic acid. a nonspecific finding that may represent trauma, infection or human papillomavirus–related disease, including invasive disease. It usually requires a biopsy for specific diagnosis. (From Apgar BS, Brotzman G, Spitzer M, eds. Colposcopy: Principles and Practice. Philadelphia, WB Saunders, 2002.)

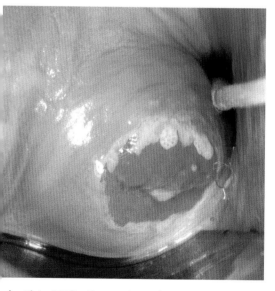

Color Plate 86-29 The cervix can be manipulated with a large Q-tip placed in the lateral fornix to maximize visualization. This adequate examination showed mild acetowhite epithelium anteriorly and a central, 12-o'clock, denser acetowhite area with coarse punctation. A biopsy of the area of punctation revealed cervical intraepithelial neoplasia, grade 2. (From Apgar BS, Brotzman G, Spitzer M, eds. Colposcopy: Principles and Practice. Philadelphia, WB Saunders, 2002.)

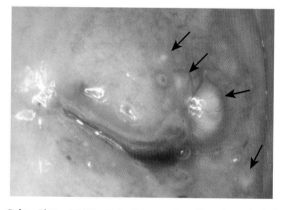

Color Plate 86-31 Nabothian cysts: dilated, occluded endocervical gland crypts indicating that squamous metaplasia has occurred. Nabothian cysts may display exaggerated vessels overlying the cyst, but there is usually normal branching, distinguishing them from atypical vessels. They provide markers of the transformation zone because they are in squamous areas but are remnants of columnar epithelium. (From Apgar BS, Brotzman G, Spitzer M, eds. Colposcopy: Principles and Practice. Philadelphia, WB Saunders, 2002.)

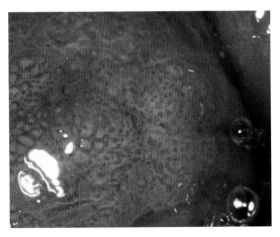

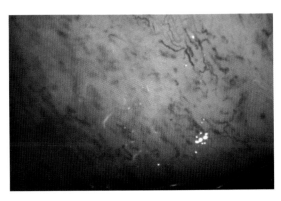

Color Plate 86-32 This is an example of punctation with a few areas of mosaicism. The caliber of the vessels vary from a fine to a coarse pattern. A relatively moderate white epithelium is present after application of acetic acid. Biopsy revealed CIN III severe dysplasia. (Courtesy of V. Cecil Wright, MD.)

Color Plate 86-34 Atypical blood vessels represent microinvasive squamous cell carcinoma of the cervix. Vessels vary from irregular, coarse caliber to coiled and bizarre branching vessels. Intercapillary distance between the vessels is greatly increased and irregular. (Courtesy of V. Cecil Wright, MD.)

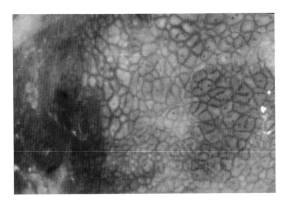

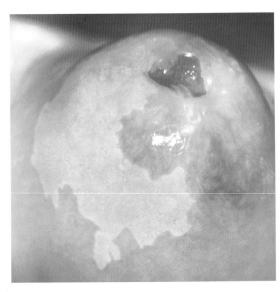

Color Plate 86-33 This is a high magnification view of mosaicism with infrequent punctation. The mosaic pattern varies only slightly in size, shape and configuration. Biopsy revealed CIN II, moderate dysplasia. (Courtesy of V. Cecil Wright, MD.)

Color Plate 86-35 This lesion represents a geographic map-like, low-grade dysplasia. The lesion itself is irregular and extends to the posterior cervical portion. (From Apgar BS, Brotzman G, Spitzer M, eds. Colposcopy: Principles and Practice. Philadelphia, WB Saunders, 2002.)

64 Restless Legs Syndrome

Max Bayard

INITIAL VISIT

Subjective

History of Present Illness

Wanda is a 58-year-old woman who complains of pain in her legs for the past 5 years. The pain is described as a "discomfort" or as a "crawling" sensation. She has trouble falling asleep because of the pain and frequently gets out of bed and walks around, which affords temporary relief. The pain bothers her only in the evenings and is particularly uncomfortable when she lies down to sleep. When she awakens in the morning, her legs feel fine. She does not experience cramps when walking. She does not have any leg weakness. She has reported these symptoms to several doctors over the last 5-year period and has been evaluated with ankle/brachial indices, magnetic resonance imaging of her lumbosacral spine, and nerve-conduction studies. According to the patient, all of these were normal. She has been treated with quinine for nocturnal leg cramps, but that was ineffective. She was told by another physician that she had fibromyalgia. She was given amitriptyline (Elavil), but it did not help her symptoms; it seemed to make them a bit worse. Occasionally, when the discomfort was very severe, she has taken hydrocodone; this has eased the pain but not completely relieved it. Three months ago, she was given clonazepam (Klonopin); although this has not completely relieved the symptoms, it has improved them significantly and has helped her to fall asleep at night.

Medical History

Wanda has chronic obstructive pulmonary disease (COPD) but has never required hospitalization. She has gastroesophageal reflux disease. She is hypertensive and has hyperlipidemia. She had ankle surgery years ago after a fracture. Her medications include albuterol metered-dose inhaler, hydrochlorothiazide, montelukast, fluticasone nasal spray, and omeprazole.

Family History

Both parents are dead. Her father died of complications of COPD. Her mother had diabetes and hypertension. Her two brothers have hypertension but are otherwise healthy.

Social History

Wanda has smoked one pack of cigarettes per day since age 15 years. She denies any alcohol use or abuse of recreational drugs. She does not exercise regularly. She is not currently employed. In the past, she worked in a school cafeteria.

Review of Systems

She has not had any weight change. She denies symptoms of depression or anxiety. She has not had any

---

chest pains or gastrointestinal complaints. She becomes short of breath with exertion secondary to her COPD, but this is chronic. She denies any endocrine diseases.

Objective

Physical Examination

Her weight is 215 pounds, and her height is 5 feet 1 inch, with a body mass index of 41. Her blood pressure is 142/86. HEENT, neck, cardiac, lung, and abdominal examinations are all normal. Straight leg–raise test is negative bilaterally. She has normal sensation and reflexes. Dorsalis pedis and posterior tibial pulses are normal bilaterally. She has no edema.

Differential Diagnosis

1. *Restless legs syndrome (RLS)* is the most likely etiology of Wanda's discomfort. Her symptoms occur in the evening and at night. She experiences improvement with activity. The difficulty describing the sensation is typical in RLS.
2. *Nocturnal leg cramps* are sudden, involuntary muscle contractions that typically occur at night. The calf muscles are most often affected. These cramps may last for seconds or minutes, and occasionally discomfort persists after the cramps. The affected muscles feel tight. The patient may experience relief by dorsiflexion of the foot or by walking around.
3. *Peripheral neuropathies* have a number of possible etiologies, including trauma, mechanical nerve compression, endocrine disorders (such as diabetes and thyroid disorders), infectious diseases, toxins, and nutritional disorders. Most commonly, neuropathies cause sensory symptoms, including burning, tingling, or numbness. Although the pain may be more noticeable at night, it is not typically relieved by activity.
4. *Peripheral vascular disease* is primarily a result of atherosclerosis. Risk factors for peripheral vascular disease are the same as those for other atherosclerotic diseases, specifically hypertension, diabetes, hyperlipidemia, and cigarette use. The dull, cramping pains of claudication usually involve the calf muscles, occur with activity, and improve with rest.
5. *Akathisia* refers to an internal need to move, but it is not necessarily associated with discomfort in the legs. Symptoms are not worse at night. It is most commonly a side effect of neuroleptic medications.

Assessment

Severity of RLS symptoms is quantified based on the rating scale developed by the International Restless Legs Syndrome Study Group (IRLSSG). Wanda's score is 24, suggesting moderate severity of symptoms.

Plan

Wanda is given a prescription for gabapentin (Neurontin). She is instructed to take 300 mg at suppertime. She is encouraged to work on weight loss and to begin a mild exercise program 3 or 4 times per week. She is encouraged to quit cigarettes. Complete blood count (CBC), basic chemistry panel, and ferritin are ordered. She will follow up in 2 weeks.

FOLLOW-UP VISIT

Wanda has had marked improvement in her symptoms. Her score on the IRLSSG rating scale is 14. Weight is unchanged. She is exercising 20 minutes per day 3 times a week. CBC results are as follows: hemoglobin, 11.4; hematocrit, 35; mean corpuscular volume, 82; and ferritin is 24. Electrolytes are normal. Blood urea nitrogen and creatinine are 14 and 0.8, respectively. She is given a prescription for iron supplementation in light of the relatively low ferritin level. Plans are to continue iron for 3 months and to reassess symptom severity in 1 month.

DISCUSSION

Epidemiology

RLS is a common condition. Its prevalence is approximately 10% of the adult population, and prevalence increases with age (Philips et al., 2000[B]). It is more common in women than in men, and increasing parity appears to increase the likelihood of RLS developing (Berger et al., 2004[C]). A recent survey reported that 24% of adult patients seen in a primary care office had symptoms consistent with RLS (Nichols et al., 2003[C]).

In spite of the high prevalence of RLS, the condition is underdiagnosed. In a survey of 23,052 patients, 2,223 (9.6%) reported weekly RLS symptoms. A subgroup of 551 had symptoms that had a significant negative impact on their lives. Of these, 357 (64.8%) had reported their symptoms to a physician, but only 46 (12.9%) reported being given a diagnosis of RLS (Hening et al., 2004). The 2001 Sleep in America Poll reported an RLS prevalence of 13% in the adult population, but only 3% of these had actually been diagnosed with RLS (National Sleep Foundation, 2001[C]).

RLS is associated with significant morbidity. Patients with RLS report sleep disturbances and daytime somnolence. Anxiety and depression are common in patients with RLS (Sevim et al., 2004[B]). RLS patients report that the symptoms have a negative impact on their quality of life (Hening et al., 2004[B]).

Although most cases of RLS are primary conditions (i.e.. no known underlying pathologic condition), RLS may be secondary to certain medical conditions or medications. Iron deficiency, even in the absence of frank anemia, may cause RLS. Ferritin levels less than 50 μg/L have been associated with RLS (Sun et al., 1998Ⓑ). Patients with spinal cord injuries have a high incidence of RLS. RLS is common in pregnancy and usually resolves after delivery. It is extremely common in patients with end-stage renal failure. Certain medications may exacerbate RLS; these include tricyclic antidepressants, selective serotonin reuptake inhibitors, lithium, dopamine antagonists, and caffeine (National Heart, Lung, and Blood Institute, 2000Ⓒ).

Pathophysiology

RLS is a neurologic movement disorder of unclear etiology. It appears to be associated with abnormalities in central nervous system dopamine and iron function. RLS runs in families, suggesting a genetic component. Although it is a separate entity from periodic limb movements of sleep (PLMSs), the majority of patients with RLS also have PLMSs. Treatments for RLS often improve PLMSs.

Clinical Findings

Patients frequently do not report symptoms of RLS, and when they do, it is frequently not diagnosed correctly. The diagnosis may be complicated by the variety of adjectives used to describe the symptoms of RLS. It is not generally described as painful; more often, it is a discomfort. It may be described as an aching, a crawling, an itching, a tingling, a moving (of the skin), or a burning (or a number of other similar adjectives). Patients may say, "I just have to move my legs," or "I don't know how to explain it." Terms patients use to describe RLS symptoms are listed in Box 64-1 (National Heart, Lung, and Blood Institute, 2000Ⓒ). It may be extremely severe, causing the patient to get out of bed and walk around. This will relieve symptoms to some degree, but only temporarily. Frequently, patients report poor sleep quality, difficulty falling asleep, and daytime somnolence. It is important to ascertain the effect of the symptoms of RLS on the patient's life. Some patients have symptoms only rarely, whereas others have symptoms daily. Some patients' symptoms are severe, whereas others' are only mild. The decision to use medications to treat RLS is dependent on the effect RLS symptoms have on the patient's quality of life.

The physical examination and laboratory evaluation serve to rule out conditions known to cause RLS and other conditions with similar presentations. A neurologic examination and vascular examination of the lower extremities should be performed.

Box 64-1	Terms Used to Describe Restless Legs Syndrome Sensations

Creeping
Crawling
Itching
Burning
Searing
Tugging
Indescribable
Pulling
Drawing
Aching
Like water falling
Like worms or bugs crawling under the skin
Like electric current
Restless
Painful

Laboratory tests that may identify secondary causes of RLS include a serum ferritin and basic chemistry panel.

The diagnosis of RLS is made based on the patient's history. Physical examination findings and laboratory studies may identify an etiology for the symptoms or other possible diagnoses, but they are not part of the criteria for the diagnosis of RLS. The criteria are listed in Box 64-2. All four criteria are required for the diagnosis (Walters, 1995Ⓒ).

The severity of restless legs symptoms can be quantified by use of the International Restless Legs Syndrome Study Group Rating Scale (Box 64-3). This 10-question survey, which is easily administered, has recently been validated (Walters et al., 2003Ⓑ). The survey assesses frequency of RLS symp-

Box 64-2	Diagnostic Criteria for Restless Legs Syndrome (Diagnosis requires all four)

1. A compelling urge to move the limbs, usually associated with paresthesias/dysesthesias
2. Motor restlessness as seen in activities such as floor pacing, tossing and turning in bed, and rubbing the legs
3. Symptoms worse or exclusively present at rest (i.e., lying, sitting) with variable and temporary relief by activity, and
4. Symptoms worse in the evening and at night

Adapted from Walters AS. Toward a better definition of restless legs syndrome. Mov Disord 1995;10:634–642.

Box 64-3	**International Restless Legs Syndrome Study Group Severity Scale Questions**

1. Overall, how would you rate the RLS discomfort in your legs or arms?
2. Overall, how would you rate the need to move around because of your RLS symptoms?
3. Overall, how much relief of your RLS arm or leg discomfort do you get from moving around?
4. Overall, how severe is your sleep disturbance from your RLS symptoms?
5. How severe is your tiredness or sleepiness from your RLS symptoms?
6. Overall, how severe is your RLS as a whole?
7. How often do you get RLS symptoms?
8. When you have RLS symptoms, how severe are they on an average day?
9. Overall, how severe is the impact of your RLS symptoms on your ability to carry out your daily affairs, for example, carrying out a satisfactory family, home, school, or work life?
10. How severe is your mood disturbance from your RLS symptoms—for example, angry, depressed, sad, anxious, or irritable?

Responses and assigned point values:

For questions 1, 2, 4, 5, 6, 8, 9, and 10, the responses and their values are as follows:
 Very severe—4 points
 Severe—3 points
 Moderate—2 points
 Mild—1 point
 None—0 points

For question 3, the responses and their values are as follows:
 No relief—4 points
 Slight relief—3 points
 Moderate relief—2 points
 Either complete or almost complete relief—1 point
 No RLS symptoms—0 points

For question 7, the responses and their values are as follows:
 6 to 7 days a week—4 points
 4 to 6 days a week—3 points
 2 to 3 days a week—2 points
 1 day a week or less—1 point
 None—0 points

Score:

31–40 Very severe
21–30 Severe
11–20 Moderate
1–10 Mild

Adapted from Walters AS, LeBrocq C, Dhar A, et al. International Restless Legs Syndrome Study Group: Validation of the International Restless Legs Syndrome Study Group rating scale for restless legs syndrome. Sleep Med 2003;4:121–132.

toms, severity of symptoms, effectiveness of activity in alleviating symptoms, effect of RLS on sleep and daytime somnolence, and the impact RLS has on the patient's daily activities and mood. Each question has a choice of answers corresponding to scores of zero (representing no symptoms or effect on quality of life) to four (representing most frequent or severe symptoms). The 10 items are totaled, yielding a score ranging from zero to 40. Higher scores are associated with more severe or frequent symptoms or both.

Treatment

Secondary Restless Legs Syndrome

Patients with RLS who have RLS secondary to another underlying medical condition or medication may improve with treatment of the condition or discontinuation of the medication. Patients with RLS who are iron deficient will likely have improvement or resolution of their symptoms with iron supplementation. Patients with end-stage renal disease may have improvement in their symptoms after renal transplant. Removal of a causative medication may also improve or eliminate symptoms.

Lifestyle

Little scientific evidence concerns the effectiveness of lifestyle interventions on the symptoms of RLS. Although it is more common in obese individuals and in individuals with sedentary lifestyles, anecdotal reports exist of both easing and worsening of symptoms with exercise. An exercise program has been shown to be beneficial in RLS/PLMS patients with spinal cord injuries, but no published studies concern the effectiveness of exercise in individuals without spinal cord injuries (deMello et al., 2004 ⓑ). Some patients may find improvement with decreasing their caffeine, alcohol, or cigarette use.

Medications

Several classes of medications are effective in the treatment of RLS. The mainstays of RLS medical treatment are dopaminergic agents and dopamine agonists, medications normally prescribed for the treatment of Parkinson's disease. Other classes of agents that have been effective in relieving the symptoms of RLS include opiates, benzodiazepines, and anticonvulsants. Ropinirole (Requip) has recently received FDA approval for treatment of moderate to severe primary RLS in adults. All other medications are used "off-label" (i.e., they are not specifically indicated for the treatment of RLS). Patients with mild or infrequent symptoms may not need medical treatment. Iron supplementation may improve symptoms in patients with iron-deficiency anemia, but it is not beneficial in individuals who are not iron deficient. Medications used to treat RLS are listed in Table 64-1.

Dopaminergic Agents Levodopa (with carbidopa or benserazide) has been used for years to treat the symptoms of RLS. It is an effective treatment for mild to moderate symptoms of RLS and improves symptoms rapidly (Benes et al., 1999 ⓐ). Side effects of levodopa include gastrointestinal upset, insomnia, and headaches. Levodopa may also cause augmentation of RLS symptoms. Augmentation refers to exacerbation of symptoms of RLS during the daytime and at other times when medication is withheld. This may limit its usefulness for patients requiring long-term daily use.

Dopamine Agonists Several dopamine agonists have been found to treat RLS effectively. Pergolide, an ergotamine dopamine agonist, has been shown to be effective in the treatment of symptoms of RLS and periodic leg movements. The PEARLS Study (Pergolide European Australian RLS study) demonstrated long-term efficacy of pergolide (Trenkwalder et al., 2004b ⓐ). Ropinirole and pramipexole are nonergotamine dopamine agonists. In the TREAT RLS 1 Study, ropinirole was associated with rapid improvement in restless legs symptoms, sleep quality, and quality of life compared with placebo (Trenkwalder et al., 2004a ⓐ).

Table 64-1 Medications Used to Treat Restless Legs Syndrome

Medication	Starting Dose	Side Effects/Disadvantages
Levodopa/ Carbidopa (Sinemet)	25/100 mg	Short half-life. Augmentation. Side effects include GI upset and headache
Pergolide (Permax) (ergotamine dopamine agonist)	0.05 mg	Side effects include hypotension. Nausea can be severe.
Non-ergotamine dopamine agonist Pramipexole (Mirapex) Ropinirole (Requip)	 0.125 mg 0.25 mg	Side effects include nausea, sleepiness, and orthostatic hypotension. Should titrate slowly
Opioids	Nightly dose varies by choice of opioid	Nausea, constipation. Potential for abuse
Benzodiazepines Clonazepam (Klonopin) Temazepam (Restoril)	 0.5 mg 15 mg	Daytime sleepiness. Increased risk of falls at night. Potential for abuse
Anticonvulsants Gabapentin (Neurontin)	 300 mg	Side effects include sedation, gastrointestinal discomfort. Long-term studies not yet available

Pramipexole was effective in treating the symptoms of RLS and remained efficacious for more than 2 years (Silber et al., 2003 B). Side effects of the dopamine agonists included nausea, headache, and orthostatic hypotension. Reports have been noted of augmentation occurring with these medications.

Benzodiazepines Clonazepam has not been shown to treat the symptoms of RLS. However, it may be beneficial in patients with RLS, as the hypnotic effects of clonazepam promote sleep in spite of the presence of symptoms. Adverse effects of clonazepam include daytime somnolence and increased risk of falls at night. Benzodiazepines also have the potential for abuse.

Anticonvulsants Patients who do not respond well to dopaminergic agents and dopamine agonists, those who have significant side effects, and those with painful restless legs may respond well to anticonvulsants. Slow-release valproic acid had similar efficacy to slow-release levodopa-benserazide in a small randomized controlled trial (Eisensehr et al., 2004 A). Gabapentin improved sensory and motor symptoms in patients with RLS; it also reduced quantity of periodic leg movements during sleep (Garcia-Borreguero et al., 2002 A). It is an effective treatment for RLS symptoms in dialysis patients (Thorp et al., 2001 A). In a head-to-head study comparing gabapentin and ropinirole, both medications were found to have similar significant

improvements in symptoms of RLS and periodic leg movements (Happe et al., 2003 B). Carbamazepine has also been shown to be more effective than placebo in treating restless legs discomfort (Telstad et al., 1984 A).

Opioids Oxycodone has been demonstrated to improve symptoms of RLS and to decrease periodic leg movements in a small trial (Walters et al., 1993 A). Small studies of other opioids have shown improvement in symptoms. Side effects of opioids include nausea and constipation. Opioids also have a potential for abuse.

Conclusion

RLS is a very common disorder associated with significant morbidity. The condition is underdiagnosed. It may be a primary condition, or it may be secondary to pregnancy, iron deficiency, spinal cord injury, end-stage renal disease, or certain medications. Treatment of the underlying condition may resolve symptoms of RLS. In patients with no apparent underlying cause for RLS, medications may significantly improve the symptoms and quality of life.

Material Available on Student Consult

Review Questions and Answers about Restless Legs Syndrome

REFERENCES

Benes H, Kurella B, Kummer J, Kazenwadel J, Selzer R, Kohnen R. Rapid onset of action of levodopa in restless legs syndrome: A double-blind, randomized, multicenter, crossover trial. Sleep 1999;22:1073–1081. A

Berger K, Luedemann J, Trenkwalder C, John U, Kessler C. Sex and the risk of restless legs syndrome in the general population. Arch Intern Med 2004;164:196–202. C

deMello MT, Esteves AM, Tufik S. Comparison between dopaminergic agents and physical exercise as treatment for periodic limb movements in patients with spinal cord injury. Spinal Cord 2004;42:218–221. B

Eisensehr I, Ehrenberg BL, Rogge Solti S, Noachtar S. Treatment of idiopathic restless legs syndrome (RLS) with slow-release valproic acid compared with slow-release levodopa/benserazid. J Neurol 2004;251:579–583. A

Garcia-Borreguero D, Larrosa O, de la Llave Y, Verger K, Masramon X, Hernandez G. Treatment of restless legs syndrome with gabapentin: A double-blind, crossover study. Neurology 2002;59:1573–1579. A

Happe S, Sauter C, Klosch G, Saletu B, Zeitlhofer J. Gabapentin versus ropinirole in the treatment of idiopathic restless legs syndrome. Neuropsychobiology 2003;48:82–86. B

Hening W, Walters AS, Allen RP, Montplaisir J, Myers A, Ferini-Strambi L. Impact, diagnosis and treatment of restless legs syndrome (RLS) in a primary care population: The REST (RLS epidemiology, symptoms, and treatment) primary care study. Sleep Med 2004;5:237–246. B

National Heart, Lung, and Blood Institute Working Group on Restless Legs Syndrome. Restless legs syndrome: Detection and management in primary care. Am Fam Physician 2000;62:108–114. C

National Sleep Foundation. The 2001 Sleep in America Poll. Washington, DC: National Sleep Foundation, 2001. C

Nichols DA, Allen RP, Grauke JH, et al. Restless legs syndrome symptoms in primary care. Arch Intern Med 2003;163:2323–2329. C

Philips B, Young T, Finn L, Asher K, Hening WA, Purvis C. Epidemiology of restless legs syndrome in adults. Arch Intern Med 2000;160:2137–2141. B

Sevim S, Dogu O, Kaleagasi H, Aral M, Metin O, Camdeviren H. Correlation of anxiety and depression symptoms in patients with restless legs syndrome: A population based survey. J Neurol Neurosurg Psychiatry 2004;75:226–230. B

Silber MH, Girish M, Izurieta R. Pramipexole in the management of restless legs syndrome: An extended study. Sleep 2003;26:819–821. B

Sun ER, Chen CA, Ho G, Earley CJ, Allen RP. Iron and the restless legs syndrome. Sleep 1998;21:371–377.🅑

Telstad W, Sorensen O, Larsen S, Lillevold PE, Stensrud P, Nyberg-Hansen R. Treatment of the restless legs syndrome with carbamazepine: A double blind study. Br Med J (Clin Res Ed) 1984;288:444–446.🅐

Thorp ML, Morris CD, Bagby SP. A crossover study of gabapentin in treatment of restless legs syndrome among hemodialysis patients. Am J Kidney Dis 2001;38:104–108.🅐

Trenkwalder C, Garcia-Borreguero D, Montagna P, et al. Ropinirole in the treatment of restless legs syndrome: Results from the TREAT RLS 1 study, a 12 week, randomized, placebo controlled study in 10 European countries. J Neurol Neurosurg Psychiatry 2004a; 75:92–97.🅐

Trenkwalder C, Hundemer HP, Lledo A, et al. Efficacy of pergolide in treatment of restless legs syndrome: The PEARLS Study. Neurology 2004b;62:1391–1397.🅐

Walters AS. Toward a better definition of the restless legs syndrome. Mov Disord 1995;10:634–642.🅒

Walters AS, Wagner ML, Hening WA, et al. Successful treatment of the idiopathic restless legs syndrome in a randomized double-blind trial of oxycodone versus placebo. Sleep 1993;16:327–332.🅐

Walters AS, LeBrocq C, Dhar A, et al. International Restless Legs Syndrome Study Group: Validation of the International Restless Legs Syndrome Study Group rating scale for restless legs syndrome. Sleep Med 2003;4:121–132.🅑

Chapter

65 Headache

Rahul Gupta

INITIAL VISIT

Subjective

Patient Identification and Presenting Problem

Mary B., a 47-year-old white woman, complains of severe headache for the past 6 hours. Mary states that she was doing well when a sudden onset of severe left-sided headache developed earlier in the day. The pain started around her left eye, gradually spread to her left temple, and soon involved the complete left side of her head. It was throbbing, 10/10 on a pain scale, and associated with nausea. The headache was worse with movement and not associated with fever. She felt somewhat better lying down in the dark. No significant improvement was achieved by taking two tablets of ibuprofen. As the pain continued, she had to take leave from her job, where she works as a bank manager, and visit her physician. This is her third visit to the physician's office in the past 12 months. On review of her chart, the past two visits have been very similar to the current one.

Mary is happily married to her husband of the past 20 years, and the couple have two children. Mary has a busy life, which she manages well. She started having headaches at age 22. Earlier she noticed that her headaches were related to her menstrual cycles, and she would be able to achieve fair control by over-the-counter medications. The headaches became somewhat less frequent after she reached menopause 5 years ago. However, she states that she thought the headaches would be better when her sons left

---

home for college 3 years ago, but her life has been more stressful. Her "bad" headaches can occur between once a month and once in 3 months, depending on "how stressed" she is. Occasionally, she gets a daily, nagging-type headache localized to the frontal area of the head, which feels like a band. The back of her neck also hurts with this type of headache, but the headache is not as severe. This headache is typically relieved with acetaminophen or ibuprofen. Her husband works as an executive and is generally supportive.

Medical History

Mary has had no major medical illnesses or surgery. Apart from her two pregnancies, she has never been hospitalized. She has never had head or other trauma. She has no allergies. Her husband has voiced concern in the past that she might be depressed, as he has occasionally observed her crying for no clear reason, and she has been sleeping less. She remembers that her headaches had improved during both pregnancies. She takes ibuprofen when she has headaches, which is once to twice a week on average. Fifteen months ago, she had to go to the local emergency department for a similar migraine episode. She was treated with intravenous medications, and the computed tomography scan of brain was normal then.

Family History

Mary's mother had migraines, as did an older sister. Her mother died of her first heart attack at age 71. Her father is alive and well at age 75.

Social History

The patient does not smoke or drink alcohol. She denies any illicit drug abuse. She has learned that some foods, including ripe bananas, avocados, chocolate, and red wine, cause her headaches to flare up, and does her best to avoid them. She also exercises daily and is absolutely sure that this has helped her control her headaches more effectively.

Review of Systems

Mary denies any recent weight gain or loss. She denies any shortness of breath, cough, palpitations, chest pain, or anxiety.

Objective

Physical Examination

Mary is a healthy-appearing, slightly overweight white woman.

General She lies comfortably in a dark room but becomes anxious during questioning.

Vital Signs
Weight, 180 pounds
Height, 5 feet 7 inches

Blood pressure, 130/72 mm Hg
Pulse, 80 beats per minute
Respirations, 14 breaths per minute

Head and Neck Mary's pupils are equal and react normally to light; both fundi are normal, as are the ocular muscles and accommodation reflex. She is tender over the left temporal area. The posterior part of the neck is tender but without any meningeal signs. No carotid bruits are heard. No lymphadenopathy is noted, and the thyroid gland is normal. Her oral cavity is normal as well.

Neurologic Mary is oriented to place, time, and person. Cranial nerves, deep tendon reflexes, motor, and sensory examinations are normal. Cerebellar functions are normal.

Chest Breath sounds are normal.

Heart Both heart sounds are normal without murmurs or clicks.

Abdomen Scaphoid and soft without tenderness. Normal bowel sounds.

Extremities Cool and sweaty.

Assessment

Working Diagnosis

The history and presentation confirm the current diagnosis of migraine. However, she reports another type of headache that may have developed recently. The following headache diagnoses should be considered.

1. Migraine without aura.
2. Tension-type headache.
3. Substance-withdrawal headache. This type of headache can be induced by prolonged use of analgesics. Patients with a predisposition to headaches often have a pharmacologic tolerance to these drugs, and a rebound headache develops as the medicine is metabolized. The headache may be diffuse or pulsating, and the onset occurs several hours after taking the analgesic.

Mary B.'s overall clinical picture includes features of all of these. The current presentation, physical examination, and the history strongly suggest an acute episode of migraine without aura. A mixed pattern of tension-type and substance-withdrawal headaches may also exist. She may be depressed, which can be contributing as well.

Plan

Diagnostic

No testing is required at this time.

Therapeutic

1. Sumatriptan (Imitrex), 50 mg, is administered via subcutaneous route to the anterior thigh area after explaining the side-effect profile. The patient's headache is reduced to 2/10 at 30 minutes. A prescription for sumatriptan is provided to the patient with directions and precautions.

2. Counseling is provided to educate the patient on the pathophysiology of migraine, tension, and withdrawal headaches. She is advised to discontinue the regular use of ibuprofen and acetaminophen.

3. A prophylaxis program is started with amitriptyline (Elavil), 25 mg at bedtime. This should further help her depression and insomnia. The side-effect profile including weight gain is explained.

4. Dietary advice is given on how to avoid all trigger factors.

5. Relaxation therapy is advised. An audiotape copy is given to the patient. The role of stress in such mixed-type headache is explained to the patient, and she agrees to try the therapy at least twice daily.

6. Daily record keeping of the headaches is emphasized. A model of a typical headache diary is provided to the patient, and she is counseled to bring her daily record on her next office visit.

Disposition

The physician and nurse educator discussed these treatment modalities with the patient. Mary was informed of the reasons to withhold analgesics and start a tricyclic antidepressant. She was given several references on available information for migraines. A strong physician/patient relationship was emphasized, and the patient seemed to understand it. A 2-week follow-up appointment was made.

DISCUSSION

Introduction and Burden of the Disease

Headache is a common clinical challenge encountered by physicians in primary care. More than 65% of Americans have a headache at some time in a given year. In the United States, migraine alone costs employers $13 billion per year because of the missed workdays and impaired work function (Johnson, 2004Ⓐ; Mannix, 2001Ⓐ).

Making the Diagnosis

A comprehensive history, including a headache history and physical examination, is the initial step. It is essential to rule out the secondary causes, including uncontrolled hypertension, infections (sinusitis, dental abscess), stroke, meningitis, brain neoplasm, subarachnoid hemorrhage, and refractory disorders

of the eye (Table 65-1 and Fig. 65-1). Danger signs or red and flags may alert the physician and generally suggest further evaluation (Box 65-1). A primary headache disorder is one that is benign, recurrent, and not associated with any underlying pathology (Headache Classification Committee, 1988Ⓒ; Headache Classification Committee, 2004Ⓒ). Primary headaches consist of migraine, tension-type headache, and cluster headache.

Migraine

Migraine is an episodic but chronic disorder that constitutes a common type of headache. The pain is typically moderate to severe and unilateral at the outset but may later become bilateral. Migraine commonly occurs without aura (common migraine); however, an aura may occur in up to 15% to 25% of the migraineurs (classic migraine). The aura can precede the headache by up to 1 hour. It includes visual symptoms like flashing lights, zig-zag lines, and a feeling of numbness or pins-and-needles around lips and hands. Migraine occurs in women 3 times as commonly as in men.

Transformed headache is the term used when the combination of tension-type and episodic migraine results in a chronic daily headache that usually occurs over a long period.

Migraine Management

The comprehensive management is an exigent task due to the chronic and episodic nature of the disease.

Table 65-1 Types of Headaches

Primary Headache Disorder
Migraine, with or without aura
Tension-type, infrequent, frequent, or chronic
Cluster and other trigeminal autonomic
   cephalgias (TACs)

Secondary Headache
Associated with head and/or neck trauma
Associated with cranial or vascular disorder, such as
   stroke
Associated with nonvascular intracranial disorder,
   such as intracranial hypertension and seizures
Associated with a substance (nitrate and alcohol)
   or its withdrawal (analgesics, caffeine,
   narcotics, and alcohol)
Associated with infection, such as meningitis and
   brain abscess
Associated with metabolic disorder, such as hypoxia,
   hypercapnia, and hypoglycemia
Associated with disorder of surrounding
   structures, including neck, eyes, ears, nose,
   sinuses, and teeth
Associated with psychiatric disorder
Cranial neuralgias

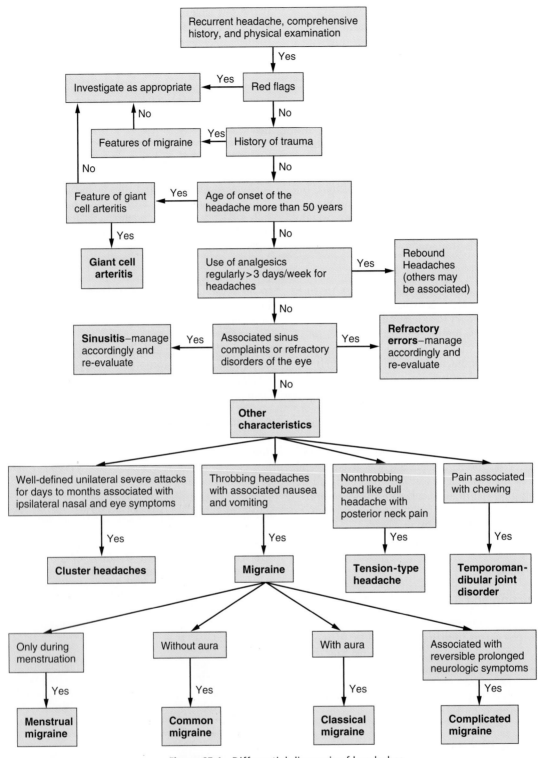

Figure 65-1 Differential diagnosis of headaches

Exclusion of a secondary headache etiology is of paramount significance and determines whether any imaging or laboratory tests are required.

The goals of migraine management involve not only improving the quality of life by reducing patient suffering in recurrent episodes but also avoiding

Box 65-1	"Red Flags" in the Diagnosis of Headache

*R*eflexes, asymmetrical or abnormal
*E*xertional, such as onset with sexual activity, coughing, or sneezing
*D*ifferent or a new headache
*F*ever, stiff neck, rash, weight loss associated
*L*oss of memory or other neurologic function such as paralysis
*A*ge older than 50 years
*G*ait abnormality
*S*everest headaches ever experienced

Box 65-2	Precipitating Factors in Migraines

*H*ormonal imbalance, such as during menses, pregnancy, and hormonal replacement therapy
*E*motional factors
*A*ccident/Trauma
*D*iet: see below
*A*lcohol and medicines such as nonsteroidal antiinflammatory drugs
*C*affeine
*H*ot or cold weather
*E*xertion
*S*moking

Migraine Dietary Restrictions

Dairy products: Aged cheeses (cheddar, Swiss), sour cream, chocolates
Meats: Beef and chicken livers, unrefrigerated dry fermented sausage, fermented bologna, salami, pepperoni, pickled fish, pickled herring, smoked fish, bacon
Beverages: Red wine, caffeinated drinks, chianti, burgundy, beer, ale, sauternes
Fruits: Avocados, overripe bananas
Vegetables: Fava beans, peanuts, snow pea pods, broad bean pods, sauerkraut
Food additives: Meat tenderizers, food containing monosodium glutamate (MSG) or brewer's yeast

medication abuse and educating the patient to avoid triggers (Silberstein, 2000Ⓐ; Snow et al., 2002Ⓒ) (Box 65-2).

To achieve these goals, the comprehensive management strategy may include the following:

1. Acute pharmacologic therapy
2. Nonpharmacologic therapy
3. Preventive therapy
4. Patient education

Acute Pharmacologic Therapy Medications used range from a wide variety of nonspecific analgesics to specific agents directed toward rectifying the cause of the migraine.

Nonsteroidal anti-inflammatory drugs (NSAIDs), such as aspirin, ibuprofen (Motrin, Advil), and naproxen (Aleve), as well as those in combination with acetaminophen, aspirin, and caffeine (Excedrin), have been proven to be superior to placebo in clinical trials for mild to moderate attacks, if used occasionally. A well-controlled study also showed the benefit of acetaminophen over placebo. Parenteral antiemetics, such as metoclopramide (Reglan) and prochlorperazine (Compazine) also have been shown to be superior to placebo in migraine headaches.

Opioids such as meperidine (Demerol) and hydrocodone (Lorcet, Lortab) are commonly prescribed for migraines but should be used sparingly. The concern for physical dependence and addiction is real.

Although ergot products are effective, their use has declined because of their significant adverse-effect profile and contraindications.

Since the introduction of triptans (Tfelt-Habsen et al., 2000Ⓐ), migraine management has been revolutionized. They have better efficacy because of their specificity for the abnormal mechanisms involved in the migraine pathophysiology. Triptans stimulate the specific serotonin receptors (5-HT1B/D) found on the cranial and meningeal vasculature and the trigeminal afferent nerves. This stimulation restores the neurovascular integrity and rectifies the ongoing secondary inflammatory reaction.

Nonpharmacologic Therapy These briefly include biofeedback (self-regulation), cognitive/behavioral (stress management) therapy, and relaxation training.

Preventive Therapy Prophylaxis is frequently required in migraineurs who continue to have frequent attacks despite the described management. A variety of preventive medications are available (Table 65-2) including antidepressants, antihypertensives, and antiseizure medications. Amitriptyline, valproate, propranolol, and timolol have been proven most efficacious in clinical trials. The drug is chosen depending on the patient's comorbidity. It is important to understand that most prophylactic agents take at least 4 to 6 weeks before their benefit can be evaluated.

Patient Education Patient education is the cornerstone of migraine management. It is imperative that the patient understand that migraines can be managed but not cured. The goal of therapy is to reduce the migraine frequency and severity to an extent at which the patient can carry out regular physical activity and daily responsibilities with a decent quality of life. This is a chronic disorder, and lifestyle modification plays a great role. Maintaining a

Table 65-2 Prophylactic Agents

Antidepressants	Tricyclic antidepressants	
	Nonsedating	Protriptyline, desipramine
	Sedating	Amitriptyline, nortriptyline, imipramine, doxepin
	Selective serotonin reuptake inhibitors	Fluoxetine, sertraline, paroxetine, fluvoxamine
	Others	Trazodone, bupropion, venlafaxine
Antihypertensives	β-Blockers	Atenolol, nadolol, propranolol, metoprolol, timolol
	Calcium channel blockers	Verapamil, nifedipine, diltiazem, nimodipine
	ACE inhibitors	Lisinopril
	Alpha agonist	Clonidine
Antiseizure	Divalproex, gabapentin, topiramate	
Others	NSAIDs, MAOIs, methysergide, cyproheptadine, ergot derivatives, magnesium	

ACE, angiotensin-converting enzyme; MAOI, monoamine oxidase inhibitor; NSAID, nonsteroidal anti-inflammatory drug.

headache diary to track the pattern of headaches is often helpful and frequently helps the patient realize that many factors are associated with headaches. Education on avoiding the triggers and focusing on protective factors is immensely important, as the patient feels more in control of his or her condition. Support groups are helpful, as patients realize they are not alone out there.

Tension-type Headache

Tension-type headaches can be episodic or chronic. This is the most common type of headache, and most of us have had them at some time in life. Female patients are more frequently affected. The pain is typically a steady, nonthrobbing, dull, and bilateral ache, which does not worsen with routine physical activity (Table 65-3). Patients commonly describe it as a bandlike constriction around the head and a sensation of heaviness and tightening at the back of the head and neck. Nausea and vomiting are absent. Posterior neck muscles may be tender as well as contracted. The headaches are commonly associated with significant life stressors and emotional lability but are usually not disabling. Concomitant depression may be an ongoing process in these patients and must be evaluated further.

Treatment

The moderate attacks are controlled well with the traditional NSAIDs (Krusz, 2004 Ⓑ). For severe attacks, triptans as well as narcotic analgesics are reserved. Muscle relaxants and osteopathic manipulative therapy also are frequently helpful because of the concomitant neck-muscle contraction associated with this type of headache. Prophylaxis may be warranted when fre-

quent urgent therapy is required. The headaches may become disabling and long lasting, interfering with performance on a daily basis. Prophylactic agents are similar to those used mostly for migraines. Tricyclic antidepressants have shown proven benefit. Management of other associated conditions, as mentioned, is helpful and should be done in all cases.

Cluster Headache

Cluster headache is the least common of the primary headaches and often causes excruciating pain, which

Table 65-3 Distinguishing Characteristics of Tension-type and Migraine Headaches

Tension-type Headache	Migraine
No aura	Aura present in 15%–25% of patients
Steady tightness or dull pain	Throbbing and pulsating pain
Not aggravated with routine physical activity	Aggravated with exertion or physical activity
Mostly bilateral	Mostly begins as unilateral but may become bilateral
Mild to moderate pain	Moderate to severe disabling pain
Usually not associated with nausea, vomiting, or photo/phonophobia	Usually associated with nausea, vomiting, photophobia, or phonophobia

peaks quickly from the onset within 15 minutes and lasts up to 4 hours. Pain commences around an orbit, radiates to the rest of the face, and is associated with lacrimation, facial flushing, conjunctival injection, and nasal congestion. It affects smoking men in their second or third decade more often than women. The headaches tend to occur at the same time of the day continuously for many days, followed by remission, only to recur later in life in similar clusters. Attacks can be triggered by alcohol consumption as well as by sudden temperature changes when a patient is within a cluster series. During an attack, the patient is restless, agitated, and can be observed pacing in pain.

Treatment

Inhalation of 100% oxygen from a tight-fitting mask at a flow rate of 5 to 10 L/min for 10 to 15 minutes during an attack is highly effective. Injectible or intranasal triptans as well as narcotic analgesics and traditional NSAIDs offer relief when given parenterally.

Summary

For the many individuals who have headaches, a primary care physician can begin by performing a comprehensive history and physical examination. This simple step helps to rule out a secondary cause for headache most of the time. The various diagnostic tests can be individualized and performed only if needed. Once a primary headache disorder is diagnosed, it becomes relatively simple to classify the headache type and treat accordingly. Often patients will have more than one primary headache type. As we understand today, considerable overlap occurs in treatment and prevention strategies of the primary headache disorders. The physician should use this fact to the advantage of the patient in the management, rather than ignoring it. Managing the chronic nature of headaches requires an ongoing healthy partnership between the physician and the patient.

> ### Material Available on Student Consult
>
> Review Questions and Answers about Headache

REFERENCES

Headache Classification Committee of the International Headache Society. Classification and diagnostic criteria for headache disorders, cranial neuralgias, and facial pain. Cephalgia 1988;8(Suppl 7):1–96.[C]

Headache Classification Committee of the International Headache Society. The International Classification of Headache Disorders, 2nd ed. Available at http://216.25.100.131/ihscommon/guidelines/pdfs/ihc_II_main_no_print.pdf. Accessed 10/7/2004.[C]

Johnson CJ. Headache in women. Prim Care 2004;31:417–428, viii.[A]

Krusz JC. Tension-type headaches: What they are and how to treat them. Prim Care 2004;31:293–311. [B]

Mannix LK. Epidemiology and impact of primary headache disorders. Med Clin North Am 2001;85:887–895.[A]

Silberstein SD. Practice parameter: Evidence-based guidelines for migraine headache (an evidence-based review): Report of the Quality Standards Subcommittee of the American Academy of Neurology. Neurology 2000;55:754–762.[A]

Snow V, Weiss K, Wall EM, Mottur-Pilson C. AAFP/ACP-ASIM Pharmacologic management of acute attacks of migraine and prevention of migraine headache. Ann Intern Med 2002;137:840–849.[C]

Tfelt-Hansen P, De Vries P, Saxena PR. Triptans in migraine: A comparative review of pharmacology, pharmacokinetics and efficacy. Drugs 2000;60:1259–1287.[A]

66 Tremor (Parkinson's Disease)

Kira Zwygart

INITIAL VISIT

Subjective

Patient Identification
John is a 62-year-old married white man.

Chief Complaint
This is a new patient on an initial visit.

History of Present Illness
John is a 62-year-old man with a history of benign prostatic hypertrophy (BPH) with an elevated prostate specific antigen (PSA), for which he is being monitored by his urologist. He has had recent biopsies for this problem, and the results indicated a benign process. He is being treated with doxazosin (Cardura), which has improved his symptoms significantly. He feels that his BPH is doing well and appears today for a complete physical examination. He has not had a complete physical in some time and is concerned about a slight hand tremor that has recently been affecting his tennis game.

John has remained very active throughout his life. He is currently working full time and playing tennis twice a week. He also works out with gym equipment. Over the past year, he has noted a slight tremor in his left hand and leg. The tremor initially began in his left leg and then moved to his left hand. It appears worse when sitting and remains constant unless he gets up and does something. John has noted that anxiety appears to worsen the symptoms. He has noted some muscle soreness and stiffness in his legs, which he has attributed to "getting older." He denies any history of similar symptoms. He has not had any weakness, tingling, headaches, dizziness, or visual changes. Other than the doxazosin (Cardura), he has not been taking any other medications. He does admit to four to five glasses of red wine per week but denies any history of alcohol abuse. He has not noted that the wine makes his tremor any better. He has no knowledge of being exposed to any toxic substances. No family history of neurologic problems or tremors is known. He has not noted any weight change, and his appetite remains good. John is concerned that the tremor is slowly worsening and would like to know if he can do anything to prevent further worsening.

Medical History
As mentioned previously, John's medical history is significant only for a history of BPH. He denies a history of coronary artery disease, diabetes mellitus, tuberculosis, hepatitis, hypertension, or thyroid disease. He has no drug allergies.

Family History
John's family history is noncontributory. His mother died at age 86 years of natural causes, and his father is still alive and well at 91 years. He has one brother who is alive and healthy. No family history of neurodegenerative illnesses or tremors is known.

Health Habits

John denies any history of smoking. He drinks four to five glasses of red wine per week with dinner. He exercises regularly and is a good tennis player.

Social History

John has been married for 42 years. He has worked in radio broadcasting for some time.

Review of Systems

Other than the complaints already mentioned, John is doing well. He denies any recurrent headaches, visual disturbances, or changes in speech or swallowing. He has no complaints of lung, cardiac, or gastrointestinal disease. His bowel movements are regular, and he has no history of melena or hematochezia.

Objective

Physical Examination

Vital Signs John's height is 67 inches; weight is 157 pounds; pulse is 51; and blood pressure is 141/77.

Head Male pattern alopecia.

Eyes Full range of motion in all quadrants with no gaze abnormality.

Nose and Ears
Clear. Hearing intact bilaterally.

Mouth Good dentition.

Neck Thyroid normal; no bruits, no thyromegaly.

Lungs Clear to auscultation.

Heart Sinus bradycardia without murmur.

Abdomen Soft, nontender, nondistended; no hernias, no organomegaly.

Genital/Rectal Normal external male genitalia, uncircumcised. Testicles descended bilaterally. No masses, no hernias. Rectal tone normal; 60-g prostate, smooth, symmetrical, without nodules. Hemoccult negative.

Extremities Muscle tone normal. Full range of motion in all extremities. No cyanosis, edema, clubbing, or joint deformities. Peripheral pulses 2+ and equal bilaterally.

Skin No rash or pigment changes.

Neurologic Oriented to person, place, and time. Affect is appropriate. Cranial nerves II through XII grossly intact. No focal motor or sensory deficit is noted. At rest, a noticeable tremor is seen in his left hand and leg. The hand tremor is fine, with a pill-rolling appearance. The tremor disappears with movement, such as picking up a magazine. The hand tremor is of slow frequency and is best noted when John is resting his hands on his lap. No rigidity is present in the larger joints, but noticeable cogwheeling is seen in his left wrist. John shows no difficulty in arising from the examining room chair when asked to sit on the examining table. His gait is appropriate, but he shows decreased arm swing with his left arm. Rapid alternating movements reveal slight bradykinesia on his left side as compared with his right. Romberg is negative. Reflexes are 2+ in all upper and lower extremities bilaterally, with no Babinski or clonus. The tremor disappears when he is asked to touch the physician's fingers.

Laboratory Tests

Office laboratory analyses ordered with the first visit included a complete blood cell count, chemistry profile, and thyroid-stimulating hormone, all of which were normal.

Assessment

Working Diagnoses

1. *Tremor.* The differential diagnosis includes various causes of tremor. Because the patient's tremor is resting, unilateral, progressive, and associated with some rigidity, the diagnosis of *idiopathic Parkinson's disease* (PD) is most likely.
2. *BPH.* Controlled with current medication. Monitored by a urologist.

Plan

Diagnostic

1. Re-address key symptoms and signs in John's history and examination to help rule in or rule out a diagnosis of PD versus benign tremor.
2. Serum chemistry laboratory work to include liver function tests to evaluate for Wilson's disease and creatinine phosphokinase to evaluate for muscle disease.
3. Magnetic resonance imaging (MRI) of the brain to evaluate for other neurodegenerative processes, although MRI is not of benefit for making the diagnosis of PD.
4. Cerebrospinal spinal fluid (CSF) analysis to evaluate for other neurologic disorders presenting with parkinsonism (optional).

Therapeutic

A full explanation of the diagnosis and treatment of PD is given to John and his wife. John is begun on selegiline (Eldepryl) at 5 mg twice a day by mouth. He is told to take it with breakfast and lunch, to limit its amphetamine-like stimulation that can interfere with sleep, and always to take it with food to limit nausea.

Patient Education

John is asked to maintain a symptom diary. He is advised to bring the symptom diary with him to all future visits. John also is encouraged to maintain a program of exercise and social activity to keep physically and mentally healthy, yet to balance these activities with the necessary rest and precautions required of patients with this disease.

Disposition

John is asked to complete the diagnostic testing, initiate the medication previously discussed, and return in 4 weeks.

FOLLOW-UP VISIT

Subjective

John has noted no difficulty with the medicine. Initially some nausea was felt, but this has resolved. His tremor is no worse, and at times it appears better. He continues playing tennis twice a week and remains active at work.

Objective

On physical examination, no change is apparent from the previous physical findings. John's resting tremor is still present, but it is less visible. The elbow and wrist joint rigidity are still present but slightly decreased.

Laboratory Tests

The serum chemistries, including liver function tests and creatinine phosphokinase, were all normal. The MRI of the brain shows mild cerebral atrophy, not unusual for his age, and otherwise is normal. CSF studies were not obtained.

Assessment

1. *Idiopathic PD in early stages.* John's history, essentially normal laboratory results, and MRI help support this diagnosis. The patient's daily activities are not yet affected by his symptoms. He is tolerating selegiline (Eldepryl) well.
2. *BPH symptoms are stable.*

Plan

The selegiline (Eldepryl) is continued at the recommended dose of 5 mg twice a day. Because John's symptoms are not affecting his activities of daily liv-

ing (ADLs), no further medication is prescribed. John is encouraged to continue with his work and routine exercises and to report any worsening of symptoms. John and his wife are given the phone number and address of the local PD support group to contact for further education and social support.

Disposition

John is scheduled to return for office follow-up in 1 month (sooner if any deterioration occurs in his condition).

DISCUSSION

The purpose of this case study is to discuss the differential diagnosis of tremors, particularly PD. Currently no laboratory or imaging tests are available that can make a definitive diagnosis of PD. Instead, these tests help rule out other neurodegenerative disorders. The diagnosis of PD is purely a clinical diagnosis and is based largely on the tremor and other symptoms (including rigidity, bradykinesia, and autonomic dysfunction). The type, onset, duration, frequency, and progression of the tremor, as well as ameliorating and aggravating factors, are all important in helping to distinguish between a parkinsonian tremor and other tremors. To aid in the diagnosis of a patient with a tremor, the tremor must first be classified. Classifications can be based either on a description or on the pathophysiology of the tremor.

Tremor Classification

Resting Tremor

This type of tremor occurs only at rest. It may worsen when the patient is engaged in mental tasks or moving an unaffected body part. It disappears quickly with muscle contraction in target-directed movements, so the patient's performance is rarely affected. Clinically, this type of tremor is associated with idiopathic PD and secondary parkinsonism. Secondary parkinsonism is a term given to conditions that mimic PD clinically but are caused by known agents. These include the following:

Postinfectious. This type of tremor is seen primarily during the convalescent phase of viral encephalitis.

Toxin-induced. This type of tremor is associated with exposure to carbon monoxide, carbon disulfide, manganese, cyanide, methanol, and the synthetic heroin analogue MPTP (1-methyl-4-phenyl-1,2,3, 6-tetrahydropyridine).

Drug-induced. This type of tremor is associated with ingestion of drugs that block dopamine receptors, especially the neuroleptic and antiemetic agents, as well as metoclopramide (Reglan) and reserpine.

Removal of the offending agent will cause resolution of symptoms within weeks to months.

Postural Tremors

These tremors are provoked by isometric contraction of the affected body segment (thus considered action tremors rather than resting tremors). They can be seen involving almost all body parts (i.e., head, neck, trunk, upper extremities, and lower extremities). They are the most common type of tremor and include both physiologic and pathologic tremors.

Physiologic tremors (normal or enhanced). These are normal tremors that occur in most individuals. The tremor is continuous, but with an irregular rate. It is usually not visible. The enhanced physiologic tremor is a more pronounced type. It is provoked by fatigue, anxiety, hypoglycemia, thyrotoxicosis, caffeine, dopaminergic agonists, β-adrenergic agonists, valproic acid (Depakene), lithium, amiodarone (which also may produce ataxia and peripheral neuropathy), and tricyclic antidepressants. It also may be seen in patients withdrawing from alcohol or benzodiazepines.

Essential tremor. This is the most prevalent pathologic postural tremor, 20 times more common than Parkinson's disease. Onset is noted in a bimodal distribution, and it is seen typically in the second and the sixth decades. A family history exists in more than 50% of patients with this disorder, whereas family history is uncommon with PD. It primarily affects the hands, followed by the head, the voice, the tongue, the lower extremities, and the trunk. In severe instances, it can appear as a resting tremor. Its progression is slow, and usually no significant change is noted for years. Often patients have noted that alcohol appears to ameliorate the tremor. β-Blockers and primidone also are effective in treatment.

Tremor with basal ganglia disease. Postural tremor also is visible in conditions affecting the basal ganglia. Therefore conditions such as Parkinson's disease, Wilson's disease, and dystonia are associated disorders in which this type of tremor is seen.

Tremor with peripheral neuropathy. These are postural tremors that occur concomitantly with a peripheral neuropathy, either acquired or hereditary. Motor-conduction velocities are slow in these patients, and β-blockers have little benefit.

Post-traumatic tremor. This may occur after a severe head injury.

Kinetic Tremor

These tremors are action (kinetic) and goal oriented (intention). They are usually the most incapacitating, and their appearance may indicate disorders of the cerebellum and related pathways. The tremors usually involve proximal muscles. They can be evoked through goal-oriented movements such as finger-to-nose or heel-to-shin testing. As the patient's finger or heel approaches the target, the tremor will increase. Kinetic and intention tremors can develop in patients with heavy-metal poisoning (lead, mercury, bismuth, thallium), carbon tetrachloride exposure, and metal chelator intoxication.

Cerebellar tremor. A cerebellar tremor is generally an intention tremor but also may occur as a postural tremor. The tremor commonly appears ipsilateral to the cerebellar lesion. The most common cause of cerebellar tremor is multiple sclerosis, but brainstem tumors, strokes, and paraneoplastic cerebellar degeneration also can be responsible. Associated symptoms and signs may include gait or speech abnormalities, defects in ocular movements, or difficulty executing rapid alternating hand movements. Chronic alcoholism also may produce this tremor.

Wilson's disease. This condition involves a defect in copper metabolism that first appears in the second or third decade and causes hepatic disease. It is treatable with chelating agents and diet. The tremor is either an intention tremor or a "wing-beating" movement seen when the patient abducts the arm.

Isometric Tremors

This tremor occurs with muscle contraction against a stationary object. An example would be a tremor while holding a heavy object.

Task-Specific Tremors

These tremors encompass both primary writing tremor and vocal tremor. They appear only with specific tasks. Primary writing tremor appears only with handwriting or a few other skilled manual tasks and, in general, is not produced by posture or goal-directed movement. Vocal tremors are apparent only when speaking. Both these types of tremors are similar to essential tremor but differ in that they are not always responsive to β-blockers, and no family history is known.

The type of tremor thus guides the physician toward the appropriate diagnosis. In John's case, the resting, unilateral tremor in a 62-year-old patient with evidence of rigidity and no other evidence of neurologic disease is most indicative of PD.

PD is the second most common neurodegenerative disorder (Alzheimer's-type dementia is more common), affecting between 300,000 and 1 million Americans. PD usually manifests itself clinically in patients of age 55 to 65 years, after 75% of the dopaminergic neurons in the substantia nigra are destroyed by mechanisms not fully understood at this time. It is a difficult disease to diagnose because many of its signs and symptoms are characteristic of several other disease entities. The classic symptoms and signs of PD include a resting tremor; rigidity, especially of the upper extremities (which is called "cogwheel rigidity" if superimposed tremors); bradykinesia or akinesia (reduced or lack of muscle movement); and postural reflex impairment causing patients to be unstable and fall. It is important to note that, the diagnosis of PD does not require all four of these symptoms and signs to be present. Balance problems are often absent in early PD. The diagnosis is made clinically, because no specific, reliable laboratory or radiologic studies confirm the diagnosis of PD. However, laboratory and radiologic studies are performed in patients with tremor to help rule out other disease entities. Other, more subtle signs and symptoms of PD include drooling due to impairment of swallowing and increased salivation; hypophonia (a soft, monotonous voice due to the loss of the ability to vary speech intensity); micrographia (very small handwriting, probably a component of bradykinesia); depression (either endogenous or reactive); and autonomic nervous system dysfunction with orthostatic hypotension.

Treatment

The treatment of PD includes not only medications but also patient and family education, as well as physical therapy to help keep the patient mobile. Various national PD organizations are available to assist patients and their families in dealing with the social and physical implications of this illness.

No established guidelines exist for the treatment of PD. Although the benefits of physical and occupational therapy, good nutrition, and education of patient and family are universally accepted, the initiation of medication is debated. Medical treatment is therefore highly individualized and symptom based. Consideration of treatment options is based on several factors: neuroprotection, or prevention of progression of the disease; treatment of motor symptoms; and treatment of nonmotor symptoms. Of course, the overall goal of treatment is to extend and improve the quality of life and maintain function.

The first concern in treating a patient with newly diagnosed PD is slowing the neuronal degeneration and progression of symptoms. Several medications have been proposed to do just that: vitamin E, selegiline, coenzyme Q_{10}, and dopamine agonists. Studies have been performed to evaluate neuroprotection in each of these cases, and none has shown irrefutable evidence of slowed disease progression. With that in mind, the first step of treatment will be to improve the motor symptoms displayed by the patient. Treatment options for this goal include selegiline (Eldepryl), amantadine, anticholinergics, levodopa, and dopamine agonists (ropinirole and pramipexole).

Selegiline is a monoamine oxidase-B inhibitor that limits the breakdown of dopamine. This results in a higher level of dopamine at the receptors, resulting in fewer symptoms. A recent meta-analysis of selegiline as compared with placebo or levodopa revealed that selegiline was effective in reducing disability and delaying the need for levodopa treatment. Recommended dosing of selegiline is 5 mg twice a day by mouth. It should be given with food to limit nausea, and it is recommended that this medication be taken with breakfast and lunch to limit its amphetamine-like stimulation, which can interfere with sleep.

Amantadine (Symmetrel) can be used for initial therapy of PD. The therapeutic benefits seem to be derived from its ability to increase dopamine release, block dopamine re-uptake, stimulate dopamine receptors, and exert possible peripheral anticholinergic properties. Studies have demonstrated a modest improvement in symptoms of tremor, rigidity, and bradykinesia. The usual dosage is 100 mg twice a day. Side effects may include edema, rash, and confusion. Alternatively, anticholinergics such as benztropine (Cogentin), trihexyphenidyl (Artane), ethopropazine (Parsidol), and procyclidine (Kemadrin) have been used in patients with predominant tremor. Their benefit is based on the balance that exists between acetylcholine and dopamine in the brain. PD patients with a depletion of dopamine have a relative excess of acetylcholine. The anticholinergic medications help limit this relative excess influence of acetylcholine. These agents are most helpful as early monotherapy in patients younger than 60 years with tremor-predominant PD. They also have been somewhat helpful in reducing bradycardia and rigidity, but because of their many side effects (including memory impairment, confusion, dry mouth, urinary retention, blurred vision, and constipation), they are limited to younger patients with minimal symptoms.

A possible choice for initial treatment in younger patients with PD is a dopamine agonist. Currently available agonists include bromocriptine, pergolide, ropinirole, pramipexole, and talipexole. These medications were initially used as adjunctive therapy to levodopa but have recently been added to the list of first-line medications. Dopamine agonists have demonstrated improvement in motor symptoms, although not to the extent that levodopa has. The agonists are also associated with more side effects (such as nausea, hypotension, edema, hallucinations, and sleep attacks), which makes them a poor option for elderly patients. The benefit of these drugs over levodopa is the decreased incidence of dyskinesia.

Levodopa is still considered the mainstay of treatment for symptoms of PD. It is the most potent of the current treatment options. It is an acceptable first-line agent, as it is inexpensive, and patients demonstrate fewer side effects than with dopamine agonists. In addition, if patients are started on any of these other medications, they will eventually require levodopa as the disease progresses (generally in 3 to 5 years).

Levodopa is converted in the brain to dopamine, although it also can be converted to dopamine outside the blood/brain barrier. If significant conversion of levodopa to dopamine occurs outside the blood/brain barrier, side effects such as nausea can be a significant problem. Carbidopa was therefore combined with levodopa, because it is able to block effectively much of the conversion of levodopa to dopamine outside the brain. A minimum of 75 mg carbidopa per day is usually necessary to block the peripheral conversion of levodopa.

Two formulations of carbidopa/levodopa are now available. The older version carbidopa/levodopa (Sinemet) is a fast-release agent; the newer version, controlled-release carbidopa/levodopa (Sinemet-CR), provides a slower sustained release of medication. PD patients taking the older, faster-release preparations are often frustrated with the short duration of action causing motor fluctuations, such as "wearing off" and "on-off" effects. The addition of controlled-release carbidopa/levodopa (Sinemet-CR) provides more stable plasma levodopa levels, helping to limit dyskinetic motor fluctuations in patients with more advanced PD. Dosing intervals can often be lengthened, although not dramatically, when PD patients are initiated on this formulation. A drawback encountered with this formulation is that achieving levodopa peak plasma levels is likewise lengthened. Use of the older, faster-acting preparations early in the morning followed by use of the newer, controlled-release formulation has been used as an answer to this therapeutic concern. Another benefit of the controlled-release formulation is its use at bedtime, which appears to improve sleep patterns in the majority of PD patients. This sustained-release preparation is available at doses of carbidopa/levodopa, 25/200 mg and 50/200 mg, and is often initially prescribed twice a day but has been used as often as 5 to 6 times a day.

To minimize nausea, it is best to give carbidopa/levodopa with food. Limiting the protein in both the breakfast and noontime meals, maximizing protein in the evening meal, and taking carbidopa/levodopa on an empty stomach after the first couple of weeks of levodopa therapy are techniques that can maximize levodopa absorption in the gastrointestinal tract. Nausea also can be limited by starting with low doses of carbidopa/levodopa combinations and building up to therapeutic doses gently. It is best to maintain a relatively low dose of 200 to 400 mg of levodopa until progressive disabling symptoms require an increase in dosage or dosing frequency. On reaching a daily dose of 600 mg of levodopa, the addition of a dopamine agonist is usually favored over further increases in levodopa.

In the majority of PD patients receiving long-term levodopa therapy, the response to therapy eventually deteriorates. After 5 years of carbidopa/levodopa therapy, in approximately 50% of patients, unstable, fluctuating response patterns to levodopa develop. The two most common types of levodopa-response deterioration that are noted are the wearing-off effect and dyskinesia. The wearing-off effect (often called end-of-dose failure) is characterized by the symptomatic benefits of each carbidopa/levodopa dose becoming more short lived than in the past, lasting only a few hours or less. This type of response is thought to be due to progressive loss of dopaminergic nigrostriatal neurons. As the disease progresses, the remaining nigrostriatal neurons are slowly depleted, limiting the brain's capacity to metabolize and store dopamine, causing a shorter response to levodopa therapy. The initial therapeutic adjustment often beneficial in limiting the wearing-off effect is to increase the frequency of doses, sometimes to as often as every 2 to 3 hours.

The other common type of levodopa-response deterioration is dyskinesia. Dyskinesias are involuntary, nonperiodic hyperkinetic movements. Several varied forms of dyskinesia can be noted as complications of levodopa therapy and include peak-dose, end-of-dose, and biphasic-pattern dyskinesias. Peak-dose dyskinesia occurs at the peak plasma drug levels or time of maximal levodopa effect. Hyperkinetic movements about 1 hour after the first daily morning levodopa dose are usually peak-dose dyskinesias. This type of dyskinesia can be limited by reducing the levodopa dose. End-of-dose dyskinesia occurs when the levodopa effect wears off. Hyperkinetic movements, especially dystonia, before the first daily levodopa dose are usually end-of-dose dyskinesias. This type of dyskinesia is best approached by shortening the interval between doses.

Biphasic-pattern dyskinesia occurs as levodopa plasma levels increase and decline. This pattern is the least common form of dyskinesia and is more commonly associated with chorea-type dyskinesia. Biphasic-pattern dyskinesias are often difficult to treat but may improve by shortening the dosing intervals. In addition to the levodopa dosage and interval adjustments discussed earlier, the addition of a dopaminergic agonist may help stabilize the response to levodopa therapy in patients with dyskinesia.

Nonmotor symptoms that may require treatment include autonomic dysfunction (leading to constipation, urinary symptoms, sexual dysfunction, and orthostatic hypotension), depression, sleep disturbances, hallucinations, and dementia. Careful attention to these symptoms and consideration of medication interactions are important in management.

Surgical treatments of PD have been used in the past but are now being studied again because of the complications of long-term levodopa treatment. The oldest successful surgical procedures have included thalamotomy and ventral pallido-tomy, which improved contralateral tremor and dyskinesia. The problem with the surgery is the possibility of permanent adverse effects, such as hemorrhage, infarct, seizures, and speech impairment. A more recent innovation is deep-brain stimulation. Electrodes are placed into the brain, and then high-frequency stimulation is performed. This procedure has been studied and performed in the thalamus, subthalamic nucleus, and globus pallidus internus. The greatest success has been at the latter two sites. Patients report significant improvement in dyskinesia, tremor, and activities of daily living. The incidence of adverse events is lower (although still present), because less trauma to the brain occurs.

The other benefit over surgery is that the electrodes can be relocated for further treatment, and the frequency can be altered to decrease adverse effects. Fetal tissue transplantation also has been studied, but it produced significant dyskinesia. Stem cell transplantation is currently under discussion, but legal and ethical debates (as well as the poor efficacy of the fetal tissue transplants) have delayed further study in this area.

Material Available on Student Consult

Review Questions and Answers about Parkinson's Disease

SUGGESTED READINGS

Bonuccelli U. Comparing dopamine agonists in Parkinson's disease. Curr Opin Neurol 2003;16(suppl 1): S13–S19. Ⓐ

Drucker-Colin R, Verdugo-Diaz L. Cell transplantation for Parkinson's disease: Present status. Cell Mol Neurobiol 2004;24:301–317. Ⓑ

Ives NJ, Stowe RL, Marro J, et al. Monoamine oxidase type B inhibitors in early Parkinson's disease: Meta-analysis of 17 randomized trials involving 3525 patients. BMJ 2004;329:593–596. Ⓐ

Jenner P. Dopamine agonists, receptor selectivity and dyskinesia induction in Parkinson's disease. Curr Opin Neurol 2003;16(suppl 1):S3–S7. Ⓑ

Minagar A, Kelley R. Movement disorders. Prim Care Clin Office Pract 2004;31:111–127.

Samii A, Nutt JG, Ransom BR. Parkinson's disease. Lancet 2004;363:1783–1793. Ⓑ

Shults CW. Treatment of Parkinson's disease. Arch Neurol 2003;60:1680–1684. Ⓐ

Sibon I, Fenelon G, Quinn NP, Tison F. Vascular parkinsonism. J Neurol 2004;251:513–524. Ⓑ

Smaga S. Tremor. Am Fam Physician 2003;68:1545–1552.

Volkman J. Deep brain stimulation for the treatment of Parkinson's disease. J Clin Neurophysiol 2004;21:6–17. Ⓐ

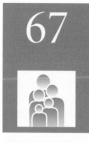

67

Clumsiness and Difficulty Walking (Brain Tumor)

Amber Barnhart

KEY POINTS

1. If unexplained neurologic symptoms occur in a patient with significant risk factors for coronary artery disease, vascular disease of the brain, stroke, and transient ischemic attack should be considered and appropriately evaluated.
2. Other clues to the causes of unexplained neurologic symptoms include
   a. Head injury and subdural hematoma
   b. Contagious infections and meningitis
   c. Recent viral infections and encephalitis
   d. Diabetes with hypoglycemia or hyperglycemia (or diabetic ketoacidosis)
   e. Medication side effects or toxicity
   f. Alcohol abuse or illicit drug use
3. Headache is the sole initial complaint in less than 20% of patients with brain tumors.
4. New-onset seizures, an abnormal neurologic examination, change in mental function, or loss of consciousness should raise concern about a possible brain tumor.
5. Brain metastases are commonly from the lung, breast, prostate, and melanomas.
6. Appropriate radiographic studies in the evaluation of a brain tumor include either computed tomography or magnetic resonance imaging. The choice depends on the suspected location of the tumor.

INITIAL VISIT

Subjective

Patient Identification and Presenting Problem

Shirley T. is a 58-year-old woman who presents to the emergency department because of "problems writing."

Present Illness

Shirley presents to the emergency department accompanied by her husband. Friends had called Shirley's husband earlier in the day because of their concern about her writing. Shirley has always been an accomplished writer and now her e-mails are filled with grammatical errors, misspellings, and incomplete sentences. Shirley has recently been fired from two housekeeping jobs because of "clumsiness." Her husband noticed that she has been unusually quiet the past several weeks, and he thought she might be depressed. The couple has just retired and moved to a new state to be close to their grandchild. Shirley's husband thought his wife seemed happy and content with their new life but had noticed this change in her recently. Because of all these concerns, he brought her to the emergency department.

Medical History

Shirley has a history of type 2 diabetes for the past 10 years. She also has a history of obesity, and with weight loss, her diabetes has been under good control. In addition, she has coronary artery disease and had a coronary artery stent inserted 2 years ago. She takes metoprolol (Lopressor), 100 mg/day; ramipril (Altace), 5 mg/day; simvastatin (Zocor), 40 mg/day; and aspirin, 325 mg/day.

Family History

Shirley is a twin; she and her twin are the youngest of 10 children. Her parents died of "undetermined causes" in their 80s. Her siblings are healthy.

Social History

Shirley is married and has worked as a housekeeper and babysitter for years. She is very active in her church, and her husband is a pastor. She has never smoked or used alcohol or drugs.

Review of Systems

Shirley denies any significant complaints, including the problems noticed by her friends and family. She

Evidence levels Ⓐ Randomized, controlled trials (RCTs), meta-analyses, well-designed systematic reviews of RCTs. Ⓑ Case-control or cohort studies, nonrandomized clinical trials, systematic reviews of studies other than RCTs, cross-sectional studies, retrospective studies, certain uncontrolled studies. Ⓒ Consensus statements, expert guidelines, usual practice, opinion.

denies seizures, dizziness, vision changes, sensation or motor changes, head pain, ear drainage, or difficulty swallowing. She denies shortness of breath, chest pain, nausea, emesis, diarrhea, or melena. She denies any unusual skin lesions or vaginal bleeding.

Objective

Physical Examination

General Shirley is a friendly woman who appears her stated age. She is in no distress.

Vital Signs Height, 5 feet 8 inches tall; weight, 230 pounds; respiratory rate, 20; pulse, 60; blood pressure, 169/83; temperature, 36.3°C (97.3°F).

Head, Eyes, Ears, Nose, and Throat Head: No signs of trauma. Eyes: Pupils equal, reactive to light and accommodation; equal ocular movement; normal without nystagmus. Sclerae and conjunctivae are clear. Fundus: No signs of papilledema, no arterio- venous nicking, no hemorrhages. Ears: Tympanic membrane normal bilaterally; canals are clear with no drainage.

Neck Neck nodes: All nonpalpable and nontender. Thyroid: Nonpalpable, no masses.

Lungs Clear without rales, rhonchi, or wheezing.

Cardiovascular Heart: Regular rhythm and rate. Normal S1 and S2. No murmurs. No carotid or renal bruits.

Abdomen Obese. Nontender in all four quadrants without masses. Liver and spleen are nonpalpable and not enlarged.

Rectal No masses and hemoccult-negative stool.

Back No costovertebral angle tenderness on right or left.

Breasts Symmetrical without masses. Supraclavicular and axillary nodes are nontender and nonenlarged.

Neurologic Cranial nerves II through XII are intact. Deep tendon reflex: Lower and upper extremities symmetrical. Sensation: Grossly normal. Strength: Normal and symmetrical in face and upper and lower extremities. Mental status: Oriented to person, place, and time. Long- and short-term memory: Grossly intact. Judgment: Grossly intact. Writing a sentence: Done correctly to oral command as well as copying.

Assessment

Working Diagnosis

This patient presents with a subtle change in a higher order of function: grammatical errors in writing. Noting the change in function should direct the physician to begin a thorough evaluation of the patient. Of course, brain tumor is high on the list of concerns and would be the working diagnosis.

Differential Diagnosis

1. *TIA or stroke.* Because of her history of diabetes, hypertension, and coronary artery disease, concerns about possible vascular disease of the brain would be appropriate. Such vascular disease could involve the small cerebral vessels with multi-infarct disease or larger arteries with transient ischemic attacks or actual stroke. Usually a transient ischemic attack or stroke presents with change to the motor and/or sensory components of the neurologic system rather than the subtle higher orders of function as seen in this patient.

2. *Non–brain tumor conditions of the brain.* Conditions such as subdural hematomas, meningitis, and encephalitis need to be considered also, but there is no history of trauma to suggest a subdural hematoma. The patient is afebrile and has no other symptoms of meningitis or encephalitis, although those may present with subtle symptoms as well.

3. *Diabetes mellitus.* The history of diabetes raises concern about the blood glucose, and possible early diabetic ketoacidosis should be considered, but this would be a very unusual presentation for diabetic ketoacidosis. Hypoglycemia should be considered if the change has been relatively acute in onset and brief, but a history of neurologic change persisting over several weeks makes this diagnosis very unlikely.

4. *Medications.* Patient use of medications and in particular narcotics, sedatives, or sleeping aids could result in subtle changes in higher level function. The medications prescribed for her chronic conditions must be evaluated. Metoprolol, ramipril, simvastatin, and aspirin were considered, but the subtle intellectual function changes that occurred in this patient have not been reported with these medications.

5. *Illicit drug or alcohol use.* The use of alcohol, illicit drugs, over-the-counter herbs and supplements, or mind-altering recreational drugs should be investigated thoroughly, although this is not relevant in this patient.

Plan

Diagnostic

Because of the importance of a brain tumor, computed tomography or magnetic resonance imaging should be ordered immediately. In addition, basic laboratory tests should be performed to exclude other possibilities given her medical history.

Therapeutics

Because the patient has subtle complaints, none of which is causing her discomfort or anxiety, no change in medications should be made at this time.

Patient Education

The patient and her family should be advised as to the various diagnostic possibilities given her symptoms. They should be encouraged to proceed with the radiographic testing. However, they should also be advised that the patient's symptoms are subtle and that it might be difficult to discover the cause of the complaints.

Disposition

A computed tomography scan is arranged for the patient (after insurance approval) for that afternoon. Blood tests are obtained as the patient completed the clinic visit. The patient and her family are given an appointment at the clinic for the next day to discuss the results of the tests.

DISCUSSION

Brain tumors are among the most feared diagnoses for a patient. Some of this fear and concern relates to the perceived inherent importance of the brain for normal function and for life. Laypeople and medical personnel alike are aware of the vital roles of the brain. Indeed, there is no simplistic "cut it out and fix it" approach for brain tumors as is possible with other tumors. Thus, treatment options are often more restricted, which makes the disease and its management difficult for both patients and physicians. In addition, simple common complaints by patients can actually herald the presence of the tumor. Although complaints such as headaches, arm weakness, or stumbling often are of no significance, they may indicate the need for further and more extensive evaluation. Conducting a careful history and physical examination is usually necessary to reassure the patient and physician that further workup is or is not necessary. The physician takes special note of any unusual features of the history or physical. Sloane and colleagues (2002) point out that "headache is the sole initial complaint in fewer than 20% of patients with brain tumor." The history of new onset seizures, an abnormal neurologic examination, a change in mental function, and loss of consciousness are hallmarks of brain tumors. Occasionally, some brain tumors, because of their distinctive location or pathology, do produce specific findings. The schwannomas, for example, cause unilateral hearing loss. Therefore, performing a complete neurologic examination is the foundation for the evaluation of brain tumors.

Brain tumors may be primary, such as the gliomas or meningiomas, or may represent metastatic disease from a distant primary malignancy. The incidence of primary brain tumors as well as of brain metastases is increasing. Brain metastases are common in lung, breast, and prostate cancers and in melanomas. When a patient presents with symptoms that suggest a brain tumor, the treating physician is usually obliged to evaluate the entire patient and not limit the investigation to the neurologic system. Fortunately, the clinical features of the patient's health will usually mandate the appropriate evaluation. Realistic and practical considerations concerning questions of medical insurance, the cost of appropriate studies, the patient's anxiety, and the need for a relatively early diagnosis and the development of an appropriate treatment plan are issues that have to be resolved with the patient in a timely fashion.

If a metastatic brain tumor is suspected, the site of the primary cancer must be determined from a thorough history and physical examination as well as appropriate comprehensive laboratory and radiographic studies of multiple organ systems (Fig. 67-1 and Box 67-1). Basic hematologic studies such as a complete blood count are indicated to evaluate for possible anemia or infection. Abnormalities in the white blood cell or platelet count may indicate lymphoma. Serum electrolytes should be assessed because electrolyte abnormalities can result in changes in mental status, and some abnormalities may suggest the primary site such as lung or adrenal cancers. Liver function tests are helpful in the investigation of possible hepatic metastases or cirrhosis. Ammonia levels may be needed if liver enzymes are normal and yet hepatic disease is suspected, because elevated ammonia levels with resultant hepatic encephalopathy often involve changes in mental status. Normal creatinine and blood urea nitrogen levels eliminate advanced renal failure as a cause of mental confusion, but renal cancer may still be a source of brain metastases even with normal creatinine and blood urea nitrogen. A thorough breast examination for both female and male patients is a requirement in the search for a primary cancer and may necessitate a mammogram as well. In addition, a digital prostate examination and a pelvic examination may be necessary in selected patients. Clinical judgment will dictate the inclusion of a prostate-specific antigen test in men. Sonograms of the uterus and ovaries, a CA 125 blood level, and a Pap smear may all be indicated in the search for a primary cancer in women. A rectal examination as well as a series of occult blood fecal tests would begin the workup for gastrointestinal cancer, which can metastasize to the brain. A chest radiograph is needed to begin the evaluation of possible lung cancer. All these were indicated for Shirley because she presented with a subtle form of confusion and with no obvious source of a primary cancer after the initial history and physical examination. In general, in the vast majority of patients the history and physical examination, and the results of the laboratory studies as well as initial radiographs, will direct the physician to the precise primary cancer involved.

If a brain tumor is suspected, a radiographic examination is the next step in the investigation. This

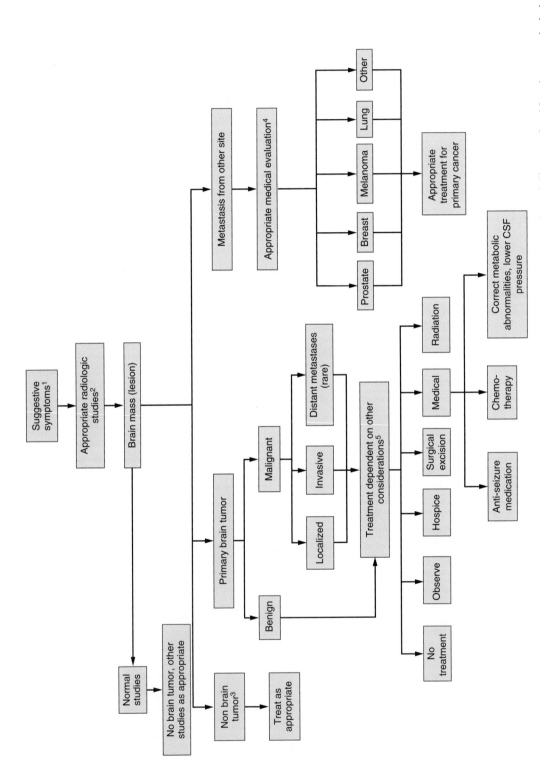

Figure 67-1 Suggested approach for the diagnosis and treatment of brain tumors. This is only a suggested approach, and, like any algorithm, it cannot include all possible variations. Although this stepwise evaluation will be helpful in the majority of patients, clinical judgment is required in selected patients. Note: Superscript numbers refer to Box 67-1, page 515. CSF, cerebrospinal fluid.

Box 67-1	**Suggested Approach for the Diagnosis and Treatment of Brain Tumor**

1. Suggestive of brain tumor
   a. Mental function changes
   b. Loss of consciousness
   c. Personality changes
   d. Seizures
   e. Sensorimotor abnormalities
2. Appropriate neurologic studies
   a. Computed tomography: most sensitive if suspected tumor is in the brain parenchyma
   b. Magnetic resonance imaging: fewer artifacts if suspected tumor is located near bony structures (e.g., base of the brain)
   c. Positron emission tomography: in selected patients
3. Non–brain tumor mass
   a. Subdural hematoma
   b. Abscess
   c. Granuloma
4. Appropriate medical evaluation for suspected metastatic brain tumors
   a. Complete blood count
   b. Liver function tests
   c. Electrolytes
   d. Renal function (creatinine, blood urea nitrogen)
   e. Prostate-specific antigen
   f. Mammogram
   g. CA 125 (and/or pelvic sonogram)
   h. Chest radiograph
   i. Hemoccult
5. Other considerations for appropriate treatment of brain tumors
   a. Patient/family decisions
   b. Location in the brain
   c. Symptoms
   d. Type of tumor/rapidity of change
   e. Size and extent of tumor
   f. Encapsulated versus invasive
   g. Comorbidities
      i. Age/state of health
      ii. Chronic obstructive pulmonary disease/congestive heart failure/other cancers, etc.

This would be the first order of testing if the physician believes a primary brain tumor is a likely diagnosis. In addition, other neurologic abnormalities such as a subdural hematoma, stroke, and brain abscess would be eliminated by this testing. There is controversy about whether computed tomography or magnetic resonance imaging is the most appropriate initial study, but the suspected location of the tumor dictates the ordering of the tests, and in many instances both studies are necessary, as are positron emission tomography scans in selected patients. Magnetic resonance imaging shows brain structures best with fewer artifacts if the tumor is adjacent to bony structures such as the base of the brain. Computed tomography is the most sensitive in the parenchyma of the brain where calcifications may be present. The addition of intravenous contrast enhancement may help "highlight" those tumors that have the same density as brain parenchyma. Positron emission tomography (PET) using fluorodeoxyglucose provides a relatively noninvasive method for studying glucose metabolism in tumors. Several studies show that PETs can assess tumor progression and response to treatment in gliomas (Padma et al., 2003⑧), glioblastoma multiforme (Tralins et al., 2002⑧), and supratentorial gliomas (Pardo et al., 2004⑧). PET will undoubtedly have greater utility in the future as the specific indications for the study become more apparent and as the technology becomes more widely available and less expensive.

Management of a brain neoplasm is based on several factors, certainly including the patient's and the family's requests and decisions. The nature of the presenting symptoms, the localization of the tumor within the brain, and the presence or absence of significant comorbidities such as heart failure, chronic pulmonary disease, and end-stage renal or hepatic disease or the presence of other malignancies or other illnesses that may limit life expectancy are critical factors that must be given consideration as an extensive workup is initiated. The cell type of origin, usually demonstrated by a brain biopsy, is critical in determining appropriate treatment. The size and extent of the tumor, the rapidity of change, and whether it is encapsulated or invasive are important factors in determining treatment. There are several cell types in the brain. Glial cells are categorized as macroglia (astrocytes, oligodendrocytes, ependyma [derived from neuroectoderm]) or microglia (derived from bone marrow). Each of these cell types can result in a different tumor type. Each tumor type requires a specific oncology treatment plan with specific outcome possibilities. Gliomas, for example, are the most common primary brain tumors. Tumors within this type of cell are further divided into astrocytomas (from astrocytes) and oligodendrogliomas (from oligodendrocytes). Within each of these cell types tumors also are graded, and each grade requires a different management plan. In addition, many brain tumors have a strong propensity to develop malignant components and have mixed cell grades. Because of the specific and extensive range of treatment plans for brain tumors, the family physician or primary care doctor will be instrumental in making the diagnosis, initiating the appropriate workup, establishing whether the brain mass is limited to the brain or represents metastatic disease, and starting initial medical management. Other members of the medical team, including a neurosurgeon and a radiation therapist or an oncologist, need to be consulted unless the patient or the family specifically requests that no aggressive therapy be provided. The initial medical management of most brain tumors includes the use of corticosteroids, such as dexamethasone. If a lymphoma with brain metastases is a possibility or the patient is HIV positive or has AIDS and is immunocompromised, the use of corticosteroids is more complex. Many tumors result in seizures, and the use of diphenylhydantoin or antiseizure medication should be strongly considered. Generally, chemotherapy is not a primary consideration for the treatment of a patient with a brain tumor because the blood-brain barrier that protects the brain in most situations is a deterrent for many chemotherapeutic agents.

The prognosis for most malignant brain tumors regardless of cell type, location, extent, and degree of invasiveness is poor, with survival measured in terms of months rather than years, but new rapidly changing developments in the treatment of brain tumors are encouraging. Recent investigational protocols combining chemotherapy, radiation, and surgery administered in varying order have shown some promising results. In addition, there are new advances in the technology of chemotherapeutic agents for treatment of brain tumors. Gliadel wafers (controlled-release 1,3-bis-(2-choroethyl)-1-nitrosourea) are inserted into the bulk of the tumor, thus bypassing the blood-brain barrier. They hold promise for the future in the treatment of brain neoplasia. Fortunately, science continues to explore options in the treatment of a deadly and very intimate disease: brain cancer.

Material Available on Student Consult

Review Questions and Answers about Brain Tumor

REFERENCES

Padma MV, Said S, Jacobs M, et al. Prediction of pathology and survival by FDG PET in gliomas. J Neurooncol 2003;64:227–237.[B]

Pardo FS, Aronen HJ, Fitzek M, et al. Correlation of FDG-PET interpretation with survival in a cohort of glioma patients. Anticancer Res 2004;24:2359–2365.[B]

Sloane PD, Slatt LM, Ebell MH, Jacques LB. Essentials of Family Medicine, 4th ed. Baltimore, Lippincott Williams & Wilkins, 2002.

Tralins KS, Douglas JG, Stelzer KJ, et al. Volumetric analysis of 18F-FDG PET in glioblastoma multiforme: Prognostic information and possible role in definition of target volumes in radiation dose escalation. J Nucl Med 2002;43:1667–1673.[B]

SUGGESTED READINGS

Becker LA, Green LA, Beaufait D, Kirk J, Froom J, Freeman WL. Detection of intracranial tumors, subarachnoid hemorrhages, and subdural hematomas in Primary care patients: A report from ASPN, part 2. J Fam Pract 1993;37:135–141.[C]

Cady R, Dodick DW. Diagnosis and treatment of migraine. Mayo Clin Proc 2002;77:255–261.[A]

68 Terminal Illness

Timothy P. Daaleman

INITIAL VISIT

Subjective

Patient Identification and Presenting Problem

Mrs. R. is an 83-year-old woman seen by her family physician after an initial consultation with a cardiologist. Mrs. R. was referred for evaluation of valvular heart disease—she underwent mitral valve replacement approximately 12 years ago—and for her chronic rate-controlled atrial fibrillation. She denies any chest pain; however, she acknowledges some dyspnea on exertion, especially when climbing stairs. During her consultation, a two-dimensional echocardiogram reveals a well-seated prosthetic mitral valve, but a markedly sclerotic aortic valve with mild regurgitation. As a result of this finding, and in consideration of Mrs. R.'s very good health and func-

tional status, the cardiologist recommends surgical replacement of her aortic valve. Mrs. R. declines the surgery and returns to her family physician for ongoing care, requesting a prognosis.

Medical History

Mrs. R. has a history of essential hypertension, urinary incontinence, macular degeneration, atrial fibrillation, valvular heart disease with mitral valve replacement, and generalized anxiety disorder with depressive symptoms. Her medications include metoprolol (Lopressor), 50 mg twice daily; bumetanide (Bumex), 0.5 mg/day; digoxin, 0.25 mg/day; amlodipine (Norvasc), 10 mg/day; sertraline (Zoloft), 25 mg/day; and warfarin (Coumadin), 5 mg/day.

Family History

Mrs. R. reports a family history of cerebrovascular and atherosclerotic heart disease; however, she states that her only daughter has no health problems.

Social History

Mrs. R. quit cigarette smoking 20 years ago and does not drink alcohol. She recently relocated to the area to be closer to her daughter, who is her primary caregiver, and resides in an apartment adjacent to her daughter's home. Mrs. R. is fully independent in all of her activities of daily living and travels to her medical appointments using public transportation. She has previously completed an advance directive and has named her daughter as having durable power-of-attorney for health-care decisions.

Review of Systems

Mrs. R. denies any syncope, orthopnea, peripheral swelling, or pain. She discloses some remorse over her recent relocation and misses her friends and other family members from her prior place of residence. She describes a functional relationship with her daughter and son-in-law, but one that is not close and intimate.

Objective

Physical Examination

The patient is a thin, anxious-appearing woman who is alert and oriented and appears her stated age. Her weight is 107 pounds, and her vital signs include blood pressure of 175/75, pulse irregular at 62, respiratory rate of 16, and temperature of 36.2°C (97.1°F). Her neck examination is without jugular venous distention, and her lungs were clear to auscultation bilaterally without wheezes, rales, or rhonchi. The cardiovascular examination is remarkable for an irregularly irregular rhythm with a loud grade 4/6 crescendo/decrescendo murmur at her right base, which radiates into neck bilaterally. In addition, a high-pitched holosystolic murmur is heard at the left sternal border and an audible mechanical valve click. Mrs. R.'s abdomen is soft and nontender, with no hepatosplenomegaly, and her extremities are without cyanosis, clubbing, or edema. Her international normalized ratio (INR) is reported at 2.6.

Assessment

Working Diagnosis

The working diagnosis is valvular heart disease and chronic atrial fibrillation, which constitutes a progressive disease leading to eventual heart failure and subsequently death. Mrs. R. chooses to forego a surgical intervention that would potentially prolong her life and has elected a palliative course of care.

Plan

Four major areas must be considered in providing palliative care to Mrs. R. as she begins to approach the end-of-life: effective communication and establishment of care goals; coordination of care; pain and symptom care; and social, spiritual, and bereavement support (Morrison and Meier, 2004).

1. *Effective communication and establishment of care goals.* Mrs. R.'s request for a prognosis for her terminal heart disease invites an open-ended discussion about the type of care that she wishes to receive and her overall goals of care. She speaks freely with her family physician and has a level of trust that has developed over several months. Mrs. R. is unambiguous about the goals of her care, predicated on a quality of life that is determined by her ability to remain independent and highly functional. Her physician reviews the existing advance directive, outlines several potential clinical scenarios regarding her disease progression, and they arrive at a care plan that includes hospitalization for symptom control, but sets limits regarding curative or aggressive treatment (EPEC, 2004). These limits include foregoing resuscitative efforts and transfer to an intensive care unit should her condition in the hospital deteriorate.

2. *Coordination of care.* Once a care plan has been established, Mrs. R.'s physician makes several copies of the advance directive for the medical record and Mrs. R.'s family members, and documents the discussion and plan within the electronic medical record that serves both the outpatient family practice clinic and the admitting hospital. The physician also contacts Mrs. R.'s daughter—who has the durable power of attorney—and reviews and verifies the care plan. The physician's pager number and direct phone line to the clinic are given to Mrs. R. and to her daughter, and a 6-week follow-up appointment is scheduled.

3. *Pain and symptom care.* Mrs. R. denies any pain but describes some dyspnea on exertion with stair climbing, but feels that supplemental oxygen is unnecessary. A greater concern is her frequent tearfulness, difficulty with sleep, and feelings of loss and distance from some family members that predated the disclosure of her terminal disease. She is maintained on sertraline, which has a low likelihood of cardiogenic side effects; however, she declines outpatient psychological therapy, such as cognitive-behavioral therapy and counseling (Morrison and Meier, 2003).

4. *Social, spiritual, and bereavement support.* Mrs. R. and her daughter would clearly benefit from a support group and the involvement of counseling or bereavement services. The patient has previously attended activities coordinated through the area agency on aging, but has no interest in returning there and considers herself too private to allow nonfamily members to be involved in her care. She comes from a Jewish faith tradition and does not draw any inner strength from her beliefs, practices, or communities of faith. Mrs. R. is offered enrollment in a hospice program but cannot see the benefit of this service at this time.

FOLLOW-UP VISIT

Subjective

Mrs. R returns for an office visit accompanied by her daughter approximately 3 months after her previous appointment and 1-week after hospitalization for upper gastrointestinal bleeding. In the emergency department, she had a 1-day history of weakness and was found to be profoundly anemic with guaiac-positive stools. Her admission INR was 2.5 (normal for therapy), and during hospitalization, she received vitamin K and fresh frozen plasma before upper endoscopy identified a bleeding site at her distal esophagus. Mrs. R. received 4 units of packed red blood cells and was started on omeprazole (Prilosec) and enoxaparin (Lovenox). Her cardiovascular status remained stable, and her weakness improved after her transfusion. She was discharged to a skilled nursing facility for interim care with an anticipated return to home. On today's visit, Mrs. R. complains of persistent shortness of breath and bilateral lower extremity swelling.

Objective

The patient's weight is 113 pounds, and her vital signs include a blood pressure of 160/72, irregular pulse of 69, respirations 20, and temperature of 36.2°C (97.1°F); her room air pulse oximetry is recorded at 90%. Her neck examination is remarkable for trace jugular venous distention, and her lungs demonstrate bibasilar crackles. The cardiovascular examination is remarkable for an irregularly irregular rhythm with a loud grade 4/6 crescendo/decrescendo murmur at her right base, a high-pitched holosystolic murmur at the left sternal border, and an audible mechanical valve click. Mrs. R.'s abdomen is soft and nontender with no hepatosplenomegaly. Her extremities show +2 nonpitting edema.

Assessment

Mrs. R. shows marked progression and exacerbation of her chronic heart failure.

Plan

1. *Effective communication and establishment of care goals.* Mrs. R.'s physician reviews the clinical impression of worsening heart failure and reassesses her understanding of the diagnosis, prognosis, and disease course (EPEC, 2004). Both disease-modifying and symptom-directed treatments, involving hospitalization, skilled nursing care, and hospice, are outlined and considered during a discussion that involves both the patient and her daughter. At the end of the discussion, Mrs. R. recognizes and accepts that her symptoms may be the beginning of a more active phase of dying and directs a care goal of symptom care only within the nursing facility.
2. *Coordination of care.* The discussion and care plan are documented within the medical record, and the advance directive is reviewed and verified. During the office visit, the physician personally contacts the medical director and director of nursing at Mrs. R.'s skilled care facility to outline and coordinate the care plan: treatment of symptoms with no hospitalization (Morrison and Meier, 2004).
3. *Pain and symptom care.* Mrs. R. has persistent dyspnea at rest, and her bumetadine is increased to 1 mg/day, and supplemental oxygen also is prescribed. She acknowledges that part of her difficulty breathing may be due to anxiety, and

lorazepam (Ativan), 0.5 mg, is prescribed at 6- to 8-hour intervals. Low-dose morphine sulfate drops are added to the treatment regimen for persistent dyspnea that is refractory to the other measures (Doyle et al., 2004).
4. *Social, spiritual, and bereavement support.* Mrs. R.'s nursing facility has an existing support group for family caregivers and a full-time chaplain on site. Both she and her daughter are open to these services and to the possibility of reconnecting with an area synagogue (National Consensus Project, 2004).

DISCUSSION

The provision of quality palliative care is an essential skill of primary care medicine. Patients consistently focus on three domains when asked about end-of-life care issues; pain and symptom management, communication and goal planning, and attention to psychosocial and spiritual needs (Morrison and Meier, 2004).

Pain and Symptom Management

A primary goal in palliative care is the relief of pain and other common symptoms, such as nausea and dyspnea, which contribute to suffering. Regular and standardized assessments of pain and symptoms are the foundation for effective treatment. Table 68-1 outlines some approaches to pain and symptom management in palliative care. The simplest, least invasive, and most effective regimen is the one that is used (Doyle et al, 2004; EPEC, 2004).

The nature, cause, and temporal component of the pain should be assessed to determine the physiologic (e.g., neuropathic or nociceptive) and contextual (e.g., psychosocial, spiritual) components composing the pain (Morrison and Meier, 2003). Pharmacologic pain medications should be scheduled on regular basis rather than waiting for symptoms to increase. Rescue dosages of immediate-release medications are generally 10% of the 24-hour required opioid dose and should be available for breakthrough pain (Doyle et al., 2004; EPEC, 2004). Dosing of both scheduled and rescue medications must be frequently reassessed and titrated according to the response to pain. Meperidine, because of low potency and the toxicity of its metabolite, in addition to antagonist agonists such as pentazocine, nalbuphine, and butorphanol, should be avoided (Doyle et al., EPEC, 2004). In addition, all patients who are taking opioids should be on a bowel regimen to prevent constipation.

Formal (e.g., nursing) and informal (e.g., family) caregivers should be directed in their routine

Table 68-1 Pain and Symptom Management in Palliative Care

Symptom	Assessment	Treatment
Pain	Visual pain analogue scales	For mild pain, consider acetaminophen or NSAIDs. For moderate pain, short-acting opioids should be titrated to pain control For severe pain, use short-acting opioids until pain is controlled Begin a long-acting opioid at equal-analgesic dosage For neuropathic pain, adjuvant analgesics include anticonvulsants or low-dose tricyclic antidepressants For bone pain, consider NSAIDs, calcitonin, or bisphosphonates
Constipation	Check bowel functioning, and review potential medication side effects	Use stool softener with stimulant until effective Consider other stimulant classes if refractory
Nausea/Vomiting	Check bowel functioning, and review potential medication side effects	Promethazine or scopolamine if mild If severe, consider haldoperidol, chlorpromazine, metoclopromide, or ondansetron
Dyspnea	Think BREATH AIR **B**ronchospasm **R**ales **E**ffusions **A**irway obstruction **T**hick secretions **H**emoglobin low **A**nxiety **I**nterpersonal issues **R**eligious concerns	Treat specific symptoms Albuterol, ipratropium, steroids Diuretics, check IV fluids Consider thoracentesis Check airway Nebulized saline, glycopyrrolate, hyoscyamine Consider transfusion Benzodiazepines, relaxation therapy, opioids Counseling Pastoral care
Anxiety	Is there panic, agitation, restlessness, insomnia, or excessive worry?	Supportive counseling, and consider benzodiazepines
Depression	Feelings of anhedonia, helplessness, hopelessness, suicidal	Psychotherapy, pharmacologic therapy, or combination
Delirium	Identify potential reversible causes; is this a terminal event?	Treat underlying causes if possible Consider atypical antipsychotics

NSAID, nonsteroidal anti-inflammatory drug.

assessments to specific symptoms (e.g., dyspnea, constipation) and away from medical parameters such as vital signs, for patients who have elected palliative care (Morrison and Meier, 2003). Table 68-1 includes common symptoms found at the end of life, which are assessed both by targeted questions to conscious patients (e.g., "are you depressed?") and by recognizing symptoms (e.g., agitation, delirium) in patients who are unable to respond (Morrison and Meier, 2004).

Communication and Goal Planning

Palliative care begins once the goals of care have been outlined and established. Arriving at a care goal requires communication skills that include open-ended questioning, empathic listening, and attention to the psychological and social contexts of the patient (Morrison and Meier, 2004). Primary care is an ideal setting to facilitate and formulate advance care planning because of an emphasis on continuity; however, adequate time must be allocated for this task.

Physicians should gauge both patient and family understanding of the disease process, prognosis, and treatment alternatives. Dying patients and their physicians frequently overestimate survival probabilities, which often influence treatment choices (Morrison and Meier, 2003). For some patients, a primary goal may be to prolong life at all costs. However, most patients approaching death want to have some quality of life that includes a closer relationship and a lessened burden to their families, treatment of their pain and other physical symptoms, and retention of a sense of control over their lives.

Advance directives are helpful in documenting and communicating care goals to other providers (e.g., first responders) and family members, once they are established. These documents verify a plan of care and treatment that the patient has designated. A durable power of attorney for health care allows a patient to identify a family member, or other individual, to make decisions regarding his or her care, and it is effective once a patient with a terminal condition no longer has the capacity to make decisions (Morrison and Meier, 2003).

Psychosocial, Spiritual, and Bereavement Support

Patients and family members who approach death have needs that cut across psychological, social, and spiritual domains (National Consensus Project, 2004). Dying is a time of tremendous stress but also offers important opportunities for growth, intimacy, reconciliation, and closure within relationships. Physicians who care for these patients should be attentive to various cues that indicate depression, familial conflict, or spiritual distress and should consider resources, such as hospice and palliative care services, that can provide care and support in these areas (National Consensus Project, 2004).

Material Available on Student Consult

Review Questions and Answers about Terminal Illness

REFERENCES

Doyle D, Hanks GW, Cherny NI, Calman K. Oxford Textbook of Palliative Medicine, 3rd ed. Oxford, England, Oxford University Press, 2004.

EPEC Project home page. Available at www. epec.net/EPEC/webpages/index.cfm. Accessed 9/30/2004.

Morrison RS, Meier DE. Geriatric Palliative Care. New York, Oxford University Press, 2003.

Morrison RS, Meier DE. Palliative care. N Engl J Med 2004;350:2582–2590.

The National Consensus Project for Quality Palliative Care home page. Available at www.nationalconsensusproject.org. Accessed 9/30/2004.

69 Pain "Everywhere" (Fibromyalgia)

Kurt A. Lindberg

KEY POINTS

1. Fibromyalgia is a distinct condition with definable findings on history and physical examination.
2. No signs of significant abnormalities are found in the peripheral tissues or the serum of patients with fibromyalgia.
3. Current theories of pathophysiology of the condition suggest abnormalities in the communication, processing, and thresholds of pain in the central nervous system.
4. Treatment of fibromyalgia includes patient education, getting regular sleep, treating comorbid conditions, and maintaining regular aerobic exercise.
5. Few medications have been shown to be helpful for this condition.

INITIAL VISIT

Subjective

Patient Identification and Presenting Problem

Jennifer C., a 55-year-old woman seen in the outpatient clinic, complains of low back pain that has been gradually worsening during the past 6 months. She attributes the pain to a day when she cared for her 2-year-old grandchild and "overdid it." Jennifer describes the back pain as a severe, dull ache that radiates into her hips. She complains of paresthesias in both lower extremities. She has difficulty falling asleep at night and wakes frequently because of her pain. Over the last several months, the pain seems to have traveled "everywhere." She now aches in her arms, her hands, and her neck. She feels severely fatigued and is unable to do even the most basic housework. She cannot even tolerate having someone touch her arm without shrinking in pain.

Medical History

Review of Jennifer's chart shows that she has a history of anxiety and depression, which has recently been under good control. She has had an appendectomy, total abdominal hysterectomy, and cholecystectomy. She carries a diagnosis of irritable bowel syndrome (IBS) and female urethral syndrome.

Medications

Jennifer takes fluoxetine (Prozac), 60 mg daily; bupropion (Wellbutrin), 150 mg twice daily; celecoxib (Celebrex), 100 mg twice daily; and conjugated estrogens (Premarin), 0.625 mg daily.

Family History

Jennifer's father died at age 65 of a sudden heart attack. Her mother was "always in the doctor's office" for various medical problems and died of a stroke at age 76. She has no siblings and two children, one of whom has depression and chronic back pain.

Social History

Jennifer has been married for 32 years. She smokes half of a pack of cigarettes per day but has been trying to "cut back." She drinks alcohol occasionally (approximately three to four drinks per week) and does not use illicit drugs.

Review of Systems

Jennifer has felt chilled and clammy but has had no fever. She has no shortness of breath or cough or significant chest pain. Her chronic IBS causes abdominal discomfort, diarrhea, and constipation, but no rectal bleeding, reflux, or nausea. She has her usual urinary frequency but no dysuria or other urologic or gynecologic symptoms. She has had no joint swelling or redness but feels as if her hands are "puffy." She has had no skin, hair, or mucous membrane abnormalities. Her mood is low because of her condition, but she denies feeling as depressed as she has been in the past. Her appetite is normal, but sleep is disturbed, as noted in the history. She often feels as if she is "in a

---

Evidence levels **Ⓐ** Randomized, controlled trials (RCTs), meta-analyses, well-designed systematic reviews of RCTs. **Ⓑ** Case-control or cohort studies, nonrandomized clinical trials, systematic reviews of studies other than RCTs, cross-sectional studies, retrospective studies, certain uncontrolled studies. **Ⓒ** Consensus statements, expert guidelines, usual practice, opinion.

fog" and is forgetful and has trouble concentrating. She has no suicidal ideations or anhedonia.

Objective

Physical Examination
Jennifer is a middle-aged Hispanic woman who appears in no acute distress. She is 5 feet 2 inches tall and weighs 160 pounds. Her temperature is 36.6°C (97.8°F), respiratory rate 16, pulse 88, blood pressure 124/78. Her head examination is normal with no mucosal lesions. Her neck is supple with no lymphadenopathy or thyromegaly. Lungs are clear to auscultation bilaterally. Her heart is regular with no murmur. Her abdomen has normal bowel sounds with generalized tenderness but no guarding or rebound. Specifically, she has no peripheral edema or joint swelling or redness. Her skin and hair are normal. Her orientation and memory appear to be intact. Objective cutaneous numbness is not found. Her muscle strength is difficult to assess because she seems to collapse because of pain when being tested. Her reflexes are normal. She is limited in spinal flexion to 45 degrees and is unable to extend backward because of pain in the lumbar musculature. The areas in which she describes pain are primarily the muscles and tendinous regions, not in bones or joints.

Assessment

Working Diagnosis
Low-back pain, diffuse myalgias, and fatigue

Differential Diagnosis
1. *Muscular strain.* Jennifer's history of low-back pain beginning after overuse could be consistent with a muscular strain. This would not explain the widespread discomfort she is experiencing, however.
2. *Polymyalgia rheumatica.* This is a condition of inflammation causing proximal muscle pains, usually seen in middle-aged patients. This condition responds well to corticosteroids and is important to identify because of rare sudden blindness due to an association with temporal arteritis. A normal erythrocyte sedimentation rate (ESR) would make this condition highly unlikely.
3. *Connective tissue disorder (e.g., lupus).* The hallmark of these disorders is objective signs of joint inflammation, objective skin or mucous membrane abnormalities, and abnormal serologies (e.g., antinuclear antibody). These conditions usually respond to immune-modulator medications and thus are important to consider in patients with generalized pain. However, this patient has mostly muscular or tendinous pain and no objective signs of joint, skin, or mucous membrane abnormalities. If signs of systemic inflammation such as sedimentation rate (ESR) or C-reactive protein are normal, these conditions can effectively be ruled out as causes of Jennifer's complaints. It should be noted that several blood tests used to diagnose connective tissue disorders (e.g., antinuclear antibody or rheumatoid factor) may be positive in a small number of normal individuals. For this reason, these tests should not be ordered unless the patient's inflammatory markers, physical examination, or history is consistent with one of these disorders. This will avoid a patient becoming overly concerned about a connective tissue disorder because of an elevated blood test that has no clinical relevance.

4. *Fibromyalgia.* Fibromyalgia is a condition of generalized pain in muscles, tendons, and skin that has no demonstrable local abnormality. Patients with fibromyalgia often are initially seen with a single area of maximal concern in the axial skeleton (spine, hips, or buttocks) and often attribute the onset to a specific event (Bradley and Alarcon, 2005Ⓐ). This diagnosis seems to fit this patient's presentation; however, further testing should be performed to rule out other conditions before arriving at this diagnosis. If fibromyalgia is suggested by the patient's history and examination, the practitioner should perform a "tender point" evaluation (Fig. 69-1). No serologic or radiologic test is available to confirm or rule out fibromyalgia (Gilliland, 2005Ⓑ).

5. *Hypothyroidism.* Patients with low levels of thyroid hormone often experience cold intolerance, fatigue, and swelling similar to Jennifer's symptoms. Hypothyroidism is common and may be easily diagnosed through testing of the serum level of thyroid-stimulating hormone (TSH). If the TSH level confirms this diagnosis, thyroid-replacement therapy would reverse any associated symptoms.

6. *Inflammatory myopathy (e.g., dermatomyositis).* Inflammation of the muscles usually results in weakness rather than pain and is ruled out if inflammatory markers and creatinine kinase are normal.

7. *Somatoform disorder.* This is a group of psychiatric diagnoses that includes somatization disorder, hypochondriasis, conversion disorder, and malingering. This group of disorders requires the assumption that no physical abnormality is present in the patient (First, 2000Ⓒ). Because fibromyalgia has no readily apparent organic abnormalities, many patients with fibromyalgia receive (formally or informally) one of these labels. However, it will be presented in the Discussion section that fibromyalgia is a distinct disorder with objective diagnostic criteria and with research findings that suggest an organic basis.

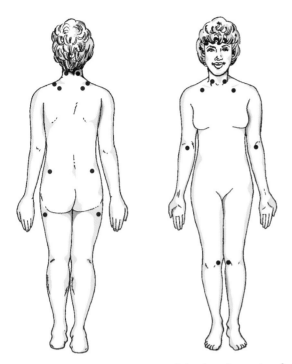

Figure 69-1 Tender points used in the diagnosis of fibromyalgia: suboccipital muscle insertion, anterior to C5–C7 intertransverse process, midpoint of the upper border of trapezius, medial origin of supraspinatus, second costochondral junction, 2 cm distal to the lateral eipcondyle, upper outer quadrant of the buttock, posterior to the trochanteric prominence, medial fat pad proximal to the knee.

9. *Worsened depression.* Depression is frequently coexistent with chronic pain conditions, and it is always appropriate to consider this in such patients. Depression or anxiety does intensify the reporting of pain. Conversely, experiencing chronic pain may lead to depression or anxiety. If screening questions reveal that a mood disorder is present, it should be appropriately treated regardless of its specific role in Jennifer's complaints.

Plan

Diagnostic
Laboratory testing to rule out these conditions should be obtained. Specifically, a complete blood count with differential, chemistry profile, ESR or C-reactive protein, TSH, and creatine kinase are most appropriate. Follow-up testing may include T_4 or free T_3 levels, antinuclear antibody (ANA), anti–double-stranded DNA, etc.

Therapeutic
It is reasonable to address Jennifer's primary concern of back pain as one would do for most musculoskeletal conditions. This includes anti-inflammatory drugs, a program of stretching, referral to physical therapy, and consideration of imaging studies if thought appropriate.

If she has abnormally painful responses on tender-point examination and the blood and radiology testing is normal, a diagnosis of fibromyalgia can be made. A patient-education brochure on fibromyalgia is then provided with information about this condition and how it can be managed (see Discussion).

She is given a prescription for amitriptyline (Elavil), 25 mg, to take at bedtime to assist with sleep. Close questioning of her husband reveals that Jennifer displays no symptoms of sleep apnea. She is strongly encouraged to institute regular aerobic exercise and specific instructions on how to do so is provided. Follow-up visits will be made on a regular basis until Jennifer becomes well accustomed to the diagnosis of fibromyalgia and its treatment strategies.

DISCUSSION

The existence of fibromyalgia has been controversial for decades. Some authors have suggested a distinct organic pathology, whereas others have repudiated this claim and insist these patients are somaticizing psychiatric problems. The current predominant opinion, however, notes that these patients have a consistent presentation of their illness, with research findings suggestive of a complex pathology involving peripheral tissues and the central nervous system. The term *fibromyalgia syndrome* (FMS) has been used to incorporate this new understanding (Bradley and Alarcon, 2005 **Ⓐ**).

In 1990 the American College of Rheumatology published its diagnostic criteria for fibromyalgia. Musculoskeletal pain must be present on both sides of the body, above and below the waist, and in the axial skeleton. Symptoms must have been present for at least 3 months. Significant pain should be evidenced in at least 11 of 18 tender points (see Fig. 69-1) with relatively low-intensity pressure. Patients with fewer than 11 tender points may still be considered for this condition outside of the research setting. The tender points are elicited with the examiner applying enough pressure (approximately 4 kg or 9 pounds) with his or her thumb to cause blanching of that thumbnail. A positive response is simply the patient's report of pain. A normal control would notice only mild pressure with the same maneuver. If malingering or exaggeration is suspected, control sites, such as the top of the patient's thumbnail, or the dorsal side of the distal forearm, may be palpated. However, it should be cautioned that patients with a formal diagnosis of fibromyalgia will have decreased thresholds for pain, even in these sites, compared with patients that do not have fibromyalgia (Bradley and Alarcon, 2005 **Ⓐ**). The hallmark of FMS is a decreased threshold for pain (allodynia) in addition to increased skin sensitivity to temperature and touch (hyperalgesia).

The pathophysiology of fibromyalgia has been difficult to identify. Consensus is building that initially a peripheral source of painful stimulus (injury, muscle microtrauma, etc.) sensitizes central nervous pain thresholds and processing. This is evidenced by documented changes in neurotransmitter levels in the blood and cerebrospinal fluid of affected patients and altered cerebral blood flow in regions of the brain known to be associated with pain processing. Malfunction of the hypothalamus/pituitary/adrenal axis, decreased secretion of growth hormone, and altered thyroid function have been documented in patients with fibromyalgia. Unfortunately, we still have no ability to rule in or rule out this condition with objective testing. However, this does not refute the growing evidence that fibromyalgia has at least some organic pathology present (Bradley and Alarcon, 2005Ⓐ).

Ninety percent of those with fibromyalgia are female patients, and the condition seems to become more common with increasing age. It is estimated that 3.4% of women in the general population and 0.5% of men fit the criteria for FMS (Gilliland, 2005Ⓑ). Reports from tertiary care centers have noted a high prevalence of psychiatric diagnoses and histories of childhood trauma in their patients with fibromyalgia. It is still debated whether psychiatric or psychosocial stressors play a role in the development of this condition, or whether they merely contribute to seeking medical attention or result in poor coping skills. Some studies have suggested that the prevalence of psychiatric diagnoses in patients with fibromyalgia who *have not* sought medical attention does not differ from controls (Bradley and Alarcon, 2005Ⓐ).

Patients with FMS consistently have difficulty with sleep. Specifically, deep-sleep deprivation has been documented and may in fact contribute to the development of symptoms of pain and the frequently reported compromises in memory and concentration. Studies also have shown a high correlation between obstructive sleep apnea and fibromyalgia. Therefore sleep testing should be considered in patients for whom this seems appropriate. Other conditions that frequently coexist in patients with fibromyalgia are listed in Box 69-1.

Severe fatigue is one of the most debilitating complaints of many fibromyalgia patients. It has been estimated that 65% to 75% of FMS patients also fit the diagnostic criteria for chronic fatigue syndrome. Fibromyalgia patients often notice worsened fatigue and pain after even minimal physical activity (e.g., doing laundry or dishes). This leads to physical deconditioning and a fear of exercise (Busch et al., 2002Ⓐ).

The treatment of fibromyalgia begins with explaining to the patient what is known about this

Box 69-1	Conditions That Frequently Coexist with Fibromyalgia

Depression
Anxiety disorders
Post-traumatic stress disorder
Migraine headaches
Tension headaches
Dysmenorrhea
Irritable bowel syndrome
Female urethral syndrome
Paresthesias/dysesthesias
Raynaud phenomenon
Sicca symptoms
Photosensitivity
Chronic pelvic pain
Multiple chemical sensitivities
Obstructive sleep apnea
Restless leg syndrome
Chronic fatigue syndrome

condition and how it can be managed. The physician should reassure the patient that the symptoms are not imaginary, empathize with the patient's suffering, and commit to working with the patient to manage symptoms. Explaining the chronic nature of this condition is essential. It has been estimated that after 5 years, up to 75% of patients have not had significant improvement of their complaints. Children and men seem to have better prognoses.

Often coexisting psychiatric problems and personality disorders inhibit patients from adopting disciplined management of the illness. Cognitive behavioral therapy may be helpful to address these issues, and coexistent mood disorders should be treated. Fluoxetine and amitriptyline have been shown to be superior to placebo in reducing symptoms of fibromyalgia in addition to their mood-altering effects. Treatment of underlying depression or sleep apnea will help to restore deep-sleep cycles, which may improve cognitive function and fatigue somewhat. Other medications that may help with sleep are tricyclic antidepressants, gabapentin, and cyclobenzaprine. Benzodiazepines have been shown to be useful when combined with ibuprofen in patients with fibromyalgia and may also assist in sleep regulation (Bradley and Alarcon, 2005Ⓐ).

Pain is best treated with regular aerobic exercise (Busch et al., 2002Ⓐ). This information is often treated with suspicion and antagonism by patients who have experienced exacerbated symptoms after exertion. In such cases, it may be helpful to have a physical therapist involved who is familiar with fibromyalgia and has access to pool therapy, which has been found to be particularly effective in treating FMS. Patients should be encouraged to start with low-impact aerobic exercise at a low intensity for only 5 minutes per day. Achieving a consistent daily routine should be stressed. Once a routine is established, the duration and intensity of the exercise can be increased.

No pain relievers have been shown to be consistently helpful in fibromyalgia patients. Acetaminophen or nonsteroidal anti-inflammatory medications may be helpful for mild cases. Tramadol (Ultram) also may be of some benefit and has few drawbacks in patients who can tolerate it. Frequently patients request opiate medications, but doctors hesitate to prescribe them. No strong research is available to help guide this decision. Most fibromyalgia experts strongly recommend against starting opiate medications in fibromyalgia patients because they rarely help reduce symptoms in the long term (Bradley and Alarcon, 2005Ⓐ; Gilliland, 2005Ⓑ). When addressing a request for pain medication from a patient with FMS, the physician should attempt to turn the focus away from depending on pills and onto adopting healthy habits such as maintaining regular exercise, getting regular sleep, and achieving emotional balance. Further study is ongoing and may soon provide a more definitive treatment for this often frustrating condition.

Material Available on Student Consult

Review Questions and Answers about Fibromyalgia

REFERENCES

Bradley LA, Alarcon GS. Fibromyalgia. In Koopman WJ, Moreland LW (eds): Arthritis and Allied Conditions: A Textbook of Rheumatology, 15th ed. Philadelphia, Lippincott Williams & Wilkins, 2005, pp 1869–1910.Ⓐ

Busch A, Schachter CL, Peloso PM, Bombardier C. Exercise for treating fibromyalgia syndrome. Cochrane Database Syst Rev 2002;(3):CD003786.Ⓐ

First MB, ed. Diagnostic and Statistical Manual of Mental Disorders–Revision (DSM-IV-TR). Washington, DC, American Psychiatric Association, 2000.Ⓒ

Gilliland BC. Fibromyalgia: Arthritis associated with systemic disease, and other arthritides. In Kasper DL, Braunwald E, Fauci AS, et al. (eds): Harrison's Principles of Internal Medicine, 16th ed. Chicago, McGraw-Hill, 2005, pp 2055–2064.Ⓑ

70 Elbow Pain (Epicondylitis)

Allan V. Abbott

INITIAL VISIT

Subjective

Patient Identification and Presenting Problem

John N. is a 48-year-old right-handed white man who works as a college English professor. John complains of pain in his right elbow for the past month and thinks that he has tennis elbow. He feels only a mild ache most of the time, but he describes a sharp pain that is brought on by certain activities. He is uncertain about the onset of the pain and states that it came on gradually but has been especially bad the past few days, when he was picking up books and boxes while moving his office. He also notices the pain when he grips and carries his briefcase or shakes hands, and he noticed it a few days before this visit

when he tried to play tennis ("that's when I decided it must be tennis elbow"). He states that the pain usually resolves within seconds or minutes after resting the arm but recurs immediately with any heavy use of the right hand.

Medical History

John has had an unremarkable medical history with no previous major illnesses or hospitalizations. He has had a few episodes of minor low back pain but has never sought medical attention.

Family History

John is an only child. His mother is living and well and is under treatment for high blood pressure. His father died 2 years ago of a myocardial infarction at the age of 75. His father was overweight and sedentary. John has a wife and two children who are in good health.

Health Habits

John takes pride in his good health. He has never smoked and only drinks a glass of wine occasionally. He follows a low-fat diet and has tried to stay thin. He jogs three mornings each week for about 3 miles and takes long hikes most weekends. He started playing tennis with a friend about 2 months ago. He takes no medications.

Objective

Physical Examination

Vital Signs His weight is 156 pounds, height is 69 inches, blood pressure is 120/70, pulse is 60 and regular, and temperature is 37.2°C (99°F) orally.

General John is pleasant and well nourished and appears physically fit. As he describes his elbow pain, he cups and holds his right elbow with his left hand. Both upper extremities appear muscular and symmetrical, and there is no apparent deformity, swelling, or inflammation of either elbow. Passive and active range of motion of both hands, wrists, elbows, and shoulders is normal. There is mild tenderness to palpation over and immediately distal to the lateral epicondyle of the right elbow. Otherwise there is no other palpable warmth, tenderness, or deformity.

John demonstrates that it hurts his elbow most when he makes a fist and extends his right wrist. Indeed, extension of his wrist against resistance causes pain near the lateral epicondyle, especially when the forearm is pronated.

Laboratory Tests
Radiographs of the elbow are normal.

Assessment

Working Diagnosis
The most likely diagnosis is lateral epicondylitis, often called tennis elbow. The onset and association of the pain with lifting and with playing tennis as well as the tenderness over the lateral epicondyle are typical.

Differential Diagnosis (Box 70-1)
In racket sports, the differential diagnosis includes lateral and medial epicondylitis, medial collateral ligament injury, bony articular injuries, and ulnar neuropathy.

Medial epicondylitis, often called golfer's elbow, occurs less often than lateral epicondylitis, but the symptoms are similar. The pain is localized to the medial epicondyle at the site of the flexor pronator tendon origins. Pain results from resisted wrist flexion and pronation. Management is similar to lateral epicondylitis. John has no medial elbow pain or tenderness.

Medial collateral ligament injury causes medial elbow pain and can overlap with other injuries such as medial epicondylitis. The medial collateral ligament receives valgus stress in tennis serves and overhead strokes. A tennis player may report medial elbow pain during vigorous overhead serves. Tenderness may be elicited over the medial collateral ligament or instability or pain may be produced when the examiner applies valgus stress to the elbow in 30 degrees of flexion.

Bony articular injuries can result from excessive articular compression during vigorous and repeated use of the elbow in racket sports. This can lead to degenerative changes, osteophytes, and loose body formation, especially in older adults. Poorly localized pain, stiffness, and limitation of motion are the most common findings. John has well-localized pain and no limitation of motion as well as normal radiographs.

Ulnar neuropathy can result from traction or compression of the nerve, direct trauma, and subluxation. Medial elbow joint instability, degenerative arthritis, and soft-tissue scarring can lead to ulnar

---

Box 70-1	Differential Diagnosis for Epicondylitis

Conditions commonly associated with racket sports
    Lateral epicondylitis (most common)
    Medial epicondylitis
    Medial collateral ligament injury
    Bony articular injuries
    Ulnar neuropathy
Other conditions
    Trauma
    Radial neck fractures
    Distal humerus fractures
    Neuropathic pain
    Radial tunnel syndrome
    Entrapment
        Of posterior interosseous nerve
        Of musculocutaneous nerve
        Of median nerve
    Inflammation
    Arthritis
    Synovitis
    Gouty arthritis
    Joint infection
    Referred pain
    Cervical radiculopathy
    Shoulder arthritis
    Carpel tunnel syndrome
    Angina pectoris
    Tumor
    Bone cyst

---

nerve compression. Numbness and tingling in the fourth and fifth fingers are common symptoms and are often associated with medial elbow pain that radiates into the forearm. Careful palpation of the ulnar nerve where it crosses the elbow and observation of the nerve in its groove as the elbow moves through its full range of motion help rule out entrapment. John has no neurologic findings.

Other differential diagnoses that are less common include the following.

Radial tunnel syndrome can closely simulate lateral epicondylitis. The radial nerve becomes compressed in the radial tunnel as it passes laterally around the posterior surface of the humerus and pierces the lateral muscular septum. Pain may be referred to the lateral epicondyle, and paresthesias may occur along the course of the superficial radial nerve. Most commonly, pain is elicited when the forearm is forcefully supinated. Tinel's sign (a distal tingling sensation in an extremity when a nerve is percussed) may be elicited over the radial head, and tenderness may be palpated in the extensor muscles more distally than 1 or 2 cm from the lateral epicondyle (as in lateral epicondylitis). Tenderness over the lateral epicondyle, as John has, would not be expected.

Entrapment of the posterior interosseous, musculocutaneous, or median nerves can lead to elbow pain. Entrapment of the posterior interosseus nerve by the supinator muscle can cause elbow pain and weakness of extension of the fifth finger, mimicking the radial tunnel syndrome. Musculocutaneous nerve entrapment can result in anterolateral elbow pain and decreased sensation in the anterior (volar) forearm. Compression of the median nerve can produce pain in the volar forearm that is worse with repeated use (pronator syndrome). Pain may be produced by resisting flexion at the third finger proximal interphalangeal joint or by resisting forearm pronation. John has none of these findings.

Fractures of the radial neck or distal humerus can be suspected if the patient has had a fall or other acute trauma. The elbow is swollen and movement is painful. The diagnosis is confirmed radiographically.

Inflammation associated with arthritis or synovitis can be suspected in cases of a swollen, painful elbow, especially in individuals with inflammation in other joints. Joint infection should be suspected if the joint is swollen, erythematous, or warm or if the patient is febrile.

Referred pain from cervical radiculopathy, shoulder arthritis, carpal tunnel syndrome, or angina pectoris can be ruled out through examination of the neck, shoulder, and wrist and careful history taking. When the history and physical examination are inconclusive, radiographic examination will rule out rare bone tumors or cysts.

Plan

Diagnostic

The diagnosis of lateral epicondylitis is based entirely on the history and physical examination. Radiographs of the elbow will be normal in lateral epicondylitis, but they may be obtained if other causes of pain are suspected by a decreased elbow range of motion or by crepitance palpated over the radiohumeral joint. Magnetic resonance imaging is rarely indicated but can be used to differentiate epicondylitis from other tendon injury, nerve entrapment, or stress fractures (Sonin et al., 1996🅑).

Therapeutic

Treatment of epicondylitis begins with patient education. The goals are to allow healing of microruptures in the tendon, to allow inflammation to resolve, and to improve muscle strength in the forearm. The patient must avoid or reduce activities that produce extensor stress on the lateral epicondyle. Racket sports should be avoided initially. Lifting of heavy objects should also be avoided; when lifting is necessary, the weight should be lifted close to the body, with the elbow extended and the forearm supinated.

Pain is aggravated most by motions of the hand and wrist; therefore, many patients find some relief with immobilization of the wrist with a Velcro wrist splint. Wrist splinting should be in neutral position and limited in duration to no more than 3 to 4 weeks if possible (Little, 1984). Tennis elbow bands wrap around the forearm, placing pressure over the attachment of the extensor tendons to the epicondyle. A tennis elbow band is likely to be helpful if the patient notices a reduction of pain when pressure is applied by fingers over the painful area while the patient performs painful arm movements. However, a systematic review of splints, bands, and other orthotic devices did not find clear benefit from any of these devices (Struijs et al., 2001🅐). Various physical therapies may be helpful in some cases, including heat, ultrasound, whirlpool, massage, and electrical stimulation.

Repeated application of ice directly to the painful area for 15 minutes every 4 to 6 hours often provides effective local anti-inflammatory treatment and pain relief. An oral nonsteroidal anti-inflammatory drug is commonly prescribed and may be continued for several weeks. Studies have shown nonsteroidal anti-inflammatory drugs to produce short-term benefit but more adverse effects than without nonsteroidal anti-inflammatory drugs (Hay et al., 1999🅐; Labelle and Guibert, 1997🅑).

Corticosteroid injections should be reserved for those patients in whom the pain is severe or persistent, and more conservative treatments are not satisfactory. Studies of these injections have yielded conflicting results (Hay et al., 1999🅐). Injection can decrease pain acutely but does not improve outcome at 1 year (Assendelft et al., 1996🅑; Hay et al., 1999🅐; Verhaar et al., 1996🅑). Injection should be in the most tender area and into the subaponeurotic space with approximately 40 mg of methylprednisolone and lidocaine. Superficial subcutaneous injection and injection into the tendon should be avoided. No more than three injections should be performed within 1 year, and repeat injections should be avoided in athletes who continue to engage in activities that aggravate the condition (Smidt et al., 2002🅐). Surgery is rarely indicated but may be considered if all else fails and symptoms have persisted for more than 1 year; however, there have been no controlled trials of effectiveness (Buchbinder et al., 2002🅐).

Rehabilitation is essential to avoid recurrences. Gentle active and passive full range of motion exercises are begun with the initial visit and should be painless. After the pain has resolved, passive stretching of the extensor forearm muscles should be performed. Beginning 3 to 4 weeks after symptoms resolve, forearm muscle strength should be restored using isometric exercise. Grip exercises are followed by exercises of wrist extension and flexion and should be continued for at least several months to prevent recurrence.

For an athlete or person who must participate in the activity that caused the lateral epicondylitis, a more formal rehabilitation and physical and occupational therapy program may be necessary. A tennis professional may be consulted to correct the backhand technique and to select the correct racket with larger head size, reduced string tension, and soft or loose grip.

DISCUSSION

Tennis elbow has been used to describe pain at or near the origin of the extensor carpi radialis brevis since 1882. It occurs most commonly in white middle-aged men and nearly always in the dominant hand. The majority of cases of lateral epicondylitis do not occur as the result of racket sports but result from repetitive movements in certain occupations. Tennis elbow affects about 50% of recreational tennis players and is related to overuse and poor technique, especially during the backhand stroke.

The exact etiology is unknown, but tennis elbow results from repeated stress on or near the lateral epicondyle by the action of the wrist extensor muscles, especially the extensor carpi radialis brevis, and the carpi radialis longus, extensor carpi ulnaris, and the brachioradialis. This causes microruptures of collagenous fibers, fibrous tendon degeneration, and an associated inflammatory response (Pfahler et al., 1998 B). Lateral epicondylitis rarely results from direct local trauma or from systemic connective tissue disease.

Lateral epicondylitis is a clinical diagnosis and, as in this patient, most cases will present with typical signs and symptoms. John typically had pain relieved by rest, and he noticed pain with gripping objects with the involved hand, especially with the right wrist extended. The pain developed gradually but was exacerbated with heavy repetitive use of his hand and arms. Morning stiffness and aching throughout the day are common symptoms.

On physical examination, tenderness over and just distal to the lateral epicondyle and pain on extension of the pronated wrist are usually diagnostic. If the patient with tennis elbow is asked to hold a 5-pound object such as a book in the affected hand with the elbow flexed at 90 degrees, there is usually little pain with the hand supinated but marked pain and associated weakness when the hand is pronated. Grip strength is usually decreased. There is normal elbow range of motion and usually no visible swelling. The presence of swelling should alert the examiner to the possibility of another etiology.

Prevention

The racket sports player who fails to follow a comprehensive conditioning program or who uses poor technique is more likely to develop lateral epicondylitis. Strengthening exercises should be done routinely using progressive resistance. Forearm extensor muscle stretching should be done consistently during the playing season and immediately before sports participation. Proper technique and equipment are also important.

> **Material Available on Student Consult**
>
> Review Questions and Answers about Epicondylitis

REFERENCES

Assendelft, WJ, Hay, EM, Adshead, R, Bouter, LM. Corticosteroid injections for lateral epicondylitis: A systematic overview. Br J Gen Pract 1996;46:209–216. B

Buchbinder, R, Green S, Bell S, et al. Surgery for lateral elbow pain (Cochrane Review). Cochrane Database Syst Rev 2002. A

Hay EM, Paterson SM, Lewis M, et al. Pragmatic randomized controlled trial of local corticosteroid injection and naproxen for treatment of lateral epicondylitis of elbow in primary care. BMJ 1999;319:964–968. A

Labelle H, Guibert R. Efficacy of diclofenac in lateral epicondylitis of the elbow also treated with immobilization. The University of Montreal Orthopaedic Research Group. Arch Fam Med 1997;6:257–262. B

Little TS. Tennis elbow: To rest or not to rest. Practitioner 1984;228:457–460.

Pfahler M, Jessel C, Steinborn M, Refior HJ. Magnetic resonance imaging in lateral epicondylitis of the elbow. Arch Orthop Trauma Surg 1998;118:121–125. B

Smidt N, van der Windt DA, Assendelft WJ, et al. Corticosteroid injections, physiotherapy, or a wait-and-see policy for lateral epicondylitis: A randomized controlled trial. Lancet 2002;359:657–662. A

Sonin AG, Tutton SM, Fitzgerald SW, Peduto AJ. MR imaging of the adult elbow. Radiographics 1996;16:1323–1336. B

Struijs PA, Smidt N, Arola H, et al. Orthotic devices for tennis elbow (Cochrane Review). Cochrane Database Syst Rev 2001. A

Verhaar JA, Walenkamp GH, van Mameren H, et al. Local corticosteroid injection versus Cyriax-type physiotherapy for tennis elbow. J Bone Joint Surg Br 1996;78:128–132. B

71 Ankle Injury (Ankle Sprain)

Trish Palmer

1. Grade I to II ankle sprains should respond well to the PRICE regimen:
   Protection: bracing or support to protect the ankle from further injury.
   Rest: limitation of activities that cause pain or swelling, relative rest of the ankle; people may continue to do exercises that do not specifically involve the ankle to keep up their aerobic fitness (e.g., weights, swimming).
   Ice: 15 minutes every 1 to 2 hours while awake; this has been shown to significantly reduce healing time (use a bucket of ice water, plastic bag of ice cubes, or bag of frozen vegetables).
   Compression: use of elastic bandage or pneumatic ankle splint while awake.
   Elevation: raise the ankle above the level of the heart.
2. Suspicion of fracture should prompt radiographs of the ankle, foot, or fibula, depending on the mechanism of injury and area of tenderness; use of Ottawa ankle rules may decrease the need for radiographs.
3. Continuation of strengthening and proprioception exercises after a grade I to II sprain is likely to decrease the risk of future injury.
4. A red, warm, swollen joint, especially with no history of trauma, is a septic joint until proven otherwise. This finding should prompt urgent aspiration of the ankle, with urgent determination of the 3 Cs—cell count, culture, and crystals—to determine whether the cause is infectious so that appropriate treatment can be immediately started.

INITIAL VISIT

Subjective

Patient Identification and Presenting Problem
Jennifer K. is a 40-year-old woman who presents to the clinic reporting a swollen right ankle. She reports that the mechanism of injury was rolling the ankle inward while playing tennis this morning, while cutting and pivoting to get at the ball. The swelling about the ankle has slowly increased since then, with some bruising below the ankle bone. She is able to bear some weight and walk several steps with a limp. This has never happened previously. She has done nothing so far to treat the ankle, including icing, bracing, or medications.

Medical History
There is none, including no history of peptic ulcers or gastrointestinal side effects to nonsteroidal antiinflammatory drugs (NSAIDs).

Family History
There is no history of arthritides.

Social History
She drinks two glasses of wine per night, does not smoke, and exercises four to five times per week.

Surgical History
There is none, including the right ankle.

Medications/Allergies
There are none.

Review of Systems
The review is negative for constitutional, other musculoskeletal, other skin, eye, and genitourinary symptoms.

Objective

Physical Examination

Inspection reveals that Ms. K's right ankle has evident moderate swelling through the talocrural joint, with ecchymosis below the lateral malleolus. There is little erythema or warmth about the joint. Palpation reveals tenderness of the anterior talofibular ligament (ATFL) but not of the calcaneofibular ligament (CFL), posterior talofibular ligament, or deltoid ligament. There is no bony tenderness at the distal lateral malleolus, medial malleolus, fifth metatarsal, navicular, or proximal fibula. Passive and active range of motion is slightly limited in both inversion and eversion compared with the unaffected left ankle. Resisted function of the peroneus longus and brevis is symmetric bilaterally but does cause some pain. The anterior drawer test is negative for laxity and positive for pain. Talar tilt testing is negative for both laxity and pain. Squeeze, external rotation, and Thompson tests are negative.

Investigations

No blood work or radiographs were ordered.

Assessment

Working Diagnosis

A first-degree sprain of the lateral right ankle (ATFL stretch) is the most likely diagnosis based on the mechanism of injury and clinical examination.

Differential Diagnosis

When there is no history of trauma, when examination reveals any concerning signs (redness and warmth with the swelling), or when the clinical findings are more than that described above, enlarge the differential diagnosis to include the following:

1. *Second- or third-degree sprain.* Examination reveals laxity of one or more of the tendons (ATFL, CFL, posterior talofibular ligament), indicating a partial to complete tear. A partial to complete tear takes a longer time to heal, and a complete tear may benefit from surgery.
2. *Syndesmotic sprain.* The syndesmosis consists of the anterior tibiofibular ligament, posterior tibiofibular ligament, and the distal interosseus membrane between the tibia and the fibula. Injury to this structure usually presents with anterior ankle pain. Examination reveals a positive squeeze test and external rotation stress test. Expect this injury to take a prolonged time to heal, from 8 to 10 weeks.
3. *Fracture.* Any bony tenderness or inability to bear weight must prompt radiographs. Specific bones to assess include the proximal fibula, navicular, fifth metatarsal, distal fibula, and tibia. Also con-

sider Salter-Harris type (growth plate) fractures in a person who is still growing (radiographs of type I may be normal).
4. *Red, warm, swollen joint.* This is a septic joint until proven otherwise, especially with no history of trauma. This finding should prompt urgent aspiration of the ankle, with urgent determination of the 3 Cs—cell count, culture, and crystals—to determine whether the cause is infectious so that appropriate treatment can be immediately started. If the joint is not septic, other diagnoses include initial presentation or flare of osteoarthritis, rheumatoid arthritis, gout, or pseudogout. This is a situation in which blood testing may also be helpful.
5. *Complex regional pain syndrome (previously termed reflex sympathetic dystrophy).* Symptoms include burning pain, hypersensitivity, allodynia, and edema, often arising after a fairly minor injury like a sprain or a fracture. The symptoms often appear to be much out of proportion to the injury and do not respond to the typical treatment regimens for the suspected cause.
6. *Osteochondritis dissecans.* This is a disorder in which a fragment of cartilage and subchondral bone separates from the articular surface, with the patient usually presenting as a teenager, many with a history of trauma or high level of athletic activity. Symptoms may include pain, effusion, and mechanical locking sensation. Diagnosis is made by radiograph, with this disorder suspected because of age and symptoms. It often responds to modification of activity if found to be a minor lesion; surgery may be necessary for larger lesions.
7. *Peroneal tendon subluxation, Achilles tendon strain or tear.* Other structures may be torn or stretched and may mimic a sprained ankle. Specific tests include eversion against resistance with palpation of the peroneal tendon moving out of place and the Thompson test, which tests the integrity of the Achilles.

Plan

Diagnostic

At this point, the diagnosis is based on the history and clinical examination. If a first-degree sprain is not improving within 3 to 4 days or if there is persistent pain, swelling, or disability, then the differential diagnosis should be expanded to include the diagnoses noted above, and consideration should be given to re-examination of the joint and a possible radiograph.

Therapeutic

The therapeutic goal is to control pain and to maintain or regain range of motion. PRICE is a mnemonic to help remember the principles of physical modalities to limit pain and swelling.

Protection: bracing or support to protect the ankle from further injury

Rest: limitation of activities that cause pain or swelling, relative rest of the ankle; people may continue to do exercises that do not specifically involve the ankle to keep up their aerobic fitness (e.g., weights, swimming)

Ice: 15 minutes every 1 to 2 hours while awake; this has been shown to significantly reduce healing time (use a bucket of ice water, plastic bag of ice cubes, or bag of frozen vegetables)

Compression: use of elastic bandage or pneumatic ankle splint while awake

Elevation: raise the ankle above the level of the heart

Medications such as acetaminophen and NSAIDs may be quite helpful in addition to physical modalities in limiting pain, while NSAIDs may also limit swelling. The use of NSAIDs in the first 24 hours in athletes has become somewhat controversial: Some believe that the decrease in swelling speeds recovery; others believe that acute use of NSAIDs may increase swelling by increasing potential bleeding through platelet inhibition. This only matters in terms of speed of recovery, which makes it an issue unique to athletes, and has not yet been studied well (Stanley and Weaver, 1998).

Immobilization may both help and hinder healing. Acute protection of the painful area is appropriate and helps to limit swelling and thus pain. Prolonged immobilization leads to muscle atrophy and loss of range of motion. Therefore, it is recommended to start gentle range-of-motion exercises (tracing of the alphabet with the foot) and weight bearing as soon as tolerable. Ankle bracing is something that is to be recommended with care and usually for short-term treatment. Taping is also effective support but is only as good as the person applying the taping and only lasts for about 20 to 40 minutes of activity (Lohrer et al., 1999; Manfroy et al., 1997).

Physical therapy has been shown to get people back to activity somewhat quicker and is used frequently with athletes for this reason. The treatment plan usually consists of regaining range of motion, strength, and proprioception. Range-of-motion exercises are the first step. Strengthening of the peroneal muscles (resisted eversion and inversion), which act as the dynamic stabilizers of the ankle, is of great importance. Proprioception can be regained through standing on the injured foot with an attempt to hold the position for longer and longer periods of time, use of a balance board, and progression through a series of cutting and pivoting exercises. This may also help prevent recurrent ankle sprains.

Patient Education

The patient needs to be reassessed if there is persistent difficulty with ambulation 3 days after the injury, the ankle is not improving, or there is an increase in pain/swelling after the first 3 days. Advice should be given about the PRICE regimen and medication in the acute phase and early mobilization progressing to proprioception rehabilitation when tolerable. The expectation is that the injury should improve over the next 3 to 4 days and not last beyond 1 to 2 weeks.

The athlete is thought to be ready to return to training and competition when a progression through activity is not painful. When the ankle is no longer painful with straight-line forward and backward walking and jogging, the athlete may progress to side-to-side jogging, then figure-of-eight jogging, and then into cutting and pivoting. Any forward progression through these steps should be painless; otherwise the athlete is not ready to progress to the next step. If all activities are now painless, the athlete may return to previous training and competition.

Continuation of strengthening and proprioception exercises should be advised to decrease the risk of future injury. Also any brace that is used needs to be tightened after bouts of activity, because braces tend to become loose.

DISCUSSION

Ankle sprain is the most common sports and non-sports injury (as many as 21% of all sports injuries), with 85% of these being lateral sprains (Garrick, 1982; Renstrom and Kannus, 1994). The normal anatomy of the ankle is shown in Figure 71-1. Inversion is the most common mechanism of injury (Fig. 71-2) because the extension of the distal end of the fibula gives the medial ankle stability by providing bony resistance to eversion. Inversion in a position of dorsiflexion puts the ATFL at its greatest tension, placing it in a likely position to sustain injury. The ATFL (laxity tested by anterior drawer test [Fig. 72-3]) is the most commonly injured ligament, followed by the CFL (laxity tested by the inversion stress or talar tilt test [Fig. 71-4]) and the posterior talofibular ligament.

Examination should begin with inspection for obvious deformity, swelling, and ecchymosis. The affected ankle should be compared in every facet of the examination to the unaffected ankle (assuming that ankle is "normal"). Examination of a first-degree sprain will likely show tenderness at the ATFL and/or CFL areas without laxity (a finding of laxity increases the grade of the sprain). The amount and area of ecchymosis often correlate with the amount of treatment (PRICE/NSAIDs) and not necessarily to the severity of injury. Pain should not be increased by a squeeze test (compression of the tibia and fibula together at midshaft, with positive tests producing pain at the distal syndesmosis [Fig. 71-5]) or by an external rotation test (external rotation of the foot

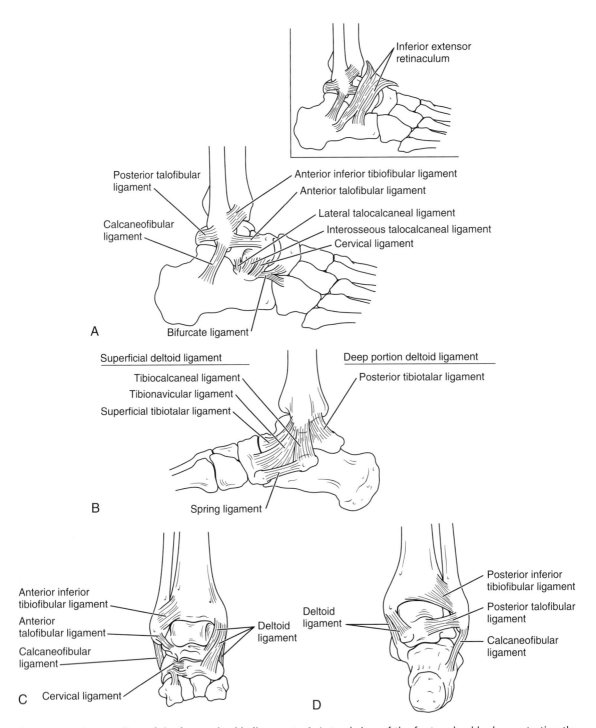

Figure 71-1 Compendium of the foot and ankle ligaments. **A,** Lateral view of the foot and ankle demonstrating the anterior talofibular ligament, calcaneofibular ligament, posterior talofibular ligament, anterior inferior tibiofibular ligament, lateral talocalcaneal ligament, inferior extensor retinaculum, interosseous talocalcaneal ligament, cervical ligament, and bifurcate ligament. **B,** Medial view of the foot and ankle demonstrating the superficial deltoid ligament, including the tibionavicular, spring ligament, tibiocalcaneal, and superficial tibiotalar components. **C,** An anterior view of the ankle and hindfoot demonstrating the deltoid ligament with its superficial and deep components, the anterior inferior tibiofibular ligament, the cervical ligament, the anterior talofibular ligament, and the calcaneofibular ligament. **D,** A posterior view of the ankle and hindfoot demonstrating the deltoid ligament with its superficial and deep components, the posterior inferior tibiofibular ligament, the posterior talofibular ligament, and the calcaneofibular ligament. (From DeLee and Drez's Orthopaedic Sports Medicine, 2nd ed. Philadelphia, Elsevier, 2003.)

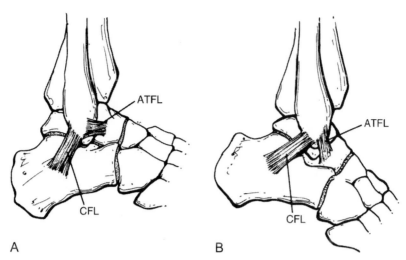

FIGURE 71-2 A, At a position of neutral dorsiflexion, the anterior talofibular ligament (ATFL) is perpendicular to the axis of the tibia, and the calcaneofibular ligament (CFL) is oriented parallel to the tibia. In this position, the CFL provides resistance to inversion stress or varus tilt of the talus. **B,** If, however, the talus is plantar flexed (the most common position for lateral ankle inversion injuries), then the ATFL is parallel and the CFL is perpendicular to the axis of the tibia, and the ATFL provides resistance to inversion stress or varus tilt of the talus. (From DeLee and Drez's Orthopaedic Sports Medicine, 2nd ed. Philadelphia, Elsevier, 2003.)

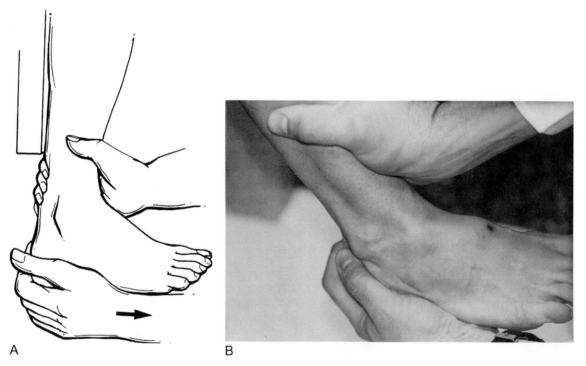

FIGURE 71-3 A and **B,** The anterior drawer test of the ankle. (From DeLee and Drez's Orthopaedic Sports Medicine, 2nd ed. Philadelphia, Elsevier, 2003.)

with the knee and foot at 90 degrees, causing pain at the distal syndesmosis [Fig. 71-6]). If pain is evoked on these tests, consider a syndesmotic sprain; more proximal pain may indicate a Maisonneuve or proximal fibula fracture. Tenderness at the deltoid (medial) ligament suggests a medial ankle sprain. The peroneal tendons are evaluated for subluxation by placing the foot in a dorsiflexed and everted position and having the patient resist inversion. If damage is present, movement of the peroneal tendon may be observed. Anterior drawer and talar tilt testing may be falsely negative in the setting of a lot of swelling.

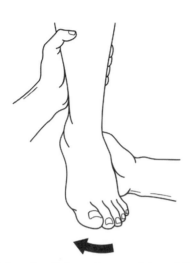

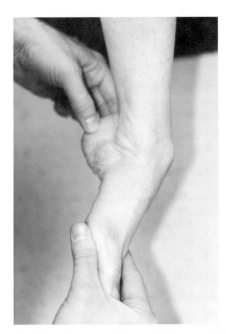

FIGURE 71-4 The talar tilt (inversion stress) test of the ankle. (From DeLee and Drez's Orthopaedic Sports Medicine, 2nd ed. Philadelphia, Elsevier, 2003.)

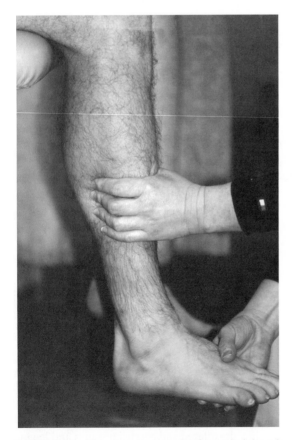

FIGURE 71-5 The squeeze test. Syndesmosis injury is suspected when compression of the midleg produces pain at the ankle syndesmosis. (From DeLee and Drez's Orthopaedic Sports Medicine, 2nd ed. Philadelphia, Elsevier, 2003.)

Ankle sprains are graded I, II, and III depending on the amount of laxity encountered on examination in addition to other factors (Table 71-1). Grade I sprains tend to heal well with little intervention, whereas grade II injuries may benefit from acute immobilization (rigid brace or casting), and treatment of grade III injuries is controversial, ranging from casting to surgery. This type of injury should probably be referred to an orthopedic surgeon for consideration of surgical repair, depending on the patient's level of function before the injury and the anticipated timing of demand on the ankle.

With a clear mechanism of injury and ability to bear weight, the likely diagnosis is an ankle sprain, which should heal within a limited amount of time. Lack of memory of a specific mechanism of injury should make the clinician suspect other diagnoses. Inability to bear weight should raise the index of suspicion for fracture, and skeletal immaturity increases the risk of an epiphyseal (growth plate) injury. History of use of anticoagulants may complicate the picture with an increased risk of bleeding into the injured site.

Bony point tenderness at the proximal fibula, lateral malleolus, medial malleolus, base of the fifth metatarsal, or midfoot bones should prompt consideration of radiographs looking for fracture of these bones. Ottawa ankle rules are used by many to determine when radiographs of the ankle are indicated (Box 71-1). These guidelines are not recommended if the patient is younger than age 18 or older than age 65, pregnant, intoxicated at the time of injury, has multiple injuries or a head injury, or has diminished sensation due to a neurologic deficit. Using these

FIGURE 71-6 The external rotation stress test of the syndesmosis. (From DeLee and Drez's Orthopaedic Sports Medicine, 2nd ed. Philadelphia, Elsevier, 2003.)

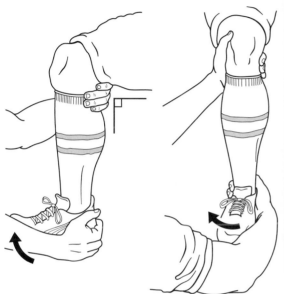
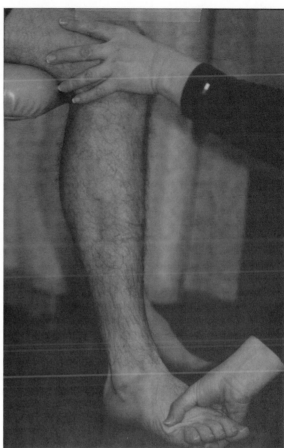

Table 71-1 Grading of Lateral Ankle Sprains

Sign/Symptom	Grade I (Stretch)	Grade II (Partial tear)	Grade III (Complete tear)
Laxity (anterior drawer test, ATFL)	None (good endpoint)	Slight (soft endpoint)	10 mm total or 3 mm greater than unaffected side on stress radiographs
Laxity (talar tilt or inversion stress test, CFL)	None (good endpoint)	Slight (soft endpoint)	20–30 degree opening or 10 degrees greater than unaffected side on stress radiographs
Loss of functional ability	Minimal	Some	Great
Pain	Minimal, localized to ATFL	Moderate, localized to ATFL, CFL	Severe, localized to ATFL, CFL, PTFL
Ecchymosis, swelling	None to slight, local	Moderate, local	Significant, diffuse
Weight-bearing ability	Full to partial	Difficult without crutches	Impossible without significant pain
Average time to return to sport	11 days	2–6 wk	4–26 wk

ATFL, anterior talofibular ligament; CFL, calconeofibular ligament; PTFL, posterior talofibular ligament.
Adapted from Wexler RK. The injured ankle. Am Fam Physician 1998;57:474–480; Renstrom PAFH, Kannus P. Injuries to the foot and ankle. Orthop Sports Med 1994;1705–1767; Gerber JP, Williams GN, Scoville CR, et al. Persistent disability associated with ankle sprains: A prospective examination of an athletic population. Foot Ankle Int 1998;19:653–660.

Box 71-1	Ottawa Ankle Rules

Ankle radiograph if pain in malleolar zone and (one of the following):
- Bony tenderness at the posterior or distal edge of the lateral malleolus
- Bony tenderness at the posterior or distal edge of the medial malleolus
- Inability to bear weight for four steps (regardless of limping) both immediately after injury and at time of medical evaluation

Foot radiograph if pain in midfoot zone and (one of the following):
- Bony tenderness at the base of the fifth metatarsal
- Bony tenderness at the navicular
- Inability to bear weight for four steps (regardless of limping) both immediately after injury and at time of medical evaluation

Adapted from Wexler RK. The injured ankle. Am Fam Physician 1998;57:474–480; Stiell IG, McKnight RD, Greenberg GH. Implementation of the Ottawa ankle rules. JAMA 1994;271:827–832.

guidelines, it is unlikely to miss a clinically significant fracture, thereby eliminating unneeded radiographs. Also consider a radiograph if the history or physical examination is suspicious for an injury other than an ankle sprain or an injury diagnosed as an ankle sprain is not improving as expected.

Special consideration must be given to patients who are still growing or have open growth plates. They may have a Salter-Harris type I fracture of the distal fibula and a normal radiograph. A finding of swelling at this spot and inability to bear weight must lead the clinician to suspect this type of fracture and treat it as such.

Suspicion of fracture should prompt radiographs of the ankle, foot, or fibula, depending on the mechanism of injury and area of tenderness. Findings to look for on radiograph include evidence of fracture, widening of the ankle mortise, and displacement or widening of the growth plate. Laboratory studies are not indicated for the diagnosis of an ankle sprain but may be considered if there is no clear mechanism of injury or rheumatologic or infectious causes are suspected (red, warm, swollen joint).

Treatment for ankle sprain in general consists of the PRICE regimen, with medications to limit pain and swelling. Once pain and swelling start to improve, usually within 1 to 2 days with a grade I ankle sprain, mobilization should begin to regain strength, range of motion, and proprioception. It is recommended to continue strengthening and proprioception to prevent future ankle sprains.

Material Available on Student Consult

Review Questions and Answers about Ankle Sprain

REFERENCES

Casillas MM. Ligament injuries of the foot and ankle. In Miller MD, ed. DeLee and Drez's Orthopaedic Sports Medicine, 2nd ed. Philadelphia, WB Saunders, 2003, pp 2323–2348.**C**

Garrick JG. Epidemiologic perspective. Clin Sports Med 1982;1:13–18.

Gerber JP, Williams GN, Scoville CR, et al. Persistent disability associated with ankle sprains: A prospective examination of an atheletic population. Foot Ankle Int 1998;19:653–660.

Lohrer H, Alt W, Gollhoffer A. Neuromuscular properties and functional aspects of tape ankles. J Sports Med 1999;27:69–75.

Manfroy PP, Ashton-Miller JA, Wojtys EM. The effect of exercise, prewrap, and athletic tape on maximal active and passive ankle resistance of ankle inversion. Am J Sports Med 1997;25:156–163.

Renstrom PAFH, Kannus P. Injuries to the foot and ankle. Orthop Sports Med 1994;1705–1767.

Stanley KL, Weaver JE. Pharmacologic management of pain and inflammation in athletes. Physician Sports Med 1998;17:375–392.

Stiell IG, McKnight RD, Greenberg GH. Implementation of the Ottawa ankle rules. JAMA 1994;271:827–832.**A**

Wexler, RK. The injured ankle. Am Fam Physician 1998;57:474–480.**C**

SUGGESTED READING

Hockenbury RT, Sammarco GJ. Evaluation and treatment of ankle sprains: Clinical recommendations for a positive outcome. Phys Sports Med 2001;29. Available at www.physsportsmed.com. Accessed 11/22/05.**C**

72 Arm Laceration (Laceration Repair)

Louis A. Kazal, Jr.

KEY POINTS

1. Lidocaine 1% is the drug of choice (~1 mL/2 cm of wound) for local anesthesia.
2. Minimize pain by injecting slowly through the opening of the wound and by using a longer needle (1.5 inches) to reduce the number of needle jabs.
3. Irrigate with a large syringe (10 to 50 mL) and an 18-gauge soft angiocatheter to provide jet stream turbulence.
4. Debride devitalized tissue whenever possible.
5. Most wounds require 4 to 5 mm of undermining, especially if there has been loss of tissue.
6. Compression applied for 5 to 10 minutes stops bleeding and prevents hematoma formation.
7. Gentle approximation of everted skin edges will produce a thinner scar that heals flatly without a ridge.
8. Simple sutures will evert the wound edges if (a) the needle enters and exits the skin at an identical distance from each edge, (b) the sutures are deeper than they are wide, and (c) the base of the loop incorporates more dermis than epidermis.
9. Stitch marks occur when sutures are (a) of too heavy a gauge, (b) too long, (c) too tight, or (d) left in too long, or (e) when they incorporate too much tissue.
10. Suture removal is performed at approximately 3 to 5 days for sutures in the face, 7 days for sutures in the scalp, 7 to 10 days for sutures on the the trunk and extremities, and 10 to 14 days for sutures on the back, hands, and feet.
11. Shaving hair around the wound increases the infection rate.
12. Antiseptics should be kept from entering open wounds because of their cytotoxic properties.

INITIAL VISIT

Subjective

Patient Identification and Presenting Problem

Gus is a 32-year-old white rancher who drove himself to the emergency department (ED) for evaluation of a 4-hour-old laceration of his arm.

Presenting Illness

Gus had dressed out a five-point bull elk, and as he hoisted one of the hindquarters onto the bed of his truck, the broken end of the elk's femur tore through the skin on the inside of his left arm. He applied pressure over the wound with a clean folded bandana, which stopped the bleeding. When Gus arrived home 3 hours later, he had no intention of seeking medical attention, but his wife insisted that he see their family physician. Once in the ED, his only concern was to confirm that he did not need stitches. He had no numbness, weakness, loss of function, or any significant pain.

Medical History

Gus has no history of a bleeding disorder or other medical illness. His last tetanus booster was 12 years ago. There are no known allergies to, or current use of, any medications.

Family History

Gus's father died of a myocardial infarction at age 48, as did his paternal grandfather at age 55. Gus's mother and two sisters are in good health.

Health Habits

Gus does not use a seat belt when driving. He has smoked two packs of cigarettes per day for 15 years. He rarely drinks alcohol.

Social History

Gus is a high school graduate who is currently a successful rancher in western Wyoming. He and his wife of 8 years have two healthy children.

Review of Systems

Gus last saw a physician 12 years ago after stepping on a rusty nail. His cholesterol level has never been checked. He coughs up yellowish phlegm every morning. There is no history of hemoptysis.

Objective

Physical Examination

Gus is alert, cooperative, and in no apparent distress. No alcohol is detected on his breath. His blood pressure is 140/92, pulse is 80, respirations are 20, and temperature is 37°C (98.6°F). He weighs 188 pounds and stands 5 feet 10 inches tall. A pack of cigarettes is in his shirt pocket.

Examination of his left arm reveals a 2.5-cm laceration of the flexor surface of the midforearm. Small portions of the wound edges are jagged. There is some dried blood over the wound. There is no weakness on resistance to flexion of his fingers or hand or on pronation of the forearm. His biceps and brachioradialis reflexes are normal. Distal sensation and circulation are intact.

Laboratory Tests

No tests are ordered.

Assessment

Diagnosis

Gus is diagnosed with what appears to be an uncomplicated 2.5-cm laceration of the left forearm. The full extent of the injury cannot be determined until it is explored.

Other Health Risk Factors

Gus has a number of other health risk factors. He does not use a seat belt, which places him at increased risk for traumatic injury or death if he is involved in a motor vehicle accident. Motor vehicle injuries are a leading cause of years of potential life lost before age 75. It is estimated that crash mortality can be reduced by 40% to 50% with the use of lap and shoulder belts.

Gus has a 30-pack-year history of smoking cigarettes (two packs a day for 15 years). Cigarettes are the leading preventable cause of death in the United States. He also has an elevated blood pressure reading. However, he is not labeled hypertensive based on one measurement. This diagnosis typically requires two or more blood pressures recorded at separate times, and then the measurements, including the initial one, are averaged.

Finally, Gus is mildly obese. His body mass index (weight in kilograms divided by height in meters squared) is 27. A body mass index of 27 or greater is associated with an increased risk for obesity-related diseases.

Plan

These findings are reviewed with Gus, who gives oral permission to assess and repair his injury. In general, lacerations of the body and extremity greater than 6 hours old should not be closed as they are prone to infection. An exception is sometimes made for lacerations of the head and neck, which have excellent blood supply and may be repaired up to 12 hours after injury.

Tetanus toxoid is administered in his nondominant arm. Tetanus prophylaxis is a priority in laceration care. If the patient has not been immunized against tetanus, 0.5 mL of toxoid is given. The injection is repeated in 6 weeks, and repeated again in 6 to 12 months. If the wound is tetanus-prone, 250 units of tetanus immune globulin (TIG) are also given intramuscularly at the initial visit. If the patient has been immunized and the wound is tetanus-prone, a booster is recommended when more than 5 years have elapsed since the last dose. For the immunized patient with a clean wound, a tetanus booster is not necessary unless it has been more than 10 years since the last dose.

The physician decides to address Gus's poor health maintenance record during the laceration repair.

Procedure

1. Two milliliters of 1% Xylocaine without epinephrine are injected with a sterile 1.5-inch, 27-gauge needle through the open wound, infiltrating the surrounding tissue in a fanlike fashion.
   a. 1% lidocaine HCl (Xylocaine) is the drug of choice as a local anesthetic in laceration repair. Approximately 1 mL is required for each 2 cm of wound. The maximum adult dose with epinephrine is 7 mg/kg, and without epinephrine it is 4.5 mg/kg. *Note:* Each milliliter of 1% Xylocaine contains 10 mg of lidocaine HCl.
   b. Aqueous epinephrine combined with lidocaine is useful in closing lacerations of the scalp and other vascular areas. In tissues with less blood supply or in dirty wounds, the routine use of lidocaine with epinephrine is discouraged because it decreases blood supply, leading to delayed healing and possible infection. Its use is contraindicated in the fingers, toes, penis, nose, and earlobes.
   c. Anesthetic solutions should not be injected into rigid fascial compartments because of potential tamponading of neurovascular bundles. Regional blocks are preferred in these circumstances *after* evaluation of sensation and function.
   d. Important cosmetic landmarks should be marked before injecting, and the least amount of local anesthetic should be used to avoid distortion and malalignment of the wound edges.
   e. Pain can be minimized by injecting (1) slowly to avoid rapid distention of the tissue (using a 27-gauge needle assists in this goal), (2)

through the opening of the wound in a fan-like fashion rather than repeatedly through the skin, (3) with a longer needle (1.5 inches), reducing the number of needle jabs, and (4) with lidocaine buffered with 8.4% sodium bicarbonate in a 1:10 solution.

f. Local anesthetic should be infiltrated 1 cm into the wound margins. (Subcutaneous fat does not need to be anesthetized.)

g. Nonsterile gloves may be worn while administering the local anesthetic but sterile gloves are used during the repair.

h. Small (1 to 2 cm) superficial lacerations requiring only a couple of sutures or staples (scalp) may be closed without an anesthetic.

i. A topical anesthetic, LET (lidocaine, epinephrine, and tetracaine), is an alternative source of analgesia for simple *open* lacerations. (The use of LET should be avoided on or near mucous membranes because of potential lidocaine toxicity or on end-arteriole regions of the body, such as digits, because of the vasoconstrictive properties of epinephrine, which may cause ischemic complications.)

2. After adequate local anesthesia is obtained, the wound is irrigated copiously with sterile saline and the skin surrounding the wound is scrubbed with Hibiclens antiseptic. The field is then draped in sterile fashion and illuminated.

a. Commonly used surgical preps are chlorhexidine gluconate (Hibiclens), povidone-iodine (Betadine), and hydrogen peroxide. Debate exists over which is the best solution because each has cytotoxic properties that interfere with wound healing and local immune response. Regardless, antiseptics should be kept from entering open wounds.

b. Irrigation is best accomplished using a large syringe (10 to 50 mL) with an 18-gauge soft angiocatheter providing jet-stream turbulence.

c. The practice of shaving hair about the wound is avoided because it may increase the risk of wound infection.

3. There is some oozing of blood, which is easily controlled with sterile 4 × 4 antiseptic pads and pressure.

4. The wound edges are slightly ragged. The laceration extends through the subcutaneous tissue and fascia without injury to the underlying musculature. No debris is seen. Digital examination using a sterile gloved finger reveals no foreign body or disruption of underlying structures.

5. Ample skin is present to permit debridement of the wound without resulting in excessive tension with closure. The damaged wound edges are trimmed with tissue scissors to produce symmetrical, freshly squared-off edges with an intact blood supply (Fig. 72-1).

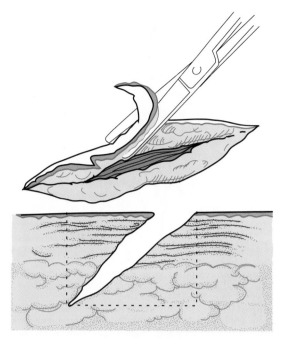

Figure 72-1 Wound revision. Jagged wound edges should be trimmed with tissue scissors or a no. 15 blade scalpel to produce a wound with even and vertical edges. Tangential wound edges, either left as such or made during revision, create a wider, more depressed scar due to retraction. (From Zuber TJ. Wound management. In Rakel RE (ed): Saunders Manual of Medical Practice. Philadelphia, WB Saunders, 1996, p 1008.)

a. Depending on the region of the body (i.e., how thick the skin is), it may be necessary to use a no. 15 blade scalpel instead of tissue scissors.

b. Debridement of devitalized tissue is essential whenever possible, except when it would compromise function or result in greater cosmetic deformity than expected if the crushed edges were closed.

c. If large areas of the wound margins are devitalized, or if the edges are too jagged, the revision may need to be more extensive. When feasible, the tension lines or wrinkles in the skin should be followed when revising a wound in order to minimize the retractive forces on the wound. An ellipse is made with a no. 15 blade scalpel parallel to the lines of tension (Fig. 72-2). It requires a length to width ratio of approximately 3:1 in order to avoid an uneven closure.

6. The new wound edges are bluntly undermined with tissue scissors (Fig. 72-3).

a. Most wounds require some degree of undermining, especially if there has been loss of tissue.

b. Undermining the edges 4 to 5 mm reduces tension on the wound by disrupting the elastic fibers that cause inversion of the skin edges.

8. Hemostasis is achieved with steady compression of the wound with a sterile 4 × 4 pad for 5 minutes. Health maintenance issues are discussed during this time.
    a. Hemostasis usually can be attained in 5 to 10 minutes with compression.
    b. Prevention of hematoma formation is critical for proper wound healing. Hematomas cause wider scars by increasing wound tension and by separating the skin edges. Wound edges also may necrose when capillary ingrowth to the skin is prevented by hematoma formation. Additionally, hematomas promote infection by providing a source of culture medium for bacteria.
9. The revised laceration is closed in layers, the *deep* layer first, using interrupted simple sutures of 4-0 Vicryl with inverted knots (Fig. 72-4).
    a. Closing all "dead space" is essential. Doing so reduces tension on the healing skin edges, decreases the chance of hematoma formation, and allows for earlier removal of skin sutures.
    b. The size of suture is dependent on the location of the laceration and degree of tension. The smaller the number, the thicker and stronger is the suture. For the deep layer, a 2-0 or 3-0 absorbable suture is used in the extremities and 4-0 or 5-0 in the face. (Subcutaneous sutures are contraindicated in facial skin flaps.)
    c. Absorbable sutures such as polyglactic acid (Vicryl), polyglycolic acid (Dexon), or chromic catgut swedged on a curved cutting needle are typically used to close the deep and subcutaneous layers.
    d. Knots should be inverted (buried), with the ends of the suture cut closely.
    e. The deeper layers should be approximated so that the skin edges come together evenly with

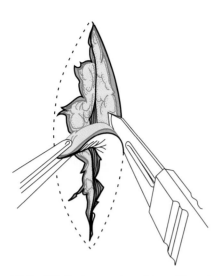

Figure 72-2 Elliptical wound revision. Wound edges with significant traumatic injury need to be revised, location permitting, by making an elliptical excision (ratio of length to width 3:1) of the wound with a no. 15 blade scalpel. (From Zuber TJ. Wound management. In Rakel RE (ed): Saunders Manual of Medical Practice. Philadelphia, WB Saunders, 1996, p 1008.)

    c. The safest level at which to undermine is just below the dermal-fat junction. Such precaution will help avoid injury to deeper blood vessels and nerves. In some lacerations of the trunk and extremities, it may be necessary to undermine at the fat-fascial level.
    d. The ends of slightly opened tissue scissors can be entered between the dermis and fat and the tissue spread apart by gently opening the scissors. The edge of a scalpel blade can also be used to tease open this tissue plane.
7. The wound is reirrigated with sterile saline.

A. Limb or Trunk

B. Face

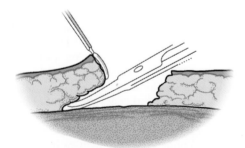 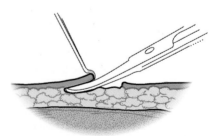

Figure 72-3 Undermining. Preparation of a laceration for repair often requires some undermining of the wound edges. Undermining disrupts elastic fibers that cause inversion of the edges and facilitates placement of deep sutures. It is performed below the subcutaneous tissue and above the muscle fascia for the limbs and trunk (**A**) and just beneath the dermal level in the face (**B**).

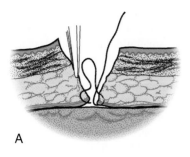

A

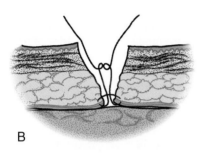

B

Figure 72-4 The inverted knot. Deep sutures should be tied so that the knots are buried below the layer being closed. This prevents the knots from interfering with the approximation of wound edges and minimizes tissue reaction to suture near the skin's surface. Start under one edge (**A**) and end underneath on the opposite side (**B**).

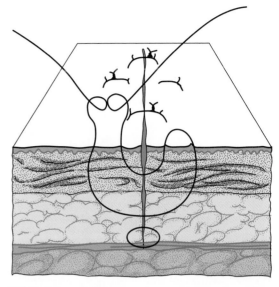

Figure 72-5 Alternating simple and vertical mattress sutures. The vertical mattress suture is an excellent technique to evert wound edges. The increased width of the deep portion of this double-layered suture also provides added wound support.

little tension. These layers include the dermal-fat and fat-fascial junctions, depending on the depth of the laceration. In this case, the skin on the inside of Gus's forearm is thin, and therefore the dermal-fat layer can be approximated with the skin closure as described below.

10. The skin is closed with a combination of alternating vertical mattress and simple sutures of 4-0 Ethilon (Fig. 72-5).

   a. A major goal in laceration repair is the gentle approximation of everted skin edges, which allows for matching of the regenerating basal layer of skin to produce a thinner scar that heals flatly without a ridge.

   b. Simple sutures will evert the wound edges if (1) the needle enters and exits the skin at identical distances from each edge, (2) they are deeper than they are wide, and (3) the base of the loop incorporates more tissue than its epidermal counterpart (Fig. 72-6).

   c. In areas of thin skin or increased tension, a vertical mattress suture effectively everts the wound edges. It is stronger than the simple suture and is often used on extremities. Alternating vertical mattress and simple sutures is a common practice. This takes some of the remaining tension off the larger vertical mattress sutures, decreasing stitch scarring.

   d. Use the smallest suture possible: 6-0 on the face, 5-0 or 4-0 on the trunk and extremities, and 4-0 on the back or other areas with thick skin.

   e. Stitch marks occur when sutures are (1) of too heavy a gauge, (2) too long (distance from entrance to exit sites), (3) too tight, or (4) left in too long, or (5) when they incorporate too much tissue.

   f. The skin layer is usually closed with nonabsorbable monofilament suture, either nylon (Ethilon or Dermalon) or polypropylene (Prolene or Surgilene) on a curved needle.

   g. Start the closure at one corner of the wound and work toward the other (unless an anatomic landmark is present, which is then approximated first). The needle should enter and exit the skin at a distance from the edge equal to the skin's thickness, usually about 3 to 4 mm. Sutures should be placed at a distance from each other equal to their length.

   h. Handle the skin as atraumatically as possible by using skin hooks or by gently grasping the fat-dermal junction with tissue forceps held parallel to the plane of the skin.

   i. Knots are tied with the needle holder by a technique known as the *instrument tie*. A surgeon's knot is made, followed by a second knot that is not squared and is incompletely tightened leaving a tiny loop. The third and fourth knots are squared. Remember to approximate, not strangulate, the tissue when tying knots.

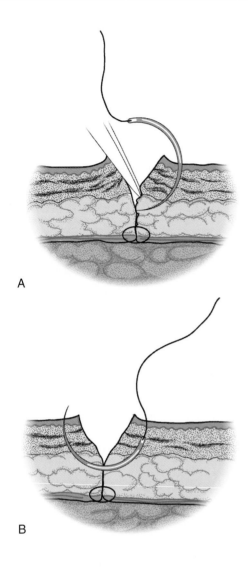

A

B

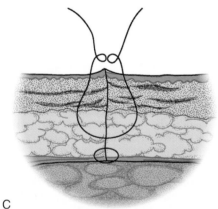

C

Figure 72-6 The simple suture. This basic suture will evert wound edges when placed correctly. Begin by piercing the skin with the needle at a right angle or greater (**A**), take a bite of tissue that is deeper than it is wide (**B**), and exit the skin symmetrically on the opposite side of the wound (**C**).

j. Cyanoacrylate tissue adhesives, such as Dermabond, are an alternative to skin sutures for closure of small superficial wounds requiring 5-0 or smaller suture. This method is a particularly attractive option in children and can be used on properly selected lacerations of the face, extremities, and torso. (The later two heal better when subcutaneous sutures are placed.)

11. The laceration repair is cleansed and dried. Benzoin is applied with a cotton swab to the skin on both sides of the closed laceration and allowed to dry. Steri-Strips are placed across the wound, and the drapes are removed. A protective nonadherent dressing is applied.

   a. Repairs are cleansed with either normal saline or hydrogen peroxide.

   b. Steri-Strips are a commonly used type of wound closure tape. They are sterile microporous tapes of various widths that add support to the repair, thus relieving some tension on the sutures. They are applied on one side of the laceration up to the skin edge, drawn across the repair, and then pressed down on the other side.

   c. Tincture of benzoin is a liquid that makes the skin more adhesive after it dries, allowing the Steri-Strips to be more effective and helping them to remain in place longer.

   d. Dressings for 24 to 48 hours serve two purposes: They keep the wound clean and help maintain a moist environment. The latter can accelerate epithelialization (sealing the wound), which protects the wound from gross contamination. After 48 hours, showering without covering the sutured laceration is permitted, but soaking and scrubbing are to be avoided.

Disposition

Gus is asked to keep the wound clean and dry and to rest and elevate his arm over the next 24 hours. Signs of infection (fever, redness, tenderness, increased local warmth, or purulent discharge) are explained. If these signs appear, he will need to return earlier than the scheduled follow-up in 2 days. The dressing is to be changed after 24 hours and hydrogen peroxide used to remove any dried blood from the sutures (unless wound closure tapes are present).

Gus is educated about the need to use a seat belt when driving and advised to stop smoking. His blood pressure will be rechecked at the time of the follow-up visit in 48 hours and again when his sutures are removed. Because of his risk factors for coronary artery disease (cigarette smoking, male sex, positive family history, and obesity), a fasting lipid profile instead of a random screening cholesterol test will be ordered. Gus is also encouraged to give consideration to a diet and exercise program.

FIRST FOLLOW-UP VISIT

Subjective

Gus returns for follow-up at the scheduled time and has no concerns about his arm. He is not aware of any fever and has had no pain or paresthesia. He is happy to report that he stopped smoking cigarettes and has already started to watch what he eats. His wife says he wore his seat belt on the way into clinic today.

Objective

Gus is afebrile, and his blood pressure is 118/78. There are no cigarettes in his pocket. The dressing is dry, and no distal edema is noted. His circulation, sensation, and function remained normal. The dressing is removed. The wound is clean and dry without signs of infection. There is no necrosis of the skin edges or hematoma formation. The wound edges are slightly everted and well approximated.

Assessment

The revised layered repair of the 2.5-cm laceration of Gus's left forearm is healing well without signs of infection. Gus's blood pressure is within normal limits today, and he has discontinued his cigarette habit.

Plan

Gus will return in 7 days for suture removal. He will continue to keep the wound clean and protect it with an adhesive bandage.

Gus is congratulated on his cessation of smoking, seat belt use, and attention to diet.

His blood pressure will be recorded by a friend (nurse) each week for 3 weeks, and he is to return to the office with these readings.

A blood sample for a lipid profile is drawn, and the results will be discussed with him at his next visit. At that time, an appropriate diet and exercise plan will be outlined.

DISCUSSION

The schedule for suture removal is approximately 3 to 5 days for the face, 7 days for the scalp, 7 to 10 days for the trunk and extremities, and 10 to 14 days for the hands, feet, back, and areas overlying joints. If a patient returns for suture removal and has a slow-healing wound with areas that may separate, partial suture removal should be considered as an option to minimize stitch scarring. Steri-Strips are placed where sutures were removed, and the remaining sutures are taken out as soon as possible. An antibiotic ointment such as Bacitracin or Polysporin is applied daily to the wound (on top of the Steri-Strips, if necessary). Antibiotic ointments may decrease the risk of infection and prevent scab formation.

Scars require 2 years to fully mature, during which time they become less erythematous and hypertrophic. Progressive collagen turnover results in retraction and produces a softer scar. Any revision should be delayed until this process of remodeling is complete.

Scarring in areas of cosmetic significance may be minimized by daily massage and protection from the sun. Massaging is started approximately 2 weeks after laceration repair and recommended daily (20 minutes qid or, more realistically, 5 minutes bid) for about 3 months (anecdotal information from plastic surgeons). Sunblock lotions and shading are used to limit sun exposure until the scar is mature. This after-laceration care may produce a softer, flatter, and less noticeable scar.

Material Available on Student Consult

Review Questions and Answers about Laceration Repair

SUGGESTED READINGS

Breitenbach KL, Bergera JJ. Principles and techniques of primary wound closure. In Snell GF (ed): Office Surgery: Primary Care Clin Office Pract. Philadelphia, WB Saunders, 1986;13:(3):411–431.

Brunds TB, Worthington JM. Using tissue adhesive for wound repair: A practical guide to Dermabond. Am Fam Physician 2000;61:1383–1388.

Dushoff IM. A stich in time. Emerg Med 1973;5:21–43.

Kundu S, Achar S. Principles of office anesthesia: Part II. Topical anesthesia. Am Fam Physician 2002;66:99–102.

Little DN. Simple and infected lacerations. In Mayhew HE, Rogers LA (eds): Basic Procedures in Family Practice. Bethany, CT, Fleschner, 1984, pp 7–12.

Moy RL, Lee A, Zalka A. Commonly used suturing techniques in skin surgery. Am Fam Physician 1991; 44:1625–1634.

Norton LW. Trauma. In Hill GJ II (ed): Outpatient Surgery, 2nd ed. Philadelphia, WB Saunders, 1980, pp 112–114.

Singer AJ, Hollander JE, Quinn JV. Evaluation and management of traumatic lacerations. N Engl J Med 1997;-337:1142–1147.

Zuber TJ. Wound management. In Rakel RE (ed): Saunders Manual of Medical Practice. Philadelphia, WB Saunders, 1996, pp 1007–1008.

Zuber TJ. The mattress sutures: Vertical, horizontal, and corner stitch. Am Fam Physician 2002;66:2231–2236.

73

Fatigue, Nausea, Breast Tenderness (Normal Pregnancy)

Randy Wertheimer

INITIAL VISIT

Subjective

Patient Identification and Presenting Problem

Rachel is a 23-year-old gravida 2, para 0, ab 1 woman who presents with a 4-week history of fatigue, nausea, and breast tenderness. She had a positive pregnancy test 2 weeks ago and is experiencing symptoms similar to those that she had 5 years ago when she was pregnant for the first time. Rachel stopped her birth control pill 3 months ago with the hope of becoming pregnant within the next year. She had a normal withdrawal menses at that time and had a few days of spotting around 8 weeks ago. She is unsure of the exact date of her last menstrual period, as the spotting episode was not typical of her menses. She expressed concern about becoming pregnant so soon after using the contraceptive pill.

Rachel has been on a multivitamin preparation with folic acid as prescribed by her family physician since she went off the birth control pill with plans to become pregnant. She has been immunized against hepatitis B with the full triple vaccine within the past 5 years. We know from her previous pregnancy that she is immune to rubella and that her blood type is B negative. She remembers having chicken pox as a child. Her last Pap smear 6 months ago was within normal limits, and she has had normal Pap smears yearly since age 18.

Ben, Rachel's husband of 3 years, is excited about this pregnancy according to Rachel. Although they have no family close by, they have been living in the area since college and have a community of close friends. Rachel plans to work part-time as a computer programmer after the baby is born, and her husband will continue to work full-time in his job as an electrical engineer.

Medical History

Menarche at age 13. Menstrual cycle 31 days, 5 days of flow. Oral contraceptives used 1990 to 1996. Pregnancy 1990: elective first-trimester termination. No complications. Rh immune globulin given after procedure. Hospitalizations: None. Allergies: None.

Family History

Maternal mother (Rachel's mother) has hypertension and hypercholesterolemia. Paternal father (Ben's

---

Evidence levels Ⓐ Randomized, controlled trials (RCTs), meta-analyses, well-designed systematic reviews of RCTs. Ⓑ Case-control or cohort studies, nonrandomized clinical trials, systematic reviews of studies other than RCTs, cross-sectional studies, retrospective studies, certain uncontrolled studies. Ⓒ Consensus statements, expert guidelines, usual practice, opinion.

father) has type 2 diabetes. No family history of congenital defects or genetic disorders.

Health Habits

Alcohol intake of one glass of wine a few times per week was stopped 3 months ago. History of occasional marijuana use. No cocaine or other substance use. No smoking.

Review of Systems

History of occasional headaches. Urinary tract infection twice in the past 10 years. No history of pyelonephritis.

Objective

Physical Examination

Rachel is a well-appearing, mildly overweight young woman. Blood pressure 110/70 mm Hg, pulse 76, regular. Height 5 feet 3 inches, weight 140 pounds. Skin: no rashes. HEENT: normal. Neck: supple. No adenopathy. Thyroid normal size. Lungs: clear. Cardiovascular: S_1 normal, S_2 normal. No murmur. Breasts: no masses, inverted nipples bilaterally. Abdomen: bowel sounds normoactive. No hepatosplenomegaly. No fetal heart tones audible by Doppler scan. Pelvic: external genitalia normal, vaginal vault has scant discharge. Cervix shows bluish discoloration. Chlamydia culture taken. Uterus is anterior, enlarged, 8 weeks in size (size of large orange). Ovaries not palpated. No adnexal masses palpated. Diagonal conjugate (distance between sacral promontory and inferior aspect of symphysis) 13 cm, distance between ischial spines 12 cm, pelvic side walls concave. Extremities: No edema.

Laboratory Tests

Urine dipstick test negative for albumin and glucose.

Assessment

Intrauterine pregnancy. History, physical examination, and laboratory data all point to an early intrauterine pregnancy. Establishing the due date is the first order of business. In addition, the physician needs to identify screening tests to diagnose and treat prenatal disease. Last, one wants to promote a healthy pregnancy by assessing the woman's home and work environment and by promoting a healthy lifestyle.

Discussion

Establishing the Due Date

The diagnosis of pregnancy in this case is relatively straightforward. Rachel has had unprotected sex, is amenorrheic, and is exhibiting many of the frequent symptoms of early pregnancy, i.e., fatigue, breast swelling and tenderness, nausea.

Her physical examination reveals changes in the cervix and the uterus, which are also consistent with early pregnancy. Her cervix has a bluish hue, know as Chadwick's sign. She has an enlarged uterus, about the size of a large orange, corresponding to 8 weeks' gestation. The physician does not hear a fetal heartbeat by Doppler ultrasound. Fetal heart tones may be audible by Doppler as early as 9 weeks' gestation, depending in part on the position of the uterus and the body habitus of the woman. By 12 weeks' gestation, fetal heart tones are audible by Doppler ultrasound in most pregnant women.

Rachel did not need a urine pregnancy test done in the office because she had a positive test that she had done at home and physical examination confirmed an intrauterine pregnancy. The commonly performed urine test measures the presence of an elevated level of human chorionic gonadotropin. Normally, nonpregnant women have low circulating levels, 0.02 to 0.08 IU of human chorionic gonadotropin. With early pregnancy, levels double every 1.3 to 2.3 days and peak at 7 to 10 weeks (100,000 IU). Elevated human chorionic gonadotropin levels are generally detected in the urine by 7 to 10 days after conception. By the time menses is missed, 89% of pregnant women have a positive test.

The most commonly used method to ascertain a pregnant woman's due date is the last menstrual period (LMP). When a woman can recall with clarity the first day of her last menstrual period and can define it as a normal period with regard to regularity and duration, and there has not been a recent use of birth control pills, then the LMP is a remarkably accurate predictor of the due date. However, in this case, Rachel's last normal menses was attached to her last cycle of oral contraceptives. The few days of spotting 4 weeks later may represent the LMP, but it is difficult to determine with accuracy by this history. Women may not ovulate regularly the first few months after stopping the pill. Her physical examination, however, with a uterus the size of an 8-week gestation, suggests that this spotting was in fact the LMP.

If the LMP were believed to be more accurate were, one could estimate the due date by using a pregnancy wheel or by applying the Nägele rule. One begins with the first day of the LMP, adds 1 year plus 7 days and subtracts 3 months. The length of human gestation is estimated at 280 days, or 40 weeks counting from the first day of the LMP. This assumes a 28-day cycle and that the time from ovulation to menses was 14 days. In women with longer cycles, as is true with Rachel who has a 31-day cycle, one should add a few days to the expected due date.

Because we are not able to estimate a due date with certainty by history and physical examination at this point, it is reasonable to order an ultrasound as an additional tool to help establish accurate dating. First-trimester scans can identify the gestational age of a pregnancy within 3 to 5 days using the crown-rump length. This method of measurement is not used after 12 weeks' gestation because of fetal spine flexion. Transvaginal scanning uses a higher frequency transducer, and structures may be seen earlier than in transabdominal screening. Fetal poles can be seen as early as 6 weeks transvaginally and 7 to 8 weeks transabdominally. It is important to note that the use of ultrasound is not recommended as a routine screening test in pregnancy. Neither early, late, nor serial ultrasounds have demonstrated an improved perinatal morbidity or mortality (U.S. Preventive Services Task Force, 1996Ⓐ). However, it is an appropriate tool to use for gestational age assessment in cases of uncertain dates.

Diagnose and Treat Prenatal Disease

Rachel did have adequate preconception care within the year before pregnancy. During this time, risk assessment, health promotion, and medical and psychosocial intervention were addressed by her family physician. We know that the greatest sensitivity to the environment for the developing fetus occurs during the 17 to 56 days after conception, yet as many as one fourth of pregnant women fail to initiate care until after the first trimester. Because healthy women are more likely to have healthier babies, the time to treat illness or change unhealthy behavior is before pregnancy.

A number of screening tests must now be ordered as part of the initial prenatal visit. Many of the tests ordered in the preconception period need not be repeated. Box 73-1 lists recommended screening laboratory tests during pregnancy.

First the hemoglobin/hematocrit level should be determined. During pregnancy, the increase in plasma volume is disproportionately greater than the red blood cell mass, causing physiologic dilution and a normal drop in hematocrit by 3% to 5%. Therefore, the definition of anemia in pregnancy is different from that in the nonpregnant adult woman. For women living at sea level, a hemoglobin of 11 g/dL in the first and third trimester, and 10.5 g/dL in the second trimester, is acceptable. Although hemoglobin values well below 10% have been associated with an increased risk of low birth weight, preterm delivery, and perinatal mortality in numerous longitudinal cross-sectional studies, most of these studies did not control for other factors such as smoking and maternal malnutrition. Whereas a large body of data suggests that iron supplements improve hematologic indices in hemoglobin levels above 10 g/dL, there is no consistent evidence that iron supplementation actually improves clinical outcomes. Therefore, there are no evidence-based outcomes to recommend routine iron supplementation in pregnant women with hemoglobin values greater than 10 g/dL.

Box 73-1	Prenatal Screening Tests

Initial Prenatal Visit

Blood pressure
Hemoglobin or hematocrit
Antibody screen
Rapid plasma reagin
HBsAg (if status unknown)
Blood group and Rh factor (if status unknown)
Rubella titer (if status unknown)
Varicella titer (if status unknown)
Urine culture (12–16 wk)
Chlamydia (if woman < 25 yr of age or high risk)
Gonococcal culture (if high risk)
Pap smear (if not done within past 6–12 mo)
Hemoglobin electrophoresis (if status unknown in at-risk racial groups)
HIV screen (counsel and offer to all)

16–18 wk

α-Fetoprotein

24–28 wk

Glucose (Glucola) screen
Antibody (if Rh negative)
Rapid plasma reagin (if high risk)

HBsAg, hepatitis B surface antigen; HIV, human immunodeficiency virus.

Testing for antibodies is done also during this first prenatal visit. One needs to know blood type (ABO/Rh) and antibodies for each pregnancy. Because Rachel was pregnant previously, we already know that she is B negative, and blood type testing need not be repeated. Antibodies must be checked with each pregnancy, however. The most prevalent antibody of concern during pregnancy is the anti-Rh (D) antibody. Rh incompatibility occurs when an Rh-negative woman is pregnant with an Rh-positive fetus. This occurs in 9% to 10% of pregnancies. Consequences for the fetus include hemolytic anemia, hyperbilirubinemia, kernicterus, and intrauterine death due to hydrops fetalis. Without preventive measures, 0.7% to 1.8% of Rh-negative women become isoimmunized antenatally and develop Rh (D) antibody through exposure to fetal blood; 8% to 15% become isoimmunized at birth; 3% to 5% become isoimmunized after spontaneous or therapeutic abortion; and 2.1% to 3.4% become isoimmunized after amniocentesis (U.S. Preventive Services Task Force, 2004Ⓐ).

Rachel's rubella status (immune) is already known, and she also has a positive hepatitis B surface antibody documented on her chart. If these results were not known as part of her medical history, they would have to be checked at the first prenatal visit. Similarly, there is no need to repeat a normal Pap smear that was done within the past 6 months in a patient with no other known risk factors and with documented yearly normal Pap smears. Rachel is not at high risk of sexually transmitted diseases. Gonorrhea is more prevalent in specific high-risk groups, i.e., in prostitutes, in women younger than 25 years of age with two or more sexual partners within the past year, and in women with recurrent episodes of sexually transmitted diseases. Routine screening for women at high risk is recommended. At this first prenatal visit, Rachel is screened for *Chlamydia*, however. Patient characteristics associated with a higher prevalence of infection include a history of a sexually transmitted disease, new or multiple sexual partners, inconsistent use of barrier contraceptives, cervical ectopy, and age younger than 25. Rachel is only 23 years old and thus fits into one of the high-risk categories.

All pregnant women need to be screened for syphilis with a rapid plasma reagin titer, even if they have been tested within the past year (U.S Preventive Services Task Force, 2004Ⓐ). The neurologic sequelae for the surviving newborn are devastating, and there is a 40% fetal or perinatal death rate in pregnancies compromised by congenital syphilis. Penicillin is an inexpensive, easily available treatment.

Rachel is advised to have human immunodeficiency virus testing, as the overall prevalence in her community of seropositive newborns has increased to greater than 0.1%. The U.S. Preventive Services Task Force (2004Ⓐ) recommends that all pregnant women from communities in which prevalence of seropositive newborns has increased be offered testing as soon as the woman is known to be pregnant. The probability of vertical transmission varies from 13% to 35%, increasing with the severity of disease in the mother, and can be significantly decreased with adequate antiviral therapy. Pregnancy is not necessarily a contraindication to the use of optimal therapeutic regimens to treat this disease in the mother as well. Other benefits of early detection include *Pneumocystis carinii* pneumonia prophylaxis, prevention of vertical transmission associated with breast-feeding, early treatment of the infant, and early accessing of social service support.

Rachel does not need hemoglobin electrophoresis, as she is not a member of one of the ethnic groups at high risk of a hemoglobinopathy, i.e., women of Caribbean, Latin American, Mediterranean, Southeast Asian, or African descent.

Promote a Healthy Pregnancy

Rachel needs to be counseled on a healthy lifestyle. She is advised to eat a diet high in calcium (1200 to 1500 mg/day) with generous amounts of protein, fruit, and vegetables. She is advised to continue her folic acid. Ninety percent to 95% of pregnancies complicated by neural tube defects occur in the absence of a positive history. It is recommended that all women planning a pregnancy take a multivitamin containing folic acid at a dose of 0.4 mg, beginning at least 1 month before conception and continuing through the first trimester to reduce the risks of neural tube defects. Rachel had been started on folic acid when she discontinued her birth control pill 3 months ago. Adequate studies have not been completed to evaluate whether adequate dietary intake without vitamin supplementation could achieve the same results.

Rachel stopped drinking her usual one glass of wine a few times a week when she stopped the birth control pill. Her physician supports that decision, although there is no proven association between occasional light drinking and adverse birth outcomes. There is a known association between problem drinking (two or more drinks per day or binge drinking) and fetal alcohol syndrome. According to the U.S. Preventive Services Task Force (2004Ⓐ), there is insufficient evidence to prove or disprove harm from occasional light drinking during pregnancy.

Fortunately, Rachel does not smoke cigarettes. Tobacco use contributes to low birth weight, placenta previa, congenital anomalies, and spontaneous abortion.

Rachel is encouraged to exercise regularly, at the same level that she was exercising before her pregnancy, providing she feels up to it. She should not work to increase her exercise stamina at this time.

Sexual activity needs to be addressed by the physician early in pregnancy. If the patient does not ask about it, the physician must feel comfortable initiating the topic. There is no contraindication to sexual intercourse in a normal health woman during her pregnancy.

We perform a screening interview to elicit any history of domestic violence, an underdiagnosed problem. Rachel was asked whether she had ever been emotionally or physically abused by her partner and if she had been hit, slapped, kicked, or otherwise physically hurt by someone within the past year. She was surprised by the questions and responded with a clearly negative answer. Surveys from women in urban clinics state that 7% to 18% of women report physical abuse or forced sex during pregnancy (Norton et al., 1995Ⓑ). Several well-controlled studies suggest detection rates improve when more than one question pertaining to violence is asked in a single interview, and with repeated questions on subsequent visits. However, there are insufficient data to recommend for or against the use of specific screening instruments, as methods have not been adequately evaluated to change behaviors once the problem is identified.

Rachel's workplace is a computer room at a college campus. No occupational hazards were discovered in review of her work site.

Plan

1. Ultrasound for dating
2. Hematocrit, antibodies, *Chlamydia,* rapid plasma reagin, human immunodeficiency virus
3. Continue multivitamins with folic acid
4. Diet, exercise, sexual activity discussed
5. Follow-up in 1 month

FIRST FOLLOW-UP VISIT

Subjective

Rachel and her husband return 4 weeks later. Ben is looking forward to hearing the fetal heartbeat today. Rachel's nausea and fatigue have passed. She has gained weight and is enjoying her pregnancy. She plans to keep working as long as possible.

Ultrasound done 4 weeks ago confirmed an 8-week-old fetus, making her 12 weeks pregnant today. She is concerned about her 5-pound weight gain over the past month. She continues to take her multivitamins with folate.

Her normal laboratory studies are reviewed. Her hematocrit is 35. Antibodies, *Chlamydia,* and human immunodeficiency virus testing are all negative.

Objective

Well-appearing gravid woman. Blood pressure 115/70 mm Hg, weight 145 pounds. Fundus palpated just above the symphysis pubis. Fetal heart audible by Doppler at 150 beats per minute.

Urine is negative for glucose and albumin.

Assessment

Normal pregnancy. Rachel's due date has been confirmed by ultrasound and she is growing well.

Discussion

A 5-pound weight gain over the past month is acceptable. Rachel has gained approximately 10 pounds from her pregravid weight, and a total pregnancy weight gain of 25 to 35 pounds, or 11 to 16 kg, is desirable in a woman of normal weight. Low prepregnant weight and inadequate weight gain are both contributors to intrauterine growth retardation. Conversely, in obese women, perinatal morbidity begins to increase with a weight gain of greater than 15 pounds (ACOG Technical Bulletin No. 179, 1993◐). Extreme obesity increases the risk of gestational diabetes, hypertension, macrosomia, shoulder dystocia, and prolonged dysfunctional labor.

At 12 weeks' gestation, Rachel may now be screened for occult bacteriuria. All pregnant women need to be screened for occult bacteriuria. The occurrence of this condition in pregnancy varies in studies between 2% and 7%. If untreated, pregnant women are at increased risk of pyelonephritis, with subsequent preterm delivery and a low birth weight infant. The timing of a urine culture may vary, although asymptomatic bacteriuria is best detected if the specimen is taken between 12 and 16 weeks' gestation. Urine dipstick testing for leukocyte esterase is not an acceptable alternative screening test in the pregnant woman. Sensitivity for dipstick testing of urine is only 50%.

The doctor notes that flu season will be starting over the next few weeks and wishes to immunize Rachel. The Advisory Committee on Immunization Practices recommends vaccination of all pregnant women regardless of stage of pregnancy if the gestation overlaps with flu season. (Harper et al., 2004◐).

Plan

Urine culture today.

1. Flu vaccine
2. Follow-up in 1 month

SUBSEQUENT FOLLOW-UP VISITS

Rachel is seen monthly over the next 24 weeks. Her uterine growth, blood pressure, and weight gain continue to be normal.

Specific objectives, e.g., screening tests, physical findings, and anticipatory guidance issues, are highlighted at subsequent visits.

1. *At 16 weeks.* Rachel is screened for potential neural tube defects with a maternal serum α-fetoprotein test. This is recommended for all women at 16 to 18 weeks' gestation. False-positive results can occur with multiple gestations, fetal demise, or incorrect gestational age. A test is considered abnormal if it is 2.0 to 2.5 times above the median value for gestational age. A very low α-fetoprotein is suggestive of Down syndrome. Rachel's results are normal.

2. *At 20 weeks.* Rachel is now at the midpoint of her pregnancy. Her physician asks her whether she has begun to feel movement. "Quickening," as it is commonly called, occurs at 18 to 20 weeks' gestation in a primipara. It is subtle at first, and Rachel describes fleeting, faint movements over the past few days. On physical examination, the fundus is at the umbilicus and measures 20 cm above the upper rim of the symphysis pubis. Over the next 12 to 16 weeks, her growth corresponds to a centimeter per week (Fig. 73-1).

3. *At 24 weeks.* Rachel expected to be screened for gestational diabetes at this visit. At 24 to 28 weeks, the goal is to identify women with glucose

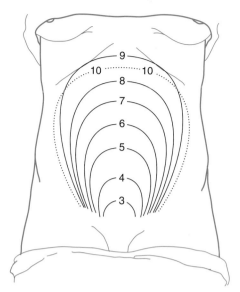

Figure 73-1 Fundal growth at various months of gestations. (From Rakel, Robert E. Textbook of Family Practice, 5th edition. Philadelphia, WB Saunders, 1996.)

Table 73-1	Leopold's Maneuvers	
Maneuver	**Action**	**Question**
First	Examine the fundus	What fetal part is in the fundus?
Second	Palpate the lateral abdomen	Where is the fetal back?
Third	Palpate the suprapubic area	Is the presenting part engaged?
Fourth (vertex only)	Find the cephalic prominence	Is the head flexed?

intolerance and treat them with diet or insulin as needed. A 50-mg glucose drink is given, and the blood sugar is checked 1 hour later. A normal reading is below 140 ng/dL. Glycosuria is not an accurate predictor of diabetes in the pregnant woman because the renal threshold for glucose is lowered. Rachel does not fit into the specified high-risk groups, including those who are obese, are age 25 or older, have a positive family history of diabetes, or are members of ethnic groups with a high prevalence of diabetes, i.e., African Americans, Asians, Native Americans, and Hispanics. Her doctor elects not to screen her as the 2003 U.S. Preventive Health Services Task Force report did not find that routine screening reduced important health outcomes for mothers or their infants, i.e., cesarean delivery, birth injury, neonatal morbidity or mortality. It does cite fair to good evidence that screening combined with diet and insulin therapy can reduce the rate of fetal macrosomia in gestational diabetes.

4. *At 28 weeks.* Antibodies are repeated at this visit because Rachel is Rh negative. She has negative results and thus is given an intramuscular injection of 300 mg of Rh immune globulin, which should prevent any isoimmunization over the third trimester.

5. *At 30 weeks and later.* Beginning at 30 weeks, the uterus is examined at each visit using Leopold's maneuvers (Table 73-1 and Fig. 73-2) to detect the baby's position. Rachel is seen weekly by her physician after 36 weeks' gestation.

Health education and risk assessment continue at each visit throughout the second and third trimesters. During the second trimester, signs of labor

are discussed and Rachel is encouraged to attend prenatal classes. In the third trimester, signs of labor are reviewed; birth plans are discussed including specifics of anesthesia and labor support. Between 35 and 37 weeks, Rachel will be screened for group B streptococcal infection via a single swab run over the skin from the vaginal introitus to the anus (Box 73-2). The vaginal and rectal areas of 10% to 30% of pregnant women may be colonized. Group B streptococcus is a leading cause of neonatal illness and death. The risk of early-onset group B streptococcal disease in the infant of a colonized mother is one infant per 50 to 100 colonized mothers. Group B streptococcal infection can also cause preterm labor, premature membrane rupture, urinary tract infections, chorioamnionitis, and postpartum endometritis (Keenan, 1998©). If Rachel's culture is positive, she will receive antibiotic prophylaxis in labor. Rachel's

Box 73-2	**High-Risk Markers for Neonatal Invasive Group B Streptococcal Infection**

Previous infant with invasive group B streptococcal disease
Maternal carrier state, especially if colonization is heavy
Maternal group B streptococcal bacteriuria
Preterm labor or preterm rupture of the membranes at an estimated gestational age of <37 wk
Rupture of the membranes for >18 h

From Centers for Disease Control and Prevention. Prevention of perinatal group B streptococcal disease: A public health persepective. MMWR Morb Mortal Wkly Rep 1996;45:679; Schuchat A, Wenger JD. Epidemiology of group B streptococcal disease. Risk factors, prevention strageties, and vaccine development. Epidermiol Rev 1994;16:374–402.

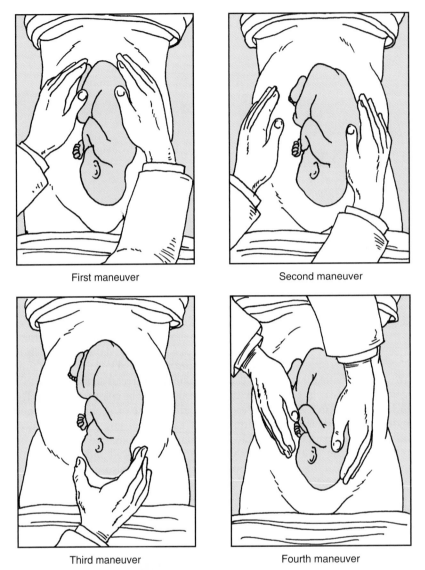

First maneuver

Second maneuver

Third maneuver

Fourth maneuver

Figure 73-2 Leopold's maneuvers for determining fetal position. (From Rakel, Robert E. Textbook of Family Practice, 5th edition. Philadelphia, WB Saunders, 1996.)

wishes for a natural childbirth are supported and documented on her prenatal form. Breast-feeding, circumcision, and postpartum contraception are also addressed, as are the plans of Ben and Rachel for help with the newborn (Table 73-2).

Material Available on Student Consult

Review Questions and Answers about Normal Pregnancy

Table 73-2   U.S. Preventive Services Task Force Recommendations for Low-Risk Pregnancies

Routine Recommendations/ Screening	Strength of Recommendation	Date of Recommendation
Folic acid supplementation (0.4–0.8 mg 1 mo before conception through 1st trimester)	A	1996
Rh incompatibility blood screening	A	2004
Syphilis screening	A	2004
Bacterial vaginosis screening in asymptomatic woman	D	2001
Routine asymptomatic bacteriuria screening at 12–16 wk	A	2004
NTD screening: maternal serum α-fetoprotein at 16–18 wk	B	1996
Gestational diabetes blood screening	I	2003
Preeclampsia screening (blood pressure measurements)	B	1996
Routine ultrasound screening in 3rd trimester	D	1996
Routine ultrasound screening in 2nd trimester	C	1996
Brief education and counseling by M.D. to promote breast-feeding	C	2003
Routine screening for intimate partner violence	I	2004

A, Good evidence that (the service) improves important health outcomes; B, at least fair evidence that (the service) improves important health outcomes and concludes that benefits outweigh harms; C, at least fair evidence that (the service) can improve health outcomes but concludes that the balance of benefits and harms is too close to justify a general recommendation; D, at least fair evidence that (the service) is ineffective or that harms outweigh benefits; I, effective evidence is lacking or of poor quality or conflicting; the balance of benefits and harms cannot be determined.

NTD, neural tube defect.

REFERENCES

ACOG Technical Bulletin No. 179: Nutrition during Pregnancy. Washington, DC, American College of Obstetricians and Gynecologists, 1993.©

Harper SA, Fukuda K, Uyeki TM, et al. Prevention and Control of Influenza: Recommendations of the Advisory Committee on Immunization Practices (ACIP). MMWR Recomm Rep 2004;53:1–40.©

Keenan C. Prevention of neonatal group B streptococcal infection. Am Fam Physician 1998;57:2713–2720.©

Norton LB, Peipert JF, Zierler S, et al. Battering in pregnancy: An assessment of two screening methods. Obstet Gynecol 1995;85:321–325.®

U.S. Preventive Services Task Force. Screening ultrasonography in pregnancy. Guide to Clinical Preventive Services, 2nd edition. Washington, DC, U.S. Department of Health and Human Services, Office of Disease Prevention and Health Promotion, 1996. Available at http://cpmcnet.columbia.edu/texts/gcps/gcps0046.html. Accessesed 4/14/2006.Ⓐ

U.S. Preventive Services Task Force. Screening for gestational diabetes mellitus. Guide to Clinical Preventive Services, 2nd edition. Washington, DC, U.S. Department of Health and Human Services, Office of Disease Prevention and Health Promotion, 2003 Available at http://www.ahrq.gov/clinic/3rduspstf/gdm/gdmrr.pdf. Accessesed 4/14/2006.Ⓐ

U.S. Preventive Services Task Force. Screening for Rh (D) incompatibility. Guide to Clinical Preventive Services, 2nd edition. Washington, DC, U.S. Department of Health and Human Services, Office of Disease Prevention and Health Promotion, 2004. Available at http://www.ahrq.gov/clinic/3rduspstf/rh/rhrs.pdf. Accessesed 4/14/2006.Ⓐ

SUGGESTED READINGS

National Institute of Health. Caring for Our Future: The Content of Prenatal Care. U.S. Department of Health and Human Services, Public Health Service, 1989. NIH publication no. 90-3182.

Connor EM, Sperling RS, Gelber R, et al. Reduction of maternal-infant transmission of HIV-1 with zidovudine treatment. N Engl J Med 1994;331:1173–1180.Ⓐ

Rakel RE. Textbook of Family Practice, 5th ed. Philadelphia, WB Saunders, 1996, pp 528–567.©

74

Short Child (Constitutional Growth Delay)

Sanford R. Kimmel

INITIAL VISIT

Subjective

Patient Identification and Presenting Problem

Johnny J. is a 5-year-old white boy seen for a prekindergarten well-child physical examination. Johnny's mother notes that he is smaller than other boys his age. His 3-year-old sister is almost as tall as he is.

Present Illness

Johnny's only recent illness has been a cold, which was treated with an over-the-counter antihistamine–decongestant medicine. His appetite and physical activity are normal. He is a picky eater who generally has cold cereal and milk for breakfast, macaroni and cheese for lunch, and a hamburger or pizza for supper. He likes apples, bananas, and corn but few green or yellow vegetables. He plays and keeps up with other boys his age.

Medical History

Johnny was the product of a full-term, uncomplicated pregnancy. His birth weight was 7 pounds 8 ounces (3.4 kg) and his length was 20 inches (51 cm). A chart of his growth is presented in Figure 74-1.

His developmental milestones include the following: he smiled at 2 months, sat without support at 6 months, said "dada" specifically at 11 months, walked alone at 13 months, and now dresses himself without supervision. He speaks in understandable sentences.

Immunizations include diphtheria–tetanus–acellular pertussis (DTaP), conjugated pneumococcal, and *Haemophilus influenzae* B vaccines at 2, 4, 6, and 15 months of age; inactivated polio vaccine (IPV) at 2, 4, and 12 months of age; and a measles–mumps–rubella (MMR) vaccine at 15 months of age. Johnny also received a hepatitis B vaccine at birth and at 2 and 6 months of age.

Johnny has had four to five upper respiratory infections per year and three lifetime episodes of otitis media. He has not had varicella, been hospitalized, or required major surgery.

Family History

Johnny's mother is 26 years old and in good health. She is 5 feet 4 inches tall and weighs 140 pounds. His 30-year-old father is 5 feet 8 inches tall and weighs 165 pounds. Johnny's father recalls being smaller than his peers as a child and being a "late bloomer." Johnny's 57-year-old paternal grandfather had a heart attack 2 years ago. His other grandparents are in their 50s and in good health. Johnny's 3-year-old sister is 37 inches tall and weighs 33 pounds.

Health Habits

Johnny uses a belted child booster seat when traveling in the car. His parents limit television viewing to 2 hours per day. He is learning to ride a bicycle.

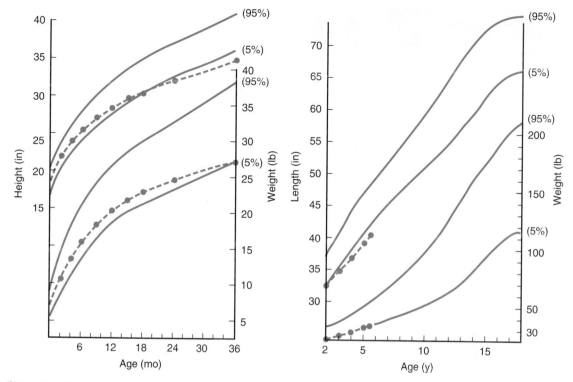

Figure 74-1 Growth curves for Johnny J. for length/height (*top curve*) and weight (*lower curve*). The 95th and 5th percentiles for each parameter are also outlined.

Social History

Johnny is currently in nursery school but will be starting kindergarten next year. His mother, who is a teacher, reports that he interacts well with other children his age. However, she and her husband, who is an executive, are concerned that his small size may place him at a disadvantage in school.

Review of Systems

Other than slight rhinorrhea, the review of systems is unremarkable.

Objective

Physical Examination

Johnny's height is 38.5 inches, weight is 33 pounds, blood pressure is 94/58, and pulse is 76 and regular. He appears normally proportioned and has no detectable deformities. Examination of the head, neck, eyes, ears, nose, and throat is normal. The cardiorespiratory and abdominal examinations are also normal. His genitalia are prepubertal (Tanner stage 1). He follows directions and can balance on one foot for 6 seconds, catch a bounced ball, and draw a man with a head, eyes, ears, nose, mouth, body, arms, and legs.

Laboratory Tests

A urinalysis demonstrates a specific gravity of 1.022, pH 6.0, with negative dipstick and microscopic examination.

Assessment

Working Diagnosis

The most likely diagnosis is constitutional growth delay (CGD) in an otherwise well child. Although Johnny's height is below the 5th percentile and his weight is at the 5th percentile, his rate of growth parallels the growth curve. His deceleration in growth occurred before age 2 and was accompanied by crossing of percentile lines. Since age 2, his linear growth has averaged 4 to 5 cm per year. Johnny's family history of delayed physical development also supports this diagnosis (Bareille et al., 1998).

Differential Diagnoses

While genetic and environmental factors often cause short stature, almost any serious chronic illness can have an adverse impact on a child's growth. Common causes of short stature are listed in Box 74-1 and are discussed later in this chapter (see Discussion section).

Box 74-1	Common or Significant Causes of Short Stature in Children

Familial

Constitutional growth delay
Familial (genetic) short stature

Congenital

Down syndrome
Noonan's syndrome
Russell-Silver syndrome
Skeletal dysplasia (dwarfism)
Turner's syndrome
Virilizing congenital adrenal hyperplasia
   (tall child, short adult)

Systemic Disorders

Cancer due to poor nutrition, chemotherapy,
   or radiotherapy
Endocrine disease
   Cushing's syndrome
   Diabetes mellitus (poorly controlled)
   Growth hormone deficiency, congenital
     or acquired
   Hypopituitarism
   Hypothyroidism
Heart disease
   Chronic heart failure
   Congenital heart disease
Gastrointestinal disease
   Celiac disease
   Inflammatory bowel disease (Crohn's dsease)
   Malabsorption syndromes
Immunologic diseases
   Acquired immunodeficiency syndrome
   Severe combined immunodeficiency
Pulmonary disease
   Asthma (poorly controlled)
   Cystic fibrosis
Renal disease
   Chronic renal failure
   Renal tubular acidosis

Environmental

Malnutrition
Psychosocial deprivation
Toxin or drug exposure (e.g., lead)

Plan

Diagnostic

1. Proper evaluation of the growth curve is the most important consideration. A normal rate of linear growth excludes most organic causes of short stature. Children younger than 2 years of age should have their length measured in the supine position. Children 2 years and older should have their shoeless standing height measured with a stadiometer. Using either method, the head should be positioned so the outer canthus of the eye is aligned with the external auditory canal and perpendicular to the measuring surface (Halac and Zimmerman, 2004). Children should wear minimal clothing when they are weighed at each visit, preferably on the same scale. Height and weight are then plotted on a growth chart developed by the National Center for Health Statistics. *Height age* is the age at which the child's height intersects the 50th percentile curve on this chart.

2. A *bone-age* radiograph of the left hand and wrist is compared with published age-specific standards (Miller and Zimmerman, 2004). Children must be at least 2 years of age for epiphyseal ossification centers to be reliably identified. Bone age films help differentiate familial short stature (FSS) from CGD and various endocrinologic disorders (Table 74-1).

3. The child's lower segment is determined by measuring the distance from the top of the symphysis pubis to the floor or surface supporting the feet. The upper segment equals this distance subtracted from the total height. The upper-to-lower segment ratio decreases from 1.7 at birth to 1.4 at 2 years of age, to 1.0 at age 10 years, and to 0.9 in adults. This ratio is increased in short-limbed dwarfism, chondrodystrophies, gonadal dysgenesis, and Klinefelter syndrome. Vertebral anomalies decrease the upper-to-lower segment ratio (Halac and Zimmerman, 2004).

4. A complete blood count with differential may reveal anemia or malignancy. An erythrocyte sedimentation rate may detect nonspecific inflammatory disorders such as inflammatory bowel disease or collagen vascular disease. Endomysial antibodies should also be considered because celiac disease is increasingly recognized. Stool specimens for fat and ova and parasites may be useful in detecting causes of malabsorption. Girls of short stature should have a karyotype evaluation (Halac and Zimmerman, 2004).

5. Serum free thyroxine and thyroid-simulating hormone determinations should be performed because hypothyroidism is easily detected and treated. Levels of insulin like growth factor 1 (IGF-1) and insulin growth factor binding protein 3 may estimate growth hormone (GH) function (Miller and Zimmerman, 2004).

6. Renal and liver function tests, blood glucose, lipid profile, calcium, phosphorus, and electrolyte determinations, and a urinalysis are useful in ruling out renal or hepatic disease, diabetes, or hyperlipidemia. Cholesterol level is important in this case because the family history is suspicious for early cardiac disease.

Table 74-1 Causes of Short Stature and Relationship to Bone Age and Growth Rate

Growth Rate	Bone Age < Chronologic Age	Bone Age = Chronologic Age	Bone Age > Chronologic Age
Initially increased (short adult)			Congenital adrenal hyperplasia Exogenous androgenic steroids Precocious puberty
Normal or slightly decreased	Constitutional growth delay	Familial short stature Skeletal dysplasias Rickets	

Decreased	Endocrine disorders
	  Cushing's syndrome
	  Growth hormone deficiency
	Chronic systemic disease
	  Crohn's disease
	  Heart failure
	  Renal failure
	Severe malnutrition
	Severe psychosocial deprivation
		Chromosomal disorders
		  Down syndrome
		  Turner's syndrome	

Therapeutic

The appropriate preschool immunizations—varicella vaccine, DTaP booster, IPV, and MMR vaccine—should be given at separate sites.

Patient (Parent) Education

The parents' concerns are acknowledged. Johnny's satisfactory rate of growth despite his small absolute size is then demonstrated on the growth curve. The parents are told that although some children are going to constitute the lower percentiles of the normal population, the family history suggests that Johnny might be a "late bloomer" like his father.

Anticipatory guidance should include injury prevention issues such as locking up poisons, medicines, dangerous tools, or firearms; teaching children to follow the proper rules of the road and to wear helmets when bicycling or rollerblading; and modeling this behavior. Children should be taught to swim, and they should be constantly supervised when in or near the water. The child should know his or her name, address, and telephone number and to say "no" to strangers. Age-appropriate chores should be encouraged at home as well as quality family time. Appropriate and consistent limit setting should balance the child's need for autonomy. Playing well with other children, taking turns, following simple directions, and dressing oneself indicate skills appropriate for school entry.

Disposition

Johnny is scheduled to return in 6 months for a follow-up of his growth parameters. Laboratory results and any subsequent necessary action will be communicated by telephone.

FIRST FOLLOW-UP VISIT

Subjective

Johnny returned 6 months later accompanied by his mother. He has been in kindergarten for several months and is adjusting well.

Objective

Johnny's height is now 39¾ inches, and his weight is 35 pounds. His bone-age film of the wrists done shortly after his first visit approximates 3 years and 6 months. His chemistry panel demonstrates normal levels of electrolytes, calcium, phosphorus, total protein, and albumin. His creatinine is normal at 0.6 mg/dL (53 μ mol/L), as is his blood urea nitrogen at 7 mg/dL (2.50 mmol/L). His alkaline phosphatase level is normal for his age at 172 U/L. Other liver enzymes are normal. Serum free thyroxine is normal at 1.4 ng/dL (17.5 pmol/L), and thyroid-stimulating hormone is 3.5 μU/L. Erythrocyte sedimentation rate is normal at 4 mm/hour. Serum cholesterol is 156 mg/dL (4.04 mmol/L).

Assessment

The delayed bone age consistent with height age and a normal growth velocity supports the diagnosis of CGD. An elevated alkaline phosphatase is appropriate for a child with active skeletal growth and should be compared to reference values for age.

Plan

Diagnostic

Continued monitoring of Johnny's growth at yearly intervals is essential. No further diagnostic testing is necessary at this time. The serum cholesterol determination may be repeated in 5 years.

Therapeutic

At this time, Johnny does not seem to be suffering any adverse psychological effects such as poor self-image or social isolation. Continued reassurance is sufficient. If a child is sustaining deleterious psychological effects, then referral to a pediatric endocrinologist to consider a trial of human GH therapy may be in order.

Patient Education

Johnny's mother is reassured that his delayed bone age indicates that he has additional time to catch up in growth. His family can expect that he will enter puberty later and be a "late bloomer" like his father.

DISCUSSION

Parents (and grandparents) are greatly interested in their child's growth. They are especially concerned if he or she is smaller than his or her peers. A careful history should include prenatal factors such as nutrition, smoking, and drug use, problems in the perinatal period, and the child's subsequent growth and development. A family history to detect short stature, delayed maturation, genetic abnormalities, and chronic diseases is also necessary. Accurate measurements of the child's height, weight, and head circumference should be made. Arm span and upper-to-lower segment ratio should also be measured if indicated, and a careful physical examination should be performed including assessment for dysmorphic features. Linear growth in children normally decreases from approximately 10 cm per year at age 2 to between 5 and 6 cm per year at age 6 until the pubertal growth spurt (Halac and Zimmerman, 2004). Growth occurs in spurts rather than continuously. Table 74-2 presents approximate growth guidelines for prepubertal children.

Constitutional Growth Delay

CGD is a variant of normal growth that occurs more frequently in boys who enter puberty and develop later than their peers. Their bone age is correspondingly delayed by 2 or more years and approximately

---

Table 74-2 Approximate Growth Guidelines for Children

Age	Length or Height	Weight
Newborn	50 cm (20 inches) average	3.4 kg (7.5 lb) average
Newborn to 3 mo		1 kg/mo (1 oz/day) average weight gain
3–12 mo		Wt (kg) = [age (mo) + 9] ÷ 2 Wt (lb) = age (mo) + 11[*]
12 mo	75 cm (30 inches) average	Triples birth weight
12–24 mo	Increases by >10 cm/yr	0.25 kg/mo
>5 yr	>5 cm (2 inches)/yr until adolescent growth spurt	2.3 kg (5 lb)/yr until adolescent growth spurt
Ages 1–6		Wt (kg) = age (yr) × 2 + 8 Wt (lb) = age (yr) × 5 + 17[*]
Ages 7–12	Height (cm) = age (yr) × 6 + 77 Height (in) = age (yr) × 2.5 + 30[*] e.g., 4 year old = 40 inches	Wt (kg) = [age (yr) × 7 − 5] ÷ 2 Wt (lb) = age (yr) × 7 + 5[*]
Puberty	8–14 cm/yr	

[*]Adapted from Needleman RD. The first year. In Behrman RE, Kliegman RM, Jenson HB (eds): Nelson Textbook of Pediatrics, 17th ed. Philadelphia, WB Saunders, 2004, p 31.

equal to their height age. Review of the growth chart demonstrates an average birth size with deceleration in the growth rate during the first 2 years of life. The growth rate subsequently returns to normal, but the child now follows a lower percentile on the growth curve. The pubertal growth spurt and adolescent development will also be correspondingly delayed. There is usually a family history of delayed growth and development (Bareille and Stanhope, 1998).

Familial Short Stature

Children with FSS usually have parents or close relatives who are short. They often have normal birth weight and length, but their growth declines during the first 2 to 3 years of life and follows a trajectory consistent with their genetic potential. Their growth curve is below the 5th percentile but then parallels the normal curve, indicating a normal growth velocity (Barielle et al. 1998). Their bone age is approximately equal to their chronologic age but less than their height age. Untreated children with FSS will have a below-normal adult height.

CGD and FSS are both characterized by a normal growth rate. The mean predicted adult height for a boy can be calculated as [father's height + (mother's height + 13 cm)] ÷ 2. If the child is a girl, the mean predicted adult height is [(father's height – 13 cm) + mother's height] ÷ 2 (Rogol, 2004). Ninety-five percent of the population will attain an adult height within 3 to 4 inches above or below their predicted height. If the child is growing at a rate that will enable him to achieve his predicted adult height, then careful observation of growth parameters is appropriate. If the child's growth rate is declining, then further investigation is warranted.

Malnutrition and Psychosocial Deprivation

Adverse nutritional or socioeconomic factors should always be considered in the evaluation of a child's growth. However, the diagnosis of psychosocial deprivation should not be made until an appropriate nutritional assessment and trial have been conducted and organic causes excluded. Some chronic illnesses that can result in poor growth are listed in Box 74-1.

Chronic Systemic Illness

Chronic systemic illness usually has an adverse effect on body mass (weight) before linear growth. Failure to grow is sometimes the only manifestation of inflammatory bowel disease or renal disease. A complete blood count, erythrocyte sedimentation rate, electrolytes, and other blood chemistries may be required if these conditions are suspected. A normal urinalysis with a specific gravity greater than 1.020 assists in ruling out diabetes insipidus, whereas a neg-

ative dipstick for glucose excludes diabetes mellitus. Poor growth due to malnutrition may be caused by malabsorption syndromes characterized by loose or foul-smelling stools and diminished caloric intake.

Endocrinologic Causes and Hypothyroidism

Endocrinologic causes of short stature are less common but are treatable diseases that must be considered. Most children with endocrine causes of poor linear growth have a normal weight for height age. *Congenital hypothyroidism* occurs in 1 in 4000 infants and is *acquired* in 1 in 1250 school-age children. Girls acquire hypothyroidism twice as often as boys. Infants may have prolonged jaundice, sluggishness, feeding difficulties, constipation, cold extremities, slow pulse, heart murmur, anemia, and developmental delay. Older children may have myxedema, cold intolerance, and significant delay in bone age. Puberty is often delayed in adolescents, but younger children may demonstrate pseudoprecocious puberty (LaFranchi, 2004). The thyroid-stimulating hormone level is elevated in primary hypothyroidism, whereas a low free thyroxine and a low thyroid-stimulating hormone suggest pituitary or hypothalamic defects. Thyroid hormone is necessary for normal GH synthesis, and levels must be assayed before GH studies are done.

Cushing's Syndrome

Cushing's syndrome is often caused by the administration of pharmacologic doses of glucocorticoids but may be due to a functional adrenocortical tumor or excess adrenocorticotropic hormone. Young children have generalized obesity, but older children often have truncal obesity, "moon" facies, "buffalo hump," purplish striae, glucose intolerance, and osteoporosis. Hypertension is present in both age groups. Children with Cushing's syndrome demonstrate excessive weight gain accompanied by growth retardation (Halac and Zimmerman, 2004).

Congenital Adrenal Hyperplasia

Undetected and untreated congenital adrenal hyperplasia ultimately leads to short stature as an adult, although the initial signs are ambiguous genitalia and virilization. Initial growth is accelerated and bone age is advanced leading to premature closure of the epiphyses.

Growth Hormone Deficiency

Infants with congenital hypopituitarism have normal or less than average birth length and poor linear growth that is apparent by 12 months of age. Prolonged neonatal conjugated and unconjugated hyperbilirubinemia is common, and apnea or severe hypoglycemia may occur. Affected boys may have micropenises (stretched length less than 2.8 cm [1.1 inch] in a term infant). Children may appear pudgy, have immature facies, underdeveloped genitalia, and secondary sexual characteristics. Fasting hypoglycemia occurs in 10% to 15% and may also be present in children with acquired GH deficiency (Parks, 2004). Acquired causes of GH deficiency include trauma, tumors such as craniopharyngioma, and central nervous system infections or irradiation. Bone age is severely delayed in children with long-standing GH deficiency, regardless of cause.

Children with classic GH deficiency fail to release normal amounts of GH in response to pharmacologic stimuli. Emotional deprivation can produce functional hypopituitarism characterized by inadequate GH response to provocative stimuli and low levels of IGH-1. Coexisting pituitary disorders must be investigated in children with suspected GH deficiency. Children with GH neurosecretory dysfunction may exhibit a normal GH response to the usual provocative tests but demonstrate a marked deficiency of pulsatile secretion of GH over a 24-hour period (Parks, 2004). Because of the variation in testing, referral to a pediatric endocrinologist is in order when GH deficiency is suspected.

Chromosomal Disorders

Children with chromosomal disorders usually have apparent dysmorphic features. Turner's syndrome should always be considered in short girls, especially if there is no family history of short stature. Characteristic features include low birth weight, webbing of the neck, low posterior hairline, broad chest with widely spaced nipples (shieldlike chest), cubitus valgus, and lymphedema of the hands and feet. If mosaicism is present, short stature may be the only manifestation. Consequently, short girls with subnormal growth rates should have banded karyotyping performed. Special growth charts are available for girls with Turner's syndrome as well as children with Down syndrome.

Skeletal Dysplasias

Skeletal dysplasias or osteochondrodysplasias are usually inherited and cause disproportionate short stature. The term dwarfism has been used to refer to this group of disorders, although there are more than 200 varieties. Skeletal dysplasias are frequently characterized by a greater than normal upper-to-lower segment ratio (Halac and Zimmerman, 2004). In contrast, children with hypogonadism have longer extremities and a less than normal ratio

caused by failure of the epiphyses to close. Complete skeletal radiographs may be required in addition to determination of serum calcium, phosphorus, protein, and alkaline phosphatase to rule out hypophosphatasia, vitamin D–resistant and vitamin D–dependent rickets. Urine screening for metabolic and storage disorders should also be considered.

Growth Hormone Treatment

Most children with CGD will reach their predicted mid-parental height. Some may remain several inches below their target height. Children with FSS will grow up to be short adults, a fact that some families may not accept. Short stature has not been shown to affect acceptance by peers among middle and high school students (Sandberg et al., 2004 Ⓑ). However, taller college graduates may earn more money and most presidents have been the taller candidate. Consequently, there has been greater pressure to give human GH to children who do not have classic GH deficiency. In addition to proven GH deficiency, recombinant human GH is now approved in the United States for the treatment of short stature in children with Turner's syndrome, intrauterine growth retardation, chronic renal insufficiency, Prader-Willi syndrome, and idiopathic short stature. Recent evidence suggests recombinant human GH treatment of children with idiopathic short stature may increase their final predicted height by 5 to 7 cm (Miller and Zimmerman, 2004), but treated individuals are still relatively short compared with their peers of normal height (Bryant et al., 2003 Ⓐ). In addition, therapy is costly ($35,000/inch), and the child must tolerate daily or thrice-weekly injections. Furthermore, it has not yet been demonstrated that GH treatment improves measured quality of life (Radcliffe et al., 2004 Ⓐ). Long-term GH use is rarely accompanied by adverse effects such as impaired glucose tolerance, pseudotumor cerebri, slipped capital femoral epiphysis, and progression of scoliosis. Children treated with GH also have a theoretical increased risk of malignancies and some with Prader-Willi syndrome have died (Miller and Zimmerman, 2004).

Material Available on Student Consult

Review Questions and Answers about Constitutional Growth Delay

REFERENCES

Bareille P, Craig F, Stanhope R. Familial short stature. In Finberg L (ed): Saunders Manual of Pediatric Practice. Philadelphia, WB Saunders, 1998, pp 733–734.

Bareille P, Stanhope R. Constitutional short stature. In Finberg L (ed): Saunders Manual of Pediatric Practice. Philadelphia, WB Saunders, 1998, pp 731–733.

Bryant J, Cave C, Milne R. Recombinant growth hormone for idiopathic short stature in children and adolescents. The Cochrane Database of Systematic Reviews 2003, Issue 2. Art. No.: CD004440. DOI: 10.1002/14651858.CD004440.🅐

Halac I, Zimmerman D. Evaluating short stature in children. Pediatr Ann 2004;33:170–176.

LaFranchi S. Hypothyroidism. In Behrman RE, Kliegman RM, Jenson HB (eds): Nelson Textbook of Pediatrics, 17th ed. Philadelphia, WB Saunders, 2004, pp 1873–1879.

Miller BS, Zimmerman D. Idiopathic short stature in children. Pediatr Ann 2004:33:177–181.

Needleman RD. The first year. In Behrman RE, Kliegman RM, Jenson HB (eds): Nelson Textbook of Pediatrics, 17th ed. Philadelphia, WB Saunders, 2004, p 31.

Parks JS. Hypopituitarism. In Behrman RE, Kliegman RM, Jenson HB (eds): Nelson Textbook of Pediatrics, 17th ed. Philadelphia, WB Saunders, 2004, pp 1847–1853.

Radcliffe DJ, Pliskin JS, Silvers JB, Cuttler L. Growth hormone therapy and quality of life in adults and children. Pharmacoeconomics 2004;22:499–524.🅐

Rogol AD. Diagnostic approach to short stature. UpToDate Online. Available at www.utdol.com/application/topic/print.asp?file=pediendo/2375&type=A&selectedTitle. Accessed 10/3/2004.

Sandberg DE, Bukowski WM, Fung CM, Noll RB. Height and social adjustment: Are extremes a cause for concern and action? Pediatrics 2004;114:744–750.🅑

Chapter

75

Behavior Problem in a 2-Year-Old Boy (Autism)

Kenneth Lin

KEY POINTS

1. Although autism remains a relatively rare disorder, the ability of early interventions to improve its prognosis mandates timely identification in the office setting.
2. Investigations continue into its genetic and environmental causes, but the measles, mumps, and rubella (MMR) vaccine does not appear to be one of them.
3. Intensive behavior modification programs seem to improve functioning, but no consensus exists about which program works best or even if there is a "best" program for all autistic children.
4. Medications are effective for controlling seizures, tantrums, and comorbid psychiatric diagnoses.

INITIAL VISIT

Subjective

Patient Identification and Presenting Problem

Adam is a 2-year-old boy who is brought to the office by his parents because they are concerned about his loss of language skills and worsening behavioral problems.

Present Illness

Adam met age-appropriate milestones on the Denver II Developmental Scale until his 9-month checkup, saying "mama" and "dada," but then he lost these words at 15 months and learned no more.

According to Adam's parents, he makes limited eye contact, has a narrow range of interests, and prefers to play alone. He also engages in unusual repetitive activities such as rocking, spinning, head

---

Evidence levels 🅐 Randomized, controlled trials (RCTs), meta-analyses, well-designed systematic reviews of RCTs. 🅑 Case-control or cohort studies, nonrandomized clinical trials, systematic reviews of studies other than RCTs, cross-sectional studies, retrospective studies, certain uncontrolled studies. 🅒 Consensus statements, expert guidelines, usual practice, opinion.

banging, and toe walking. Certain sounds, such as the vacuum and lawn mower, cause him great distress. He is impulsive and has frequent tantrums that are extremely difficult to manage.

Medical History

Adam was hospitalized for pneumonia at 10 months of age and uses twice-daily inhaled budesonide for mild persistent asthma.

Adam has never had significant head trauma and has no history of seizures.

Immunizations are up to date for his age, including the first dose of the MMR vaccine at 14 months.

Birth History

Adam was born at term to a primigravida mother by spontaneous vaginal delivery after an 18-hour labor. The pregnancy was complicated by maternal tobacco use. Adam's birth weight was 7 pounds, 2 ounces. Apgar scores were 9 and 9. His newborn nursery course was uneventful. He passed the hearing screen. There was no neonatal jaundice. Newborn screening results are not available.

Family History

There is no family history of mental retardation, developmental disorders, or other childhood illnesses except for attention-deficit/hyperactivity disorder in a maternal cousin. A paternal uncle was diagnosed with bipolar disorder in his 20s.

Social History

Adam lives with his father, mother, and 7-month-old brother in a single-family home built in 1957. His father was recently laid off from his job as a machine operator at a chemical plant, and his mother has not worked outside the home since Adam was born. As a result, the family now depends on public assistance for income, which both parents say has been "stressful." Adam's father smokes cigarettes at home. They have no pets.

Review of Systems

Adam's head circumference, height, and weight have been within normal limits for age at his previous well-child visits. The remainder of the review of systems is otherwise unremarkable.

Objective

Physical Examination

General Adam is a nontoxic-appearing toddler who is unable to sit still or follow instructions for any part of the examination.

Vital Signs Temperature 37°C (98.6°F) orally, with height, weight, and head circumference all in the Vital Signs 75th percentile for age.

Head, Eyes, Ears, Nose, and Throat Normocephalic, atraumatic. Pupils are equal, round, and reactive to light. Extraocular movements are intact. Mucous membranes are moist. No deformities of the ears or prominence of facial features. Palate is intact. Oropharynx is without erythema or exudate.

Neck No lymphadenopathy or thyromegaly.

Pulmonary Clear to auscultation bilaterally.

Cardiovascular Regular rate and rhythm, without murmurs, rubs, or gallops.

Abdomen Soft, nontender, with normoactive bowel sounds. No hepatomegaly or splenomegaly.

Extremities No clubbing, cyanosis, or edema.

Genitourinary Normal male genitalia, testes descended bilaterally, Tanner stage 1.

Skin No rashes or lesions.

Musculoskeletal Moves all four extremities symmetrically. Walks, runs, and climbs on to the examination table without difficulty. Can stack two blocks.

Neurologic Cranial nerves II through XII are grossly intact. Occasionally vocalizes but makes no understandable speech. Does not repeat words or imitate behaviors of his parents or the examiner. Does not follow simple directions or respond to requests to identify his parents or familiar objects. Exhibits no recognition when shown a photograph of himself.

Assessment

Working Diagnosis

Autistic spectrum disorder (ASD), most likely autistic disorder with associated mental retardation.

Differential Diagnoses

A hallmark of ASDs, distinguishing them from conditions such as cerebral palsy caused by prenatal or perinatal insults, is a period of normal growth and development followed by stagnation or regression. Common conditions that may mimic ASDs in their clinical presentation are lead intoxication, fragile X syndrome, and hearing impairments (Simms and Schum, 2000).

Plan

Diagnostic

Adam's parents and physician complete the Checklist for Autism in Toddlers, which consists of nine yes/no questions for the parents, followed by five questions for the physician based on observations of the child at play. The answers are consistent with the working diagnosis of autism.

The physician orders a lead level, chromosomal analysis, and formal audiology evaluation, all of which are normal.

Therapeutic

Adam is referred to an intensive, 40 hours per week behavioral modification therapy program with a 2:1 student-to-teacher ratio. His parents are given information about support groups for parents of autistic children.

Patient and Parental Education

The physician explains to Adam's parents that autism is a neurodevelopmental disorder, the cause of which is unknown. Although it was originally thought to be secondary to problem parenting (mothers who did not demonstrate physical affection), it is now thought to be the result of a complex genetic predisposition triggered by uncertain environmental influences. Nearly half of all children with autism will never develop communicative speech, and fewer than 5% will be completely self-sufficient as adults. Early, intensive behavioral interventions do appear to improve the prognosis. Studies of siblings of autistic children predict that Adam's younger brother Nathan has a 5% chance of being diagnosed with autism in the future.

DISCUSSION

Definition/Epidemiology

Autism is not a single disease but rather a spectrum of behaviorally defined disorders (Table 75-1) distinguished by impaired social interactions, impaired communication, and restricted, repetitive, or stereo-typed patterns of behavior, interests, and activities (Volkmar and Pauls, 2003). Box 75-1 describes some common behaviors in autistic children. Although not essential for the diagnosis, autism is associated with mental retardation (75%), epilepsy (35%), behavioral problems, and depression and anxiety disorders (Rapin, 1997). Although the skills of "autistic savants" were well publicized in the 1988 movie *Rain Man* and by the protagonist of Oliver Sacks's *An Anthropologist on Mars*, these persons are rarities. In fact, almost 50% of autistic children will never develop communicative speech. Although one-third will eventually achieve some degree of independent living, fewer than 5% are completely self-sufficient as adults.

ASDs affect approximately six in 1000 children, with a 4:1 male-to-female ratio (Baird et al., 2003). Their prevalence appears to be on the rise; from 1992 to 1993 to 2000 to 2001, the U.S. Department of Education reported a more than sevenfold increase in the number of autistic children served under the Individuals with Disabilities Education Act (Vastag, 2004). Although part of the observed increase may be secondary to increased recognition, the reasons for the remainder are unknown and have been the subject of much speculation.

The sharp rise in prevalence of ASDs, along with its typical age of diagnosis between the ages of 18 months and 3 years, prompted concerns that some element of the MMR vaccine, administered between 12 and 15 months of age, could be responsible. These concerns received support from a case series by Wakefield and colleagues published in *Lancet* in 1998 that described 12 patients with gastrointestinal complaints who developed autistic symptoms within 1 month after receiving the MMR vaccine. These investigators hypothesized that a component of the MMR vaccine causes small intestinal inflammation, increasing gastrointestinal absorption of encephalopathic proteins, which leads to the development of autism in these children. Several well-controlled retrospective cohort studies, as well as a recent systematic review,

---

Table 75-1 The Autistic Spectrum Disorders

Autistic disorder: "classic" autism
Asperger's syndrome: social withdrawal without cognitive or language delays
Rett's syndrome: young girls lose previously acquired motor and cognitive skills between 6 and 18 months
Childhood disintegrative disorder: 2–10 years of normal development followed by regression
Pervasive developmental disorder—not otherwise specified: milder form of autistic disorder that does not satisfy *Diagnostic and Statistical Manual of Mental Disorders IV* criteria

Modified from American Psychiatric Association. Diagnostic and Statistical Manual of Mental Disorders, 4th ed. Washington, DC, American Psychiatric Association, 1995, pp 65–78.

Box 75-1 Behaviors Associated with Autism

Clumsiness
Hand flapping, rocking, pacing, spinning
Head banging
Inadequate or nonexistent expressive language
Inflexibility
Preference for playing alone
Sensitivity to loud noises
Toe walking

Data from Rapin I. Clinical crossroads. An 8-year-old boy with autism. JAMA 2001;285:1749–1757.

have since refuted this hypothesis (Madsen et al., 2002Ⓑ; Makela et al., 2002Ⓓ; Smeeth et al., 2004Ⓑ; Wilson et al., 2003Ⓓ). In April 2004, Wakefield and colleagues retracted the interpretation of their original study, admitting that "no causal link was established between MMR and autism as the data were insufficient" (Murch et al., 2004). In the United States, the National Immunization Safety Review Committee (2004Ⓒ) subsequently concluded that the overwhelming evidence "favors rejection of a causal relationship" between the MMR vaccine and autism.

Genetics and Neuroanatomy

Autism is in part a genetic disorder. Identical twin studies have demonstrated that the twin of an autistic child has a 60% chance of developing autism and a 92% chance of developing an ASD. Fraternal twins and siblings have approximately 50 times the incidence of the general population, as much as 5%. Multiple chromosomal abnormalities have been linked to autism in studies of affected families, but because the most common accounts for only 1% to 3% of cases, experts believe that there are many genetic pathways to autism (Veenstra-Vanderweele and Cook, 2003).

If genes predispose a child to autism, then prenatal, perinatal, and neonatal factors may serve as triggers. In multiple studies, "unfavorable events" such as maternal tobacco use, contraceptive use at the time of conception, prolonged second stage of labor, and neonatal hyperbilirubinemia have been associated with an increased risk of being diagnosed with an ASD (Juul-Dam et al., 2001Ⓑ). More sophisticated analyses, however, have cast doubt on the hypothesis that these associated events actually *cause* autism (Zwaigenbaum et al., 2002Ⓑ).

Investigators have also sought to understand what brain structures may be abnormal in autistic children. Some believe that autism results from the disruption of a "neural network" of distinct brain areas that are responsible for social cognition; for example, the amygdala is thought to mediate the process of facial recognition (Tuchman, 2003). This theory of "underconnectivity" recently received support from a functional magnetic resonance imaging study sponsored by the National Institute of Child Health and Human Development of the National Institutes of Health (Koshino et al., 2005Ⓑ).

Diagnosis

Although universal screening is not recommended, any suspicion of autism should prompt investigation. The commonly used Denver II Developmental Scale fails to reliably detect children with ASDs; in contrast, the presence of parental concerns about a child's development has both reasonable sensitivity (75% to 83%) and specificity (79% to 81%) for ASDs (Filipek et al., 2000Ⓒ). Several developmental "red flags," listed in Box 75-2, should automatically prompt screening.

The Checklist for Autism in Toddlers screening instrument was published in 1992 and has been validated in multiple prospective studies of children older than 18 months of age. It does not require specific training and takes 5 to 10 minutes to administer and score. Although it is not a diagnostic instrument, the Checklist for Autism in Toddlers has been shown to effectively differentiate children with ASDs from children with other types of developmental delays (Scambler et al., 2001Ⓑ).

Box 75-3 outlines the expert consensus for further testing of a child with suspected autism (American Academy of Pediatrics Committee on Children with Disabilities, 2001Ⓒ; Filipek et al., 2000Ⓒ).

Box 75-2	Developmental "Red Flags"

No babbling, pointing, or other gestures by 12 months
No single words by 16 months
No two-word spontaneous phrases by 24 months
Loss of previously learned language or social skills at *any* age

From Prater CD, Zylstra RG. Autism: A medical primer. Am Fam Physician 2002;66:1667–1674,1680.

Box 75-3	Evaluation for Suspected Autism

Recommended
  Formal audiology evaluation
  Lead level
  Chromosomal analysis for fragile X syndrome if mental retardation is present
Not recommended
  Routine metabolic testing
  Routine neuroimaging
  Routine electroencephalography

Data from Filipek PA, Accardo PJ, Ashwal S, et al. Practice parameter. Screening and diagnosis of autism. Report of the Quality Standards Subcommittee of the American Academy of Neurology and the Child Neurology Society. Neurology 2000;55:468–479; American Academy of Pediatrics Committee on Children with Disabilities. The pediatrician's role in the diagnosis and management of autistic spectrum disorder in children. Pediatrics 2001;107:1221–1226.

Management

Few treatments for autism have proven to be effective. The best studied are intensive, individualized behavior modification programs that reward positive behaviors such as appropriate social responses. These range from the classic conditioning techniques pioneered by UCLA's Lovaas to North Carolina's school-based TEACCH (Treatment and Education of Autistic and Related Communication Handicapped Children). Both programs have documented short-term gains, but long-term results are not well studied (Rapin, 2001).

The treatment plan for autism includes controlling seizures and comorbid psychiatric disorders, including schizophrenia, mood disorders, and attention-deficit/hyperactivity disorder. As many as 35% of patients with autistic disorder develop epilepsy by adolescence, with increasing risk corresponding to increasing degrees of mental retardation. Baseline electroencephalography and prophylactic antiepileptic medication are not recommended for autistic children without a history of seizures. It is uncertain whether certain medications are more effective than others (Tuchman and Rapin, 2002). Atypical antipsychotic agents such as risperidone have been effective in controlling serious behavioral problems in autistic children (McCracken and the Research Units on Pediatric Psychopharmacology Autism Network, 2002Ⓐ).

The limited benefit of proven therapies has often led parents of autistic children to turn to untested medications or supplements popularized on the Internet or in the lay press. The perils of this approach are well illustrated in the case of secretin, a peptide hormone that stimulates pancreatic secretion. A single case report of a 3-year-old child with autism who underwent endoscopy for chronic diarrhea, received intravenous secretin, and then showed dramatic improvements in behavior and language skills led to secretin being hailed as a "miracle cure" for ASDs. However, a subsequent double-blind, placebo-controlled trial of 60 children with ASDs found that secretin administration was not associated with improvement in functioning or decreases in any associated symptoms (seizures, behavioral problems, sleep disorders) (Sandler et al., 1999Ⓐ).

Material Available on Student Consult

Review Questions and Answers about Autism

SELECTED AUTISM RESOURCES ONLINE

Centers for Disease Control and Prevention Autism Information Center: www.cdc.gov/ncbddd/dd/ddautism.htm

National Institutes of Health, National Institute of Child Health and Human Development: www.nichd.nih.gov/autism/

MEDLINE Plus: Autism: www.nlm.nih.gov/medlineplus/autism.html

Autism Society of America: www.autism-society.org

Cure Autism Now: www.cureautismnow.org

REFERENCES

American Academy of Pediatrics Committee on Children with Disabilities. The pediatrician's role in the diagnosis and management of autistic spectrum disorder in children. Pediatrics 2001;107:1221–1226.Ⓒ

American Psychiatric Association. Diagnostic and Statistical Manual of Mental Disorders, 4th ed. Washington, DC, American Psychiatric Association, 1995, pp 65–78.

Baird G, Cass H, Slonims V. Diagnosis of autism. BMJ 2003;327:488–493.

Filipek PA, Accardo PJ, Ashwal S, et al. Practice parameter: Screening and diagnosis of autism: Report of the Quality Standards Subcommittee of the American Academy of Neurology and the Child Neurology Society. Neurology 2000;55:468–479.Ⓒ

Immunization Safety Review Committee of the Institute of Medicine. Vaccines and autism. Washington, DC, National Academy of Sciences, 2004. Available at http://books.nap.edu/catalog/10997.html. Accessed 1/12/06.Ⓒ

Juul-Dam N, Townsend J, Courchesne E. Prenatal, perinatal, and neonatal factors in autism, pervasive developmental disorder-not otherwise specified, and the general population. Pediatrics 2001;107:767(E63).Ⓑ

Koshino H, Carpenter PA, Minshew NJ, et al. Functional connectivity in an fMRI working memory task in high-functioning autism. Neuroimage 2005;24:810–821.Ⓑ

Madsen KM, Hviid A, Vestergaard M, et al. A population-based study of measles, mumps, and rubella vaccination in autism. N Engl J Med 2002;347:1477–1482.Ⓑ

Makela A, Nuorti JP, Pelota H. Neurologic disorders after MMR vaccination. Pediatrics 2002;110:957–963.Ⓑ

McCracken JT, the Research Units on Pediatric Psychopharmacology Autism Network. Risperidone in children with autism and serious behavioral problems. N Engl J Med 2002;347:314–321.Ⓐ

Muhle R, Trentacoste SV, Rapin I. The genetics of autism. Pediatrics 2004;113:e472–e484.

Murch SH, Anthony A, Cassen DH, et al. Retraction of an interpretation. Lancet 2004;363:750.

Prater CD, Zylstra RG. Autism: A medical primer. Am Fam Physician 2002;66:1667–1674,1680.

Rapin I. Autism. N Engl J Med 1997;337:97–104.

Rapin I. Clinical crossroads: An 8-year-old boy with autism. JAMA 2001;285:1749–1757.

Sandler AD, Sutton KA, DeWeese J, et al. Lack of benefit of a single dose of synthetic human secretin in the treatment of autism and pervasive developmental disorder. N Engl J Med 1999;341:1801–1806.Ⓐ

Scambler D, Rogers SJ, Wehner EA. Can the Checklist for Autism in Toddlers differentiate young children with autism from those with developmental delays? J Am Acad Child Adolesc Psychiatry 2001;40:1457–1463.Ⓑ

Simms MD, Schum RL. Preschool children who have atypical patterns of development. Pediatr Rev 2000; 21:147–158.

Smeeth L, Cook C, Fombonne E, et al. MMR vaccination and pervasive developmental disorders: A case-control study. Lancet 2004;364:963–969.Ⓑ

Tuchman R, Rapin I. Epilepsy in autism. Lancet Neurol 2002;1:352–358.

Tuchman R. Autism. Neurol Clin 2003;21:915–932.

Vastag B. National autism summit charts a path through a scientific, clinical wilderness. JAMA 2004;291:29–31.

Veenstra-Vanderweele J, Cook EH. Genetics of childhood disorders: XLVI. Autism, part 5: Genetics of autism. J Am Acad Child Adolesc Psychiatry 2003;42:116–118.

Volkmar FR, Pauls D. Autism. Lancet 2003;362:1133–1141.

Wakefield AJ, Murch SH, Anthony A, et al. Ideal-lymphoid-nodular hyperplasia, non-specific colitis, and pervasive developmental disorder in children. Lancet 1998; 351:637–641.

Wilson K, Mills E, Ross C, McGowan J, Jadad A. Association of autistic spectrum disorder and the measles, mumps, and rubella vaccine: A systematic review of current epidemiological evidence. Arch Pediatr Adolesc Med 2003;157:628–634.Ⓑ

Zwaigenbaum L, Szatmari P, Jones MB, et al. Pregnancy and birth complications in autism and liability to the broader autism phenotype. J Am Acad Child Adolesc Psychiatry 2002;41:572–579.Ⓑ

Chapter

76

Difficulty Paying Attention (Attention-Deficit/Hyperactivity Disorder)

Lloyd A. Darlow

KEY POINTS

1. Not every child with an attentional disorder has attention-deficit/hyperactivity disorder (AD/HD).
2. Success in treating AD/HD starts with a proper diagnosis.
3. Comorbid disorders must be ruled in or out.
4. Psycho-educational assessment must be performed to rule out learning disabilities.
5. The initial workup should entail (a) a physical examination, including assessments of hearing, vision, and airway patency; (b) mental status testing; (c) administration of parent-teacher rating scales for AD/HD and comorbid disorders; and (d) administration of a child rating scale for depression.
6. The follow-up schedule is monthly until the condition is stable, then at least every 3 months.

INITIAL VISIT

Subjective

Patient Identification and Presenting Problem

Phillip is a 12-year-old white male in the sixth grade. A teacher at his middle school recommended an assessment. The presenting complaint, offered by Phillip's mother, is "difficulty paying attention in class." The initial assessment is performed midway through the fall semester. Phillip's mother is present during the interview.

History of Present Illness

A problem with Phillip's attention span was first noted in kindergarten, when his teacher observed that he had difficulty staying on task. Historically, he has had more trouble with math and the sciences from grades one through five, and homework in these subject areas usually takes him longer than homework in his other classes. He typically has been a B or C student, with higher grades in courses he likes (art, social studies) than in those he does not (math, science). His mother notes that he sustained some injuries early in childhood due to impulse control, and she continues to worry about his safety: "He leaps before he looks." She does not note any specific problems with extreme physical hyperactivity, purposeless movements, or difficulty sitting in his chair in school or at the dinner table.

From time to time, Phillip's behavior at home has been an issue, and he can get angry, but his mother tends to associate these outbursts with frustration. For instance, after he had difficulty with a homework assignment, he kicked a hole in the bathroom door. He recently had an altercation at school during which he said some hurtful words to another child, but he has never been in trouble for fighting, and he is always remorseful after such episodes. There have never been any instances of vandalism, theft, or cruelty to animals. In general, he has had no problems complying with requests unless schoolwork is involved, and in these situations he can occasionally become outwardly defiant. His mother notes that he helps out a lot at home. Mornings are not a problem for him, nor are weekends or school holidays; his difficulty seems to be confined to school hours and the after-school homework period.

Socially, Phillip has several friends and plays soccer and basketball. He likes to do things with his hands. His parents do not feel that he is worried, depressed, or preoccupied, and there are no reported problems with getting him to sleep, although as a young child he reportedly had some nightmares. This is the first time he has been evaluated for any educational or behavioral disorder. No academic assessments have been done by his public school, but his parents have never been told that he was more than a grade level behind where he should be for his age.

Medical History

Phillip is the younger of two children. He was born after a normal pregnancy, with labor complicated by premature rupture of the membranes; he was discharged home with his mother on the third postpartum day. Developmental milestones were achieved uneventfully: his mother reports no delays in speech, language development, motor skills, or toilet training. Phillip has no active medical problems and has never undergone surgery. He is not currently taking medication and has no known allergies.

Family History

An uncle has a bipolar disorder.

Social History

Phillip lives at home with both parents and his older brother. There is no exposure to cigarette smoke in the home. Both parents are college educated. Phillip's father is an engineer and his mother is an administrative aide at a local college.

Review of Systems

No problems are noted with snoring. Phillip's vision and hearing have been checked recently as part of a school screening; no abnormalities were found. He has no problem with seasonal or perennial allergies. He has no exertional dyspnea or chest pain, no abdominal complaints or weight loss, no joint pains, no dizziness, and no fatigue.

Objective

Physical Examination

Phillip is a well-developed, well-nourished white male adolescent in no distress. His blood pressure is 108/62, pulse is 82 and regular, and respiratory rate is 18, with unlabored breathing. His height is 60 inches (60th percentile) and weight is 95 pounds (61st percentile). On eye examination the pupils are equally reactive to light and accommodation, and extraocular movements are intact. Visual acuity is 20/20 in both eyes without correction. Ear examination shows clear tympanic membranes and hearing within normal limits to whisper. The nares are patent. The throat is clear, with a class I airway. The neck is supple. Lungs are clear to auscultation, with good respiratory effort. Heart rate and rhythm are regular, without murmurs. The extremities show no edema, cyanosis, or clubbing. Muscle strength is 5/5; deep tendon reflexes are 2+ (normal). The neurologic examination shows entirely nonfocal findings; gross motor function is intact, fine motor control is adequate.

Mental Status Examination

1. *Attention.* Phillip can do forward digit spans to four, but transposes the last two digits at five places. He repeats a phrase ("No ifs, ands, or buts") without errors and can execute a four-step command in correct order.
2. *Concentration.* Phillip can do a verbal math problem (money calculation) without errors and can do backward digit spans to four places. He spells "world" backward as d-l-o-r-w.
3. *Short-term memory/four-word recall.* Phillip recalls four out of four words at 10 minutes, in order.
4. *Speech.* His articulation and rate are age-appropriate.
5. *Language.* His language is coherent and organized.
6. *Mood.* Phillip's mood is stable and his affect is bright; he is cooperative during the evaluation.

Working Diagnosis

The working diagnosis is attention-deficit/hyperactivity disorder (AD/HD), probably the inattentive type rather than the hyperactive/impulsive or combined type. Oppositional-defiant disorder seems doubtful. It is also possible that Phillip has a learning disability.

DISCUSSION

The prevalence of AD/HD is in the range of 2% to 9% in the general population and 3% to 5% of all school-aged children. Although many causative factors have been proposed, recent evidence seems to point to a genetic defect in the process of dopamine transport in the frontal lobes (Dougherty et al., 1999). Media bias has led some in the general public to conclude that AD/HD is a phenomenon of the late 20th century, yet the first mention of this condition dates back to the pre–Civil War era. Various terms for AD/HD have been used over the years in the medical literature, many of them unfortunate, including brain damage syndrome, minimal brain disorder, and organic behavior syndrome. The first analysis of the effects of psychostimulants on schoolchildren with attentional deficits took place in 1937 by Charles Bradley, who demonstrated that children taking these medications attended and focused better in class and caused fewer disruptions socially. For those who choose to believe that AD/HD is merely a social phenomenon and the result of bad parenting or relaxed social expectations, it may be worth the physician's time to note that the diagnosis and treatment of AD/HD predate the use of penicillin.

The initial office visit consists of a thorough history, including identification of who initiated the referral of the child to the physician. The diagnostic criteria set forth in the *Diagnostic and Statistical Manual of Mental Disorders* (DSM-IV-TR) mandate that the patient's symptoms be present in more than one clinical setting. If the child shows no significant signs of impairment at home but is having considerable difficulty at school, alternative explanations for the attention difficulty should be sought. The physical examination should include an evaluation of the child's hearing and vision, as well as the patency of the upper airway; sleep disorders, including sleep apnea, will not cause AD/HD but, if not addressed, will make an existing attentional deficit more difficult to treat successfully. Some assessment of mental status and function should be performed, taking into account distant and short-term memory and the ability to follow instructions.

Comorbid disorders are conditions that can mimic or masquerade as an attentional deficit and must be ruled in or out during the initial evaluation (Box 76-1). The main comorbid disorders to consider in a workup for AD/HD are oppositional-defiant disorder, conduct disorder, depression, anxiety, bipolar disorder, and learning disabilities. Thirty-three percent of children with AD/HD have one or more comorbid conditions; "pure" AD/HD (that is, AD/HD without a comorbid condition) is seen in only 30% of cases. Oppositional-defiant disorder is the most common comorbidity, with up to 33% of AD/HD patients (60% of males and 30% of females) exhibiting this condition (Agency for Healthcare Research and Quality, 1999).

The rating scale has become the staple of the diagnostic process for AD/HD and its common comorbid conditions (Box 76-2). The Connors scale has been the gold standard over the years, but only recently has this scale begun to factor in the comorbid conditions. In reality, it does not matter which scale or combination of scales the physician uses. Any number of rating scales can be used, and the choice should be

---

Box 76-1	Attention-Deficit/Hyperactivity Disorder: Comorbid Conditions

Oppositional-defiant disorder
Conduct disorder
Childhood depression
Anxiety
Bipolar disorder
Learning disabilities

Box 76-2	Rating Scales on the Internet

www.addwarehouse.com
www.help4adhd.org
www.addvance.com (for girls)
www.therapeuticresources.com
www.fpnotebook.com (depression scales)

based on factors such as cost, comorbid consideration, and ease of interpretation. A separate scale should be given to the parents and one other person, usually in the school setting, who knows the child well. Both inattentive and hyperactive/impulsive types of AD/HD require six positive responses out of nine possible criteria; for oppositional-defiant disorder, four positive responses out of eight are necessary (American Psychiatric Association, 2000●). In addition to the parent/teacher rating scales, the child should be given a scale that addresses mood disorders.

A final piece of information that is of critical necessity, but is often overlooked, is a formal educational assessment to rule out learning disabilities, to be done by the school the child attends. Comorbid learning disorders (Box 76-3) occur in 12% to 30% of children with AD/HD (Agency for Healthcare Research and Quality, 1999). If the student attends a private school, the public school that child would have attended must perform this evaluation. If a learning disability is present, the student will qualify for academic interventions under the Individuals with Disabilities Education Act; if no formal learning disability is found, the child with AD/HD may still be eligible for accommodations under the learning disability category of "Other Health Impaired." A full discussion of the physician's role in the educational process is beyond the scope of this chapter, but Matthew Cohen's excellent article (2004) on this subject should be mandatory reading for all physicians who evaluate and treat patients for AD/HD.

The second office visit should begin with a review of the rating scales and a discussion of the findings, which should enable the physician to make a formal diagnosis. The treatment plan is formulated, including recommendations for medication (if appropriate), further educational testing (if necessary), writing of 504 Plans or Individualized Educational Plans (IEPs), and referrals for counseling. The physician should encourage the parents to read about their child's condition on physician-approved, refereed sites (Box 76-4). The patient and parents should make plans to return for follow-up in 1 month's time, at which point the physician should request some form of written communication from school regarding the child's progress. Reviewing assignments, tests, progress notes and report cards are essential for assessing the efficacy of the treatment plan. If necessary, the plan should be modified at subsequent visits, and the schedule of follow-up appointments from this point forward should be monthly until the situation is stable, then every 3 months thereafter.

A thorough addressing of AD/HD pharmacotherapy can be a textbook chapter unto itself. In 2001 the American Academy of Pediatrics (AAP) provided a clinical practice guideline to aid in the decision-making process (AAP, 2001●), but the development of new medications and a greater body of research have only complicated the issue. Briefly, the treatment options for AD/HD can be broken down into two classes: stimulants and nonstimulants. As a group, the stimulants have been shown to have greater overall efficacy than the nonstimulants (Faraone, 2003 ●). Classic stimulants, such as methylphenidate and dextroamphetamine, primarily block the reuptake of dopamine at the postsynaptic neuron in the prefrontal cortex and have been shown to have excellent long-term efficacy (Centre for Reviews and Dissemination, 2002). Within the stimulant group, the medications differ in duration of action; short-acting stimulants typically last up to 4 hours, intermediate-acting agents are effective for approximately 5 hours, and sustained-release preparations can improve focus and attention for 6 to 12 hours. It is common practice to give a child attending

---

Box 76-3	Common Learning Disorders

Disorders of Developmental Speech and Language

Developmental articulation disorder
Developmental expressive language disorder
Developmental receptive language disorder

Academic Skills Disorders

Developmental reading disorder
Developmental writing disorder
Developmental arithmetic disorder

Nonverbal Learning Disabilities

Visual-spatial
Visual motor
Sensory deficits
Motor deficits

Central Auditory Processing Deficit

Box 76-4	Resources for Parents on the Internet

www.chadd.org (Children and Adults with Attention-Deficit/Hyperactivity Disorder, CHADD)
www.ADHD.com
www.additudemag.com (ADDitude magazine)
www.ldonline.org (for learning disabilities)

school a longer-acting preparation to minimize the social stigma of having to receive medication daily from the nurse, as well as to smooth the transitions that occur between doses of the shorter-acting formulations. However, some students metabolize these medications faster than others and may require a dose of a short-acting preparation when they get home from school in order to complete their homework in a timely manner. The physician must be aware of the side effects typical of the class, including suppression of appetite and insomnia, when recommending dosing of these medications later in the day.

For decades, the nonstimulants have been utilized for the approximately 20% of patients who, because of existing contraindications, intolerance, or lack of efficacy, could not take a stimulant. This group of medications includes tricyclic antidepressants; SSRI antidepressants; a$_2$-receptor agonists; buspirone; bupropion; and the selective norepinephrine reuptake inhibitor, atomoxetine. Of the nonstimulants, only atomoxetine is currently approved by the U.S. Food and Drug Administration (FDA) for the treatment of AD/HD in children and adults. The nonstimulants differ radically from the stimulants in their mechanism of action, primarily blocking the reuptake of neurochemicals other than dopamine, and they may also last up to 24 hours, double the duration of any of the stimulant preparations. For this reason, persons who require a longer duration of action, such as a child who has significant difficulty in the morning (before the stimulant takes effect) or evening (after the stimulant has worn off), may benefit from the primary use of a nonstimulant.

It is of critical importance for the physician to identify the patient's core symptoms during the initial part of the workup. By clarifying the hours during the day when the patient's function is impaired by the attentional deficit, the physician can then decide which pharmacologic approach offers the best chance for a successful outcome. At each successive visit, these core symptoms should be revisited, with emphasis placed on whether the symptoms are better, worse, or the same under the current treatment plan. If a patient has not improved on a given medication in a specific class, another medication in that same class may be tried (AAP, 2001⊙). However, if a second trial of medication produces unsatisfactory results, the prudent physician will go back to the beginning and reconsider the diagnosis. Further testing or referral to a psychologist, psychiatrist, or educational specialist may reveal a comorbid diagnosis that had not previously been considered.

Behavioral modifications for AD/HD and its comorbid conditions are an integral part of the treatment algorithm (National Institute of Mental Health, 2000). It should never be only about pills; the approach must consist of "pills and skills," and the physician has to provide guidance to the child and family in both areas. Counseling may be recommended for the child, family, or both. List making should be taught as a means of organizational skill building. Parents should be instructed to develop reasonable expectations and goals for their child, set clearly defined limits, and construct a reward and punishment system to help the child attain those goals. This system should be based on privileges rather than monetary rewards. Statistically speaking, three out of four children diagnosed with AD/HD will not take medication for this condition into adulthood, and since AD/HD is a lifelong disorder, it is only through the integration of behavior modification into the patient's daily life that the need for medication becomes secondary.

At the conclusion of the first visit, the physician should distribute rating scales (Connors or equivalent) for parent and teacher to complete; the physician should also request that these scales be sent to the office before their next appointment. The Children's Depres-sion Index should be completed by the patient at home. A written request should be made to the school for a complete psycho-educational assessment, to be done within 6 calendar weeks, with a copy of the findings to be sent to the physician's office upon completion.

SECOND OFFICE VISIT

Interval History

Phillip returns to the office in 10 days, accompanied by his mother and father. No change in his history is noted since his previous visit.

During this visit the physician reviews the rating scales filled out by Phillip, his parents, teachers, and the school's trained evaluator.

Parental Rating Scale
The rating scales filled out by the parents show six positive responses out of nine possible for AD/HD, inattentive type; one positive response out of nine possible for AD/HD, hyperactive/impulsive type; one positive response out of eight criteria for oppositional-defiant disorder; and no positive responses on criteria for conduct disorder.

Teacher Rating Scale
The rating scales filled out by the teacher show eight positive responses out of nine possible for AD/HD, inattentive type; one positive response out of nine possible for AD/HD, hyperactive/impulsive type; two positive criteria out of eight possible for oppositional-defiant disorder; and no positive responses on criteria for conduct disorder.

Children's Depression Index

The score on this instrument is 2 (low probability of depression).

Psycho-educational Assessment

The psycho-educational assessment has not yet been completed by the school.

Impression

The rating scales imply a diagnosis of AD/HD, inattentive type. Learning disability is a possible comorbid diagnosis.

Plan

1. *Medication.* Recommend starting a stimulant, given that Phillip's difficulties are confined to school and homework time. He is not in favor of taking medication at school because of the social stigma of doing so; therefore, a longer-acting stimulant is recommended. Phillip and his parents are not in favor of him taking medication on the weekends, and as long as he has nothing planned that would require an intense intellectual or educational effort, this is felt to be an acceptable option. Side effects are discussed, including but not limited to appetite suppression, stomach upset, headache, insomnia, and emotional lability.
2. *Behavior modification.* Advice is given to Phillip regarding list making for organization. Reasonable goals are established: he agrees to make lists of things he has to accomplish the following day, including specifically assigning his after-school homework hours. Reward–punishment methods are discussed for compliance and noncompliance with these goals. Phillip and his parents mutually decided on a points system that he could redeem each night for extra television or computer game time.
3. *School intervention.* Phillip's parents will continue to urge the school to complete his educational testing expediently. His mother will be in touch with his teachers, who will be asked to notify her in writing at the end of each week as to how Phillip is doing in their classes.
4. A follow-up visit is scheduled in 4 weeks' time.

THIRD OFFICE VISIT

Interval History

Phillip returns with his mother. He has had no side effects from his long-acting stimulant. His teachers have noted a significant improvement in his ability to focus on his work, even in math and science; he has achieved several good test grades in these subjects. He

has been completing his homework on time according to his lists, although his mother notes that he doesn't always like to fill out the lists. The medication effect seems to be lasting about 8 hours. He has done a good enough job completing his homework on time so that he has been able to do "pretty much whatever he wants to do" at night. He does not take his medication on weekends. Vital signs show no appreciable change in pulse, blood pressure, or weight from his first visit. His psycho-educational assessment has been completed, and no learning disabilities were found during the evaluation by the school psychologist, who found him to be "helpful and friendly," with intellectual testing in the superior range.

Impression

The physician's impression is AD/HD, inattentive type, stable on a long-acting stimulant.

Plan

A follow-up visit is scheduled in 1 month.

FOURTH OFFICE VISIT

Interval History

Phillip and his parents return for this visit. He continues to do well. He has brought his grades up to a mix of Bs and As and has made the honor roll. He continues to experience no side effects from his medication. Vital signs are again unchanged significantly from his prior visits. He has no objections to taking his medications. Behavior modification is working well, and he likes being rewarded for completing his homework before his father gets home; this has increased the amount of time the family can spend together.

Assessment

The assessment is AD/HD, inattentive type, stable on a long-acting stimulant.

Plan

A follow-up visit is scheduled in 3 months' time. The parents are to call if the condition changes or worsens in any way.

SUBSEQUENT VISITS

Phillip has been followed for 3 years. He continues to take the long-acting stimulant on school days only, and not on weekends or during school holidays or vacations unless he has an activity that requires him to maximally focus his attention. He experienced a brief decrease in the medication's efficacy in the second year, and the dose was increased to the next level, with good improvement in his core symptoms. His weight and height have continued to increase, with percentile ranks in the 80th and 85th range, respectively; no significant increases in his blood pressure or pulse have been noted. He returns to the office every 3 months for a follow-up visit, at which time an interval history is taken, his progress in school is reviewed, his vital signs are checked, and a medication refill is prescribed.

Material Available on Student Consult

Review Questions and Answers about Attention-Deficit/Hyperactivity Disorder

EVIDENCE-BASED MEDICINE SOURCES

Source: National Institute of Mental Health

URL: www.nimh.nih.gov/events/mtaqa.cfm

Recommendation: The optimal treatment approach for children with AD/HD is medication plus behavior modification.

Summary: The recommendation is based on the findings of the MTA (Multimodal Treatment Study of Children with AD/HD) study, which included nearly 600 children ages 7 to 9 years, randomly assigned to one of four treatment groups: (1) medication alone, (2) psychosocial/behavioral treatment alone, (3) a combination of medication and behavioral modification, or (4) routine community care. Long-term combination treatments and management by medication alone were both shown to be significantly superior to intensive behavior therapy in reducing AD/HD symptoms. The combined approach was also demonstrated to be superior in other areas of functioning, including anxiety, academic performance, oppositional behavior, parent-child interaction, and social skills. The combined approach allowed children to be treated with lower doses of medication than were used in the medication-only group.

Source: Centre for Reviews and Dissemination

URL: nhscrd.york.ac.uk/online/dare/20013548.htm

Recommendation: Methylphenidate is a safe, long-term therapeutic option for treating AD/HD.

Summary: The recommendation was made based on a review of 29 studies with 551 participants, including 8 crossover trials. All studies reported statistically significant improvements after treating with methylphenidate. The drug appeared to be well tolerated, with side effects reported to be dose dependent, and virtually nonexistent at lower doses.

Source: Agency for Healthcare Research and Quality (formerly Agency for Health Care Policy and Research)

URL: www.ahrq.gov/clinic/epcsums/adhdsutr.htm

Recommendation: Comorbid conditions must be actively considered in the evaluation and treatment processes for any child with a working diagnosis of AD/HD.

Summary: The evidence on AD/HD prevalence and diagnosis reported here was gathered from 87 published articles and 10 behavioral scale manuals. The prevalence rates for comorbid educational and behavioral disorders with AD/HD are high; up to 33% of children with AD/HD have more than one comorbid condition. The most common comorbid condition is oppositional-defiant disorder (ODD), with approximately one-third of children diagnosed with AD/HD meeting criteria for this condition. Approximately one-quarter of children diagnosed with AD/HD meet some criteria for conduct disorder. In general, anxiety is more common than depression in ADHD children. More than 10% of students with AD/HD also have a comorbid learning disability.

REFERENCES

American Academy of Pediatrics. Clinical practice guideline: Diagnosis and evaluation of the child with attention-deficit/hyperactivity disorder. Pediatrics 2001;105:1158–1170.🅒

American Psychiatric Association. Diagnostic and Statistical Manual of Mental Disorders, 4th ed., Text Revision. Bethesda, MD, American Psychiatric Press, 2000.🅒

Cohen M. Section 504 and IDEA: Limited vs. substantial protections for children with AD/HD and other disabilities. Available at www.chadd.org/pdfs/Section_504_and_IDEA_by_Matt_Cohen.pdf. Accessed 4/27/2004.

Dougherty DD, Bonab AA, Spencer TJ, Rauch SL, Madras BK, Fischman AJ. Dopamine transporter density in patients with attention deficit hyperactivity disorder. Lancet 1999;354:2132–2133.

Faraone SV. Understanding the effect size of AD/HD medications: Implications for clinical care. Medscape Psychiatry & Mental Health 2003;8. Available at www.medscape.com/viewarticle/461543. Accessed 3/2/2004.🅐

77

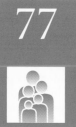

Third-Trimester Vaginal Bleeding (Placenta Previa)

Melissa Nothnagle

KEY POINTS

1. Because of the high rate of blood flow to the placenta in the second part of pregnancy, conditions resulting in bleeding can be life threatening to both the mother and fetus.
2. Vaginal examinations are contraindicated in patients presenting with third-trimester bleeding until the placental location is determined using ultrasound and placenta previa is excluded.
3. Maternal stabilization should be the first priority in managing third-trimester bleeding and may be life preserving for both the mother and fetus.
4. Conservative management of early third-trimester bleeding to prolong gestation may be possible depending on the rate of bleeding and maternal and fetal stability.

INITIAL EVALUATION

Subjective

Patient Identification and Presenting Problem

Elena is a 24-year-old gravida 2 para 1 at 37½ weeks' gestation who presents at obstetric triage with vaginal bleeding for the previous 3 hours. She reports that she has had no major problems in her pregnancy but mentions that she had an ultrasound when she was about 4 months pregnant and was told that her placenta was over the cervix. At that time her physician advised her to have a repeat cesarean section (which is scheduled for next week), avoid sexual intercourse, and come to the hospital immediately if she experienced any bleeding.

Further history is deferred until maternal hemodynamic status has been assessed.

Objective

Physical Examination

Vital Signs Blood pressure, 110/70 mm Hg; pulse, 88; temperature, 36.9°C (98.4°F).

General Appearance Well-appearing pregnant woman; somewhat anxious.

Cardiovascular Regular rate and rhythm, no murmurs.

Pulmonary Lungs clear to auscultation bilaterally.

Abdomen Gravid; fundal height, 38 cm. Uterus is nontender. Leopold's maneuvers: fetus in vertex position; estimated fetal weight, 6.5 pounds.

Pelvic Examination Deferred. External examination shows a small amount of bleeding from the vagina, and the patient has soaked through one sanitary pad since the onset of the bleeding.

Extremities Warm and well perfused; trace edema to the mid-calf bilaterally.

External Fetal Monitoring Fetal heart rate baseline 140 beats per minute with several reactive accelerations and no decelerations.

Tocometry Uterine contractions every 8 to 10 minutes.

Further history is obtained while intravenous fluids are started, blood for laboratory tests drawn, and ultrasound done.

History of Present Illness

Elena was at home making dinner for her family when she felt a leakage of fluid. The amount of bleeding is similar to the first day of her period. She has been having mild contractions for the past 2 days. She denies any recent trauma.

Prenatal History

Elena reports that she started prenatal care early in pregnancy and denies any complications during this pregnancy, including diabetes, vaginal or urinary infections, anemia, or high blood pressure.

Obstetric and Gynecologic History

One previous pregnancy 3 years ago. She delivered a healthy male infant weighing 3270 g at 38 weeks by cesarean section for breech presentation. She had no bleeding during her first pregnancy.

Menarche at age 14. No history of infections or abnormal Pap smears. No miscarriages or abortions.

Medical History

Hospitalized at age 8 with pneumonia. Migraine headaches that have been rare during her pregnancy.

Medications Prenatal vitamins daily, acetaminophen as needed for headaches.

Family History

Elena's mother has type 2 diabetes. Her father has hypertension. She has two healthy siblings.

Social History

Elena lives with her husband and 3-year-old son. She works part time at a hair salon. Her mother, who lives in the apartment upstairs, helps care for her son. Elena does not smoke, drink alcohol, or use drugs. She denies domestic violence. This pregnancy was planned. She intends to breast-feed, and she plans to use an intrauterine device for postpartum birth control.

Review of Systems

No fevers or chills. No lightheadedness. No headaches. No vision changes. No abdominal pain or back pain. No dysuria. No vaginal itching or discharge. Good fetal movement. Mild swelling of both ankles for several weeks. As noted above, mild contractions for several days.

Assessment

Working Diagnosis

Because of the potential for maternal and fetal morbidity from hemorrhage in pregnancy, the first priority in assessing a patient with third-trimester bleeding is not to establish a diagnosis but rather to assess maternal hemodynamic status and institute resuscitative measures if necessary. This patient's vital signs appear normal, and her bleeding appears mild. Initial vital signs should be interpreted with caution, however, as the increased blood volume of pregnancy may blunt early signs of shock. After ensuring stability of the mother, attention can be turned to the fetus. The fetal heart tracing in this case is reassuring. Fetal bradycardia, tachycardia, or prolonged or late decelerations would suggest fetal compromise and warrant expedited delivery.

Based on the patient's reported ultrasound and her presentation with painless bleeding, the most likely diagnosis is placenta previa, meaning that part of the placenta has implanted over the internal os of the cervix. The diagnosis of placenta previa is confirmed by localization of the placenta on ultrasound. Vaginal examinations of patients with third-trimester bleeding must be avoided until placenta previa has been ruled out, as disruption of the placenta can result in large-volume hemorrhage.

Differential Diagnosis

1. *Placental abruption* refers to premature separation of the placenta from the uterus. The most common symptom of abruption is pain, which may vary from mild cramping to severe pain. Vaginal bleeding and uterine tenderness may be present. Fetal distress will be evident with moderate to severe abruption. A history of risk factors for abruption, including hypertension, trauma, smoking, and crack cocaine use, should be sought.

2. *Ruptured vasa previa* is a rare event that may occur in the presence of a low-lying placenta or a velamentous cord insertion, in which umbilical vessels insert into the membranes rather than directly into the placenta. Vessels crossing the internal os rupture, usually at the time of rupture of the membranes. Because fetal blood is lost, fetal heart monitoring may show a rapid deterioration, and immediate cesarean section is indicated. Pediatric personnel should be prepared for volume resuscitation of the infant at delivery. Fetal mortality in cases of ruptured vasa previa approaches 50%. If vasa previa is suspected in the context of a normal fetal heart tracing, the Apt test may be used to rapidly diagnose fetal blood. A sample of vaginal blood is collected and mixed with a small amount of tap water to lyse the red blood cells. The sample is centrifuged for 5 minutes, and the pink supernatant is removed and mixed in a 5:1 ratio with 1% sodium hydroxide. Persistent pink color of the resulting mixture indicates fetal hemoglobin; adult hemoglobin turns brown within 2 minutes.

3. Other causes of bleeding in the latter part of pregnancy include *lower genital tract lesions* such as cervicitis, cervical ectropion, cervical polyps, cervical cancer, or vaginal trauma. The most benign and probably most common cause of bleeding in the third trimester is bleeding from cervical dilation in early labor. This "bloody show" is generally a small volume of blood with a mucous consistency.

Plan

Diagnostic

Complete blood count, blood type, and antibody screen are ordered. Vital signs are assessed frequently, and continuous external fetal monitoring is used. No vaginal examinations are performed. An ultrasound is done to determine location of the placenta.

Therapeutic

Because of the potential for large-volume hemorrhage, two large bore IV catheters are placed and crystalloid solution infused. Four units of packed red blood cells are cross-matched.

Patient Education

Elena is informed that close monitoring of her and her fetus are needed and that an urgent cesarean delivery may be necessary if there is increased blood loss or signs of fetal compromise.

Disposition

The patient is hemodynamically stable, and the fetal heart tracing remains reassuring.

Initial laboratory test results are normal except for hemoglobin of 10.5 and hematocrit of 32. Ultrasound shows a single fetus in cephalic presentation. The placenta is anterior and the lower border overlies the internal os. The cervix appears 75% effaced and 1 cm dilated. Ongoing bleeding is noted. Because Elena is at more than 36 weeks' gestation, there is low risk of fetal lung immaturity. She gives consent for a cesarean section and delivers a 3230 g baby with Apgar scores of 8 and 9.

DISCUSSION

Third-trimester bleeding occurs in 6% of pregnancies. Placental abruption and placenta previa account for as many as half of these cases. Because of the high rate of uterine blood flow during the third trimester (25% of the cardiac output or 500 mL/min), these conditions are potentially life threatening for both the mother and fetus.

Approach to the Patient

Initial evaluation of third-trimester bleeding should include a rapid assessment and stabilization of maternal hemodynamic status. Assessment should begin with basic components of advanced cardiac life support, including status of the patient's airway, breathing, and circulation, followed by identification of the amount and character of bleeding. Large-bore IV access should be obtained and volume replacement initiated (if indicated) with crystalloid solution while blood products are ordered. Transfusion of

packed red blood cells should be considered early to ensure adequate oxygen delivery to the fetus. If evidence of disseminated intravascular coagulation is observed, platelets and fresh frozen plasma should be administered. Ongoing monitoring of maternal and fetal well-being is essential. In the context of maternal shock, fetal distress may not be an indication for delivery. Maternal stabilization results in improved placental perfusion and oxygen delivery to the fetus. Often apparent fetal distress will resolve with these measures, and unnecessary delivery of a preterm fetus and the increased maternal morbidity due to blood loss from emergent surgery can be avoided.

After maternal hemodynamic stability has been established, the cause of bleeding should be investigated. History should include an assessment of pain and any recent trauma. Patients in normal active labor do not have pain between contractions. Ultrasound should be used to exclude placenta previa before speculum or digital examinations. Any Rh-negative woman with antepartum bleeding should be treated with a full dose of Rh immune globulin (Wible-Kant and Beer, 1983 Ⓑ).

Placenta Previa

Placenta previa occurs in one of 250 livebirths. Current classifications of placenta previa include *complete*, in which the placenta directly overlies the internal os, and *marginal*, in which the placental border lies within 2 to 3 cm of the os. Risk factors include previous cesarean delivery, previous uterine instrumentation, multiparity, advanced maternal age, maternal smoking, and multiple gestation. With access to high-resolution ultrasonography, most cases of placenta previa are detected prenatally, and this has greatly reduced maternal and fetal mortality from this condition. However, most placentas that appear to cover the os in the second trimester will have a normal location at term. This is likely due to differential growth of the lower uterine segment and limitations of ultrasound to precisely localize the placental border early in pregnancy. For patients whose second trimester ultrasound shows placenta previa, repeat ultrasound should be scheduled between 24 and 28 weeks to re-evaluate placental location. Bleeding episodes before this repeat study should be treated presumptively as placenta previa. Patients with documented placenta previa after 24 weeks can be managed expectantly but must avoid sexual intercourse and digital examination. Early in gestation, cervical cerclage may reduce the incidence of delivery before 34 weeks and of low birth weight (Neilson, 2003 Ⓒ).

Placenta previa classically presents with painless bleeding at the end of the second trimester or early third trimester. The bleeding may be associated with contractions, although pain between contractions should raise suspicion for placental abruption. Placenta previa rarely causes large-volume hemorrhage unless instrumentation or digital examination is performed.

Because most perinatal morbidity from placenta previa results from preterm birth, management depends on gestational age, in light of the severity of bleeding and maternal and fetal well-being. Before term in a stable patient, tocolysis with magnesium sulfate or beta agonists may be considered as a way to prolong gestation (Sharma et al., 2004 **B**; Towers et al., 1999 **C**). Tocolysis before 34 weeks may also provide a sufficient time to administer corticosteroids to promote fetal lung maturation. Patients should be monitored closely for signs of hemodynamic instability or disseminated intravascular coagulation. Indications for delivery include ongoing bleeding, documented fetal lung maturity, and signs of fetal distress.

At term, cesarean delivery is indicated for ongoing bleeding or nonreassuring fetal heart tracing after maternal stabilization. In cases of marginal placenta previa, vaginal delivery may be possible because the fetal head may tamponade the bleeding from the placental border. Vaginal delivery should be attempted only under conditions of a "double setup" in the operating room, with immediate availability of blood products and surgical and anesthesia personnel to perform a cesarean section in case of rapid blood loss.

Placental Abruption

Bleeding due to placental abruption is usually associated with abdominal or back pain. Although most patients will present with vaginal bleeding, abruption may also occur behind the placenta or into the myometrium without vaginal bleeding (concealed or occult abruption). Risk of placenta abruption is increased with maternal trauma, cocaine use, hypertension, smoking, multiparity, and history of abruption. In cases of third-trimester bleeding, if placenta previa is not seen on ultrasound and lower genital tract lesions or labor have been ruled out, placental abruption is the most likely diagnosis.

Treatment of placental abruption depends on the degree of placental separation (Box 77-1). Grade 1 abruption is mild and may be managed conservatively with Pitocin induction at term or tocolysis for the stable preterm patient. Expeditious delivery, generally by cesarean section, is indicated for signs of

Box 77-1	Classification of Placental Abruption

Grade 1: Small abruption with minimal maternal or fetal symptoms
Grade 2: Bleeding, contractions, and uterine tenderness with a live fetus (usually with a nonreassuring fetal heart tracing)
Grade 3: Moderate to severe bleeding with intrauterine fetal demise, high risk of maternal coagulopathy

fetal distress or ongoing bleeding. Grade 2 abruption is more severe and usually requires emergent cesarean section unless vaginal delivery is imminent. In cases of grade 3 abruption, in which fetal death is confirmed, expeditious vaginal delivery is preferable to operative delivery because of risks from coagulopathy (Sher and Statland, 1985 **C**).

Conclusion

Third-trimester bleeding involves potentially life-threatening conditions for both mother and fetus. In cases of significant hemorrhage, maternal stabilization is always the first priority. No vaginal examinations should be done until placenta previa has been ruled out by ultrasound. Management of third-trimester bleeding depends on severity of bleeding, maternal and fetal well-being, and length of gestation. Urgent delivery should be considered if there is evidence of fetal compromise or fetal maturity. With minor amounts of bleeding from placenta previa or placental abruption before 36 weeks' gestation, conservative management may be possible. Attempts to prolong gestation with tocolysis should be made only after careful consideration of maternal and fetal risks and benefits and informed consent of the patient. Any Rh-negative woman with bleeding in pregnancy should receive Rh immune globulin.

Material Available on Student Consult

Review Questions and Answers about Placenta Previa

REFERENCES

Neilson JP. Interventions for suspected placenta praevia. Cochrane Database Syst Rev 2003(2):CD001998. **A**

Sharma A, Suri V, Gupta I. Tocolytic therapy in conservative management of symptomatic placenta previa. Int J Gynaecol Obstet 2004;84:109–113. **B**

Sher F, Statland BE. Abruptio placentae with coagulopathy: A rational basis for management. Clin Obstet Gynecol 1985;28:15–23. **C**

Towers CV, Pircon RA, Heppard M. Is tocolysis safe in the management of third trimester bleeding? Am J Obstet Gynecol 1999;180:1572–1578. **C**

Wible-Kant J, Beer AE. Antepartum Rh immune globulin. Clin Perinatol 1983;10:343–355. **B**

78 Abdominal Pain (Endometriosis)

Kenneth J. Grimm

KEY POINTS

1. Endometriosis is found in up to 65% of adolescents with pelvic pain and 30% to 50% of women undergoing laparoscopy for pelvic pain or infertility.
2. There is a tenfold increased risk of endometriosis in patients who have a first-degree relative with endometriosis.
3. Ultrasound can eliminate other causes of pelvic pain but a definitive diagnosis can be made only by direct visualization, such as with laparoscopy.
4. Treatment of endometriosis includes non-steroidal anti-inflammatory drugs (NSAIDs), oral contraceptives, progesterone, danazol, gonadotropin-releasing hormone (GnRH) agonists, and surgery (either laparoscopically or by hysterectomy).

INITIAL VISIT

Subjective

Patient Identification and Presenting Problem

Amanda E. is a 17-year-old who complains of abdominal pain.

Present Illness

Amanda says the pain began about 9 months ago and has been steadily worsening since then. It is located in her lower abdomen, midline. She notes a near-constant dull ache, but she has worsening cramping pain typically beginning the day before her menses and lasting for 4 to 5 days. She has missed approximately 10 days of school this year because of the pain. When the pain is at its worst, she often experiences constipation and painful defecation. She denies diarrhea or blood in her stool. She has not traveled recently. She has no history of fever, changes in her appetite, weight loss, upper abdominal pain, nausea, or vomiting. She has had no dysuria, hematuria, or increase in urinary frequency. She has never been sexually active and denies vaginal discharge. The pain is partially relieved by ibuprofen, 400 mg, taken every 6 hours.

Medical History

Amanda is a healthy young woman. She is not taking any medications, and her only hospitalization was for the surgical correction of an imperforate hymen at menarche. Her immunizations are up to date.

Developmental History

Amanda reached all of her developmental milestones at the appropriate ages. Menarche was at age 13, and her menses have been regular since, occurring every 28 to 30 days and lasting for 6 days with normal flow.

Family History

Amanda's parents and younger brother are healthy. She has a maternal aunt with ulcerative colitis. No family history of depression is known.

Social History

Amanda is a well-adjusted, happy teenager. She is in 12th grade and excels academically. She is looking forward to studying at a local college next year. She has been an avid skier and tennis player, and she has continued to participate in these activities. She denies smoking, alcohol, or illicit drug use. Her parents have no concerns regarding her peer group. No history of physical or sexual abuse is known.

Review of Systems

Gastrointestinal and genitourinary symptoms as mentioned, otherwise unremarkable. Her last menstrual period was normal in timing and duration and began 3 weeks ago.

Evidence levels ⒶRandomized, controlled trials (RCTs), meta-analyses, well-designed systematic reviews of RCTs. Ⓑ Case-control or cohort studies, nonrandomized clinical trials, systematic reviews of studies other than RCTs, cross-sectional studies, retrospective studies, certain uncontrolled studies. Ⓒ Consensus statements, expert guidelines, usual practice, opinion.

Objective

Physical Examination

Amanda is a well-appearing adolescent in no distress. Her temperature is 98.4°F, her pulse is 76, her respiration rate is 12, her blood pressure is 112/64, her weight is 120 pounds, and her height is 5 feet 5 inches. She is alert and oriented with a full affect. She displays no psychomotor retardation and is appropriately interactive, with good eye contact throughout the interview and examination. Heart and lung examinations are normal. Abdominal examination shows normally active bowel sounds. Her abdomen is soft with moderate tenderness, worse in the suprapubic area and radiating to the right lower quadrant, with no guarding or rebound tenderness. No masses are appreciable. Pelvic examination reveals normal, Tanner stage 4 external genitalia. The vaginal discharge is normal, and no blood is seen. The cervix appears unremarkable. She has moderate cervical motion tenderness. The uterus is normal size, midline, and retroverted but mobile. Her right adnexal area is moderately tender with no palpable mass. She has no anterior tenderness. Rectovaginal examination reveals tender nodularity in the rectovaginal septum.

Impression

Working Diagnosis

This patient has chronic pelvic pain. Chronic pelvic pain is defined as pain lasting 6 or more months that localizes to the anatomic pelvis (ACOG, 2004Ⓒ). This patient has both a cyclic and a noncyclic component that localizes on examination to the uterus and right adnexa and is significant enough to cause her to miss school.

Differential Diagnosis

The differential diagnosis of chronic pelvic pain is complex and includes both gynecologic and nongynecologic etiologies (Table 78-1). Endometriosis can cause both cyclic and noncyclic pain, especially in adolescents. The absence of a history of sexual activity rules out pelvic infection and pregnancy complications. The pattern of her pain makes ovulation an unlikely etiology. Her pelvic examination is not suggestive of leiomyomata or an ovarian cyst or neoplasm. She denies any voiding symptoms and has no anterior tenderness on examination, making a urologic etiology unlikely. Her bowel symptoms warrant considering inflammatory bowel disease in the differential diagnosis, especially with a family history of ulcerative colitis. However, with no diarrhea, hematochezia, or weight loss, this is unlikely to be the cause of her symptoms. Gastrointestinal and urologic symptoms are common in adolescent patients with endometriosis. Finally, no history suggests physical abuse, and she has no other symptoms of depression. Endometriosis seems to be the most likely diagnosis.

Plan

Diagnostic

A urinalysis, obtained to rule out urinary tract infection and interstitial cystitis, was normal. A urine pregnancy test was negative. Given the lack of a palpable mass on pelvic examination, the yield from an

Table 78-1 Differential Diagnosis of Chronic Pelvic Pain	
Gynecologic Causes	**Nongynecologic Causes**
Endometriosis	Urologic disease
Ovulatory pain (mittelschmertz)	Interstitial cystitis
Ovarian cyst	Urethral syndrome
Gynecologic neoplasia	Bladder malignancy
Pelvic inflammatory disease	Chronic urinary tract infection
Leiomyomata	Gastrointestinal
Adhesions	Inflammatory bowel disease
Primary dysmenorrhea	Irritable bowel syndrome
Adenomysosis	Diverticular disease
Pelvic congestion syndrome	Gastrointestinal neoplasia
Chronic ectopic pregnancy	Constipation
	Musculoskeletal source
	Other
	Porphyria
	Shingles
	Depression
	History of abuse

ultrasound would be very low. If an adequate pelvic examination had not been possible, an ultrasound would have been important in ruling out various pelvic abnormalities as the cause of her pain.

A definitive diagnosis of endometriosis requires laparoscopic visualization of the ectopic endometrial implants. For this reason, it is widely acceptable to treat suspected endometriosis empirically, especially in the adolescent population, when other causes of pelvic pain have been reasonably well ruled out.

Therapeutic

After discussing the diagnostic and therapeutic options, Amanda and her parents elect initial empiric treatment. Because she has received some relief from over-the-counter dosing, ibuprofen 800 milligrams three times per day was prescribed.

FOLLOW-UP VISIT

Subjective

After 2 months of treatment, Amanda returns to the office for re-evaluation. Her symptoms are significantly improved with regular use of ibuprofen. The continuous pain has mostly resolved, but she continues to have significant pain beginning just before her menses. She wishes to try something else for relief of her pain.

Objective

Unchanged from previous examination.

Impression

Amanda has had an inadequate response to a trial of a nonsteroidal anti-inflammatory drug (NSAID). She desires further treatment but still wishes to avoid surgery unless it is necessary.

Plan

A trial of low-dose combined oral contraceptive pills is prescribed. If this is not effective, Amanda agrees to a referral for laparoscopy before more aggressive medical management is started.

DISCUSSION

Endometriosis is a common cause of chronic pelvic pain and infertility. Endometriosis has been reported in up to 32% and 48% of women undergoing laparoscopy for pelvic pain and infertility, respectively (Sangi-Haghpeykar and Poindexter, 1995❸). In adolescents with pelvic pain, the prevalence may be as high as 65% (Chatman and Ward, 1982❸). The ectopic endometrial glands and stroma can be found throughout the pelvis (ovaries, fallopian tubes, broad ligament, uterosacral ligaments, bladder) as well as in extrapelvic locations (bowel, omentum, kidneys, abdominal wall, diaphragm, pleura/lung), and even in nasal mucosa and skin.

The etiology of endometriosis is not known with certainty. Ectopic endometrial tissue can result from retrograde menstruation (supported by an increased incidence in patients with outflow tract obstruction, such as in this case), hematologic or lymphatic spread, or metaplasia of undifferentiated coelomic cells in the peritoneal cavity. Observational data demonstrate an association between endometriosis and other autoimmune diseases, suggesting that a component of immune system alteration may allow the ectopic endometrial tissue to grow (Sinaii et al., 2002❸). Some genetic component to the disease exists, with up to a tenfold increase risk in patients with first-degree relatives with endometriosis (ACOG, 2000❸).

Although endometriosis is often asymptomatic, it can cause significant morbidity related to pain and infertility. Patients often have deep pelvic pain and dyspareunia. The pain is often cyclic, being worse immediately before or during menses, but the pain can be noncyclic as well, especially in adolescents. Involvement of the bladder can cause urinary symptoms such as dysuria, urgency, and hematuria, and bowel involvement can result in constipation, painful defecation, and rectal bleeding. Adolescent patients are more likely to have these bowel and bladder symptoms. The relation between endometriosis and fertility is complex. Although anatomic alterations from the scarring of severe endometriosis can clearly lead to tubal factor infertility, controversy exists over the role milder forms of endometriosis can play in infertility.

The diagnosis of endometriosis is typically a clinical one. History and physical examination can suggest the diagnosis, while helping to rule out other causes of pelvic pain. Ultrasound can be helpful in eliminating other potential causes for pain, particularly if the physical examination is abnormal or limited. It also has a role in the diagnosis of endometriomas (chocolate cysts), blood-filled cystic lesions that may complicate endometriosis.

A definitive diagnosis of endometriosis can be made only after direct visualization of the lesions in the operating room. Laparoscopy allows confirmation of the diagnosis and staging into categories of minimal, mild, moderate, and severe, based on the location and severity of the disease (American Society for Reproductive Medicine, 1997❸). Interestingly, no correlation appears to exist between the amount of ectopic endometrium found at laparoscopy and the severity of pain that women experience.

When deciding on treatment for endometriosis, it is important first to determine the goals of treatment for a particular patient. For some patients, the goal may be treatment of the pain associated with the disease; for others, it may be treatment for infertility. The treatment can include both medical and surgical modalities, and the approach may be different, depending on which of these problems is being addressed.

If the primary treatment goal is relief of pain, then many medical options can be considered (Mahutte and Arici, 2003 Ⓒ). NSAIDs are commonly prescribed for various forms of pain, including pelvic pain. They have a well-established role in the treatment of primary dysmenorrhea, a prostaglandin-mediated disease. Whereas they have no direct effect on the pathophysiology of endometriosis, they have been extensively used for first-line symptomatic relief of pain. They are inexpensive, and most physicians are very familiar with their use. Side effects from NSAIDs include gastrointestinal problems (gastritis, peptic ulcer disease) and a rare incidence of renal failure. Despite the commonness of their use, data supporting the effectiveness of NSAIDs in endometriosis are relatively scarce. At least one older placebo-controlled crossover trial demonstrated a benefit over placebo (Kauppila and Ronnberg, 1985 Ⓐ). A systematic review of the use of NSAIDs in endometriosis is currently under way and is expected to be published sometime in 2005 (Allen et al., 2004 Ⓐ).

Because of the role of ovarian hormones in supporting the growth of the endometrium, treatments that decrease production of these hormones have been used extensively for endometriosis. These treatments attempt to mimic either pregnancy or menopause, two physiologic states associated with improvement in this disease. Options in this category include oral contraceptive pills, progesterones, danazol, and gonadotro-pinreleasing hormone (GnRH) agonists. Oral contraceptives have been extensively used to treat the pain associated with endometriosis. A common strategy is to use continuous low-dose combination agents (i.e., no "placebo" week, unlike their normal use for birth control.) A systematic review found only one randomized controlled trial supporting their efficacy against pain (Moore et al., 2004 Ⓐ). Side effects include nausea, breast tenderness, hypertension, and a small risk of thromboembolic disease. Progesterone-only therapy also has been widely used. Medroxyprogesterone can be used either orally (50 to 100 mg daily), or the depo-formulation can be given intramuscularly (150 mg every 3 months). The effectiveness of progesterone therapy is supported by a recent systematic review (Prentice et al., 2004 Ⓐ). Side effects include weight gain, irregular menses or amenorrhea, and a small risk of thromboembolic disease. Danazol is a weak androgen that is used to treat endometriosis by decreasing estrogen production through negative feedback at the hypothalamic and pituitary level. Its effectiveness in reducing endometriosis-associated pain also has been supported by a recent systematic review (Selak et al., 2004 Ⓐ). Danazol has significant side effects, including menopausal symptoms, acne, hirsutism, liver disease, and thromboembolic disease. GnRH agonists decrease ovarian function by acting at the level of the pituitary. Normally, pulsatile secretion of GnRH stimulates the pituitary to produce follicle-stimulating hormone and luteinizing hormone. Continuous GnRH stimulation has the opposite effect, decreasing pituitary gonadotropin production and creating a sort of "medical menopause." Although they are effective in treating endometriosis pain, a recent systematic review found no evidence that they are superior to other medical treatments (Prentice et al., 2000 Ⓐ). Significant side effects relating to estrogen deficiency occur, including a decrease in bone mineral density. These can be improved with the concurrent use of add-back estrogen/progesterone therapy at levels sufficient to reduce hormonal withdrawal symptoms, but low-enough not to stimulate the ectopic endometrial tissue. It is important to realize that medical treatments, although effective for pain, have not been shown to improve fertility in patients with endometriosis (Hughes et al., 2003 Ⓐ).

The role of surgery in the management of endometriosis includes definitively diagnosing the disease and both conservative and definitive treatment options. Conservative treatment involves destruction of endometriosis lesions and restoration of normal anatomy through lysis of adhesions created by the disease. This is typically accomplished laparoscopically. A recent systematic review identified only one randomized controlled trial evaluating the effectiveness of conservative surgery on the pain of endometriosis (Jacobson, 2001 Ⓐ). This study showed a significant decrease in pain 6 months after surgery. Unlike medical therapy, surgery has been shown to have some effectiveness against infertility associated with endometriosis (Jacobson, 2002 Ⓐ). If future fertility is not desired, definitive surgery (hysterectomy, often with oophorectomy) can be used to treat endometriosis pain that has not adequately responded to other treatment options. It should be noted, however, that even this is not 100% effective in refractory disease.

Material Available on Student Consult

Review Questions and Answers about Endometriosis

REFERENCES

Allen C, Hopewell S, Prentice A. Non-steroidal Anti-inflammatory Drugs for Pain in Women with Endometriosis (Protocol for a Cochrane Review). Chichester, The Cochrane Library, 2004.Ⓐ

American College of Obstetricians and Gynecologists. Medical management of endometriosis: ACOG Practice Bulletin No. 11. Int J Gynecol Obstet 2000;71:183–196.Ⓒ

American College of Obstetricians and Gynecologists. Chronic pelvic pain: ACOG Practice Bulletin No. 51. Obstet Gynecol 2004;103:589–605.Ⓒ

American Society for Reproductive Medicine Revised classification of endometriosis, 1996. Fertil Steril 1997;67:817–821.Ⓒ

Chatman D, Ward A. Endometriosis in adolescents. J Reprod Med 1982;27:156–160.Ⓒ

Hughes E, Fedorkow D, Collins J, et al. Ovulation Suppression for Endometriosis (Cochrane Review). Chichester, UK, The Cochrane Library, 2003.Ⓐ

Jacobson T, Barlow DH, Garry R, et al. Laparoscopic Surgery for Pelvic Pain Associated with Endometriosis (Cochrane Review). Chichester, UK, The Cochrane Library, 2001.Ⓐ

Jacobson T, Baklow DH, Koninckx P, et al. Laparoscopic Surgery for Subfertility Associated with Endometriosis (Cochrane Review). Chichester, UK, The Cochrane Library, 2002.Ⓐ

Kauppila A, Ronnberg L. Naproxen sodium in dysmenorrhea secondary to endometriosis. Obstet Gynecol 1985; 65:379–383.Ⓐ

Mahutte N, Arici A. Medical management of endometriosis-associated pain. Obstet Gynecol Clin North Am 2003;30:133–150.Ⓒ

Moore J, Kennedy S, Prentice A. Modern Combined Oral Contraceptives for Pain Associated with Endometriosis (Cochrane Review). Chichester, UK, The Cochrane Library, 2004.Ⓐ

Prentice A, Deary A, Bland E. Progestagens and Anti-progestagens for Pain Associated with Endometriosis (Cochrane Review). Chichester, UK, The Cochrane Library, 2004.Ⓐ

Prentice A, Deary EJ, Goldbeck-Wood S, et al. Gonadotropin-releasing Hormone Analogues for Pain Associated with Endometriosis (Cochrane Review). Chichester, UK, The Cochrane Library, 2000.Ⓐ

Sangi-Haghpeykar H, Poindexter A. Epidemiology of endometriosis among parous women. Obstet Gynecol 1995;85:983–992.Ⓑ

Selak V, Farquhar C, Prentice A, et al. Danazol for Pelvic Pain Associated with Endometriosis (Cochrane Review). In. Chichester, UK, The Cochrane Library, 2000.Ⓐ

Sinaii N, Cleary SD, Ballweg ML, et al. High rates of autoimmune and endocrine disorders, fibromyalgia, chronic fatigue syndrome and atopic diseases among women with endometriosis: A survey analysis. Hum Reprod 2002;17:2715–2724.Ⓑ

79

Severe Menstrual Cramps (Primary Dysmenorrhea)

Melissa Nothnagle

INITIAL VISIT

Subjective

Patient Identification and Presenting Problem

Marta R. is a 16-year-old girl with painful cramps in her back and lower abdomen that have occurred with her menses for the past 2 years.

History of Present Illness

For the past 2 years, Marta has experienced severe cramps in her back and lower abdomen during the first 2 days of her period. She occasionally has nausea and loose stools when she has the pain. She has tried taking ibuprofen, 200 mg every 6 hours, without much relief. Sometimes she misses school because her pain is so severe. Her last period was 2 weeks ago.

Medical History

Marta states that her periods began when she was 13 years old. They occur every 30 days with moderate bleeding, lasting 4 to 5 days. Marta had her tonsils and adenoids removed at age 5. She uses albuterol for exercise-induced asthma. She is otherwise healthy.

Family History

Marta has two younger brothers. Her mother, who is with her today, reports mild cramps with her own menstrual periods. Marta's maternal grandmother had a hysterectomy at age 40 for uterine fibroids.

Social History

Marta denies smoking, alcohol, or drug use. She is an honor-roll student in the 10th grade. She has never been sexually active.

Review of Systems

She denies vaginal discharge, weight loss, constipation, and fever. She denies midcycle pain or bleeding.

Objective

Physical Examination

Marta appears well. Her blood pressure is 110/70 mm Hg, pulse is 72 and regular, height is 5 ft 3 inches, and weight is 120 pounds. Abdominal examination: normal bowel sounds, soft, nontender, nondistended. No masses are palpated. Pelvic examination reveals normal external genitalia, normal cervix and vagina. Her uterus is normal size, anteverted, and nontender. Adnexal examination shows normal ovaries with no masses or tenderness.

Assessment

Working Diagnosis

The most likely diagnosis in this case is primary dysmenorrhea. This syndrome generally appears during adolescence, within 1 to 2 years of menarche, when ovulatory cycles are established. Patients report sharp, intermittent suprapubic pain that may radiate to the lower back or the back of the legs. Associated

---

symptoms may include nausea, vomiting, diarrhea, fatigue, or headache. Pain usually begins on the first day of menses and peaks in the first or second day of menses, during the heaviest flow. Uterine prostaglandins appear to have a causative role in primary dysmenorrhea. During menstruation, the disintegrating endometrial cells release prostaglandins, which stimulate myometrial contractions and ischemia. Higher levels of prostaglandins have been found in the menstrual fluid of women with more severe dysmenorrhea (Chan, 1978 Ⓑ). In addition, nonsteroidal anti-inflammatory drugs (NSAIDs), which inhibit prostaglandin synthesis, are effective in relieving symptoms of dysmenorrhea.

Differential Diagnosis

Secondary dysmenorrhea is defined as painful menses that are associated with an identifiable pathologic condition. Such conditions can often be identified by history and physical examination. Patients should be asked about age of menarche, onset of symptoms, and timing of the pain in relation to the menstrual cycle. Secondary causes of dysmenorrhea may be suggested by abnormal findings on physical examination or poor response to NSAIDS or combined hormonal contraceptives. Secondary dysmenorrhea also should be suspected in women who report onset of symptoms after puberty or who have associated infertility, irregular menses, or dyspareunia. Treatment for many causes of secondary dysmenorrhea is surgical, so these patients may need referral to a gynecologist for evaluation.

1. *Endometriosis.* This condition is characterized by growth of endometrial tissue outside the uterine cavity. Cyclic stimulation of the ectopic endometrial tissue causes pelvic pain. Women with endometriosis classically appear with cyclic pelvic pain, infertility, and dyspareunia, especially with deep penetration. Physical examination findings suggestive of endometriosis include cervical motion tenderness, uterosacral nodularity, and decreased uterine mobility. However, the physical examination has low sensitivity and specificity for endometriosis. The diagnosis should be suspected in patients who report midcycle and perimenstrual pain, especially those with a history of fertility problems. The gold standard for diagnosis of endometriosis is laparoscopy. However, the extent of the disease at laparoscopy does not correlate well with severity of symptoms. Many patients with a history suggestive of endometriosis will respond to empirical treatment with combined oral contraceptives or gonadotropin-releasing hormone agonists.
2. *Cervical stenosis.* A less-common cause of dysmenorrhea than was previously believed, cervical stenosis may result from infection or from trauma

due to instrumentation, cryotherapy, or surgery for cervical dysplasia.
3. *Cervical or endometrial polyps.* These are benign growths of the endocervical canal or endometrium. Cervical polyps often have postcoital bleeding and are visible protruding from the cervix on speculum examination. Endometrial polyps may be diagnosed with ultrasound or hysteroscopy.
4. *Pelvic inflammatory disease.* Pelvic inflammatory disease (PID) is a polymicrobial infection of the upper genital tract that usually occurs with lower abdominal pain and fever. Examination findings include purulent cervical discharge, cervical motion tenderness, and adnexal tenderness. A subacute infection could cause symptoms similar to dysmenorrhea, but differences in timing of symptoms, examination findings, and cervical cultures would likely point to infection. Pelvic adhesions resulting from a previous episode of PID may be associated with subsequent dysmenorrhea.
5. *Ovarian cysts.* Cyclic pain may be associated with functional ovarian cysts or hemorrhagic cysts. However, symptoms are unlikely to occur only during the initial days of the menses. Pelvic ultrasound is helpful in diagnosing ovarian cysts, but given the high prevalence of asymptomatic ovarian cysts, it may be difficult to establish that these are the cause of a patient's pain.
6. *Leiomyomata (uterine fibroids).* These benign tumors of the uterine muscle are uncommon in adolescents and may be associated with heavy, painful menses. Nodularity or enlargement of the uterus may be noted on bimanual examination. Pelvic ultrasound is useful in confirming this diagnosis.
7. *Adenomyosis.* Rarely seen in women younger than 30 years, this condition involves penetration by endometrial glands and stroma deep into myometrial tissue. This is associated with increased menstrual bleeding and dysmenorrhea. Mild uterine enlargement may be noted on examination. The diagnosis can be made with magnetic resonance imaging or at the time of hysterectomy.
8. *Intrauterine devices.* Some intrauterine devices are associated with increased volume of menstrual flow, which may result in higher incidence of dysmenorrhea.

Plan

Diagnostic

Because Marta has a history typical of primary dysmenorrhea and a normal physical examination, no further testing is indicated. A poor response to empirical treatment would suggest a secondary cause of dysmenorrhea, warranting further evaluation.

Therapeutic

The patient is prescribed naproxen, 500 mg, twice daily. She is encouraged to start the medicine the day before her anticipated onset of menses and to continue through the first 3 days of menses.

Patient Education

Marta's mother is concerned that the cause of Marta's severe pain could be associated with future fertility problems. Marta and her mother are informed about the high prevalence of primary dysmenorrhea among adolescents and the lack of a relation between dysmenorrhea and future problems with fertility. She is told that if her pain is not adequately relieved with these higher-dose NSAIDs, combined oral contraceptives are an effective second-line treatment.

Disposition

Marta is instructed to make a follow-up appointment in 2 months to review her response to NSAID therapy.

FOLLOW-UP VISIT

Subjective

Marta returns for her follow-up visit 2 months later. She reports taking naproxen as instructed, starting the day before her anticipated period. She describes some reduction in pain, although on her first day of menses this month, the pain was still severe enough that she left school early. She has not had any pain between her periods.

Objective

Her vital signs are normal.

Assessment

Marta's partial response to NSAID therapy is still consistent with the diagnosis of primary dysmenorrhea.

Plan

Combined oral contraceptives were recommended to Marta, given her inadequate response to NSAID therapy. In addition to preventing pregnancy, benefits of treatment with combined oral contraceptives include improvement in acne, menstrual regularity, reduced risk of anemia, prevention of ovarian cysts, and prevention of PID (Fraser and Kovacs, 2003 Ⓑ Ⓒ). While taking oral contraceptives, she can continue to use NSAIDs to relieve any discomfort during her menses.

DISCUSSION

Primary dysmenorrhea is the most common gynecologic problem in menstruating women. Reported prevalence rates are as high as 90% (Jamieson and Steege, 1996 Ⓑ). Dysmenorrhea is a major cause of activity restriction and absence from work and school. Further, this problem is underreported as well as undertreated in primary care.

The diagnosis of primary dysmenorrhea can generally be made based on a typical history and a normal physical examination. Primary dysmenorrhea usually is first seen within 2 years of menarche, and onset of the pain coincides with the onset of menses and resolves after 2 to 3 days. Table 79-1 lists features suggestive of primary or secondary dysmenorrhea.

Physical examination findings may suggest a secondary cause of dysmenorrhea, although several causes of secondary dysmenorrhea such as endometriosis or ovarian cysts may not be detectable by physical examination. Laboratory testing and imaging studies are not needed to make the diagnosis of primary dysmenorrhea.

Treatment of Primary Dysmenorrhea

Nonsteroidal Anti-inflammatory Drugs

The efficacy of NSAIDs for primary dysmenorrhea has been demonstrated in randomized controlled trials, although insufficient evidence exists to evaluate

Table 79-1 Features Suggestive of Primary or Secondary Dysmenorrhea

Primary Dysmenorrhea	Secondary Dysmenorrhea
Onset in early adolescence	Onset after adolescence
Duration of symptoms, 2–3 days	Duration of symptoms, >3 days
Onset of pain coincides with menses	Pain before menses or midcycle pain
Normal pelvic exam	Abnormal findings on pelvic exam
Relief with NSAIDs or OCPs	Lack of response to NSAIDs or OCPs
	Infertility
	Irregular bleeding

NSAID, nonsteroidal anti-inflammatory drug; OCP, oral contraceptive.

differences in efficacy among various NSAIDs (Marjoribanks et al., 2003 Ⓐ). Possible adverse effects of NSAIDs include nausea, epigastric pain, and gastrointestinal bleeding. Contraindications include history of peptic ulcer disease or gastrointestinal bleeding and renal or hepatic insufficiency.

Combined Oral Contraceptives

The efficacy of combined oral contraceptive pills for primary dysmenorrhea has been demonstrated in laboratory and observational studies, as well as a few small randomized controlled trials (Davis and Westhoff, 2001 Ⓑ; Hendrix and Alexander, 2002 Ⓑ). No data are available comparing different formulations. Treatment with oral contraceptives is ideal for women with dysmenorrhea who desire effective contraception, or for those who do not respond adequately to a trial of NSAIDs.

Combined oral contraceptives inhibit ovulation, which reduces stimulation of endometrial tissue. As a result, menstrual volume decreases, as does prostaglandin release. Newer combined hormonal delivery systems such as the contraceptive patch and vaginal ring should have similar effects on the endometrium. Possible adverse effects of combined hormonal contraceptives include nausea, breakthrough bleeding, amenorrhea, headache, and thromboembolic events. Smokers older than 35 years and women with breast cancer, cerebrovascular or coronary artery disease, thromboembolic disorders, or undiagnosed abnormal vaginal bleeding should not use combined hormonal contraceptives.

Other hormonal contraceptives also are beneficial in treating primary dysmenorrhea (Fraser and Kovacs, 2003 Ⓑ Ⓒ). Extended-cycle oral contraceptives may be helpful for patients with severe dysmenorrhea. They may reduce the frequency of menstruation to 4 times per year, in addition to preventing ovulation and reducing menstrual volume. Specific products are marketed for this purpose, but any combined oral contraceptive can be prescribed for extended cycles by instructing patients to use only the active pills for 3 months, followed by a week of placebo pills. Progestin-only hormonal contraceptives, including progestin-only pills, injectable progestins and progestin-releasing intrauterine devices (IUDs), alleviate primary dysmenorrhea through their inhibitory effects on the endometrium. Both injectable progestins and the progestin-releasing IUDs may induce amenorrhea in some users, which may be of benefit to women with severe menstrual symptoms.

In summary, primary dysmenorrhea is a common but undertreated condition in primary care. Once secondary causes have been ruled out from the history and physical examination, dysmenorrhea is usually managed successfully with medications.

> ### Material Available on Student Consult
>
> Review Questions and Answers about Primary Dysmenorrhea

REFERENCES

Chan WY, Hill JC. Determination of menstrual prostaglandin levels in nondysmenorrheic and dysmenorrheic subjects. Prostaglandins 1978;130:83.Ⓑ

Davis AR, Westhoff CL. Primary dysmenorrhea in adolescent girls and treatment with oral contraceptives. J Pediatr Adolesc Gynecol 2001;14:3–8.Ⓑ

Fraser IS, Kovacs GT. The efficacy of non-contraceptive uses for hormonal contraceptives. Med J Aust 2003;178:621–623.Ⓑ Ⓒ

Hendrix SL, Alexander NJ. Primary dysmenorrhea treatment with a desogestrel-containing low-dose oral contraceptive. Contraception 2002;66:393–399.Ⓑ

Jamieson DJ, Steege JF. The prevalence of dysmenorrhea, dyspareunia, pelvic pain, and irritable bowel syndrome in primary care practices. Obstet Gynecol 1996;87:55–58.Ⓑ

Marjoribanks J, Proctor ML, Farquhar C. Nonsteroidal anti-inflammatory drugs for primary dysmenorrhoea. Cochrane Database Syst Rev 2003;CD001751.Ⓐ

80 Back Pain (Osteoporosis)

Kenneth J. Grimm

KEY POINTS

1. Vertebral compression fractures, seen with new-onset back pain radiating to the anterior abdominal wall ("girdle of pain"), are a common presentation of osteoporosis.
2. It should be recognized that vertebral compression fractures are a sign of generalized osteoporosis and are associated with a three-fold increase in the risk of hip fractures.
3. Risk factors for osteoporosis include age, female sex, sex hormone deficiency, family history, being white, poor calcium and vitamin D intake, inactivity, smoking, low body weight, excessive caffeine intake, hyperthyroidism, diabetes, inflammatory bowel disease, and the use of corticosteroids, anxiolytics, anticonvulsants, and neuroleptics.
4. The risk of fracture is increased by conditions that increase the general risk of falling.
5. Osteoporosis is a common condition, resulting in significant morbidity, mortality, and health care expenditure.
6. Osteoporosis is defined by the World Health Organization as resulting in a T-score of −2.5 or less.
7. Osteopenia is defined as resulting in a T-score of between −1.0 and −2.5.
8. Screening for osteoporosis with dual-energy x-ray absorptiometry should be offered to all women older than 65 years, and all high-risk women older than 60 years.
9. Adequate calcium and vitamin D intake should be recommended to all women, regardless of age, to protect against the development of osteoporosis.
10. Bisphosphonates have the best evidence that they are effective at preventing fractures and should be used as first-line therapy. Other treatments that have been shown to affect bone density include calcitonin, calcium and vitamin D, and hormone replacement therapy.

INITIAL VISIT

Subjective

Patient Identification and Presenting Problem

Mrs. M. is a 74-year-old white woman complaining of back pain.

Present Illness

Mrs. M. reports that she awoke with pain in her back approximately 2 weeks ago. She denies fall, trauma, and unusual or new activities. She has had no previous problems with her back. The pain is midline in the upper lumbar area. It does not radiate to either leg, but it does extend to her anterior abdomen on both sides. It was initially sharp and severe, significantly limiting her activities for the first 4 or 5 days. Since then it has lessened somewhat, and she now describes it as a constant ache. It has affected her sleep, and she has been using acetaminophen regularly for the past 2 weeks with some relief. She denies fever, dysuria, hematuria, changes in bowel or bladder function, or incontinence. She has no lower-extremity weakness, pain, or numbness. The pain does not change with position.

Medical History

Mrs. M. has a long history of asthma, for which she has required five hospital admissions since childhood. Her last admission was 2 years ago. She is seen in the office for an exacerbation of her asthma approximately twice per year and has required short courses of oral prednisone every 1 to 2 years. Her asthma is well controlled with a combination of inhaled corticosteroid and long-acting β₂-agonist twice daily, with a short-acting β₂-agonist as needed for symptoms approximately once a week. She also has a history of Parkinson's disease, which is treated with a dopamine agonist. She is otherwise healthy and uses no other medications. She had a negative mammogram 6 months ago and a normal colonoscopy within the past 5 years.

Evidence levels Ⓐ Randomized, controlled trials (RCTs), meta-analyses, well-designed systematic reviews of RCTs. Ⓑ Case-control or cohort studies, nonrandomized clinical trials, systematic reviews of studies other than RCTs, cross-sectional studies, retrospective studies, certain uncontrolled studies. Ⓒ Consensus statements, expert guidelines, usual practice, opinion.

Family History

Mrs. M.'s father died at age 75 of complications of diabetes. He had asthma as well. Her mother is age 92 and healthy except for obesity.

Social History

Mrs. M. has a significant smoking history of 60 pack-years. She was finally convinced to quit after her last hospitalization 2 years ago. She denies alcohol or drug use, and she only occasionally drinks caffeinated beverages. She lives with her husband of 55 years in a senior apartment complex.

Review of Systems

She is thin but denies changes in her appetite or weight. She has tremor and difficulty with ambulation initially in the morning, which improves after taking her Parkinson's medication. She has fallen twice in the past 6 months without injury. Aside from her back pain, she denies musculoskeletal complaints. Review of other systems is noncontributory.

Objective

Physical Examination

Mrs. M. appears to be a thin, healthy woman, sitting in a chair in no distress. She has some clear discomfort when moving about the examination room. Her temperature, pulse, and blood pressure are normal. Her weight is 98 pounds, which is unchanged from her last visit. Her height is 61 inches, which is 2 inches less than the last recorded height from 2 years ago. Head and neck, cardiovascular, and pulmonary examinations are normal. Abdominal examination reveals normally active bowel sounds with no tenderness, organomegaly, or mass. Her aorta is easily palpable, nontender, and not enlarged. She has normal femoral pulses. Inspection of her back reveals loss of lumbar lordosis and some mild thoracic kyphosis. She has no muscular atrophy. No significant tenderness or spasm is noted in the thoracic or lumbar paraspinal muscles. She has midline tenderness on palpation of the spine at the upper lumbar level. Her straight-leg raise shows no sign of radiculopathy. Her neurologic examination reveals minimally increased tone in all extremities, with mild cogwheel rigidity. She is slow to arise from her chair and has mild difficulty in initiating movement, but her gait is normal once she has started walking. She has some difficulty turning to climb onto the examination table. Lower-extremity strength, sensation, and deep tendon reflexes are normal with no Babinski sign.

Assessment

Mrs. M is a 72-year-old woman with asthma and Parkinson's disease with a 2-week history of midline back pain with no warning symptoms to suggest neurologic compromise or malignancy. She is tender over her upper lumbar spine and has lost 2 inches of height in the past 2 years.

Working Diagnosis

Spinal compression fracture secondary to osteoporosis.

Differential Diagnosis

Back pain is a common problem, usually resulting from muscular strain or osteoarthritis of the facet joints. More significant spinal causes of back pain include disc herniation, spondylolisthesis, spinal stenosis, infections (osteomyelitis or epidural infection), and malignancy. In an elderly patient, spinal stenosis with neurologic compromise and cancer must be seriously considered, but Mrs. M. has no "alarm" symptoms or signs to suggest the presence of these more serious causes of back pain.

Plan

Diagnostic

Plain films of her back show generalized osteopenia and the presence of a spinal compression fracture of the L2 vertebral body. Bone mineral density (dual-energy x-ray absorptiometry [DEXA]) scan reveals a T-score of -2.8 at the hip and -3.0 in the lumbar spine. The diagnosis of an osteoporotic spinal compression fracture is confirmed.

Therapeutic

She is prescribed calcium, vitamin D, and antiresorptive therapy with a once-weekly dose of a bisphosphonate. Additionally, she is started on daily nasal calcitonin to help with pain and advised to increase the dosage of acetaminophen to 1000 mg every 6 hours, if needed. Her Parkinson's regimen is adjusted to decrease her risk of falling.

Patient Education

The high risk of hip fracture from falling is stressed to Mrs. M. She is asked to use a cane, and the use of hip-protective padding is discussed. Interventions aimed at decreasing her risk of falling at home, such as removing throw rugs and installing shower handles, are suggested.

DISCUSSION

Vertebral fractures are the most common manifestation of osteoporosis (Genant et al., 1999 Ⓑ). This patient's pain is typical for spinal compression fracture, with its abrupt onset and its radiation to the anterior abdominal wall (the "girdle of pain"). Although vertebral fractures can cause significant and disabling pain in some patients, their larger significance is that they denote a threefold increase in the risk of the more serious osteoporotic hip fracture (Black et al., 1999🅑). Failure to diagnose the systemic disease of osteoporosis in a patient with a spinal compression fracture is common, occurring more than 60% of the time (Neuner et al., 2003🅑).

Osteoporosis is a disease characterized by decreased bone strength and increased risk of fracture. Whereas bone strength is affected by both bone density and bone quality, the latter factor, determined by the microarchitectural structure, is difficult to determine. Therefore the World Health Organization defines osteoporosis as a decrease in bone mineral density of more than 2.5 standard deviations below what would be expected for the average young white woman (a T-score of less than − 2.5). Approximately 7% of women older than 50 years meet this definition. A T-score between −1.0 and −2.5 is defined as osteopenia, and this occurs in 40% of women aged 50 and older (Siris et al., 2001 🅑). Osteoporosis results in approximately 1.3 million fractures (Consensus Development Conference, 1993🅒) and costs between $10 and $15 billion every year in the United States (National Institutes of Health, 2001🅒). Common sites for osteoporotic fractures include the vertebrae, the wrist, and the hip, with the majority of the morbidity, mortality, and cost resulting from hip fractures. Approximately one third of patients with hip fractures are unable to return to independent living, and 20% die within the first year (National Institutes of Health, 2001🅒).

Risk factors for osteoporosis can be divided into those that decrease peak bone mass and those that lead to accelerated bone loss. Peak bone mass is reached by the mid-30s. Genetic factors are the most important determinants of peak bone mass. Gender is an important factor, as women have lower peak bone mineral densities than men. Race also is an important factor, with African-American women achieving higher peak bone mass than whites. Environmental factors also play a role in determining peak bone mass. These factors include calcium and vitamin D intake, as well as activity level. Certain diseases, such as celiac disease, cystic fibrosis, and the female-athlete triad (amenorrhea, disordered eating, and osteoporosis) are risk factors for failure to achieve optimal peak bone mass. Factors known to accelerate bone loss include age, low levels of sex hormones, smoking, inactivity, low body weight, high caffeine intake, certain medical conditions (hyperthyroidism, diabetes, and inflammatory bowel disease), as well as certain medications (steroids, anxiolytics, anticonvulsants, and neuroleptics) (Cummings et al., 1995🅑). Finally, factors that increase the risk of falling will result in a higher incidence of fractures at any level of bone density, but this effect is especially important in

patients with osteoporosis. In our case, Mrs. M.'s risk factors for osteoporosis include her age, her race, her smoking history, and previous steroid use. Furthermore, her neurologic condition increases her risk of falling.

Screening for osteoporosis can be an effective strategy for decreasing the morbidity and mortality associated with fractures. Screening is generally considered to be beneficial when the target condition is common and carries significant morbidity or mortality, when a reasonably accurate and affordable screening test is available, and when treatment offers additional benefit when it is initiated during an early, asymptomatic stage of the disease. Although no studies have directly looked at the effect of screening, it is reasonably clear from the literature that treatment of patients identified as having high fracture risk can decrease this risk. The United States Preventive Services Task Force has evaluated the evidence related to screening and recommended that DEXA at the femoral neck be offered to all women age 65 and older, and to high-risk women between the ages of 60 and 65. Testing should not be repeated more often than every 2 years because of limitations in the precision of bone mineral density measurements, and no clear data exist to suggest at which age screening should be discontinued (United States Preventive Services Task Force, 2002🅑).

Strategies for the prevention and treatment of osteoporosis include modification of risk factors for bone loss and for falls, increase in physical activity, and the use of pharmacologic agents. If modifiable risk factors exist, these should be addressed. Patients should be advised to stop smoking and to limit caffeine intake. Medical conditions associated with increased bone loss should be controlled, and the use of medications that increase the risk of osteoporosis should be minimized. The use of external hip protectors to prevent fracture has been evaluated in several studies. A recent systematic review of this literature shows no benefit for the use of these devices in community-dwelling elderly patients at risk for falls and fractures. The reviewed studies give conflicting results regarding the benefit of these devices when used in nursing homes. Finally, compliance with use of these devices is poor (Parker et al., 2004🅐).

The effect of exercise on the prevention of osteoporosis has been evaluated in several studies. A Cochrane review of 18 randomized controlled trials concluded that aerobic, weight-bearing, and resistance exercises can have positive effects on bone mineral density. However, no data exist to show a decreased risk of fracture from any form of exercise (Boniauti et al., 2002🅐).

Pharmacologic agents commonly used for the prevention and treatment of osteoporosis include calcium with vitamin D, bisphosphonates, calcitonin, and hormone replacement therapy (HRT). Calcium and vitamin D are the most commonly used agents for the prevention of osteoporosis. Although their combined use has been shown to increase bone mineral density in several different populations, studies have shown only a modest trend toward decreasing fracture risk that did not reach statistical significance (Cranney et al., 2002Ⓐ). Calcium, 1200 to 1500 mg/day, and vitamin D, 400 IU/day, should be recommended for primary prevention of osteoporosis in all women. They are also used as adjuvant to other osteoporosis treatments but should not be used alone for the treatment of established osteoporosis.

Bisphosphonates have more high-quality evidence (Cranney et al., 2002Ⓐ) supporting their use in the prevention and treatment of osteoporosis than does any other category of drug. The use of bisphosphonates has been clearly shown to increase bone mineral density. Their effectiveness for prevention of fractures also has been shown. Alendronate has been shown to reduce the risk of both vertebral and nonvertebral fractures by approximately half, whereas risedronate decreases the risk of vertebral fractures by one third and the risk of nonvertebral fractures by one fourth. Bisphosphonates are the only agents that have direct evidence for a decrease in the risk of hip fractures in high-risk patients. The magnitude of the effect bisphosphonates have on fracture risk can be expressed by the number of patients who would need to be treated with the drugs for 2 years to prevent one fracture, also known as the number needed to treat (NNT). For low-risk patients, approximately 2000 patients would need to be treated to prevent one vertebral fracture. For high-risk patients (those with a previous fracture, or those with a bone mineral density less than −2.5), between 75 and 100 patients would need to be treated to prevent one vertebral fracture, and 25 to 50 patients would need to be treated to prevent one nonvertebral fracture. These NNTs are well within the range of what is commonly considered acceptable for pharmacologic therapy.

Some evidence exists for the effectiveness of calcitonin in the treatment of osteoporosis (Cranney et al., 2002Ⓐ). Calcitonin has been shown to increase bone mineral density in the wrist and spine. Studies also have shown a strong, but not statistically significant, trend toward increased bone density in the hip. The evidence for an actual decrease in fracture risk is less clear. Some, but not all, studies have shown a decrease in the risk of vertebral fractures, but no effect seems to exist on the risk for nonvertebral fractures, including fractures of the hip. Therefore, calcitonin is considered a second-line agent for the prevention and treatment of osteoporosis, usually used for patients for whom more effective bisphosphonates either fail or cannot be tolerated. In addition to preserving bone density, calcitonin can be used to decrease the pain resulting from a vertebral fracture.

Because of the significant decrease in bone mineral density in the first 10 years after menopause, HRT was once recommended as the primary means of preventing osteoporosis and fracture. Initial observational studies demonstrated a 50% reduction in vertebral fractures and a 25% to 50% reduction in hip fractures from HRT (Cranney et al., 2002Ⓐ). The Women's Health Initiative (Rossouw et al., 2002Ⓐ), the largest prospective clinical trial evaluating the risks and benefits of HRT, confirmed a 35% reduction in the risk of hip fractures. In this population at relatively low risk for fracture, this corresponded to an NNT of approximately 2000 over a 5-year period. However, because the study also showed that HRT resulted in an increased risk of cardiovascular disease and breast cancer, the long-term use of HRT for the prevention of osteoporosis and fractures is no longer recommended.

Material Available on Student Consult

Review Questions and Answers about Osteoporosis

REFERENCES

Black DM, Arden NK, Palermo L, et al. Prevalent vertebral deformities predict hip fractures and new vertebral deformities but not wrist fractures: Study of Osteoporotic Fractures Research Group. J Bone Miner Res 1999;14:821–828.Ⓑ

Bonaiuti D, Shea B, Iovine R, et al. Exercise for preventing and treating osteoporosis in postmenopausal women Cochrane Database Syst Rev 2002;CD000333Ⓐ

Consensus Development Conference. Diagnosis, prophylaxis, and treatment of osteoporosis. Am J Med 1993;94:646–650.Ⓒ

Cranney A, Guyatt G, Griffith L, et al. Summary of meta-analyses of therapies for postmenopausal osteoporosis. Endocr Rev 2002;23:570–578.Ⓐ

Cummings SR, Nevitt MC, Browner WS, et al. Risk factors for hip fractures in white women: Study of Osteoporotic Factures Research Group. N Engl J Med 1995;332:767–773.Ⓑ

Genant HK, Cooper C, Poor G, et al. Interim report and recommendations of the World Health Organization Task Force for Osteoporosis. Osteoporos Int 1999; 10:259–264.Ⓑ

Neuner J, Zimmer J, Hamel M. Diagnosis and treatment of osteoporosis in patients with vertebral compression fractures. J Am Geriatr Soc 2003;51:483–491.**Ⓑ**

National Institutes of Health (NIH). NIH Consensus Development Panel on osteoporosis prevention, diagnosis, and treatment. JAMA 2001;285:785–795.**Ⓑ**

Parker M, Gillespie L, Gillespie W. Hip protectors for preventing hip fractures in the elderly. Cochrane Database Syst Rev 2004;(3):CD001255.**Ⓐ**

Rossouw JE, Anderson GL, Prentice RL, et al. Risks and benefits of estrogen plus progestin in healthy postmenopausal women. JAMA 2002;288:321–333.**Ⓐ**

Siris E, Miller P, Barrett-Connor E, et al. Identification and fracture outcomes of undiagnosed low bone mineral density in postmenopausal women: Results from the National Osteoporosis Risk Assessment. JAMA 2001; 286:2815–2822.**Ⓑ**

United States Preventive Services Task Force. Screening for osteoporosis in postmenopausal women: Recommendations of the United States Preventive Services Task Force. Ann Intern Med 2002;137:526–528.**Ⓑ**

Chapter

81

Vaginal Discharge (Vulvovaginal Candidiasis)

Karl E. Miller

KEY POINTS

1. Vulvovaginal candidiasis usually presents with intense pruritus on the external and internal genitalia with a discharge that is thick cottage cheese–like in appearance.
2. The treatment for bacterial vaginosis includes both oral and intravaginal routes, which have similar cure rates.
3. The use of fluoroquinolones in the treatment of uncomplicated gonorrhea should be avoided in individuals that live in Asia, the Pacific Islands, and California.
4. Uncomplicated genital chlamydia can be treated either with a one-time, 1-g dose of azithromycin or with doxycycline, 100 mg twice daily for 7 days.
5. The Centers for Disease Control and Prevention recommends empiric treatment for pelvic inflammatory disease if the patient has cervical motion tenderness or uterine/adnexal tenderness and is at risk for sexually transmitted diseases.

INITIAL VISIT

Subjective

Patient Identification and Presenting Problem
Mrs. P. is a 45-year-old woman whose main complaint is a vaginal discharge for the past 3 weeks. She describes the discharge as thick, cottage cheese–like material. She also states that she is having severe itching on her external genitalia. Her last menstrual period was 3 weeks ago and was normal. She does complain of pain during intercourse but it occurs only during initial penetration. She denies any pelvic or abdominal pain. She also denies any fevers, chills, or sweats. She currently takes no medications or supplements and no recent antibiotics. She has been in a monogamous relationship for the last 25 years, and her partner has no symptoms and no known sexual contact outside of their relationship.

Medical History
She has had no prior medical illnesses or hospitalization other than for two pregnancies and a postpartum tubal ligation.

Evidence levels Ⓐ Randomized, controlled trials (RCTs), meta-analyses, well-designed systematic reviews of RCTs. **Ⓑ** Case-control or cohort studies, nonrandomized clinical trials, systematic reviews of studies other than RCTs, cross-sectional studies, retrospective studies, certain uncontrolled studies. **Ⓒ** Consensus statements, expert guidelines, usual practice, opinion.

Family History
Mother and father have type 2 diabetes.

Social History
She has been married for 23 years and works as an administrative assistant. She denies any alcohol, tobacco, or illicit drug use.

Review of Systems
Her only other complaint is increased urine output and excessive thirst over the last 6 months.

Objective

Her height is 5 feet 3 inches; her weight is 180 pounds, with a body mass index of 32. She is afebrile, and her vital signs are normal. Her abdomen is non-tender to palpation with no rebound or guarding, and no masses or organomegaly. Genital examination reveals an inflamed-appearing introitus, some minor swelling of the labia, and no lesions. Examination with a speculum finds a normal-appearing cervix with no discharge from the os; the posterior vaginal vault has a thick, cottage cheese–like discharge with no odor. A wet preparation and potassium hydroxide sample are performed. The bimanual examination reveals no tenderness or abnormalities.

Laboratory Tests
The pH of the discharge is 5.0, with budding yeast and hyphae noted on the potassium hydroxide portion of the slide. The wet preparation has epithelial cells present and no white blood cells (WBCs). The "whiff" test is negative.

Assessment

Vaginal discharge: vulvovaginal candidiasis.

Plan

The patient requests an oral agent, so fluconazole (Diflucan), 150 mg, one-time dose is prescribed. Her random blood sugar is 205.

Differential Diagnosis
1. *Vulvovaginal candidiasis.* This is the most likely diagnosis because the patient has external pruritus with erythema and swelling of the labia. The presence of the characteristic thick, cottage cheese–like discharge with no odor in the vaginal vault also supports this diagnosis. Budding yeast and hyphae on the potassium hydroxide portion of the slide, no other abnormalities on the wet preparation, and a vaginal pH between 4.5 and 5.5 make this the most likely diagnosis.
2. *Bacterial vaginosis.* The characteristic discharge in patients with bacterial vaginosis has an off-white appearance and is adherent to the vaginal wall. The discharge usually does not cause any external symptoms. Other findings include clue cells present microscopically, a vaginal pH greater than 4.5, and a positive "whiff" test when potassium hydroxide is added to the sample of the discharge.
3. *Trichomoniasis.* This organism causes a thin, frothy, green-yellow or gray malodorous vaginal discharge. Dyspareunia or vaginal soreness may be present. The cervix has a "strawberry" red appearance, or some erythema of the vagina or external genitalia may be seen. The laboratory findings include a vaginal pH of more than 5.0, more than 10 WBCs per high-power field, and mobile trichomonads on the wet preparation.
4. *Chlamydia and gonorrhea.* Any time a female patient has a vaginal discharge during her reproductive years, these two infections must be considered. Risk factors for these infections include being younger than 25, history of multiple sexual partners, previous sexually transmitted diseases (STDs), and nonbarrier contraception. The discharge is mucopurulent and comes from the cervical os.
5. *Pelvic inflammatory disease (PID).* Because this infection can have such a negative long-term impact on women, it should be considered in women in their reproductive years who have vaginal discharge. The history and physical examination were not consistent with what would be expected in patients with PID.

DISCUSSION

The accurate diagnosis of vaginal discharge is based on signs, symptoms, and microscopic examination of the discharge. The presence of pruritus, the odor of the discharge, and presence of inflammation provide information that can assist in establishing the correct diagnosis. Office microscopy provides the most accurate laboratory test (Anderson et al., 2004 Ⓑ).

Vulvovaginal Candidiasis

Vulvovaginal candidiasis is one of the most common causes of vaginitis; *Candida albicans* is the most common etiologic agent, but infections also can result from *C. tropicalis* or *C. glabrata.* This form of vaginal discharge usually is first seen with intense pruritus on the external and internal genitalia. The discharge characteristics are odorless, thick, cottage cheese–like appearance. Risk factors for developing vulvovaginal candidiasis include recent antibiotic use, oral contraception use, pregnancy, receptive oral sex, diabetes mellitus, or a partner with candidiasis.

Physical examination usually reveals erythema and edema of the vulvovaginal area. The speculum examination reveals a normal-appearing cervix with a thick, cottage cheese–like discharge present in the vaginal vault. The discharge has a pH of 4.5 to 5.5, and the microscopic examination shows budding yeast or hyphae after applying potassium hydroxide to the slide.

Some treatment regimens for vulvovaginal candidiasis are available over the counter. In some instances with a potential for resistant infections, the use of terconazole (Terazol) in a 3- or 7-day intravaginal course may improve the cure rate. Fluconazole (Diflucan), 150 mg orally, in one dose, is available to treat vulvovaginal candidiasis. Oral and vaginal treatments have similar cure rates, with more side effects with the oral regimens (Watson et al., 2002Ⓐ).

Complicated vulvovaginal candidiasis is defined as four or more infections during 1 year. In these cases, the intravaginal treatment should be expanded to 10 to 14 days. If oral fluconazole is used, a repeated tablet must be given 3 days after the initial dose. This regimen for fluconazole also can be used in women with severe infections.

Women with recurrent infections of vulvovaginal candidiasis must be assessed for underlying causes. This may include a screen for glucose intolerance or for immunocompromise, such as human immunodeficiency virus testing.

Bacterial Vaginosis

Bacterial vaginosis develops when the normal flora of the vagina is replaced with high concentrations of anaerobic bacteria. This is one of the most common causes of vaginal discharge. Most women will be seen initially with a malodorous vaginal discharge, but approximately half will be asymptomatic.

The Centers for Disease Control and Prevention (CDC) established criteria for the diagnosis of bacterial vaginosis (Workowski and Levine, 2002 Ⓐ) (Box 81-1). Clue cells are epithelial cells that are coated with bacteria. The "whiff" test is performed by adding 10% potassium hydroxide to the vaginal secretion. A positive test is the emission of a fishy odor. Cultures of the vaginal discharge are not needed because they are not specific and do not usually assist establishing the diagnosis. A DNA probe tests for high concentrations of *Gardnerella vaginalis*.

The CDC recommends a different treatment regimen for bacterial vaginosis than that used for vulvovaginal candidiasis (Workowski and Levine, 2002Ⓐ) (Box 81-2). Both oral and intravaginal regimens provide similar cure rates (Hanson et al., 2000Ⓐ). Patients taking metronidazole should be advised to avoid alcohol consumption during treatment and for 24 hours after completing the course. Clindamycin cream is oil based and has the potential to weaken latex condoms and diaphragms.

Box 81-1	Criteria for the Diagnosis of Bacterial Vaginosis

Homogeneous, white noninflammatory vaginal discharge
Discharge coats vaginal wall
Clue cells present on microscopic examination
Vaginal fluid pH, >4.5
Positive "whiff" test

Adapted from Workowski KA, Levine WC. Sexually transmitted diseases treatment guidelines 2002: Centers for Disease Control and Prevention. MMWR Morb Mortal Wkly Rep 2002;51:1–80.

Bacterial vaginosis has been shown to cause adverse outcomes in women who are pregnant. These include premature rupture of membranes, preterm labor, preterm birth, and postpartum endometritis. The treatment of bacterial vaginosis during pregnancy has had inconsistent outcomes. The CDC currently recommends that women who are at high risk for preterm delivery should be treated (Workowski and Levine, 2002Ⓐ). Both metronidazole and clindamycin can be used during pregnancy.

Chlamydia Infection

More than 800,000 new cases of *Chlamydia trachomatis* infections were reported in 2002. The majority of the time, women with *Chlamydia* infec-

---

Box 81-2	Treatment Recommendations for Bacterial Vaginosis

Recommended Regimens

Metronidazole (Flagy l), 500 mg orally, twice per day for 7 days
Metronidazole gel, 0.75%, one applicator intravaginal, once per day for 5 days
Clindamycin (cleocin) cream 2%, one applicator intravaginally at bedtime for 7 days

Alternative Regimens

Metronidazole, 2 g orally, in a one-time dose
Clindamycin, 300 mg orally, twice per day for 7 days
Clindamycin ovules, 100 g intravaginally once at bedtime for 3 days

Adapted from Workowski KA, Levine WC. Sexually transmitted diseases treatment guidelines 2002: Centers for Disease Control and Prevention. MMWR Morb Mortal Wkly Rep 2002;51:1–80.

tions have no or minimal symptoms, but in some cases, the infection will ascend the genitourinary tract and cause PID.

If women are symptomatic with *C. trachomatis* infections, the most common symptom is a mucoid vaginal discharge that has little or no odor. In addition, they can have vaginal bleeding or spotting, lower abdominal pain, and irregular or heavy menses. A rare presentation for this infection is pleuritic right upper quadrant abdominal pain with or without pelvic pain. The cervix will appear inflamed and will have a yellow or cloudy mucoid discharge from the os. The cervix tends be friable and bleeds easily. Chlamydia infections in the lower genital tract do not cause vaginitis.

Currently two techniques are available to detect *C. trachomatis* infections—culture and nonculture. Culture techniques are considered the gold standard but have been replaced in some instances by the nonculture techniques. The new nonculture technique is nucleic acid amplification tests (NAATs). These tests have good sensitivity and specificity when compared with cultures. NAAT techniques can be used to diagnose urogenital chlamydia by either an endocervical or a urine specimen.

Patients who have signs and symptoms suggestive of salpingitis or PID should be evaluated by a white blood cell count with a differential. In addition, a serum pregnancy test and pelvic ultrasound should be performed if ectopic pregnancy is a possibility.

The current recommended treatment according to the CDC for uncomplicated genital chlamydia infections includes azithromycin or doxycycline (Workowski and Levine, 2002Ⓐ) (Box 81-3). Both regimens are acceptable because they have similar cure rates and adverse effects (Lau and Qureshi, 2004Ⓐ). Azithromycin has the benefit of being able to provide the patient with the one-time dose in the office. For patients who may not be able to tolerate either azithromycin or doxycycline, the CDC has published alternative regimens (Workowski and Levine, 2002Ⓐ) (see Box 81-3).

The CDC currently does not recommend rescreening for chlamydia after completion of an antibiotic course unless the patient has persistent symptoms or is pregnant (Workowski and Levine, 2002Ⓐ). Because reinfection is a common problem, the CDC recommends that women with chlamydia infections should be rescreened 3 to 4 months after antibiotic completion. The CDC also recommends that women seen within 12 months after treatment who have not been screened should be reassessed for chlamydia infection.

Gonorrhea Infection

Neisseria gonorrhoeae is one of the more common STDs in the United States. The normal incubation time between exposure and infection is 3 to 5 days.

Box 81-3	**Treatment Regimens for Uncomplicated Urogenital *Chlamydia***

Recommended

Azithromycin (Zithromax), 1 g orally in a single dose
Doxycycline (Vibramycin), 100 mg, twice per day for 7 days

Alternative

Erythromycin base, 500 mg orally, 4 times per day for 7 days
Erythromycin ethylsuccinate, 800 mg orally, 4 times per day for 7 days
Ofloxacin (Floxin), 300 mg, twice per day for 7 days
Levofloxacin (Levaguin), 500 mg, once per day for 7 days

Adapted from Workowski KA, Levine WC. Sexually transmitted diseases treatment guidelines 2002: Centers for Disease Control and Prevention. MMWR Morb Mortal Wkly Rep 2002;51:1–80.

The most common site for gonococcal infections is the endocervix. Symptoms include vaginal discharge, dysuria, abnormal vaginal bleeding, or pelvic pain. The majority of women have few or no symptoms. The cervix on examination may appear normal or may be inflamed with a mucopurulent discharge from the os.

In addition to infecting the lower genital tract, gonorrhea also can develop at other sites, either through direct or contiguous spread or by dissemination through the bloodstream. These include anorectal gonorrhea, conjunctivitis, perihepatitis (Fitz-Hugh-Curtis syndrome), pharyngitis, and PID. Anorectal gonorrhea can result from direct sexual contact or contiguous spread from the vagina. Patients with this infection can be asymptomatic, have mild pruritus and mucoid discharge, or have severe proctitis. Pharyngeal gonorrhea is asymptomatic the majority of the time, but if symptoms are present, the patient tends to have a mild sore throat. Physical findings usually are an erythematous pharynx, but in some cases, an exudative pharyngitis with oral ulcers may be seen. Gonococcal conjunctivitis develops after direct contact and tends to have copious amounts of purulent secretions from the eye.

Left untreated, gonococcal infections can develop into a disseminated infection. This occurs in two stages, with the first being bacteremic, in which patients will have fever, chills, and typical skin lesions. The skin lesions develop on the volar aspect of the hands and plantar aspect of the feet, initially as small vesicles and then developing into pustules with a hemorrhagic base and central necrosis. During this stage, patients also will have joint stiffness and pain. The second stage is the septic arthritis stage, in which patients have a purulent synovial effusion more commonly occurring in the knees, ankles, and wrist.

There are two different methods for detecting *N. gonorrhoeae*—culture and nonculture. The new nonculture technique is NAAT, and in women with urogenital gonorrhea, NAAT can be performed on either endocervical or urine specimens.

Treatment recommendations by the CDC for uncomplicated gonococcal infections of the cervix, urethra, and rectum include oral and parenteral options (Workowski and Levine, 2002Ⓐ) (Box 81-4). Because of the increase in the incidence of fluoroquinalone-resistant *N. gonorrhoeae* in individuals who live in Asia, the Pacific Islands (including Hawaii), and in California, the CDC recommends that fluoroquinalones should not be used. A substantial increase of fluoroquinalone-resistant *N. gonorrhoeae* has been seen in men who have sex with men, so fluoroquinalones should not be used as first-line treatment in these cases (CDC, 2004Ⓐ).

Patients with suspected disseminated gonococcal infections should be hospitalized for their initial parenteral treatment. Parenteral antibiotics should be continued for 24 to 48 hours after clinical improvement begins and then switched to oral regimens for at least 1 week (Workowski and Levine, 2002Ⓐ) (see Box 81-4).

Pelvic Inflammatory Disease

In women with infections in the lower genital tract, an ascending infection may cause acute salpingitis with or without endometritis, also known as PID. Symptoms tend to have a subacute onset and usually develop during menses or the first 2 weeks of the menstrual cycle. Symptoms may range from none to severe abdominal pain with high fevers. Other symptoms include dyspareunia, prolonged menses, and intramenstrual bleeding. Women in whom PID develops have significant increase in the risk for developing infertility.

The CDC recommends that physicians maintain a low threshold for diagnosing PID (Workowski and Levine, 2002Ⓐ). It recommends empiric treatment in women at risk for STDs if they have any of the minimal criteria (Box 81-5). Additional and specific criteria to assist physicians in establishing the diagnosis of PID have been published (see Box 81-5).

A patient with PID can be treated as an outpatient if the patient does not meet any of the criteria for hospitalization (Workowski and Levine, 2002Ⓐ) (Box 81-6). The options for outpatient treatment include two regimens that are equally efficacious with regard to cure rates (Table 81-1). If patients with PID meet any of the criteria for hospitalization, parenteral antibiotic therapy is indicated.

Trichomoniasis

The protozoan *Trichomonas vaginalis* is the etiologic agent for trichomoniasis, which is considered an STD. The incubation period is 3 to 21 days after exposure. Women with a history of multiple sex partners or sexual activity, or who are currently pregnant or menopausal, are at increased risk for this infection.

The majority of women with trichomoniasis have no symptoms. If symptoms are present, they include a diffuse, malodorous, yellow-green vaginal discharge, vaginal soreness, and dyspareunia. Because the vaginal pH changes around the time of menses, women are at risk for trichomoniasis developing during that period. The discharge may start during or immediately after menses and may be exacerbated during this time.

Box 81-4	Treatment Guidelines for Uncomplicated Gonococcal Infections

Uncomplicated

Cefixime (Suprax), 400 mg orally, as a single dose
Ceftriaxone (Rocephin), 125 mg IM, as a single dose
Ciprofloxacin (Cipro), 500 mg orally, as a single dose
Levofloxacin (Levaguin), 250 mg orally, as a single dose
Ofloxacin (Floxin), 500 mg orally, as a single dose

Disseminated

Recommended parenteral
    Ceftriaxone, 1 g IM or IV, q24h
Alternative parenteral
    Cefotaxime (Claforan), 1 g IV, q8h
    Ciprofloxacin, 400 mg, q12h
    Ofloxacin, 400 mg IV, q12h
    Levofloxacin, 250 mg IV, daily
    Spectinomycin (Trobicin), 2 gm IM, q12h
Oral Regimen: Can be started 24–48 hr after improvement begins, and ≥1 week of antimicrobial therapy must be completed
    Cefixime, 400 mg, twice daily
    Ciprofloxacin, 500 mg, twice daily
    Ofloxacin, 400 mg, twice daily
    Levofloxacin, 500 mg, once daily

Adapted from Workowski KA, Levine WC. Sexually transmitted diseases treatment guidelines 2002: Centers for Disease Control and Prevention. MMWR Morb Mortal Wkly Rep 2002;51:1–80.

Box 81-5	Diagnostic Criteria for Pelvic Inflammatory Disease

Minimum Criteria

Cervical motion tenderness or
Uterine/adnexal tenderness

Additional Criteria

Abnormal cervical or vaginal mucopurulent
  discharge
Documentation of gonorrhea or chlamydia
  infection
Elevated C-reactive protein
Elevated erythrocyte sedimentation rate
Oral temperature >38.3°C (>101°F)
White blood cells present on saline
  preparation of vaginal secretions

Specific Criteria

Endometrial biopsy with evidence of endometritis
Laproscopic abnormalities consistent with
  pelvic inflammatory disease
Transvaginal ultrasound or MRI showing
  thickened, fluid-filled tubes with or without
  free pelvic fluid or tubo-ovarian complex

Adapted from Workowski KA, Levine WC. Sexually transmitted diseases treatment guidelines 2002: Centers for Disease Control and Prevention. MMWR Morb Mortal Wkly Rep 2002;51:1–80.

Box 81-6	Hospitalization Criteria for Pelvic Inflammatory Disease

Unresponsive to oral antimicrobial therapy
Pregnancy
Severe illness (i.e., nausea, vomiting or high
  fever)
Surgical emergencies cannot be excluded
Tubo-ovarian abscess present
Unable to follow or tolerate outpatient oral
  regimen

Adapted from Workowski KA, Levine WC. Sexually transmitted diseases treatment guidelines 2002: Centers for Disease Control and Prevention. MMWR Morb Mortal Wkly Rep 2002;51:1–80.

Physical findings consistent with trichomoniasis include a copious vaginal discharge that is yellow-green or gray, frothy, and malodorous. The cervix can be inflamed and have a "strawberry" appearance, red and inflamed with punctations. The vaginal pH will be 5 or greater, and on microscopic examination, 10 white blood cells per high-power field will be seen, with mobile trichomonads. Cultures are indicated only when the diagnosis of trichomoniasis is uncertain.

The current CDC treatment recommendation is metronidazole, 2 g, in a single dose (Workowski and Levine, 2002 Ⓐ). For those who cannot tolerate the one-time dose, the alternative is metronidazole, 500 mg, twice a day for 7 days. Follow-up after treatment is not necessary unless symptoms persist. If the infection persists or recurs, the recommendation is to treat with metronidazole, 500 mg twice per day, for 5 days. Those who experience treatment failure

Table 81-1	PID Treatment Regimens	
Parenteral	Cefotetan (Cefotan), 2 g IV, q12h	
	or	
	Cefoxitin (Mefoxin), 2 g IV, q6h	
	and	
	Doxycycline (Vibramycin) 100 mg orally or IV, q12h	
Oral Regimen A	Ofloxacin (Floxin), 400 mg orally, twice daily	
	or	
	Levofloxacin (Levaquin), 500 mg, once daily	
	with or without	
	Metronidazole (Flagyl), 500 mg, bid	
Oral Regimen B	Ceftriaxone (Rocephin), 250 mg IM, in a single dose	
	or	
	Cefoxitin (Mefoxin), 2 g IM, plus Probenecid, 1 g orally, in a single dose	
	and	
	Doxycycline, 100 mg orally, twice daily	
	with or without	
	Metronidazole, 500 mg, twice daily	

All oral regimens must be given for 14 days.
Adapted from Workowski KA, Levine WC. Sexually transmitted diseases treatment guidelines 2002: Centers for Disease Control and Prevention. MMWR Morb Mortal Wkly Rep 2002;51:1–80.

after this course should be given metronidazole, 2 g orally, once per day for 3 days. Because this is an STD, it is important to treat the patient's partner (Forna, and Gulmezoglu, 2003 Ⓐ).

REFERENCES

Anderson MR, Klink K, Cohrssen A. Evaluation of vaginal complaints. JAMA 2004;291:1368–1379. Ⓑ

Centers for Disease Control and Prevention. Increases in fluoroquinalone-resistant *Neisseria gonorrhoeae* among men who have sex with men: United States, 2003, and revised recommendations for gonorrhea treatment, 2004. MMWR Morb Mortal Wkly Rep 2004;53: 335–338. Ⓐ

Forna F, Gulmezoglu AM. Intervention for treating trichomoniasis in women. Cochrane Database Syst Rev 2003;CD000218. Ⓐ

Hanson JM, McGregor JA, Hillier SL, et al. Metronidazole for bacterial vaginosis: A comparison of vaginal gel vs. oral therapy. J Reprod Med 2000;45:889–896. Ⓐ

Lau CY, Qureshi AK. Azithromycin versus doxycycline for genital chlamydia infections: A meta-analysis of randomized clinical trials (structured abstract). In The Cochrane Library, Issue 2, 2004. DARE 2002217. Ⓐ

Watson MC, Grimshaw JM, Bond CM, Mollison J, Ludbrook A. Oral versus intra-vaginal imidazole and triazole anti-fungal agent for the treatment of uncomplicated vulvovaginal candidiasis (thrush): A systematic review. Br J Obstet Gynecol 2002;109:85–95. Ⓐ

Workowski KA, Levine WC. Sexually transmitted diseases treatment guidelines 2002: Centers for Disease Control and Prevention. MMWR Morb Mortal Wkly Rep 2002;51:1–80. Ⓐ

Chapter

82
Lower Abdominal Pain (Pelvic Inflammatory Disease)

Ann M. Aring

KEY POINTS

1. Failure to isolate a sexually transmitted agent from the cervix does not rule out pelvic inflammatory disease (PID). PID is a polymicrobial infection whose causative agents may include gram-positive and gram-negative anaerobic organisms, gram-positive and gram-negative rods, and cocci, as well as sexually transmitted pathogens such as *Chlamydia trachomatis* and *Neisseria gonorrhoeae*.

2. A high index of suspicion is essential for diagnosing PID. No single physical examination finding can be used to suggest PID. No individual blood test or combination of blood tests can reliably diagnose PID.

3. According to the 2002 guidelines from the Centers for Disease Control and Prevention, empirical treatment of PID should be initiated in sexually active women if the following minimum criteria are present and no other cause for the illness can be identified: uterine/adnexal tenderness or cervical motion tenderness.

4. The recommended drug regimens for the treatment of PID require two or more agents. The data are insufficient to recommend azithromycin in the treatment of PID.

5. Fertility is better preserved when patients are treated within 48 hours of symptom onset.

Evidence levels Ⓐ Randomized, controlled trials (RCTs), meta-analyses, well-designed systematic reviews of RCTs. Ⓑ Case-control or cohort studies, nonrandomized clinical trials, systematic reviews of studies other than RCTs, cross-sectional studies, retrospective studies, certain uncontrolled studies. Ⓒ Consensus statements, expert guidelines, usual practice, opinion.

INITIAL VISIT

Subjective

Patient Identification and Presenting Problem

Gabrielle W. is a 19-year-old white teenager who presents to the clinic reporting lower abdominal pain for 1 week. Her last menstrual period occurred 3 weeks ago.

Medical History

Ms. W. entered menarche at age 12. Her menses are regular, with 28- to 30-day cycles. Her age at first intercourse was 15 years. She had her first baby at age 16 years and a second baby at age 18. Cultures for *Chlamydia* were positive during both pregnancies. The infections were treated successfully, with two documented negative cultures for cure. She delivered vaginally at term with both pregnancies. She did not breast-feed or use contraceptives. Her surgical history includes the removal of four impacted wisdom teeth last year. She does not have any chronic medical problems and does not take any prescription medications.

Family History

Ms. W.'s mother has type 2 diabetes mellitus and hypertension, and underwent a hysterectomy for cervical cancer. Her father has type 2 diabetes and hypercholesterolemia. She has three sisters and one brother, who are all healthy. There is no family history of breast cancer or colon cancer. Ms. W.'s children are healthy.

Health Habits

Ms. W. started smoking at age 14. She currently smokes half a pack of cigarettes daily. She also reports weekly marijuana use "to relax." She drinks one to two beers each week. Ms. W. estimates that she has had more than 30 lifetime sexual partners. She has had three sexual partners within the past month. She does not use condoms.

Social History

Ms. W. lives with her mother, three younger siblings, and her own two children. She dropped out of high school but did earn her GED certificate. She is currently unemployed. She enjoys spending time with her friends and watching television.

Review of Systems

Ms. W. reports pelvic pain, dyspareunia, vaginal discharge, and low-grade fever. She denies abnormal vaginal bleeding, dysuria, nausea, vomiting, diarrhea, constipation, or back pain.

Objective

Physical Examination

Ms. W. is a well-developed, thin, older adolescent. Her blood pressure is 124/82, pulse is 72 and regular, weight is 130 pounds, and height is 5 feet 4 inches. Abdominal examination reveals normal bowel sounds, mild diffuse lower abdominal tenderness, no hepatosplenomegaly, no rebound, and no guarding. Gynecologic examination shows Tanner stage 5 external genitalia with several external genital warts noted, normal vaginal tissue, and a multiparous cervical os. A mucopurulent discharge is seen. The cervix is friable and bleeds easily with manipulation. Her uterus is anteverted and of normal size. She does have cervical motion tenderness. Adnexal examination reveals bilateral tenderness. Her rectal examination is normal, with a negative fecal occult blood test.

Assessment

Working Diagnosis

The working diagnosis is pelvic inflammatory disease (PID), most likely from a sexually transmitted disease (STD).

Differential Diagnosis

The differential diagnosis includes appendicitis, ovarian torsion, hemorrhagic or ruptured cyst, endometritis, irritable bowel syndrome, ectopic pregnancy, and PID (Box 82-1).

Discussion Pelvic inflammatory disease manifests with infection and inflammation of the upper female genital tract, including any combination of endometritis, salpingitis, tubo-ovarian abscess, and pelvic peritonitis (Centers for Disease Control and Prevention [CDC], 2002**C**). PID is a common condition that affects about 8% of women during their reproductive years (Ness et al., 2002**A**). Recent estimates from the CDC indicate that approximately 780,000 cases of acute PID are diagnosed annually in the United States (Beigi and Wisenfeld, 2003**B**). Several demographic, behavioral, and contraceptive factors are identified as risk factors for PID (Box 82-2).

Box 82-1	Differential Diagnosis of Pelvic Inflammatory Disease

Appendicitis
Ectopic pregnancy
Ovarian torsion
Hemorrhagic or ruptured ovarian cyst
Endometriosis
Irritable bowel syndrome

Box 82-2	**Risk Factors for Pelvic Inflammatory Disease**

Young age at first intercourse
Multiple sexual partners
Increased frequency of sexual intercourse
Prior history of PID
Sexually transmitted infection
No barrier contraceptive use

Adapted from Beigi RH, Wisenfeld HC. Pelvic inflammatory disease: New diagnostic criteria and treatment. Obstet Gynecol Clin North Am 2003;30: 777–793.

There is considerable overlap between the risk of acquiring an STD and the risk for PID. Women younger than age 25 years account for more than 75% of all cases of PID and have a 10 times greater incidence compared with older women (Peipert et al., 2000Ⓐ). Sexually active adolescents are more than three times more likely to have PID than women of similar activity who are 25 to 29 years old (CDC, 2002Ⓒ). Studies have also shown at least a twofold increase in the risk for PID with a history of prior tubal infection (Beigi and Wisenfeld, 2003Ⓑ). Physiologically, the risk of infection with PID is accelerated in adolescents by the columnar epithelium exposure found in the adolescent cervix and the greater permeability of the cervical mucous plug. The risk of acquiring PID from insertion of an intrauterine device (IUD) occurs primarily in the first 3 months after insertion (Beigi and Wisenfeld, 2003Ⓑ).

PID is thought to arise from an ascending infection of the female genital tract. PID is a polymicrobial infection whose causative agents may include gram-positive and gram-negative anaerobic organisms, gram-positive and gram-negative rods, and cocci, as well as sexually transmitted pathogens such as *C. trachomatis* and *N. gonorrhoeae*. Approximately two thirds of all proven cases of PID involve either *C. trachomatis* or *N. gonorrhoeae* (Beigi and Wisenfeld, 2003Ⓑ). Bacterial vaginosis–associated microflora are also identified in the upper genital tract in most cases of PID (Beigi and Wisenfeld, 2003 Ⓑ; CDC, 2002Ⓒ). Therefore, PID cannot be ruled out even if a sexually transmitted organism is not isolated.

Barrier contraception reduces the risk for PID because it protects against some cervical infections. Oral contraceptive users also have a lower risk for developing PID. This may be explained by the fact that there is a higher detection rate associated with oral contraceptive users and consequently earlier treatment (Beigi and Wisenfeld, 2003Ⓑ; Eschenbach et al., 1977Ⓑ).

Menses also may increase the risk of PID since retrograde flow may spread infection from the uterus to the fallopian tubes. Classically, gonococcal PID occurs within a week of the onset of menses (Eschenbach et al., 1977Ⓑ). The relationship between PID and douching has also been evaluated, with one study showing that twice as many women with PID had douched recently (Scholes et al., 1993 Ⓑ). The mechanical pressure of douching was postulated to contribute to upper genital tract infections. In addition, a change in the pH may also contribute to an environment that allows an infection to flourish.

Plan

Diagnostic

N. gonorrhoeae and *Chlamydia* cultures were obtained. KOH and wet prep slides showed 10 white blood cells (WBCs) per high power field. No trichomonas, buds, or hyphae were observed under the microscope. A urine pregnancy test was negative. A complete blood cell (CBC) count, erythrocyte sedimentation rate (ESR), and C-reactive protein (CRP) level were determined. In addition, Ms. W. was scheduled for pelvic computed tomography (CT).

Discussion The diagnosis of PID is often difficult to establish. A high index of suspicion is essential for optimizing patient outcomes. In the past, the CDC recommended diagnosis and treatment of women who met all three major criteria (lower abdominal tenderness, cervical motion tenderness, and bilateral adnexal tenderness) plus one of the minor supporting criteria (temperature >38.3°C [101°F] orally, mucopurulent cervicitis, elevated ESR or CRP level, documented cervical infection with *C. trachomatis* or *N. gonorrhoeae*, or the presence of an inflammatory mass on pelvic ultrasound) (CDC, 1998Ⓒ). Since many women with PID have subtle signs and symptoms, the 2002 guidelines are less stringent. The 2002 CDC guidelines state that empirical treatment of PID should be initiated in sexually active women if the following minimum criteria are present and no other cause for the illness can be identified: uterine/adnexal tenderness or cervical motion tenderness. A recent study showed that when the CDC's new criteria for diagnosing PID were used, the prevalence doubled and the incidence tripled (Risser et al., 2004Ⓑ).

PID is suggested in the patient's history by lower abdominal pain, fever, vaginal discharge, onset of symptoms after the menstrual cycle, and abnormal vaginal bleeding. No single finding on physical examination can be used to suggest PID. Many laboratory studies have been evaluated for their usefulness in predicting PID. The CDC makes no specific recommendation for the use of a specific blood test in the diagnosis of PID (CDC, 2002**C**).

No individual blood test or combination of blood tests can reliably diagnose PID (Hall et al., 2004**A**). Individual tests do not appear to significantly improve diagnostic accuracy (Hall et al., 2004**A**). The WBC count is a nonspecific indicator of infection and is elevated in less than half of women with PID (Beigi and Wisenfeld, 2003**B**). In addition, the ESR and CRP level have been studied in PID, with the CRP level having a slightly higher sensitivity and specificity (Beigi and Wisenfeld, 2003**B**). The absence of WBCs on a vaginal wet smear has a high negative predictive value (94.5%) (Beigi and Wisenfeld, 2003**B**; Peipert et al., 2000**A**). Three or more WBCs per high power field on a vaginal wet smear has a sensitivity of 87% to 91% (Beigi and Wisenfeld, 2003**B**; Yudin et al., 2003**B**). The combination of WBC count, CRP level, ESR, and vaginal WBCs can reliably exclude PID if results on all four tests are normal. Combining CRP and ESR is helpful in excluding PID (Hall et al., 2004**B**).

The definitive diagnosis of PID requires more invasive testing with transvaginal ultrasound (US), endometrial biopsy, or laparoscopy. US features consistent with PID include large, dilated fallopian tubes or the presence of a tubo-ovarian abscess. Pelvic US has been well studied in PID and is useful for identifying tubal and ovarian pathology. In one study, endovaginal US showing a thickened, fluid-filled fallopian tube with or without free pelvic fluid had a sensitivity of 85%, a specificity of 100%, and a predictive value above 95% for the diagnosis of endometritis (Boardman et al., 1997**B**). Another study reported that endovaginal US had a high specificity (97%) but a low sensitivity (32%) in the diagnosis of upper genital tract infection (Beigi and Wisenfeld, 2003**B**; Boardman et al., 1997**B**).

Endometrial biopsy is helpful for making a diagnosis of PID but has limited clinical use because of a delay in reading and reporting results. One published study showed that the presence of five or more neutrophils per 400 power field and one or more plasma cells per 120 power field had a sensitivity of 92% and a specificity of 87% for the prediction of upper genital tract microbial infection (Beigi and Wisenfeld, 2003**B**).

Clinical diagnosis has a positive predictive value of 65% to 90% compared with laparoscopy (CDC, 2002**C**; Hall et al., 2004**C**). Most experts agree that laparoscopy is still the gold standard for establishing the diagnosis of PID (Beigi and Wisenfeld, 2003**B**). Findings consistent with PID on laparoscopy include edema and erythema of the fallopian tubes, purulent exudate in the fallopian tubes, and peritubal adhesions. Because of cost and surgical risk, laparoscopy is not a practical screening tool. However, laparoscopy is an important technique when the diagnosis of PID is in question or when the patient

does not improve as expected. Although computed tomography is not specifically mentioned in the CDC guidelines, this imaging technique can also identify pathology consistent with PID.

Therapeutic

Ms. W. is started on ofloxacin (Floxin), 400 mg orally twice a day for 14 days, and metronidazole (Flagyl), 500 mg orally twice a day for 14 days.

Discussion A high index of suspicion and a low threshold for treatment are important for managing patients with PID. The CDC has established treatment guidelines for patients that provide broad-spectrum coverage. According to the CDC, all regimens should be effective against *N. gonorrhoeae* and *C. trachomatis*, and should also include coverage for anerobic organisms and gram-negative rods (CDC, 2002**C**). Because no single drug meets these requirements, the recommended drug regimens for the treatment of PID require two or more agents

Table 82-1	Oral Treatment of Pelvic Inflammatory Disease
Regimen A	**Regimen B**
Oflaxacin (Floxacin), 400 mg PO bid for 14 days	Ceftriaxone (Rocephin), 250 mg IM in a single dose
or	*or*
Levofloxacine (Levaquin), 500 mg PO qd for 14 days	Cefoxitin (Mefoxin), 2 g IM in a single dose, and
with or without	Probenecid, 1 g PO in a single concurrent dose
Metronidazole (Flagyl), 500 mg PO bid for 14 days	*or*
	Other parenteral third-generation cephalosporin (e.g., ceftizoxime [Cefizox] or cefotaxime [Claforan])
	plus
	Doxycycline (Vibramycin), 100 mg PO bid for 14 days
	with or without
	Metronidazole, 500 mg PO bid for 14 days

Adapted from CDC. 2002 guidelines for treatment of sexually transmitted diseases. MMWR Morb Mortal Wkly Rep 2002;51:48–52.

Table 82-2	Parenteral Treatment of Pelvic Inflammatory Disease
Regimen A	**Regimen B**
Cefotetan (Cefotan), 2 g IV q12h *or* Cefoxitin (Mefoxin), 2 g IV q6h *plus* Doxycycline (Vibramycin), 100 mg PO or IV q12h	Clindamycin (Cleocin), 900 mg IV q8h *plus* Gentamicin (Garamycin), loading dose IV or IM (2 mg/kg body weight), followed by a maintenance dose of 1.5 mg/kg q8h

Adapted from CDC. 2002 guidelines for treatment of sexually transmitted diseases. MMWR Morb Mortal Wkly Rep 2002;51:48–52.

(Tables 82-1 and 82-2). Several recent studies have evaluated the use of azithromycin (Zithromax) in the treatment of PID. However, the data are not sufficient to recommend azithromycin in the treatment of PID (CDC, 2002©). Results from the Pelvic Inflammatory Disease Evaluation and Clinical Health (PEACH) trial showed no difference in outcomes between inpatient and outpatient treatment in women with mild to moderate PID (Ness et al., 2002Ⓐ). Fertility is better preserved when patients are treated within 48 hours of symptom onset (Beigi and Wisenfeld, 2003Ⓑ; Hollie and Workowski, 2003Ⓑ).

Patient Education

The patient is counseled regarding safer sex practices, STDs, and the use of barrier contraceptives. Hepatitis B vaccination is offered, as well as syphilis and HIV testing. No douching is also discussed because douching may flush bacteria higher into the genital tract and mask the discharge that may signal a problem. The importance of a 48-hour follow-up visit to check the response to treatment is emphasized.

FOLLOW-UP VISIT

Subjective

Ms. W. returns for her follow-up visit in 2 days. She reports continuing lower abdominal pain, low-grade fever, and nausea. She has tried to take the oral antibiotics but cannot keep them down.

Objective

Physical Examination

Her blood pressure is 132/85 mm Hg, pulse is 100 and regular, and temperature is 38°C (100.5°F) (measured orally). She has moderate lower abdominal tenderness on palpation. No rebound tenderness is noted. She does have some involuntary guarding. Pelvic examination shows bilateral adnexal tenderness and cervical motion tenderness. Copious purulent discharge is seen in the vaginal vault.

Laboratory Tests

Cultures performed earlier for *N. gonorrhoeae* and *Chlamydia* are negative. A CBC count showed WBCs at 17.0 (normal, 4.5 to 11) with 66% neutrophils, 27% lymphocytes, 4% monocytes, and 2% eosinophils. Hemoglobin is 13.5 (normal, 12.0 to 16.0 g/dL), CRP is 12.0 (normal, 0 to 10.0 mg/L), and ESR is 18 (normal, 0 to 15 mm/hr). A hepatitis B screen was negative. Results of a rapid plasma reagin test and HIV test are also negative. The pelvic CT scan shows free fluid in the pelvis and dilated fallopian tubes bilaterally, which suggests PID (Figs. 82-1 to 82-3). The radiologist recommends pelvic US to better assess for PID.

Assessment and Plan

Since Ms. W. has nausea and vomiting and is unable to tolerate outpatient therapy, she is admitted to the hospital and started on cefoxitin (Mefoxin), 2 g intravenously (IV) every 6 hours, and doxycycline (Vibramycin), 100 mg IV every 12 hours. The pelvic US shows inflammation of the fallopian tubes, normal ovaries, and purulent peritoneal free fluid (Figs. 82-4 and 82-5), but no evidence of a tubo-ovarian abscess. Since Ms. W.'s condition is not responding clinically to treatment, laparoscopy is performed and shows a tubo-ovarian abscess and peritoneal free fluid (Figs. 82-6 and 82-7). The abscess is drained surgically.

Discussion

Close follow-up of outpatients within 24 to 48 hours after treatment is started is crucial. Patients who fail to improve after initiation of therapy require hospitalization, additional diagnostic testing to reconfirm the diagnosis, and possibly surgical intervention (Beigi and Wisenfeld, 2003Ⓑ; CDC, 2002©). Additional criteria for hospitalization include pregnancy, nausea and vomiting, tubo-ovarian abscess, and inability to tolerate outpatient therapy (Box 82-3). Women older than 35 years who are hospitalized with PID are more likely to have a complicated course (CDC, 2002©; Jamieson et al., 2000Ⓑ). Only

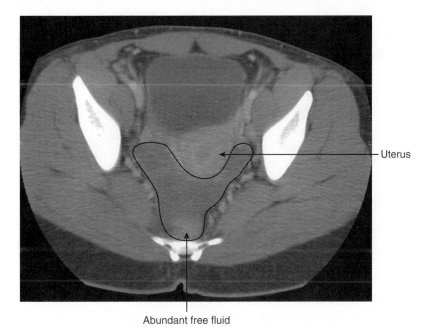

Figure 82-1 Pelvic CT scan showing abundant free fluid around the uterus.

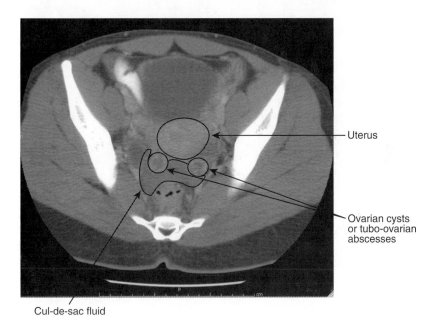

Figure 82-2 Pelvic CT scan shoping enlarged fallopian tubes and cul-de-sac fluid.

20% to 25% of PID patients treated in the United States are hospitalized (Hollie and Workowski, 2003❸).

Tubo-ovarian abscess (TOA) is a serious acute complication of PID and is estimated to occur in 33% of women hospitalized with acute PID (Beigi and Wisenfeld, 2003❸). Tubo-ovarian abscesses are also polymicrobial, with anaerobic organisms predominating. They may manifest with atypical abdominal pain, low-grade fevers, and weight loss.

Another acute complication of PID is perihepatitis (Fitz-Hugh-Curtis syndrome). The presenting

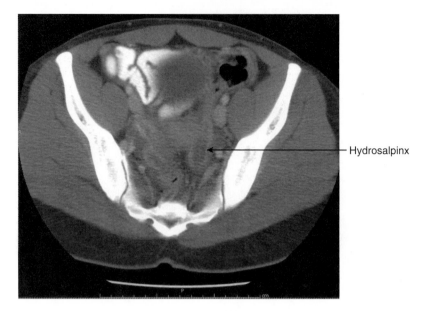

Figure 82-3 Pelvic CT scan showing hydrosalpinx.

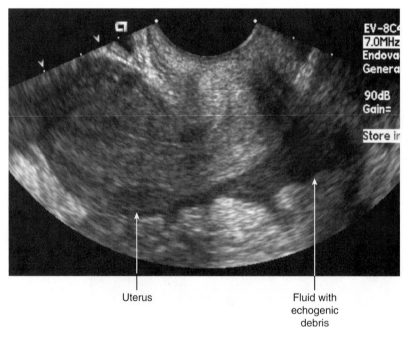

Figure 82-4 Longitudinal endovaginal pelvic ultrasound image showing the uterus and surrounding echogenic free fluid.

complaint is right upper quadrant pain, which is due to perihepatic inflammation and adhesions between the liver and anterior abdominal wall. Liver function test results may also be elevated. This complication is seen in 5% to 20% of all women with PID (Beigi and Wisenfeld, 2003❸). Characteristic stringlike adhesions are seen on laparoscopy.

The long-term sequelae of PID include tubal factor infertility, ectopic pregnancy, pelvic adhesions, and chronic pelvic pain. A study by Westrom

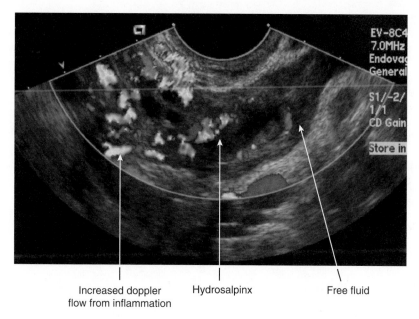

| Increased doppler | Hydrosalpinx | Free fluid |

Increased doppler flow from inflammation   Hydrosalpinx   Free fluid

Figure 82-5 Longitudinal endovaginal pelvic ultrasound image with increased Dopper flow from inflammation, hydrosalpinx, and free fluid.

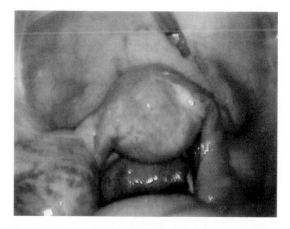

Figure 82-6 An enlarged fallopian tube corresponding to tubo-ovarian abscess was seen on laparoscopy.

(1980) showed a 10 times greater risk of infertility in women who had had PID compared with controls. In addition, the risk of infertility is directly related to the number of episodes of PID. With one episode of PID, a woman's risk of infertility is 11%. After two episodes, the risk rises to 34%, and with three or more episodes the risk rises to 54% (Hollie and Workowski, 2003Ⓑ). Scarring of the fallopian tubes also increases the risk for ectopic pregnancy, with a 7 to 10 times greater rate of ectopic pregnancy seen in women with a prior history of PID (Beigi and Wisenfeld, 2003Ⓑ). Rates of ectopic pregnancy also increase with successive episodes of PID. Increasing severity of infection also seems to predict a higher chance of ectopic pregnancy (Beigi and Wisenfeld, 2003Ⓑ). Scarring from PID can

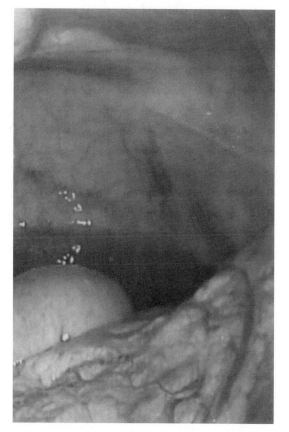

Figure 82-7 Abundant free fluid was also seen on laparoscopy.

Box 82-3	Criteria for Hospitalization for Pelvic Inflammatory Disease

Surgical emergencies such as appendicitis cannot be excluded

Pregnancy

No response to oral antibiotics

Unable to follow or tolerate oral antibiotic regimen

Nausea, vomiting, high fever, and severe illness

Tubo-ovarian abscess present

Adapted from CDC. 2002 guidelines for treatment of sexually transmitted diseases. MMWR Morb Mortal Wkly Rep 2002;51:48–52.

produce pelvic adhesions that may result in chronic pelvic pain. Approximately one third of women with PID develop chronic pelvic pain and associated depression, dyspareunia, postcoital pain, and vaginismus (Haggerty et al., 2003Ⓐ).

Material Available on Student Consult

Review Questions and Answers about Pelvic Inflammatory Disease

REFERENCES

Beigi RH, Wisenfeld HC. Pelvic inflammatory disease: New diagnostic criteria and treatment. Obstet Gynecol Clin North Am 2003;30:777–793.Ⓑ

Boardman LA, Peipert JF, Brody JM, et al. Endovaginal sonography for the diagnosis of upper genital tract infection. Obstet Gynecol 1997;90:54–57.Ⓑ

Centers for Disease Control and Prevention, 1998 guidelines for treatment of sexually transmitted diseases. MMWR Morb Mortal Wkly Rep 1998;47:1–116.Ⓒ

Centers for Disease Control and Prevention, 2002 guidelines for treatment of sexually transmitted diseases. MMWR Morb Mortal Wkly Rep 2002;51:48–52.Ⓒ

Eschenbach DA, Harnisch JP, Holnes KK. Pathogenesis of acute pelvic inflammatory disease: Role of contraception and other risk factors. Am J Obstet Gynecol 1977;128:838–850.Ⓑ

Haggerty CL, Schulz R, Ness RB. Lower quality of life among women with chronic pelvic pain after pelvic inflammatory disease. Obstet Gynecol 2003;102 (5 Pt 1):934–939.Ⓐ

Hall MN, Leach L, Beck E. Which blood tests are most helpful in evaluating pelvic inflammatory disease? J Fam Pract 2004;53:326, 330–331.Ⓐ

Hollie LM, Workowski K. Treatment of sexually transmitted diseases in women. Obstet Gynecol Clin North Am 2003;30:751–775.Ⓑ

Jamieson DJ, Duerr AM, Macasaet MA, et al. Risk factors for a complicated clinical course among women hospitalized with pelvic inflammatory disease. Infect Dis Obstet Gynecol 2000;8:88–93.Ⓑ

Ness RB, Soper DE, Holley RL, et al. Effectiveness of inpatient and outpatient treatment strategies for women with pelvic inflammatory disease: Results from the Pelvic Inflammatory Disease Evaluation and Clinical Health (PEACH) Randomized Trial. Am J Obstet Gynecol 2002;186:929–937.Ⓐ

Peipert JF, Ness RB, Soper DE, Bass B. Association of lower genital tract inflammation with objective evidence of endometritis. Infect Dis Obstet Gynecol 2000;8:83–87.Ⓐ

Risser WL, Cromwell PF, Bortot AT, Risser JMH. Impact of new diagnostic criteria on the prevalence and incidence of pelvic inflammatory disease. J Pediatr Adolesc Gynecol 2004;17:39–44.Ⓑ

Scholes D, Daling JR, Stergachis A, et al. Vaginal douching as risk factor for acute pelvic inflammatory disease. Obstet Gynecol 1993;81:601–606.Ⓑ

Westrom L. Incidence, prevalence, and trends of acute pelvic inflammatory disease and its consequences in industrialized countries. Am J Obstet Gynecol 1980; 138:880–892.

Yudin MH, Hillier SL, Wisenfeld, HD, et al. Vaginal polymorphonuclear leukocytes and bacterial vaginosis as markers for histologic endometritis among women without symptoms of pelvic inflammatory disease. Am J Obstet Gyencol 2003;188:318–323.Ⓑ

Chapter

83 Breast Cancer

Virginia D. Aguila

KEY POINTS

1. A new palpable mass in a patient with advanced age, a history of exposure to exogenous estrogen, a weak family history of breast cancer despite several annual negative mammograms and a clinical breast examination should increase our index of suspicion for malignancy.
2. Mammography and clinical breast examinations remain the cornerstone for the screening of breast cancer.
3. Minimally invasive breast biopsy (MIBB), the least surgical procedure, provided the patient with a diagnosis and tumor marker status and aided in treatment planning.
4. Sentinel node mapping, now the standard of care for axillary nodal status in patients with breast cancer, was positive; therefore, full axillary node dissection had to be done.
5. Accurate staging of cancer remains the most important factor in planning treatment and prognostication; therefore, early diagnosis is essential in patients with breast cancer.
6. The multidisciplinary approach done in this patient greatly enhanced the overall quality of care to the patient with breast cancer.
7. Vigilant surveillance is a must in follow-up of all patients with breast cancer.

INITIAL VISIT

Subjective

Patient Identification and Presenting Problem

Mrs. Rossalyn P., a 62-year-old white woman G4, P3, Ab1, comes into the clinic for her annual physical examination. She denies any complaints.

Medical History

Mrs. P. had menarche at age 11, first pregnancy at age 20, and last pregnancy at age 26. She used oral contraceptives from ages 27 to 35 and had a tubal ligation at age 35. She was menopausal at 53 and took Prempro for 5 years. At age 58, she underwent total abdominal hysterectomy with bilateral salpingo-oophorectomy with removal of large left benign ovarian mucinous cystadenoma. Subsequently, she was started on Premarin but discontinued use a year ago. She has yearly physical examinations and mammograms and performs monthly self-breast examinations. Last year's mammogram was normal. Other medical conditions include hypertension, hypercholesterolemia, type 2 diabetes mellitus, and asthma.

Medications

Enalapril, 20 mg; Pravachol, 40 mg; albuterol metered-dose inhaler as needed.

Family History

Her mother had lung cancer and uterine cancer. A maternal aunt was diagnosed with breast cancer at age 43. Her father died of a myocardial infarction at age 57.

Review of Systems

Unremarkable.

Objective

Physical Examination

Well-developed, well-nourished white female in no acute distress. Vital signs: weight, 205 pounds; height, 64.5 inches; blood pressure, 130/80; temperature, 98.1°F (36.7°C); pulse, 92; and RR, 18. Head, eyes, ears, nose, and throat: normal. Lungs: clear. Heart: regular rate and rhythm without murmurs or gallop. Breast examination: left breast reveals a 0.75-cm firm, nonmovable mass in the upper outer quadrant without notable tenderness, erythema, skin changes, nipple discharge, or induration; right breast normal. Abdominal examination: no palpable masses, no hepatosplenomegaly. Pelvic examination: normal external genital and vaginal vault, no pelvic masses or tenderness. Rectal examination: no masses, hemoccult negative. Neurologic examination: intact. Lymph nodes: axilla and supraclavicular nodes reveal no lymphadenopathy.

Assessment

Working Diagnosis

A new breast mass in a 62-year-old menopausal woman, after total abdominal hysterectomy with bilateral salpingo-oophorectomy with a weak family history of breast cancer on maternal side. Malignancy cannot be ruled out.

Differential Diagnosis

1. *Breast cancer* is commonly seen with advanced age and exogenous estrogen exposure. Most women with breast cancer do not have identifiable risk factors. Early findings include nontender, firm, ill-defined masses, whereas late findings include skin changes and lymph node involvement.
2. *Fibrocystic disease* is the most common disease of the breast, peaking before menopause and rarely seen before adolescence or after menopause. Fibrocystic disease includes several disease processes associated with risks for cancer development. These processes are divided into three broad categories: (1) nonproliferative lesions, (2) proliferative lesions without atypia, (3) atypical hyperplasia. The first category shows no increased risk of cancer development, whereas the second and third show a relative risk of 1.6% and 4.4%, respectively.
3. *Fibroadenoma,* the most common benign tumor of the breast in younger women, peaks in the late 20s and early 30s. The tumors are composed of fibrous and glandular tissue and do not increase the risk of breast cancer.
4. *Solitary intraductal papillomas,* occurring between the ages of 30 and 50, are papillary proliferations of epithelial cells in the main lactiferous duct. Patients often present with bloody nipple discharge and occasionally have a palpable mass that is smaller than 1 cm but that can be as large as 4 to 5 cm. These tumors rarely increase the patient's risk of developing breast cancer.
5. *Fat necrosis,* difficult to distinguish from cancer, both clinically and mammographically, is often associated with trauma, surgical intervention, or radiation therapy. Histologically, it consists of walled-off, lipid-laden macrophages, and neutrophils and can occur in the subareolar region.
6. *Duct ectasia,* commonly seen in the fifth and sixth decades of life, is a palpable mass characterized by dilation of subareolar ducts with debris accumulation and inflammation. It is often associated with thick, "cheesy" nipple secretion.
7. *Mammary abscess* is typically painful and erythematous, often associated with *Staphylococcus aureus.* It can clinically mimic inflammatory breast cancer.
8. *Granulomatous mastitis* accounts for fewer than 1% of all breast masses. It can be associated with sarcoidosis, Wegener's granulomatosis, or infectious agents like *Mycobacteria* or fungal organisms.
9. *Hematomas* can mimic carcinoma clinically and mammographically. They are most common post-traumatically.
10. Miscellaneous nonbreast tissue benign tumors include lipomas, leiomyomas, hemangiomas, and neurofibromas (Schnitt et al., 1991).

Plan

Diagnostic

Mrs. P. underwent mammography that showed a 1 × 1-cm irregular mass with indistinct margins in the outer upper quadrant of the left breast. Ultrasound imaging of the mass showed a 1.3 × 1.3-cm irregular, hypoechoic mass with posterior shadowing. The suspicious results of the mammogram and ultrasound were discussed with the patient, and she was referred for surgical consultation. The patient was seen in a multidisciplinary breast clinic that included the involvement of a surgical oncologist, diagnostic radiologist, medical oncologist, radiation oncologist, and social worker. An ultrasound-guided fine needle aspiration was done. The biopsy showed poorly differentiated infiltrating ductal adenocarcinoma. Simultaneously, vacuum-assisted core biopsy of the mass confirmed the same histopathologic findings. The tumor was estrogen receptor and progesterone receptor negative and negative for HER2/NEU.

Staging and Therapeutic

The patient underwent a left breast lumpectomy with sentinel node mapping. The sentinel node was identified and was positive for malignancy. A full axillary node dissection was performed. With the exception of the sentinel node, 21 axillary lymph nodes were negative for malignancy. The final staging of the tumor was T1C, N1, and M0. The patient underwent adjuvant chemotherapy with four cycles of epirubicin and Cytoxan, followed by radiation therapy for 6 weeks. Except for some nausea and vomiting with chemotherapy, the patient did well with this treatment.

DISCUSSION

Breast cancer remains the most common nonskin cancer in women in the United States, with its incidence continuing to increase since the 1980s (Fig. 83-1). The U.S. Breast Cancer Statistics 2004 showed 215,999 new cases of invasive cancer,

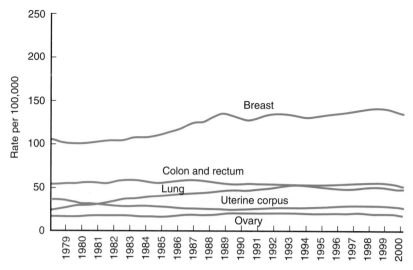

Figure 83-1 Cancer incidence rates for women in the United States, 1979–2000. Age-adjusted to the 2000 U.S. standard population. (From U.S. Surveillance Epidemology, 1970–2000.)

accounting for 32% of all cancer diagnoses in women, and 59,390 new cases of in situ breast cancers due to better screening (Jemal et al., 2004 ⊙). The lifetime probability that a woman will develop invasive breast cancer is 13.36%, that is, the illness will strike one in every seven women (Table 83-1). Despite the increase in incidence, there has been a decrease in mortality, with a mortality rate of 2.2% per year from 1990 to 2000, most likely due to earlier detection and improvement in the various treatment modalities now available (Fig. 83-2).

Breast cancer is a progressive, hormonally driven disease. It is extremely important that early diagnosis be made because early arrest can lead to

improved survival. Five-year survival rate for stage 0 is 99%, and for stage IV it is 14% (Table 83-2 and Fig. 83-3). Those with certain risk factors have a higher incidence (Box 83-1). A positive family history, regardless of paternal/maternal lineage, is present in less than 10% of women with breast cancer but remains an important risk factor. The presence of genetic gene mutation in BRCA1 and BRCA2 increases the risk *immensely* but accounts for only 5% to 10% of all diagnosed breast cancer (National Institutes of Health Consensus Development Panel, 2001 ⊙).

Mammography is currently the most valuable and important screening test for early detection. It is widely available, has more than 90% sensitivity, is inexpensive, and can detect two to six cancer cases per 1000 mammograms done. Limitations include very dense breasts, such as in young women, breast-feeding women, and those on hormone replacement therapy, for whom both sensitivity and specificity are reduced (Linver, 2005). Clinical breast examination by a physician is the other cornerstone for early detection. Many studies have shown that self-breast examination is not an effective screening tool (Mincey and Perez, 2004 ⊙). Current guidelines for screening are outlined in Box 83-2.

Ultrasonography should be used as an adjunct to mammography, detecting whether a lesion is solid or cystic, and can be used to further categorize the solid lesion. Generally recommended for women with very dense breasts, it has an overall lower sensitivity, especially in detecting calcifications and lower specificity than mammography (Smith et al., 2003 ⊙).

Magnetic resonance imaging of the breast, now available in many centers, is currently not recommended as a screening test because of expense and

Table 83-1	Lifetime Probability of Developing Cancer, by Site, U.S. Women, 1998–2000
Site	**Risk**
All sites	1 in 3
Breast	1 in 7
Lung and bronchus	1 in 17
Colon and rectum	1 in 18
Uterine corpus	1 in 38
Non-Hodgkin's lymphoma	1 in 57
Ovary	1 in 59
Pancreas	1 in 83
Melanoma	1 in 82
Urinary bladder	1 in 91
Uterine cervix	1 in 128

From DevCan. Probability of Developing or Dying of Cancer Software, Version 5.1. Statistical Research and Applications Branch. Available at http://srab.cancer.gov/devcan.

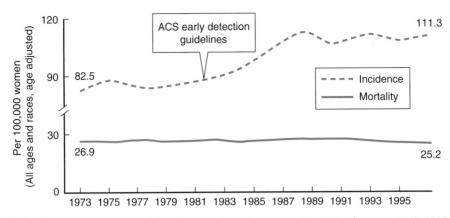

Figure 83-2 Rising incidence, falling mortality. Invasive breast cancer in the United States, 1973–1995. (From SEER Cancer Statistics Review, 1973–1995 [1998].)

Table 83-2 Breast Cancer Survival Rates

Stage	5-Year Relative Survival Rate
0	99%
I	92%
IIA	82%
IIB	65%
IIIA	47%
IIIB	44%
IV	14%

Data from National Cancer Institute SEER (Surveillance, Epidemiology, and End Results) Program, 2004. Available at http://seer.cancer.gov.

lack of both availability and physician expertise as compared to mammography (Smith et al., 2003⦿). More trials of this test are currently under way. Its use is mainly in high-risk patients or when mammograms with ultrasonographic results are inconclusive. Magnetic resonance imaging does not replace mammography as the preferred screening test for detecting breast cancer.

Diagnosis

Once an abnormality (i.e., a palpable mass, abnormal mammogram, abnormal ultrasound scan, abnormal magnetic resonance imaging scan) is found, a breast biopsy is performed. Seventy to 80% of breast biopsies are benign (Hall et al., 1988). Traditionally, a breast biopsy is done with open excisional biopsy, and if malignancy is found, definitive surgery is recommended and performed.

Excisional breast biopsies have been replaced with MIBBs. MIBBs include stereotactic biopsy, ultrasound-guided fine needle aspiration, and ultrasound-guided core biopsy. MIBB has 90% sensitivity and

100% specificity (Fuhrman et al., 1998⦿). Stereotactic biopsy is often used in calcifications, whereas ultrasound-guided biopsies, fine-needle aspirations, and core biopsies are used in most masses detectable by ultrasonography. With MIBBs, diagnosis and treatment planning can be done in advance of any surgical intervention, permitting all surgical treatment to be completed in a single surgical procedure.

Once the diagnosis of breast cancer is established, further treatment is discussed with the patient, family, and, ideally, a multidisciplinary team. Treatment will depend on the stage of the disease, age and general health of the patient, menopausal status, estrogen-receptor status, progesterone-receptor status, and presence of HER2/NEU gene amplication. The presence of estrogen receptor and/or progesterone receptor is a good prognostic indicator, but the presence of HER2/NEU is a negative prognostic factor (Lippman, 2005). Of all the above prognostic factors, the stage of the tumor, characterized by size, nodal involvement, and presence of distant metastasis, is most important in planning treatment and prognostication.

Staging

Currently, breast cancer staging uses the American Joint Committee on Cancer TNM system. This system classifies cancers based on their tumor size, nodal status, and metastases (Table 83-3 and Box 83-3). This classification has been refined with the use of sentinel node mapping. Sentinel node mapping has now become the standard of care in axillary staging of breast cancer. This is based on the concept that lymphatic spread to the axilla occurs in an orderly manner. The sentinel node is defined as the first lymph node to receive drainage from a breast cancer (Fig. 83-4). This is identified using a radioisotope tracer and blue dye using one of several protocols. The sentinel node is localized with an intraoperative gamma probe and identified by its blue color. If the sentinel node is nega-

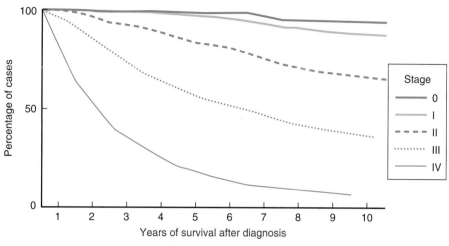

Figure 83-3 Survival by stage at diagnosis.

Box 83-1	Risk Factors for Breast Cancer Development

Advanced age
Family history of breast cancer (paternal or
    maternal risk)
Presence of genetic mutations (BRCA1, BRCA2)
Early menarche
Late menopause
Nulliparity
Absence of history of breast-feeding
Birth of first child after age 30

Data from American Cancer Society, 2005. Available
    at www.cancer.org.

Box 83-2	Screening Guidelines for the Early Detection of Breast Cancer, American Cancer Society, 2003

- Yearly mammograms are recommended starting at age 40 and continuing for as long as a woman is in good health.
- A clinical breast examination should be part of a periodic health examination, about every 3 years for women in their 20s and 30s, and every year for women 40 and older.
- Women should know how their breasts normally feel and report any breast changes promptly to their health care providers. Breast self-examination is an option for women starting in their 20s.
- Women at increased risk (e.g., family history, genetic tendency, past breast cancer) should talk with their doctors about the benefits and limitations of starting mammography screening earlier, having additional tests (i.e., breast ultrasound and Magnetic resonance imaging), or having more frequent examinations.

From Smith AR, Saslow D, Sawyer KA, et al. American Cancer Society guidelines for breast cancer screening: Update 2003. CA Cancer J Clin 2003;53:141–169

tive for malignancy, no further axillary dissection is needed. If the sentinel node is positive or not found, a full axillary node dissection is performed. This approach has significantly reduced the number of full axillary node dissections and long-term postoperative complications and morbidity, i.e., lymphedema and pain of involved upper extremity (Green et al., 2002©).

Treatment

Breast cancer is commonly treated by a combination of surgery, systemic therapy in the form of either chemotherapy and/or hormonal therapy, and radiotherapy.

Surgical Treatment

Breast conservation therapy (BCT) is preferred over the more deforming mastectomy. Multiple studies have shown that BCT provides survival rates similar to those of mastectomy. BCT offers the patient a cosmetically acceptable result and the psychological benefit that goes with it. Not all patients are candidates for BCT. Conditions that preclude BCT include multicentric breast tumors, patients requesting a mastectomy, tumors larger than 5 cm, and tumors

Table 83-3 Summary of Breast Cancer Stages

Stage	Description
Stage 0: Tis, N0, M0	Ductal carcinoma in situ (DCIS) is the earliest form of breast cancer. In DCIS, cancer cells are located within a duct and have not invaded the surrounding fatty breast tissue, or lobular carcinoma in situ (LCIS), which is sometimes classified as stage 0 breast cancer, but most oncologists believe it is not a true breast cancer. In LCIS, abnormal cells grow within the lobules or milk-producing glands, but they do not penetrate through the wall of these lobules or is Paget's disease of the nipple. In all cases, the cancer has not spread to lymph nodes or distant sites.
Stage I: T1, N0, M0	The tumor is ≤2 cm (~4/5 inch) in diameter and has not spread to lymph nodes or distant sites.
Stage IIA: T0, N1, M0/T1, N1, M0/T2, N0, M0	No tumor is found in the breast but it is in one to three axillary lymph nodes, or the tumor is <2 cm and has spread to one to three axillary lymph nodes or found by sentinel node biopsy as microscopic disease in internal mammary nodes but not on imaging studies or by clinical examination, or the tumor is >2 cm in diameter and <5 cm but has not spread to axillary nodes. The cancer has not spread to distant sites.
Stage IIB: T2, N1, M0/T3, N0, M0	The tumor is >2 cm in diameter and <5 cm and has spread to one to three axillary lymph nodes or found by sentinel node biopsy as microscopic disease in internal mammary nodes, or the tumor is >5 cm and does not grow into the chest wall and has not spread to lymph nodes. The cancer has not spread to distant sites.
Stage IIIA: T0–2, N2, M0/T3, N1–2, M0	The tumor is <5 cm in diameter and has spread to four to nine axillary lymph nodes, or found by imaging studes or clinical examination to have spread to internal mammary nodes, or the tumor is >5 cm and has spread to one to nine axillary nodes or to internal mammary nodes. The cancer has not spread to distant sites.
Stage IIIB: T4, N0–2, M0	The tumor has grown into the chest wall or skin and may have spread to no lymph nodes or as many as nine axillary nodes. It may or may not have spread to internal mammary nodes. The cancer has not spread to distant sites.
Stage IIIC: T0–4, N3, M0	The tumor is any size, has spread to ≥10 nodes in the axilla or to one or more lymph nodes under the clavicle (infraclavicular) or above the clavicle (supraclavicular) or to internal mammary lymph nodes, which are enlarged because of the cancer. All these are on the same side as the breast cancer. The cancer has not spread to distant sites.
Inflammatory breast cancer	Classified as stage III, unless it has spread to distant organs or lymph nodes that are not near the breast, in which case it would be stage IV.
Stage IV: T0–4, N0–3, M1	The cancer, regardless of its size, has spread to distant organs such as bone, liver, or lung, or to lymph nodes far from the breast.

Data from American Cancer Society, 2005. Available at www.cancer.org.

involving the nipple areola complex and persistent positive margins. If a mastectomy is chosen, the most common type is the modified radical mastectomy with or without breast reconstruction using implants or autogenous tissue. Frequently, both procedures can be done at the same time. BCT is always followed by radiation therapy (Mincey and Perez, 2004☻; Lippman, 2005).

Adjuvant Systemic Therapy

This includes chemotherapy and/or hormonal therapy. The treatment goal is prevention of recurrence and increased survival.

Hormonal Therapy For postmenopausal women, hormonal adjuvant therapy for invasive breast cancer that is estrogen and/or progesterone receptor positive is 5 years of therapy with tamoxifen, an estrogen receptor antagonist. A new form of hormonal ablation is aromatase inhibitors. These work by inhibiting aromatase, the enzyme responsible for the conversion of androstenedione to estrone and testosterone to estradiol in the adrenal gland. Hormonal ablation is the most powerful adjuvant therapy available today.

Chemotherapy Combination chemotherapy is recommended for invasive breast cancer in premenopausal

Box 83-3	The 2002 American Joint Committee on Cancer TNM System

The most common system used to describe the stages of cancers is the American Joint Committee on Cancer TNM system. This staging system classifies cancers based on their T, N, and M stages:

- **T** stands for **tumor** (its size and how far it has spread within the breast and to nearby organs).
- **N** stands for spread to lymph **nodes** (bean-shaped collections of immune system cells that help fight infections and cancers).
- **M** is for **metastasis** (spread to distant organs).

The approach to staging used here is based on the findings after surgery, when the pathologist has looked at the breast mass and lymph nodes (the pathologic stage).

Additional letters or numbers appear after T, N, and M to provide more details about the tumor, lymph nodes, and metastasis:

- The letter T followed by a number from 0 to 4 describes the tumor's size and spread to the skin or chest wall under the breast. Higher T numbers indicate a larger tumor and/or wider spread to tissues near the breast.
- The letter N followed by a number from 0 to 3 indicates whether the cancer has spread to lymph nodes near the breast and, if so, how many lymph nodes are affected.
- The letter M followed by a 0 or 1 indicates whether the cancer has spread to distant organs, for example, the lungs or bones, or to lymph nodes that are not next to the breast, such as those above the collarbone.

Once the T, N, and M categories have been determined, this information is combined in a process called stage grouping to determine your disease stage. This is expressed as stage 0 and in Roman numerals from stage I (the least advanced stage) to stage IV (the most advanced stage).

Data from Green FL, Page DL, Fleming ID, et al. AJCC Cancer Staging Handbook. In American Joint Committee on Cancer (eds): AJCC Staging Manual, 6th ed. New York, Springer-Verlag, 2002.

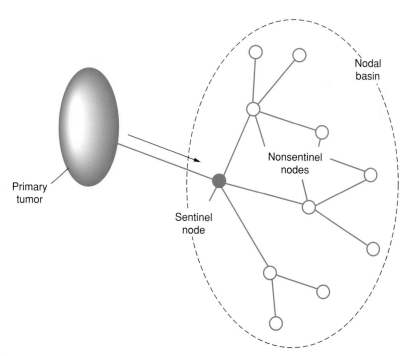

Nodal basin

Nonsentinel nodes

Primary tumor

Sentinel node

Figure 83-4 Drainage to one node before others. (From Kapteijn BA. Biopsy of the Sentinel Node in Melanoma Penile Carcinoma and Breast Carcinoma, Enschede, The Netherlands, Print Parters Ipskamp, 1997.)

and selected postmenopausal patients. Anthracyclines (doxorubicin or epirubicin), cyclophosphamide, methotrexate, and 5-fluorouracil are mainly used. Antimetabolites (capecitabine, gemcitabine) and anti-tubulin agents like taxanes (paclitaxel, docetaxel, and vinorelbine) have also been used. The most common side effects of chemotherapy are nausea, vomiting, myelosuppression, alopecia, and mucositis. Chemotherapy treatment is individualized for each patient (Mincey et al., 2002 ⊙). For current guidelines of drugs used to treat breast cancer, see Table 83-4.

Radiation Therapy

Radiation therapy is currently delivered using external beam radiation to the whole breast as part of the standard local treatment. It is also used in metastatic bone lesions for relief of symptoms. Radiation therapy is administered over a 5- to 6-week period. If recommended with chemotherapy, radiation is given after chemotherapy.

Neoadjuvant chemotherapy consists of chemotherapy given before surgery to shrink and downstage tumors so that BCT can be performed.

Table 83-4 Drugs of Choice for Breast Cancer

Drugs of Choice	Some Alternatives or Additional Drugs
Risk reduction: Tamoxifen	
Adjuvant[2] Doxorubicin + cyclophosphamide ± fluorouracil (AC or CAF) ± followed by paclitaxel or docetaxel Cyclophosphamide + methotrexate + fluorouracil (CMF) Tamoxifen for hormone receptor positive	**Adjuvant[2]** Cyclophosphamide + epirubicin[3] + fluorouracil (CEF) Anastrazole for postmenopausal hormone receptor positive[4]
Metastatic Doxorubicin + cyclophosphamide ± fluorouracil (AC or CAF) Cyclophosphamide + methotrexate + fluorouracil (CMF)	**Metastatic** Capecitabine; paclitaxel; docetaxel; vinorelbine; mitoxantrone; epirubicin; fluorouracil by continous infusion
For hormone receptor positive: Letrozole,[5,6] anastrozole,[5,7] exemestane,[5,8] tamoxifen, toremifene, or fulvestrant[9]	*For hormone receptor positive:* Megestrol acetate Fluoxymestrone
For tumors overexpressing HER2 protein: Trastuzumab[10] + vinorelbine or + paclitaxel	*For tumors overexpressing HER2 protein:* Trastuzumab[10] + docetaxel Pegylated lipsomal doxorubicin + trastuzumab[10] or gemcitabine

[1] Available in the United States for investigational use only.
[2] Adjuvant treatment with chemotherapy and/or hormone therapy is generally recommended node-positive patients, and for node-negative patients with tumors >1 cm in size or other unfavorable prognostic features. Use of hormone therapy is limited to patients with tumors that are hormone receptor positive or unknown and should begin after completion of chemotherapy (KS Albain et al. Proc Am Soc Clin Oncol 2002; 21:37a, abstract 143). If radiation therapy is used, it is probably best to have a similar delay. An anthracycline-containing regimen is preferred in patients with node-positive disease.
[3] Med Lett 2000;42:12.
[4] For adjuvant therapy of postmenopausal women with tumors that are hormone receptor positive, initial data suggest that anastrozole may be more effective than tamoxifen but longer follow-up is needed (ATAC Trialists' Group, Lancet 2002;359:2131). Anastrozole can be considered as an alternative to tamoxifen for postmenopausal women.
[5] For premenopausal hormone receptor-positive women, a luteinizing hormone releasing hormone agonist (goserelin, leuprolide, or tritorelin) should be given in combination with an aromatase inhibitor (anastrozole, letrozole, or exemestane).
[6] Mouridsen H, et al. J Clin Oncol 2001;19:2596.
[7] Bonneterre J, et al. J Clin Oncol 2000;18:3748; Nabholtz JM, et al. J Clin Oncol 2000;18:3758.
[8] Med Lett 2000;42:35.
[9] Med Lett 2002;44:65.
[10] Slamon DJ et al. N Engl J Med 2001;344:783; liposomal doxurubicin is being studied because concurrent trastuzumab increases the cardiac toxicity.
Data from Med Lett 2003;1(7):42.

Commonly Used Treatment Options

Stage 0 Carcinoma in situ is where the tumor cells are confined to the ducts or the lobules. Ductal carcinoma in situ is a preinvasive lesion. If left untreated, it can potentially progress to invasive cancer. Current recommendations include BCT + radiation therapy ± tamoxifen; total mastectomy ± tamoxifen. Lobular carcinoma in situ is also an indicator lesion for potential increased risk of invasive cancer of 1% per year (Recht, 2003). Close observation of both breasts after diagnostic biopsy is recommended. Treatment with tamoxifen in patients with lobular carcinoma in situ has shown to decrease the incidence of subsequent breast cancer.

Early Invasive Breast Cancer Stage I (tumor < 2 cm, axillary nodes negative) and stage II (ipsilateral movable axillary nodes positive, tumor > 2 cm, or a tumor < 5 cm that is node negative) are considered early stage. BCT and radiation therapy or mastectomy ± breast reconstruction and adjuvant systemic therapy (chemotherapy ± hormonal therapy) are recommended (Mincey and Perez, 2004 ©; Lippman, 2005).

Locally Advanced Breast Cancer Stage III (extensive axillary node involvement, supraclavicular node involvement, direct extension to chest wall or skin, or inflammatory breast cancer): neoadjuvant chemotherapy, surgery, and radiation are recommended.

Inflammatory Breast Cancer This is an aggressive form of locally advanced breast cancer. A multimodality approach, combining induction chemotherapy, surgery, and radiation, is used.

Metastatic Breast Cancer Stage IV tumors are unlikely to be cured. Multimodality approaches, including local and systemic treatment, may provide those with oligometastatic disease (limited metastasis) with improved survival rates. For positive HER2/NEU cases, use of trastazumab (monoclonal antibody) with other drugs has shown improved survival. Currently, more aggressive approaches, such as high-dose chemotherapy plus autologous stem cell transplantation, do not appear to improve survival (Green et al., 2002 ©).

Follow-up Surveillance

Current recommendations from the American Society of Clinical Oncology include history and routine physical examination every 2 to 6 months during the first 3 years after primary therapy, every 6 to 12 months for the next 2 years, then annually. Visits should focus on signs of local recurrence as well as evidence of metastasis, which occurs primarily in the bone, liver, and lungs. A pelvic examination, including a Pap smear and endometrial ultrasound scan, should be obtained annually, especially for those patients using tamoxifen. Yearly mammography cannot be overemphasized, with more frequent mammography if needed.

Advances in Breast Cancer Screening and Treatment

Advances in breast cancer screening in mammography, including digital imaging and computer-aided devices, have increased cancer detection. Trials are under way on the use of magnetic resonance imaging with contrast to enhance the detection of breast cancer. Newer techniques on evaluating partial breast irradiation (brachytherapy) are being studied; in these radiation is administered to the tumor bed and the area surrounding the margin, allowing tumoricidal doses of radiation with a shortened course of treatment duration. Furthermore, advances in genetics continue, and these will help physicians detect high-risk patients and will lead to advances in prevention and treatment

Material Available on Student Consult

Review Questions and Answers about Breast Cancer

REFERENCES

Fuhrman GM, Bolton JS, Cederbom GJ, et al. Image-guided core-needle breast biopsy is an accurate technique to evaluate patients with nonpalpable imaging abnormalities. Ann Surg 1998;227:932–939.©

Green FL, Page DL, Fleming ID, et al. AJCC Cancer Staging Handbook. In American Joint Committee on Cancer (eds): AJCC Staging Manual, 6th ed. New York, Springer-Verlag, 2002.©

Hall FM, Storella JM, Silverstone DZ, Wyshak G. Nonpalpable breast lesions: Recommendations for biopsy based on suspicion of carcinoma at mammography. Radiology 1988;167:353–358.

Jemal A, Tiwari RC, Murray T, et al. Cancer statistics, 2004. CA Cancer J Clin 2004;54:8–29.©

Linver MN. The medical audit. In Bassett LW, Jackson VP, Jahan R, Fu YS, Gold RH (eds): Diagnosis of Diseases of the Breast, 2nd ed. Philadelphia, Saunders, 2005, pp 141–143.

Lippman ME. Breast cancer. In Kasper DL, Fauci AS, Longo DL, Braunwald E, Hauser SL, Jameson JL (eds): Harrison's Principles of Internal Medicine, 16th ed. New York, McGraw-Hill, 2005, pp 516–523.

Mincey BA, Palmieri FM, Perez EA. Adjuvant therapy for breast cancer: Recommendations for management based on consensus review and recent clinical trials. Oncologist 2002;7:246–250.**ⓒ**

Mincey BA, Perez EA. Advances in screening, diagnosis, and treatment of breast cancer. Mayo Clin Proc 2004; 79:810–816.**ⓒ**

National Institutes of Health Consensus Development Panel. National Institutes of Health Development Conference Statement: Adjuvant therapy for breast

cancer, November 1–3, 2000. J Natl Cancer Inst 2001; 93:979–989.**ⓒ**

Recht A. Integration of systemic therapy and radiation therapy for patients with early-stage breast cancer treated with conservative surgery. Clin Breast Cancer 2003;4:104–113.

Schnitt SJ, Connolly JL, Sclafani L, Smith BL, Morrow M, Eberlein TJ. Benign breast disorders. In Harris JR, Hellman S, Handerson IC, Kidney DW (eds): Breast Diseases. Philadelphia, Lippincott, 1991, pp 15–50.

Smith RA, Saslow D, Andrews-Sawyer K, et al. American cancer society guidelines for breast cancer screening: Update 2003. CA Cancer J Clin 2003;53:141–169.**ⓒ**

Chapter

84 Vaginal Bleeding (Endometrial Cancer)

Giang T. Nguyen

KEY POINTS

1. Endometrial cancer is a common malignancy in women.
2. Postmenopausal women with vaginal bleeding should be evaluated for endometrial cancer.
3. Prognosis is determined by histologic type, grade, and stage of the disease.
4. Racial disparities exist in the prognosis of endometrial cancer, with African-American and Asian-Pacific Islander patients having poorer outcomes than Caucasian patients.
5. Treatment of endometrial cancer consists of hysterectomy and may also include radiation therapy, hormonal therapy, and palliative chemotherapy.
6. Annual screening with endometrial biopsy starting at age 35 is recommended for women with or at risk for hereditary nonpolyposis colon cancer.

INITIAL VISIT

Subjective

Patient Identification and Presenting Problem

Huong N. is a 66-year-old Vietnamese woman who presents for a new patient visit with the complaint of vaginal bleeding.

History of Present Illness

Mrs. N. is accompanied today by her husband and her adult son. She speaks minimal English but refuses professional interpretation, choosing to use her son for translation instead. You explain to the son that he will need to translate everything verbatim during the visit, and he agrees to do this. Mrs. N. complains of vaginal bleeding that started 1 week ago and ended 3 days before this visit. She describes it as thick clots and heavy flow that was more than an average menstrual period. She experienced menopause at

---

Evidence levels **Ⓐ** Randomized, controlled trials (RCTs), meta-analyses, well-designed systematic reviews of RCTs. **Ⓑ** Case-control or cohort studies, nonrandomized clinical trials, systematic reviews of studies other than RCTs, cross-sectional studies, retrospective studies, certain uncontrolled studies. **Ⓒ** Consensus statements, expert guidelines, usual practice, opinion.

age 50. She has not had any pain and denies bleeding or bruising anywhere else on her body. She admits that she did have another similar bleeding episode several months ago, but it was mild and self-limited, and she did not tell anyone. The episode that prompted today's visit, however, was much more severe, which is why she decided to tell her family. She was reluctant to go today since the problem has stopped already, but her family insisted that she see a doctor.

Mrs. N. has never used birth control pills or hormonal therapy. She had a normal Pap smear and normal mammogram about 10 years ago.

Medical History

No major medical problems, hospitalizations, surgeries, cancer, tuberculosis, blood clotting disorders, chronic conditions, or allergies. No other history of gynecologic problems. Four uncomplicated full-term vaginal deliveries between ages 20 and 28. No medications except for occasional acetaminophen for mild headaches.

Family History

No family history of breast, colon, or gynecologic cancer. Her parents died in their 80s of natural causes.

Social History

The patient is married. She is a retired secretary. No alcohol, tobacco, or illicit drug use. She does have passive exposure to smoke from her husband and sons. No history of sexually transmitted infections and no sexual intercourse for several years.

Review of Systems

She denies weight loss, fatigue, fever, night sweats, chest pain, shortness of breath, bowel changes, melena, bloody stool, dysuria, myalgias, arthralgias, depression, and neuralgias.

Objective

Physical Examination

Mrs. N. is an obese Asian woman in no acute distress. Vital signs: height, 62 inches; weight, 185 pounds; temperature, 99.0°F (37.2°C); respiratory rate, 18; blood pressure, 100/63; heart rate, 90. Cardiac examination is unremarkable. Lungs are clear bilaterally. Abdomen is nontender with no hepatosplenomegaly or masses. Gynecologic examination shows no inguinal lymphadenopathy and normal female genitalia. There is a large blood clot in the vagina, but no active bleeding. No lesions, lacerations, or polyps are noted. Bimanual examination reveals no cervical tenderness, no adnexal masses, and no uterine mass. Rectal examination shows normal tone, no masses, and guaiac-negative stool. A Pap smear is sent to the

laboratory for evaluation. After discussion of risks and benefits of the procedure, the patient consents to having an endometrial biopsy as well, and this specimen is also sent to the laboratory. A blood sample for complete blood count is also sent.

Assessment

Working Diagnosis

The working diagnosis is abnormal vaginal bleeding in an obese postmenopausal Asian female.

Differential Diagnosis

There are a number of conditions that can result in vaginal bleeding in a postmenopausal woman.

1. *Atrophic vaginitis.* This is more common in older women. Atrophic vaginal tissue may be more at risk for irritation. Severely atrophic tissue can very rarely be associated with bleeding (Pandit and Ouslander, 1997). Physical examination can suggest this diagnosis.
2. *Cervical lesions.* This may be due to cervicitis, cervical polyps, or cervical cancer. When cervical polyps cause bleeding, it is often in the setting of postcoital bleeding. Cervicitis can cause bleeding in rare instances. Other causes of bleeding include submucosal myomas and condylomata acuminata (Beers and Berkow, 1999). During the examination, attention should be paid to the presence of any lesions on the cervix or cervical tenderness. Routine Pap smears should be performed to screen for cervical cancer, which is a highly treatable malignancy when diagnosed early.
3. *Uterine polyp, fibroid, or adenomyosis.* Benign uterine tumors are a frequent cause of dysfunctional uterine bleeding. Endometrial polyps can account for 25% of abnormal bleeding; they can be treated with curettage. Fibroids (leiomyomas) can cause bleeding and pelvic pressure. In general, they do not require surgery unless they cause persistent bleeding problems, pain, or deleterious mass effects on neighboring structures. Adenomyosis is a benign condition in which endometrial tissue is present within the myometrium and can result in hypertrophy of the surrounding myometrium (Feldman and Stewart, 1999).
4. *Endometrial hyperplasia.* Like endometrial cancer, endometrial hyperplasia most commonly presents with dysfunctional uterine bleeding. Although hyperplasia without atypia usually has a benign course, atypical hyperplasia has a high risk of developing into cancer (Montgomery et al., 2004).
5. *Endometrial/uterine cancer.* Uterine cancers develop as endometrial carcinomas and uterine sarcomas. Uterine sarcomas (including leiomyosarcomas, endometrial stromal sarcomas, and mixed müllerian sarcomas) represent only 2% of

uterine malignancies. The overwhelming majority of uterine cancers are endometrial carcinomas (Feldman and Stewart, 1999).

Plan

Diagnostic

Preliminary laboratory studies were ordered (Pap smear, endometrial biopsy, complete blood count).

Therapeutic

The patient is not currently bleeding and is clinically stable (vital signs and symptoms are not worrisome at this time). Therefore, no acute management is necessary at this point. Further therapeutic approaches will be determined based on test results and clinical course.

Patient Education

Mrs. N. is instructed to follow up in 2 weeks to discuss the results of her tests and to see how she is doing clinically. She is also instructed to call if any new or recurrent symptoms develop in the meantime. She is provided with counseling and education about the potential diagnoses, and the importance of good follow-up is emphasized. In addition, noting that she has had no consistent health care, you advise her that to maintain her health, she should also consider other matters for her general health, including cholesterol testing, vaccinations (including pneumonia, influenza, and tetanus), mammography, and other screening.

FOLLOW-UP VISIT

Mrs. N. returns with her husband and son for the 2-week follow-up visit. She reports no recurrent bleeding and no new symptoms. She is eager to learn about her test results. Review of the laboratory tests show evidence of endometrial carcinoma in the biopsy specimen. The Pap smear is normal, as is the complete blood count.

Mrs. N. is counseled about the results of the tests. She and her family are frightened about the diagnosis, but they are willing to proceed with whatever the doctor recommends. Mrs. N. is referred to gynecologic oncology specialists for further workup and surgical evaluation.

DISCUSSION

Endometrial cancer is the fourth most common malignancy in women in the United States and the most common gynecologic malignancy (American Cancer Society, 2004 ©). One in every 50 women in the United States will develop this disease (Stenchever,

2001). The median age at diagnosis is 61 years, with only 5% of cases being diagnosed at less than 40 years of age (Feldman and Stewart, 1999). Death rates from endometrial cancer have dropped dramatically over the past century (American Cancer Society, 2004 ©). Endometrial carcinoma generally has a survival rate of 65% or better (Stenchever, 2001), with an 89% 5-year survival reported in cases that are limited to the mucosa (Abeler and Kjorstad, 1991 ®). Some racial disparities do exist. Cox proportional hazards models derived from Surveillance, Epidemiology, and End Results (SEER) data showed an unadjusted hazard ratio of 2.57 for death from endometrial cancer for African-American women as compared to white women. African-American women were significantly less likely to undergo primary surgery and had shorter survival than white women (Randall and Armstrong, 2003 ®). Among Asian Americans, some evidence suggests that women born in the United States have higher rates of endometrial cancer than their Asian-born counterparts (Liao et al., 2003 ®). A multivariate analysis of data from the Department of Defense tumor registry showed that the Asian-Pacific Islander race also independently predicts poor outcome for endometrial cancer (Kost et al., 2003 ®).

The majority of cases of endometrial cancer are diagnosed as the result of an evaluation for abnormal vaginal bleeding (Canavan and Doshi, 1999). Vaginal bleeding in a postmenopausal woman (i.e., after 1 year without menses) should prompt an evaluation. The differential diagnosis of abnormal vaginal bleeding includes endometrial/uterine cancer, endometrial hyperplasia, uterine polyp or fibroid, cervical disease, and atrophic vaginitis.

Risk

Risk factors for endometrial cancer include a history of colon cancer (especially hereditary nonpolyposis colon cancer), unopposed estrogen therapy, late menopause, tamoxifen therapy, nulliparity, infertility or failure to ovulate, obesity, diabetes, and hypertension (National Guideline Clearinghouse, 2001 ©). A family history of endometrial cancer may also increase risk (Parslov et al., 2000 ®), but there is insufficient evidence to suggest that a family history of breast cancer affects endometrial cancer risk (Kazerouni et al., 2002 ®).

In addition to being linked to endometrial cancer, increased estrogen exposure is also associated with endometrial hyperplasia with atypia, which is a premalignant disease (Feldman and Stewart, 1999). Estrogen exposure can occur through increased endogenous production, particularly in patients with obesity, estrogen-secreting tumors, and anovulatory cycles (Canavan and Doshi, 1999). Patients with polycystic ovary syndrome are therefore at increased risk (Lobo and Carmina, 2000). Obesity increases production as well as bioavailability of estrogen. Women who are overweight by up to 22.7 kg have a threefold increase in risk of endometrial cancer, and those more than 22.7 kg overweight have a ninefold increase in risk (Feldman and Stewart, 1999). Women with early menarche (before age 12), late menopause (after age 52), or nulliparity also have increased exposure to estrogen throughout their lifetimes and are at increased risk (Canavan and Doshi, 1999). Clinicians should therefore be particularly aware of this in the case of patients who are lesbians or who practice lifelong celibacy.

Unopposed estrogen can also come from exogenous sources. A Danish case-control study of 237 endometrial cancer patients and 538 controls demonstrated an odds ratio of 3.1 (95% confidence interval 1.4 to 7.0) for women younger than age 50 who received estrogen-only hormone replacement therapy for 1 to 5 years (Parslov et al., 2000 Ⓑ). The use of combined estrogen and progestin therapy, however, produced endometrial cancer rates similar to placebo; the hazard ratio for this regimen in the Women's Health Initiative was 0.81 (95% confidence interval 0.48 to 1.36). Although the combined therapy did not appear to increase endometrial cancer rates, it was associated with increased rates of endometrial biopsies to assess vaginal bleeding (Anderson et al., 2003 Ⓐ). Like HRT, tamoxifen (commonly used for breast cancer chemoprevention) has estrogenic properties in the female genital tract (Canavan and Doshi, 1999). When compared to placebo, tamoxifen is associated with increases in endometrial cancer risk, particularly in women 50 years of age and older (Kinsinger et al., 2002 Ⓐ).

Some evidence suggests that the use of oral contraceptives for 1 to 5 years decreases the risk of endometrial cancer (odds ratio 0.2; 95% confidence interval 0.1 to 0.3) (Parslov et al., 2000 Ⓑ). Smoking also reduces the risk of endometrial cancer. The mechanism may be related to higher serum androstenedione levels and, among overweight women, lower estradiol levels (Austin et al., 1993 Ⓑ). However, this benefit is clearly surpassed by the other risks associated with smoking.

Because women with endometrial cancer tend to present with symptoms at an early, favorable stage, the American Cancer Society does not recommend screening for endometrial cancer, even in women with "increased risk" (e.g., obesity, nulliparity, tamoxifen therapy) (National Guideline Clearinghouse, 2001 Ⓒ). The U.S. Preventive Services Task Force does not have any recommendations for routine endometrial cancer screening either. A consensus conference in Europe also concluded that repeat endometrial biopsies in women on tamoxifen therapy are of little value, and transvaginal ultrasonography is likely to yield many false-positive results (Neven and Vergote, 1998 Ⓒ).

Women classified as at high risk of endometrial cancer are those known to carry mutations associated with hereditary nonpolyposis colorectal cancer, women who have a substantial likelihood of being a mutation carrier for it (i.e., family history), and women from families with an autosomal dominant predisposition to colon cancer in the absence of genetic testing results. For these women, the American Cancer Society recommends annual endometrial biopsy starting at age 35. In addition, those high-risk women who are no longer considering child-bearing and who are undergoing surgery for colorectal cancer should be offered prophylactic hysterectomy (National Guideline Clearinghouse, 2001 Ⓒ). This recommendation is supported by reports of occult endometrial cancer identified by prophylactic hysterectomy in patients with hereditary nonpolyposis colorectal cancer (Chung et al., 2003).

Initial Evaluation

The majority of patients with endometrial cancer present initially with abnormal vaginal bleeding. Occasionally, older patients may present with pelvic pain associated with retained blood in the uterus due to stenosis of the cervical os. Asymptomatic patients may also present with abnormal Pap smears showing atypical endometrial cells. On physical examination, clinicians should carefully examine the external genital structures and note the size, shape, position, and mobility of the uterus as well as any abnormalities in the adnexal regions (to determine the presence of possible estrogen-secreting ovarian tumors) (Canavan and Doshi, 1999). Patients presenting with abnormal vaginal bleeding should receive a Pap smear because cervical bleeding is often difficult to differentiate from uterine bleeding (Feldman and Stewart, 1999).

Evaluation of any suspected case of endometrial cancer should include endometrial biopsy for histologic examination. Endometrial sampling can be accomplished in the outpatient setting, and this is an appropriate skill for family physicians to have. It is a blind procedure performed using sterile technique with the patient in lithotomy position. Local anesthesia can be used in addition to oral nonsteroidal anti-inflammatory medications. A detailed description of this procedure is provided in Zuber (2001).

Some recent work has suggested that a negative transvaginal ultrasound (showing endometrial thickness ≤ 4 mm) with or without a normal Pap smear may negate the need for an endometrial biopsy (Gull et al., 2000 Ⓑ; 2003 Ⓑ). The sensitivity of transvaginal ultrasonography has been reported to be 90% for endometrial disease (Langer et al., 1997 Ⓑ) and 100% for endometrial cancer (Gull et al., 2003 Ⓑ). However, because endometrial biopsies are fairly simple and only minimally invasive, it is still prudent to proceed with endometrial sampling in cases of suspected cancer. Table 84-1

Table 84-1   Response to Biopsy Results

Pathologic Finding on Biopsy	Response
Endometrial carcinoma	Referral for hysterectomy Progestin therapy if surgery is contraindicated Possible role for radiation or chemotherapy
Endometrial hyperplasia with atypia	High risk of progression to cancer Offer hysterectomy (especially if child-bearing is complete) or treat with progestin and closely monitor with endometrial biopsy every 3 months
Endometrial hyperplasia without atypia	Low risk of progression to cancer Often regresses to normal tissue in 1 year Treat with progestin and repeat biopsy in 3 months Consider hysterectomy for persistent hyperplasia despite hormone treatment
Atrophic endometrium	Treat with progestin and reevaluate
Normal endometrium	Treat abnormal bleeding with progestin Additional workup if continued suspicion of cancer (transvaginal ultrasound, fractional dilation and curettage, hysteroscopy).

See Canavan and Doshi (1999), Zuber (2001), Triwitayakorn and Rojanasakul (1999), Weinberg et al. (1999).

lists recommended responses to pathologic findings on biopsy.

After Diagnosis

On detection of endometrial cancer, further evaluation should include a complete history and examination, a complete blood count (to rule out anemia), liver function tests (to screen for occult metastatic disease), and a chest radiograph (to rule out pulmonary metastases) (Feldman and Stewart, 1999).

Definitive treatment of endometrial cancer requires surgery (total abdominal hysterectomy, bilateral salpingo-oophorectomy, and surgical evaluation for metastatic disease). Staging can be determined at the time of surgery (Canavan and Doshi, 1999). For patients who cannot tolerate surgery, staging can be attempted through use of transvaginal ultrasonography or magnetic resonance imaging (Feldman and Stewart, 1999). Table 84-2 shows basic grading and staging schemata. Patients beyond stage IB grade 2 should also be offered postoperative radiation therapy. Cytotoxic chemotherapy is reserved only for palliative therapy because tumor response is generally poor. Progestin therapy is another option, but it also is not highly effective against endometrial cancer (Canavan and Doshi, 1999).

Patients diagnosed with endometrial cancer should also be screened routinely for colorectal cancer. A retrospective cohort analysis of the Surveillance, Epidemiology, End Results (SEER) program database demonstrated a standardized incidence ratio for colorectal cancer of 3.39 (95% confidence interval 2.73 to 4.17) among women diagnosed with endometrial cancer before the age of 50 (Tabata et al., 2001 Ⓑ).

Table 84-2   Grade and Staging of Endometrial Cancer

Grade		Stage	
1	Well differentiated	I	Corpus uterus only
2	Intermediate differentiation	II	Corpus uterus and cervix only
3	Poorly differentiated	III	Extending beyond the uterus but confined to the pelvis
		IV	Extending outside the pelvis or into bladder or rectal mucosa

Histologic grade and stage affect the prognosis for endometrial cancer. Patients with higher grade and stage have worse prognosis (Stenchever, 2001).

In summary, endometrial cancer is a common malignancy. While routine screening is not recommended for most women, any occurrence of abnormal vaginal bleeding, particularly in a postmenopausal woman, should prompt an evaluation for this diagnosis. Early stages of endometrial cancer have a very good prognosis, and primary care physicians play an important role in the prompt diagnosis of this disease.

Material Available on Student Consult

Review Questions and Answers about Endometrial Cancer

REFERENCES

Abeler VM, Kjorstad KE. Endometrial adenocarcinoma in Norway. A study of a total population. Cancer 1991;67:3093–3103.🅑

American Cancer Society. Cancer Facts and Figures 2004. Atlanta: American Cancer Society, 2004.🅒

Anderson GL, Judd HL, Kaunitz AM, et al. Effects of estrogen plus progestin on gynecologic cancers and associated diagnostic procedures: The Women's Health Initiative randomized trial. JAMA 2003;290:1739–1748.🅐

Austin H, Drews C, Partridge EE. A case-control study of endometrial cancer in relation to cigarette smoking, serum estrogen levels, and alcohol use. Am J Obstet Gynecol 1993;169:1086–1091.🅑

Beers MH, Berkow R. Menstrual abnormalities and abnormal uterine bleeding. In Beers MH, Berkow R (eds): The Merck Manual of Diagnosis and Therapy, 17th ed. Rahway, NJ, Merck, 1999, Section 18, Chapter 235.

Canavan TP, Doshi NR. Endometrial cancer. Am Fam Physician 1999;59:3069–3076.

Chung L, Broaddus R, Crozier M, Luthraa R, Levenback C, Lu K. Unexpected endometrial cancer at prophylactic hysterectomy in a woman with hereditary nonpolyposis colon cancer. Obstet Gynecol 2003; 102:1152–1155.

Feldman S, Stewart EA. The uterine corpus. In Ryan KJ, Kistner RW (eds): Kistner's Gynecology and Women's Health, 7th ed. St. Louis, Mosby, 1999. pp 121–142.

Gull B, Carlsson S, Karlsson B, Ylostalo P, Milsom I, Granberg S. Transvaginal ultrasonography of the endometrium in women with postmenopausal bleeding: Is it always necessary to perform an endometrial biopsy? Am J Obstet Gynecol 2000;182: 509–515.🅑

Gull B, Karlsson B, Milsom I, Granberg S. Can ultrasound replace dilation and curettage? A longitudinal evaluation of postmenopausal bleeding and transvaginal sonographic measurement of the endometrium as predictors of endometrial cancer. Am J Obstet Gynecol 2003;188:401–408.🅑

Kazerouni N, Schairer C, Friedman HB, Lacey JV, Jr, Greene MH. Family history of breast cancer as a determinant of the risk of developing endometrial cancer: A nationwide cohort study. J Med Genet 2002;39: 826–832.🅑

Kinsinger LS, Harris R, Woolf SH, Sox HC, Lohr KN. Chemoprevention of breast cancer: A summary of the evidence for the U.S. Preventive Services Task Force. Ann Intern Med 2002;137:59–69, I62.🅐

Kost ER, Hall KL, Hines JF, et al. Asian-Pacific Islander race independently predicts poor outcome in patients with endometrial cancer. Gynecol Oncol 2003;89:218–226.🅑

Langer RD, Pierce JJ, O'Hanlan KA, et al. Transvaginal ultrasonography compared with endometrial biopsy for the detection of endometrial disease. Postmenopausal Estrogen/Progestin Interventions Trial. N Engl J Med 1997;337:1792–1798.🅑

Liao CK, Rosenblatt KA, Schwartz SM, Weiss NS. Endometrial cancer in Asian migrants to the United States and their descendants. Cancer Causes Control 2003;14:357–360.🅑

Lobo RA, Carmina E. The importance of diagnosing the polycystic ovary syndrome. Ann Intern Med 2000;132: 989–993.

Montgomery BE, Daum GS, Dunton CJ. Endometrial hyperplasia: A review. Obstet Gynecol Surv 2004;59: 368–378.

National Guideline Clearinghouse. American Cancer Society guidelines on testing for early endometrial cancer detection—Update 2001. In American Cancer Society Guidelines for the Early Detection of Cancer. Available at www.guideline.gov. Accessed 9/24/2004.🅒

Neven P, Vergote I. Should tamoxifen users be screened for endometrial lesions? Lancet 1998;351:155–157.🅒

Pandit L, Ouslander JG. Postmenopausal vaginal atrophy and atrophic vaginitis. Am J Med Sci 1997;314:228–231.

Parslov M, Lidegaard O, Klintorp S, et al. Risk factors among young women with endometrial cancer: A Danish case-control study. Am J Obstet Gynecol 2000;182:23–29.🅑

Randall TC, Armstrong K. Differences in treatment and outcome between African-American and white women with endometrial cancer. J Clin Oncol 2003;21:4200–4206.🅑

Stenchever MA. Neoplastic diseases of the uterus. In Stenchever MA (ed): Comprehensive Gynecology, 4th ed. St. Louis, Mosby, 2001, pp 919–954.

Tabata T, Yamawaki T, Yabana T, Ida M, Nishimura K, Nose Y. Natural history of endometrial hyperplasia: Study of 77 patients. Arch Gynecol Obstet 2001;265:85–88.🅑

Triwitayakorn A, Rojanasakul A. Management of endometrial hyperplasia: A retrospective analysis. J Med Assoc Thailand 1999;82:33–39.🅑

Weinberg DS, Newschaffer CJ, Topham A. Risk for colorectal cancer after gynecologic cancer. Ann Intern Med 1999;131:189–193.🅑

Zuber TJ. Endometrial biopsy. Am Fam Physician 2001; 63:1131–1135, 1137–1141.

85

Cervical Cancer Screening

Wendy Brooks Barr

INITIAL VISIT

Subjective

Patient Identification and Presenting Problem

Altagracia L., a 32-year-old Latina, comes to the office for her annual gynecologic examination. She has no complaints and reports good general health.

Gynecologic and Obstetric History

Ms. L. entered menarche at age 13 and began having intercourse at age 16. She reports her periods as regular and occurring approximately every 28 days, with the flow lasting 5 to 6 days. Her last period was 2 weeks ago. She has no previous history of abnormal Papanicolaou (Pap) smears. Her last Pap smear was 1 year ago. She has a distant history of *Chlamydia* infection when she was 18 that was treated. She has

no other history of sexually transmitted diseases (STDs).

Her obstetric history includes four previous pregnancies resulting in two spontaneous vaginal deliveries without complications, one miscarriage in the first trimester, and one first-trimester induced abortion. Her last delivery was 2 years ago with you as her provider. She underwent a tubal ligation immediately post partum for future contraception. Tests for HIV were negative at the time of delivery of her last child.

Social and Family History

Ms. L. reports having one current male sexual partner whom she has been with for 9 months. She thinks he is monogamous with her. She states she does not use tobacco, alcohol, or drugs. Her family history is significant for diabetes in both her mother and father. Her mother did not take diethylstilbestrol.

Review of Systems

Ms. L. states she has not had any vaginal discharge or discomfort, or any irregular bleeding. She has not noticed any changes or masses in her breasts or any nipple discharge.

Objective

On physical examination, the patient has normal external female genitalia without any evidence of external or perianal warts. The speculum examination discloses no abnormalities of the introitus, vagina, or cervix. The cervix is not friable. The external cervical os is slightly open, consistent with previous vaginal deliveries. No abnormal discharge is noted in the posterior fornix. A Pap smear is obtained, along with a swab for *Neisseria gonorrhoeae* and *Chlamydia* testing. On bimanual examination, no abnormalities are noted on palpation of the vagina, and there is no cervical motion tenderness. The uterus is of normal size and anteverted. No

---

Evidence levels Ⓐ Randomized, controlled trials (RCTs), meta-analyses, well-designed systematic reviews of RCTs. Ⓑ Case-control or cohort studies, nonrandomized clinical trials, systematic reviews of studies other than RCTs, cross-sectional studies, retrospective studies, certain uncontrolled studies. Ⓒ Consensus statements, expert guidelines, usual practice, opinion.

adenexal tenderness or masses are noted. Examination of the breasts reveals no dimpling or thickening of the skin on visual inspection, no masses on palpation of the breast or adenexal lymph nodes, and no nipple discharge.

Assessment

This is a normal female gynecologic examination.

Plan

Provide anticipatory guidance by discussing the use of condoms to prevent STDs, including HIV and human papillomavirus (HPV) infection. Also discuss HIV testing for Ms. L. and her partner, and discuss her risk for cervical dysplasia and HPV infection and whether she should have yearly versus every third year cervical cancer screening.

DISCUSSION

Cervical Cancer Screening: The Pap Smear

The Pap smear is a screening test designed to detect precancerous lesions of the cervical epithelium that, if left untreated, could develop into invasive cervical cancer. These precancerous lesions are known as cervical intraepithelial neoplasia (CIN). Most intraepithelial lesions and cervical cancer lesions contain HPV. There are many types of HPV, which vary in their ability to transform cervical epithelium into CIN and cancerous lesions. The high-risk types most frequently associated with moderate to severe dysplasia (CIN II or III) and carcinoma in situ are types 16, 18, 31, 33, and 35 (Cannistra and Niloff, 1996ⓒ).

The Pap smear does not diagnose CIN but rather samples for abnormal-appearing cells from the cervical epithelium. It is ideal to sample from the epithelial transformation zone (t-zone) where normal endocervical columnar cells change into normal squamous cells of the exocervix. The t-zone is the area of the cervix where dysplasia is most likely to occur. The test can be performed at any time during the menstrual cycle except during menstruation itself, since the red blood cells can obscure the epithelial cells on the smear. Ideally, specimen collection for the Pap smear should be done before bimanual examination or other manipulation of the cervix is performed to avoid lubricant artifact and disruption of cells on the surface of the cervix. After the speculum has been placed and the cervix is visualized, a dry swab can be used to remove any obscuring cervical mucus, and then the specimen should be obtained. Currently, Pap smear specimens can be collected directly onto slides (traditional slide method) or the cells can be placed in a liquid medium and later placed on a slide by the pathologist (liquid-based cytology, e.g., ThinPrep).

The traditional slide method typically involves collecting squamous cells from the cervix using a spatula and then collecting endocervical cells with a cytobrush placed into the cervical os. The cells are then spread onto a slide from both the spatula and cytobrush and quickly sprayed with a cell fixative to prevent drying artifact. With the liquid-based cytology method the sample typically is collected using a cytologic broom placed into the cervical os and turned to obtain both the squamous and endocervical cells or by using an extended-tip plastic spatula. The collection instrument is then placed into the fixative and agitated to release the cells into the liquid medium. Liquid-based cytology has a slightly higher sensitivity than the traditional slide sample technique but is more expensive and has not been shown to be cost-effective in improving patient-oriented outcomes (U.S. Preventive Services Task Force [USPSTF], 2003ⓒ). For this reason, current guidelines do not recommend for or against the use of the liquid-based cytology technique over the conventional slide-based Pap smear technique (American College of Obstetricians and Gynecologists [ACOG], 2003 ⓒ; USPSTF, 2003ⓒ). The advantage of liquid-based cytology is that it is useful for colposcopy triage. Reflex HPV testing can be done with the Pap sample without the need for a second collection at a later date.

The Bethesda system, a uniform system for reading and reporting Pap smear results, was developed by a consortium of groups involved in cervical cancer screening. The most recent revision of the Bethesda system occurred in 2001. The accepted Bethesda 2001 terminology for cervical epithelial cell abnormalities is given in Table 85-1 (Solomon, 2002ⓒ). Table 85-2 presents the known epidemiology for abnormal epithelial and glandular cell Bethesda categories for CIN and cervical cancer (Wright et al., 2001ⓒ).

HPV Testing

A recent addition to Pap smear testing for cervical cancer screening has been molecular testing for high-risk types of HPV. This testing can be done directly from the liquid medium for liquid-based cytology smears, or the specimen can be collected separately along with a traditional slide-based Pap smear specimen. The testing can be done at the same time as Pap smear testing (routine testing) or it can be performed after the processing of a Pap smear that is read as atypical squamous cells of undetermined significance (ASC-US) (reflex testing). The current preferred approach (of the three currently approved approaches) for managing ASC-US includes using reflex HPV testing to determine who should proceed to colposcopy versus retesting in 12 months (Wright et al., 2002ⓒ). Table 85-3 gives the 2001 recommendations of the American Society of Colposcopy and Cervical Pathology (ASCCP) for managing patients

Table 85-1 The 2001 Bethesda System (Abridged)

Specimen Adequacy
Satisfactory for evaluation (note presence/absence of endocervical/transformation zone component)
Unsatisfactory for evaluation (specify reason)
Specimen rejected/not processed (specify reason)
Specimen processed and examined, but unsatisfactory for evaluation of epithelial abnormality because of (specify reason)

General Categorization (Optional)
Negative for intraepithelial lesion or malignancy
Epithelial cell abnormality
Other

Interpretation/Result
Negative for Intraepithelial Lesion or Malignancy
Organisms
  Trichomonas vaginalis
  Fungal organisms morphologically consistent with *Candida* species
  Shift in flora suggestive of bacterial vaginosis
  Bacteria morphologically consistent with *Actinomyces* species
  Cellular changes consistent with herpes simplex virus
Other non-neoplastic findings (optional to report)
  Reactive cellular changes associated with:
    Inflammation (includes typical repair)
    Radiation
    Intrauterine contraceptive device
  Glandular cells status post hysterectomy
  Atrophy

Epithelial Cell Abnormalities
Squamous cell
  Atypical squamous cells (ASC)
    Of undetermined significance (ASC-US)
    Cannot exclude HSIL (ASC-H)
  Low-grade squamous intraepithelial lesions (LSIL)
    Encompassing: human papillomavirus, mild dysplasia, CIN I
  High-grade squamous intraepithelial lesions (HSIL)
    Encompassing: moderate and severe dysplasia, carcinoma in situ, CIN II, and CIN III
  Squamous cell carcinoma
Glandular cell
  Atypical glandular cells (AGC) (specify endocervical, endometrial, or not otherwise specified)
  Atypical glandular cells, favor neoplasia (specify endocervical or not otherwise specified)
  Endocervical adenocarcinoma in situ (AIS)
  Adenocarcinoma

Automated Review and Ancillary Testing (Include as Appropriate)
Educational Notes and Suggestions (Optional)

CIN, cervical intraepithelial neoplasia; HSIL, high-grade squamous intraepithelial lesions.
From Solomon D, Davey D, Kurman R, et al. The 2001 Bethesda system: Terminology for reporting results of cervical cytology. JAMA 2002;286:2114–2119.

with abnormal screening cytology results (Wright, 2002©). For women older than 30, the National Cancer Institute, the ASCCP, and the American Cancer Society have recommended combined testing with cytology (Pap smear) and HPV testing, with the advantage of prolonging the testing interval to every 3 years if the results of both are negative (Wright et al., 2004©). Table 85-4 provides the recommenda-

tions from this group for managing results based on simultaneous cytologic and HPV testing.

Cervical Cancer Screening Intervals

There is increasing controversy over the interval at which women should have Pap smears done as part of a routine gynecologic examination. Traditionally,

Table 85-2 Risk of Significant Cervical Dysplasia or Invasive Cancer Based on Cervical Cytology Result

Bethesda Abbreviation	Bethesda Description	Identified as CIN II or III (%)	Identified as Invasive Cancer (%)
ASC-US	Atypical squamous cells of undetermined significance	10–20	0.1
ASC-H	Atypical squamous cells—cannot exclude HSIL	24–94	N/D
LSIL	Low-grade squamous intraepithelial lesion (includes HPV, mild cervical dysplasia, CIN I)	15–30	N/D
HSIL	High-grade squamous intraepithelial lesion (includes moderate and severe dysplasia, carcinoma in situ, CIN II, CIN III)	70–75	1–2
AGC	Atypical glandular cells	9–54	<1–8
AGC—favor neoplasia	Atypical glandular cells, favor neoplasia	27–96 (includes AIS and invasive cancer)	N/D
AIS	Endocervical adenocarcinoma in situ	48–69 (with AIS)	38

CIN, cervical intraepithelial neoplasia; HPV, human papillomavirus; N/D, no data reported.
Data from Solomon D, Davey D, Kurman R, et al. The 2001 Bethesda system: Terminology for reporting results of cervical cytology. JAMA 2002;286:2114–2119; Wright TC, Cox JT, Massad LS, et al. 2001 consensus guidelines for the management of women with cervical cytological abnormalities. JAMA 2002;287:2120–2129.

Table 85-3 Management of Cervical Cytology Results: Bethesda/ASCCP 2001 Guidelines

Pap (Cytology) Result	Follow-up Test	Follow-up Timing
Negative	Pap (cytology)	12 mo[¶]
ASC-US[*] (no reflex HPV[†] test)	Pap (cytology)	4–6 mo
ASC-US (negative reflex HPV)	Pap (cytology)	12 mo
ASC-US (positive reflex HPV)	Colposcopy	Immediately
ASC-H	Colposcopy	Immediately
AGC	Colposcopy and endometrial sampling	Immediately
LSIL[‡,§]	Colposcopy	Immediately
HSIL	Colposcopy	Immediately

[*]ASC-US in postmenopausal women can be triaged using intravaginal estrogen therapy for 1 week and repeat cytology. If the study is negative, the Pap smear can be repeated in 4 months; otherwise, colposcopy is required.
[†]HPV testing is molecular testing for high-risk types of HPV DNA.
[‡]LSIL in postmenopausal women with evidence of atrophy can be managed similarly to ASC-US (see first note above).
[§]LSIL in adolescents can be managed as indicated or with repeat cytologic examination in 6 months or with HPV testing in 12 months, with colposcopy after repeat testing if the result remains abnormal.
[¶]See text for discussion of testing intervals for routine screening.
HPV, human papillomavirus.
Data from Wright TC, Cox JT, Massad LS, et al. 2001 consensus guidelines for the management of women with cervical cytological abnormalities. JAMA 2002;287:2120–2129.

many patients and physicians have believed that the annual Pap smear was an essential part of routine care for women to prevent cervical cancer. Indeed, the Pap smear has been a success story for cancer screening and prevention. The incidence of cervical cancer decreased by 70% in the United States after the introduction of mass screening programs (Cannistra and Niloff, 1996ⓒ). Today, approximately 50% of women found to have invasive cervical cancer never had a Pap smear prior to diagnosis, and 10% did not have a Pap smear

Table 85-4 Management of Combined Cervical Cytology and HPV Testing

Pap (Cytology) Result	HPV Result	Follow-up Test	Follow-up Timing
Negative	Negative	Pap/HPV	36 mo
Negative	Positive	Pap/HPV	6-12 mo*
ASC-US	Negative	Pap/HPV	12 mo
ASC-US	Positive	Colposcopy	Immediately
ASC-US or worse	Positive	Colposcopy	Immediately
ASC-US or worse	Negative	Colposcopy	Immediately
AGC	Positive or negative	Colposcopy and endometrial sampling	Immediately

*If follow-up testing is both cytology and HPV negative, the woman can return to routine screening every 3 years. If follow-up testing is ASC-US and HPV negative, the woman can undergo rescreening with both tests in 12 months. Otherwise, any HPV positive findings or any cytology ASC-US or worse requires immediate colposcopy.

HPV, human papillomavirus.

Data from Wright TC, Schiffman M, Solomon D, et al. Interim guidance for the use of human papillomavirus DNA testing as an adjunct to cervical cytology for screening. Obstet Gynecol 2004;103:304–309.

Table 85-5 Summary of Cervical Cancer Screening Recommendations

	ACOG	ASCCP	ACS	USPSTF
Start screening	Within 3 years of first intercourse or age 21 (whichever comes first)	18 or the onset of sexual activity	Within 3 years of first intercourse or age 21 (whichever comes first)	Within 3 years of first intercourse or age 21 (whichever comes first)
Screening interval	Every year if <30 years. Every 3 years if >30 years and previous three Pap smears were normal or if combined testing was negative and patient has low risk for disease	Same as ACOG	Same as ACOG	Screen at least every 3 years
Stop screening	No set age; instead, should base on individual risk	Same as ACOG	Age 70 if 3 previous Paps normal and no abnormal Pap in 10 years	Age 65 if has previous normal Paps and low risk for disease
Screening patients with total hysterectomy for benign disease	Screening not needed	Same as ACOG	Same as ACOG	Same as ACOG

Data from American of Obstetricians and Gynecologists (ACOG). Cervical Cytology Screening. ACOG Practice Bulletin no. 45. Obstet Gynecol 2003;102:417–425; Saslow D, Ranowicz CD, Solomon D, et al. American Cancer Society guidelines for the early detection of cervical neoplasia and cancer. CA Cancer J Clin 2002;52:342–362; U.S. Preventative Services Task Force. Screening for cervical cancer: Recommendations and rationale. 2003. Available at www.preventativeservices.ahrq.gov. Accessed 1/26/2006; Wright TC, Cox JT, Massad LS, et al. 2001 consensus guidelines for the management of women with cervical cytological abnormalities. JAMA 2002; 287:2120–2129.

in the previous 5 years. There is agreement that every woman should have some type of regular Pap smear screening for some portion of her life. The disagreements concern when screening should start, how often women should have Pap smears done, and when they should stop. The introduction of testing for high-risk types of HPV has also complicated this picture and may affect recommendations for screening intervals and cessation of screening. Interim guidelines state that for women older than 30, routine screening can occur every 3 years if the patient has both negative cytology and negative high-risk HPV results (Wright et al., 2004ⓒ). They do not recommend using combined testing routinely, but only if a patient is interested and it is appropriate to increase the screening interval to every 3 years. If there is any reason why the patient would want to continue with yearly screening (such as a previous history of abnormal cytology), then only cytology with reflex HPV testing for ASC-US results should be performed. These guidelines specifically recommend against using combined testing to lengthen screening intervals to every 3 years in women in several categories: (1) women less than 30 years old, because of the high prevalence of transient HPV infection; (2) women who are immunosuppressed, including HIV-positive women, because of their high risk for rapidly progressive cervical dysplasia, which mandates frequent screening; and (3) women who have undergone a total hysterectomy for benign disease, who, because of their very low risk of disease, do not need screening. The age cutoff of 30 years for combined testing is based on the age strata prevalence of HPV, which decreases after age 30; the fact that very few cases of cervical cancer occur before age 25; and the observation that most clinical trials investigating the use of HPV testing have been conducted in women more than 30 years old. The underlying assumption is that by age 30, most women in the United States are engaging in lower-risk sexual behaviors (i.e., they have fewer changes in partners or fewer new partners, and there is a lower prevalence of STDs in the sexual cohort). This may not be true for all patient populations, which means these guidelines may need to be modified based on the particular patient or patient population. For example, longer screening intervals with combined testing may be appropriate for a non-sexually active 25-year-old woman until she becomes sexually active but may not be appropriate for a 35-year-old woman with multiple sexual partners or a new sexual partner in a population with a high incidence of cervical dysplasia. Table 85-5 summarizes current cervical cancer screening recommendations, including when to start, how often to screen, and when to stop routine screening.

Discussion of Case

Our patient, Altagracia L., is at lower risk for cervical dysplasia in that she has no known history of abnormal Pap smear results and is older than 30 years, but because she has recently changed sexual partners and is a Latina (a population at higher risk for cervical dysplasia compared to non-Latin white women), she may want to proceed with yearly screening instead of combined screening at 3-year intervals. Even if Ms. L. opts for combined testing, with a plan to repeat in 3 years if all testing is normal, she should be informed that she should still return yearly for annual gynecologic examinations, including an internal pelvic examination and breast examination (ACOG, 2003ⓒ).

Material Available on Student Consult
Review Questions and Answers about Cervical Cancer Screening

REFERENCES

American College of Obstetricians and Gynecologists (ACOG). Cervical Cytology Screening. ACOG Practice Bulletin no. 45. Obstet Gynecol 2003;102:417–425.ⓒ

Cannistra SA, Niloff JM. Cancer of the uterine cervix. N Engl J Med 1996;334:1030–1038.ⓒ

Saslow D, Ranowicz CD, Solomon D, et al. American Cancer Society guidelines for the early detection of cervical neoplasia and cancer. CA Cancer J Clin 2002;52:342–362.

Solomon D, Davey D, Kurman R, et al. The 2001 Bethesda system: Terminology for reporting results of cervical cytology. JAMA 2002;286:2114–2119.ⓒ

U.S. Preventive Services Task Force. Screening for cervical cancer: Recommendations and rationale. 2003. Available at www.preventiveservices.ahrq.gov. Accessed 1/26/2006.ⓒ

Wright TC, Cox JT, Massad LS, et al. 2001 consensus guidelines for the management of women with cervical cytological abnormalities. JAMA 2002;287:2120–2129.ⓒ

Wright TC, Schiffman M, Solomon D, et al. Interim guidance for the use of human papillomavirus DNA testing as an adjunct to cervical cytology for screening. Obstet Gynecol 2004;103: 304–309.ⓒ

86

Cervical Dysplasia: Diagnosis and Management

Jon C. Calvert

KEY POINTS

1. Routine Pap smear screening has markedly reduced the incidence of cervical cancer.
2. Currently, half of those who develop cervical cancer either never had a Pap smear or have not had a Pap smear within the past 5 years.
3. Risk factors for cervical cancer include human papillomavirus (HPV), smoking, and human immunodeficiency virus (HIV).
4. To optimize Pap smear test sensitivity and specificity, adequate numbers of cells need to be collected from the squamocolumnar junction and the transition zone.
5. New liquid-based Pap smear preparation techniques overcome some of the causes of false negative results associated with the traditional methods of cervical cell collection and processing.
6. Of the three conventional Pap smear methods, the endocervical brush/spatula method transfers the most cells to the slide.
7. The correct timing of a Pap smear collection improves the quality of the Pap smear.

8. Several groups have published guidelines recommending when and from whom to obtain Pap smears.
9. HPV-DNA testing is playing an increasingly important role in the diagnosis and management of cervical dysplasia and cervical cancer.
10. The Bethesda system 2001 revision clarifies and redefines Pap smear interpretation.
11. Approximately one third of high-grade squamous intraepithelial lesions (HSILs) regress to normal in 2 years, and most women infected with HPV do not develop significant cervical abnormality.
12. Management has changed for the Pap smear with absent endocervical cells.
13. Management of atypical squamous cells has changed. It is different for ASC-H and for ASC-US (with and without HPV-DNA testing).
14. Colposcopy is a skill that can be mastered by the practicing family physician.

INITIAL VISIT

Subjective

Patient Identification and Presenting Problem

Aletha W. is a 24-year-old single woman who returns today to discuss the results of her abnormal Pap smear.

Present Illness

Aletha has been sexually active since age 14, with a total of at least 11 different male partners. Currently

she lives with her boyfriend and has been in a monogamous relationship with him for the past 2 years. She is aware that during these 2 years her boyfriend has had other sexual encounters outside their relationship. She has had previous Pap smears; the last one was 6 years ago at the time of her last pregnancy. To her knowledge, all of her Pap smears have been normal. She has been treated twice in the past at the health department, once for gonorrhea (3 years ago) and then for *Trichomonas vaginitis* (last year). She did not keep her posttreatment test-of-cure appointments. She has been treated at the health department with cryoablation for genital warts. She

---

Evidence levels Ⓐ Randomized, controlled trials (RCTs), meta-analyses, well-designed systematic reviews of RCTs. Ⓑ Case-control or cohort studies, nonrandomized clinical trials, systematic reviews of studies other than RCTs, cross-sectional studies, retrospective studies, certain uncontrolled studies. Ⓒ Consensus statements, expert guidelines, usual practice, opinion.

has been pregnant three times, has one child, and has had two elective abortions, both prior to her third pregnancy. She is currently using oral contraceptive pills as a method of birth control.

Four months ago she had an abnormal Pap smear, ASC-H, and was scheduled for colposcopy 3 months ago but did not keep her appointment. After several missed appointments she presents today for colposcopy.

Medical History

Aletha has had no major medical illnesses. She had an appendectomy at age 8. She has been admitted to a hospital for the appendectomy and for the delivery of her child.

Family History

Aletha does not know the family medical history on her father's side because he left home when she was 4 years old. Her mother has previously been diagnosed with cervical dysplasia and has been treated. Aletha does not know the type of treatment. There is no family history of breast cancer, cervical cancer, uterine cancer, colon cancer, hypertension, diabetes mellitus, or heart disease.

Social History

Aletha lives with her boyfriend and works as a waitress at a local restaurant. She has smoked one to two packs of cigarettes per day since age 14. She occasionally drinks alcohol and has used marijuana in the past, but not for the past 4 years.

Review of Systems

The review of systems is unremarkable except as described above.

Objective

Colposcopy is performed. Examination of the external genitalia and vagina does not reveal any evidence of condylomata or dysplasia. The cervix is visualized in its entirety. There is a small, 2- to 3-mm area of leukoplakia at 10 o'clock, just proximal to the new squamocolumnar junction in the transition zone (Color Plate 86-1). Three percent acetic acid is applied. The area of leukoplakia becomes a denser white without mosaicism or punctation or abnormal blood vessels, with and without the use of a green filter. Two areas of acetowhite are identified, at 12 o'clock and at 6 o'clock, in the transition zone between the new squamocolumnar junction and the old squamocolumnar junction. Linear and geographic in shape, each demonstrates fine punctation and mosaicism without evidence of abnormal blood vessels. The previously identified area of leukoplakia becomes a deeper white after acetic acid is applied but does not exhibit punctation or mosaicism. Each

of the acetowhite lesions is seen in its entirety. The entire transition zone can be visualized. Biopsy specimens are obtained from each of the three lesions. Because the colposcopy is satisfactory, endocervical curettage is not done.

Assessment

The Pap smear is ASC-H, with colposcopy findings suggestive of cervical intraepithelial neoplasia (CIN) and cervical condylomata acuminata.

Plan

Aletha is asked to make a follow-up appointment to review the results of the biopsies and discuss future management.

Discussion

According to the new Bethesda guidelines (Table 86-1), the Pap smear finding of ASC-H (a new designation) requires that a colposcopy be performed. With colposcopy and biopsy, 5% to 15% of ASC-H Pap smears will be either CIN 2 or CIN 3.

FOLLOW-UP VISIT

Subjective

Aletha returns to review her colposcopy findings. She has been quite concerned and is apprehensive that she may have cancer. She says she had some spotting for 2 days following the procedure but is not currently experiencing vaginal spotting or discharge.

Objective

You review with her the pathology findings: mild dysplasia or CIN 1 (6 and 12 o'clock biopsies) and human papillomavirus (HPV) (10 o'clock biopsy).

Assessment

The assessment is CIN 1 in a 24-year-old woman who is a smoker, has genital HPV, and is living with a partner who has been and is sexually active with multiple individuals.

Plan

There are two management options. The first is to repeat the Pap smears every 4 to 6 months four times. It is explained to Aletha that 60% to 70% of cases of CIN 1 resolve. Of those that do not regress, about half progress to a higher grade of dysplasia and half remain unchanged. If follow-up Pap smears indicate that the CIN 1 is staying the same or worsening, another

Table 86-1 Comparison of the 1991 Bethesda System for Reporting Cervical/Vaginal Cytologic Diagnoses and the Bethesda (2001) Revision

1991 Bethesda System Specimen Adequacy	2001 Revision of Bethesda System Specimen Adequacy
Satisfactory for evaluation	Satisfactory for evaluation (describe presence or absence of endocervical T zone component and any other quality indicators)
Satisfactory for evaluation but limited [reason specified]	[category eliminated*]
Unsatisfactory for evaluation [reason specified]	Unsatisfactory for evaluation (specify reason) Specimen may be processed and unsatisfactory or unprocessed
General Categorization (Optional)	
Within normal limits	Negative for intraepithelial lesion or malignancy (NIL)
Benign cellular changes; see descriptive diagnosis	[category eliminated†]
Epithelial cell abnormality; see descriptive diagnoses	Epithelial cell abnormality; see interpretation/result (specify squamous or glandular) Other (see interpretation/result)
Descriptive Diagnoses ***Benign Cellular Changes*** Infection *Trichomonas vaginalis* Fungal organisms morphologically consistent with *Candida* species Predominance of coccobacilli consistent with shift in vaginal flora Bacteria morphologically consistent with *Actinomyces* species Cellular changes consistent with Herpes simplex virus Other	**Interpretation/Result** ***Negative for Intraepithelial Lesion or Malignancy*** Organisms *Trichomonas vaginalis* Fungal organisms morphologically consistent with *Candida* species Shift in vaginal flora suggestive of bacterial vaginosis Bacteria morphologically consistent with *Actinomyces* species Cellular changes associated with Herpes simplex virus Other non-neoplastic findings (optional to report; list not inclusive)
Reactive and reparative changes	Reactive cellular changes associated with inflammation (includes typical repair), radiation, intrauterine contraceptive device
Reactive cellular changes associated with inflammation (includes typical repair), atrophy with inflammation (atrophic vaginitis), radiation, intrauterine contraceptive device, or other	Atrophy, benign-appearing glandular cells post hysterectomy

Epithelial Cell Abnormalities
Squamous cells
 Atypical squamous cells of undetermined significance
	Epithelial Cell Abnormalities
	Squamous cells
	 Atypical squamous cells
	  Of undetermined significance
	  Cannot exclude HSIL‡

Low-grade squamous intraepithelial lesion encompassing human papillomavirus/mild dysplasia/CIN 1	Low-grade squamous intraepithelial lesion encompassing human papillomavirus/mild dysplasia/CIN 1
High-grade squamous intraepithelial lesion encompassing moderate and severe dysplasia, CIN 2, and CIN 3/CIS	High-grade squamous intraepithelial lesion encompassing moderate and severe dysplasia, CIS/CIN 2, and CIN 3 With features suspicious for invasion (if invasion is suspected)
Squamous cell carcinoma	Squamous cell carcinoma

Table 86-1 Comparison of the 1991 Bethesda System for Reporting Cervical/Vaginal Cytologic Diagnoses and the Bethesda (2001) Revision (Continued)

1991 Bethesda System Specimen Adequacy	2001 Revision of Bethesda System Specimen Adequacy
Glandular cells	Glandular cells
Endometrial cells, cytologically benign in postmenopausal women	Category reported as NIL (above)
Atypical glandular cells of undetermined significance	Atypical endocervical cells, endometrial cells, glandular cells
	Atypical glandular/endocervical cells, favor neoplastic
	Endocervical adenocarcinoma in situ
	Adenocarcinoma
Endocervical adenocarcinoma	Endocervical
Endometrial adenocarcinoma	Endometrial
Extrauterine adenocarcinoma	Extrauterine
Adenocarcinoma not otherwise specified	Not otherwise specified
Other Malignant Neoplasms	*Other Malignant Neoplasms (specify)*
Hormonal evaluation (applies to vaginal smears only)	*Educational Notes*
Hormonal pattern compatible with age and history	
Hormonal pattern incompatible with age and history [reason specified]	
Hormonal evaluation not possible owing to [reason specified]	

*These smears are categorized as satisfactory and the limiting factors are described.

†These smears are categorized as either NIL if they are clearly negative or as ASC-US if an epithelial abnormality is suspected.

‡New category.

CIN, cervical intraepithelial neoplasia; CIS, carcinoma in situ.

From Apgar BS, Brotzman G, Spitzer M (eds). Colposcopy: Principles and Practice. Philadelphia, WB Saunders, 2002.

colposcopy will be recommended. If the results of the four follow-up Pap smears are all satisfactory and negative, she can return to annual Pap smears.

The second option is cryotherapy. This procedure entails freezing the skin of the cervix, causing it to slough off, taking with it the abnormal cells. The healing that follows replaces the abnormal skin with normal skin. After cryotherapy, Aletha would be asked to have four follow-up Pap smears obtained every 4 to 6 months.

DISCUSSION

Pap Smears and Cervical Dysplasia in Perspective

The impact of Pap smear technology on the reduction of cervical cancer rates is impressive. If Pap smear screening were implemented in a group of women never before tested, the rate of cancer would be reduced by 60% to 90% within 3 years and the mortality from cervical cancer would be reduced by 20% to 60%. The early detection of cervical cancer significantly improves survival. Localized cervical

cancer (early detection) is associated with a 5-year survival rate of 92%, whereas with late detection, when distant disease is present at the time of diagnosis, the 5-year survival rate is 13%.

In the 1930s, cervical cancer was the leading cause of cancer death in women. Today, worldwide, cervical cancer is the third most common neoplastic disease (9.8%) in women, after breast cancer (21%) and colorectal cancer (10.1%). In the United States, cervical cancer is the eighth most common female malignancy.

George Papanicolaou first proposed evaluation of cervical/vaginal cells for purposes of diagnosing cervical cancer in 1948. Refining and improving the cell collection technique, J. Ernest Ayre introduced the use of a wooden spatula to harvest cells directly from the cervical transition zone. In 1954 Papanicolaou introduced the cytologic classification system dividing Pap smear results into five classes (I, II, III, IV, and V), a system still used by some pathologists today. With the development of these cytologic criteria, the World Health Organization embraced this classification system in the late 1950s. Using histologic criteria based on the microscopic assessment of the cervical biopsy specimen, Richart

Table 86-2 Papanicolaou Smear Nomenclature

Papanicolaou Class System (1954)	Descriptive (1968)	CIN (1978)	Bethesda System (1988)
Class 1	Negative for malignant cells	Negative	Within normal limits
Class 2	Inflammatory atypia		Reactive and reparative changes
	Squamous atypia		Atypical squamous cells of undetermined significance
	Koilocytotic atypia		Low-grade SIL; includes condyloma
Class 3	Mild dysplasia	CIN 1	Low-grade SIL; includes condyloma
	Moderate dysplasia	CIN 2	High-grade SIL
	Severe dysplasia	CIN 3	High-grade SIL
Class 4	Carcinoma in situ	CIN 3	High-grade SIL
Class 5	Invasive carcinoma	Invasive carcinoma	Invasive carcinoma

CIN, cervical intraepithelial neoplasia; SIL, squamous intraepithelial lesion.
Modified from Apgar BS, Brotzman G, Spitzer M (eds). Colposcopy: Principles and Practice. Philadelphia, WB Saunders, 2002.

introduced the concept of cervical intraepithelial neoplasia, with the CIN 1, 2, and 3 classification system in 1978 (Table 86-2). In an effort to develop a Pap smear classification system more broadly accepted by pathologists, an expert panel was convened in 1988. The result was the proposal and adoption of the Bethesda system. This system remains in use today and has undergone two revisions, the latest in 2001.

The introduction of the Pap smear as a screening tool has had a major impact on the incidence of cervical cancer in the United States. It is largely as a result of Pap smear screening that the mortality from cervical cancer has fallen by more than 70% over the past 50 years. In the United States in the year 2004 it was estimated that there were 11,520 new cases of cervical cancer and 3,900 cervical cancer-related deaths. In 1998 there were 8 new cases of cervical cancer per 100,000 women, compared with 44 new cases per 100,000 women in 1947.

Work remains to be done in the area of cervical cancer detection. Currently, more than one-half of all new cervical cancer cases identified each year fall into two subgroups. Fifty percent of the new cases are in women who have never had a Pap smear (Nuovo et al., 2001 ⓒ). Ten percent of new cases are in women who have not had a Pap smear test during the preceding 5 years.

Risk Factors

There are several risk factors for cervical cancer (Table 86-3). HPV infection is the most important of these risk factors. Among U.S. women, the mean age for occurrence of HPV is in the mid-20s. Most HPV infections are transient, but one of the high-risk

HPV virus types, type 16, has been shown to persist in the same host for at least 5 years. HPV is incorporated into the host DNA. Factors affecting this incorporation include age, nutritional status, immune function, smoking, and genetic polymorphism. HPV has been identified in 75% to 95% of high-grade squamous intraepithelial lesions (HSILs) and in 95% to 100% of squamous cell cervical cancers. There are currently more than 60 viral types of HPV (Table 86-4). The four types that carry the highest risk for cervical cancer are 16, 18, 31, and 45. With the advent of hybrid capture technology and clarification of the role of intermediate-risk HPV virus types in the development of cervical cancer, some groups combine the high- and intermediate-risk groups into one group and call it "high risk."

Table 86-3 Risk Factors for an Abnormal Pap Smear Result

History of human papillomavirus
Exposure to diethylstilbesterol
History of an abnormal Pap smear result
Initiation of early sexual activity
More than one sexual partner (ever)
Partner with history of human papillomavirus (HPV)
Illicit drug use
Smoking habit
Infection with HIV
Having never had a Pap smear
Having had no Pap smear for preceding 5 years

Modified from Apgar BS, Brotzman G, Spitzer M (eds). Colposcopy: Principles and Practice. Philadelphia, WB Saunders, 2002.

Table 86-4 Human Papillomavirus Types	
High risk	16, 18, 31, 45
Intermediate risk	33, 35, 39, 51, 56, 58, 59, W13B
Low cancer risk	6, 11, 53, 54, 66, PAP 155, PAP 291

Modified from Apgar BS, Brotzman G, Spitzer M (eds). Colposcopy: Principles and Practice. Philadelphia, WB Saunders, 2002.

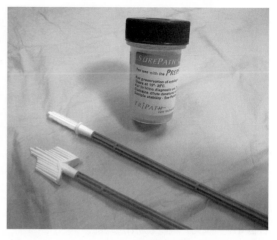

Figure 86-1 There are several providers of liquid thin prep Pap smear technology. A "paint brush" tip (lower brush) can be used to obtain the specimen when the squamocolumnar junction is visible. The narrow tip (upper brush) can be used to obtain the specimen when the squamocolumnar junction has moved deeper in the endocervical canal and cannot be visualized. Either the collected materials are deposited in the liquid container with a rapid movement or the tip is dislodged and dropped into the container.

In addition to HPV, other risk factors include smoking and human immunodeficiency virus (HIV) infection. There is a two- to fourfold increase in abnormal Pap smears in woman who smoke. Women with HIV have a higher prevalence of dysplasia. Contrary to initial assumptions, recent findings suggest that the speed with which dysplasia progresses to cervical cancer does not appear to be increased in women with HIV.

Cytologic Screening Method

The goal of cytologic screening is to sample superficial cells (shed or mechanically dislodged) from the surface of the transformation zone. To optimize the test sensitivity and specificity, cells need to be collected at the point of physiologic cell transformation (squamous metaplasia) from endocervical columnar cells to ectocervical squamous cells (Nuovo et al, 2001☉). An optimal cytologic cell sample would contain three cell types: endocervical cells, squamous cells, and squamous metaplastic cells (cells transforming from endocervical to ectocervical cell types). Recognizing the squamocolumnar junction (the point at which endocervical cells meet squamous cells) and collecting cells from this line of transformation increases the sensitivity of the Pap smear test by reducing the number of false negative test results.

The sensitivity of the conventional Pap smear test is 57% (95% confidence interval [CI]: 37% to 66%) with a specificity of 98% (95% CI: 97% to 99%). The major causes of false negative results include inadequate sampling (i.e., not obtaining adequate numbers of cells from appropriate areas of the cervix) and inappropriate sample transfer through traditional methods (e.g., drying artifact on slides, inappropriate application of collected specimen to slide, inappropriate fixation of slide). It is apparent that the transfer of cells to the slide is a random event.

New liquid-based preparation techniques promise to overcome some of these deficiencies (Fig. 86-1). Two current liquid-based techniques, ThinPrep and Autocyte Prep, have been approved by the U.S. Food and Drug Administration (FDA) with labeling stating that they are equivalent to or superior to the conventional Pap smear slide technology for the detection of cervical cancer precursor lesions (Wright and Cox, 2004☉). With improved sensitivity (decreased false negative interpretations) there is decreased specificity (increased percentage of false positive interpretations). With liquid-based methods there appears to be improved identification of glandular cells associated with atypical glandular cells of undetermined significance associated with adenocarcinoma of the cervix. As of early 2004, there were no published prospective studies comparing the new liquid-based technology with conventional Pap smear prep technology.

The optimal conventional method for collecting and transferring cervical cells has been studied. The area from which cell samples should be obtained is the transformation zone and the endocervical canal, using a spatula and a brush (Fig. 86-2). The transformation zone is that surface of the portion of the cervix that lies between the old squamocolumnar junction and the new squamocolumnar junction. Whether a spatula is used, as in the conventional Pap smear collection method, or a brush, as in the liquid-based technology, harvesting cells from the transition zone markedly improves the detection of cervical cancer and precervicalcancer changes.

Of the three conventional Pap smear methods studied—swab/spatula, endocervical brush/spatula, and the use of a broomlike device—the endocervical brush/spatula method transferred more than twice

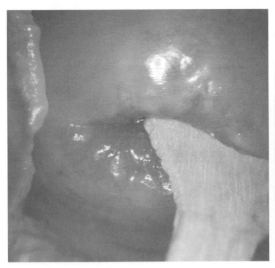
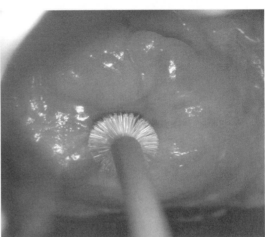

Figure 86-2 Traditional Pap smear. Note that the spatula is positioned to collect cells from the squamocolumnar junction and transition zone (*left*). The brush (cytobrush) is used to collect cells from the squamocolumnar junction that is not easily visualized within the external os of the endocervical canal (*right*). (From Apgar BS, Brotzman G, Sptizer M (eds). Colposcopy: Principles and Practice. Philadelphia, WB Saunders, 2002.)

as many cells, 18%, versus 7% and 8% for the other methods. When the spatula is used, cells collected from the transformation zone should be placed on a properly labeled glass slide with a single stroke, using moderate pressure to thin out the clumps of cells and mucus. To decrease the amount of blood collected and to lessen the risk of cells air-drying before they can be fixed, the cytobrush is used after the spatula. The cytobrush is rotated 180 degrees in the endocervical canal, then removed, and the cells are transferred from the brush to the slide by rolling the bristles across the slide by twisting the brush handle (Fig. 86-3). Fixative should immediately be applied before the cells have had a chance to air dry.

When spraying on fixative, the preparer should hold the container far enough away from the slide that the force of the spray does not disrupt the cells on the slide and cause them to pile up.

There are several other techniques to optimize collection of cells. Cells should be collected before the bimanual examination is performed. Recent studies suggest that a small amount of water-based lubricant can be used on the speculum when collecting a Pap smear specimen without adversely affecting the interpretation (Amies et al., 2002 Ⓐ; Harer et al., 2002 Ⓐ). Cells for cytologic study should be collected before cervical specimens are obtained for culture. The entire portion of the cervix should

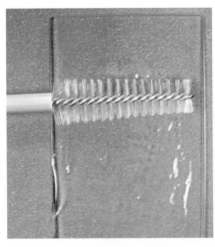
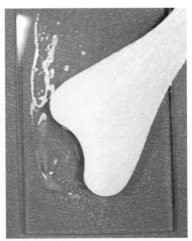

Figure 86-3 Cells are obtained from the transformation (transition) zone and the squamocolumnar junction (Fig. 86-2) with a wooden spatula and then a cytobrush. The collected cells are applied to the slide in a thin layer using the spatula in a firm, steady stroke from one end of the slide to the other. The bristles of the brush are then gently rolled across the same slide from one end of the slide to the other. Finally, fixative is applied.

be visualized and the transition zone identified before a sample is obtained. Routine swabbing of discharge from the cervix may result in a cytologic sample of scant cellularity. Normally, less than 20% of the cells collected are transferred to the slide. Too few cells may result in a true false negative interpretation. Air-drying artifact can be avoided by transferring and fixing the specimen as quickly as possible. Rapid transfer is important whether a liquid-based method or a conventional method is used.

The correct timing of the collection of a Pap smear improves the quality of the Pap smear. Although some liquid-based technology is capable of separating out red blood cells, it is best not to collect a specimen during menses. The following should be avoided for 48 hours prior to collection: vaginal medications, vaginal contraceptives, and douches. Intercourse should be avoided the night prior to and the day of sample collection. Allow for reparative changes to be complete by obtaining Pap smears no sooner than 6 to 8 weeks after delivery. In postmenopausal woman, when a Pap smear identifies atrophy and inflammation or when endocervical cells are lacking, a 3-week course of vaginal estrogen should precede a repeat Pap smear.

Pap Smears: When and for Whom

More frequent Pap smears (e.g., yearly or every other year) have a more favorable impact on the reduction of invasive cervical cancer than less frequent Pap smears (e.g., every 3, 5, or 10 years). As noted previously certain risk factors or risk behaviors also affect the incidence of abnormal pap smears. In 1987 the American Cancer Society (ACS) and the American College of Obstetricians and Gynecologists (ACOG) presented a joint statement in an effort to quell controversy and establish an optimal interval for cervical cytology. In summary, all sexually active women (past or present) or women 18 years old or older should have annual Pap smears; after three or more consecutive negative annual Pap smears, a Pap smear may be performed less frequently, at the discretion of the woman's physician.

More recently, in an effort to incorporate current research data, several groups have published their individual guidelines for obtaining Pap smears. Some of these groups include the American Academy of Family Physicians, the U.S. Preventive Services Task Force (2003ⓒ; 2004ⓒ), ACS (Schroeder, 2003ⓒ), and ACOG (2003ⓒ). A combined summary of these recommendations follows. As with any health care guidelines, they should be applied at the discretion of the physician and with patient understanding and agreement.

1. Obtain annual Pap smears as long as the individual is at risk or is involved in high-risk behavior (see Table 86-3).

2. Have the first Pap smear done 3 years after becoming sexually active or at age 21, whichever occurs first.

3. Once begun, continue conventional Pap smears annually or liquid-based Pap smears every other year until age 30.

4. If the woman is 30 years old or older and three previous annual Pap smears have been negative, and in the absence of high risk behavior, then, regardless of method (conventional or liquid), screening can be performed every 2 to 3 years.

5. If the woman is HIV positive, screen twice the first year and then annually.

6. If there is a history of diethylstilbestrol exposure while in utero or an immunocompromised state, Pap smears should be done annually.

7. If there is a past history of CIN 2, CIN 3, or a DNA test positive for HPV, annual Pap smears are indicated.

8. If the woman has had a hysterectomy for a benign condition, a Pap smear is no longer indicated. If the hysterectomy was supracervical (the cervix was not removed), manage as if uterus were still present.

9. If the woman has had a hysterectomy for CIN 2, CIN 3, or cervical cancer, or if the reason for the hysterectomy cannot be documented, or the absence of a history of CIN 2 or CIN 3 cannot be documented, continue annual Pap smears. If then three consecutive annual Pap smears are negative and no abnormal or positive test in past 10 years can be documented, annual Pap smears may be stopped.

10. If a Pap smear is normal but endocervical cells are absent and there is no history of an abnormal Pap smear or high-risk behavior, repeat the Pap smear in 1 year; otherwise repeat in 4 to 6 months.

11. If the individual is pregnant and the Pap smear is negative but there are no endocervical cells, repeat the Pap smear postpartum.

12. If the Pap smear is negative, repeat in 6 months if (a) there is a recent abnormal Pap smear (ASC-US or worse), (b) the abnormal result is incompletely evaluated, (c) the cervix was incompletely visualized, (d) the individual is in an immunocompromised state, or (e) there is a history of a poor prior screening.

13. If the individual is 65 to 70 years old and has had three consecutive, annual normal Pap smear and no positive test within the past 10 years, stop Pap smears.

14. If the individual is 65 to 70 years old and involved in at-risk behavior (see Table 86-3), continue annual Pap smears.

15. Screening in woman 70 years or older is recommended if no previous screening has been performed or is unlikely to have been performed, or

if information about previous screening is not available.

16. Testing may be stopped in women who have severe comorbid or life-threatening illness.

17. As with any set of guidelines, the physician should assess the clinical situation and adjust the guideline accordingly.

When Is HPV Testing Appropriate?

The application of liquid film Pap smear technology and the development of HPV testing by Hybrid Capture II technology allow for specific HPV typing from the same cellular material that was obtained for the Pap smear. The FDA has approved liquid-based preparation technology for cervical cancer screening. The FDA has also approved Hybrid Capture II technology for the screening of cells obtained from the cervix for HPV DNA. Using the cells present in the liquid prep medium, the presence or absence of high-risk or intermediate-risk HPV types is determined (see Table 86-4).

There currently are two situations in which HPV-DNA typing is called for (Wright and Cox, 2004⊙). The first is in the presence of Pap smears read as atypical squamous cells of undetermined significance (ASC-US). With the liquid film preparation and ASC-US there is an automatic "reflex testing" to Hybrid Capture II. Current guidelines recommend colposcopy for ASC-H when identified by Pap smear only. Colposcopy is also recommended if there is an ASC-US Pap smear with a high-risk test positive for HPV. This situation carries a 79% to 98% sensitivity for identification of CIN II/III at colposcopy.

A second application of HPV DNA testing is when a Pap smear identifies ASC-US, ASC-H, or low-grade squamous intraepithelial lesions (LSIL) and both the colposcopy and the colposcopically directed biopsy are negative (Wright et al., 2002⊙). At the time of the next Pap smear (in 6 or 12 months), HPV typing should be obtained. If the typing is positive for high-risk HPV, even if the Pap smear is normal, colposcopy should be considered.

The Bethesda System of Pap Smear Reporting

First proposed in 1988 and revised in 1991 and 2001, the Bethesda system is most widely used in the United States (Apgar et al., 2003⊙). A comparison of the 1991 Bethesda system for reporting cervical/vaginal cytologic diagnoses and the 2001 revision of the Bethesda system is given in Table 86-1. Several important changes occurred with the 2001 revision (Solomon et al., 2002⊙).

The Bethesda system 2001 revision is divided into two large categories: Specimen Adequacy and Interpretation/Result. In turn, the category Interpretation Result is divided into three subcategories: Negative for Intraepithelial Lesion or Malignancy, Epithelial Cell Abnormalities (squamous cells and glandular cells), and Other Malignant Neoplasms (specified).

With regard to adequacy of the specimen, the phrase "satisfactory but limited by . . ." is no longer used. Slides are not to be reported "satisfactory" or "unsatisfactory." If the specimen is unsatisfactory for evaluation, a specific reason is to be given.

The category Negative for Intraepithelial Lesion or Malignancy does not include slides with evidence of neoplasm. It may include findings specific either for infection or for reactive cellular changes associated with inflammation, radiation therapy, an intrauterine contraceptive device (IUD), or atrophy. Endometrial cells found in women age 40 years or older will be placed in this category. In women younger than 40, the presence of endometrial cells will not be reported.

In the subcategory Epithelial Cell Abnormalities (squamous cells and glandular cells), under the subheading squamous cells there is a significant change in atypical cell terminology that impacts management decisions (Wright et al., 2002⊙). The term "atypical squamous cells of undetermined significance, favor reactive" (ASCUS, favor reactive) has been replaced with "atypical squamous cells of undetermined significance" (ASC-US). Depending on the presence or absence of risk factors, this finding may or may not require colposcopy. If there are no risk factors, a Pap smear may be repeated in 12 months. If there are risk factors, a Pap smear may be repeated in 6 months. If HPV DNA testing is performed and high-risk HPV is also present, colposcopy is indicated.

The term "atypical squamous cells of undetermined significance, favor dysplasia" (ASCUS, favor dysplasia), is no longer used. It has been replaced with "atypical squamous cells, cannot exclude HSIL" (ASC-H). Because 5% to 15% of women with ASC-U Pap smears will have CIN 2/3 by colposcopic examination/biopsy, women with ASC-H should be scheduled for colposcopy.

In the subcategory Epithelial Cell Abnormalities (squamous cells and glandular cells), under glandular cells the term "atypical glandular cell" has replaced the term "atypical glandular cells of undetermined significance." The finding atypical glandular cell (AGC) is more likely to be associated with both glandular and squamous abnormalities than the term ASC-US. The three types of AGC reported are endocervical, endometrial, and glandular cells not otherwise specified. The addition of the term "favor neoplastic" AGC has been retained, but "favor reactive" has been dropped. The third and fourth categories listed under glandular cells are endocervical adenocarcinoma in situ and adenocarcinoma.

The category of AGC is less clearly defined (Levine et al., 2003 ©; Solomon et al., 2002©). Unlike in squamous disease, there are no intermediary categories between AGC and adenocarcinoma. Therefore, there is an intermixing of benign causes of AGC with premalignant and malignant causes. Benign causes of AGC include polyps, IUD use, cervical endometriosis, previous cervical conization, tubal metaplasia, inflammatory changes, microglandular hyperplasia, and pregnancy-associated changes. Unlike ASC-US cytology, AGC cytology carries with it a very high rate of invasive and preinvasive cancer, although the incidence of AGC cytology is low, varying from 0.1% to 0.4% of all smears.

Progression from Dysplasia to Cervical Cancer

The progression of HSIL to invasive cancer is 1.44%. In 35% of cases, HSIL regresses to normal in 2 years. Even though HPV is necessary to foster the development of cervical dysplasia, most women infected with HPV do not develop significant cervical abnormality. HPV is transmitted during intercourse, and once infection with HPV takes hold, the viral load is reduced to undetectable levels in 8 to 24 months. In the development of dysplasia, in addition to HPV two other cofactors may include smoking and a compromised immune system. Though many consider there to be a continuum in the development of dysplasia from CIN 1 to CIN 3, this is currently being debated.

Absence of Endocervical Cells

Recent data have led to a reevaluation regarding the management of Pap smears reported unsatisfactory because of the absence of endocervical cells. The assumption has been that when endocervical cells are present, the cell population sampled represents the transition zone of the cervix. This is also assumed to be true if metaplastic squamous cells are present (squamous metaplasia occurs at the interface of the squamous cells with the columnar endocervical cells-new squamocolumnar junction). ACOG suggests the following guideline for the management of Pap smears where endocervical cells are reported absent.

If a recent Pap smear is negative and there are no findings of ASC-US or worse, repeat the Pap smear in 1 year. In the absence of endocervical cells, the Pap smear should be repeated in 6 months if (1) a recent Pap smear is not normal (finding of ASC-US or worse), (2) there is an incompletely evaluated abnormal test result, (3) the cervix was incompletely visualized, (4) the woman has an immunocompromised status, or (5) there is a history of poor prior screening. During pregnancy a Pap smear that does not contain endocervical cells should be repeated 6 to 10 weeks postpartum.

Management of the Pap Smear Result

The Pap smear test has been performed and the report is back. Now, what to do? Various groups have recommended guidelines (Levine et al., 2003©; Wright et al., 2002©). If the Pap smear is satisfactory and negative, schedule the patient for the next appropriate Pap smear according to age and risk factors (see subsequent discussion under Pap Smears: When and for Whom).

If the Pap smear is ASC-US, repeat in 6 to 12 months, depending on level of risk. If there are risk factors (see Table 86-3), repeat in 6 months. If there are no risks, repeat in 1 year. If the Pap smear is ASC-US and liquid cytology was performed with reflex to HPV DNA typing and the HPV type is high risk, schedule the patient for colposcopy.

If the Pap smear is ASC-H or LSIL or HSIL, schedule the patient for a colposcopy. If colposcopic results identify CIN 1 and this finding matches the Pap smear findings, follow-up Pap smears can be performed every 4 to 6 months until three negative results are noted; after three negative results are found, return to routine Pap smears according to the individual patient's particular level of risk. Cryotherapy also can be performed, followed by Pap smears every 4 to 6 months until three negative tests are noted, and then return to routine Pap smears according to the individual patient's particular level of risk.

If the colposcopic biopsy reveals CIN 2, cryotherapy or cone biopsy can be performed, depending on the practitioner's level of confidence in his or her ability to identify by colposcopy the area of most advanced dysplastic involvement. If the colposcopic biopsy reveals CIN 3 or the endocervical curettings reveal CIN 2 or CIN 3, a cone biopsy (loop electrosurgical excision procedure [LEEP] or cold-knife-cone) is the next step.

If the Pap smear is interpreted as invasive squamous cell cancer, refer the patient to a gynecologist or gynecologic oncologist. If the Pap smear is interpreted as AGC, a colposcopically directed evaluation and biopsy with endocervical curettage should be performed (Wright et al., 2002©). If the result is negative, monitor with a Pap smear every 4 to 6 months until a minimum of three normal Pap smears have been obtained. If the Pap smear identified glandular abnormality recurs, a cone biopsy should be performed. If the patient with AGC is postmenopausal or perimenopausal and has irregular bleeding or is otherwise at risk for endometrial cancer, an endometrial biopsy should be performed.

If the Pap smear is interpreted as AGC, favor neoplasia, a colposcopy with endocervical curettage should be performed. If this is positive for adenocarcinoma in situ (AIS), referral to an appropriate specialist is the next step. If the colposcopy and endocervical curettage (ECC) are negative, a cervical conization is the next step because there is a 50% false negative rate in this situation. If the patient is postmenopausal, many recommend an endometrial biopsy along with colposcopy and endocervical curettage.

COLPOSCOPY: GETTING STARTED

Colposcopy: The Equipment

To perform colposcopy, certain forms or documents are helpful, and proper equipment is necessary. A patient colposcopy information sheet (Fig. 86-4), an informed consent form for biopsies of the cervix, endocervix, vagina, introitus, perineum, or anus (Fig. 86-5), a comprehensive patient intake form to be completed by the patient before the colposcopy is performed (Fig. 86-6), and an example of a form that can be used to record colposcopic findings, results, and management plans (Fig. 86-7).

The equipment and instruments necessary to perform colposcopy need not be expensive. Most of them can be purchased used. The primary consideration should be the colposcope (Fig. 86-8), and in particular the optics. Good optics are available on

pre-owned scopes and even inexpensive new scopes. Good colposcopy can be done without a lot of bells and whistles. For instance, the scope need not have more than two magnification settings (for example, 8× and 13× are sufficient) (Fig. 86-9). An expensive zoom lens is not needed. Most colposcopy is performed around 8× magnification; only rarely is a higher magnification needed. A green or blue filter should be available to facilitate identification of abnormal blood vessel patterns. Gross focus is achieved by moving the entire scope toward and away from the cervix. This can be achieved with the colposcope on rollers or on a stationary stand with an elbow where the support rod attaches to the floor plate. Selection of one or the other is usually a personal preference, so it is helpful to try out different stands before making a purchase. The mechanism for fine focus takes various forms and is found on the colposcope head (see Fig. 86-9).

A supply and equipment setup for colposcopy is demonstrated in Figure 86-10. Because it is wider than a Pederson speculum, a metal Graves speculum is most commonly used to optimize visualization of the cervix. Sometimes it is necessary to use a Pederson speculum or even a large pediatric speculum when the vaginal opening does not allow com-

Colposcopy Information Sheet

What is colposcopy? It is a close-up examination of the cervix using a special microscope called a colposcope.

Why do I need it? It will help identify the cause of your abnormal Papanicolaou (Pap) smear. An abnormal Pap smear may indicate cancerous and precancerous conditions, as well as some relatively harmless conditions. The Pap smear alone, however, cannot give a definitive diagnosis. The cervix must be magnified many times by the colposcope to look for the source of the abnormal cells. A small segment of each of these areas is then obtained for study by a pathologist. This is called a biopsy.

Is any preparation necessary? You should not douche, use any vaginal creams, or have intercourse 2 days before the examination. It is ideal to perform the colposcopy just after your period has ended. Many women find it helpful to take three ibuprofen tablets 1 to 2 hours before their appointment to reduce any cramping associated with a biopsy (do not use ibuprofen if you are allergic to it or to aspirin or if you are pregnant).

What is the examination like? It is like a regular pelvic examination, except that instead of looking at the cervix with the naked eye, the clinician will be looking through the colposcope. The entire examination takes approximately 20 to 30 minutes. If a biopsy is obtained, a slight pinching sensation may be experienced. The final step is to do a scraping of the inside of the cervix. This is called an endocervical curettage. This part of the examination lasts only about 15 seconds and is usually associated with some cramping.

What happens after the examination? You will be given a sanitary napkin to wear. No time off from work is needed. Intercourse should be avoided until all bleeding stops. No other limitation of activities is needed. The biopsy results will be back within 2 weeks, at which time your clinician will contact you to discuss treatment plans, if necessary, as well as what follow-up is needed. Please contact your clinician if she or he has not contacted you within 2 weeks of your appointment. If your phone number or address changes, please inform_____ at _____ so that we can update your chart.

Figure 86-4 Colposcopy information sheet. (From Apgar BS, Brotzman G, Spitzer M (eds). Colposcopy: Principles and Practice. Philadelphia, WB Saunders, 2002.)

Informed Consent for Colposcopy with Biopsy of Cervix, Endocervix, Vagina, Introitis, Perineum, or Anus

_____ or his/her assistant has explained to me the procedures and local anesthesia necessary to diagnose my condition or my dependent's condition. I understand the nature of the procedure summarized below and I request and authorize the performance of biopsy of the cervix, endocervix and possibly the vagina, vulva, perineum or anus.

I have been informed and understand that the following are possible risks associated with the procedure:
— Light bleeding that may require a sanitary napkin
— Heavy bleeding (rare) that may require a stitch or hospitalization
— Pain during the procedure (usually mild)
— Infection of biopsy site or uterine lining

I have also been informed of the following benefits of the procedure:
— Can be done in the office
— Helps diagnose cause of abnormal Pap smear
— Helps plan future therapy

I understand that the procedure to be performed will be done under the guidance of a colposcope (a special microscope). I consent to the administration of such local anesthesia as is considered necessary. I understand that video or photographic equipment may be used during my procedure for later educational purposes.

The procedure of biopsy of the cervix, endocervix, vagina, vulva, perineum, and anus has been explained to me. I have read and understand this information, and I have had all questions answered to my satisfaction. I consent to the procedures outlined in this form.

(Adult patient): _____

Signature: _____ Date: _____

Witness: _____ Time: _____ Date: _____

(Minor patient accompanied by parent or guardian): _____

I, the parent or legal guardian of the above-named minor, an unemancipated minor, do hereby consent to the procedures described above.

Signature (parent/guardian): _____ Date: _____

Witness: _____ Time: _____ Date: _____

Telephone authorization for unaccompanied minors:

Parent/guardian name: _____ Telephone: _____
_____

Caller (clinician) signature: _____ Date: _____
_____

Figure 86-5 Informed consent for colposcopy with biopsy of cervix, endocervix, vagina, introitus, perineum, or anus. (From Apgar BS, Brotzman G, Spitzer M (eds). Colposcopy: Principles and Practice. Philadelphia, WB Saunders, 2002.)

---

fortable passage of a larger speculum. In some women the lateral side walls of the vagina collapse inward and partially or completely obscure visualization of the cervix. Two methods are available to improve visualization. One is the use of a lateral wall retractor. The second is using a condom, which is less expensive and usually just as satisfactory (Fig. 86-11).

When the new squamocolumnar junction is difficult to visualize in the endocervical canal or when trying to visualize the full extent of an acetowhite lesion into the endocervical canal, an endocervical speculum can be used (Fig. 86-12).

Several types of punch biopsy forceps are available. The handles vary in length and the biopsy teeth

Patient Intake Form

Referred by: _____ Your name: _____

Your address: _____ City/State: _____ Zip code: _____

Home telephone: _____ Work telephone: _____

Your age now: _____ Date of your last menstrual period: _____

Please answer the following questions. Your answers will remain strictly confidential.

Reason(s) for referral: _____ Abnormal Pap smear

                _____ Vaginal discharge

                _____ Vaginal bleeding

                _____ DES exposure

                _____ Warts   For how long?_____

                _____ Other _____

Any prior treatment for abnormal Pap smears? _____ Yes _____ No

If yes, please list date and type of treatment: _____

Martial status: _____ Married _____ Single _____ Divorced

Age at first intercourse: _____ (0 = not applicable)

Total number of sexual partners in your lifetime: _____

Total # of pregnancies: _____ # of miscarriages or abortions: _____

Type of birth control currently used: _____ Birth control pill

                _____ IUD

                _____ Tubal ligation

                _____ Norplant

                _____ Vasectomy in partner

                _____ Barrier method

                _____ Other   What? _____

Do you smoke cigarettes? _____ Yes _____ No

   If yes, how many packs a day? _____ For how many years? _____

Have you ever been treated for any of the following:

_____ Herpes   _____ Chlamydia   _____ Trichomoniasis   _____ Other _____

_____ Gonorrhea   _____ Syphilis   _____ Warts   _____ No

Has your sexual partner ever been treated for the following:

_____ Herpes   _____ Chlamydia   _____ Trichomoniasis   _____ Other _____

_____ Gonorrhea   _____ Syphilis   _____ Warts   _____ No

Have you ever taken an AIDS test? _____ Yes_____ No

   If yes, was the result _____ positive or _____ negative?

Do you use intravenous drugs presently? _____ Yes _____ No

   In the past? _____ Yes _____ No

Do you have a history of a bleeding disorder? _____ Yes _____ No

Figure 86-6 Patient intake form. (From Apgar BS, Brotzman G, Spitzer M (eds). Colposcopy: Principles and Practice. Philadelphia, WB Saunders, 2002.)

Colposcopy Form

Patient ID#: _____

Examiner name(s): _____ Date: _____ Primary care physician: _____

Reason(s) for colposcopy: _____

_____

Colposcopic findings: LK — leukoplakia, WE — white epithelium, PN — punctation, MO — mosaic, AV — atypical vessel, SCJ — squamocolumnar junction, X — biopsy sites

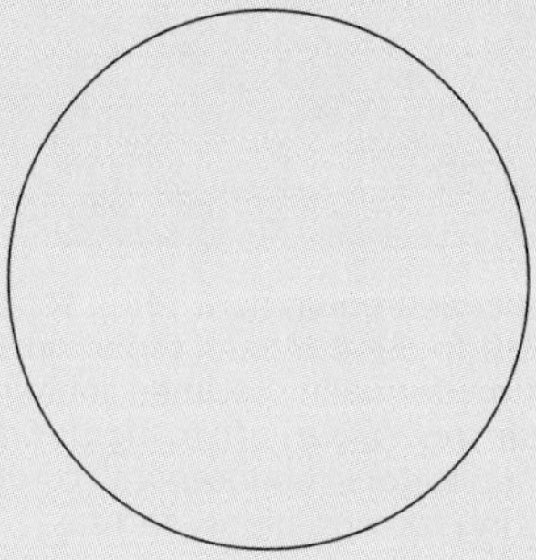

Pap smear done: _____ Yes _____ No

_____ ECC _____ Biospy of _____ Cervix _____ Vagina _____ Vulva

_____ HPV testing _____ Wet prep _____ Other _____

Colposcopy findings:

*Vulva, vagina, perineum, perianal area normal: _____ Yes _____ No

If no, describe:_____

*Entire SCJ seen: _____ Yes _____ No

*Limits of lesion seen: _____ Yes _____ No _____ NA

*Invasive cancer seen: _____ Yes _____ No

Colposcopic diagnosis: _____

Cytology diagnosis: _____

Biopsy diagnosis: _____

Final impression:

_____ Low-grade CIN

_____ High-grade CIN

_____ Invasive carcinoma

_____ Condyloma acuminatum

_____ Ectropion

_____ Squamous metaplasia

_____ Endocervical polyp _____ Endometrial polyp

_____ Other _____

Remarks: _____

_____

• Results and plan discussed with patient: _____ Yes _____ No

by _____ Phone _____ Letter _____ Other ( ) Date: _____

• Treatment options discussed, including:

_____ LEEP _____ LEEP cone _____ Laser _____ Cryo _____ CKC _____ TCA _____ Observation _____ Other

Management option selected: _____

• Follow-up date: _____

• Note sent to primary care physician: _____ Yes Date: _____ _____

Colposcopist signature

Figure 86-7 Colposcopy form. (From Apgar BS, Brotzman G, Spitzer M (eds). Colposcopy: Principles and Practice. Philadelphia, WB Saunders, 2002.)

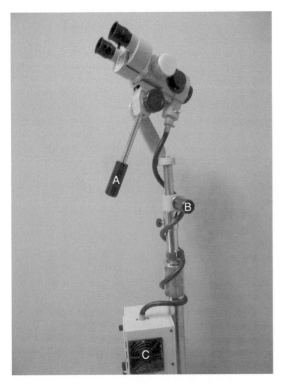

Figure 86-8 Colposcope on a stand. A, Twisting this handle moves the body of the colposcope toward or away from the object being viewed, allowing for fine focus. B, Twisting this handle moves the head of the scope vertically to allow for best visualization of the cervix. C, This box contains the light source, an on-off switch, and a rheostat to adjust the brightness of the light.

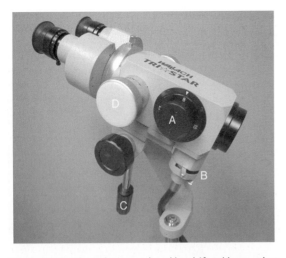

Figure 86-9 The colposcope head has bifocal lenses that adjust for varying intraocular distance and have an individual adjustment for focal length. A, This dial allows for selection of various lens magnifications. B, This is the green filter. It is in place at this time; flipping the silver handle horizontally will remove the green filter from the light source path. C, This handle moves the colposcope to allow for fine focus. D, When this white cap is removed, a camera can be attached to allow colposcopic pictures to be taken.

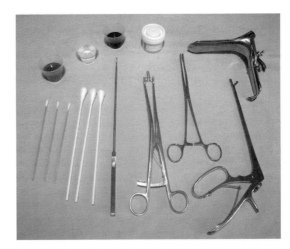

Figure 86-10 Basic supply and equipment setup for colposcopy. *Top row from left to right:* Monsel's solution, 3% acetic acid, Lugol's solution, formalin specimen container, Graves speculum. *Bottom row from left to right:* Small and large cotton tip applicators, endocervical curette, endocervical speculum, ring forceps, biopsy forceps.

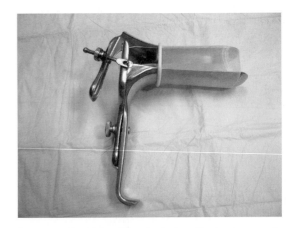

Figure 86-11 Although a lateral wall retractor can be used, it is usually sufficient to use a condom placed on a Grave's speculum to retract collapsing vaginal side walls.

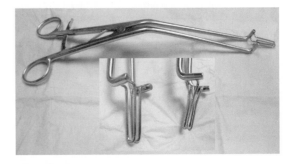

Figure 86-12 An endocervical speculum is helpful in opening the external os of the cervix to evaluate the full extent of the squamocolumnar junction or to determine the distance an acetowhite lesion extends into the endocervical canal. Inset: The tip of the endocervical speculum comes in two sizes to accommodate various endocervical canal openings.

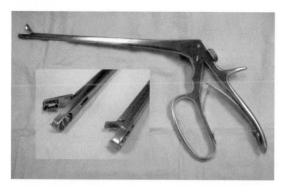

Figure 86-13 Biopsy forceps come in different lengths and with a variety of tips, varying in shape and size. This is a Tischler punch biopsy forceps. *Inset:* The two tips demonstrated here are the regular size Tischler and the baby Tischler.

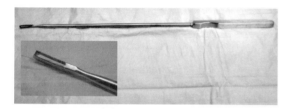

Figure 86-14 Endocervical curette. These come in various lengths and with various curette tips, some with a "basket" and some without. The inset shows a curette tip without a basket.

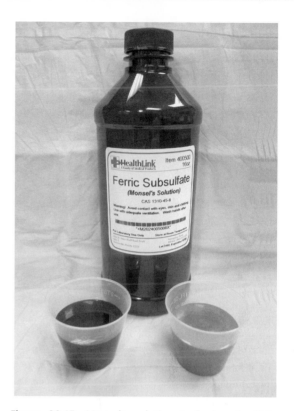

Figure 86-15 Monsel's solution is ferric subsulfate. Straight out of the bottle it is a dark watery liquid. When allowed to sit in a container that is open to the air for several days it will gradually thicken and change to a yellow-brown color. If it becomes too thick, it can be thinned by adding a small amount of ferric subsulfate straight out of the bottle.

vary in size and shape (Fig. 86-13). Because the focal length of most colposcopes is 30 cm, punch biopsy instruments with long handles may be difficult to maneuver. Again, personal preference comes into play. The endocervical curette also comes in various lengths and various tip configuration (with and without a basket) (Fig. 86-14). Some prefer a basket to help collect the curettings, others do not.

After a punch biopsy is performed, the biopsy site will bleed. Ferric subsulfate (Monsel's solution) is commonly used to achieve hemostasis (Fig. 86-15). To control bleeding, place Monsel's solution (Fig. 86-16) on a small, cotton-tipped swab and apply pressure to hold the swab to the biopsy site defect. Though this is almost always sufficient to stop bleeding, rarely it may be necessary to place a suture to stop the bleeding. For this purpose long instruments (needle driver, forceps, scissors) with needle and suture should be sterilized and available.

Colposcopy: The Examination

Vulua

Because condylomata and dysplasia can occur anywhere in the lower reproductive tract, colposcopy should include examination of the vulva, vagina, and

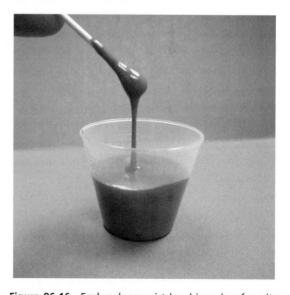

Figure 86-16 Each colposcopist has his or her favorite consistency of Monsel's solution for "best" application to the biopsy site to stop the bleeding. When it comes in contact with blood, the solution changes to a dark brown or black color. It is wise to warn the patient that she will have a colored discharge for several days following the application of Monsel's solution.

Table 86-5 Site-Specific Colposcopy: Vulva

Steps in Colposcopic Assessment	The Kinds of Observations You Can Expect to Make at This Step of the Examination	
	Normal Findings	*Abnormal Findings*
1. Assess before the application of 3%–5% acetic acid.	Hart's line Hair-bearing and non–hair-bearing squamous epithelium Sebaceous hyperplasia	Benign epithelial abnormalities (lichen selerosus, lichen planus, squamous cell hyperplasia) Lentigo maligna Bartholin's cyst/abscess Epithelial cysts
2. Assess with 3% acetic acid.	Micropapillomatosis labialis Nonspecific acetowhite epithelium	Condyloma acuminatum Acetowhite epithelium specific for preinvasive disease or invasion VIN 1, 2, 3 Vulvar carcinoma
3. Perform colposcopic-directed biopsy* (local anesthesia, punch, excision).		
4. Perform hemostasis (direct pressure, Monsel's solution [small amount, wipe away excess]).		
5. Apply protective dressing.*		

*Not required.
VIN, vulvar intraepithelial neoplasia.

cervix. Before a speculum is placed in the vagina begin with examination and colposcopy of the vulva (Table 86-5). Before applying acetic acid, begin the examination with the hair-bearing mons pubis and labia major lateral to Hart's line. Move medially evaluating the clitoral area outer aspect of labia minora and inner aspect. Continue to move the examination medially to and including the hymenal ring. Then examine the skin of the fourchette and move down to include the perineum and perianal area. Sebaceous hyperplasia is a common normal finding. Abnormal vulvar findings prior to application of acetic acid may include: vulvar atrophy, psoriasis (Color Plate 86-2), lichen simplex chronicus (Color Plate 86-3), lichen sclerosis (Color Plates 86-4 and 86-5), and lichen planus (Color Plate 86-6).

To apply 3% to 5 % acetic acid, fold 4 × 4-inch gauze in fourths, soak with acetic acid, gently spread the labia minora, and place the gauze just distal to the hymenal ring between the labia minora. Leave in place for 3 to 5 minutes (acetowhite changes take longer to manifest in the less moist vulvar epithelium than in the more moist cervical epithelium). Normal findings include micropapillomatosis labialis (Color Plate 86-7), nonspecific acetowhite epithelium (Color Plate 86-8) and lentigo simplex (Color Plate 86-9). Abnormal findings include condylomata acuminata (Color Plate 86-10), vulvar intraepithelial neoplasia (VIN) 1, 2, and 3 (Color Plates 86-11 to

86-14), and vulvar squamous cell carcinoma (Color Plates 86-15 and 86-16).

Suspicious areas should be biopsied using local anesthesia (topical application followed by injection) and punch biopsy. Hemostasis is achieved using direct pressure, a silver nitrate stick, and/or Monsel's solution. Rarely, suture placement may be necessary to achieve hemostasis. A protective dressing may or may not be applied. A topical broad-spectrum antibiotic can be applied.

Vagina

Colposcopy of the vagina is achieved in two steps (Table 86-6). The lateral walls of the vagina are examined after the speculum has been placed and opened. The cervix is gently moved in all directions with the open speculum to promote complete visualization of the anterior, posterior, and lateral fornices representing the cervical-vaginal junction. The anterior and posterior walls of the vagina can be examined as the speculum is removed slowly, allowing visualization of the vaginal epithelium as it rolls over the ends of the speculum. These steps will need to be repeated while applying acetic acid and after application of Lugol's solution. Lugol's iodine solution can be applied, with the normal glycogenated epithelium staining a dark mahogany. In comparing the appearance before and after application of Lugol's solution, the abnormal epithelium will not stain (Color Plate 86-17).

Table 86-6 Site-Specific Colposcopy: Vagina

Steps in Colposcopic Assessment	The Kinds of Observations You Can Expect to Make at This Step of the Examination	
	Normal Findings	*Abnormal Findings*
1. Clean the vagina with saline* and assess.	Squamous epithelium (no glands)	Adenosis Vaginal polyps Vaginal cysts DES morphology
2. Assess the vagina with a green filter before the application of 3%–5% acetic acid.*		Abnormal vascular patterns (punctation) Atypical vessels Patches of superficial erosions (strawberry spots caused by vaginitis)
3. Assess the vagina after the application of 3%–5% acetic acid.	Nonspecific acetowhite epithelium	Acetowhite epithelium specific for preinvasive or invasive disease VAIN 1, 2, 3 Vaginal carcinoma
4. Assess the vagina after the application of diluted Lugol's iodine solution.	Dark, mahogany staining (glycogenated epithelium)	Nonstaining (nonglycogenated epithelium) Variegated
5. Perform colposcopic-directed biopsy* (vaginal biopsy punch, local anesthesia, excision).		
6. Perform hemostasis (pressure, Monsel's solution, silver nitrate).		

*Not required.
DES, diethylstilbestrol; VAIN, vaginal intraepithelial neoplasia.
From Apgar BS, Brotzman G, Spitzer M (eds). Colposcopy: Principles and Practice. Philadelphia, WB Saunders, 2002.

Before the application of acetic acid, abnormal findings may include adenosis, vaginal polyps, vaginal cysts, diethylstilbestrol (DES) morphology such as adenosis (Color Plate 86-18), atrophy with petechial hemorrhages (Color Plate 86-19), and endometriosis. Examination using the green filter will accentuate punctation and other atypical vascular pattern such as the "strawberry" pattern (Color Plate 86-20) associated with infection. Application of 3% to 5% acetic acid will identify acetowhite areas with or without abnormal vascular patterns, which may represent squamous metaplasia, human papillomavirus (Color Plate 86-21), VIN 1, 2, and 3 (Color Plates 86-22 and 86-23), or vaginal squamous cell carcinoma (Color Plate 86-24).

After application of local anesthetic, a cervical punch biopsy instrument can be used to obtain a tissue sample. Hemostasis is achieved by applying direct pressure with Monsel's solution. If bleeding is light, a brief application of silver nitrate is sufficient. Rarely, suture placement may be necessary to achieve hemostasis.

Cervix

With the exception of use of the terms "satisfactory" or "unsatisfactory," colposcopy of the cervix is similar in many respects to colposcopy of the vulva and vagina (Table 86-7). The focus of the colposcopic examination is the ectocervix (Color Plate 86-25). For the colposcopic examination to be satisfactory all of the transition zone must be visualized and the full extent of any cervical lesion must be visualized. For example if an acetowhite lesion is present at the cervical os and it extends up into the endocervical canal such that the deep margin within the endocervical canal cannot be visualized, the examination would be referred to as unsatisfactory. The transition zone is the area of the cervix located between the old squamocolumnar junction (Color Plate 86-26) and the new squamocolumnar junction. The new squamocolumnar junction may be near the endocervical canal os (Color Plate 86-27) or may be separated from the endocervical os by the presence of ectropion (Color Plate 86-28).

The entire transition zone should be visualized, since this is where dysplasia begins. A large "Texas

Table 86-7 Site-Specific Colposcopy: Cervix

Steps in Colposcopic Assessment	The Kinds of Observations You Can Expect to Make at This Step of the Examination	
	Normal Findings	*Abnormal Findings*
1. Clean the cervix with saline.*	Mature squamous and columnar epithelia	Leukoplakia Polyps Nabothian cysts
2. Assess the cervix with a green filter before the application of 3%–5% acetic acid.*		Abnormal vascular patterns Atypical vessels
3. Assess the cervix after the application of 3%–5% acetic acid.	Gland openings Squamous metaplasia Squamocolumnar junction Nonspecific acetowhite changes	Condyloma acuminatum Acetowhite changes specific for preinvasive and invasive disease CIN 1, 2, 3 Cervical carcinoma Abnormal vascular patterns Atypical vessels
4. Assess the cervix after the application of diluted Lugol's iodine solution.*	Dark, mahogany staining (glycogenated epithelium)	Nonstaining Variegated (nonglycogenated epithelium)
5. Perform endocervical sampling* (ECC, cytobrush).		
6. Perform colposcopic-directed biopsy* (cervical biopsy punch).		
7. Perform hemostasis (pressure, Monsel's solution, silver nitrate).*		

*Not required.
CIN, cervical intraepithelial neoplasia; ECC, endocervical curettage.
From Apgar BS, Brotzman G, Spitzer M (eds). Colposcopy: Principles and Practice. Philadelphia, WB Saunders, 2002.

swab" can be used to apply acetic acid and move the cervix, allowing complete visualization of the transition zone (Color Plate 86-29). Before 3% to 5% acetic acid is applied, the colposcopic examination should be completed, first without using the green filter and then with the green filter. Acetic acid is applied for 1 to 2 minutes to allow the acetowhite areas to become evident. Without continuous application of acetic acid, the acetowhite lesions will fade. Not all colposcopists use Lugol's solution. If it is used, it is applied after all other examinations are completed.

Prior to application of acetic acid, abnormal findings might include leukoplakia (Color Plate 86-30), polyps, and nabothian cysts (Color Plate 86-31). Abnormal vascular patterns include mosaicism and punctation (Color Plates 86-32 and 86-33) and atypical blood vessels (Color Plate 86-34). After application of 3% to 5% acetic acid, condylomata acuminata, CIN I, II, or III, cervical cancer, abnormal vascular patterns, and atypical vessels may be seen. Acetowhite changes tend to occur in a geographic maplike pattern that can extend across the entire transition zone from the new squamocolumnar junction to the old squamocolumnar junction (Color Plate 86-35). The presence of a cervical collar or a coxcomb anterior lip suggests prior exposure to DES and increases the risk for adenosis and related cancer.

If the colposcopy is unsatisfactory, an endocervical sampling should be obtained using either an endocervical curette or a cytobrush. The endocervical curette is used to pull endocervical cells from a depth of 1 to 1.5 cm in a circumferential fashion to the external cervical os. The sample of cells is deposited there and once the sampling is complete, a ring forceps is used to gather the accumulated cell sample and place it in formalin. Following endocervical sampling the biopsy forceps are used to obtain as many biopsies as are indicated. In most situations anesthesia is not necessary prior to obtaining the biopsy. A general rule of thumb is, if a lesion is suspicious or you are not certain what it represents, biopsy it. Hemostasis is achieved using direct pressure and Monsel's solution. Rarely, suture placement may be necessary to achieve hemostasis.

Material Available on Student Consult

Review Questions and Answers about Cervical Dysplasia

REFERENCES

American College of Obstetricians and Gynecologists. ACOG Practice Bulletin: Clinical management guidelines for obstetrician-gynecologists. No. August 2003. Cervical cytology screening. Obstet Gynecol 2003;102: 417–427.ⓒ

Amies AE, Miller L, Lee SK, Koutsky L. The effect of vaginal speculum lubrication on the rate of unsatisfactory cervical cytology diagnoses. Obstet Gynecol 2002;100: 889–892.Ⓐ

Apgar BS, Zoschnick L, Wright, TC. The 2001 Bethesda system terminology. Am Fam Physician 2003;68: 1992–1998.ⓒ

Harer WB, Valenzuela G, Lebo D. Lubrication of the vaginal introitus and speculum does not affect Papanicolaou smears. Obstet Gynecol 2002;100: 887–888.Ⓐ

Levine L, Lucci III JA, Dinh TV. Atypical glandular cells: New Bethesda terminology and management guidelines. Obstet Gynecol Surv 2003;58:399–406.ⓒ

Nuovo J, Melnikow J, Howell LP. New tests for cervical cancer screening. Am Fam Physician 2001;64: 780–786.ⓒ

Schroeder BM. ACS Updates: Guidelines for the early detection of cervical neoplasia and cancer, Am Fam Physician 2003;67:2011–2016.ⓒ

Solomon D, Davey D, Kurman R, et al. The 2001 Bethesda System: Terminology for reporting results of cervical cytology. JAMA 2002;287:2116–2119.ⓒ

U.S. Preventive Services Task Force. Screening for cervical cancer: Recommendations and rationale. Am Fam Physician 2003;67:1759–1766.ⓒ

U.S. Preventive Services Task Force. Screening for cervical cancer. Rockville, MD, Agency for Healthcare Research and Quality, 2003. Available at www.ahrq.gov/clinic/uspstf/uspscerv2.htm. Accessed 11/6/2004.ⓒ

Wright TC, Cox JT. Clinical Uses of Human Papillomavirus (HPV) DNA Testing. American Society for Colposcopy and Cervical Pathology, 2004, pp 1–26.ⓒ

Wright TC, Cox JT, Massad LS, Twiggs LB, Wilkinson EJ. 2001 Consensus guidelines for the management of women with cervical cytologic abnormalities. JAMA 2002;287:2120–2129.ⓒ

Chapter

87

Feeling Depressed (Drug Dependency)

Timothy Scanlan

KEY POINTS

1. Screen all adult patients for drug problems.
2. The CAGE questions are effective and easy to remember.
3. It's easy to miss a drug problem through focusing on the chief complaint. Be sure to ask specifically about drug use.
4. A brief intervention may help to reduce or eliminate drug use.
5. Adjunct medication can be helpful to some patients in stopping drug use.

INITIAL VISIT

Subjective

Patient Identification and Presenting Problem

Lisa is a 35-year-old white woman complaining of feeling "terribly depressed" and wondering if an antidepressant "would help me feel better." Lisa states that she has been feeling really depressed for the last couple of weeks and has lost interest in everything, even things she previously enjoyed. She believes her symptoms started about a year ago but have become worse recently. She states that she has been "stressed

Evidence levels Ⓐ Randomized, controlled trials (RCTs), meta-analyses, well-designed systematic reviews of RCTs. Ⓑ Case-control or cohort studies, nonrandomized clinical trials, systematic reviews of studies other than RCTs, cross-sectional studies, retrospective studies, certain uncontrolled studies. Ⓒ Consensus statements, expert guidelines, usual practice, opinion.

out" since her divorce 3 years ago. Lisa complains of loss of energy, difficulty sleeping, poor concentration at work, and pervasive sadness. She has experienced decreased appetite and some weight loss, but she is pleased about that. She denies any thoughts of harming herself but really wants to feel better. She usually sees you about every 2 years for her well-woman examinations.

Medical History

Lisa has no history of medical problems and no prior surgery. She takes oral contraceptives. She has had only one pregnancy, when she was 18, but terminated it. She has no history of sexually transmitted diseases (STDs).

Family History

Lisa's parents are divorced; both are alive and well. There is no family history of depression. Her mother is an alcoholic. She has two siblings, a brother and a sister, with no known health problems.

Social History

Lisa was married for 10 years but divorced 3 years ago. She has no children. She denies being physically abused but states that her ex-husband used cocaine. She is not currently in a relationship. Lisa is employed as a secretary. She reports no legal problems but admits she is having financial difficulties.

Health Habits

Lisa states she has smoked half a pack of cigarettes a day since age 15 and has never attempted to quit. She drinks alcohol when out socially with friends, usually only two to three drinks or beers once a week. After some hesitation in answering questions regarding drug use, she admits to using cocaine. She states she experimented a few times when she was married, with her husband's encouragement, and then started using cocaine on her own to party after her divorce. She initially snorted but now smokes crack cocaine. She uses cocaine at least 5 to 7 days a week if she can afford it. She uses a lot on weekends when out with her friends. She says she likes the way it makes her feel, and it makes her depression go away for a while. Recently, she has been using every day. She doesn't seem to think it's a big problem. Her main concern is getting into legal trouble if caught. She says she can quit anytime she wants. She admits that cocaine makes her promiscuous, and she feels guilty about that sometimes. Her last use of cocaine was last night. Lisa denies using other substances and denies intravenous (IV) drug use.

Review of Systems

The review of systems is unremarkable for any additional symptoms.

Objective

Physical Examination

On physical examination, blood pressure is 130/75, pulse is 90, respirations are 20/min, and temperature is 37.2°C (99°F). Weight is 110 pounds; height, 5 feet 4 inches.

The ear, nose, and throat examination is normal, including an intact nasal septum. The chest is clear to auscultation. The cardiac examination shows normal sinus rhythm; no murmur is detected. The extremities show no needle tracks. The abdomen is nontender on palpation, and no organomegaly is detected.

In appearance, Lisa is thin but well nourished and well hydrated. She exhibits sad affect and a depressed mood, and is guarded in conversation. She expresses no suicidal ideation or thought disorder.

Assessment

Lisa clearly is having problems with cocaine and meets criteria for cocaine dependence. She might not have been so open about her cocaine use if she were not depressed and if you were not her family physician. Her openness is not an indication of understanding, acceptance, or readiness to quit on her part. In all likelihood her depression is due in part to her cocaine use and her susceptibility to drug problems is in part due to genetic susceptibility. To diagnose major depression as an independent condition, she would need to have persistent symptoms after being drug-free for 2 to 4 weeks. Lisa urgently needs treatment for cocaine dependence and symptoms of depression.

Other concerns are her high-risk sexual behavior and her smoking while taking oral contraceptives. It is probable that her sexual behavior is directly linked to her drug use and will stop when her drug problem is adequately treated. She likely is not ready to quit smoking right now, but this issue needs to be addressed with her. Her weight loss is evident (current weight, 110 pounds) and is probably due to her cocaine use.

Plan

Diagnostic

A urine drug screen (UDS) can be helpful when it is not clear whether someone is using a specific drug, and it can also be used to rule out use of other drugs. Urine drug testing can detect the common drugs of abuse, such as cocaine, opiates, marijuana, amphetamines, and phencyclidine (PCP). Urine drug testing does not routinely test for benzodiazepines or barbiturates. Also, a routine UDS can have false positive results from prescription and over-the-counter medications.

Obtaining a complete blood cell count, comprehensive metabolic profile, and thyroid-stimulating hormone level can help rule out other contributing factors to her depression. Given Lisa's history, an evaluation for STDs is appropriate.

Therapeutic

Lisa needs referral to a drug treatment program for further evaluation and treatment. It is helpful and reinforcing for the physician to assist with this referral appointment, even discussing your concerns with the treatment professional in the patient's presence.

Starting antidepressant medication is also appropriate. Lisa's depression is likely to improve with treatment of her drug dependence, but she would benefit more from that treatment if she experienced some relief of her depressive symptoms. Tricyclic antidepressants (TCAs) and selective serotonin reuptake inhibitors (SSRIs) seem to have equal efficacy in the treatment of depression. Some considerations are the incidence of side effects and the mechanism of action. Since depression from cocaine abuse is thought to be due to dopamine depletion, TCAs might be the drug of choice, and in fact there is some evidence that desipramine works well for both the depression associated with cocaine use and the relief of craving. SSRIs may also have some benefit in treating the depression, especially if TCAs are not tolerated.

Patient Education

This patient needs support and encouragement and firm advice to follow through with treatment. You should be clear about your concern for her well-being. The FRAMES format for a brief intervention (Box 87-1) provides a helpful guide to thinking about what to discuss in these situations, even though this case is not ideal for brief intervention because of the severity of the problem. You should discuss the relationship between her cocaine use and her symptoms of depression, her weight loss, and her financial problems. Making the connections explicit will help her understand that treatment will help her return to full function and satisfaction with her life and help her resolve her current problems.

This is also an opportunity to discuss other healthy lifestyle changes, such as smoking cessation (especially since she is taking oral contraceptives) and increasing exercise, while recognizing that she may not be ready to address these issues right now.

DISCUSSION

Patients should always be asked about drug use. While this is a fairly typical presentation for cocaine use in a family practice setting, it would have been easy to overlook drug use given the other potential factors that may have contributed to Lisa's symptoms, such as a prior abortion, divorce, and financial problems. The clues that lead you to at least suspect the possibility of drug use are her age, her ex-husband's use, the pattern of symptoms (depression, weight loss, smoker), and a family history of alcoholism. Drug use often masquerades as psychological problems. Depending on the drug, patients may present with depression, anxiety, psychosis, or delirium in the office or emergency department. Checking for drug use by asking is the best way to screen. A UDS can also be helpful. The CAGE questions are useful in the presence of drug use to evaluate the extent of the problem (Box 87-2). Differentiating between drug abuse and drug dependence is not as clear-cut as with alcohol use, although the criteria are the same (Box 87-3). The health risks of drug abuse increase significantly as the amounts used and the frequency of use increase, and also increase with the onset of IV drug use.

Some patients are "unsafe" users of illicit drugs but do not meet abuse or dependence criteria. The social use of illegal drugs is a nebulous area and not one easily addressed. Insofar as there is no known safe use of illicit drugs, brief intervention involves discussing with the patient the health risks of drug use and recommending abstinence.

Box 87-1	FRAMES: Outline for a Brief Intervention

Feedback—regarding concerns, risks, problem indicators
Responsibility—emphasize choice and personal control to change
Action—advice/recommendations about appropriate steps
Menu—options or strategies
Empathy—warm, reflective understanding
Support—optimize self-empowerment

Box 87-2	CAGE Questions (for Drugs)

1. Have you ever felt you should _cut down_ on your drug use?
2. Do you ever feel _annoyed_ when others criticize your drug use?
3. Have you ever felt bad or _guilty_ about your drug use?
4. Have you ever used drugs the next day to relieve symptoms from the previous day's drug use ("_eye-opener_")?

Adapted from Ewing JA. Detecting alcoholism: The CAGE questionnaire. JAMA 1984;252:1905–1907. Cited in

Box 87-3	DSM-IV Criteria for Diagnosing Substance Abuse and Substance Dependence

Substance Abuse

A maladaptive pattern of substance use leading to clinically significant impairment or distress, as manifested by one (or more) of the following within a 12-month period:
1. Failure to fulfill major role obligations
2. Use that is physically hazardous
3. Recurrent legal problems
4. Continued use despite persistent adverse social or interpersonal problems/consequences

Substance Dependence

A maladaptive pattern of substance use leading to clinically significant impairment or distress, as manifested by three (or more) of the following within a 12-month period:
1. Tolerance
2. Withdrawal
3. Using larger amounts or over a longer period than intended
4. A persistent desire or unsuccessful efforts to cut down or quit
5. Spending a great deal of time to obtain, use, and/or recover from the drug
6. Giving up social, occupational, or recreational activities because of substance use
7. Continued use despite persistent or recurrent physical or psychological problems

Data from American Psychiatric Association. Diagnostic and Statistical Manual of Mental Disorders, 4th ed., Text Revision (DSM-IV-TR). Bethesda, MD, American Psychiatric Association, 2000.

This patient clearly shows very disturbing patterns of her drug use. Her use is accelerating, and she is depressed and losing weight. She is not likely to respond to an antidepressant alone. Her sexual behavior is very risky. Her denial is currently being supported by the positive reinforcement of the euphoria that cocaine produces. Knowing she needs to quit using drugs and being willing to do so are vastly different things. It is important to consider a backup plan should she refuse to see a substance abuse counselor. Some alternatives include monitoring her in your office with UDSs and insisting she at least attend Cocaine Anonymous (CA) meetings. She could also still be treated with antidepressants. She may not see the need for more formal treatment until her problems become more severe.

Cocaine is not the only drug of abuse seen in family medicine. Marijuana and methamphetamines are also commonly used. It is important to note that prescription drug abuse is becoming more common than illicit drug use in the United States. Table 87-1 shows the most recent statistics from the National Household Survey on the prevalence of drug use in American communities. Past month use as described in this table is more descriptive of current use than is past year use. The prevalence of drug use by patients in our practices may be higher than is indicated in the table because drug users tend to use primary health care services more than nonusers do.

Patients who are advised by their family physician about their alcohol or drug use are more likely to attend and complete a treatment program than patients who do not have that discussion. Family physicians should show care and concern, be open about the issues, and give firm, sensible advice. It is also important to recognize that patients who attempt to stop drug use with a treatment program may still use drugs intermittently during or after treatment. An understanding approach that does not instill guilt will help patients through this period of early recovery.

The evaluation of patients with possible alcohol or drug problems should include an evaluation of medical and psychiatric stability, as well as the risks associated with withdrawal.

Table 87-1 Common Drugs of Abuse

Drug	Percent Who Reported Use in Past Year/ Past Month
Marijuana	11.0 / 6.2
Cocaine, methamphetamines	3.2 / 1.2
Heroin	0.2 / 0.1
Hallucinogens	2.0 / 0.5
Inhalants	0.9 / 0.3
Psychotherapeutics (prescription)	6.2 / 2.6

Data from U.S. Department of Health and Human Services, Substance Abuse and Mental Health Services Administration. 2002 National Survey on Drug Use and Health. Bethesda, MD, U.S. Department of Health and Human Services Adminstration, 2002.

Treatment

The treatment of drug problems may include formal inpatient or outpatient treatment, depending on the severity of the problem. Attending meetings of self-help groups such as CA or Narcotics Anonymous (NA) is an important component of recovery. The emphasis of treatment is on abstinence from all mood-altering substances; even modest alcohol use can lead back to drug use. Some narcotic addicts with addiction unresponsive to other forms of therapy might benefit from methadone or buprenorphine therapy.

Monitoring patients in recovery helps motivate them and ensure their adherence. Urine and hair drug testing are accurate and useful. Patients who have been IV drug users should also be tested for hepatitis and HIV.

Great care should be taken when prescribing medications for patients with a history of drug problems because they are at risk for developing abuse of or dependence on scheduled drugs. Avoid these medications whenever possible and use noncontrolled alternatives.

The management of drug withdrawal is also an important consideration. Although most drug withdrawal syndromes, with the exception of alcohol and benzodiazepine withdrawal, are not life-threatening, drug withdrawal is very uncomfortable and is typically associated with drug craving. Failure to manage these symptoms often leads to resumption of drug use. Two excellent resources for help with withdrawal management are noted in the list of suggested readings.

Material Available on Student Consult

Review Questions and Answers about Drug Dependency

SUGGESTED READINGS

Giannini A J. An approach to drug abuse, intoxication and withdrawal. Am Fam Physician 2000;61:2763–2774.

A Guide to Substance Abuse Services for Primary Care Physicians (Treatment Improvement Protocol Series No. 24, DHHS Publication No. 97-3139). Bethesda, MD, U.S. Department of Health and Human Services, Substance Abuse and Mental Health Services Administration, 1997. Available at www.ncbi.nlm.nih.gov/books. Accessed 11/15/2004.●

Schuckit M. Drug and Alcohol Abuse: A Clinical Guide to Diagnosis and Treatment, 5th ed. New York, Plenum, 2000.

Weaver M, Jarvis M. Overview of the recognition and management of the drug abuser. UpToDate, Jan. 9, 2004. Available at www.patients.uptodate.com/topic.asp?file=genr_med/21475. Accessed 11/15/2004.●

Wilford B. Principles of Addiction Medicine, 3rd ed. Chevy Chase, MD, American Society of Addiction Medicine, 2003.

88

Chest Pain and Fatigue (Anxiety Disorder)

Katherine Margo

INITIAL VISIT

Subjective

Patient Identification and Presenting Problem

Susan M. is a 32-year-old woman who presents for the first time with chest pain and fatigue.

Present Illness

Susan started having chest pains in the past week, which is why she finally decided to come in. She was in the emergency department two nights ago where they did several tests and told her it was not her heart. She does not understand what it could be and is very worried. Her pain is sharp and on the left side of her chest. It comes and goes, and nothing really helps it. Susan also says that she has been feeling more and more tired over the past few months. She does admit that she is having trouble sleeping and

often wakes up early. She has no history of psychiatric illness including panic attacks. She denies any recent changes in her work, life, or marriage. However, on careful questioning, she is able to recall feeling worried over the past 7 to 8 months, but it has become such a constant part of her daily experience that she did not think to mention it.

Medical History

Susan is generally healthy with no hospitalizations except for childbirth. She does not like taking medicine but does take vitamins and some herbs from a local health food store. She denies alcohol, cigarettes, or illicit drug use.

Family History

Her father is an alcoholic, and she does not see him much. Her mother's health is fair, but her mother has no specific disease that Susan knows about.

Social History

Susan is married and has one child, age 3. She works full time as an account executive in an advertising agency. She is a hard worker but reports that recently she is not as productive as she would like to be because she functions less efficiently when she feels so stressed. When asked about this, she says that her concentration is not what it used to be and she worries that something is seriously wrong.

Review of Systems

She has no history of diabetes, hypertension, or thyroid disease. She denies problems with her eyes, ears, or mouth but does get headaches from time to time. She has no trouble with her heart, although she does notice that her heart beats fast. She has no trouble breathing and no cough or history of asthma. She does not have urinary problems but does have loose stools. She has no joint problems. Her periods have been normal.

Evidence levels Ⓐ Randomized, controlled trials (RCTs), meta-analyses, well-designed systematic reviews of RCTs. Ⓑ Case-control or cohort studies, nonrandomized clinical trials, systematic reviews of studies other than RCTs, cross-sectional studies, retrospective studies, certain uncontrolled studies. Ⓒ Consensus statements, expert guidelines, usual practice, opinion.

Objective

Physical Examination

Susan is a healthy-appearing woman who looks anxious. Vital signs: height, 5 feet 7 inches tall; weight, 140 pounds; temperature, 36.9°C (98.5°F); respiratory rate, 18; pulse, 100; blood pressure, 110/70. Head, eyes, ears, nose, and throat are all normal. Pupils are equal and reactive with normal extraocular muscle function. Neck: thyroid is normal and symmetrical. No bruit or lymphadenopathy. Her lungs are clear and her heart has a regular rate and rhythm with a grade 1/6 systolic flow murmur. Her chest wall is tender diffusely. Her breast examination is normal. Neurologic examination is normal, including deep tendon reflexes throughout, sensation, and muscle strength. Abdominal examination is nontender, with no masses or organomegaly.

Assessment

Working Diagnosis

Generalized anxiety disorder (GAD). This is one of a number of conditions collected under the heading of anxiety disorders. The *Diagnostic and Statistical Manual of Mental Disorders, 4th Edition*, criteria for diagnosing GAD are listed in Box 88-1. Susan has been feeling anxious for more than 6 months, even though she has not used this term to describe her feelings. This differentiates it from panic attacks that are brief, intense attacks of anxiety. The anxiety has been sufficient to disrupt her work functioning and she feels that something is seriously wrong. Her sleep has been disturbed lately, leaving her tired and irritable during the day. The chest pain that brought her to medical attention seems to be from muscle soreness of her chest wall.

Differential Diagnosis

Anxiety can be considered a symptom as well as an illness. All conditions, both psychological and somatic, that include anxiety as an associated symptom should be considered in the differential diagnosis.

1. *Psychiatric illnesses.* Other anxiety disorders are agoraphobia and other phobias, social phobia, panic disorder, obsessive-compulsive disorder, and post-traumatic stress disorder, in addition to the anxiety disorder associated with medical conditions and substances noted earlier. However, any psychiatric illness in which patients feel that something frightening is happening to them will have an anxiety component. Such a list includes depression, schizophrenia and other psychoses, and even early dementia. These, especially depression, should be specifically assessed for to determine whether they are also present.

Box 88-1	Diagnostic Criteria for Generalized Anxiety Disorder (GAD)

The following criteria describe GAD

1. Excessive anxiety and worry about several events or activities, occurring most of the time for at least 6 months, and which seem out of proportion.
2. The worry is pervasive and difficult to control.
3. The anxiety and worry are associated with three (or more) of the following six symptoms:
   Restlessness or feeling on edge
   Being easily fatigued
   Trouble concentrating
   Irritability
   Muscle pain or tightness
   Sleep disturbance (difficulty falling or staying asleep, or restless sleep)
4. The anxiety, worry, or physical symptoms cause effects on social, occupational, or other important areas of functioning.
5. There is no other explanation, such as drug use, prescribed or abused, or a medical condition that explains the symptoms.

Adapted from American Psychiatric Association. Diagnostic and Statistical Manual for Mental Disorders, 4th Edition. Washington, DC, American Psychiatric Association, 1994.

2. *Drugs*, prescribed (sympathomimetics) or not (caffeine, cocaine, amphetamines), can produce anxiety, as can alcohol and sedative-hypnotic withdrawal.
3. *Metabolic and endocrine diseases* associated with anxiety include hyperthyroidism, pheochromocytoma, hypoadrenalism, hypoglycemia, and hypokalemia.
4. *Heart disease.* Anxiety is commonly seen in coronary artery disease, especially during myocardial infarction, when the anxiety is an expression of the fear that the patient has of dying. The common cardiac illnesses that are often associated with anxiety include coronary artery disease, heart failure of any cause, rhythm disturbances, and mitral valve prolapse.
5. *Respiratory illness* associated with dyspnea can have associated anxiety. This includes common illnesses such as asthma and chronic obstructive pulmonary disease as well as uncommon conditions like pulmonary embolism and scleroderma.

Plan

Susan's history and physical examination show no evidence of other psychiatric or substance abuse conditions or any major medical illness including cardiac or pulmonary disease. Her electrocardiogram is normal. Laboratory studies confirm normal electrolyte and glucose levels and normal thyroid status. Because there are no clinical findings pointing to other potential anxiety-associated nonpsychiatric diseases, additional testing is not indicated. However, in the course of the slow and careful history taking, it is evident that Susan is facing a number of emotionally troubling issues. She is bothered that she has to leave her young daughter in day care for a long day. She is particularly sensitive to perceived criticism at work for not being more productive, and in a counterproductive way, her anxiety leads to increasing irritability at home, alienating her usually supportive husband. Her alcoholic father is doing badly, and she avoids him but feels guilty for doing so.

DISCUSSION

GAD is the most common anxiety disorder. The prevalence in primary care is approximately 5% (Roy-Byrne and Katon, 1997Ⓐ).

It is more common in women than men: 60% to 40%. It tends to follow a chronic course and fluctuates in intensity over time. There is often a familial pattern to anxiety, but whether this is genetic or learned is not clear (American Psychiatric Association, 1994Ⓒ).

Medical conditions can produce anxiety as part of their symptom picture. More common examples include hyperthyroidism and mitral valve prolapse (Gliatto, 2000Ⓑ). Medical conditions typically associated with stress, such as irritable bowel syndrome and headache, can have concurrent GAD. As noted in the differential diagnosis section, there are multiple possibilities to consider. GAD is also often seen with other anxiety disorders, depression, and substance abuse (Brawman-Mintzer et al., 1993Ⓐ). Patients with GAD tend to be high utilizers of medical services and to have poorer health.

A discussion of GAD is complicated by multiple connotations of the word *anxiety*. Anxiety, as it is used in this case, refers to one of a group of psychiatric disorders. The word is also used in common language to refer to psychological distress of a worried or fearful kind and as such is seen widely in all illnesses and in any aspect of human life. In this sense, an anxiety disorder would not be diagnosed. The formal designation of "anxiety disorder" is given when the experience of anxiety reaches a certain level of severity, interferes with function, and lasts for a period of time. This distinction is more than just philosophical. Unless the distinction is understood, we may find ourselves overtreating our patients, medicating the ups and downs of life rather than listening to a story of real but limited distress.

Treatments of GAD can be primarily psychological or pharmacologic. In practice, it is common for patients, especially those with more severe symptoms, to receive combined psychological and pharmacologic treatment.

Psychological treatments can be broadly divided into those aimed primarily at symptom control through cognitive and behavioral methods and those aimed at exploring the psychological meaning of the symptom followed by working through and resolution of underlying psychological issues. Examples of the first approach are supportive counseling and cognitive-behavioral therapy. Supportive work includes psychoeducational efforts directed at reducing symptoms by educating the patient about the disorder and the generally good outcome. Cognitive-behavioral therapy takes this further by identifying unrealistic or distorted thinking patterns behind the anxiety, and learning new ways to solve problems and cope with symptoms (Gliatto, 2000Ⓑ).

Exploratory or psychodynamic therapies work on the assumption that the anxiety arises as a signal of underlying psychological distress, such as that caused by conflicts, disrupted relationships, and so on. The anxiety is relieved by identifying the psychological causes of distress, looking at the issues in therapy, and finding new ways or meanings that allow for a new psychological equilibrium (Gabbard, 2000Ⓑ). Psychodynamic psychotherapy receives little attention in the family medicine literature, and the common perception is that the approach has no sound evidence base. This is not correct, and a full discussion is beyond the scope of this case. However, an unusual study warrants a mention as a beginning of discussion of this topic. Consumers Union, the publishers of *Consumer Reports*, studied a self-selected sample of 3079 of their readers who had sought help for anxiety, depression, or a combination of both. In general, patients who received psychotherapy for periods of 13 weeks or more did as well as or better than those receiving drugs alone. The therapy is described as "talk therapy," a phrase used to describe an exploratory approach to treatment (*Consumer Reports*, 2004Ⓑ).

Pharmacologic treatments follow from the idea that anxiety symptoms are the result of a disordered response of the neurotransmitters norepinephrine, serotonin, and γ-aminobutyric acid to stress. The mainstay of anxiety medication management has been the benzodiazepines (Gliatto, 2000Ⓑ). While these drugs do not cure anxiety, they effectively reduce or eliminate the experience of anxiety. Short-acting benzodiazepines are effective but must be taken every 2 to 3 hours for continued symptom control. In addition to this practical disadvantage, the shorter-acting benzodiazepines tend to be more addictive than the longer-acting forms. Some patients like the rapid onset and "buzz" of alprazolam, but the problems of addiction and subsequent struggles over withdrawal cause many practitioners to avoid it. Lorazepam (Ativan) has the advantage of quick onset, especially when used sublingually, and longer duration of action (4 to 5 hours). Clonazepam (Klonopin) is a particularly advantageous benzodiazepine for ongoing use in that it requires only twice-daily dosing. Dosing starts at 0.25 to 0.5 mg twice daily with a maximum daily dose of 3 to 4 mg. The rule is to start low and titrate upward slowly to reach acceptable symptom control. Drowsiness is the most significant adverse effect. Withdrawal must be done slowly, cutting 10% of the dose per week, and adding imipramine if necessary to make the taper easier. Given this information, it is reasonable to avoid these drugs in patients with anxiety associated with chronic illnesses, in addicts, and in those with a severe personality disorder.

Buspirone (BuSpar) is also an effective antianxiety agent but with a slow onset of action over several weeks. It is not addictive and can be withdrawn without difficulty. Doses range between 15 and 30 mg twice daily (Davidson et al., 1999Ⓐ).

Many antidepressant drugs are effective for treatment of GAD. Tricyclics, selective serotonin reuptake inhibitors, and venlafaxine (Effexor) have all been shown to be useful (Kapczinski et al., 2003Ⓐ). Tricyclics tend to be used less often nowadays because of their side effect profile and greater risk of overdose. However, there is no difference in efficacy that would make one choose one antidepressant over another in GAD other than considerations of side effects and cost. It is important to remember two clinical pearls: response to these drugs is variable among individuals, so that an unsuccessful trial of 3 to 4 weeks of one drug should be followed by a different drug, preferably of a different class; and, second, although the new antidepressants are promoted as being better tolerated than the old tricyclics, there is no one drug that is uniformly well tolerated.

GAD can be regarded as a diagnosis of exclusion in that anxiety is the dominant symptom without specific precipitants as found, for example, in phobias, and without the severe dominant physical symptoms such as seen in panic attacks. Likewise, GAD is diagnosed when no obvious medical illness or substance abuse or withdrawal is causing the anxiety symptoms. Although the focus here is on GAD, it is important to be able to differentiate between the major anxiety disorders. Correct diagnosis is important in tailoring treatment for the patient. The following review of the diagnostic criteria for the various anxiety disorders allows the practitioner to place an anxious patient into the appropriate category (American Psychiatric Association, 1994Ⓒ). Even though anxiety disorders have much in common in terms of treatment, some key differences from the treatment of GAD are noted.

In *phobias*, there is a clearly recognizable precipitant for the anxiety. The most common phobia, *agoraphobia*, arises from the fear of being exposed or trapped in a situation perceived as dangerous or embarrassing. In its severe form, such patients tend to stay at home or in familiar places or may only venture out accompanied by a friend or relative. Other phobias such as fear of dogs and snakes are easily recognized. Cognitive-behavioral therapy is most helpful for phobias, with the addition of an antidepressant in agoraphobia.

Social phobia is also known as social anxiety disorder; this is probably a better name because "phobia" usually refers to a specific precipitant, whereas in social anxiety disorder, a whole range of social exposure leads to crippling anxiety. Such patients avoid interactions with others to the extent that they may be unable to eat in a social setting or work with colleagues. They often end up in solitary jobs, often on the night shift. This disorder is particularly difficult to treat. Selective serotonin reuptake inhibitors are the mainstay of treatment, often combined with behavior therapy.

Panic disorder is diagnosed when *panic attacks* are recurrent and are followed by at least a month of anxiety about another attack or about the effect of the attacks. Panic attacks are a particular variant of anxiety characterized by severe, discrete episodes of sympathetic discharge with symptoms such as sweating, palpitations, shortness of breath, trembling, choking, chest pain, dizziness, paresthesias, nausea, as well as a fear of dying or of losing control. Tricyclics, selective serotonin reuptake inhibitors, and venlafaxine are used in treatment.

Obsessive-compulsive disorder is a severe, complex illness characterized by recurrent obsessive thinking and/or compulsive behavior. These patients suffer from anxiety usually provoked by any factor that may interfere with the expression of their compulsions or obsessions. It not possible to do justice to the complexity and morbidity of obsessive-compulsive disorder here. It is the least anxiety disorder-like of the group and probably deserves a diagnostic category all its own. Both cognitive-behavioral therapy and antidepressants (clomipramine and the selective serotonin reuptake inhibitors) are primary treatment modalities.

Post-traumatic stress disorder follows for some people after a real or potential life-threatening experience. The symptoms can be considered in three groups: anxiety-associated with recurrent, intrusive recollections of the event; nightmares of the traumatic event and waking re-experiencing the event; avoiding situations that remind the patient of the traumatic experience and a general numbing of responsiveness; and symptoms of increased arousal such as hypervigilance, exaggerated startle, and irritability. Acute stress disorder refers to the development of a stress disorder within a month of the experience, whereas post-traumatic stress disorder is used for a disorder that persists longer than a month. Treatment is difficult and combinations of psychotherapy of all types, antianxiety agents, and antidepressants are all used.

FOLLOW-UP VISIT

Susan and her physician discuss the material presented here. This psychoeducational approach helps her gain a perspective on what at first were puzzling and frightening symptoms. She is psychologically minded but initially felt embarrassed to acknowledge that "my mind could play such tricks on me." Once she overcomes that hurdle, she is intrigued at the range of treatment options. Because she prefers to avoid taking medicine and because she is curious about the idea of understanding where her anxiety is coming from, she accepts a referral to a psychodynamic psychotherapist. When she returns to the office some months later, she is happy to report that the pieces in her life are falling into place. For example, she had not consciously realized how difficult it was for her to leave her child for as long a day as she was doing. She felt that she had to show that she was tough and capable in the work world. As she looked at this, she realized that she could make some changes that allowed for a better compromise between her wish to pursue her career and desire to be a loving mother. She also allowed herself to ask for, and to accept, more help from her husband. He was delighted, and their relationship found a new and better balance. She says that now for the first time in years, she is ready to take another look at her relationship with her father, whose drinking had had a significantly adverse effect on her life. She thanks her physician for discussing the full range of treatment options and for encouraging her to make her own choices once she had the information.

Material Available on Student Consult

Review Questions and Answers about Anxiety Disorder

REFERENCES

American Psychiatric Association. Diagnostic and Statistical Manual of Mental Disorders, 4th ed. Washington, DC, American Psychiatric Association, 1994, pp 432–436. Ⓒ

Brawman-Mintzer O, Lydiard RB, Emmanuel N, et al. Psychiatric comorbidity in patients with generalized anxiety disorder. Am J Psychiatry 1993;150:1216–1218. Ⓐ

Consumer Reports. Drugs vs. talk therapy. Consumer Rep 2004:69:22–29. Ⓑ

Davidson JR, DuPont RL, Hedges D, Haskins JT. Efficacy, safety, and tolerability of venlafaxine extended release and buspirone in outpatients with generalized anxiety disorder. J Clin Psychiatry 1999;60:528–535. Ⓐ

Gabbard GO. Psychodynamic Psychiatry in Clinical Practice, 3rd ed. Washington, DC, American Psychiatric Association, 2000, pp 233–266. Ⓑ

Gliatto MF. Generalized anxiety disorder. Am Fam Physician 2000;62:1591–1602. Ⓑ

Kapczinski F, Lima MS, Souza JS, Schmitt R. Antidepressants for generalized anxiety disorder. Cochrane Database Syst Rev 2003:CD003592. Ⓐ

Roy-Byrne PP, Katon W. Generalized anxiety disorder in primary care: The precursor/modifier pathway to increased health care utilization. J Clin Psychiatry 1997; 58(Suppl 3):34–38. Ⓐ

89

Multiple Somatic Complaints (Generalized Anxiety Disorder)

Michael G. Kavan

INITIAL VISIT

Subjective

Patient Identification and Presenting Problem

Katherine M. is a 36-year-old single white woman who works as a receptionist for a medical clinic. She is referred by a medical staff member at her place of employment because of her various somatic complaints, which have worsened over the past 3 months. This is her first visit to this clinic.

Katherine reports that she has been experiencing shakiness, shortness of breath, rapid heart rate, chest pain, light-headedness, sleep difficulties, and weight loss. She has also been worrying excessively about several issues in her life, and this worrying in turn has resulted in concentration difficulties at work and home. Although her symptoms have been present over the past year, she says they have worsened considerably over the past 3 months.

Present Illness

Katherine initially believed she was hyperthyroid based on a conversation with a nurse at her medical clinic. However, when queried further, Katherine thinks her symptoms are more likely related to her tendency to "worry about everything"—specifically, her health, her son's academic problems, and finances.

Medical History

Katherine reports a history of migraine headaches that began at age 15 years. She has had excessive absenteeism from work due to her migraine headaches and physical symptoms. She denies any other significant medical history.

Family and Social History

Katherine is single and has a 15-year-old son who lives with her. She has been living with her boyfriend, who is employed as a cabinet maker, for the past 8 years. Katherine describes her relationships with her boyfriend and son as "fine" and supportive.

Health Habits

Katherine admits to smoking one-half pack of cigarettes per day. She had quit for several months but recently reinitiated the habit to cope with her "nervousness." She states she consumes a few alcoholic beverages per week but denies problems when queried with the CAGE questions (Box 89-1) (Ewing, 1984). She says she drinks six or seven cans of caffeinated cola per day. Katherine denies any other substance use at this time but reports a history of intermittent cocaine use when she was younger. She reports consuming a normal diet but says she does not get any regular exercise.

Box 89-1 **Cage Questionnaire**

C Have you ever felt you ought to CUT down on your drinking?

A Have people ANNOYED you by criticizing your drinking?

G Have you ever felt bad or GUILTY about your drinking?

E Have you ever had a drink first thing in the morning to steady your nerves or get rid of a hangover (EYE-opener)?

Answering yes to two or more items is indicative of an alcohol problem and should be investigated further by the physician.

From Ewing JA. Detecting alcoholism: The CAGE Questionnaire. JAMA 1984;252:1905-1907.

Review of Systems

Katherine reports a weight loss of 15 pounds over the past 3 months. She states she does not currently suffer from headaches, shortness of breath, or any aches or pains but does experience nervousness. She has no known allergies.

Objective

Physical Examination

Katherine is well developed, slightly underweight, cooperative, and friendly. She is 5 feet 6 inches tall and weighs 118 pounds. Her blood pressure is 104/76, respiratory rate is 16, and oral temperature is 36.9°C (98.4°F). Her heart rate is 72 with a normal rhythm. Breast and abdominal examinations are normal. The patient exhibits no distress, other than fidgeting, and shows normal affect.

Laboratory Tests

Laboratory testing includes thyroid function (serum TSH, free T_4, and serum T_3), serum glucose, electrolytes, and a complete blood cell count. All results are within normal limits.

Psychological Screening

Katherine is given the Sheehan Panic Disorder Scale (SPDS), formerly the Sheehan Patient Rated Anxiety Scale (SPRAS) (Sheehan and Harnett-Sheehan, 1990) (Table 89-1) and the Zung Self-Rating Depression Scale (ZSRDS) (Zung, 1965 **B**) (Table 89-2) to complete. The SPDS is a 35-item self-report screening measure for anxiety. Katherine's score is 83, indicating a high degree of anxiety, with physical complaints and excessive worrying being most prominent. The ZSRDS is a 20-item self-report screening measure for depression. Katherine's score is 54, which suggests a

mild level of depression. Most of her points accrued from symptoms associated with anxiety. During the interview she mentions occasionally feeling sad but states she is not depressed.

Assessment

Working Diagnosis

The working diagnosis for Katherine's presenting complaint is generalized anxiety disorder, since she has been worrying excessively about many issues, including her health, her son, and finances. Her worrying is longstanding and has affected her performance at work.

Plan

The initial plan is to educate Katherine about anxiety and stress and how to better cope with these through psychological and behavioral strategies. The provider gives her an educational handout on these topics. Because of her score on the ZSRDS instrument, Katherine is asked about suicidal ideation, which she denies, referring to the impact it would have on her son. The provider asks her to return in 1 week for assessment of her status and to further discuss treatment strategies.

Differential Diagnosis

Based on Katherine's presenting complaints and history, the following diagnoses may be considered by the physician.

1. *Generalized anxiety disorder.* The most likely diagnosis for Katherine is generalized anxiety disorder. She admits to a tendency to "worry about everything," including her health, her son, and finances. She also reported excessive worrying on the SPDS instrument. Her anxiety and worry appear to be associated with numerous physical symptoms (e.g., shakiness, shortness of breath, rapid heart rate, chest pain, light-headedness, weight loss) and difficulties with sleep. Katherine's anxiety and physical concerns have resulted in work-related problems (absenteeism). Therefore, she meets the *Diagnostic and Statistical Manual of Mental Disorders* (DSM-IV) criteria for generalized anxiety disorder (Box 89-2) (American Psychiatric Association [APA], 1994).

2. *Anxiety disorder due to a general medical condition.* Anxiety may be directly related to the physiologic effects of various medical conditions (APA, 1994). These conditions should be considered in the differential diagnosis and ruled out as appropriate. They include endocrine disorders, cardiovascular problems, respiratory conditions, metabolic conditions, and neurologic conditions (Table 89-3).

Table 89-1 Sheehan Panic Disorder Scale (SPDS)*

Instructions: Below is a list of problems and complaints that people sometimes have. Indicate how you have felt during THE PAST WEEK. Mark only one box for each problem and do not skip any items.

During the past week, how much did you suffer from:	Not at all	A little	Moderately	Markedly	Extremely
1. Difficulty in getting your breath, smothering, or overbreathing					
2. Choking sensation or lump in throat.					
3. Skipping, racing, or pounding of your heart.					
4. Chest pain, pressure, or discomfort.					
5. Bouts of excessive sweating.					
6. Faintness, lightheadedness, or dizzy spells.					
7. Sensation of rubbery or "jelly" legs.					
8. Feeling off balance or unsteady like you might fall.					
9. Nausea or stomach problems.					
10. Feeling that things around you are strange, unreal, foggy, or detached from you.					
11. Feeling outside or detached from part or all of your body, or a floating feeling.					
12. Tingling or numbness in parts of your body.					
13. Hot flashes or cold chills.					
14. Shaking or trembling.					
15. Having a fear that you are dying or that something terrible is about to happen.					
16. Feeling you are losing control or going insane.					
17. *Situational Anxiety Attack*: Sudden anxiety attacks with 4 or more of the symptoms (listed previously) that occur when you are in or about to go into a situation that is likely, from your experience, to bring on an attack.					
18. *Unexpected Anxiety Attack*: Sudden unexpected anxiety attacks with 4 or more symptoms (listed previously) that occur with little or no provocation (i.e., when you are not in a situation that is likely, from your experience, to bring on an attack).					
19. *Unexpected Limited Symptom Attack*: Sudden unexpected spells with only one or two symptoms (listed previously) that occur with little or no provocation (i.e., when you are not in a situation that is likely, from your experience, to bring on an attack).					

Continued

Table 89-1   Sheehan Panic Disorder Scale (Continued)

During the past week, how much did you suffer from:	Not at all	A little	Moderately	Markedly	Extremely
20. *Anticipatory Anxiety Episode*: Anxiety episodes that build up as you anticipate doing something that is likely, from your experience, to bring on anxiety that is more intense than most people experience in such situations.					
21. Avoiding situations because they frighten you.					
22. Being dependent on others.					
23. Tension and inability to relax.					
24. Anxiety, nervousness, restlessness.					
25. Spells of increased sensitivity to sound, light, or touch.					
26. Attacks of diarrhea.					
27. Worrying about your health too much.					
28. Feeling tired, weak, and exhausted easily.					
29. Headaches or pains in neck or head.					
30. Difficulty in falling asleep.					
31. Waking in the middle of the night, or restless sleep.					
32. Unexpected waves of depression occurring with little or no provocation.					
33. Emotions and moods going up and down a lot in response to changes around you.					
34. Recurrent and persistent ideas, thoughts, impulses, or images that are intrusive, unwanted, senseless, or repugnant.					
35. Having to repeat the same action in a ritual, e.g., checking, washing, counting repeatedly, when it's not really necessary.					

Not at all   = 0
A little   = 1
Moderately = 2
Markedly   = 3
Extremely = 4

25–37	37–57	57–77	>77
Mild	Moderate	Severe	Very severe

Although originally developed for use with panic disorder, the SPDS has extensive breadth of symptom coverage. Scores may range from 0 to 140.

*Formerly Sheehan Patient Rated Anxiety Scale.
From Sheehan JV. The Sheehan Patient Rated Anxiety Scale. J Clin Psychiatry 1999;60(Suppl 18):63–64.

Table 89-2   Zung Self-Rating Depression Scale

Name_____ Age____Sex____Date_____	None or a little of of the time	Some of the time	Good part the time	Most or all of the time
1. I feel downhearted, blue and sad.				
2. Morning is when I feel the best.				
3. I have crying spells or feel like it.				
4. I have trouble sleeping through the night.				
5. I eat as much as I used to.				
6. I enjoy looking at, talking to and being with attractive women/men.				
7. I notice that I am losing weight.				
8. I have trouble with constipation.				
9. My heart beats faster than usual.				
10. I get tired for no reason.				
11. My mind is as clear as it used to be.				
12. I find it easy to do the things I used to.				
13. I am restless and can't keep still.				
14. I feel hopeful about the future.				
15. I am more irritable than usual.				
16. I find it easy to make decisions.				
17. I feel that I am useful and needed.				
18. My life is pretty full.				
19. I feel that others would be better off if I were dead.				
20. I still enjoy the things I used to do.				

Key for Scoring the Self-Rating Depression Scale (SDS)

SDS item number	Responses			
	None or a little of the time	Some of the time	Good part of the time	Most or all of the time
1	1	2	3	4
2	4	3	2	1
3	1	2	3	4
4	1	2	3	4
5	4	3	2	1
6	4	3	2	1
7	1	2	3	4
8	1	2	3	4

Continued

Table 89-2 Zung Self-Rating Depression Scale (Continued)

SDS item number	Responses			
	None or a little of the time	Some of the time	Good part of the time	Most or all of the time
9	1	2	3	4
10	1	2	3	4
11	4	3	2	1
12	4	3	2	1
13	1	2	3	4
14	4	3	2	1
15	1	2	3	4
16	4	3	2	1
17	4	3	2	1
18	4	3	2	1
19	1	2	3	4
20	4	3	2	1

Patients are requested to rate themselves (from "None or a little of the time" to "Most or all of the time") on various items related to depression. Scores range from 0 to 80, with scores of 50 or more indicating depression.
From Zung, WW. A self-rating depression scale. Arch Gen Psychiatry 1965;12:63–70.

Box 89-2 **DSM-IV Diagnostic Criteria for Generalized Anxiety Disorder**

A. Excessive anxiety and worry (apprehensive, expectation), occurring more days than not for at least 6 months, about a number of events or activities (such as work or school performance).
B. The person finds it difficult to control the worry.
C. The anxiety and worry are associated with three (or more) of the following six symptoms (with at least some symptoms present for more days than not for the past 6 months). Note: Only one item is required in children.
  1. Restlessness or feeling keyed up or on edge
  2. Being easily fatigued
  3. Difficulty concentrating or mind going blank
  4. Irritability
  5. Muscle tension
  6. Sleep disturbance (difficulty falling or staying asleep, or restless unsatisfying sleep)
D. The focus of the anxiety and worry is not confined to features of an Axis I disorder (e.g., the anxiety or worry is not about having a panic attack [as in panic disorder], being embarrassed in public [as in social phobia], being contaminated [as in obsessive-compulsive disorder], being away from home or close relatives [as in separation anxiety disorder], gaining weight [as in anorexia nervosa], having multiple physical complaints [as in somatization disorder], or having a serious illness [as in hypochondriasis]), and the anxiety and worry do not occur exclusively during posttraumatic stress disorder.
E. The anxiety, worry, or physical symptoms cause clinically significant distress or impairment in social, occupational, or other important areas of functioning.
F. The disturbance is not due to the direct physiological effects of a substance or a general medical condition and does not occur exclusively during a mood disorder, a psychotic disorder, or a pervasive developmental disorder.

From American Psychiatric Association: Diagnostic and Statistical Manual of Mental Disorders, 4th ed., Text Revision (DSM-IV-TR). Bethesda, MD, American Psychiatric Association, 1994.

Table 89-3 Potential Medical Diagnoses in Patients with Anxiety

Endocrine
Hyperthyroidism (thyrotoxicosis)
Hypothyroidism
Hypoglycemia
Hyperadrenocorticism
Graves' disease

Cardiovascular
Angina pectoris
Cardiomyopathy
Congestive heart failure
Pulmonary embolism
Arrhythmia
Mitral valve prolapse
Myocardial infarction

Respiratory
Chronic obstructive pulmonary disease
Pneumonia
Hypoxia

Metabolic Conditions
Acidosis
Electrolyte abnormalities
Pernicious anemia

Neurologic
Neoplasms
Vestibular dysfunction
Encephalitis
Parkinson's disease

Intoxication
Caffeine
Alcohol
Amphetamines
Cannabis
Cocaine
Hallucinogens
Inhalants
Phencyclidine
Sympathomimetics

Withdrawal
Alcohol
Cocaine
Sedatives
Opiates
Hypnotics
Anxiolytics (e.g., benzodiazepines)
Nicotine

Nutritional Deficiencies
Vitamin B_{12}
Pyridoxine
Folate

Medications
Corticosteroids
Herbal medicines (e.g., ginseng)
Over-the-counter sympathomimetics
SSRIs
Digoxin
Thyroxine
Theophylline

SSRIs, selective serotonin reuptake inhibitors.

Katherine presented with symptoms similar to those indicative of hyperthyroidism, including weight loss, nervousness, a rapid heart rate, light-headedness, and sleep problems. The results of laboratory tests suggested that Katherine's thyroid functioning, as measured by serum thyroid-stimulating hormone, free T_4, and serum T_3, is normal. These results, in combination with physical findings, rule out medical disorders.

3. *Panic disorder.* For a diagnosis of panic disorder to be made, a person must experience recurrent and unexpected panic attacks, with at least one of these attacks followed by persistent concern regarding a future attack, worrying about the implications of such an attack, and significant behavioral change due to the attacks. A panic attack is characterized by a discrete period of intense fear or discomfort that is accompanied by symptoms such as palpitations, sweating, shaking, shortness of breath, choking sensations, chest pain, nausea, and dizziness; derealization or depersonalization; fear of losing control, dying, or going crazy; paresthesias; and/or hot flushes or cold chills that peak within 10 minutes of their onset (APA, 1994). Katherine reports physical symptoms; however, her symptoms do not occur abruptly and do not peak within 10 minutes of their onset. She also denies persistent concern about such attacks. Therefore, this disorder may be ruled out.

4. *Major depressive disorder.* Katherine describes various symptoms associated with depression, including weight loss, sleep problems, and difficulty concentrating. In addition, her ZSRDS score suggests mild levels of depression. However, in order to be diagnosed with major depressive disorder, a person must experience at least five of the following nine symptoms nearly every day for at least 2 weeks: (a) depressed mood, (b) markedly diminished interest or pleasure in all or nearly all activities, (c) significant weight loss or gain, or a decrease or increase in appetite, (d) insomnia or hypersomnia, (e) psychomotor agitation or retardation,

(f) fatigue or loss of energy, (g) feelings of worthlessness or excessive or inappropriate guilt, (h) diminished ability to think or concentrate, or indecisiveness, and/or (i) recurrent thoughts of death, recurrent suicidal ideation without a specific plan, or a suicide attempt or a specific plan for committing suicide (APA, 1994). Katherine does not meet the full criteria since she experiences only a limited number of these symptoms and does not experience those consistently (Box 89-3 gives the SIG E CAPS + Mood mnemonic for major depressive episode).

5. *Adjustment disorders (with anxiety or with mixed anxiety and depressed mood).* To be diagnosed with an adjustment disorder, a person must experience emotional or behavioral symptoms within 3 months of the onset of a particular stressor or stressors. Either the person must experience marked distress, in excess of what would be expected, or the symptoms must result in significant social or occupational (or academic) impairment (APA, 1994). Although Katherine is experiencing emotional symptoms that cause occupational impairment, there does not appear to be a specific stressor or stressors responsible for her symptoms. In addition, her symptoms are better accounted for by a diagnosis of generalized anxiety disorder.

6. *Substance-induced anxiety disorder.* This diagnosis is considered when there is evidence from the history, physical examination, or laboratory findings that the patient's anxiety developed during or within 1 month of substance intoxication or withdrawal or when medication is etiologically related to the anxiety (APA, 1994) (see Table 89-3). Although Katherine describes cocaine use in the past, she denies current use of cocaine or other substances and denies significant alcohol use. Therefore, this diagnosis is not likely.

Box 89-3	**SIG E CAPS + Mood Mnemonic**

S Sleep (insomnia or hypersomnia)
I Interests (diminished interest or pleasure in activities)
G Guilt (excessive or inappropriate guilt; feelings of worthlessness)
E Energy (loss of energy or fatigue)
C Concentration (diminished concentration or indecisiveness)
A Appetite (decrease or increase in appetite; weight loss or gain)
S Suicide (recurrent thoughts of death, suicidal ideation, or suicide attempt)
+ Mood (depressed mood or sadness)

FOLLOW-UP VISITS

A week later Katherine returns to the clinic for her first follow-up visit. She reports having difficulty focusing on the patient education material. She notes that her mind continues to wander onto various topics of worry. The provider then raises medication as a management option, with the hope that it will allow her to focus more effectively on the cognitive and behavioral strategies provided to her. Katherine is interested in giving it a try; therefore, she is prescribed the selective serotonin reuptake inhibitor (SSRI) escitalopram oxalate (Lexapro) for her generalized anxiety. The starting dose is 10 mg/day. The provider asks Katherine to try again to read the patient education materials given to her previously and asks her to return to the clinic in 2 weeks.

At her second follow-up visit, Katherine reports that her symptoms have lessened and her concentration has improved enough that she could read and understand the materials. She is continued on escitalopram oxalate.

Over the next several visits, Katherine is instructed in relaxation techniques, cognitive strategies such as thought stopping, and the importance of initiating a regular exercise regimen. Smoking cessation and caffeine reduction are also broached with her.

DISCUSSION

Prevalence of the Disorder

Generalized anxiety disorder is a common problem in the United States. According to results from the U.S. National Comorbidity Survey (Kessler et al., 1994), the 12-month prevalence rate for generalized anxiety disorder is 3.1% and the lifetime prevalence rate is 5.1%. The lowest rates occurred in the 15- to 24-year-old age group (2.0%) and the highest rates occurred in the 45- to 55-year-old age group (6.9%). Women are almost twice as likely as men to be diagnosed with generalized anxiety disorder over their lifetime (6.6% vs. 3.6%) (Wittchen et al., 1994), and whereas the prevalence of the disorder decreases with age in men, it increases in women (Halbreich, 2003).

Wittchen (2002) reported that 5.3% of patients seen in primary care settings have generalized anxiety disorder. The highest incidence was found in patients aged 35 to 60 years. It is the most frequently seen anxiety disorder in primary care, and only 28% of patients with generalized anxiety disorder are correctly diagnosed. Of these, many are improperly managed with pharmacologic or nonpharmacologic treatments.

There is also a high degree of comorbidity with generalized anxiety disorder, with 66.3% of patients having an additional concurrent psychiatric diagnosis and 90.4% having a lifetime history of another psychiatric disorder. Studies suggest that major depressive disorder, panic disorder, and alcohol abuse are the three most common diagnoses associated with generalized anxiety disorder (Fricchione, 2004; Wittchen, 2002).

Diagnostic Criteria and Clinical Presentation

The essential feature of generalized anxiety disorder is excessive anxiety and worry (apprehensive, expectation) that occurs persistently for at least 6 months and is directed toward a number of events or activities, such as work or school performance (see Box 89-2). In the clinical setting, patients with generalized anxiety disorder typically do not present with anxiety as their primary complaint. More often, patients present with rather general, vague, or nonspecific somatic complaints such as headaches, low back pain, gastrointestinal distress, fatigue, and insomnia (Anxiety Disorders Association of America, 2004). Patients with generalized anxiety disorder use health care services to a greater extent for these symptoms. Whereas most visit primary care physicians, gastroenterologists are the most frequently seen specialists (Kennedy and Schwab, 1997❸).

Management of Generalized Anxiety Disorder

Medical conditions, psychosocial issues, and personality factors all must be considered before any treatment plan for generalized anxiety disorder can be developed (Katon and Geyman, 2002). Once this occurs, the physician and patient should work collaboratively to develop a treatment plan. Physician interventions may include psychosocial interventions, pharmacologic interventions, or combined therapy.

Psychosocial Management

Several psychosocial interventions are available to the physician when treating a patient with chronic anxiety. A useful way to organize one's approach to interventions is the REST mnemonic, which cues the physician to address several important areas (Box 89-4). The R stands for *reassurance and support*. Patients with chronic anxiety, especially those presenting with physiologic symptoms, are often worried about health problems and related issues. Therefore, assurances that an appropriate history, physical examination, and laboratory testing will be completed to rule out medical disease is necessary. The E represents *education* of the patient and possibly family members about anxiety, factors that may cause it, and how the body responds. A discussion of the neuroendocrine response to stress (i.e., the fight-

---

Box 89-4	**Psychosocial Management of Anxiety: REST Mnemonic**

R *Reassurance and support* provided to patient regarding the physician's ability to conduct an appropriate history, physical examination, and laboratory testing in order to rule out medical disease. This should be done in a supportive manner.

E *Education* provided to the patient and possibly family members on anxiety, its etiology, the neuroendocrine response (fight-or-flight response), and how this may lead to psychological, physiological, and behavioral problems.

S *Stress management* techniques are introduced and taught to the patient. These include:
- Deep breathing (teach the patient how to belly breathe and to take slow breaths)
- Relaxation training (teach the patient how to participate in progressive muscle relaxation, imagery, and so forth; provide a relaxation tape to the patient)
- Thought-stopping strategies (talk to the patient about the role of negative thinking

in causing anxiety; teach the patient how to monitor his or her thoughts and then to catch the negative thinking that leads to stress, "stop" it, and replace it with more rational or positive thinking)
- Exercise (encourage the patient to begin a reasonable exercise program such as walking, riding a bicycle, or jogging)
- Time management (help the patient understand how to break large tasks into smaller tasks, make lists, prioritize, learn to say no)
- Social support (encourage the patient to talk to and to participate in activities with others)
- Habit reduction (assist the patient to reduce nicotine, caffeine, and so on)

T *Therapy* may be necessary for patients who continue to experience significant anxiety despite the use of the above interventions. For these patients, referral to a psychologist or psychiatrist for formal therapy may be necessary.

or-flight response) and how this may lead to various physiologic symptoms is helpful. All information should be presented at the patient's level of comprehension. The S stands for *stress management* interventions. These interventions include (1) deep breathing and relaxation, (2) exercise, (3) positive self-talk, (4) time management, (5) social support, and (6) habit reduction strategies. Information should be supplemented with patient education handouts, once again keeping in mind the comprehension level of the patient (Box 89-5). In addition, patients will likely benefit from other resources such

---

Box 89-5	A Patient's Guide to Anxiety and Stress Management

Background

Anxiety and stress are very common problems. Generalized anxiety involves excessive worrying about a variety of issues or events. Worrying typically results in various physical symptoms that include restlessness, fatigue, difficulty concentrating, muscle tension, and sleep problems. Some persons may develop other physical problems such as headaches (typically in the back of the neck area or a bandlike effect around the head), low back pain, indigestion, constipation, diarrhea, and bruxism (grinding one's teeth). In addition to physical symptoms, persons may experience increased irritability, frustration, and impatience. Eventually, these symptoms may result in excessive tardiness and absenteeism from school or work, withdrawal from social activities, and isolation from others.

Anxiety Management

There are several strategies available to assist in the management of anxiety. The more effective techniques for dealing constructively with anxiety include time management, cognitive strategies, and relaxation techniques.

Time management. Key here is to break large tasks into smaller tasks. Don't put off til tomorrow what you can do now. Schedule important events, prioritize, and say no if you are feeling overwhelmed.

Cognitive strategies attempt to change how you think about events in your life, knowing that how you think determines how you feel. Many people will look at an upcoming examination or interview as a terrible event that they are doomed to fail. They then catastrophize by thinking about how this failure will lead to additional problems, and so forth, until a mountain is made from a molehill. Thought-stopping strategies can be used to stop or at least minimize this process. The first step is recognizing your unproductive self-talk ("There is so much to study, I'm going to fail miserably"),

stopping it immediately—you can either say aloud "stop" or think it to yourself— and replacing the unproductive self-talk with more rational self-talk ("I have a lot to study, but if I focus on one section at a time, I should be OK"). The key is to notch it down and keep the catastrophizing to a minimum.

Relaxation training begins by assuming a comfortable position (such as relaxing in a reclining chair) and taking slow, deep belly breaths. Think of these as taking 7-second breaths (breathe in to a mental count of one one-thousand, two one-thousand, three one-thousand, then pause for a count of one one-thousand, then exhale for a count of one one-thousand, two one-thousand, three one-thousand), all the time making sure that as you breathe in your belly goes out and as you exhale your belly goes back in. You can then accompany this breathing with cue words such as "relax" or "let go," along with muscle relaxation and imagery. Imagery involves putting yourself in any place that is comfortable or peaceful for you (in your family room by a fireplace, on a quiet beach). Continue with the breathing and imagery for 20 minutes and end your relaxation session by saying something positive about yourself. Allow this relaxation and accompanying affirmation to carry you through your day.

Watch Those Habits

There are a variety of substances that people take that can make their anxiety worse. These include the excessive use of caffeine, nicotine, or any other stimulant. Decreasing or eliminating these substances from your daily routine will have a positive impact on your psychological and physical health. Also, avoid using substances such as alcohol or marijuana to calm down, since their use can lead to abuse and dependency problems. More productive coping involves using the techniques described above. They may take more time to work, but in the end, they will be much more effective.

Box 89-5	A Patient's Guide to Anxiety and Stress Management (Continued)

Final Suggestions

If you recognize early when anxiety and stress is impacting you negatively, you are wise to use the strategies mentioned above and then to take action. More appropriately, it is better to take a proactive approach by doing things that will buffer you against the anxiety and stress that everyone encounters naturally as part of daily life. These include a regimen of positive thinking, socializing, relaxation, and exercise. If you find that you need more help, seek professional assistance.

Organizations and Internet Site Resources

A variety of resources are available to persons interested in learning more about anxiety and stress. These include the following:

Anxiety Disorders Association of America (ADAA)—www.adaa.org

International Association of Anxiety Management—www.anxman.org

American Psychiatric Association—www. psych. org

American Psychological Association—www.apa. org

as books, Web sites, and self-help groups. If these strategies are not totally effective, the physician may consider referring the patient for T, or formal *therapy* with a psychologist or psychiatrist.

In Katherine's case, medical factors were ruled out and it was determined that her physiologic symptoms were due mainly to her tendency to worry about various life issues. During her first visit she was provided with reassurance and support and was then educated about anxiety and stress. At her first follow-up visit she continued to complain of concentration difficulties, so medication was prescribed. In subsequent sessions, Katherine was further instructed in deep breathing and relaxation strategies. A relaxation training cassette tape was given to her and she was instructed to practice with the tape at least once daily. In addition, she was taught thought-stopping strategies that entail catching negative thinking or "self-talk," immediately stopping it, and then replacing those thoughts with more rational thinking. Katherine was also instructed to begin an exercise program of walking 3 days per week for 20 minutes each time. When she returned to the clinic, Katherine noted that she did practice relaxation several times each week and walked almost daily as part of her new exercise program. She continued to have difficulty with catching negative thinking and worrying. She was commended for her progress with relaxation and exercise and was further assisted with thought-stopping strategies. Medication was also prescribed.

Pharmacologic Management

Three major classes of pharmacologic agents are available for the treatment of generalized anxiety disorder: SSRIs, nonbenzodiazepines, and benzodiazepines.

SSRIs SSRIs are now considered first-line agents for treating anxiety disorders (Augustin, 2005). Various

SSRIs are available in the United States for the treatment of generalized anxiety disorder (Table 89-4). Escitalopram oxalate (Lexapro), which received FDA approval for the treatment of generalized anxiety disorder in 2003, was prescribed for Katherine. It is a pure S-enantiomer (single isomer) of the racemic bicyclic phthalane derivative citalopram. Its action results from inhibiting serotonin (5-HT) reuptake and neuronal firing rate.

The initial starting dose of escitalopram oxalate is 10 mg once daily in either the morning or evening. It may be increased to 20 mg after a minimum of 1 week. Major side effects include headache (24%), nausea (18%), ejaculation disorder (14%), somnolence (13%), and insomnia (12%).

Some patients taking SSRIs may experience a decrease in symptoms during the first 2 weeks; however, most respond gradually with continued improvement for 8 to 12 weeks or for as long as 6 months. Therefore, optimal trials of SSRIs for generalized anxiety disorder should be at least 8 weeks of adequate dosing before other options are considered by the physician. Because of the potential for a delayed response, it is not uncommon to use benzodiazepines in combination with antidepressant medication during the initial treatment of an anxiety disorder (Augustin, 2005).

A major advantage of the SSRIs is that they seem to be more effective than the benzodiazepines in ameliorating cognitive symptoms (i.e., excessive worry) of generalized anxiety disorder. They also have less potential for abuse and dependence.

Nonbenzodiazepines Buspirone (Buspar) is considered a first-line treatment for generalized anxiety disorder. It is the only nonbenzodiazepine available and is thought to exert its influence by acting as an agonist at presynaptic serotonin (5-HT$_{1A}$) receptor sites. Its onset of action is slower than that of the benzodiazepines and it may take several days to 2 weeks

Table 89-4 Pharmacologic Agents Used in the Management of Generalized Anxiety Disorder

Agent	Usual Starting Dose (mg)	Total Dosage Range (mg/day)	Half-life (hr)
Selective Serotonin Reuptake Inhibitors			
Citalopram (Celexa)	20 qd	20–60	35
Escitalopram oxalate (Lexapro)	10 qd	10–20	27–32
Fluoxetine (Prozac)			24–384[†]
Obsessive-compulsive disorder	20 qd	20–80	
Panic disorder	10 qd	10–60	
Paroxetine (Paxil)			
Generalized anxiety disorder	20 qd	20–50	21
Obsessive-compulsive disorder	20 qd	20–60	
Panic disorder	10 qd	10–60	
Post-traumatic stress disorder	20 qd	20–50	
Social anxiety	20 qd	20–60	
Paroxetine (Paxil CR)			15–20
Panic disorder	12.5 qd	12.5–75	
Social anxiety	12.5 qd	12.5–37.5	
Sertraline (Zoloft)			
Panic disorder, post-traumatic stress disorder, social anxiety disorder	25 qd	25–200	26
Nonbenzodiazepines			
Buspirone (BuSpar)	7.5 bid	15–60	2–3
Benzodiazepines*			
Alprazolam (Xanax)	0.25–0.5 tid	0.75–4	6–27
Chlordiazepoxide (Librium)	5 bid, tid, or qid	10–100	6–20
Clonazepam (Klonopin)	0.5 tid	1.5–20	18–50
Chlorazepate (Tranxene)	7.5–15 qd	7.5–60	48
Diazepam (Valium)	2 bid–qid	4–40	>20
Lorazepam (Ativan)	1–3 qd in divided doses	1–10	12–18
Oxazepam (Serax)	10 tid	30–90	6–11
Serotonin/Norepinephrine Reuptake Inhibitors			
Venlafaxine (Effexor)	75 qd in 2–3 divided doses	75–225	3–13[‡]
Venlafaxine (Effexor XR)	75 qd (some patients may be started on 37.5 mg for 4–7 days)	37.5–225	3–13[‡]
Heterocyclic Antidepressants			
Trazodone (Desyrel)	150 qd in divided doses	150–600	3–9
Tricyclic Antidepressants			
Clomipramine (Anafranil)	25 qd	25–250	19–77[§]
Desipramine (Norpramin)	25 bid to qid	50–300	21
Imipramine (Tofranil)	75 qd	75–200	30
Nortriptyline (Aventyl)	25 tid or qid	75–150	26

* Rate of onset for benzodiazepines: alprazolam, diazepam, and chorazepate—fast; chordiazepoxide, lorazepam, and clonazepam—intermediate; oxazepam—slow.
† Includes both fluoxetine and norfluoxetine.
‡ Includes both venlafaxine and *N*-desmethylvenlafaxine.
§ Includes both clomipramine and desmethylclomipramine.

or longer to reach full therapeutic benefit. Buspirone lacks general central nervous system depressant effects and is relatively free from any significant abuse or dependence potential. Therefore, buspirone is preferred over benzodiazepines in persons with a substance abuse/dependency history and in persons who are elderly or medically ill. Reported side effects include dizziness, drowsiness, nausea, and headaches.

Benzodiazepines Benzodiazepines are still the most widely used anxiolytic for anxiety disorders. The benzodiazepines are believed to influence four types (α_1, α_2, α_3, and α_5) of $GABA_A$, with anxiolytic effects occurring on the α_2 $GABA_A$ receptors within the CNS. Overall, the benzodiazepines are safe and well-tolerated medications, with sedation, fatigue, cognitive impairment, and psychomotor impairment being their major side effects. Sedation and psychomotor impairment typically resolve within a few weeks of ongoing treatment. Withdrawal symptoms are usually associated with a quicker rate of cessation, larger doses, longer-term use, and higher-potency medications. Although abuse of benzodiazepines is a concern, misuse and abuse are typically limited to persons with a history of substance abuse.

Other Medications Other medications used in the treatment of generalized anxiety disorder include serotonin/norepinephrine reuptake inhibitors, heterocyclic antidepressants, and tricyclic antidepressants. Monoamine oxidase inhibitors, beta blockers, and antihistamines have also been used for symptoms related to anxiety.

Summary

Generalized anxiety disorder is a common problem characterized by chronic, excessive anxiety and worry about a number of events or activities, difficulty controlling the worry, associated physical symptoms, and functional impairment. Generalized anxiety disorder is frequently seen in primary care; however, it often goes undiagnosed or improperly managed. Once medical disease is ruled out, the physician may use psychosocial strategies and/or pharmacologic interventions. SSRIs, nonbenzodiazepines, and benzodiazepines have proved effective in the management of generalized anxiety disorder. A combination of psychosocial and pharmacologic interventions is most effective in the long-term management of this disorder.

Material Available on Student Consult

Review Questions and Answers about Generalized Anxiety Disorder

REFERENCES

American Psychiatric Association. Diagnostic and Statistical Manual of Mental Disorders, 4th ed., Text Revision (DSM-IV-TR). Bethesda, MD, American Psychiatric Association, 1994.

Anxiety Disorders Association of America. Improving the Diagnosis and Treatment of Generalized Anxiety Disorder: A Dialogue Between Mental Health Professionals and Primary Care Physicians. Silver Spring, MD, Anxiety Disorders Association of America, 2004.

Augustin SG. Anxiety disorders. In Koda-Kimble MA, Young LY, Kradjan WA, Guglielmo BJ (eds): Applied Therapeutics: The Clinical Use of Drugs, 8th ed. Philadelphia, Lippincott Williams & Wilkins, 2005, pp 76-1–76-47.

Ewing JA. Detecting alcoholism: The CAGE Questionnaire. JAMA 1984;252:1905–1907.

Fricchione G. Generalized anxiety disorder. N Engl J Med 2004;351:675–682.

Halbreich U. Anxiety disorders in women: A developmental and lifecycle perspective. Depression Aging 2003;17:107–110.

Katon W, Geyman JP. Anxiety disorders. In Rakel RE (ed): Textbook of Family Practice, 6th ed. Philadelphia, WB Saunders, 2002, pp 1438–1453.

Kennedy BL, Schwab JJ. Utilization of medical specialists by anxiety disorder patients. Psychosomatics 1997;38: 109–112.

Kessler RC, McGonagle KA, Zhao S, et al. Lifetime and 12-month prevalence of DSM-III-R psychiatric disorders in the United States: Results from the National Comorbidity Survey. Arch Gen Psychiatry 1994;51: 8–19.

Sheehan JV. The Sheehan Patient Rated Anxiety Scale. J Clin Psychiatry 1999;60(Suppl 18):63–64.

Sheehan DV, Harnett-Sheehan K. Psychometric assessment of anxiety disorders. In Sarorius N, Andreoli V, Cassano G, et al. (eds): Anxiety: Psychobiological and Clinical Perspectives. Washington, DC, Hemisphere, 1990, pp 85–98.

Wittchen H-U. Generalized anxiety disorder: Prevalence, burden, and cost to society. Depression Anxiety 2002;16:162–171.

Wittchen H-U, Zhao S, Kessler RC, Eaton WW. DSM-III-R generalized anxiety disorder in the National Comorbidity Survey. Arch Gen Psychiatry 1994;51:355–364.

Zung WW. A self-rating depression scale. Arch Gen Psychiatry 1965;12:63–70.

90 Delirium (Hypomagnesemia)

Robert S. Freelove

INITIAL VISIT

Subjective

Patient Identification and Presenting Problem

George B. is a 66-year-old man who is brought to the emergency department (ED) of a rural hospital by ambulance for confusion and agitation. His wife accompanies him and states that everything started 3 hours earlier, when she found Mr. B. urinating in the kitchen sink. When she asked him what he was doing, he seemed confused and mumbled nonsensically. She helped him back to bed and reawakened 2½ hours later to find him pacing about the bedroom, shouting and talking to people who were not there. She tried to calm him, and he pushed her down. She subsequently called emergency medical services. Mrs. B. notes that Mr. B. went to his bowling league earlier that evening and came home acting normally. She had not smelled alcohol on his breath. Mr. B. pays no attention to questions and provides no history.

Medical History

Mrs. B. provides Mr. B.'s medical history. To her knowledge, he has no medical illnesses, is not taking any medications, and is not allergic to any medications. His only surgery was an inguinal herniorrhaphy at age 31.

Family History

Mr. B. was adopted and never indicated to Mrs. B. that he knew anything about his biological parents.

Social History

Mr. B. is a retired city maintenance worker who now runs a small family farm. He smokes two to four cigars daily and has a history of alcoholism but has been sober for 18 years. There is no history of illegal drug use, to his wife's knowledge. He is married and has three children and seven grandchildren.

Review of Systems

The review of systems cannot be performed because the patient does not respond to questions. He continues to moan, mumble words that have no relation to the questions asked, and call out names. His wife indicates that the names are those of deceased friends and family members. He becomes agitated when approached or touched.

Objective

Physical Examination

Mr. B. is sitting upright, awake, hypervigilant, and startled when touched. His temperature is 37.4°C (99.3°F), pulse is 106, blood pressure is 162/88, respiratory rate is 22. Examination of the head reveals no evidence of trauma. He does not allow evaluation of the ears, nose, or throat. His pupils are equally round and reactive to light, and there is no scleral icterus. He does not allow palpation of the neck. His lungs are clear to auscultation. Cardiac auscultation reveals normal S_1 and S_2 without a murmur, rub, or heave. The abdomen is soft, without guarding. He is unable to follow directions for a neurologic examination, but there are no obvious gross motor deficits. As the physical examination progresses, he becomes more agitated and eventually tries to strike anyone who touches him.

Assessment

Working Diagnosis

The working diagnosis is delirium, etiology unknown.

Underlying Medical Conditions

Delirium is a generally reversible syndrome of disturbed consciousness, attention, and cognition or perception that develops acutely, fluctuates during the course of the day, and is attributable to a physical disorder. The presence of delirium indicates an underlying medical condition that should be aggressively investigated and treated, because the mortality associated with any serious disease increases if delirium ensues (Cole and Primeau, 1993❸; McCusker et al., 2002❸). There are many potential causes to consider (Box 90-1), and often more than one source is discovered.

Infection of the central nervous system (CNS)—for example, encephalitis, meningitis, syphilis, CNS abscess—may manifest with delirium and should be

Box 90-1	Possible Causes of Delirium

Acute metabolic disturbances (uremia, liver failure)
Acute vascular disease (stroke, vasculitis, subarachnoid hemorrhage, sagittal vein thrombosis)
Central nervous system (CNS) disease (tumor, space-occupying lesions, seizure)
Dehydration
Electrolyte disturbances (hypo- or hypernatremia, hypoglycemia, acidosis, hypercalcemia, hypomagnesemia)
Endocrinopathy (hypo- or hyperthyroid, adrenal crisis)
Environmental exposure (hypo- or hyperthermia, sleep deprivation, unfamiliar surroundings)
Heavy metals (lead, mercury)
Hypoxia
Infection (encephalitis, meningitis, syphilis, CNS abscess, sepsis)
Intoxication (alcohol, amphetamines, cocaine)
Medication
Nutritional deficiencies (vitamin B_{12}, niacin, thiamine, malnourishment)
Pain (fractures, burns, surgery)
Toxins (pesticides, carbon monoxide, cyanide, solvents)
Trauma (intracranial hemorrhage, closed head injury)
Withdrawal (alcohol, barbiturate, benzodiazepene, opiate)

Note: Causes are listed in alphabetical order.
Data from Gleason OC. Delirium. Am Fam Physician 2003;67:1027–1034.

rapidly identified and treated. Similarly, infection of the urinary tract, respiratory tract, or skin and soft tissues or sepsis from any source may also produce acute alterations in consciousness. Usually, the physical examination and simple laboratory tests, including a complete blood cell (CBC) count and urinalysis with culture, will identify a focus of infection. Routine lumbar puncture is not necessary; however, if headache or meningismus is present or if an infectious focus is not readily identified, lumbar puncture should be performed.

Withdrawal from substances with sedative properties often results in delirium. A history of alcohol, barbiturate, benzodiazepine, opiate, or other sedative hypnotic use should be elicited and quantified. Occasionally, previously unrecognized alcoholism is diagnosed when a patient admitted for another reason subsequently goes through withdrawal. Signs and symptoms of withdrawal typically include restlessness, tachycardia, tremor, nausea, sweats, tactile and visual hallucinations, and occasionally seizures. *Intoxication* with alcohol or street drugs, such as amphetamines or cocaine, also induces delirium. Blood alcohol level determination and urine or serum drug screening corroborate suspected intoxication.

Fluid and electrolyte disturbances and other *acute metabolic disturbances* may cause delirium, including dehydration, hypo- or hypernatremia, hypoglycemia, acidosis, hypercalcemia, hypomagnesemia, uremia, and liver failure. A complete metabolic profile (CMP) and serum calcium and magnesium levels should be obtained in patients when a cause is not immediately evident. Special attention should be paid to fluid balance and hydration status during the physical examination. In addition to hydration status, the nutritional status should be determined, because general malnutrition, as well as specific *nutritional deficiencies* (vitamin B_{12}, niacin, thiamine), may play a role.

Intracranial hemorrhage or other closed head injury from *head trauma* may be the underlying cause. Patients with delirium and evidence of a head injury should undergo immediate computed tomography (CT). *Pain* from other forms of trauma, including fractures, burns, or surgery, can cause delirium. Postoperative pain is especially troublesome because it may be unclear whether the symptoms are due to the pain or to the opioid analgesic medication used to treat the pain. This uncertainty may lead to inadequate pain management and worsening delirium.

Delirium may accompany many *CNS diseases*. Focal neurologic deficits suggest the presence of a tumor or other space-occupying lesion. Focal deficits should be assessed with CT. Other *acute vascular diseases* such as stroke, vasculitis, subarachnoid hemorrhage, sagittal vein thrombosis, and hypertensive emergency must be ruled out if they are suggested by the overall clinical picture.

Environmental exposure should be taken into account, and hypo- or hyperthermia should be readily recognized and treated. A common iatrogenic cause is the so-called ICU psychosis that can occur in critically ill patients on closed units who are not exposed to diurnal cues or are sleep deprived. Other environmental considerations, including exposure to *toxins* such as pesticides, industrial *poisons* (carbon monoxide, cyanide, solvents), or *heavy metals* (lead, mercury), are generally elicited in the history.

Hypoxia causes fluctuations in consciousness, attention, and cognition characteristic of delirium. This occurs with acute hypoxia from respiratory failure, worsening of chronic lung disease, or hypotension and decreased cerebral perfusion.

Up to 30% of cases of delirium are attributable to *medication toxicity* (Francis, 1996). Many medications can cause delirium (Box 90-2). Medication lists

---

Box 90-2 | **Commonly Prescribed Medications That Can Cause Delirium**

Antibiotics
  Clarithromycin
  Fluoroquinolones
Anticholinergics
  Antiemetics
  Antihistamines
  Antiparkinsonian agents
  Antipsychotics
  Antispasmodics
  Tricyclic antidepressants
Anticonvulsants
Anti-inflammatories
  Corticosteroids
  Nonsteroidal anti-inflammatory drugs
  Salicylates
Benzodiazapines
Cardiovascular drugs
  β-blockers
  Antidysrhythmics
  Antihypertensives
  Digoxin
H_2-receptor antagonists
Lithium
Narcotic analgesics

Note: Drugs are listed in alphabetical order.
Data from Francis J. Drug-induced delirium: Diagnosis and treatment. CNS Drugs 1996;5:103.

---

should be carefully reviewed and potential drug-drug interactions considered, including over-the-counter drugs and any other medications the patient may have access to in the household. Drugs with levels that can be checked (digoxin, lithium, certain anticonvulsants) should be checked because they may cause symptoms even in the therapeutic range.

Endocrinopathies (thyroid storm, myxedema coma, adrenal crisis) are uncommon but serious causes of delirium. Myxedema coma is a rare complication of severe hypothyroidism, often induced by an underlying infection, with severe hypothermia, hypoventilation, hypoxia, hyponatremia, hypotension, and hypercapnia. Thyroid storm is a very rare form of thyrotoxicosis manifested by delirium, tachycardia, vomiting, diarrhea, dehydration, and high fever. A thyroid-stimulating hormone (TSH) level is usually adequate to screen for thyroid dysfunction. Acute adrenal insufficiency, or adrenal crisis, most commonly occurs following stress or illness in a patient with latent insufficiency or treated insufficiency if steroid replacement is not increased to account for increased stress. A cosyntropin stimulation test establishes the diagnosis, and an elevated plasma adrenocorticotropic hormone (ACTH) level distinguishes primary adrenal disease from secondary.

Plan

Diagnostic

Mr. B. is too combative to allow blood to be drawn or other testing. So, before further testing is undertaken, he is given 2 mg of haloperidol intramuscularly (IM). His agitation does not improve after 30 minutes, so he is given a repeat dose of 2 mg. He calms significantly, and blood is drawn for a CMP, CBC, blood culture, and TSH and blood alcohol level determination. A fingerstick blood glucose level is normal at the bedside. Urine is collected for urinalysis and drugs of abuse screen. An electrocardiogram (ECG) and chest radiograph (using portable equipment) are obtained while the patient is cooperative.

Therapeutic

Intravenous (IV) access is obtained, and 100 mg of thiamine is administered. Physical restraints are not employed, as he is cooperative after the haloperidol.

ED Course

Mr. B. remains calm but does not respond appropriately to questions. He occasionally points and says the names of dead family and friends. Other than being calmer, there is no significant change in his physical examination.

Laboratory/Special Studies

The CBC, CMP, TSH, urinalysis, blood alcohol level, and urinary drug screen are normal. The ECG shows sinus tachycardia but is otherwise unremarkable. The chest radiograph shows poor inspiratory effort but no infiltrate or increased vascular markings.

Further Testing

More blood is drawn for serum magnesium and B_{12} level determination. Arterial blood gas values are normal. Mr. B. allows a head CT to be performed, which is normal. A lumbar puncture performed after sedation with 1 mg of midazolam (Versed) reveals clear fluid with a normal cell count and normal protein and glucose levels, and no organisms are seen on Gram stain. The remaining test results show a normal B_{12} level but a low magnesium level at 0.8 mg/dL.

Assessment

Mr. B. suffers from delirium secondary to hypomagnesemia. Mrs. B. returns from the house with a bottle of hydrochlorothiazide prescribed for her husband 2 weeks earlier. Hypomagnesemia is an adverse reaction to hydrochlorothiazide, although it usually does not occur in isolation.

Plan

Mr. B. is admitted to the hospital and given 2 g of magnesium sulfate intravenously over 30 minutes; followed by 6 g of magnesium sulfate in 1 liter of normal saline over 24 hours. He is placed on haloperidol, 5 mg every 8 hours scheduled and 2 mg every 2 to 4 hours as needed for agitation, to prevent him from removing his IV line and monitors.

FOLLOW-UP

The next morning, Mr. B.'s magnesium level is 1.5 mg/dL. The haloperidol is tapered to 2 mg every 8 hours, and Mr. B. is back to normal mentation. He remembers nothing of the previous 2 days. Atenolol, 50 mg/day, replaces the hydrochlorothiazide. The IV magnesium is continued for another 24 hours and oral magnesium replacement is started. The haloperidol is tapered further and discontinued after 48 hours.

DISCUSSION

Delirium is a serious problem that is encountered in up to 30% of elderly hospitalized patients (Francis, 1992) and 10% of elderly ED patients (Lewis et al., 1995®). Elderly patients who develop delirium have longer hospital stays (Ely et al., 2001®), a more rapid deterioration in function, and an increased risk of institutionalization (Inouye et al., 1998®). Both 1-month and 6-month mortality double for patients with delirium versus those without (Cole and Primeau, 1993®). Mortality remains increased for up to a year (McCusker et al., 2002®). Risk factors include advanced age, preexisting dementia or cognitive impairment, severe chronic medical illness, multiple medical conditions, polypharmacy, sensory impairment, and sleep deprivation (Gleason, 2003).

Box 90-3 lists the diagnostic criteria for delirium (American Psychiatric Association, 2000). The hallmark characteristic is an acute change in level of consciousness and in ability to focus, sustain, or shift attention. Initially these changes may be subtle and tend to fluctuate, making early recognition a challenge. Short-term memory deficits and disorientation to date, place, or situation are very common. Patients with delirium may be agitated or apathetic and withdrawn, resulting in hyperactive, hypoactive, and mixed subtypes of delirium. Perceptual disturbances commonly accompany delirium. Auditory hallucinations are more typical than tactile or visual, but all three can occur. Most important, delirium is caused by an underlying medical illness and will not improve if the underlying illness is not addressed.

Delirium often goes unrecognized (Lewis et al., 1995®). The Confusion Assessment Method (CAM) (Box 90-4) can be used as a diagnostic tool. It has a sensitivity of 94% to100% and a specificity of 90% to 95% in medical and surgical settings (Inouye et al., 1990®).

Evaluation of a patient with delirium starts with a thorough history and physical examination, including a careful review of the medication list. Special attention should be paid to signs and symptoms implicating one of the underlying causes listed in Box 90-1. Often, the initial assessment identifies the cause, and focused laboratory testing verifies the diagnosis. When a cause is not readily apparent, a CMP, a CBC, and a urinalysis are appropriate initial testing. Fingerstick blood glucose testing rapidly assesses glycemic status in diabetics. Chest radiography and lumbar puncture should be performed if infection is suspected and a source is not readily found. Evidence of head trauma, focal neurologic deficits, or severe impairment of consciousness warrants neuroimaging with CT. Further studies should be performed as indicated by the history and physical examination findings.

Treatment is aimed at correcting the underlying medical condition causing the problem, including discontinuation of any medication known to cause delirium. Supportive needs should be addressed, including hydration, nutrition, mobility, pain relief, and aspiration precautions. Thiamine is safe and inexpensive and should be administered to all patients prior to glucose- or dextrose-containing solutions to decrease the risk of precipitating Wernicke's encephalopathy in those with unrecognized thiamine deficiency or chronic alcoholism.

Box 90-3	DSM-IV Diagnostic Criteria for Delirium

A. Disturbance of consciousness (i.e., reduced clarity of awareness of the environment) with reduced ability to focus, sustain, or shift attention.
B. A change in cognition (such as memory deficit, disorientation, language disturbance) or the development of a perceptual disturbance that is not better accounted for by a pre-existing, established, or evolving dementia.
C. The disturbance develops over a short period (usually hours to days) and tends to fluctuate during the course of the day.
D. Evidence from the history, physical examination, or laboratory findings indicates that the disturbance is caused by the direct physiologic consequences of a general medical condition.

Adapted from American Psychiatric Association. Diagnostic and Statistical Manual of Mental Disorders, 4th ed., Text Revision (DSM-IV-TR). Bethesda, MD, American Psychiatric Association, 2000.

Box 90-4	The Confusion Assessment Method (CAM) Diagnostic Algorithm

Feature 1—Acute onset and fluctuating course

This feature is usually obtained from a family member or nurse and is shown by positive responses to the following questions: Is there evidence of an acute change in mental status from the patient's baseline? Did the (abnormal) behavior fluctuate during the day, that is, tend to come and go, or increase and decrease in severity?

Feature 2—Inattention

This feature is shown by a positive response to the following question: Did the patient have difficulty focusing attention, for example, being easily distractible, or have difficulty keeping track of what was being said?

Feature 3—Disorganized thinking

This feature is shown by a positive response to the following question: Was the patient's thinking disorganized or incoherent such as rambling or irrelevant conversation, unclear or illogical in flow of ideas, or unpredictable and switching from subject to subject?

Feature 4—Altered level of consciousness

This feature is shown by any answer other than "alert" to the following question: Overall, how would you rate this patient's level of consciousness (alert [normal], vigilant [hyperalert], lethargic [drowsy, easily aroused], stupor [difficult to arouse], or coma [unarousable])?

Note: CAM positive for delirium if patient has *both* features 1 and 2 *and either* feature 3 or 4.
Adapted from Inouye SK, vanDyck CH, Alessi CA, Balkin S, Siegal AP, Horwitz RI. Clarifying confusion: The Confusion Assessment Method, a new method for detection of delirium. Ann Intern Med 1990;113:941–948.

Symptomatic treatment for agitation, hallucinations, or disruptive behaviors is accomplished with the antipsychotic haloperidol (Haldol). Most adults will respond to 1 to 2 mg administered orally (PO) or IM and repeated every 2 to 6 hours as needed. The dosage can range from 0.5 to 10 mg PO or IM every 1 to 4 hours as needed. Haloperidol can be given IV, but patients should be on a cardiac monitor, because IV administration can cause QTc prolongation. Benzodiazepines generally worsen confusion and sedation, and their use is limited to the treatment of delirium due to withdrawal from alcohol or sedative hypnotics or as an adjunct for sedation for diagnostic procedures.

Nonpharmacologic interventions can be helpful in managing patients with delirium (Meagher, 2001). Many of these interventions are common sense and easily accomplished. Family members should remain with the patient and provide orientation. Family members can also bring familiar objects from home to place in the room. It is important to ensure that eyeglasses and hearing aids are available and easy to locate. A clock and a calendar with large, easy-to-read numbers placed conspicuously in the room help maintain orientation to time. The facility should maintain consistency in nursing staff and avoid having the patient change rooms. Uninterrupted sleep during the night can be maximized by arranging treatments, phlebotomy, and recording of vital signs to occur during waking hours. Physical restraints should be used only in extreme cases after other methods have failed to manage disruptive behaviors and patient safety is of concern.

Delirium is a serious condition that significantly increases morbidity and mortality when present. Recognizing delirium and rapidly assessing for the underlying cause are crucial. Information gleaned from the history, physical examination, medication review, and focused laboratory and imaging studies usually reveals the cause. Treatment is primarily aimed at correcting the underlying medical problem. Both pharmaceutical and nonpharmaceutical treatments help manage symptoms to facilitate evaluation or treatment of the underlying problem. Most patients will experience complete resolution if the correct cause of the delirium is identified and treated appropriately; however, symptoms of delirium can persist for several months.

Material Available on Student Consult

Review Questions and Answers about Hypomagnesemia

REFERENCES

American Psychiatric Association. Diagnostic and Statistical Manual of Mental Disorders, 4th ed., Text Revision (DSM-IV-TR). Bethesda, MD, American Psychiatric Association, 2000.

Cole MG, Primeau FJ. Prognosis of delirium in elderly hospital patients. CMAJ 1993;149:41–46. [B]

Ely EW, Bautam S, Margolin R, et al. The impact of delirium in the intensive care unit on hospital length of stay. Intensive Care Med 2001;27:1892–1900. [B]

Francis J. Delirium in older patients. J Am Geriatr Soc 1992;40:829–838.

Francis J. Drug-induced delirium: Diagnosis and treatment. CNS Drugs 1996;5:103.

Gleason OC. Delirium. Am Fam Physician 2003;67:1027–1034.

Inouye SK, Rushing JT, Foreman MD, Palmer RM, Pompei P. Does delirium contribute to poor hospital outcomes? A three-site epidemiologic study. J Gen Intern Med 1998;13:234–242. [B]

Inouye SK, van Dyck CH, Alessi CA, Balkin S, Siegal AP, Horwitz RI. Clarifying confusion: The Confusion Assessment Method, a new method for detection of delirium. Ann Intern Med 1990;113:941–948. [B]

Lewis LM, Miller DK, Morley JE, et al. Unrecognized delirium in ED geriatric patients. Am J Emerg Med 1995;13:142–145.

McCusker J, Cole M, Abrahamowicz M, Primeau F, Belzile E. Delirium predicts 12-month mortality. Arch Intern Med 2002;162:457–463. [B]

Meagher DJ. Delirium: Optimizing management. BMJ 2001;322:144–149.

91

Chest Pain and Shortness of Breath (Panic Disorder)

Layne A. Prest

INITIAL VISIT

Subjective

Patient Identification and Presenting Problem

Andy B. is a 41-year-old white man who comes to the clinic with chest pain, shortness of breath, and a fear that he was having a heart attack and dying. He also reports some mild nausea and feeling hot or flushed. Andy says he came to the clinic this morning because he is afraid of what these symptoms might mean, especially since this isn't the first time he has experienced them. The symptoms come on relatively suddenly and usually unexpectedly, although he is more likely to experience one or more of them when he is exerting himself emotionally or physically, especially at work.

Present Illness

Andy reports that he has had increasing problems that he first noticed on Super Bowl weekend 3 weeks ago. In addition to the symptoms mentioned above, Andy is concerned about dizziness with exercise, hyperventilation, numbness and tingling in his hands, chest pain that extends up into the side of his face, the perception of a rapid heart rate, and subsequent anticipatory anxiety when he detects the onset of similar symptoms. Because the symptoms begin with and are exacerbated by activity, he has stopped exercising and has stopped all sexual activity. After the initial onset of these symptoms, he experienced a diminished appetite and weight loss of 15 pounds. He reports that in his capacity as an emergency department (ED) nurse, he had recently taken care of several men around his age who "had a look of panic in their eyes before they died." They had been complaining of symptoms similar to his own. Because of these concerns, over the past 2 months he has obtained through colleagues at work several electrocardiograms, a treadmill test, 24-hour Holter monitoring, and blood tests for cardiac enzymes. The results of all these tests were negative.

Medical History

Andy takes atorvastatin for hypercholesterolemia and ibuprofen as needed for chronic back pain due to an old injury. He also has a history of gastroesophageal reflux, but this is not currently a regular problem and is not being treated. He has no known allergies. His immunizations are up to date.

Family History

Andy is the second of three children. His parents, who divorced when he was 20, are still alive. His father has coronary artery disease, hypertension, and hyperlipidemia. The latter two conditions seem to be well controlled by medication at this point. Andy's mother is in fairly good health for her age. She has some minor osteoarthritic pain that is well controlled with medication.

Social History

Andy is married and has one daughter. He is an ED nurse. Although he finds his work challenging, he is somewhat dissatisfied because he had hoped to become a flight nurse. Andy's wife is a data manager for an insurance company. The two of them are considering adopting her cousin's 2-year-old son (the

---

cousin has been imprisoned on theft and drug charges; the identity of the biological father is unknown). Andy reports being ambivalent about this adoption because of financial concerns and his fear that they would be "taking on someone else's problems." Andy is an ex-smoker (he quit 10 years ago). Although he has drunk socially since college, Andy reports that he has recently noticed he has been drinking more than usual (12 to 15 beers per day), in part to cope with his worries about his health. But he has wondered if the alcohol intake might actually be contributing to his cardiac symptoms. As a result, in the past 2 weeks he has made largely unsuccessful attempts to cut down. Andy's last attempt to quit began 2 days ago. He reports not having had a drink for 48 hours. He denies symptoms of withdrawal. He denies illegal drug use.

Review of Systems

Andy reports some general muscle aches and weakness of a couple of months' duration, as well as fatigue. He denies cough, orthopnea, or paroxysmal nocturnal dyspnea. He reports occasionally having some epigastric pain after eating meals, but he does not identify any specific food intolerance and says he does not vomit. He denies nocturia or any other genitourinary symptoms. He says he has no vision or hearing disturbance, vertigo, tinnitus, or ataxia. He does describe some low back pain when he engages in activity involving lifting, bending, or twisting. The review of systems is otherwise negative.

Objective

Physical Examination

General Andy is a well-developed, well-nourished man. He appears somewhat agitated, trembling, and in some emotional distress. His speech is goal-directed and well organized, but somewhat pressured. He is well oriented. His height is 6 feet 2 inches and his weight is 210 pounds (with a body mass index of 27).

Vital Signs His temperature 36.9°C (98.4°F), pulse is 75 and regular, and respiratory rate is 25. His blood pressure is 156/109 initially and 135/85 on repeat testing. Blood pressure and pulse readings remain unchanged on orthostatic testing. Pulse oximetry yields a value of 99%.

Head, Eyes, Ears, Nose, and Throat Andy's head is normocephalic and without signs of trauma. Extraocular movements are intact. Pupils are equal, round, and reactive to light and accommodation. Funduscopic examination is normal. The external ears, canals, and tympanic membranes are normal bilaterally. Conversational hearing is normal. The nose is normal. The conjunctivae are pink. The oropharynx is moist, with no erythema or exudate noted. His dental hygiene is good.

Neck Examination of the neck discloses no lymphadenopathy, thyromegaly, venous distention, or cervical bruits.

Lungs Andy appears to be slightly tachypneic, but respirations are quiet and the lungs are clear to auscultation bilaterally.

Abdomen The abdomen is soft, nontender, and nondistended. No masses or organomegaly is present. Bowel sounds are normal.

Extremities No tenderness, weakness, muscle atrophy, deformity, edema, ischemic changes, or cyanosis is present.

Laboratory Tests

A complete blood cell count, comprehensive metabolic panel, erythrocyte sedimentation rate, thyroid-stimulating hormone level, and creatinine kinase level are within normal limits. Fasting lipids are at goal levels. A review of the tests he previously had obtained through his colleagues confirms that all results were normal.

Assessment

Working Diagnosis

The working diagnoses for Andy's presenting complaint are (1) panic attacks and (2) alcohol withdrawal–induced anxiety.

Differential Diagnosis

The patient in this case presents with symptoms consistent with panic attacks. However, the presence of panic attacks does not necessarily indicate a diagnosis of panic disorder, since they are a commonly associated feature of several other disorders. Therefore, the clinician must differentiate between panic disorder and other entities.

Panic attacks can result from certain medical conditions (e.g., hyperthyroidism, cardiac arrhythmias), the ingestion of various central nervous system (CNS) stimulants (cocaine, caffeine), or the withdrawal from CNS depressants (alcohol, barbiturates). If the attacks occur only during the medical illness or substance use/withdrawal, panic disorder is not diagnosed. Consequently, after the onset of panic attacks, all patients should be evaluated by a physician to rule out the presence of medical factors. As a result of considerable discussion about panic disorder in the popular media, increasing numbers of patients are self-diagnosing and presenting directly to mental health professionals. Although this is beneficial in that appropriate treatment can occur more quickly, the therapist now has the added responsibility of ensuring that all patients have been medically evaluated.

Once organic causes are ruled out, panic disorder must be differentiated from other DSM-IV disorders that include panic attacks. In order to arrive at an accurate diagnosis, it is necessary to understand the context and pattern of the symptoms. Panic attacks that occur in the context of panic disorder are not associated with a situational stimulus but instead appear to occur "out of the blue" (*unexpected or uncued panic attacks*). Those that almost always occur on exposure to, or in anticipation of, a specific stimulus are referred to as *situationally bound* (*cued*) *panic attacks*. Panic attacks that are likely to occur on exposure to a specific stimulus but are not invariably associated with that stimulus are referred to as *situationally predisposed panic attacks*. Both of these types of panic attacks are associated with other anxiety disorders. Patients who experience panic attacks only when in uncomfortable social settings (social phobia), in response to trauma-associated stimuli (posttraumatic stress syndrome), in response to specific stimuli (specific phobia), or as the object of obsessions and compulsions (obsessive-compulsive disorder) should not be given a diagnosis of panic disorder. Although patients with panic disorder may experience situationally bound and situationally predisposed attacks following the development of agoraphobia (e.g., a patient with panic disorder always experiences a panic attack when getting into an elevator), for the diagnosis of panic disorder to be warranted, the initial attacks had to have been unexpected.

It is possible for a person to have more than one disorder (that is, comorbid conditions). The majority of people with panic disorder do have a comorbid disorder, usually an additional anxiety disorder or depression. A diagnosis of panic disorder does not preclude the diagnosis of other anxiety disorders as well. Approximately 25% have generalized anxiety disorder and specific phobia. Slightly fewer have social phobia. On the other hand, obsessive-compulsive disorder and post-traumatic stress disorder are infrequently diagnosed. The diagnosis of panic disorder usually takes priority, but the other conditions need to be treated as well.

One of the more common conditions occurring along with panic attacks and panic disorder is agoraphobia. Specific or social phobias can be distinguished from agoraphobia by taking a careful history. If the avoidance of certain situations (e.g., driving, flying, public transportation, enclosed places) preceded the onset of the panic attacks, then specific or social phobia is likely a more appropriate diagnosis. However, if the patient began having panic attacks unexpectedly and subsequently began avoiding those situations for fear of having another panic attack (anticipatory anxiety), then he or she should be diagnosed with panic disorder with agoraphobia.

Although most people with panic disorder experience some symptoms of depression, dysthymia is more common than major depression. If the panic disorder remains untreated, however, the comorbid depression worsens over a lifetime because of the debilitating effects of this anxiety disorder. Patients with panic disorder and a current or past history of major depression have a chronic course, more severe symptoms, more frequent panic attacks, and more extensive phobic avoidance.

Plan

The plan for helping Andy manage his symptoms includes four recommendations. First, recommendations for medication are made. The provider suggests that a short course of a medication (e.g., a benzodiazepine) might help to alleviate the most problematic physical symptoms. A selective serotonin reuptake inhibitor (SSRI) is suggested for long-term management. Second, Andy is encouraged to consider cognitive-behavioral therapy and stress management training. Third, he is counseled to slowly work back into an exercise regimen. Last, he is counseled on behavior change regarding his alcohol use.

Andy's initial response to reassurance about not being in a life-threatening situation is a mixture of relief and disbelief. He states that he has been reassured before and is glad to know it is not his heart, but he asks about the possibility of having more extensive or repeat testing done to make sure. When he is told that further tests are not necessary except to reassure him, he acknowledges that he gets very anxious about these issues. The provider then begins to discuss anxiety and the flight-or-fight response, and makes the recommendations about medications, cognitive-behavioral therapy, stress management, and exercise. The provider also asks more about Andy's alcohol use. Andy is judged to be in the action stage of readiness for change but lacks a cogent plan for doing so. The provider commends Andy for his decision to quit and recommends that he consider regular attendance at Alcoholics Anonymous (AA) meetings, rely on stress management and social support, and take the medication as prescribed to treat the anxiety that seems to fuel his alcohol intake. Andy agrees to try the breathing exercise and to take the medication. He will consider the other recommendations and come back in 1 week.

FOLLOW-UP VISITS

At his first follow-up visit, Andy reports that he has had another attack but that it wasn't as serious as previous episodes. He has taken the medication as prescribed and reports that it seems to help. He has not tried exercising because his symptoms have been triggered in the past by physical exertion. He has tried the breathing exercise a few times, but he does not think it helps. He went to AA with a friend from work, but he didn't like the atmosphere. He is not sure he needs the meetings and would prefer a meeting where there was less religious talk. During this conversation he appears more receptive to the idea of cognitive-behavioral psychotherapy, so a referral is made. He is also given a handout on the management of panic disorder, including the role of stress management and exercise. The provider recommends that Andy consider starting a slow build-up to a regular aerobic exercise program. An appointment is made for another follow-up visit in 2 weeks.

At the 2-week follow-up visit, Andy reports that he drank on two occasions. He states that he felt initially better but later felt worse. As a result, he went back to AA (a different meeting) and made an appointment with the counselor. His next meeting is in 2 days. A release for exchange of information is signed by Andy so that the provider may discuss the treatment plan with the cognitive-behavioral therapist. Andy and his wife both read the handout on panic disorder management. He believes the diagnosis fits him very well, so he is encouraged to continue with this treatment plan. He reports not having any more symptoms and is overall a bit calmer, which supports the likelihood of withdrawal. He is reluctant to stop the short-term medication altogether, so it is agreed that he will cut the dose in half for the next 2 weeks. Further education about the different roles of benzodiazepines and SSRIs is provided.

At a follow-up appointment 2 weeks later, Andy reports that he has begun feeling better and did not use the benzodiazepine on several different days. He has discontinued attending AA meetings but has decided the counseling will work well for him, especially since his wife agreed to the therapist's request that she attend as well (in order to become educated about the issues, provide support and accountability, and address marital and family issues that have been contributing to Andy's stress). It is agreed that Andy can rely on the stress management, support, and cognitive-behavioral therapy to handle day-to-day pressures at this point. The benzodiazepine is discontinued. He agrees to take the SSRI regularly. He has remained abstinent from alcohol. The provider and Andy agree to follow up in 3 months, or sooner if needed.

DISCUSSION

Millions of people throughout the world experience panic disorder in their lifetime (American Psychiatric Association [APA], 2000©). Twice as many women as men, beginning as early as in adolescence, experience the debilitating effects of this disorder. Many of these individuals are likely to seek help from physicians in a variety of settings, most notably the ED and outpatient primary care clinics. In fact, they are more likely than patients with depression to visit a physician for help (Kessler et al., 1999©). Panic disorder is one of the more distressing mental health problems experienced by patients visiting primary care physicians. As many as 80% of primary care patients with this disorder present with alarming physical symptoms such as chest pain, dyspnea, and tachycardia (Roy-Byrne et al., 2002©). Panic attacks can be so distressing that a significant number of people become suicidal.

According to the American Psychiatric Association's *Diagnostic and Statistical Manual of Mental Disorders—Fourth Edition,* the defining characteristic of panic disorder is recurrent, unexpected panic attacks. Panic attacks can occur several times a day or only a few times during a year. A panic attack is defined as a discrete period of intense fear or discomfort that develops abruptly and reaches a peak within 10 minutes and is accompanied by at least four of the following 13 somatic and cognitive symptoms: shortness of breath, dizziness, palpitations, trembling, sweating, feeling of choking, nausea/abdominal distress, depersonalization, paresthesias (numbness/tingling), flushes/chills, chest pain, fear of dying, and fear of going crazy or fear of doing something uncontrolled. An individual must experience at least two unexpected panic attacks followed by at least 1 month of concern about having another panic attack in order to be diagnosed with panic disorder (APA, 2000©). Panic disorder may or may not be accompanied by agoraphobia, or the experience of anxiety in situations in which escape might be difficult or where help may not be immediately available in the event of the occurrence of a panic attack (e.g., on airplanes, buses, trains, or elevators; being alone; being in a crowd of people) (Sanderson and Rego, 2002©).

Andy presents with the classic symptoms of panic attacks. After obtaining a detailed history, it is clear that Andy is also experiencing comorbid problems as a result of alcohol abuse. Both need to be treated aggressively, since the outcome for each is poor if untreated; in addition, they exacerbate each other.

Material Available on Student Consult

Review Questions and Answers about Panic Disorder

REFERENCES

American Psychiatric Association, Committee on Nomenclature and Statistics. Diagnostic and Statistical Manual of Mental Disorders, 4th ed., Text Revision. Washington, DC, American Psychiatric Association, 2000.Ⓒ

Kessler RC, Zhao S, Katz SJ, et al. Past-year use of outpatient services for psychiatric problems in the National Comorbidity Survey. Am J Psychiatry 1999;156: 115–123.Ⓑ

Roy-Byrne P, Russo J, Dugdale DC, Lessler D, Cowley D, Katon W. Under-treatment of panic disorder in primary care: Role of patient and physician characteristics. J Am Board Fam Pract 2002;15:443–450.Ⓑ

Sanderson WC, Rego SA. Empirically supported psychological treatment of panic disorder and agoraphobia. Psychiatry MedPulse, 2002. Available at www.medscape.com/psychiatryhome. Accessed 3/1/2005.Ⓑ

Chapter

92 Bizarre Behavior (Schizophrenia)

Leslie Brott

KEY POINTS

1. Schizophrenia is a psychotic disorder with an onset usually during adolescence or early adulthood.
2. Cognitive impairment is a key element in the course of schizophrenia.
3. Diagnosis of schizophrenia involves ruling out a general medical condition or substance abuse that could cause the symptoms.
4. A psychiatrist's assistance in the management of schizophrenia is invaluable.
5. Treatment of schizophrenia includes antipsychotic medications, life-skills training, and family education and support.

INITIAL VISIT

Subjective

Patient Identification and Presenting Problem

Juan A. is a 19-year-old man first seen with his father, who is concerned about Juan's abnormal behavior and the possibility of a head injury.

Present Illness

Juan's father reports that Juan has not been acting normally for the last 6 to 8 months. Over the last 4-week period, his bizarre behavior has intensified. Juan has not been talking much unless he is asked a question. He sits much of the time, doing nothing. Often he seems to smile or laugh for no particular reason. His parents have been concerned about his depression for months and have considered taking him to a counselor. His father has been taking Juan to work with him, as he is concerned about leaving Juan home alone. Matters worsened acutely 3 weeks ago when Juan left home alone for several hours. On his return he was behaving strangely, speaking incoherently, and acting confused. His parents were concerned that he might have hit his head. They noticed no seizure activity or abnormal movements. Juan's father does not believe that alcohol or drugs are an issue, and Juan denies any use of them. Juan initially denies auditory or visual hallucinations or feelings of depression or anxiety.

Medical History

The patient's history is unremarkable except for episodes of gastroesophageal reflux disease.

Family History

Juan's parents and siblings are alive and well. No family history of mental illness is known.

Evidence levels Ⓐ Randomized, controlled trials (RCTs), meta-analyses, well-designed systematic reviews of RCTs. Ⓑ Case-control or cohort studies, nonrandomized clinical trials, systematic reviews of studies other than RCTs, cross-sectional studies, retrospective studies, certain uncontrolled studies. Ⓒ Consensus statements, expert guidelines, usual practice, opinion.

Social History

Juan lives with his parents, two younger brothers, and one younger sister. He dropped out of high school last year, before graduation. He has never held a job. He denies use of tobacco, alcohol, or illicit drugs.

Review of Systems

Juan has had no recent fevers, chills, fatigue, or malaise. His weight has not significantly changed in the last 6 months. He experiences epigastric and chest pain occasionally, and his symptoms are relieved with antacids. He denies palpitations, shortness of breath, and dyspnea on exertion. No nausea, vomiting, diarrhea, or constipation has occurred.

Objective

Physical Examination
Vital Signs
Blood pressure, 128/88
Heart rate, 95
Temperature, 36.4°C (97.6°F)
Respiratory rate, 18
Weight, 177 pounds

General Patient is a well-developed, slightly disheveled young man in no acute distress.

Head, Eyes, Ears, Nose, and Throat Normocephalic, no evidence of trauma. Pupils are equal, round, and reactive to light. Extraocular muscles intact. No nystagmus. Fundoscopic examination is normal. Tympanic membranes and oropharynx are within normal limits.

Neck Supple, no lymphadenopathy or thyromegaly.

Heart Regular rate and rhythm, no murmurs.

Lungs Clear.

Abdomen Normal bowel sounds, no hepatosplenomegaly.

Extremities No clubbing, cyanosis, or edema.

Neurologic Cranial nerves II to XII intact. Brachial and patellar reflexes are brisk and symmetrical. Upper and lower extremity strength is grossly symmetrical. Gait is within normal limits. Romberg is negative. No pronator drift.

Psychiatric Juan appears his stated age. He is dressed in faded jeans and a torn T-shirt. He sits quietly making exaggerated facial expressions. He smiles and laughs for no particular reason, and he appears to be attending to internal stimuli. He does not speak sponta-neously. Questions are answered with brief one-word answers, if at all. He does not maintain any eye contact. He is oriented to the day, date, month, year, and place, but he declines to answer a question about why he is in the clinic today. He is able to subtract serial 7s. He will not answer questions regarding judgment (i.e., *What would you do if you found a sealed, stamped envelope on the sidewalk?*) and abstraction (i.e., *What does the phrase "People who live in glass houses should not thrown stones" mean?*). On persistent questioning, Juan admits to hearing voices. Sometimes he thinks the voices are coming from the television in his house, but at other times he senses the voices are inside his head. He cannot associate the voices with anyone he knows and often cannot understand what they are saying. He denies visual hallucinations.

Assessment

Working Diagnosis

Juan is diagnosed with a psychotic disorder, as evidenced by his hallucinations and disorganized speech and behavior. His symptoms are consistent with disorders in the schizophrenia spectrum, including schizophrenia and schizophreniform disorder.

Schizophrenia is defined by positive and negative symptoms as well as social and occupational dysfunction. The positive symptoms include those that are classified as psychotic: delusions and hallucinations. Delusions are defined as thoughts that are completely disconnected from reality. In schizophrenia, the delusions may be paranoid, grandiose, or persecutory. The hallucinations in schizophrenia are most commonly auditory but occasionally can be visual or olfactory. Disorganized speech and grossly disorganized or catatonic behavior are other positive symptoms identified in schizophrenics. The untreated schizophrenic patient has difficulty holding a normal conversation and has trouble making sense of everyday input.

Negative symptoms are those of apathy, avolition, and social withdrawal. Schizophrenic patients have a flat affect and have trouble expressing emotions. They lack the motivation to initiate and complete everyday tasks, including self-care duties. As a result, they often demonstrate social withdrawal and isolation.

For a diagnosis of schizophrenia, a patient must have positive or negative symptoms with evidence of functional decline for at least 6 months. In those 6 months, the patient must exhibit two or more positive symptoms for at least 1 month. Only one positive symptom is needed for the diagnosis if the delusions are bizarre or if the auditory hallucinations include two or more voices or one voice making a running commentary. The patient's symptoms must not be due to a medical condition or to drug or alcohol use. An associated mood disorder may be included in the diagnosis of schizophrenia.

If an individual has symptoms as described for schizophrenia but has had them for less than 6 months, then a diagnosis of schizophreniform disorder is made. Individuals with schizophreniform disorder do not exhibit the marked social and occupational dysfunction, likely because of the brief period of symptoms. Schizophreniform patients have a complete remission of symptoms, without the benefit of medication, before 6 months. If the symptoms persist beyond 6 months, a diagnosis of schizophrenia may be made.

Juan exhibits symptoms consistent with schizophrenia. His social dysfunction has lasted more than 6 months. His positive symptoms—hallucinations and disorganized behavior and speech—have lasted for at least 1 month. He has no underlying medical condition or substance abuse that would better explain his symptoms.

Differential Diagnosis

Psychosis, a loss of contact with reality, occurs in several mental conditions. The following are the most common conditions, in addition to the schizophrenia spectrum, considered in the workup of psychosis. Some argue that the various disorders lie on a continuum of mental disease and that diagnoses overlap. Nevertheless, the differential diagnoses are listed as outlined in the *Diagnostic and Statistical Manual of Mental Disorders*, 4th edition (DSM-IV).

Schizoaffective disorder. Some patients meet the criteria for schizophrenia but also meet criteria for a mood disorder such as major depressive disorder or generalized anxiety disorder. In this case, a diagnosis of schizoaffective disorder is assigned, and patients are treated for both disorders.

Schizotypal personality disorder. This disorder is an axis II diagnosis with characteristics similar to those of schizophrenia but without hallucinations or delusions. Schizotypal patients exhibit social detachment and isolation. They are often socially inept and prefer to be alone. Unlike schizophrenics, they do not exhibit chronic psychosis, and their clinical course is stable over time.

Bipolar disorder. Recurrent episodes of depression and mania with intervening periods of euthymia characterize bipolar disorder. In the throes of a depressive or manic period, patients may have hallucinations or delusions. It can be differentiated from schizophrenia by the presence of psychosis which occurs only in the setting of depression or mania. Usually the depressive or manic symptoms will precede the onset of psychotic behavior. Delusions, if present, are mood congruent in bipolar disorder, whereas in schizophrenia, the delusions tend to be unrelated to mood. In any event, at the time of the manic or depressive exacerbation, it may be very difficult to distinguish bipolar disorder from schizophrenia.

Obsessive-compulsive disorder. Classified as an anxiety disorder, obsessive-compulsive disorder (OCD) is characterized by delusions. Patients with OCD have persistent and recurrent thoughts that cause distress or dysfunction in their lives. They perform repetitive behaviors in response to their obsessive thoughts. These patients have insight into their disorder; however, they recognize that their thoughts are irrational. Their behaviors, however, may mimic the disorganized behavior found in schizophrenics. Interestingly, a large percentage of patients with schizophrenia exhibit obsessive-compulsive behaviors. A significant number of patients initially diagnosed with OCD will later have a psychotic decompensation and meet criteria for schizophrenia.

Alcoholic hallucinosis. Patients with an addiction to alcohol can develop psychotic symptoms, especially paranoid delusions, which mimic symptoms of schizophrenia. Schizophrenic patients likewise may have a dependence on alcohol. Distinguishing the two can be problematic unless the full history of a patient is known. Schizophrenic individuals will exhibit psychosis before, or early in, the development of alcohol abuse. Differentiation also can be made when abstinence occurs. If the delusions resolve after 6 months of abstinence, then alcoholic hallucinosis is the diagnosis.

Delusional disorder. Some patients have delusions that are not bizarre. Their delusions are plausible but without any basis in reality. If such nonbizarre delusions last for at least 1 month, the other criteria for schizophrenia are not met, and the patient is able to function, a diagnosis of delusional disorder is made.

Plan

Diagnostic

To confirm that no medical condition or substance use better explains Juan's symptoms, laboratory and radiologic studies are performed. A complete metabolic panel and complete blood count, as well as thyroid studies and a urine drug screen, are performed. A head computed tomography (CT) is performed as well. The results of all studies are normal.

Therapeutic

Once the results of laboratory and radiologic studies are obtained, Juan and his parents return to the clinic. Juan is started on an atypical antipsychotic at a low dose: risperidone (Risperdal), 1 mg nightly. He is referred to the county health department's psychiatrist for further evaluation and treatment.

Patient Education

The patient and his parents are informed that schizophrenia is a chronic condition that requires lifelong care. Literature describing the disorder is given to the family. The need for family education and support is emphasized.

Disposition

An appointment is made with the psychiatrist, and chart notes and evaluation results are forwarded. Juan's parents are informed of the signs of acute decompensation and are directed to take Juan to the local emergency department should they occur.

DISCUSSION

Demographics

Schizophrenia has a 1% lifetime prevalence. The onset in male patients is earlier than that in female patients, but overall an even sex distribution is found. Its onset is usually in adolescence or early adulthood but can range from ages 13 to 40.

Etiology

Clearly a genetic component to schizophrenia exists. Studies of monozygotic twins demonstrate a 50% concordance rate. Those individuals with a first-degree family member with schizophrenia have a 5% prevalence rate of schizophrenia versus the 1% for the general population. Although it is known that schizophrenia has a strong genetic component, it has not yet been linked to a specific gene.

In addition to the strong genetic component, environmental factors play a role in the development of schizophrenia. Schizophrenia is thought to be a neurodevelopmental disorder characterized by defective neuronal migration. This is evidenced by the fact that patients with schizophrenia have cortical atrophy and dilated ventricles on brain CT and magnetic resonance imaging at the *onset* of the disease. The defective neuronal migration is postulated to have been caused by either obstetrical/birth trauma or by an *in utero* viral infection. Evidence for the latter lies in the preponderance of winter births among schizophrenics. In any event, it is clear that both genetic and environmental forces are at work in the development of schizophrenia.

Natural History

Although schizophrenia can have an insidious or acute onset, four phases have been identified. A *prodromal period* usually precedes the development of active disease. During this period, patients demonstrate unusual behaviors, social withdrawal, and a generalized decline in function. Individuals will experience failure in academic and occupational endeavors.

The *acute phase* is characterized by the onset of psychotic symptoms. The positive symptoms of delusions, hallucinations, and bizarre, disorganized behavior become evident. It is at this point that the diagnosis of schizophrenia is established. This is followed by the *recovery phase* in which the positive symptoms begin to wane, but the disorganization and confusion continue. A *residual phase* ensues, in which the negative symptoms of schizophrenia predominate.

Schizophrenia can be divided into four subtypes, with the prognosis affected by the subtype. The subtypes are characterized as paranoid, catatonic, disorganized, or simple. Patients who do not fit into any category are characterized as undifferentiated. Paranoid and catatonic subtypes tend to demonstrate a fluctuating course throughout their lifetimes, whereas disorganized and simple subtypes tend to be more chronic.

One marked feature of schizophrenia, regardless of subtype, is cognitive impairment. Cognitive deficits persist throughout the phases of schizophrenia. They are evident both during and after psychotic episodes and are progressive throughout the schizophrenic's lifetime. The specific cognitive deficits include impairment in working memory (ability to remember information for a short time and then use it to perform a task), executive function (ability to plan actions, problem solve), attention and information processing, long-term memory, and ability to learn.

Diagnosis and Treatment

No diagnostic test will confirm the diagnosis of schizophrenia. The workup essentially serves to rule out medical conditions or substance use as the cause of symptoms. The history and physical examination should guide the workup. Basic laboratory studies should include complete blood count, serum chemistries, thyroid function, urinalysis, and drug and alcohol screens. Imaging studies and electroencephalograms should be ordered as needed based on the history and physical.

A psychiatrist's assistance with the diagnosis and treatment of schizophrenia is extremely helpful. The treatment of schizophrenia includes antipsychotic medications, psychotherapy, and social skills training. Patients may be initially hospitalized, especially if their psychosis creates a dangerous environment for themselves or others. Those with severe delusions or hallucinations, those who cannot take care of themselves, and those who are suicidal warrant inpatient hospitalization. Some patients may be repeatedly hospitalized throughout their lives, whereas others may be managed well at home or in group or foster home settings.

Antipsychotic medications are a mainstay of schizophrenia treatment. Medication is started during the acute phase to curb the psychosis and then

Table 92-1   Antipsychotic Medications

Typical	Atypical
Chlorpromazine (Thorazine)	Aripiprazole (Abilify)
Fluphenzine (Prolixin)	Clozapine (Clozaril)
Haloperidol (Haldol)	Olanzapine (Zyprexa)
Perphenazine (Trilafon)	Quetiapine (Seroquel)
Thioridazine (Mellaril)	Risperidone (Risperdal)
Thiothixene (Navane)	Ziprasidone (Geodon)
Trifluoperazine (Stelazine)	

continued as maintenance therapy. The medications are divided into older "typical" antipsychotics and the newer "atypical" ones (Table 92-1). The older, typical antipsychotics include haloperidol, chlorpromazine, and fluphenazine. These agents tend to be much less expensive than the newer drugs. Haloperidol and fluphenazine are uniquely available in injectable, long-acting formulations. A high potential exists for extrapyramidal side effects including dystonia, akathisia, and parkinsonism with the older medications, especially haloperidol.

The newer atypical antipsychotics tend to have fewer extrapyramidal side effects than the older medications. They are as effective for positive symptoms and perhaps better for negative symptoms than their older counterparts. The newer medications include clozapine, risperidone, olanzapine, quetiapine, ziprasidone, and aripiprazole. These agents antagonize the dopamine and serotonin neurotrans-mitter systems, whereas the typical antipsychotics are purely dopamine antagonists (Table 92-2).

Once the pharmacotherapy has been established, therapy turns to cognitive-behavioral treatment for the patient and supportive therapy for the patient's family. Schizophrenics benefit from social-skills training, including self-care and independent-living skills. Insight-based psychotherapy is contraindicated in these patients as it can exacerbate their illness. Family therapy includes instruction in the course of the disease, its treatment, and realistic expectations for the patient's future. Family support groups can provide much of this information. It has been shown that family intervention results in reduced relapse rates for the schizophrenic as well as improved well-being in the family.

Prognosis

Schizophrenia is a lifelong condition for the majority of patients. Complete remission does occur, but this is unusual. Although the positive and negative symptoms can be moderately controlled with medication, it is the ongoing cognitive and functional impairment that debilitates the schizophrenic. Only 10% are employed on a full-time basis, and only 20% succeed with part-time employment. Meaningful interpersonal relationships are rare.

Material Available on Student Consult

Review Questions and Answers about Schizophrenia

Table 92-2   Common Side Effects of Antipsychotic Medications

Side Effect	Characteristics	Associated Medications
Extrapyramidal side effects	Dystonia (muscle spasms), akathisia (restless, jittery), parkinsonism (tremors, bradykinesia)	Predominantly typical antipsychotics but can occur with any
Tardive dyskinesia	Writhing movements of hands, mouth and tongue. Associated with long-term use of medication	Predominantly typical antipsychotics
Anticholinergic symptoms	Dry mouth, blurred vision, urinary retention, constipation, confusion	Low-potency typical antipsychotics
Neuroleptic malignant syndrome	Hyperthermia, catatonic rigidity, unstable blood pressure, dyspnea. Mortality rate $\leq 20\%$	All antipsychotics, predominantly typical antipsychotics
Galactorrhea	Elevated prolactin	Atypical antipsychotics
Agranulocytosis	Severe leukocytopenia	Clozapine
Diabetes mellitus	Elevated fasting blood glucose levels	Atypical antipsychotics
Weight gain	Associated with development of diabetes and hyperlipidemia	Atypical antipsychotics
Cardiac dysrhythmia	Prolonged QT	Atypical antipsychotics

SUGGESTED READINGS

Adler CM, Strakowski SM. Boundaries of schizophrenia. Psychiatr Clin North Am 2003;26:1–23.

American Academy of Child and Adolescent Psychiatry. Practice parameter for the assessment and treatment of children and adolescents with schizophrenia. J Am Acad Child Adolesc Psychiatry 2001;20:4S–23S.Ⓒ

American Psychiatric Association. Diagnostic and Statistical Manual of Mental Disorders, 4th ed. Washington, DC, American Psychiatric Association, 1994.Ⓒ

Flashman LA, Green MF. Review of cognition and brain structure in schizophrenia: Profiles, longitudinal course, and effects of treatment. Psychiatr Clin North Am 2004;27:1–18.

Lehman AF, Buchanan RW, Dickerson FB, et al. Evidence-based treatment for schizophrenia. Psychiatr Clin North Am 2003;26:939–954.

Moore DP, Jefferson JW. Schizophrenia: Handbook of Medical Psychiatry, 2nd ed. St. Louis, Mosby, 2004, pp 115–124.

Expert consensus treatment guidelines for schizophrenia: A guide for patients and families. J Clin Psychiatry 1996;57(Suppl 12B):51–58.

Chapter

93

Cold and Numb Hands and Feet (Frostbite)

Stephen G. Cook

KEY POINTS

1. Frostbite is the result of actual freezing of tissue.
2. Exposure to cold (such as through winter outdoor activities or homelessness) and decreased awareness of cold and numbness (due to alcohol, drugs, or psychiatric illness) are the main factors contributing to frostbite.
3. Frostbitten tissue is extremely fragile and should never be rubbed in an attempt to thaw it.
4. Careful tissue rewarming in warm water slightly above body temperature is the mainstay of initial therapy.
5. Recovery typically is quite prolonged. Surgery, especially amputation, should be delayed until it becomes absolutely necessary.

INITIAL VISIT

Subjective

Patient Identification and Presenting Problem

Joe C. is a 19-year-old college student brought to the emergency department with hands and feet that are cold, white, and numb.

Present Illness

Joe was attending a late November college football game with his friends. Despite the weather forecast predicting snow, they wore body and face paint and no shirts during the game. Joe's friends say they kept warm by drinking vodka from a large wineskin; they had also had "a bunch" of beer before going to the game. As the sun dropped in the late afternoon, Joe began to say that his hands felt funny. His friends

Evidence levels Ⓐ Randomized, controlled trials (RCTs), meta-analyses, well-designed systematic reviews of RCTs. Ⓑ Case-control or cohort studies, nonrandomized clinical trials, systematic reviews of studies other than RCTs, cross-sectional studies, retrospective studies, certain uncontrolled studies. Ⓒ Consensus statements, expert guidelines, usual practice, opinion.

noticed that he became clumsier and was unable to open a bag of peanuts or get money out of his pocket. His friends thought his clumsiness was due to Joe's being drunk, and they all stayed at the game until the end. After they returned home, Joe's friends noted that his hands remained very white and cold. When he complained that he still could not feel anything in his hands or his feet, they brought him to the school's health center.

Medical History

Joe was treated 1 year ago for a broken wrist sustained when he fell from a fraternity porch during a party; his blood alcohol level at the time was 0.29. He has no history of chronic illness and is taking no medications. His immunizations are all up to date, according to college health service records. He has no history of prior cold exposure injury.

Family History

Joe's father is 48 and is a recovering alcoholic; he has hypertension and hypercholesterolemia. Joe's mother is in excellent health at age 45. He has two younger siblings who have no health problems.

Social History

Joe is a C student in his sophomore year at the college. His friends report that he "parties hard" at least 3 days per week. He smokes tobacco, one-half pack per day, and occasionally uses marijuana, but denies other illicit drug use.

Review of Systems

There are no recent acute illnesses. He reports no pain in his hands and feet, only numbness.

Objective

Physical Examination

General Joe appears very drowsy on the gurney and smells strongly of alcohol, but he opens his eyes in response to voice command and gives simple answers to questions.

Vital Signs His temperature (measured rectally) is 32°C (89.6°F), blood pressure is 92/50, pulse is 48, and respiratory rate is 10. Weight and height are reported at 195 pounds and 71 inches, respectively, but Joe is unable to stand on the scale.

Skin Green paint is noted on Joe's face, chest, and upper arms, but his forearms and hands are white, cold, and pulseless. When his wet shoes are removed, his feet are also white, cold, and pulseless.

Head, Eyes, Ears, Nose, and Throat The tip of the nose and both earlobes appear waxy and white and are very cold to the touch. Tympanic membranes are unremarkable. Oral mucous membranes are dry.

Neck No masses or adenopathy is noted.

Lungs The lungs are clear to auscultation bilaterally.

Heart The heart exhibits a bradycardic regular rhythm without a murmur.

Abdomen Bowel tones are absent. No tenderness or masses are noted.

Neurologic There is decreased sensation to pinprick, light touch, and vibration below the ankles and in the hands. Patellar and ankle jerk reflexes are absent. Romberg's sign cannot be tested for, as Joe is unable to stand without assistance.

Assessment

Working Diagnosis

Frostbite is injury due to the actual freezing of tissues. The condition was historically seen mainly in soldiers but has become more common in recent years as winter sports and outdoor activities have become more popular and as an increasing number of people become homeless (Murphy et al., 2000**B**). Generally, frostbite occurs at temperatures from −4°C to −10°C (25°F to 14°F) or lower. Wind, decreased mobility, venous stasis, malnutrition, and occlusive arterial disease all increase the risk for frostbite (Tierney et al., 2004**B**). Lack of awareness of cold exposure contributes significantly to cold injury. Psychiatric illness is quite common among frostbite victims, with prevalences estimated as high as 61% to 65%. Alcohol use is also highly correlated with frostbite (Murphy et al., 2000**B**). Alcohol decreases a person's awareness of cold and numbness, thus leading to prolonged exposure. Alcohol also inhibits heat generation through shivering and can accelerate heat loss due to its vasodilatory effects (Biem et al., 2003**B**). Nicotine use exacerbates peripheral vasoconstriction and may worsen tissue injury. It may also be associated with preexisting peripheral vascular disease. Patients with peripheral neuropathy from diabetes or other causes are at increased risk for frostbite injury owing to their decreased ability to sense cold, particularly in the extremities, where frostbite is most likely to occur (Murphy et al., 2000**B**). Hypothyroidism, adrenal insufficiency, hypoglycemia, and central nervous system abnormalities also may predispose to frostbite (Biem et al., 2003**B**).

Frostbite occurs when skin is exposed to subfreezing temperatures for time sufficient to allow ice crystals to form within tissue. Extracellular ice crystals form initially, damaging the cell membrane, changing its permeability, and leading to intracellular dehydration and dramatic changes in cell electrolyte concentrations. With longer exposure and further cooling, intracellular ice forms; as these ice crystals expand, they cause mechanical destruction of cells (Murphy et al., 2000B). Rewarming and thawing of ice crystals leads to further damage due to cellular and tissue edema, red cell and platelet aggregation, thrombosis, and skin bleb formation. Tissue death is caused by ischemia and thrombosis of smaller vessels, as well as by actual freezing of tissue at the cellular level. Tissue injury is worst when cooling is slow, cold exposure is lengthy, rewarming is prolonged, and especially when tissue is thawed and then refreezes (Mechem, 2005B).

The severity of frostbite injury generally correlates more with the duration of cold exposure than with the temperature to which skin is exposed. Although skin freezes more quickly at lower temperatures, once frozen, it is the length of time the tissue remains frozen that determines the degree of irreversible damage. Hands and feet account for 90% of all injuries. Other commonly involved sites include the ears, nose, cheeks, and penis (Murphy et al., 2000B).

Like burns, frostbite can be classified by degree. First-degree injury may manifest with hard white plaques on waxy-looking skin, along with some early sensory deficits. Progressively deeper levels of freezing lead to worsening symptoms, including paresthesia and stiffness; the skin becomes increasingly white or yellowish, inelastic, and immobile. In second-degree frostbite, clear blisters form that are typically high in thromboxane; many experts advocate debridement of these blisters to avoid thromboxane-mediated tissue injury. Third-degree injury blisters usually are filled with blood; owing to the risk of infection, these blisters should generally be left intact. Fourth-degree injury denotes full-thickness freezing, including freezing of the muscles, tendons, and bones (Mechem, 2005B).

Differential Diagnosis

Frostnip is the mildest form of cold exposure, involving only the subcutaneous tissue. It may manifest with numbness, prickling, and itching, and there may be visible whitening of the skin, commonly at the tips of the fingers, ears, and nose. It is rapidly reversible with removal from the cold exposure and does not cause long-term damage (Tierney et al., 2004B).

Chilblain, or *erythema pernio*, occurs when prolonged cold exposure does not cause actual freezing of the tissues. It is a mild form of cold injury and most often manifests with red, itchy plaques. There may be some degree of blistering or edema, but no necrosis of tissue occurs (Tierney et al., 2004B).

Immersion syndrome, or *trench foot*, represents a more serious exposure. It is caused by prolonged contact of the extremity with cold or cool, but not freezing, liquid. Temperatures from 0°C to 10°C (32°F to 50°F) are typically enough to cause immersion syndrome; damp exposure as mild as 12.8°C (55°F) for 10 hours has been sufficient to cause this disorder. Typical stages in immersion syndrome can include:

1. A prehyperemic stage, characterized by cold and numbness without pain
2. A hyperemic stage with intense burning and shooting pains
3. A posthyperemic stage with pallor or cyanosis and decreased pulsations

Immersion syndrome can present with a wide variety of visible changes, including blistering, swelling, redness, heat, ecchymosis, hemorrhage, necrosis, and gangrene (Tierney et al., 2004B). Though some of these skin changes may be apparent at presentation, as with frostbite, the degree of tissue necrosis may take weeks or months to fully assess.

Peripheral vascular disease can lead to absent pulses and a cool or cold extremity, but it is unlikely to be of rapid onset with a symmetric distribution. Other systemic illnesses, including diabetes and other causes of neuropathy, may exacerbate the problems caused by frostbite but would be unlikely to present with the acute changes seen in this case.

Plan

Diagnostic

Although the full extent of freezing injury is often difficult to assess clinically, imaging modalities such as triple-phase bone scanning and magnetic resonance angiography have been used to assess the severity of injury and to discriminate viable from nonviable tissue (Tierney et al., 2004B). However, controlled trials establishing the effectiveness of these techniques are lacking (Biem et al., 2003B). Laboratory studies are rarely helpful in the diagnosis, though they may show hemoconcentration and decreased liver function (Mechem, 2005B).

Therapeutic

Rapid thawing of tissue at temperatures slightly above body heat can help decrease or limit tissue necrosis. However, if there is any possibility of refreezing, thawing should be delayed until long-term warmth can be assured, as refreezing leads to a marked increase in tissue death (Tierney et al., 2004B). Frostbitten skin is extremely fragile, and rubbing the affected areas can markedly worsen tissue damage (Biem et al., 2003). Rewarming is best done by immersion in a moving water bath at 40°C to 42°C (104°F to 108°F); dry heat is much more difficult to regulate, and excessive heat can further damage tissue. Once the distal part of the frozen area flushes, thawing can be considered complete. At that point, external heat should be removed and the affected body parts should be elevated and left uncovered. During the recovery period, contact with blistered skin should be minimal (Mechem, 2005Ⓑ).

As skin and deeper tissues thaw, pain can be quite severe. Morphine or similar analgesics should be employed liberally in the early stages of treatment. Ibuprofen, 200 to 400 mg taken four times per day, and aloe vera applied to blistered skin, have been used to prevent dermal ischemia. Due to the extensive tissue disruption, tetanus immunization boosters are recommended in cases of frostbite. Patients who have not previously been fully immunized should also receive tetanus immune globulin. Some experts advocate prophylactic antibiotics, but this is not universally recommended (Mechem, 2005Ⓑ). Local infection can be treated with soaks in soapy water or application of povidine-iodine. Whirlpool therapy can help with cleaning and debridement of sloughing tissue (Tierney et al., 2004Ⓑ). In all cases, rubbing or scrubbing must be avoided.

Surgical management to debride or amputate tissue may be needed eventually but should be delayed as long as possible. The one exception in which early surgery would be needed is when fasciotomy is called for in the case of compartment syndrome (Mechem, 2005Ⓑ). Frostbitten tissue may appear dead but can still prove viable even 6 to 8 weeks after cold injury. Even with obvious overlying necrosis and black eschar formation, underlying tissue can still heal over a period of months. Therefore, amputation should be put off until absolutely indicated (Tierney et al., 2004Ⓑ).

Patient Education

After a frostbite injury, the affected part is often very cold sensitive and usually remains increasingly susceptible to recurrent cold injury (Tierney et al., 2004Ⓑ). Neuropathic changes may include pain, numbness, tingling, anhydrosis or hyperhydrosis, cold sensitivity, and nerve conduction abnormalities, and may persist for years after the cold injury (Mechem, 2005Ⓑ).

Material Available on Student Consult

Review Questions and Answers about Frostbite

REFERENCES

Biem J, Koehncke N, Classen D, Dosman J. Out of the cold: Management of hypothermia and frostbite. Can Med Assoc J 2003;168:305–311.Ⓑ

Mechem CC. Frostbite. Available at www.emedicine.com. Accessed 3/21/2006.Ⓑ

Murphy JV, Banwell PE, Roberts AHN, McGrouther DA. Frostbite: Pathogenesis and treatment. J Trauma 2000;48:171–178.Ⓑ

Tierney LM, Jr, McPhee SJ, Papadakis MA. 2004 Current Medical Diagnosis and Treatment, 43rd ed. New York, McGraw-Hill, 2004, pp 1530–1531.Ⓑ

94 Disorientation (Heat Stroke)

Scott Kinkade

INITIAL VISIT

Subjective

Patient Identification and Presenting Problem

Mr. K. is a 52-year-old white man whom you have been seeing for many years. He is brought to the clinic by his wife, who noticed he was disoriented this morning.

Present Illness

Piecing the history together from Mr. K. and his wife, it seems he came in from baling hay because he felt dizzy, fatigued, and nauseated. He had been baling hay on his open-air tractor from 7 AM to 10 AM. Mr. K. does not remember parking his tractor and coming inside. His wife says she noticed him standing in the kitchen having trouble remembering where the drinking glasses were kept. She also noticed that he was very hot and was sweating, so she helped him take off his shirt, had him lie on the couch, and got him a glass of water. Although he kept telling her, "I'm fine," he could not recall whether he had finished baling his hay and what else he was going to do today. She estimates that his mental status seemed to return to normal after about 45 minutes.

It is now about 1 PM, and Mr. K. is able to tell you that he feels fine, except he is a little tired and has some muscle soreness. He was in his usual state of health this morning when he started working on his tractor. He had a half-gallon water jug that he says he drank from frequently because of the hot, humid conditions. He remembers feeling dizzy and nauseated and thinking he should head back to the house to rest. The next thing he can recall is that he was lying on his couch with his shirt off and his wife standing over him. He urinated once this morning, before going to the fields, and has not had an urge to urinate since. He cannot recall ever having any significant problems because of the heat. He does note that during prolonged work in the summer, when he is sweating quite a bit, he occasionally gets some cramps in his legs and arms. They resolve if he rests and drinks some Gatorade.

Medical History

Hypertension well controlled with hydrochlorothiazide, 25 mg daily, and lisinopril, 10 mg daily. Diet-controlled diabetes.

Family History

He has a brother who is alive and well and a sister who had breast cancer several years ago. His father died of cardiac disease, and his mother died of complications of Parkinson's disease and Alzheimer's dementia.

Social History

Mr. K. lives in the country with his wife, owns a small business, and raises cattle. He uses smokeless tobacco and drinks an average of one or two beers every day. He denies any illicit drug use.

Review of Systems

The patient denies headache, blurred vision, nasal congestion, or sore throat. He denies chest pain, palpitations, or shortness of breath. He has not had any emesis, diarrhea, or abdominal pain. His last bowel movement was last night. He has not noticed any

Evidence levels Ⓐ Randomized, controlled trials (RCTs), meta-analyses, well-designed systematic reviews of RCTs. Ⓑ Case-control or cohort studies, nonrandomized clinical trials, systematic reviews of studies other than RCTs, cross-sectional studies, retrospective studies, certain uncontrolled studies. Ⓒ Consensus statements, expert guidelines, usual practice, opinion.

blood in his stool or dark stool. He denies any dysuria or change in his urine. He has not noticed any weakness or dysequilibrium before this morning.

Objective

Physical Examination

Mr. K. is a well-developed white man in no apparent distress.

Vital Signs

Height, 5 feet 10 inches
Weight, 205 pounds
Temperature, 99.3°F
Respirations, 16
Blood pressure, 138/84
Pulse, 92

No significant orthostatic change occurs in pulse or blood pressure.

Head and Neck Eyes are clear, nares without discharge, oropharynx appears slightly dry, but no lesions or drainage. The neck is supple without lymphadenopathy. The thyroid is not palpable.

Heart and Lungs Normal cardiac rate and rhythm without any murmurs. The lung fields are clear.

Abdomen Normal bowel sounds, nontender and nondistended.

Extremities Pulses are strong in all extremities, with no edema.

Neurologic Alert and oriented; no deficiencies on mental-status testing. Motor strength, 5/5 in all extremities. Cerebellar function intact. Sensation is intact to light touch and vibration. Cranial nerves are intact. Deep tendon reflexes in the upper and lower extremities are normal.

Assessment

Working Diagnosis

Mr. K. probably has a heat-related illness, most likely heat stroke. Heat stroke is characterized by a core temperature greater than 40°C (104°F), acute mental-status changes, and other organ dysfunction (renal, cardiac, hepatic, hematologic). In severe heat stroke, the central nervous system symptoms can include coma and seizures. Heat stroke is a medical emergency. However, the spectrum ranges from mild heat exhaustion to severe heat stroke, and some cases can be difficult to differentiate, particularly when mental-status changes are resolving and cooling has been instituted. Heat stroke usually implies that the body's normal thermoregulatory mechanisms are overwhelmed, and therefore these patients do not cool spontaneously. Whether his core temperature was greater than 40°C when he came inside and his wife began modest cooling measures is unknown.

Differential Diagnosis

Other heat-related illnesses, such as heat syncope or heat exhaustion, are possible. Heat syncope is loss of consciousness with prolonged standing or on standing in hot environments. This is unlikely, given that no loss of consciousness was reported. It is due to mild-volume dehydration, peripheral vasodilation, lack of acclimatization, and orthostasis. It is fairly common with prolonged standing in outdoor warm events (marching band rehearsals, military formations, concerts, and spectator sports). Recovery is spontaneous once the individual is in the horizontal position, and treatment involves hydration and modest cooling measures.

One of the distinctions between heat exhaustion and heat stroke is that no significant neurologic impairment is found with heat exhaustion. The 45 or more minutes of disorientation Mr. K. exhibited are not typical of heat exhaustion. Patients with heat exhaustion may have mild neurologic symptoms such as irritability, confusion, impaired judgment, dizziness, and headache. Sweating, thirst, fatigue, weakness, muscle cramps, and myalgias are common, often with nausea and sometimes vomiting. Temperature can be elevated, but is still less than 40°C. If the thermoregulatory mechanisms are not overwhelmed, spontaneous cooling can occur, but if untreated, heat exhaustion can progress to heat stroke.

Hyperthermia with mental status changes is concerning for infectious diseases such as sepsis and meningitis. Given the lack of preceding or residual symptoms and the resolution of the hyperthermia without antipyretics, infectious diseases are unlikely. However, even milder infections (sinusitis, strep pharyngitis, pneumonia, etc.), although not causative of the heat illness, may be predisposing factors and make an individual more susceptible.

Hyper- or hypoglycemia is possible. Hyperglycemia usually does not resolve on its own or with one glass of water. Hypoglycemia, besides being uncommon in someone not taking any hypoglycemic medicines, usually does not resolve until treated.

A cerebrovascular accident, such as a transient ischemic attack, is a possibility. Given the lack of focal weakness at the time and the current normal examination, it is hard to confirm. At this time, it would be part of the differential, but most likely a diagnosis of exclusion.

Mr. K. may have had cardiac ischemia or arrhythmia. Although these are possible, without symptoms of palpitations or chest discomfort, they are unlikely.

Drug ingestion either (illicit or too much of a usual medicine) or toxins can cause mental-status changes and hyperthermia. Farmers would be susceptible to organophosphate poisoning. Additionally, drug or toxin ingestion may not be the direct etiology but may make an individual more susceptible to heat injury.

Plan

Diagnostic

One important aspect of diagnosing heat stroke is measuring core temperature. Ideally this should be done early in the course of treatment. In this case, Mr. K. is now afebrile and has cooled on his own. Because heat stroke can cause multiorgan failure, testing directed at finding organ dysfunction is warranted. Ruling out predisposing infectious diseases may be necessary. Finally, heat illnesses usually involve electrolyte imbalances and some degree of dehydration. Diagnostic testing will be directed by the severity of the symptoms and initial laboratory findings. Because the laboratory values cannot be obtained in the office, Mr. K. is admitted to the hospital across the street.

A basic starting point would include blood urea nitrogen and creatinine to look for renal dysfunction and degree of dehydration. Urinalysis typically shows elevated specific gravity and sometimes casts and red blood cells (RBCs). The urine also can be checked for the presence of myoglobin, which would indicate rhabdomyolysis and would increase the risk of acute renal failure. In instances in which a urine myoglobin is not readily available, the presence of myoglobin can be assessed with a routine urine dipstick and microscopic urine sediment examination. With true hematuria, the microscopic analysis of the urine will show RBCs or fragmented RBCs in addition to changing the color of the urine dipstick. With rhabdomyolysis and myoglobinuria, no RBCs will appear in the microscopic examination, but because the dipstick cannot distinguish between hemoglobin and myoglobin, it will still register as positive. It is important to check electrolytes, with particular attention to sodium and potassium in addition to calcium and phosphate, which are often low. The complete blood count typically shows hemoconcentration and often a leukocytosis related to the inflammatory response. Persistently elevated white blood cell counts should prompt an investigation for infection. Low platelet levels would be concerning for disseminated intravascular coagulation (DIC). Measurement of the prothombin time, and activated partial thromboplastin time, D-dimer, and fibrin split products also may be necessary to rule out DIC. Liver transaminases are almost always elevated.

A chest radiograph may be obtained to rule out pneumonia, acute respiratory distress syndrome, and pulmonary edema, which is sometimes a complication of vigorous intravenous rehydration. A patient with ongoing mental-status changes or other neurologic deficits should undergo computed tomography scanning of the head. Patients with respiratory distress or pulmonary edema should have an echocardiogram to assess ventricular function.

Laboratory Data

Na: 131
K: 3.3
Cl, bicarb, Ca, Mg are normal
Glucose, 135
BUN, 42
Cr, 1.5
Complete blood count is normal
Urine: tea colored, specific gravity, >1030; trace RBC, trace protein. The remainder of the urinalysis including microscopy is negative. Urine myoglobin is positive.
AST: 142
ALT: 185
Lactate dehydrogenase, Alk phos, and bilirubin: normal
CPK, 3500
ECG and chest radiograph are normal.

Therapeutic

Beyond the lifesaving ABCs (airway, breathing, and circulation), cooling is the most important immediate intervention. This patient is no longer hyperthermic and therefore does not need aggressive cooling. Heat-stroke patients typically do not need large amounts of IV fluids. Mr. K. is given 1 L of normal saline via IV. Because his nausea has resolved, he is able to continue rehydration with oral fluid intake. His urine output is monitored to confirm adequate hydration and within 6 hours is averaging more than 50 mL urine per hour. Laboratory tests are repeated the next morning and have normalized. His urine is clear, and no myoglobin is detected. His examination is unchanged and still within normal limits.

Patient Education

Mr. K. is discharged home the next morning. He is advised to avoid strenuous activity for 72 hours and to avoid prolonged exposure to the heat for 1 week. Unfortunately, an area in which research is severely lacking is in the prognosis of heat-stroke patients and their potential for recurrence. Some heat-stroke patients seem more susceptible to recurrent heat injuries than others who have not had any heat-related illnesses. How to discern who is more susceptible or how long they are more susceptible has not been well studied.

Mr. K. is counseled about fluid and electrolyte intake, early warning signs of heat illness, and avoidance measures such as mandatory rest breaks and cooling techniques. He is instructed to consider any future heat-exhaustion or heat-stroke symptoms as an emergency.

DISCUSSION

Heat-related illness ranges from the mild to severe, although only heat stroke requires emergency treatment. Heat-related illnesses include the following, in order of severity.

Heat edema is benign and self-limited swelling of the hands and feet. It is due to vasodilation. Treatment is with elevation of the affected extremities or compression stockings or both. Diuretics should be avoided because they can cause volume depletion.

Heat cramps are painful spasms of skeletal muscles. They are usually due to a combination of physical activity, salt loss, and dehydration. They can be prevented with adequate fluid and salt intake. Most people obtain enough salt in foods or from sports drinks and do not need to use salt pills, which are available over the counter.

Heat syncope and *heat exhaustion* were described previously.

Heat stroke is defined as a core temperature greater than 40°C with signs of organ dysfunction and mental-status changes. Commonly, tachycardia, hyperventilation, and anhidrosis (lack of sweating) are noted, although many heat-stroke patients will still be found to be sweating.

Although a distinction is made between classic heat stroke and exertional heat stroke, the ultimate treatment measures are the same. The classifications have different epidemiologic characteristics, and possibly different pathophysiology. Classic heat stroke is due to exposure to high environmental temperatures and occurs more commonly in the very young or elderly, the poor or socially isolated, those with chronic medical conditions (cardiovascular disease, psychiatric disorders, obesity), and those without access to air conditioning. Exertional heat stroke is due to strenuous activity that may or may not be in a hot environment, although hot humid conditions confer higher risk. It generally occurs in young, otherwise healthy individuals (Box 94-1).

The mortality for heat stroke ranges from 5% to more than 50% (Bouchama, 2002, Rav-Acha, 2004), depending on how rapidly and effectively it is treated. When heat stroke is anticipated and medical personnel are prepared, such as in military training or sporting events, the mortality should be less than 10%. For patients in whom the diagnosis is not recognized promptly (such as heat waves leading to classic heat stroke) or if medical care is not readily available (i.e., religious pilgrimages to Mecca), the mortality may exceed 50%. For survivors of heat stroke, usually complete recovery ensues, with no long-term neurologic sequelae.

Treatment of heat stroke begins with prompt recognition and attention to the ABCs of resuscitation. All clothing should be removed from a heat-

Box 94-1	Risk Factors for Heat Stroke

Drugs: cocaine, phenothiazines, diuretics, stimulants (including ephedra, ma huang, pseudoephedrine), anticholinergics, antihistamines
Improper work/rest cycles
Dehydration
Lack of fitness or acclimatization
High environmental temperature and high humidity
Heavy equipment or too much clothing (over-bundled babies, firemen's protective gear, football gear).
Alcohol
Obesity
History of heat illness
Illness, particularly febrile illnesses, gastroenteritis, or hyperthyroidism

stroke patient, and the temperature should be measured rectally. This can help with the diagnosis and be used to monitor cooling. Start immediate cooling measures, preferably by using cool mist and fans. Other methods include ice baths, ice packs in the groin and axilla, ice-water gastric or peritoneal lavage, and cooling blankets. Ice baths can be technically difficult because it is difficult to record rectal temperatures and perform procedures including possible cardiac defibrillation. Because many of these methods can cause peripheral vasoconstriction, vigorous massage of the skin is usually required to help promote heat loss. Cooling measures can be stopped when the core temperature is less than 38°C (100.4°F). Antipyretics and dantrolene are ineffective. Frequent monitoring is required to avoid hypothermia. Shivering (or seizures), which can generate additional body heat, can be treated with benzodiazepines.

Heat-stoke patients should be resuscitated with normal saline, but typically do not require more than 1 or 2 L of IV fluids unless they are hypotensive. Initial laboratory studies include electrolytes, glucose, calcium, complete blood count, prothrombin time and activated partial thromboplastin time, blood urea nitrogen, creatinine, liver panel, arterial blood gases, urinalysis and urine myoglobin, and creatine phosphokinase. Observe the patient for evidence of rhabdomyolysis; renal, cardiac, or hepatic failure; disseminated pulmonary edema, or adult respiratory distress syndrome, and treat accordingly.

Material Available on Student Consult

Review Questions and Answers about Heat Stroke

REFERENCES

Bouchama A, Knochel JP. Heat stroke. N Engl J Med 2002;346:1978–1988.

Rav-Acha M, Hadad E, Epstein Y, et al. Fatal exertional heat stroke: A case series. Am J Med Sci 2004;328:84–87.

SUGGESTED READINGS

Coris EE, Ramirez AM, Van Durme DJ. Heat illness in athletes: The dangerous combination of heat, humidity, and exercise. Sports Med 2004;34:9–16.

Hadad E, Rav-Acha M, Heled Y, Epstein Y, Moran DS. Heat stroke: A review of cooling methods. Sports Med 2004;34:501–511.©

Lugo Amador NM, Rothenhaus T, Moyer P. Heat-related illness. Emerg Med Clin North Am 2004;22:315–327.

Wexler RK. Evaluation and treatment of heat-related illnesses. Am Fam Physician 2002;65:2307–2314.

Yeo TP. Heat stroke: A comprehensive review. AACN Clin Issues 2004;15:280–293.©

Chapter

95   Spider Bites

Jeffery Alan May

KEY POINTS

1. The staple of spider bite management is supportive, *primum non nocere*, with RICE—rest, ice, compression, and elevation. Prudent use of tetanus + diphtheria immunization, antihistamines, and antibiotics (if the bite is deemed infected) is the best recognized plan and holds the least potential for worsening the patient's condition.

2. In severe circumstances (e.g., in patients with disseminated intravascular coagulation) steroids are useful; antibiotics or even inhibitors of polymorphonuclear leukocyte migration, such as dapsone, may be considered.

3. Without an obvious perpetrator (a spider or remnants thereof), the clinician should think of other causes of the lesion.

INITIAL VISIT

Subjective

Patient Identification and Presenting Problem

On a typical spring day in our large rural practice, on average three people present with "spider bites." These patients have lesions consistent with an insect bite, which is ubiquitous in the human experience. The typical signs of inflammation—rubor, dolor, calor, and tumor—as well as pruritus are likely to be associated in all cases.

A 20-year-old woman comes to the office complaining that something bit her on the right lower back 3 days earlier. The lesion is approximately 1.5 cm, erythematous, macular, pruritic, and slightly papular. It blanches on pressure, indicating a nonvasculitic lesion. She is given a tetanus + diphtheria (Td) booster and diphenhydramine, and released.

Our patient later returns to the office complaining of headaches, myalgias, and chills. By this time a 1-cm necrotic lesion on her right lower back has formed. Two other individuals seen on the same day also have lesions, which they attribute to spiders, but only one actually saw and killed a spider, which was in a pair of pants he was putting on. He was bitten on the thigh. These pants had lain on the floor overnight. This young man also has a lesion similar to the young woman's, but other than ensuing local necrosis, requiring 4 weeks' healing time, he suffered no further sequelae. The other patient's wounds did not progress, nor were there other problems.

Assessment

On her return visit to our office, the young woman is now moderately ill. The wound has grown to an ulcer 3 by 5 cm in circumference and 1 cm deep near the original lesion. She also reports darkening of her urine for 3 to 4 days. A complete blood cell count shows a hemoglobin value of 7 g/dL and a hematocrit of 20%, with a white blood cell count of 13,000/mm³. There is a neutrophilic predominance with five to seven band cells (a left shift). Her reticulocyte count is 16% with a positive indirect Coomb's test. The INR, or international normalization ratio, of her prothrombin time is 1.2; her activated partial thromboplastin time is 31 (i.e., both of these coagulation parameters are elevated, revealing a mild coagulopathy); and her erythrocytic sedimentation rate is 132.

Treatment

She is hospitalized and treated with corticosteroids and intravenous fluids, with prompt relief of symptoms. She is treated with a high dose of prednisone (60 mg) every day for 3 weeks and seen in the office once a week. She has no further complications. At the end of 5 weeks the wound has healed, with no need of revision or grafting.

DISCUSSION

Two of our patients probably sustained envenomation by the brown recluse spider (*Loxosceles reclusa*). It is the primary culprit in significant cases of necrotic arachnidism in the United States. Of lesser significance are the black widow (*Latrodectus mactans*), the hobo spider (*Tegenaria agrestis*), and the tarantula. To place the problem of spider bites in perspective, it should be recognized that of the 60,000 members of the phyllum Arthropoda, class Arachnida, 30,000 are spiders. We are seldom more than a few feet from a member of these groups whether we are indoors or outside, and so, luckily, our topic narrows to only a few significant exemplars. They are discussed here in order of priority to their bite, prevalence, severity, and U.S. geographic locale.

Brown Recluse Bites

Brown recluse envenomation may result in local necrosis and sometimes a more generalized systemic response, which may range from local necrosis to intravascular hemolysis and even disseminated intravascular coagulation. Although other *Loxosceles* species exist in the United States, *L. reclusa* is of greatest significance. The spiders' habitat range centers on the mid-South, the Southeast, and parts of the Southwest, including more than 16 states extending to the Midwest (Fig. 95-1).

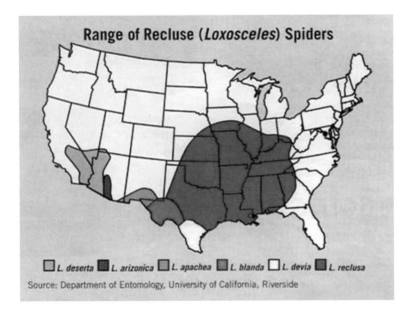

Figure 95-1 Range of recluse (*Loxosceles*) spiders. (Courtesy of Rick Vetter, www.spiders.ucr.edu.)

The arachnid prefers temperatures above 40°F, enjoys the dry environment of woodpiles and outbuildings, and particularly likes attics, basements, closets, and storage areas. It is a nocturnal hunter and can be aggressive, although its general behavior befits its name.

The leg spread of the adult is commonly 3 to 4 cm, with a body length of about 5 mm. It is dark to medium brown with a characteristic violin shape (the neck of which points caudad) on the dorsal cephalothorax. This marking is more prominent in some species than in others, but *L. reclusa* in its mature form usually has the marking (Fig. 95-2).

The clinical presentation of a brown recluse bite is called loxoscelism or necrotic arachnidism (Fig. 95-3). Although all spiders possess some venom designed to immobilize and begin digestion of their prey, few species have the mouthparts and fangs to penetrate and envenomate human skin (Table 95-1). Most encounters with humans are caused by spiders nesting or foraging in clothes that are put on by the unsuspecting victim. Bites of the brown recluse are probably more numerous than once suspected because the vast majority probably result only in minimal inflammatory responses and thus are unreported. To some extent, people who have been bitten several times may develop neutralizing antibodies.

Brown recluse venom is both cytotoxic and hemotoxic and contains a complex mixture of enzymes, the most well-known constituent of which is sphingomyelinase-D. The clinical presentation varies dramatically from a small, local phenomenon to coagulopathy and, rarely, death. In the worst of lesions there is an aching, painful lesion with redness

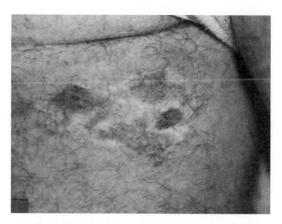

Figure 95-3 Clinical appearance of a brown recluse bite. (From Sams H. *Cortland Forum*, July 2000, p 35.)

at the site, followed by a bluish bleb, usually occurring within 12 to 24 hours. This necrotic bleb is often surrounded by a white ischemic halo, which may then have an erythematous margin. The classic dermonecrotic lesion is red, white, and blue and may be extremely pruritic. The bleb usually drains within a day, leaving an ulcer. In more severe cases, the erythematous ulceration may progress. Areas with abundant adipose deposits, such as the thigh, abdomen, and buttocks, may be more severely affected. By the third or fourth day, if no spreading has occurred, the envenomation will probably not be

Table 95-1	**Differential Diagnosis of Possible Necrotizing Arachnidism Lesions**

Vascular ulcers (arterial or venous insufficiency)
Diabetic ulcer
Infection
    Bacterial (e.g., *Streptococcus, Staphylococcus,* anthrax)
    Mycobacterial (e.g., *Mycobacterium ulcerans*)
    Fungal
    Viral (?)
Foreign body
Focal vasculitis
Injection of toxin (accidental or deliberate)
Drug reaction
Physical/mechanical trauma (may be deliberate)
Burns (especially chemical burns)
Pyoderma gangrenosum
Neoplasm
Immunosuppression
α-Antitrypsin deficiency
Fat herniation with infarction

From Hawdon GM, Winkel KD. Venomous marine creatures. *Aust Fam Phys* 1997;26:1369.

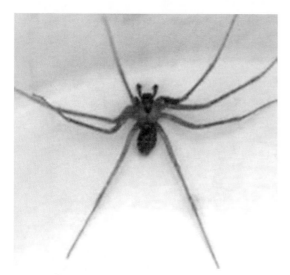

Figure 95-2 Brown recluse spider. (From Crown LA, Loftin B, Magill E. Successful treatment of hemolytic anemia secondary to brown recluse bite. *Family Practice Recertification* 1998;20:22–29.)

significant. Ulcers have progressed to as much as 30 cm in diameter and have taken months to heal. Systemic responses may also occur, including fever, chills, nausea, vomiting, headache, malaise, myalgias, arthralgias, and maculopapular rashes. Severe reactions are rare and usually affect very young, very old, or immunocompromised individuals. Treatment of these very ill patients includes systemic steroids and supportive measures aimed at ameliorating the symptoms.

Management of the noncritically ill or milder cases of loxoscelism is problematic. There are no current practical tests for envenomation and there is no antivenom available. Local wound care, tetanus prophylaxis, and, rarely, antibiotics (if the wound is truly infected) may be considered. Antibiotics are not routinely of use; however, the antileprosy drug dapsone has been advocated by some. As mentioned earlier, sphingomyelinase-D is a relatively large and well-studied constituent of brown recluse venom. It is a potent chemotactic agent for polymorphonuclear leukocytes, whose proteolytic enzymes are then responsible for probably most of the inflammation and tissue destruction. Inhibition of this migration might be useful in diminishing the extent of the necrosis; thus is the theoretical utility of the drug dapsone derived. The downside is that at doses high enough to gain this utility (the suggested dose is 50 to 200 mg/day), many patients will suffer some degree of hemolysis (especially those with glucose-6-phosphate dehydrogenase deficiency) or methemoglobinemia (if they have NADH reductase deficiency). Testing for both prior to initiating treatment complicates use of the drug. Furthermore, there are no studies that validate its use.

Methods of dealing with these necrotic lesions have included local excision, oxygen, electric shock, antihistamines, isotretinoin, nicotine patches, phentolamine, dextran, low molecular weight heparin, and meat tenderizer, among others. Ice and diphenhydramine, as well as problem-focused wound care, are the only modalities that do not risk worsening or confounding the condition. Laboratory work is also focused on any specific systemic symptoms the patient develops.

Black Widow Bites

Black widow spiders (*Latrodectus*) are endemic to nearly all of the United States except the extreme ecological niches of deserts, glaciers, and areas above the mountain tree lines. The female body length is up to 1.5 cm with a leg span of 4 to 5 cm. The male is approximately one-third that size. The male cannot envenomate humans and suffers a grim fate after mating with the female black widow. Only the female has fangs that are capable of penetrating human epidermis. Several species exist in the United States, but only three are black. *Latrodectus mactans* is shiny black and has the classic red hourglass figure on the ventral abdomen (Fig. 95-4).

Most victims are bitten on the hand while reaching into the spider's web lair. The bite usually causes a pinprick sensation but may go totally unrecognized. The venom consists primarily of neurotoxins, and therefore necrotic local tissue damage is unlikely. Latrodectism is the syndrome produced by the black widow venom. These neurotoxins exert, via acetylcholine release, extremes of either pallor or hyperemia at the site. This may then spread locally and, in larger envenomations, systemically. Presynaptic acetylcholine release is increased and uptake is inhibited postsynaptically, resulting in myriad symptoms that are proportional to the quantity of envenomation but may also to some extent be idiosyncratic, based on size, age, and immunocompetence of the victim. Symptoms may manifest as severe cramping usually occurring within 30 to 90 minutes and proceeding in a migratory fashion from the inoculation site. Cramping may involve the entire body, although children particularly exhibit abdominal musculature contractions. Confusion and mixed autonomic dysfunction follow: nausea, vomiting, diaphoresis, dizziness, headache, extreme restlessness or agitation and even motor paralysis may occur. Seizures and hypertensive crises with tachycardia and tachypnea are indicators of severe envenomation. Except in the special populations of the very old, young, immunocompromised, or pregnant women, complications are rare. Recovery is the rule. Peak symptoms usually occur during the few hours after the bite and subside

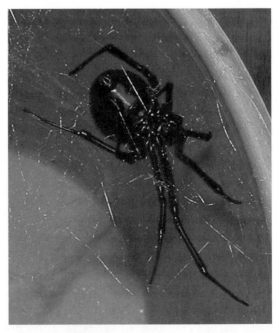

Figure 95-4 Black widow spider.

Table 95-2	Systemic Signs and Symptoms of Black Widow Spider Bite	
Common	**Occasional**	
Abdominal rigidity	Arrhythmia	
Agitation	Bradycardia	
Cutaneous	Convulsion	
hyperesthesia	Hypertension	
Headache	Mild fever	
Muscle cramps	Priapism	
and spasms	Psychosis	
Nausea	Shock	
Pain	Tachycardia	
Perspiration	Tachypnea and	
Restlessness	dyspnea	
Vomiting		

From Koh WL. When to worry about spider bites: Inaccurate diagnosis can have serious, even fatal, consequences. Postgrad Med 1998;103:235.

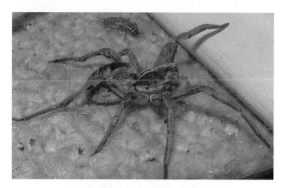

Figure 95-5 Wolf spider.

within a day or so. Some residual subjective complaints such as paresthesias, weakness, and malaise, as well as headaches, joint pain, and insomnia, may persist for weeks (Table 95-2). Management of severe envenomation from the black widow consists primarily of supportive care with attention to airway, breathing, circulation, appropriate laboratory tests, and interventions to counteract symptoms. The primary goal is to relieve the spasms and associated pain. Intravenous calcium gluconate has been used for some time but may be of limited use. If used, 10 mL of a 10% solution is given over 20 minutes and may be repeated every 2 to 4 hours. Dantroline (a skeletal muscle relaxant) given intravenously may prove to be useful for severe envenomations. Analgesics and narcotics, either parenteral or oral, are appropriate. Antivenom use is problematic; although it is very effective, up to 9% of patients will develop a serum sickness from the equine-based product, and hypersensitivity reactions are also a risk. Authorities recommend that the use of antivenoms be restricted to situations involving life-threatening manifestations such as cardiovascular collapse, severe hypertension, or in pregnant woman with severe symptoms. If available, antivenom is given at a dose of 1 to 2 vials over 20 to 60 minutes. Skin testing should be performed before administration.

Other Spiders

Less frequent, and hence less important clinically, are the hobo spider (*Tegenaria agrestis*), wolf spider (*Lycosidae* species), and the tarantula. *Tegenaria agrestis*, the hobo spider, also known as the Northwestern brown spider, a European immigrant of the 20th century to Washington, Idaho, and Oregon, may contribute to cases of necrotic arachnidism similar to *Loxosceles reclusa*. Because experience is minimal and cases are few, it is to date managed similarly.

The wolf spider's moniker *Lycosidae* developed because the Greeks thought these spiders hunted in packs (Fig. 95-5). Its most famous member, *Lycosa tarantula*, was credited with causing stuporous intoxication and wild dancing. However, a different European spider, *Latrodectus tredecimguttatus*, was found to be the real culprit of this syndrome. In reality, *Lycosa tarantulas* are not true tarantulas and do little more than cause trivial stinging pain.

The last spiders of clinical importance in North America are the 40 species of large, slow, and long-lived tarantulas (Fig. 95-6). These somewhat fearsome-appearing spiders are not aggressive, although they possess potent tissue-toxic venom. The geometry of their jaws is more vertical than that of the other spiders discussed here, and this puts them in a different suborder, Orthognatha, and requires that they must strike their victims after assuming a raised position anteriorly. To date, treatment is purely supportive. No human demise from envenomation of these arachnids in the United States is known.

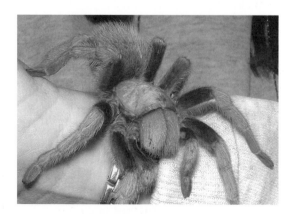

Figure 95-6 Tucson blonde tarantula.

Summary

The much maligned spiders usually are problematic for humans only during mutually unexpected encounters. The brown recluse is the most significant member with the most frequently seen bites. It and others mentioned here, with the exception of *Latrodectus*, use mostly cytotoxic and hemotoxic poisons, and their bites are ultimately best treated with supportive care only. This care may include cool compresses, limb immobilization, tetanus prophylaxis, and diphenhydramine, as deemed appropriate. The black widow and its *Latrodectans* ilk use neurotoxins and may cause broader and more serious symptoms, but they are much less frequently encountered. Although antivenom exists, its use is problematic and necessary only in the most severe circumstances.

The primary job for practitioners when patients present with an assumed bite is to attempt to ascertain whether the lesion was caused by the accused. As clinicians, we should never immediately accept a diagnosis purely on a hunch. The differential diagnosis of a necrotic lesion is extensive and depends on the setting, circumstances, presence of an eight-legged perpetrator, and progress of the lesion (see Table 95-1).

Material Available on Student Consult

Review Questions and Answers about Spider Bites

SUGGESTED READINGS

Auerbach PS (ed). Wilderness Medicine: Management of Wilderness and Environmental Emergencies, 3rd ed. St. Louis, Mosby, 1995, pp 769–782.

Crown LA, Loftin B, Magill E. Successful treatment of hemolytic anemia secondary to brown recluse bite. Family Practice Recertification 1998;20:22–29.

Family Practice News, Clinical Rounds, April 10, 2004, p 15.

Hardman J (ed). Goodman and Gilman's The Pharmacological Basis of Therapeutics, 10th ed. New York, McGraw-Hill, 2001, pp 1288–1289.

Treatment varies for severe *Loxosceles* spider bite. Family Practice News, May 1, 2004, p 15.

96 Upper Extremity Numbness and Pain (Double Crush Syndrome)

James M. Daniels

KEY POINTS

1. The key to identifying patients with numbness in the upper extremity is a careful history and physical examination.
2. Physical examination and history should focus first on elementary central nervous system lesions and then progress peripherally to peripheral nerve entrapments to rule out systemic processes that are associated with peripheral neuropathy.
3. A differential diagnosis of the upper extremity may include stroke, focal seizures, multiple sclerosis, or some type of spinal cord tumor. It may include entrapment of the cervical spine, thoracic outlet syndrome, or peripheral nerve entrapment.
4. Patients with confusing physical examination findings may be considered for the diagnosis of "double crush" syndrome or thoracic outlet syndrome.
5. Nerve root entrapment of the cervical spine may cause bilateral upper extremity symptoms. The sixth cervical nerve root can cause the same sensory changes that are associated with carpal tunnel syndrome. Cervical spondylosis is common, and the diagnosis should be considered in evaluating patients for carpal tunnel syndrome.
6. The thoracic outlet can be divided into four specific anatomic areas and nerve root

entrapment can be traced back to our embryologic development.
7. A number of populations are at increased risk of thoracic outlet syndrome and include patients involved in strenuous upper extremity work, female patients, patients with diabetes, patients involved in long work in a slumped over position such as office computer work.
8. The hallmark of carpal tunnel syndrome is nocturnal pain and paresthesias.
9. The clinical course of patients with carpal tunnel syndrome can be separated into three distinct groups: those with neurapraxia who have mild symptoms; those with axonotmesis who often have burning pain in their hands as a major complaint; and those with neurotmesis, which causes pronounced thenar wasting.
10. Double crush syndrome involves a nerve entrapment at multiple sites. Patients may present with symptomatic nerve compression and have negative electromyographic nerve conduction studies. One single site may not be sufficient to cause the patient to have symptoms, but when a second site is compressed, the patient may become symptomatic. Once identified, patients can be treated conservatively and symptoms can greatly improve in 3 to 4 months.

INITIAL VISIT

Subjective

Patient Identification and Presenting Problem
Tish S. is a 45-year-old white right-hand dominant computer analyst who presents to your clinic complaining of right hand numbness.

History of Present Illness
Approximately 2 years ago, Tish S. underwent endoscopic surgery on her left hand for carpal tunnel syndrome. Her symptoms abated slowly over 1 month. For the past 3 months, she has been waking at approximately 2 AM complaining of a "pins and needles" feeling in both hands. Her symptoms are relieved if she lets her arms hang over the edge of the

bed. In the morning, both of her hands feel numb and clumsy. She has trouble putting on her makeup; after this she is okay for the rest of the day. She recently started an aerobics fitness program and her symptoms have worsened. She is now having difficulty completing her exercise program because of these symptoms. Over the past week her symptoms have started affecting her work.

Medical History

Allergies: none. Medications: venlafaxine (Effexor XR), 75 mg at bedtime for depression; ramipril (Altace), 10 mg every morning for blood pressure; glyburide and metformin (Glucovance), 1.25 mg/250 mg every morning for diabetes; 81 mg coated aspirin every morning for stroke/myocardial infarction prevention; calcium and vitamin D (Citracal: 315 mg of calcium + 200 IU of vitamin D), two in the morning and two at night, for osteoporosis prevention.

Social History

She has been treated for depression for approximately 3 years. She is married with three children. Tish drinks about three glasses of wine per week; she smokes socially, approximately eight cigarettes per week.

Surgeries

Her last child was born by cesarean section. She has had a laparoscopic cholecystectomy. She had the endoscopic carpal tunnel surgery on her left wrist performed by a board-certified hand surgeon at the nearby regional medical center a few years ago.

Review of Systems

The patient has been in good health her whole life except for her diabetes, which was diagnosed 3 to 4 years ago. Tish was a gymnast in college, and she had a vaulting accident in which she fractured her right clavicle. Two months ago, she saw the surgeon who previously operated on her. The surgeon ordered electromyographic nerve conduction studies of her upper extremities, and they were normal. He prescribed neutral wrist night splints and placed her on pyridoxine (vitamin B$_6$), 200 mg daily. He diagnosed her with a very mild case of carpal tunnel syndrome but felt that she was not a candidate for surgery at that time. She recently started perimenopausal symptoms, including hot flashes and worsening of her depression.

The numbness in her hand is located in the thumb and index finger, but she occasionally feels that her whole hand will fall asleep. A year ago she was involved in a motor vehicle accident and underwent chiropractic manipulative therapy for approximately 3 months. The patient plays the violin in the local municipal symphony. She has difficulty with her violin technique and feels she no longer has the control of her hands that she once had. The only thing that seems to help her is sleeping in a recliner at night. During a recent vacation to the Caribbean with her husband, her symptoms greatly improved. Her job involves the use of a computer at work and a laptop at home. She spends approximately 6 hours per day on a computer. When she was in the Caribbean, she was without any type of computer.

Objective

Physical Examination

The patient is a 5 feet 4 inch, 164-pound white woman sitting on the examination table. She is tearful with her head down and sits in a "slumped over" position. Her blood pressure is 120/80. Her pupils are equal, round, and reactive to light and accommodation. She has complete range of motion of her neck. Spurling's maneuver does not reproduce any of her symptoms. Figure 96-1 illustrates this test. There is symmetry of her shoulders except for a large bone callus over the middle of her right clavicle. She has indentations on her shoulders where her brassiere is resting.

Her lungs are clear to auscultation and heart sounds are within normal limits. There are no bruits noted.

A modified Roos maneuver reproduces the patient's symptoms in approximately 8 seconds. Figure 96-2 illustrates this maneuver. The Valsalva maneuver does not reproduce any of the symptoms in her extremities. There is no evidence of any increased spasticity in her extremities or clonus and her deep tendon reflexes are +2 and symmetrical. She can extend and flex her elbow without any difficulty and reports no symptoms with resisted pronation of the forearm. She has a negative Tinel's sign of the proximal forearm and negative Phalen's test in the proximal forearm. Median nerve compression tests at the wrist are done bilaterally for 1 minute. Figure 96-3 illustrates this tests. The patient complains that her hands feel swollen, but her physical examination is normal. Her hands are warm to touch, and there is no increase in perspiration or evidence of any type of weakness in the upper extremities. The patient has a well-healed surgical scar on her left wrist from her previous surgery. There is no redness or inflammation of any of her joints.

She has a negative Tinel's sign at the cubital tunnel, and flexion of both elbows for 60 seconds does not reproduce any symptoms. Flexion of both wrists for 60 seconds does not reproduce any of the patient's symptoms.

Assessment

Differential Diagnosis

1. *Central nervous system lesions* can produce numbness in the upper extremities. A stroke or some type of focal seizure could cause these symptoms. The patient has diabetes and does smoke. Her blood pressure has been under good control. She

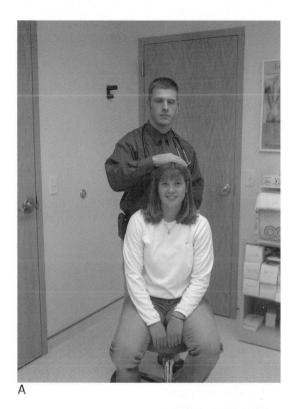

A

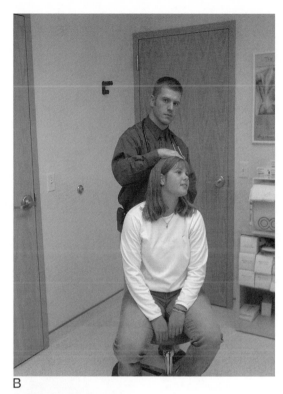

B

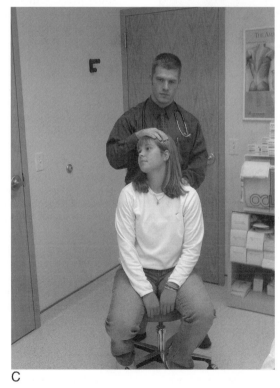

C

Figure 96-1 Spurling's maneuver. **A,** Axial load being applied to the top of the patient's head with the neck in a neutral position. **B,** The patient rotating her neck to approximately 45 degrees while slightly extending her neck. The physician then places an axial load to the patient's head, which causes compression of the ipsilateral nerve root. A positive test results in the patient complaining of reproduction of the symptoms in the affected extremity. Pain or discomfort in the neck is not considered a positive test. **C,** The patient rotated to the opposite direction at a 45-degree angle with her chin in extension. An axial load should not reproduce symptoms.

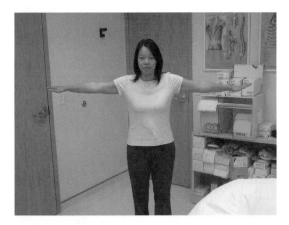

Figure 96-2 Roos maneuver. The patient abducts her arms to 90 degrees. It is considered a positive test if there is reproduction of the patient's symptoms in the affected extremity within 1 minute.

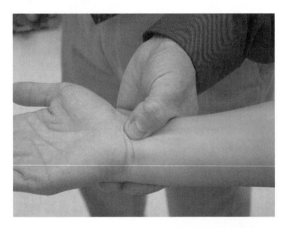

Figure 96-3 Median nerve compression test. This test is shown to be more reproducible than Phalen's test. It requires the examiner to place pressure on the volar aspect of the wrist on the affected extremity. The thumb is placed just proximal to the distal radial crease in the central part of the wrist. If the patient has palmaris longus tendon, intersection of these structures may act as a landmark for the examiner to place his or her thumb. A positive test results in the patient's symptoms being reproduced within 60 seconds of compression.

does have some risk factors for cardiovascular disease, but her physical examination is not consistent with this problem.

2. *Syringomyelia, multiple sclerosis,* or some type of spinal cord tumor may also produce these symptoms. The patient's symptoms have been intermittent and not constant. She also lacks any long track signs that would go along with any cord lesion.

3. *Nerve root entrapment of the cervical spine* can cause bilateral upper extremity symptoms. The

sixth cervical nerve root exits the central nervous system between the C5 and C6 vertebrae. Sixth cervical nerve root entrapment causes weakness of biceps and wrist extension. The patient has neither of these findings. The sixth cervical nerve also innervates the brachioradialis reflex and is partially responsible for the biceps reflex. Sixth cervical nerve entrapment can also cause sensory changes in the forearm and thumb similar to that of carpal tunnel syndrome. Cervical spondylolysis commonly occurs in middle-aged or elderly patients and can have almost identical symptoms to those of a median nerve pathology. The patient did not have symptoms with the Valsalva maneuver, and she had a negative Spurling's test. Cervical spine films and magnetic resonance imaging of the neck can be ordered to help identify cervical spine lesions.

4. *Thoracic outlet syndrome.* Pancoast's tumor can cause myosis, ptosis, and anhydrosis of the ipsilateral side of the face. This diagnosis should always be considered in a smoker. A chest radiograph or, if necessary, computed tomography of the chest can rule out this condition. The thoracic outlet consists of a triangle of muscle and bone in the shoulder and neck region in which the cervical spine nerve roots and brachial plexus transition into the upper extremity. The thoracic outlet can be divided into four sections. The first is the sternocostovertebral space, which can be occupied by Pancoast's tumor. The second is the scalene triangle bordered by the scalene muscles. These muscles can become taut or traumatized such as in a whiplash injury. They can then scar and exert pressure on the plexus. The third division of the thoracic outlet is the costoclavicular space. This is the space between the clavicle and the first rib. This space can be compromised if there is a history of trauma to the mid-clavicle and there is a large bone callus formation.

The fourth space is the coracopectoral space, which can be compromised if there is tightness in the anterior shoulder. This often happens in middle-aged people or people who have a job that requires them to be in a bent or stooped-over position for long periods of time. The anterior musculature of the chest hypertrophies while the posterior musculature of the upper back stretches. The long dynamic tunnel of the thoracic outlet is greatly affected by posture. Rare anatomic abnormalities can cause symptoms in this area. Approximately 1% of the population has a congenital abnormality of the cervical spine that can be seen on a radiograph. An unusually long transverse process of the seventh cervical vertebra is associated with a fibrotic band. This band originates at the transverse process of C7 and inserts on the body of T2. A cervical rib on the C7 vertebrae may be associated with one of these bands but can impinge on the brachial plexus itself.

Thoracic outlet syndrome can be traced back to our embryologic development. During development of the forelimb, buds must rotate 270 degrees to produce the position of the upper extremity at our side as opposed to the forward flexed position of quadrupeds. This rotation of the brachioplexus causes it to be circumducted between the clavicle and the first rib. As we age, the clavicle has a tendency to "sag" and cause more imbalance between the anterior and posterior thorax. This patient participates in a number of activities that can predispose her to thoracic outlet syndrome. Playing the violin causes the patient to work with her arm in an abduction position, which causes increased tension of the scalene muscle and the superior trapezius. These muscles become activated and will sometimes fire inappropriately during breathing. Usually these muscles have only a secondary function when one is breathing. In some individuals, an abnormal pattern can develop and these muscles become primarily responsible for breathing instead of the usual diaphragmatic pattern. In a relaxed position with arms at the side, the diaphragm accounts for most of the effort in breathing by approximately a 3:1 magnitude. In females, the medial third of the clavicle is lower than in males, thus shrinking the costoclavicular space. In addition to this, in women, the second dorsal vertebra is more caudad to the top of the sternum compared with men. This particular patient has what is referred to as "droopy shoulder syndrome." Patients hold their head in a slightly flexed position and the shoulders are flexed forward. This causes scapular ptosis, especially in females with larger breasts. The breasts attach to the pectoralis major muscles and exert a downward pull on the medial aspect of the clavicle. The problem is accelerated when brassiere straps are located more laterally further increasing forward flexion of the shoulders.

The patient also has some endocrine issues that can affect neural physiology. She has diabetes and recently has experienced perimenopausal symptoms. The patient received relief when she went on vacation, decreasing the amount of physical work that she did with her violin as well as the computer keyboard. Many patients with thoracic outlet syndrome will notice that if they do any type of strenuous work during the day, that evening they will "pay the price." The patients may eventually realize that after a few days of a "lazy holiday," their symptoms improve.

Controversy exists about thoracic outlet syndrome, and in the past only patients with vascular compromise were considered to have this entity. Neurogenic thoracic outlet syndrome is much more common, and tests performed to detect change in the patient's pulse such as Addison's and Wright's maneuver are not particularly helpful. This condition usually responds to conservative therapy in the form of specialized stretching and strengthening exercises of the neck and shoulder coupled with diaphragmatic breathing exercises. Over time, this often leads to complete resolution, if not great improvement of the patient's symptoms. The process, however, usually takes 3 to 4 months to complete.

5. *Pronator teres syndrome.* The proximal median nerve courses through the anterior part of the forearm. As it does so, it passes through a number of structures in the elbow in which it can become trapped (Fig. 96-4). This syndrome can be differentiated from carpal tunnel syndrome by a number of aspects. There is usually more pain in the forearm than in the hand. Symptoms can be brought on by wrist movement. There may be a positive Tinel's sign of the forearm. Resisted pronation and passive supination bring on symptoms.

6. *Anterior interosseous syndrome.* The anterior interosseous nerve arises from the median nerve approximately 5 to 8 cm distal to the lateral epicondyle. It is a pure motor nerve. This nerve innervates the flexor pollicis longus, the flexor

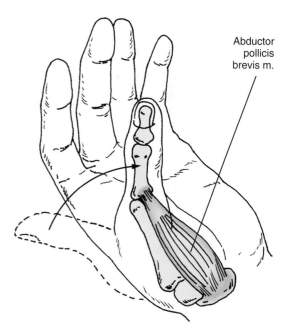

Abductor
pollicis
brevis m.

Figure 96-4 Manual abductor pollicis brevis testing for median nerve injury. Weakness manifests as a decreased ability to abduct the thumb, making it difficult to grasp a large object. Eventually an adduction deformity of the thumb may result (ape hand). (From Saidoff DC, McDonough AL. Critical Pathways in Therapeutic Intervention: Upper Extremity. St. Louis, Mosby Yearbook, 1997, p 28.)

digitorum profundus, and the pronator quadratus muscle. These patients may have specific problems with pincer grip. The pronator quadratus muscle can be tested with the elbow in flexion and the forearm in pronation, while one stretches the pronator quadratus into extreme supination.

7. *Diabetic neuropathy.* This usually manifests itself by symmetrical "stocking glove" distribution and is caused by a decreased blood supply to the nerve or the nerve trunks. It usually happens in the lower extremities and would be rare to present only in the upper extremities.

8. *Carpal tunnel syndrome.* The most commonly entrapped nerve in the upper extremity is the median nerve at the carpal tunnel. The nerve enters the osteofibrous tunnel, which is dorsally and laterally bounded by the bony carpus and superiorly bounded by a thick transverse carpal ligament. The median nerve shares this tunnel with nine other flexor tendons covered by two layers of synovium. This syndrome often affects patients between the ages of 40 and 60.

There can be a number of causes for this syndrome: (1) increased volume of the tunnel content secondary to nonspecific tenosynovitis of the flexor tendon; (2) thickening or fibrosis of the transverse carpal ligament; (3) alteration of the margins of the carpus caused by fractures, dislocations, or arthritic changes; (4) tumors; or (5) systemic disease. This patient has no history of any type of injury to her wrist or any evidence that would make us think that she has any type of tumor in her wrist.

The hallmark of this clinical syndrome is nocturnal pain and paresthesia. The patients are often awakened with a burning pain or tingling in their hand. It is relieved with shaking or wringing of their hands. In some cases, the patient's symptoms can be relieved by running their hands under hot or cold water. The median nerve has both sensorimotor branches, and usually the sensory abnormalities are noted first. Later they progress into motor involvement, and clinical findings are proportional to the degree of nerve damage.

The clinical course of this disorder can be predicted by placing the patient into one of three groups: those with neurapraxia, those with axonotmesis, and those with neurotmesis. Group 1 patients (those with neurapraxia) would have mild symptoms including weakness or clumsiness brought on by manual labor or by computer work. Symptoms are sporadic but increase over time, and there are usually no abnormal findings on clinical examination. Group 2 patients (those patients with axonotmesis) often have burning pain in their hands, and this is usually the major complaint. There may also be some thenar weakness and atrophy, sensory loss, and loss of dexterity. These patients will lose two-point discrimination (most

patients can discriminate two points at 5 mm or greater at their fingertips). Group 3 patients (those with neurotmesis) are characterized by pronounced thenar wasting. The thenar eminence can be easily evaluated by having the patient put his or her hands together in a "praying position." There could be noted loss of thenar mass when compared with the opposite hand. These patients have poor prognosis regardless of treatment.

9. *Double crush syndrome.* Double crush syndrome was first described by Nakomis, who proposed that patients could become symptomatic with nerve compression if the nerve was compressed at multiple levels. One single site may not be sufficient to cause the patient to have symptoms, but when a second site is compressed, the patient may become symptomatic. This syndrome can explain why some patients continue to have symptoms or will have recurrent symptoms after nerve decompression surgery. Although each site in isolation may not be sufficient to completely relieve symptoms or electrical diagnostic abnormalities, multiple compression sites may together produce these symptoms. Patients may be mislabeled with the diagnosis of somatization or malingering when in reality they have double crush syndrome. Figure 96-5 shows potential sites of "double crush" of the median nerve. Figure 96-6 shows the most common areas of nerve injury to the upper extremity. It is only through a thorough history and physical examination that this entity can be diagnosed.

Clinical Course

A radiograph of the patient's cervical spine shows a rudimentary C7 cervical rib (Fig. 96-7). In addition to this finding, the seventh spinous process is twice the length of the other spinous processes. At this time the patient is diagnosed with double crush syndrome because of her congenital abnormalities of her cervical spine and her posture.

The patient is referred for physical and occupational therapy. The occupational therapist reviews her workspace and helps her make some adjustments, such as repositioning her computer at her desk and chair. The physical therapist recommends postural re-education, selective muscle strengthening, and selective soft-tissue stretching. The treatment plan consists of a 90-day program aimed at controlling her symptoms, restoration of shortened tissue, restoration of muscle balance, improvement of posture, and development of stress management techniques.

The insurance company denies the physical therapist's treatment plan and recommends that Tish be evaluated by a neurologist. The neurologist repeats her electromyographic nerve conduction studies, which remain normal, and obtains a magnetic resonance imaging scan of the cervical spine.

NERVE GLIDING PROGRAM
For Median Nerve Decomposition at the Wrist

Exercises to be done_____times each,_____times a day.
Hold position to a count of_____.

Starting position 1

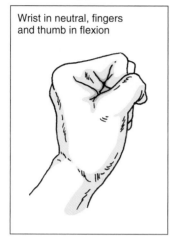

Wrist in neutral, fingers and thumb in flexion

Position 2

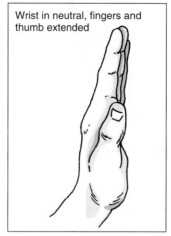

Wrist in neutral, fingers and thumb extended

Position 3

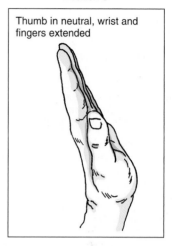

Thumb in neutral, wrist and fingers extended

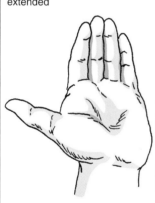

Wrist, fingers, and thumb extended

Position 4

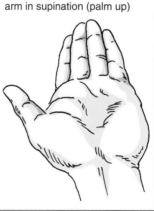

Same as position 4, with forearm in supination (palm up)

Position 5

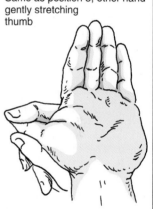

Same as position 5, other hand gently stretching thumb

Position 6

Figure 96-5 Nerve-gliding exercises permit mobilization of the median nerve. (From Hunter JM, Schneider LH, Mackin EJ, Callahan AD (eds): Rehabilitation of the Hand: Surgery and Therapy, 3rd ed. St. Louis, Mosby, 1990.)

The scan shows degenerative changes in the cervical spine but no evidence of any type of nerve root impingement or cord tumor. The neurologist agrees with the assessment of the physical therapist. The patient is instructed on the "rest position" for scapular abduction and elevation (Fig. 96-8). The patient is also instructed on cervical retraction exercises (Fig. 96-9) and a brachioplexus gliding program. The occupational therapist advises the patient to switch to a sports-type brassiere, which gives the patient support without depressing her distal clavicle.

In approximately 1 month, the patient's symptoms improve, but she continues to have symptoms toward the end of the work week. The patient is referred to a counselor with background in biofeedback techniques and is instructed on diaphragmatic breathing exercises (Fig. 96-10). At the end of her prescribed program, the patient continues to have some intermittent symptoms but is very pleased with the result of the program. She describes her symptoms now as "manageable."

Material Available on Student Consult

Review Questions and Answers about Double Crush Syndrome

The most frequently encountered causes of damage at the various sites are indicated

C7 Root
By far the most frequent "acute cervical disc lesion" occurs at this level. C6 and C5 less often. Other levels very rarely

Axillary nerve
Fracture of humeral neck
Dislocation of the humerus
Intramauscular injections

Radial nerve in spiral groove
Direct blow laterally. During anesthesia medially. While drunk medially ("Saturday night palsy"). Fractures of the humerus-immediate or delayed

Radial nerve
(Posterior interosseus nerve) Nerve enters forearm through supinator muscle. Occupational overuse of muscle may damage nerve. Also occurs idiopathically. Extensors of thumb and index finger mainly affected

C5 and C6 Roots
Most frequently involved roots in cervical spondylosis. C7 involved occasionally. Others very rarely

Lower trunk of the brachial plexus
Cervical rib syndrome. Altered anatomy (outlet syndrome). Pancoast tumor of lung apex

Radial nerve in the axilla
Incorrect use of a crutch

Ulnar nerve
Damage from repeated minor trauma
Prolonged bed rest
Delayed after fractures

Median nerve
At elbow. Rarely damaged by direct trauma or fracture

(Anterior interosseus nerve)
Rarely damaged nerve lies very deep Flexors of thumb and index finger are affected by damage to nerve

Median nerve
(Carpal tunnel syndrome) Nerve damaged by swelling of infiltration of tunnel it transverses. Transiently seen in pregnancy. Idiopathically in females. Complicates rheumatoid arthritis. Rarely seen in other systemic diseases

Ulnar nerve
(deep branch) Trauma to heel of the hand. Idiopathically (often a ganglion found on exploration) No sensory loss in typical cases

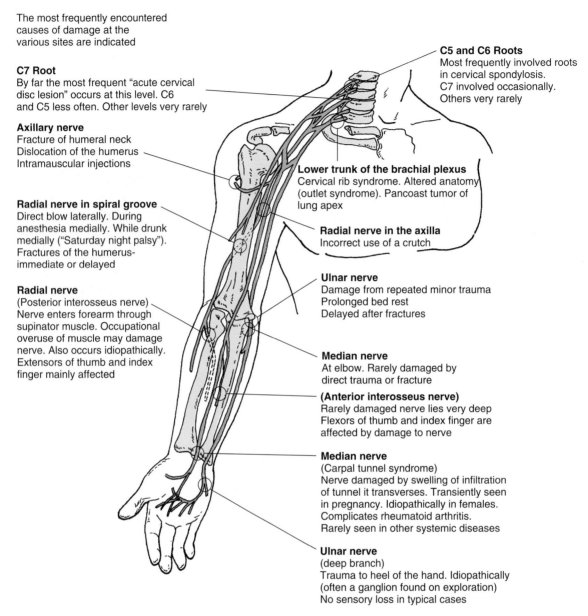

Figure 96-6 Common sites of nerve injury in the upper extremity. (From Patten J. Neurologic Differential Diagnosis. London, Springer-Verlag, 1996.)

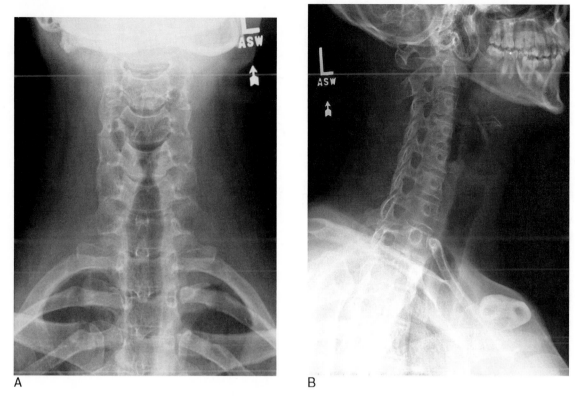

A   B

Figure 96-7 Radiographs of the patient's cervical spine show rudimentary C7 cervical rib.

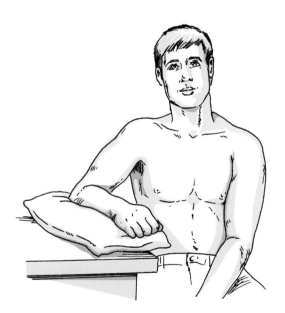

Figure 96-8 Sitting rest position using a pillow to support the arm. (From Saidoff DC, McDonough AL. Critical Pathways in Therapeutic Intervention: Upper Extremity. St. Louis, Mosby Yearbook, 1997, p 226.)

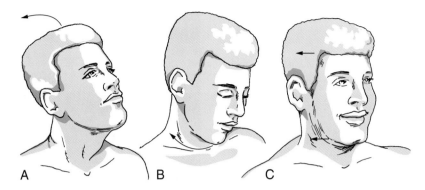

Figure 96-9 Cervical retraction exercises. **A,** Poor technique: elevated chin. **B,** Poor technique: depressed chin. **C,** Good technique. (From Saidoff DC, McDonough AL. Critical Pathways in Therapeutic Intervention: Upper Extremity. St. Louis, Mosby Yearbook, 1997, p 227.)

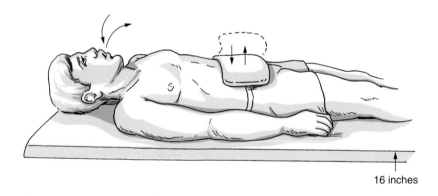

16 inches

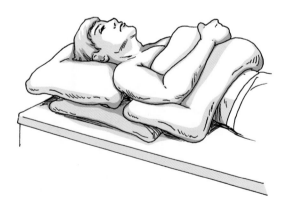

Figure 96-10 Rest position in supine. Pillows or use of a triangle foam wedge should be used to support the thoracic spine, scapula, and arm. (From Saidoff DC, McDonough AL. Critical Pathways in Therapeutic Intervention: Upper Extremity. St. Louis, Mosby Yearbook, 1997, p 230.)

SUGGESTED READINGS

Cherniack M, Warren N. Ambiguities in office-related injury: The poverty of present approaches. Occup Med 1999;14:1–18 **B**

Derebery VJ. Determining the cause of upper extremity complaints in the workpace. Occup Med 1998;13:569–582. **B**

Kasdan ML. Occupational Hand and Upper Extremity Injuries and Diseases, 2nd ed. Philadelphia, Hanley & Belfus, 1998. **A**

Magee DJ. Orthopedic Physical Assessment, 2nd ed. Philadelphia, WB Saunders, 1992.

Saidoff DC, McDonough AL. Critical Pathways in Therapeutic Intervention: Upper Extremity. St. Louis, Mosby Yearbook, 1997. **C**

Index

Note: Page numbers followed by f indicate figures; those followed by t indicate tables; those followed by b indicate boxed material.